ROSEN'S DIAGNOSIS OF
Breast Pathology
By Needle Core Biopsy

FIFTH EDITION

ROSEN'S DIAGNOSIS OF Breast Pathology By Needle Core Biopsy

FIFTH EDITION

▲ Syed A. Hoda, MD
Professor of Clinical Pathology
Weill Medical College of Cornell University
Chief of Breast Pathology, and Attending Pathologist
New York Presbyterian Hospital–Weill Cornell Medical Center
New York, New York

▲ Raza S. Hoda, MD
Assistant Professor of Pathology
Cleveland Clinic Lerner School of Medicine
Staff Pathologist
Cleveland Clinic
Cleveland, Ohio

▲ Elaine W. Zhong, MD
Assistant Professor of Pathology
Zucker School of Medicine at Hofstra–Northwell
Hempstead, New York
Staff Pathologist
Northwell Health
New Hyde Park, New York

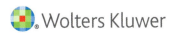

Philadelphia • Baltimore • New York • London
Buenos Aires • Hong Kong • Sydney • Tokyo

Acquisitions Editor: Nicole Dernoski
Senior Product Development Editor: Ariel S. Winter
Editorial Coordinator: Anju Radhakrishnan
Production Project Manager: Frances M. Gunning
Manager, Graphic Arts & Design: Stephen Druding
Manufacturing Coordinator: Lisa Bowling
Prepress Vendor: S4Carlisle Publishing Services

Fifth Edition

Copyright © 2025 Wolters Kluwer.

Copyright © 2017 Wolters Kluwer. Copyright © 2010 Wolters Kluwer Health | Lippincott Williams & Wilkins. Copyright © 2006, 1999 Lippincott Williams & Wilkins. All rights reserved. This book is protected by copyright. No part of this book may be reproduced or transmitted in any form or by any means, including as photocopies or scanned-in or other electronic copies, or utilized by any information storage and retrieval system without written permission from the copyright owner, except for brief quotations embodied in critical articles and reviews. Materials appearing in this book prepared by individuals as part of their official duties as U.S. government employees are not covered by the above-mentioned copyright. To request permission, please contact Wolters Kluwer at Two Commerce Square, 2001 Market Street, Philadelphia, PA 19103, via email at permissions@lww.com, or via our website at shop.lww.com (products and services).

9 8 7 6 5 4 3 2 1

Printed in Mexico

Library of Congress Cataloging-in-Publication Data

ISBN-13: 978-1-975198-36-7
ISBN-10: 1-975198-36-0

Cataloging in Publication data available on request from publisher.

This work is provided "as is," and the publisher disclaims any and all warranties, express or implied, including any warranties as to accuracy, comprehensiveness, or currency of the content of this work.

This work is no substitute for individual patient assessment based upon healthcare professionals' examination of each patient and consideration of, among other things, age, weight, gender, current or prior medical conditions, medication history, laboratory data, and other factors unique to the patient. The publisher does not provide medical advice or guidance and this work is merely a reference tool. Healthcare professionals, and not the publisher, are solely responsible for the use of this work including all medical judgments and for any resulting diagnosis and treatments.

Given continuous, rapid advances in medical science and health information, independent professional verification of medical diagnoses, indications, appropriate pharmaceutical selections and dosages, and treatment options should be made and healthcare professionals should consult a variety of sources. When prescribing medication, healthcare professionals are advised to consult the product information sheet (the manufacturer's package insert) accompanying each drug to verify, among other things, conditions of use, warnings and side effects and identify any changes in dosage schedule or contraindications, particularly if the medication to be administered is new, infrequently used or has a narrow therapeutic range. To the maximum extent permitted under applicable law, no responsibility is assumed by the publisher for any injury and/or damage to persons or property, as a matter of products liability, negligence law or otherwise, or from any reference to or use by any person of this work.

shop.lww.com

Dedication

Syed A. Hoda
to Rana
and all other Hodas
—*sine qua non*

~

Raza S. Hoda
to Dalia, Jude, and Sehyr
—the ethereal three

~

Elaine W. Zhong
to my parents
and other mentors

Contributors

Judith A. Ferry, MD
Professor of Pathology
Harvard Medical School
Nancy Lee Harris M.D. Endowed Chair in Pathology
Director of Hematopathology, and Attending Pathologist
Massachusetts General Hospital
Boston, Massachusetts

Raza S. Hoda, MD
Assistant Professor of Pathology
Cleveland Clinic Lerner School of Medicine
Staff Pathologist
Cleveland Clinic
Cleveland, Ohio

Syed A. Hoda, MD
Professor of Clinical Pathology
Weill Medical College of Cornell University
Chief of Breast Pathology, and Attending Pathologist
New York Presbyterian Hospital–Weill Cornell Medical
Center
New York, New York

Aliyah R. Sohani, MD
Professor of Pathology
Harvard Medical School
Director of Surgical Pathology, and Attending Pathologist
Massachusetts General Hospital
Boston, Massachusetts

Elaine W. Zhong, MD
Assistant Professor of Pathology
Zucker School of Medicine at Hofstra–Northwell
Hempstead, New York
Staff Pathologist
Northwell Health
New Hyde Park, New York

Foreword

PASSING THE TORCH

In 1997, during the Vietnam War, I was finishing my 2 years of residency in Clinical Pathology at the New York Veterans Administration Hospital with Sigmund Wilens, and began to consider whether a Pathology Fellowship might be beneficial. At the time, my Resident colleagues, Dennis Daut and George Green, expressed an interest in applying for an Oncologic Pathology Fellowship at Memorial Hospital. So, I followed them in applying to Memorial Hospital. Having spent a year studying Surgical Pathology at Columbia Presbyterian Hospital with Raphael Lattes and Nathan Lane, I naively considered myself an expert in the diagnosis of oncologic pathology and not in need of further training. George and Dennis were promptly accepted to the Fellowship but my application was on hold until I scheduled an interview with Frank Foote, Chairman of the Pathology Department. The circumstances surrounding this interview, which led eventually to my acceptance to the Memorial Hospital National Institutes of Health (NIH)-sponsored Oncologic Pathology Fellowship, were described in my preface entitled *On the Shoulder of Giants* in the fifth edition of *Rosen's Breast Pathology*. This preface also describes the opportunity that opened up for me to develop my interest in breast pathology that had sparked during my residency at Columbia Presbyterian Hospital with Lattes, Lane, and especially Cushman Haagensen, the pre-eminent breast surgeon and student of breast pathology, who maintained an office in the Surgical Pathology Division. Of course, the spiritual leader of the Surgical Pathology Division was its founder, Arthur Purdy Stout, who was then afflicted with advanced prostatic cancer. My interactions with Stout came mostly in the second half of my residency, as described in detail in the aforementioned preface.

It was during my 6-month residency at the Delafield Hospital, a New York City cancer hospital, affiliated with Columbia Presbyterian Hospital, that I also met Sheldon Sommers, Chairman of the Delafield Hospital Pathology Department. It was through Sommers that I was introduced to the pathology publishing industry, which proved to be in great flux in the following years.

The senior staff had been depleted when I was accepted as an Oncologic Fellow in the Pathology Department by the departure of Bob McDivitt to become Director of Surgical Pathology at New York Hospital as well as Robert Hutter who became the Director of Pathology at Yale University Hospital. To fill this gap in the staff, three of the Pathology Fellows from the previous year (1967) were offered the opportunity to remain for a second year in a Chief Resident/ Junior Staff capacity with sign-out responsibility. In 1969, Tom Sparrow and I became the Chief Residents; 1969 was also the year in which the Pathology Department moved from the second floor of the Old Memorial Hospital to the sixth floor of what was then the Outpatient Clinic Building. Tom and I were assigned room 609, which we shared. The following year (1970) when Tom returned to Texas, room 609 became my office when I joined as an Assistant Attending Pathologist at Memorial Hospital and Assistant Professor of Pathology at the Weill Cornell Medical College. Initially, my responsibilities involved Surgical Pathology, but several years later I joined the Cytology Service after which I signed out in Cytology on Wednesday afternoons and covered Surgical Pathology including frozen sections and aspiration cytology related to surgical procedures all day on Thursdays starting at 7:30 AM and ending when the OR closed for the day.

By 1990, I had been on the Pathology Department Staff for 20 years and had been promoted from Assistant Attending Pathologist to Associate Attending Pathologist with a comparable appointment at Weill Cornell Medical College. Subsequently, I was promoted to the level of Attending Pathologist and was honored with the title of Member of Memorial Sloan-Kettering Cancer Center for my contributions to the study of breast pathology.

It was in 1990 that Dr. Syed Hoda joined the Pathology Department as a Fellow on the Cytology Service where he served until 1991, after which he was a Fellow in the Oncologic Pathology Service until 1992. During these 2 years, I had many opportunities to observe Dr. Hoda's diagnostic work, which I found to be of the highest quality. At the conclusion of his 2 years as a Fellow, there being no openings at the Staff level in the Pathology Department at Memorial Hospital, Dr. Hoda was recruited by the Pathology Department at New York Hospital (now New York Presbyterian Hospital-Weill Cornell Medical Center) and joined the faculty at Weill Cornell Medical College (now Weill Medical College of Cornell University) in 1992.

Dr. Syed Hoda was still in the Pathology Department of New York Hospital when I was recruited by the then Chairman, Daniel Knowles, to bring my breast pathology consultation practice to his Department after I had retired from Memorial Hospital in 1998 and had been invited to move that service to White Plains Hospital near where I was living at that time in Croton-on-Hudson. I was receiving an average of 10 cases a day at White Plains Hospital and Dr. Knowles expected me to use this material to provide one-on-one training for residents.

ix

My office was next to Dr. Syed Hoda's and in time he began to assist me in writing the third edition of *Rosen's Breast Pathology*. He was very much involved in teaching medical students, residents, and fellows, signing out surgicals, and writing articles based on his research that were published in peer-reviewed journals.

When it was time to assemble the fourth and fifth editions of *Rosen's Breast Pathology*, Dr. Syed Hoda assumed an increasingly important role in getting the books ready for publication (although I read and edited most of the chapters). Now I feel that it is time to pass the torch to him and am grateful to him for taking on this challenge. It was my suggestion that he invite Dr. Elaine Zhong and Dr. Raza Hoda to contribute to this effort by updating portions of the book. Dr. Judith Ferry has worked with us to clarify the mysteries of lymphoproliferative and hematopoietic diseases in the breast and, as in the past, her contributions are masterful. We welcome Dr. Aliyah Sohani who has worked with Dr. Ferry to produce an exceedingly useful chapter in this edition.

I am very grateful that Dr. Syed Hoda has taken on this challenge and have passed the torch to him. I have not read and edited any of the chapters in this book in manuscript form but am confident the product will be of the highest standard. At present, I suffer from long COVID that has taken the form of posttraumatic stress disorder and look forward to seeing the fifth edition of a book that I began to write more than 25 years ago.

Paul Peter Rosen, MD
Emeritus Professor of Pathology
Weill Medical College of Cornell University
Formerly, Chief of Breast Pathology
New York Presbyterian Hospital–
Weill Cornell Medical Center
New York, New York

Preface

The use of needle core biopsies (NCBs) for the diagnosis of palpable as well as non-palpable lesions of the breast is a valuable, and increasingly employed, procedure. The technique epitomizes the complexity of the interaction between pathologists, radiologists, surgeons, and oncologists in the management of mammary diseases—often before any therapeutic intervention.

It is obvious that the diagnosis rendered on an NCB specimen can only be based on the sample made available to the pathologist. This "challenge" is summarized in the three principles enunciated by Dr. Paul Peter Rosen in the Preface to the First Edition of this book. First, anything can turn up. Second, what you see is what you have, and it may not be all there is. Third, what you have may be all there is. The pathologist must always keep these precepts in mind when rendering a diagnosis based on NCB samples.

In some cases, NCB sampling offers "equivocal" or "negative" findings when the clinical level of "suspicion" is high. This is an inherent limitation of the procedure—and ought not to be viewed as a failure on the part of the pathologist or of the radiologist. When such a circumstance arises, it is necessary for all physicians caring for the patient to consider the clinical, physical, and radiologic situation. Such collaborative reflection is referred to as "clinicopathologic correlation." The latter process can be disregarded only at one's peril.

The diagnostic breast pathology report, even for NCB specimens, has evolved over the last few decades from one- or two-line statements to a catalog of data often spanning multiple pages. Results of estrogen receptor, other biomarkers, oncogene expression, etc., are now integral to the "positive" report (please see the newly minted Chapter 27). Notwithstanding myriad evolutionary (and revolutionary) advances, the hematoxylin and eosin (H&E)-stained section remains the most effective method to render a diagnosis. This edition of the book, which appears 7 years after the publication of its precursor, continues to focus on histopathology. Much of the text and illustrative material has been either updated or revised or otherwise augmented. Pertinent immunohistochemical and molecular pathology information is included. There is incorporation of newer disease classifications, recent clinicopathologic guidelines, and evolving advances in management. Related clinical, surgical, and imaging details are included *pro re nata*. Despite assorted additions, and owing to ample pruning, the book has gained only a few pages.

The antecedent editions of the book benefited from several distinguished contributors. The latter's work added enduring value, and every effort has been made to retain their immutable words of wisdom. Elaine Zhong and Raza Hoda, the two coeditors inducted into this edition, bring innovative and inventive (yet cautious and conservative) perspectives to the book.

The monumental contributions of Dr. Paul Peter Rosen to breast pathology are legendary. Dr. Rosen is the nonpareil begetter of the book, and his name is embedded in its title. The team of contributors to this edition realize that it is neither possible to equal Dr. Rosen's vast experience nor to match his unique writing style—and consider the opportunity to be associated with it to be an exceptional professional honor. This team has done its best and earnestly hopes that the latest edition of the book will continue to provide aid in the always exacting (and often exhilarating) task of diagnosing breast lesions on limited sampling.

Syed A. Hoda, MD

LEGENDS FOR COVER IMAGES

Clockwise from top left: Liesegang-like rings in a dilated duct with lactational-like change, breast carcinoma with amplification of human epidermal growth factor receptor 2 (HER2) on fluorescent in situ hybridization (FISH) preparation, atypical ductal hyperplasia, invasive metaplastic matrix-producing carcinoma, microinvasive carcinoma associated with ductal carcinoma in situ on cytokeratin AE1/AE3 immunostain, invasive carcinoma with intraneural and perineural involvement, Gram-positive bacilli in cystic neutrophilic granulomatous mastitis, and microinvasive tubular carcinoma.

Acknowledgments

All contributors to this book are indebted to the countless anonymous patients with various breast disorders who contributed precious material to this book. The incalculable (subliminal) input of countless pathologists, surgeons, oncologists, radiologists, radiation oncologists, and other specialists is appreciated. The earnest support of our colleagues and trainees, including Oliver Michaud, Anne Moore, Alexander Swistel, and Diana Vulcain, is recognized. Serine Baydoun, Melanie Chellman, and Paulette Turk, all staff radiologists at Cleveland Clinic, provided invaluable details and images. Patricia Kuharic of Medical Arts at Weill Cornell Medical College assiduously and expertly processed all the images in the book. The excellent endeavors of the publishing team, especially those of Nicole Dernoski, Samson Premkumar Charly, Anju Radhakrishnan, and Ariel Winter, are saluted. Finally, the book has immeasurably benefited from the benevolent guidance and inestimable encouragement of Dr. Paul Peter Rosen.

Contents

Contributors vii

Foreword ix

Preface xi

Acknowledgments xiii

List of Abbreviations xvii

1 Embryology, Development, Histology, and Physiologic Morphology 1
Raza S. Hoda and Syed A. Hoda

2 Inflammatory and Reactive Lesions 14
Raza S. Hoda and Syed A. Hoda

3 Specific Infections and Infestations 34
Raza S. Hoda and Syed A. Hoda

4 Benign Papillary Tumors 41
Elaine W. Zhong and Syed A. Hoda

5 Adenomyoepithelial and Myoepithelial Neoplasms 71
Raza S. Hoda and Syed A. Hoda

6 Adenosis and Microglandular Adenosis 82
Raza S. Hoda and Syed A. Hoda

7 Fibroepithelial Neoplasms 105
Raza S. Hoda and Syed A. Hoda

8 Ductal Hyperplasia, Atypical Ductal Hyperplasia, and Ductal Carcinoma In Situ 128
Raza S. Hoda and Syed A. Hoda

9 Invasive Ductal Carcinoma 183
Raza S. Hoda and Syed A. Hoda

10 Tubular Carcinoma 208
Raza S. Hoda and Syed A. Hoda

11 Papillary Carcinoma 224
Elaine W. Zhong and Syed A. Hoda

12 Medullary Carcinoma and Related Carcinomas 241
Raza S. Hoda and Syed A. Hoda

13 Metaplastic Carcinomas, Including Low-Grade Adenosquamous Carcinoma 250
Raza S. Hoda and Syed A. Hoda

14 Mucinous Carcinoma 269
Raza S. Hoda and Syed A. Hoda

15 Apocrine Carcinoma 285
Elaine W. Zhong and Syed A. Hoda

16 Adenoid Cystic Carcinoma 299
Elaine W. Zhong and Syed A. Hoda

17 Other Special Types of Invasive Breast Carcinoma 310
Elaine W. Zhong and Syed A. Hoda

18 Lobular Carcinoma In Situ and Atypical Lobular Hyperplasia 332
Elaine W. Zhong and Syed A. Hoda

19 Invasive Lobular Carcinoma 359
Elaine W. Zhong and Syed A. Hoda

20 Mesenchymal Lesions 375
Elaine W. Zhong and Syed A. Hoda

21 Lymphoid and Hematopoietic Tumors 421
Aliyah R. Sohani and Judith A. Ferry

22 Metastases From Nonmammary Malignant Neoplasms 443
Elaine W. Zhong and Syed A. Hoda

23 Pathologic Effects of Therapy 455
Elaine W. Zhong and Syed A. Hoda

24 Men and Children 468
Elaine W. Zhong and Syed A. Hoda

25 Pathologic Changes and Clinical Complications Associated With Needling Procedures 483
Elaine W. Zhong and Syed A. Hoda

26 Processing, Examining, and Reporting of Needle Core Biopsy Specimens 497
Raza S. Hoda and Syed A. Hoda

27 Biomarker, Molecular, and Other Ancillary Testing 518
Elaine W. Zhong and Syed A. Hoda

Index 527

List of Abbreviations

ACC	adenoid cystic carcinoma
ADH	atypical ductal hyperplasia
AFB	acid-fast bacilli
AJCC	American Joint Committee on Cancer
ALH	atypical lobular hyperplasia
ALN	axillary lymph node
AME	adenomyoepithelioma
AR	androgen receptor
ASCO	American Society of Clinical Oncology
BDA	blunt duct adenosis
BI-RADS	Breast Imaging-Reporting and Data System
BnPT	benign phyllodes tumor
CAP	College of American Pathologists
CCH	columnar cell hyperplasia
CEA	carcinoembryonic antigen
CHH	cystic hypersecretory hyperplasia
CIS	carcinoma in situ
CK	cytokeratin
CT	computed tomography (imaging)
DCIS	ductal carcinoma in situ
DFS	disease-free survival
EGFR	epidermal growth factor receptor
EMA	epithelial membrane antigen
ER	estrogen receptor
FA	fibroadenoma
FCC	fibrocystic changes
FEA	flat epithelial atypia
FISH	fluorescence in situ hybridization
FNA	fine needle aspiration
FS	frozen section
GCDFP-15	gross cystic disease fluid protein 15
H&E	hematoxylin and eosin
HER2	human epidermal growth factor receptor 2
HPF	high-power field
IDC/IFDC	invasive (infiltrating) ductal carcinoma
IHC	immunohistochemistry
JP	juvenile papillomatosis
LCIS	lobular carcinoma in situ
LGASC	low-grade adenosquamous carcinoma
LOH	loss of heterozygosity
LVI	lymphovascular involvement
MALT	mucosa-associated lymphoid tissue
MGA	microglandular adenosis
MLL	mucocele-like lesion
MPT	malignant phyllodes tumor
MRI	magnetic resonance imaging
MSA	muscle-specific actin
NACT	neoadjuvant chemotherapy
NCB	needle core biopsy
NOS	not otherwise specified
OS	overall survival
PAS (-D)	periodic acid–Schiff (-diastase)
PASH	pseudoangiomatous stromal hyperplasia
PCR	polymerase chain reaction
PET	positron emission tomography (imaging)
PLH	pregnancy-like hyperplasia
PR	progesterone receptor
RFS	relapse-free survival (or recurrence-free survival)
RR	relative risk
RSL	radial sclerosing lesion (synonym: radial scar)
SA	sclerosing adenosis
SCC	squamous cell carcinoma
SEER	Surveillance, Epidemiology, and End Results
SLN	sentinel lymph node
SMA	smooth muscle actin
s/p	status post
SMMHC	smooth muscle myosin heavy chain
SSDH	subareolar sclerosing duct hyperplasia
TDLU	terminal duct lobular unit
TNM	tumor (size), regional node (involvement), (distant) metastases
TRAM	transverse rectus abdominis myocutaneous
TTF1	thyroid transcription factor 1
UDH	usual ductal hyperplasia
US	ultrasound (imaging)
VNPI	Van Nuys Prognostic Index
WHO	World Health Organization
WT1	Wilms tumor 1

Embryology, Development, Histology, and Physiologic Morphology

RAZA S. HODA AND SYED A. HODA

EMBRYOLOGY AND DEVELOPMENT

The mammary glands develop from **mammary ridges** (or "milk lines"). The latter are thickenings of the epidermis that appear on the ventral surface of the 5-week fetus. The bilateral mammary ridges extend from the axilla to the vulva. In humans of either gender, the ridges largely disappear during normal fetal development, except for a pair of thickenings, one on either side of the pectoral region. Persistence of other segments of the milk line results in the development of **ectopic mammary glandular tissue**, which occurs most often at the extreme ends of the mammary ridge, that is, in the axilla and vulva (1). The aforementioned thickenings are caused by epithelial buds that form around condensed mesenchymal tissue. Columns of epithelial cords grow downward, branch, canalize, and transform into ducts and, ultimately, lobules. Each column eventually forms a lobe of the breast. At this time, the roles of stem cells and molecular mechanisms in mammary development remain unclear (2,3).

In most girls, functional breast development does not begin until puberty. **Premature thelarche** is the unilateral or bilateral appearance of a discoid subareolar thickening before puberty (4). The incidence in female infants and children up to 7 years of age in the United States in 1980 was 20.8 per 100,000 (5). Its prevalence, as reported in 2010, among 318 female children aged between 1 and 4 years in a midwestern American hospital, was calculated to be 4.7% (6). The nodular breast tissue formed in premature thelarche can measure up to 6.5 cm and tends to slowly regress over a period of 6 months to 6 years. Premature thelarche has been associated with precocious puberty (7) but not with a predisposition to develop breast carcinoma (8). Histologically, the breast glandular tissue in premature thelarche resembles gynecomastia. Both lesions are characterized by ductal epithelial hyperplasia with solid and micropapillary configurations. Branching of proliferating ducts results in an increased number of ducts. The latter are surrounded by variably cellular stroma. Excisional biopsy, or overzealous sampling via needle core biopsy, of prematurely developed breast tissue is inappropriate, because it could result in impairment of subsequent physical development of the breast or even complete failure of the breast to develop.

With the onset of the cyclical production of estrogen and progesterone at puberty, adolescent female breast development begins **(Fig. 1.1)**. Growth of ducts and periductal stroma is estrogen dependent (9). As stated previously,

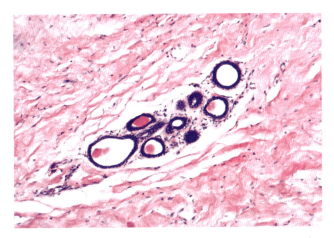

FIGURE 1.1 Immature Breast. Breast tissue at the onset of puberty in an 11-year-old girl showing early lobular differentiation with glandular secretions and developing intralobular stroma.

mammary lobules are derived from solid masses of cells that form at the ends of terminal ducts. Breast glandular differentiation occurs mostly during puberty, but this process can continue into the third decade of life and is enhanced by pregnancy (3). The bulk of lobules in the mature breast are embedded in fibrous tissue; however, normal lobules may also be located amid mammary adipose tissue—particularly in postmenopausal women **(Fig. 1.2)**.

HISTOLOGY

The functional lobular and ductal elements of the breast are embedded in fibrous or adipose tissues. These tissues form the bulk of the mammary gland. The relative proportions of fibrous and fatty stroma vary greatly among individuals and with age, and the ratio of stromal and glandular components is largely responsible for the radiologic appearance of breast structure in normal and pathologic states. Magnetic resonance imaging (MRI) provides a relatively precise method for discriminating between fatty and fibroglandular tissue in the breast. By comparing images obtained with mammography and MRI, Lee et al (10) found a mean fat content of 42.5% (SD ± 30.3%) in mammograms and 66.5% (SD ± 18%) in MRI images.

Breast "density" refers to the proportion of relatively dense (fibroconnective and glandular) to less dense (adipose)

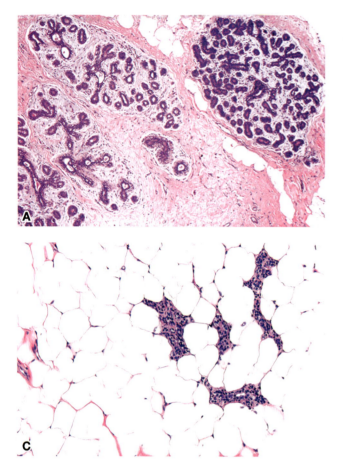

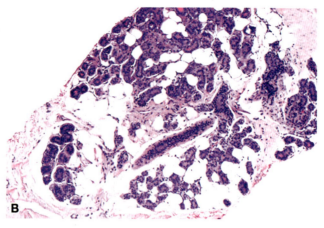

FIGURE 1.2 **Normal Lobules. A:** A lobule in fibrocollagenous stroma. **B:** A lobule in mammary adipose tissue. **C:** An atrophic lobule amid mammary adipose tissue in a 75-year-old woman.

tissues, as evidenced on mammography. There has been considerable interest in the genetic and hormonal basis of such density and its relationship to the detection, incidence, and even prognosis of breast carcinoma (11,12). Greater breast density has been associated with advanced tumor stage at diagnosis and increased risk of both local recurrence and second primary cancers. At this time, understanding of the biologic pathways that modulate mammographic density (and its variability during various phases of the menstrual cycle) is evolving.

Approximately 20 lactiferous (collecting) ducts terminate in, and exit from, the breast at the nipple (13). Each lactiferous duct drains a mammary lobe **(Fig. 1.3)**. The lobes vary in extent and are arranged in a spoke-like manner radiating from the nipple. The individual lobes do not constitute grossly discrete structures and may overlap with adjacent ones around the edges. The structure of the **mammary lobe** is simple: the lactiferous duct extends distally from the nipple through a series of branches that diminish in caliber from the nipple to the terminal duct lobular units (TDLU). The squamocolumnar junction in the lactiferous ducts, where the squamous epithelium joins the glandular duct epithelium, is normally distal to a dilated segment of the lactiferous duct, the lactiferous sinus, located just beneath the surface of the nipple. Extension of squamous epithelium into or below the lactiferous sinus represents metaplasia of the lining ductal epithelium. This process, when exuberant, may result in obstruction of the affected duct. Lactiferous ducts in the nipple are surrounded by circular and longitudinal arrays of smooth muscle fibers rooted in dense fibrous stroma.

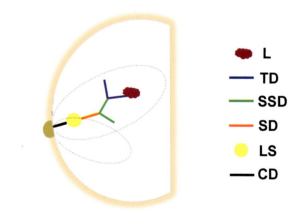

FIGURE 1.3 **Diagrammatic Representation of the Glandular Structure of the Adult Female Breast.** The lobules (violet) open into terminal ducts (blue). The lobules and terminal ducts together constitute the terminal duct lobular unit (TDLU). Terminal ducts connect in sequence to subsegmental ducts (green), segmental ducts (orange), lactiferous sinus (yellow), collecting duct (red), and nipple. Two (of the 20 or so) lobes are depicted in stippled outline. Note the variable size of lobes. CD, collecting duct; L, lobules; LS, lactiferous sinus; SD, segmental ducts; SSD, subsegmental ducts; TD, terminal ducts.

The branching mammary ductal system is embedded in specialized, hormonally responsive, stroma. The extralobular ducts are lined mainly by a single layer of epithelium, with underlying myoepithelial cells and basement membrane. In the nonlactating breast, the major ducts cut in cross section have contours marked by numerous folds that create a stellate structure with a serrated contour. The epithelium in the bay-like pouches of the duct lumen can give rise to ductular branches. Fully formed lobules originate directly from these pouches in the more distal segments of the mammary ductal system—and more rarely in its more proximal segments, that is, the lactiferous ducts of the nipple (14).

Most of the **epithelial cells** that form the lining of the mammary glandular system (ducts and lobules) are cuboidal or columnar cells. Their cytoplasm is endowed with abundant organelles involved in secretory functions. **Myoepithelial cells** lie between the epithelial layer and the basal lamina **(Fig. 1.4)**. The cytoplasm of myoepithelial cells, distributed in a network of slender processes that invest the overlying epithelial cells, is rich in myofibrils. The histologic appearance and immunoreactivity of myoepithelial cells are variable, especially in pathologic conditions, and depend on the degree to which their myoid or epithelial phenotype is accentuated in a particular situation. Myoepithelial cells are typically spindle shaped ("bipolar"), but they may become cuboidal, or undergo "myoid" or clear cell change in certain proliferative or pathologic conditions **(Fig. 1.5)**. Myoepithelial cells display nuclear reactivity for p63, p40, and DOG-1 (15);

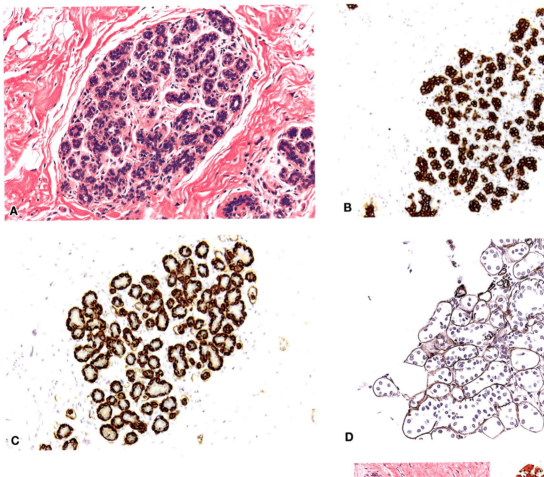

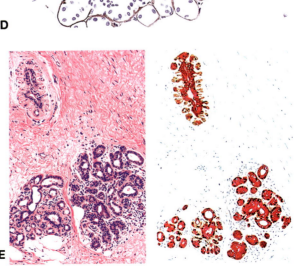

FIGURE 1.4 Topography of Myoepithelial Cell Layer and Basement Membrane. A: Typical inactive lobule in a patient of childbearing age. Note the relatively inconspicuous myoepithelial cell layer on H&E stain. **B:** A cytokeratin AE1/AE3 immunostain highlights the mammary epithelium in the luminal aspect of the glands. **C:** A smooth muscle myosin immunostain shows the myoepithelial cell layer in the abluminal aspect of the gland. **D:** Laminin immunostain highlights the basement membrane lining the glands. **E.** Terminal duct lobular unit (TDLU) decorated by ADH5 immunostain highlights the topographic relationship between epithelial and myoepithelial cell layer. CK7 and CK18 stain epithelial cytoplasm red; CK5 and CK14 stain the myoepithelial cytoplasm brown, and p63 stains the myoepithelial nuclei also brown.

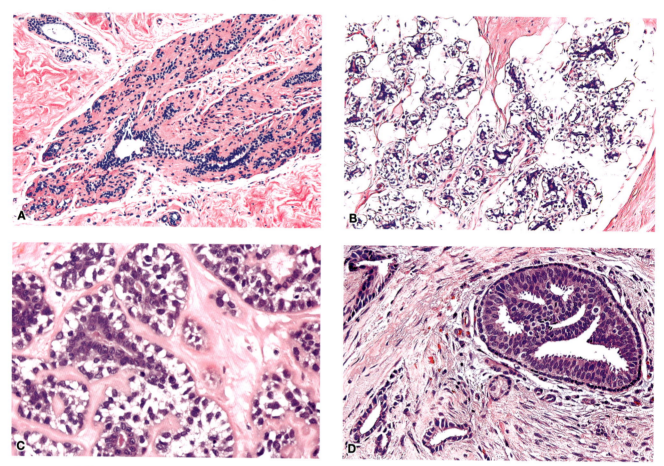

FIGURE 1.5 Variations in Myoepithelial Cells. A: Myoepithelial cells appear "myoid," that is, with prominently plump cytoplasm, in atrophic ducts. **B:** Clear cell change in myoepithelial cells in adenosis. **C:** Typical adenomyoepithelioma with clear cell change in the myoepithelial cell component. **D:** Myoepithelial cells appear prominent in the intraductal carcinoma associated with tubular carcinoma.

and cytoplasmic reactivity for calponin, CD10, smooth muscle actin, and smooth muscle myosin heavy chain, among others. Epithelioid (cuboidal) myoepithelial cells can have reduced (or even absent) p63 reactivity. Glands lined by apocrine epithelia (inactive, hyperplastic, or noninvasive malignant) may also occasionally show diminished or absent myoepithelial cells, as evident via immunostains (16-18).

The normal **periductal stroma** contains fibroblasts and elastic fibers, as well as scattered sparse lymphocytes, plasma cells, mast cells, and histiocytes. **Ochrocytes** are histiocytes with a cytoplasmic accumulation of lipofuscin pigment **(Fig. 1.6)**. These pigmented cells become numerous in association with inflammatory or proliferative conditions—especially in the postmenopausal breast (19). In addition to being present in the duct lumen and periductal stroma, ochrocytes are found in the ductal epithelium, where they can show a "pagetoid-like" distribution. These cells are distinguished from pagetoid and invasive carcinoma cells by immunostains that typically yield the following results: CK7 (−), CK20 (−), and CD68 (+). When restricted to an intraepithelial position, ochrocytes may be confused with epithelioid myoepithelial cells, but they are not immunoreactive with myoepithelial markers.

Secretion of milk originates in lobules—the distal-most portion of the mammary glandular system. Lobules are composed of alveolar glands encased in specialized vascularized stroma. They are drained by terminal ducts, which in turn open into the extralobular ductal system. The resting lobular gland is lined by a single layer of cuboidal epithelial cells supported by loosely connected myoepithelial cells and a basement membrane.

PHYSIOLOGIC MORPHOLOGY

The "normal" microscopic anatomy of the lobules is inconstant. This histologic inconsistency is caused by physiologic changes therein by the menstrual cycle, pregnancy, lactation, exogenous hormone administration, aging, and menopause. Furthermore, there is variation in the functional state of individual lobules regardless of physiologic circumstances, an observation that suggests that individual lobules or regions of the breast have intrinsic differences in response to hormonal and other stimuli. This is reflected in the substantial variability in proliferation indices, indicating different multiplication rates among lobules (20). Immunoreactivity for estrogen and progesterone receptors (ER and PR) is also variable in the epithelial cells of "normal" lobules and ducts.

Histologic alterations occur in the normal breast during the menstrual cycle (21-23). Some have stated that the **proliferative phase**, days 3 through 7, features a high rate

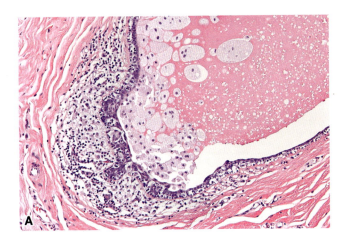
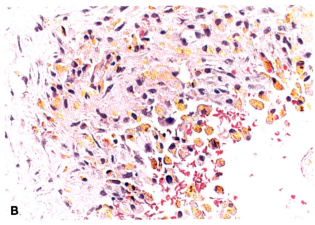
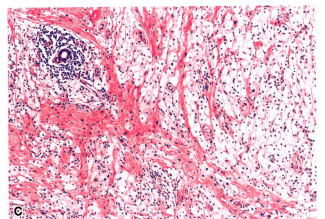

FIGURE 1.6 Clear Cells (Histiocytes and Ochrocytes).
A: Histiocytes with clear and finely granular cytoplasm within ductal lumen and in periductal stroma in duct ectasia.
B: Ochrocytes (from Greek, ochre: yellow-red/rust color) replace ductal epithelia and infiltrate periductal stroma in another example of duct ectasia. **C:** Histiocytes with clear cytoplasm in the "tumor bed" after complete pathologic response to neoadjuvant chemotherapy for invasive breast carcinoma.

of epithelial mitoses and of apoptosis (23); however, other investigators who defined this phase as days 0 to 5 report that "apoptosis and mitosis are by and large absent in this phase" (22). Be that as it may, lobular glands in this phase are lined by crowded epithelial cells with little or no lumen formation or secretions. Myoepithelial cells are inconspicuous and difficult to distinguish from epithelial cells. During this stage of the cycle, the lobular stroma is relatively dense and hypovascular, with plump fibroblasts ringing the glands.

Mitoses and apoptotic bodies are inconspicuous in the **follicular phase** (days 8-14). At this stage, the myoepithelial cells have a polygonal shape and clear cytoplasm and become more apparent. Epithelial cells become columnar, with increasingly basophilic cytoplasm and basally oriented, darkly staining nuclei. An acinar lumen without secretion is evident.

During the **luteal phase**, comprising days 15 through 20, myoepithelial cells become more prominent with increased glycogen accumulation, resulting in cytoplasmic clearing. The glandular lumen is clearly defined by epithelial cells with basophilic cytoplasm. Luminal secretion is present in a few glands. Edema and a mixed inflammatory cell infiltrate appear in the intralobular stroma. Mitoses and apoptotic bodies are infrequent.

The **secretory phase** corresponding to days 21 through 27 features increased secretory activity with distention of glandular lumina. The epithelium consists of columnar cells, and myoepithelial cells display progressively clearer cytoplasm. It is at this stage that mitoses and apoptotic bodies are most conspicuous with maximal intralobular edema associated with a minimal inflammatory cell infiltrate.

In the **menstrual phase**, comprising days 28 through 2, the mammary stroma becomes compact with loss of intralobular edema. At this stage, lymphocytes, macrophages, and plasma cells are most conspicuous in the lobular stroma (22). Some glandular lumina persist, whereas others collapse. Mitotic activity is absent.

The ability to recognize menstrual cycle–related histopathologic changes in the breast is useful—especially for the assessment of proliferative changes. Parenthetically, evidence suggesting that surgery performed during the luteal phase is prognostically advantageous remains controversial (24-28). Also, it is believed that premenopausal women could benefit from higher sensitivity if screening mammography and MRI is scheduled during the first week of the menstrual cycle (29).

Estrogen and progesterone receptors are variably expressed in the nuclei of epithelial cells in the normal breast. Immunostaining reveals a higher proportion of ER and PR reactivity in lobular than in ductal cells. Notably, ER and PR expression is generally higher in older women (30). Considerable heterogeneity exists in ER and PR immunoreactivity in lobules. Maximal expression of ER and PR is typically observed in the follicular phase (31); however, no consistent menstrual cycle–related pattern has been found in the expression of ER and PR in breast carcinomas in premenopausal women (32,33).

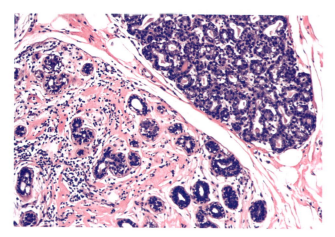

FIGURE 1.7 Lactational Hyperplasia. This needle core biopsy specimen from a 34-week pregnant 31-year-old woman shows lactational hyperplasia in one lobule (upper right) and another unaltered lobule with fibroadenomatoid change (sclerosing ductal hyperplasia).

Secretory changes associated with **pregnancy** occur unevenly throughout the breast **(Fig. 1.7)**. There is progressive recruitment of lobules with advancing stages of pregnancy. Earlier in pregnancy, lobules grow rapidly, resulting in lobular enlargement with relative depletion of the fibrofatty stroma (34). Stromal vascularity increases, accompanied by infiltration by mononuclear inflammatory cells. During the second and third trimesters, lobular growth progresses through epithelial hypertrophy (enlargement of cells) as well as epithelial hyperplasia (proliferation of cells). The cytoplasm of lobular epithelial cells becomes vacuolated, and secretion accumulates in lobular glands (35) **(Fig. 1.8)**. In later stages, there is distention of lumens of lobular glands. The lobular nuclei become hyperchromatic, with prominent nucleoli **(Fig. 1.9)**.

Hormonal alterations that occur during and after **menopause** are manifested by a decrease in the cellularity and number of lobules, that is, atrophy. Coincidentally with the loss of glandular epithelium, there is a tendency toward thickening of basement membranes and collagenization of intralobular stroma. The process of menopausal atrophy occurs in a heterogeneous fashion, often leaving some lobules relatively unaffected. Most lobular glands appear to collapse and shrink, but cystic distention may also occur. Calcifications can form in atrophic lobules **(Fig. 1.10)**. In some elderly women, glandular integrity is lost to such a degree that erstwhile glandular-based calcifications appear to lie embedded directly in fibrocollagenous stroma. Atrophy tends to spare lobular myoepithelial cells. Thus, the latter become

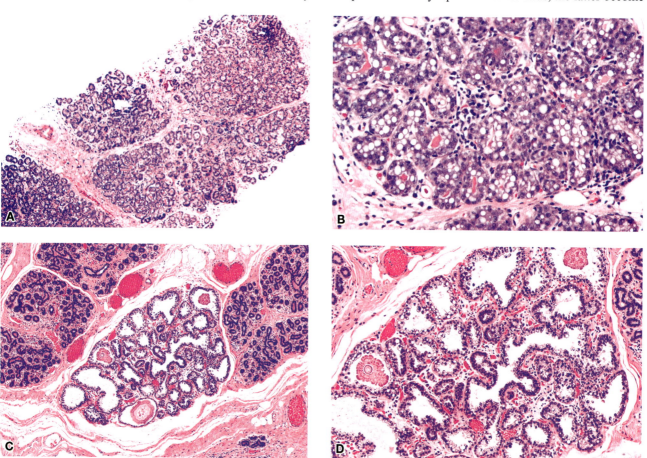

FIGURE 1.8 Lactational Hyperplasia in a Pregnant and in a Nonpregnant and Nonlactating Patient.
A, B: The patient was 8 months pregnant when this needle core biopsy was performed for a mass that proved to be nodular lactational hyperplasia. The markedly enlarged lobules are composed of a greatly increased number of glands that should not be mistaken for carcinoma. **C, D:** The patient was an adult nonpregnant and nonlactating woman with lactational-like hyperplasia in a lobule (center). The enlarged lobule shows prominent secretory change. Note unaltered lobules in the immediate vicinity of the affected lobule.

EMBRYOLOGY, DEVELOPMENT, HISTOLOGY, AND PHYSIOLOGIC MORPHOLOGY

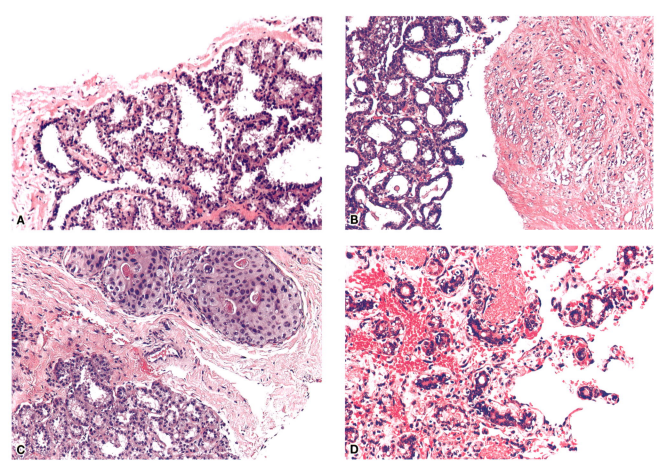

FIGURE 1.9 Uncommon Findings in Lactating Breast. A: This needle core biopsy specimen was obtained from an 8-month postpartum 36-year-old nursing woman. The lactating glands shown here are larger and more irregular in shape than in lactational hyperplasia. The cytoplasm has prominent apical blebs and a frayed appearance at the luminal border. Nuclei are condensed and hyperchromatic. **B:** A portion of this needle core biopsy (right) shows ischemic necrosis in lactational hyperplasia. **C:** This patient was 6-month pregnant when this needle core biopsy was performed for a mass that proved to be ductal carcinoma in situ (DCIS) of the solid type with high-grade nuclei. **D:** Angiosarcoma in a pregnant woman. Note interanastomosing dilated vascular channels that dissect native mammary glands. The latter show secretory change (top right).

relatively prominent. The relative proportions of fat and stroma vary in the atrophic breast; however, in most cases fat is dominant. In advanced atrophy, pronounced elastotic change in the stroma can be a source of calcifications **(Fig. 1.11)**. The extent of TDLU involution has been linked to a lower risk of breast carcinoma; however, this matter has not been fully studied (36).

Mammographic changes suggestive of physiologically induced proliferative alterations have been observed in women receiving **postmenopausal hormone replacement therapy** (37,38). The effect of hormone replacement therapy on the mammographic appearance of the breast is substantially less in women who have undergone breast radiation (39). In the nonirradiated breast, the effect of hormone replacement is manifested mainly by increased parenchymal density. This has been observed after treatment with estrogen alone and with an estrogen–progesterone combination therapy. Histologic examination does not reveal a consistent pattern. Some patients have lobular differentiation comparable to the premenopausal state, whereas others have prominent cystic or proliferative alterations of ducts and lobules. The findings suggest that the existing epithelial status of the breast is accentuated by exogenous hormone administration.

Pregnancy-like change (pseudolactational metaplasia) is usually a focal microscopic alteration characterized by lobules that resembles the physiologic process of lactation. It occurs in breast tissue from women who are neither pregnant nor lactating. Many such patients are parous and either pre- or postmenopausal. Similar changes have been observed in nulliparous women (40). The reported frequency of pregnancy-like change is 1.7% to 3% (40,41). The etiology of pregnancy-like change remains unknown. Glands and terminal ducts with pregnancy-like change usually contain little or no secretions, although they may be dilated **(Fig. 1.12)**. The glandular cells are swollen with abundant pale-to-clear, finely granular, or vacuolated cytoplasm. The nuclei are typically relatively uniformly round. The luminal cytoplasmic borders of glandular cells are frayed, and minute cytoplasmic blebs

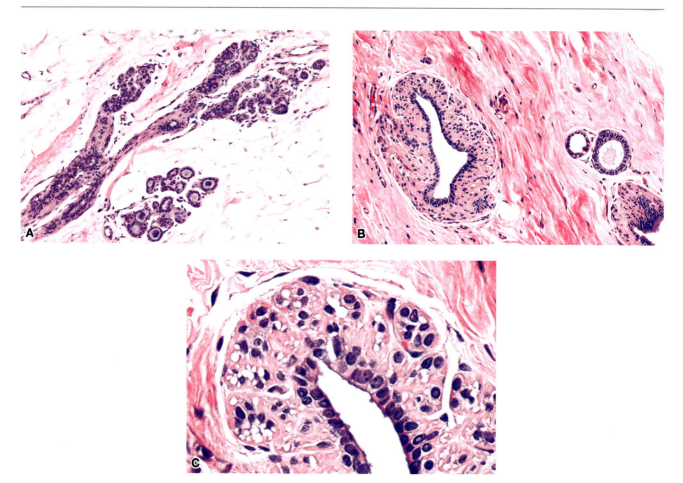

FIGURE 1.10 Atrophy. A: An atrophic lobule with a calcification in inactive glands (lower center). The needle core biopsy was performed on a 73-year-old woman with mammographically detected calcifications. **B, C:** Myoid metaplasia of myoepithelial cells is evident around the atrophic duct in this biopsy specimen.

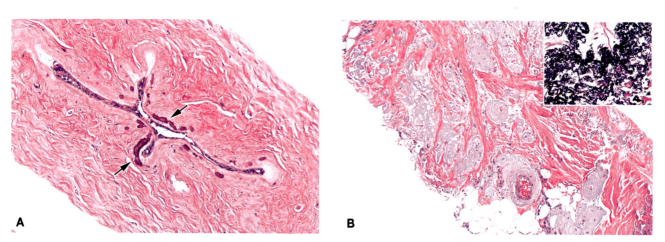

FIGURE 1.11 Atrophy. A: Calcifications (arrows) are shown in the periductal stroma in a needle core biopsy specimen from a postmenopausal woman. **B:** Diffuse stromal elastosis in a needle core biopsy from an elderly woman with a breast mass. Inset highlights elastic fibers on Verhoeff van Gieson stain.

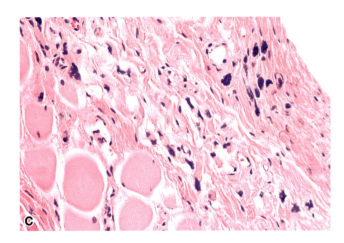
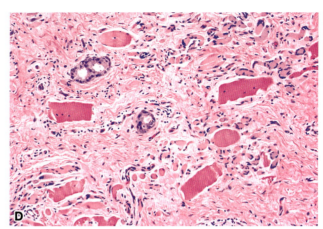
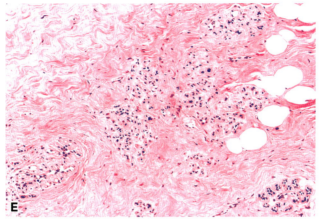

FIGURE 1.11 (*continued*) **C:** Needle core biopsy performed to evaluate a "seroma" (s/p mastectomy) showing atrophy of chest wall skeletal muscle. The altered skeletal muscle fibers appear largely clumped with aggregates of pyknotic nuclei (right). Relatively less affected muscle fibers are seen on left. **D:** Atrophic skeletal muscle fibers around recurrent invasive carcinoma (center and upper -left), status-post mastectomy and radiation. **E:** Marked mammary glandular atrophy, status-post radiation. Note preservation of lobular architecture of the atrophic glands.

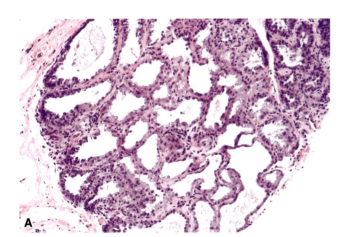
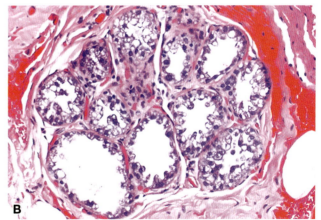

FIGURE 1.12 **Pregnancy-Like Change. A:** This lobule was present in a needle core biopsy specimen from a 49-year-old woman with invasive carcinoma. The enlarged lobule is composed of irregularly shaped glandular acini that contain small amounts of secretion. **B:** Pregnancy-like change in the lobule of a 74-year-old woman who had a needle core biopsy performed for calcifications that were localized to columnar cell change.

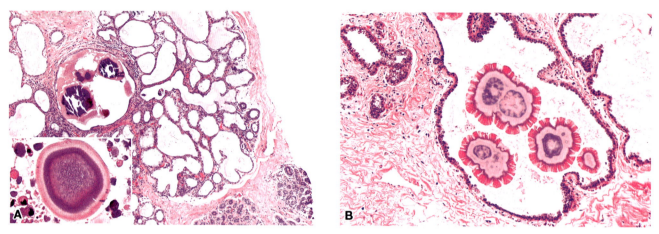

FIGURE 1.13 Pregnancy-Like Change, With Calcification. A, B: Characteristic intraluminal laminated calcifications are present in pregnancy-like change shown in these two-needle core biopsy specimens from adult nonpregnant, nonlactating women with mammographically detected calcifications. Inset (in **A**) shows details of calcifications around a Liesegang-like structure.

are formed that protrude into the glandular lumen. Calcifications, occasionally of the psammomatous type (or with Liesegang-like features), can be formed in pregnancy-like change **(Fig. 1.13)**. Diastase-resistant granules that stain positively with periodic acid–Schiff (PAS) are present in the cytoplasm. The affected cells are immunoreactive for α-lactalbumin and S-100 protein (41).

In most instances, the epithelium in lobules altered by pregnancy-like change remains one or two cell layers thick. **Pregnancy-like hyperplasia** represents the occurrence of pregnancy-like change in hyperplastic epithelium. The hyperplastic epithelial tissue usually assumes papillary or micropapillary configurations **(Fig. 1.14)**. The epithelium is arranged in irregular fronds composed entirely of glandular cells. Although the cytologic appearance may duplicate the findings of pregnancy-like change, some lesions feature nuclear atypia, manifested mainly by nuclear pleomorphism. Rarely, these atypical cytologic changes may warrant a diagnosis of **atypical pregnancy-like hyperplasia (Fig. 1.15)**. Atypical changes are more likely to be present when pregnancy-like hyperplasia coexists with **cystic hypersecretory hyperplasia** (42) **(Fig. 1.16)**. Rarely, carcinoma has been found to arise from pregnancy-like hyperplasia, usually in combination with cystic hypersecretory hyperplasia (43).

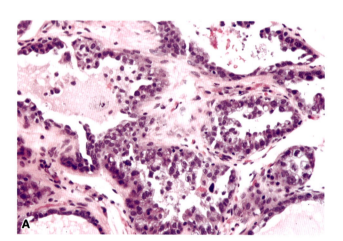
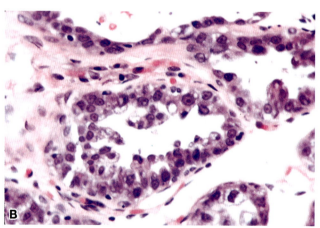

FIGURE 1.14 Pregnancy-Like Hyperplasia. A, B: Micropapillary fronds composed of hyperplastic epithelium protrude into some gland lumina. Note the slightly uneven, crowded distribution of nuclei. Some nuclei have prominent nucleoli. Pale eosinophilic secretion is present. This appearance resembles cystic hypersecretory carcinoma in a lobule, but the epithelium does not have the appearance of micropapillary carcinoma, and the secretion lacks the intense eosinophilia and linear parallel cracks that characterize a cystic hypersecretory lesion.

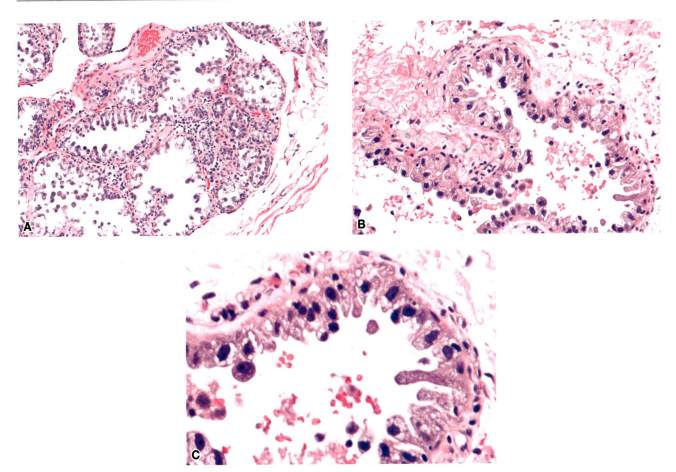

FIGURE 1.15 Atypical Pregnancy-Like Hyperplasia. A: The cells lining the affected glands are elongated and tend to be distributed in a single layer. **B, C:** Enlarged, hyperchromatic, and pleomorphic nuclei in pregnancy-like change from a needle core biopsy specimen in a 48-year-old woman. Despite the cytologic atypia, the cells tend to be distributed in a single layer. Near-extrusion of nuclei is shown at the luminal border.

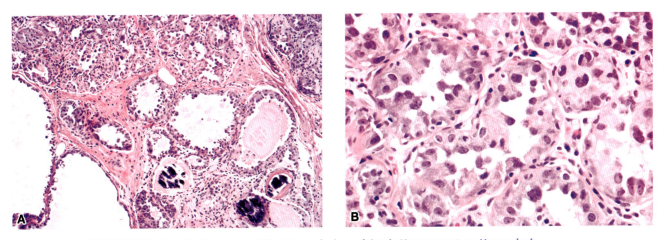

FIGURE 1.16 Atypical Pregnancy-Like Hyperplasia and Cystic Hypersecretory Hyperplasia. A: This needle core biopsy specimen was obtained for calcifications that proved to be at the junction between cystic hypersecretory hyperplasia (below) and atypical pregnancy-like hyperplasia (above). **B:** Magnified view of lobular glands in atypical pregnancy-like hyperplasia.

METAPLASIA

Apocrine metaplasia is a common "normal" finding in the glandular epithelia of the adult female breast. Apocrine metaplastic cells of the breast are histologically akin to the apocrine cells that are normally present in cutaneous glands, especially in the axillary, periareolar, and perineal regions. On hematoxylin and eosin (H&E) stain, apocrine cells may appear to be either uniformly pink with extremely fine vacuoles or coarse granules. The granules are birefringent and tend to accumulate in the luminal aspect of cells. Apical snouts can be a prominent feature. In general, the nuclei of apocrine cells are round and centrally placed with distinct nucleoli. Nucleoli may not be evident in flattened or cuboidal apocrine epithelium. Apocrine cells typically show some nuclear variability, even in putatively inactive cells; however, overt nuclear atypia, mitotic activity, and necrosis are harbingers of apocrine carcinoma. It is notable that radiation-related nuclear changes are relatively more evident in apocrine metaplastic cells. Apocrine metaplastic cells are immunoreactive for epithelial membrane antigen (EMA), cytokeratins 8 and 18, and androgen receptors (AR). They usually do not express ER or PR. Apocrine cells are also immunoreactive with proteins found in mammary cyst fluids, namely, gross cystic disease fluid protein (GCDFP) 15, 24, and 44 (44).

Clear cell (change) metaplasia is a cytologic alteration in lobular and terminal duct epithelium that has also been referred to as *hellenzellen* (German: clear or bright cells) (45). The etiology of clear cell change remains unknown. The affected lobules tend to be larger than adjacent uninvolved lobules. Some glands have dilated lumina in which there is PAS-positive, diastase-resistant secretion, but more often, the lobular gland lumina are obliterated by the swollen cells (46). The lobular gland epithelium is composed of swollen cells with abundant clear or pale cytoplasm **(Fig. 1.17)**. The cells have well-defined borders. The relatively small, round, and dark nuclei are often displaced toward the center of the gland. Calcifications are uncommon in clear cell change. The clear cells are immunoreactive for cytokeratin but not for actin. This type of change is encountered in pre- and postmenopausal women, and there is no association with pregnancy or with exogenous hormone use (46,47). Foci of clear cell change have been identified retrospectively in breast tissue obtained before exogenous hormones were available. This type of change is usually multifocal and can be bilateral. Viña and Wells (41) reported finding clear cell change in 15 of 934 (1.6%) biopsies. Specimens that contain clear cell change may harbor carcinoma or a variety of benign or atypical changes (41). Rarely, clear cell and pregnancy-like changes may coexist in the same breast (47). The differential diagnosis of

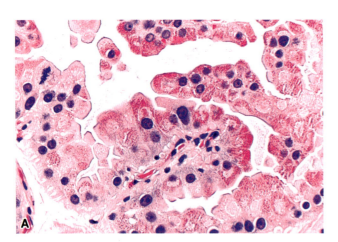

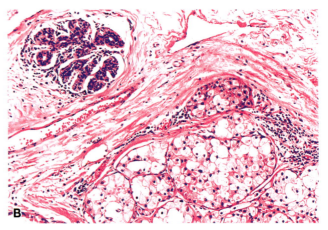

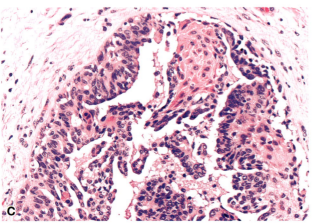

FIGURE 1.17 Metaplastic (Apocrine, Clear Cell, and Squamous) Changes in Breast Epithelia. A: Apocrine metaplasia is characterized by uniformly pink cytoplasm with relatively fine granules. **B:** Clear cell change in the lower lobule is composed of cells with optically clear cytoplasm and minute dark nuclei in this needle core biopsy from a 54-year-old woman. **C:** Squamous metaplasia (lower right) involves a duct adjacent to duct ectasia.

clear cell change includes pregnancy-like change as well as cytoplasmic clearing in apocrine metaplastic cells and in myoepithelial cells and clear cell forms of carcinoma—such as some cases of lobular carcinoma, glycogen-rich carcinoma, and metastatic renal clear cell carcinoma. Pregnancy-like change is readily distinguished from clear cell change by the presence of "decapitation" secretion at the luminal borders of the cells in the former. Cytoplasmic clearing in apocrine metaplasia is usually a focal change in epithelium that otherwise has the typical features of apocrine metaplasia. Myoepithelial cells with clear cell change retain their position between the epithelium and basement membrane.

Squamous metaplasia of the mammary epithelium occurs in association with inflammatory, reactive, and ischemic conditions; however, in current practice it is most commonly encountered as an iatrogenic reparative change in epithelium damaged by an antecedent procedure. De novo squamous metaplasia may, inexplicably, be associated with intraductal papilloma (48), phyllodes tumor, and gynecomastia.

REFERENCES

1. Marinho-Soares C, Pulido-Valente M. Axillary mass after delivery. *N Engl J Med*. 2021;385:450.
2. Spina E, Cowin P. Embryonic mammary gland development. *Semin Cell Dev Biol*. 2021;114:83-92.
3. McNally S, Stein T. Overview of mammary gland development: a comparison of mouse and human. *Methods Mol Biol*. 2017;1501:1-17.
4. Codner E, Román R. Premature thelarche from phenotype to genotype. *Pediatr Endocrinol Rev*. 2008;5:760-765.
5. van Winter JT, Noller KL, Zimmerman D, Melton LJ. Natural history of premature thelarche in Olmsted County, Minnesota, 1940 to 1984. *J Pediatr*. 1990;116:278-280.
6. Curfman AL, Reljanovic SM, McNelis KM, et al. Premature thelarche in infants and children: prevalence, natural history and environmental determinants. *J Pediatr Adolesc Gynecol*. 2011;24:338-341.
7. Pasquino AM, Pucarelli I, Passeri F, Segni M, Mancini MA, Municchi G. Progression of premature thelarche to central precocious puberty. *J Pediatr*. 1995;126:11-14.
8. Adriance MC, Inman JL, Petersen OW, Bissell MJ. Myoepithelial cells: good fences make good neighbors. *Breast Cancer Res*. 2005;7:190-197.
9. Topper YJ, Freeman CS. Multiple hormone interactions in the developmental biology of the mammary gland. *Physiol Rev*. 1980;60:1049-1106.
10. Lee NA, Rusinek H, Weinreb J, et al. Fatty and fibroglandular tissue volumes in the breasts of women 20-83 years old: comparison of x-ray mammography and computer-assisted MR imaging. *AJR Am J Roentgenol*. 1997;168:501-506.
11. Huo CW, Chew GL, Britt KL, et al. Mammographic density—a review on the current understanding of its association with breast cancer. *Breast Cancer Res Treat*. 2014;144:479-502.
12. Maskarinec G, Pagano IS, Little MA, Conroy SM, Park SY, Kolonel LN. Mammographic density as a predictor of breast cancer survival: the multiethnic cohort. *Breast Cancer Res*. 2013;15:R7.
13. Zucca-Matthes G, Urban C, Vallejo A. Anatomy of the nipple and breast ducts. *Gland Surg*. 2016;5:32-36.
14. Rosen PP, Tench W. Lobules in the nipple: frequency and significance for breast cancer treatment. *Pathol Annu*. 1985;20(pt 1):317-322.
15. Cheng H, Yang S, Qu Z, Zhou S, Ruan Q. Novel use for DOG1 in discriminating breast invasive carcinoma from noninvasive breast lesions. *Dis Markers*. 2016;2016:5628176. doi:10.1155/2016/5628176
16. Cserni G. Lack of myoepithelium in apocrine glands of the breast does not necessarily imply malignancy. *Histopathology*. 2008;52:253-255.
17. Tramm T, Kim JY, Tavassoli FA. Diminished number or complete loss of myoepithelial cells associated with metaplastic and neoplastic apocrine lesions of the breast. *Am J Surg Pathol*. 2011;35:202-211.
18. Cserni G. Benign apocrine papillary lesions of the breast lacking or virtually lacking myoepithelial cells—potential pitfalls in diagnosing malignancy. *APMIS*. 2012;120:249-252.
19. Davies JD. Pigmented periductal cells (ochrocytes) in mammary dysplasias: their nature and significance. *J Pathol*. 1974;114:205-216.
20. Christov K, Chew KL, Ljung B-M, et al. Proliferation of normal breast epithelial cells as shown by in vivo labeling with bromodeoxyuridine. *Am J Pathol*. 1991;138:1371-1377.
21. Ramakrishnan R, Khan SA, Badve S. Morphological changes in breast tissue with menstrual cycle. *Mod Pathol*. 2002;15:1348-1356.
22. Longacre TA, Bartow SA. A correlative morphologic study of human breast and endometrium in the menstrual cycle. *Am J Surg Pathol*. 1986;10:382-393.
23. Ferguson DJP, Anderson TJ. Morphological evaluation of cell turnover in relation to the menstrual cycle in the "resting" human breast. *Br J Cancer*. 1981;4:177-181.
24. Donegan W, Shah D. Prognosis of patients with breast cancer related to the timing of operation. *Arch Surg*. 1993;128:309-313.
25. Badwe R, Mittra I, Havaldar R. Timing of surgery during the menstrual cycle and prognosis of breast cancer. *J Biosci*. 2000;25:113-120.
26. Milella M, Nisticò C, Ferraresi V, et al. Breast cancer and timing of surgery during menstrual cycle: a 5-year analysis of 248 premenopausal women. *Breast Cancer Res Treat*. 1999;55:259-266.
27. Nomura Y, Kataoka A, Tsutsui S, Murakami S, Takenaka Y. Lack of correlation between timing of surgery in relation to the menstrual cycle and prognosis of premenopausal patients with early breast cancer. *Eur J Cancer*. 1999;35:1326-1330.
28. Grant CS, Ingle JN, Suman VJ, et al. Menstrual cycle and surgical treatment of breast cancer: findings from the NCCTG N9431 study. *J Clin Oncol*. 2009;27:3620-3626.
29. Miglioretti DL, Walker R, Weaver DL, et al. Accuracy of screening mammography varies by week of menstrual cycle. *Radiology*. 2011;258:372-379.
30. Santandrea G, Bellarosa C, Gibertoni D, et al. Hormone receptor expression variations in normal breast tissue: preliminary results of a prospective observational study. *J Pers Med*. 2021;11:387.
31. Fabris G, Marchetti E, Marzola A, Bagni A, Querzoli P, Nenci I. Pathophysiology of estrogen receptors in mammary tissue by monoclonal antibodies. *J Steroid Biochem Mol Biol*. 1987;27:171-176.
32. Markopoulos C, Berger U, Wilson P, Gazet JC, Coombes RC. Estrogen receptor content of normal breast cells and breast carcinoma throughout the menstrual cycle. *Br Med J*. 1988;296:1349-1351.
33. Smyth CM, Benn DE, Reeve TS. Influence of the menstrual cycle on the concentrations of estrogen and progesterone receptors in primary breast cancer biopsies. *Breast Cancer Res Treat*. 1988;11:45-50.
34. Collins LC, Schnitt SJ. Breast. In: Mills SE, ed. *Histology for Pathologists*. Raven Press; 2020:69-87.
35. Heymann JJ, Halligan AM, Hoda SA, Facey KE, Hoda RS. Fine needle aspiration of breast masses in pregnant and lactating women: experience with 28 cases emphasizing Thinprep findings. *Diagn Cytopathol*. 2015;43:188-194.
36. Figueroa JD, Pfeiffer RM, Patel DA, et al. Terminal duct lobular unit involution of the normal breast: implications for breast cancer etiology. *J Natl Cancer Inst*. 2014;106(10):dju286.
37. Rand T, Heytmanek G, Seifert M, et al. Mammography in women undergoing hormone replacement therapy: possible effects revealed at routine examination. *Acta Radiol*. 1997;38:228-231.
38. Laya MB, Gallagher JC, Schreiman JS, Larson EB, Watson P, Weinstein L. Effect of postmenopausal hormonal replacement therapy on mammographic density and parenchymal pattern. *Radiology*. 1995;196:433-437.
39. Margolin FR, Denny SR, Gelfand CA, Jacobs RP. Mammographic changes after hormone replacement therapy in patients who have undergone breast irradiation. *AJR Am J Roentgenol*. 1999;172:147-150.
40. Kiaer HW, Andersen JA. Focal pregnancy-like changes in the breast. *Acta Pathol Microbiol Scand A*. 1977;85:931-941.
41. Viña M, Wells CA. Clear cell metaplasia of the breast: a lesion showing eccrine differentiation. *Histopathology*. 1989;15:85-92.
42. Shin SJ, Rosen PP. Pregnancy-like (pseudolactational) hyperplasia: a primary diagnosis in mammographically detected lesions of the breast and its relationship to cystic hypersecretory hyperplasia. *Am J Surg Pathol*. 2000;24:1670-1674.
43. Shin SJ, Rosen PP. Carcinoma arising from preexisting pregnancy-like and cystic hypersecretory hyperplasia lesions of the breast: a clinicopathologic study of 9 patients. *Am J Surg Pathol*. 2004;28:789-793.
44. Wells CA, El-Ayat GA. Non-operative breast pathology: apocrine lesions. *J Clin Pathol*. 2007;60:1313-1320.
45. Skorpil F. About the occurrence of so-called light cells in the mammary gland. *Beitr Pathol Anat*. 1943;108:378-393.
46. Barwick KW, Kashgarian M, Rosen PP. "Clear-cell" change within duct and lobular epithelium of the human breast. *Pathol Annu*. 1982;17 (pt 1):319-328.
47. Tavassoli FA, Yeh IT. Lactational and clear cell changes of the breast in nonlactating, nonpregnant women. *Am J Clin Pathol*. 1987;87:23-29.
48. Ginter PS, Hoda SA, Ozerdem U. Exuberant squamous metaplasia in an intraductal papilloma of breast. *Int J Surg Pathol*. 2015;23:125-126.

Inflammatory and Reactive Lesions

RAZA S. HODA AND SYED A. HODA

Needle core biopsy (NCB) of the breast is usually performed to evaluate lesions that are either palpable or detected via various imaging modalities, including mammography, sonography, and magnetic resonance imaging (MRI). Thus, NCBs yield a wide variety of neoplastic and inflammatory/reactive conditions. Many of the latter are described in this chapter.

FAT NECROSIS

Mammary fat necrosis may occasionally result from incidental trauma; however, currently, the most common causes are previous needling procedures (eg, fine needle aspiration [FNA] or NCB), surgery, and radiation therapy (1,2). Patients with fat necrosis typically present with a painless superficial mass, occasionally associated with retraction or dimpling of the overlying skin. Any part of the breast may be affected. At presentation, the typically solitary mass spans approximately 2 cm. Fat necrosis in the male breast is usually traumatic in origin and can also be diagnosed on NCB (3). Hemorrhagic and fat necrosis of subcutaneous and breast tissue, occasionally progressing to gangrenous necrosis, has been associated with warfarin (Coumadin) anticoagulant treatment (4); however, with better therapeutic monitoring, this iatrogenic complication is now uncommon (5).

The clinical and radiologic problem of distinguishing fat necrosis from recurrent carcinoma is especially difficult in patients who have undergone breast-conserving surgery and various modalities of radiation therapy (6-8). Mammography of fat necrosis usually reveals a spiculated mass that may contain irregular, punctate, or coarse calcifications (9,10). Less frequently, the lesion appears as an "oil cyst": a circumscribed, oil-filled, partly calcified cyst (11). Both patterns may coexist in a single lesion. Ultrasonography and MRI features of fat necrosis are also variable and may be indistinguishable from carcinoma (10).

The initial histologic change in fat necrosis is adipocyte injury (diminished size, fine vacuolization, and dropout) associated with a neutrophilic infiltrate **(Fig. 2.1)**. Further evolution of the lesion is marked by the progressive appearance of histiocytes, eosinophils, lymphocytes, and plasma cells—occasionally with deposition of hemosiderin **(Fig. 2.2)**. Some histiocytes that accompany fat necrosis can simulate lipoblasts. Unlike lipoblasts, histiocytes are of relatively uniform size with fine intracytoplasmic vacuoles that do not indent the generally round nucleus. A giant cell granulomatous reaction may develop over time. Fibrosis develops peripherally, demarcating the region of necrotic fat, cellular debris, and calcifications **(Fig. 2.3)**. In late lesions, the reactive inflammatory components are replaced by fibroplasia, which evolves into a dense scar. An exaggerated histiocytic response to fat necrosis that can be encountered post NCB may take the form of a "cellular spindled histiocytic pseudotumor" (12) (arguably, an innovative term for "inflammatory pseudotumor," IPT), wherein the mitotically active histiocytic spindle cell proliferation has the potential to be mistaken for spindle cell neoplasm, including metaplastic carcinoma. Reactive squamous metaplasia may develop in ducts and lobules in the vicinity of fat necrosis. Loculated necrotic fat ("oil cysts") may persist for years, and dystrophic calcifications are permanent. Among patients who develop fat necrosis after radiotherapy, the characteristic histopathologic effects of radiation on stromal, vascular, and epithelial tissues can be identified in the native mammary tissue.

A peculiar form of individual fat necrosis is manifested by histiocytes encircling necrotic adipocytes. These histiocytes form a "crown-like structure" **(Fig. 2.4)**. The structures can be found, de novo, in mammary adipose tissue of patients who are obese and those with breast carcinoma and may be indicative of insulin resistance (13).

NCB is indicated in all instances wherein clinical and radiologic diagnosis of fat necrosis is uncertain. Careful microscopic examination is warranted in every NCB of fat necrosis because the process may mask a histologically occult invasive carcinoma **(Fig. 2.5)**. The use of epithelial (cytokeratin) and histiocytic (CD68, CD163, etc.) immunostains can be helpful in this regard.

Erdheim–Chester Disease

Erdheim–Chester disease (also known as *sclerosing non-Langerhans cell histiocytosis* and as *polyostotic fibrosing histiocytosis*), an extremely infrequent xanthomatous form of histiocytosis of uncertain etiology, rarely involves the breast (14,15). Histologically, the disease can be mistaken for fat necrosis, especially if the initial clinical manifestation is a breast mass (14). Typically, there are synchronous cutaneous, osseous, and orbital lesions that are characterized by infiltrates of histiocytes, Touton-type giant cells (with wreath-like arrangement of nuclei at the perimeter of the giant cell), plasma cells, and infrequent epithelioid granulomata. The lesional histiocytes are immunoreactive

INFLAMMATORY AND REACTIVE LESIONS **15**

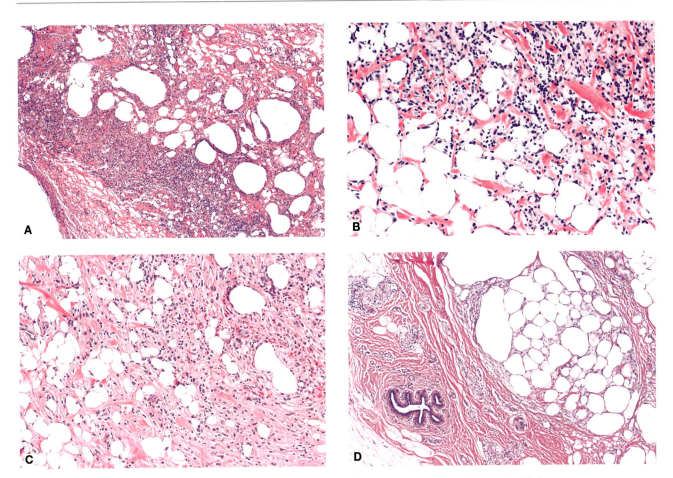

FIGURE 2.1 Fat Necrosis, Earlier Phases. A, B: Early fat necrosis manifested by a mixed inflammatory cell infiltrate with associated hemorrhage. The inciting injury was sustained a few days back. **C:** Fat necrosis, subacute phase. Note the presence of lymphocytes and eosinophils amid necrotic adipocytes. The instigating trauma was suffered 2 weeks back. **D:** Early organizing fat necrosis: Histiocytes are prominent, and there is fibroplasia. This NCB of a breast mass followed a sports injury 4 weeks earlier.

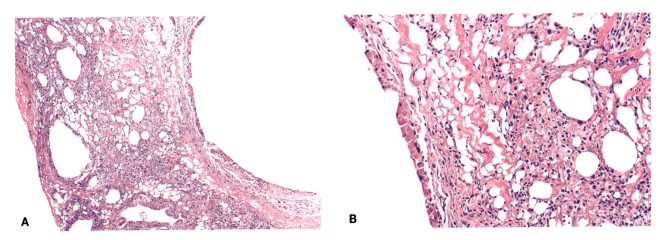

FIGURE 2.2 Fat Necrosis, Later Phases. A, B: Note cystic change (created by liquefactive necrosis of adipocytes) amid fat necrosis. The cystic space is lined by histiocytes.

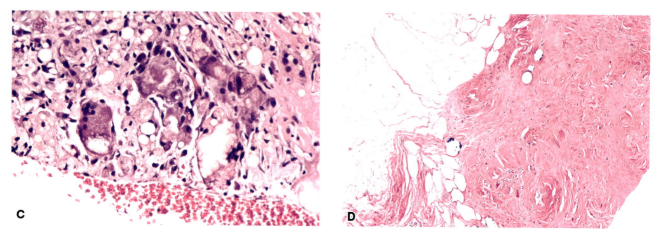

FIGURE 2.2 (*continued*) **C:** Multinucleated giant cells of the foreign body material are present amid the process. **D:** Fibrotic scarring following fat necrosis. Note stromal-based calcification (fractured) amid fibrosis.

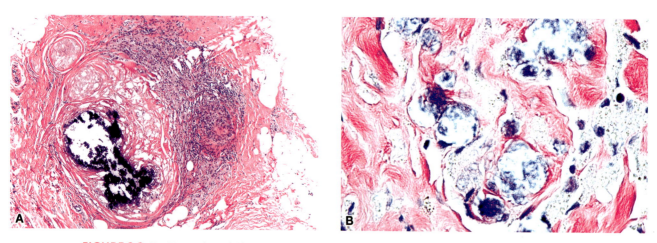

FIGURE 2.3 Fat Necrosis, Calcifications. **A:** Coarse calcification and fibrosis are evident around this focus of healed fat necrosis. The section shows "knife scoring" artifact (top right) resulting from damage to the microtome knife caused by the dense deposit of calcification. **B:** Stromal-based particulate-type calcifications that seem to have deposited onto necrotic adipocytes.

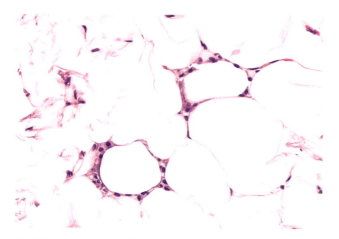

FIGURE 2.4 "Crown-Like Structure" in Fat Necrosis. Histiocytes encircle necrotic adipocytes forming "crown-like structures." These structures can be found, de novo, in mammary adipose tissue of patients who are obese and those with breast carcinoma.

for CD68 but are negative for S-100 protein, CD1a, and cytokeratins (14). The disease is usually interpreted as a benign histiocytic proliferation on NCB—unless the clinical setting is known, and Touton-type giant cells are recognized (15).

BREAST INFARCT

Breast infarct (ischemic necrosis) typically occurs during pregnancy or in the postpartum period and usually presents as a solitary, discrete, and firm mass that can clinically suggest carcinoma. Pain and tenderness are common. Hemorrhage and ischemic degeneration with minimal inflammatory cell infiltrate characterize the histologic appearance of early lesions. Later stages feature fully developed necrosis (ie, infarct), usually of the coagulative type. Bilateral and multifocal infarcts involving lactational breast tissue have been reported (16). Infarcts can occur spontaneously in fibroadenomas (17-19) and in benign proliferative lesions. Foci of necrosis may be found in florid sclerosing adenosis, usually

INFLAMMATORY AND REACTIVE LESIONS

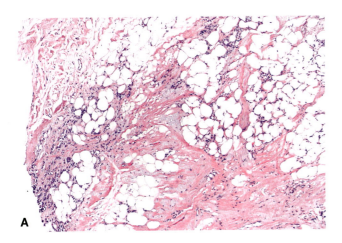
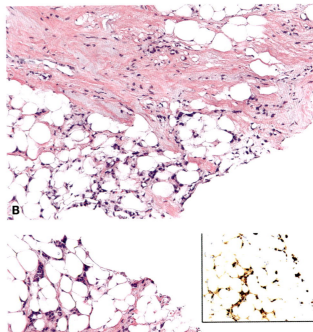

FIGURE 2.5 Invasive Carcinoma in Needle Core Biopsies Simulating Fat Necrosis. A-C: Three examples of invasive lobular carcinoma, all without a history of antecedent trauma or prior needling procedure, are shown. Cursory microscopic examination can misleadingly suggest fat necrosis in each case. Inset in **(C)** shows estrogen receptor positivity in the malignant cells.

during pregnancy. Reactive cytologic atypia can be striking in FNA of breast infarcts (20,21).

Papillomas are susceptible to partial or complete infarction, especially those that occur in major lactiferous ducts. Infarcts can occur in papillomas at any age but tend to be more frequent in postmenopausal women, and there is no known association with pregnancy. Bloody nipple discharge is the most frequent sign of an infarcted papilloma. Acute infarcts in papillomas exhibit ischemic degeneration that progresses to coagulative necrosis. Despite increasing loss of cytologic detail, the architectural integrity of the papilloma is usually maintained **(Fig. 2.6)**. At a later stage, fragmentation of infarcted papillomas occurs. Occasionally, such necrotic papillomas convert to inflammatory polyps. The latter comprise mainly granulation tissue with little or no epithelium. Healing of infarcts is marked by fibrosis, which may cause sclerosing entrapment of residual epithelium, producing a pattern that could be mistaken for carcinoma (22). Squamous metaplasia sometimes develops in the proliferating reparative epithelium within an infarcted papilloma (23,24). The latter may develop calcifications.

Infarcted carcinoma can be distinguished from infarction of a benign lesion if there is residual viable in situ or invasive carcinoma (25) **(Fig. 2.7)**. In such cases, one can display the "ghost" architecture of the lesion upon reticulin staining. In some instances, immunoreactivity for epithelial and myoepithelial markers (especially CK-AE1/AE3 and p63) is surprisingly well preserved. When this occurs, it may be possible to "resurrect" the structure of the original lesion to a considerable degree. If a papillary structure can be demonstrated in this circumstance, the lesion was more likely a papilloma rather than a papillary carcinoma because infarcts occur considerably more often in benign papillary tumors than in papillary carcinomas.

NCB can be diagnostic of a mammary infarct. In most cases, recognition of the underlying condition hinges on finding a residual histologically viable (ie, noninfarcted) component. As noted earlier, a reticulin stain and myoepithelial immunostains (particularly p63) may be useful. Rarely, the diagnosis of a totally infarcted lesion remains enigmatic.

Before diagnosing a breast infarct, particularly on NCB sampling, it is prudent to exclude the presence of a centrally necrotizing carcinoma. These carcinomas typically harbor a large central acellular zone (26). Clinical and radiologic correlation is helpful in this regard.

GALACTOCELE

A galactocele is a cystically dilated major duct, typically filled with degenerated milky contents. The lesion is encountered in younger women who are either pregnant or lactating. At presentation, the lesion typically spans about

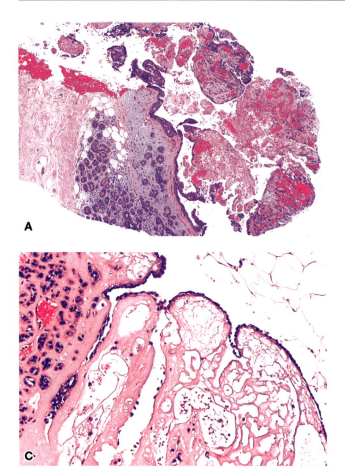

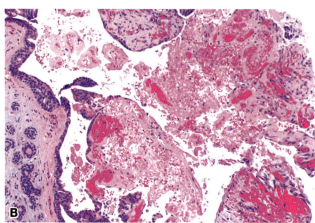

FIGURE 2.6 **Infarcted Papilloma. A, B:** A needle core biopsy specimen showing focal infarction (and associated hemorrhage) in a papilloma. **C:** Excised partially necrotic papilloma showing focal intact papillary structures with viable cells (top left).

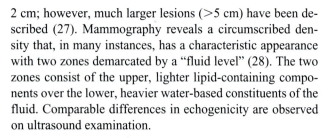

2 cm; however, much larger lesions (>5 cm) have been described (27). Mammography reveals a circumscribed density that, in many instances, has a characteristic appearance with two zones demarcated by a "fluid level" (28). The two zones consist of the upper, lighter lipid-containing components over the lower, heavier water-based constituents of the fluid. Comparable differences in echogenicity are observed on ultrasound examination.

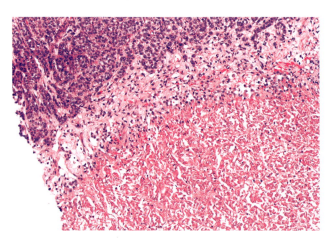

FIGURE 2.7 **Infarct in Invasive Carcinoma.** This needle core biopsy specimen shows ischemic type necrosis (ie, infarct) in an invasive solid-type of lobular carcinoma. The necrotic portion of the tumor is rimmed by reactive granulation tissue (center).

Clinically, the firm and usually painless lesion may suggest carcinoma. Necrotic cells and debris, accompanied by inflammatory cells, are present in FNA-derived cytology preparation (29,30). Viable cells with reactive hyperchromatic nuclei may be present and could be mistaken for carcinoma. Excisional biopsy is diagnostic and provides adequate therapy if the lesion does not resolve after the aspiration of cyst contents.

Histologically, a galactocele is composed of a cyst, or an aggregate of cysts, lined by simple cuboidal epithelium **(Fig. 2.8)**. The cysts contain milky inspissated secretions in the form of soft caseous material. Intact cysts are encompassed by a variably thick fibrous wall with little or no inflammatory reaction. Leakage from a cyst elicits a chronic inflammatory cell reaction that may be accompanied by fat necrosis and a xanthogranulomatous reaction (31). Peri-implant galactocele formation has been described after breast augmentation procedure (32) and also after an NCB procedure (33).

DUCT ECTASIA

Duct ectasia (ie, dilatation) is usually encountered in the breasts of premenopausal women as a localized reaction to inspissated secretions in larger ducts (34). The earliest symptom of the disease is spontaneous, intermittent, mainly watery nipple discharge. Upon disease progression, subareolar induration may lead to the formation of a mass and turbid

INFLAMMATORY AND REACTIVE LESIONS   19

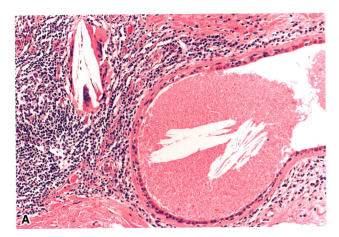
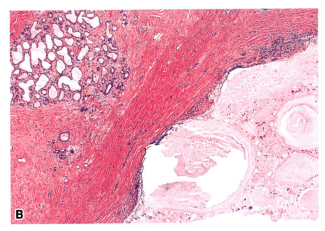

FIGURE 2.8 **Galactocele. A, B:** Cystically dilated glands, with "milky" contents, are lined by flattened epithelial cells. Cholesterol crystals are present within and outside the galactocele (**A**). Note pregnancy-related change in the native breast tissue adjacent to this galactocele (**B**).

greenish nipple discharge. Nipple retraction and inversion are generally associated with periductal fibrosis and contracture. In some cases, squamous metaplasia of the terminal lactiferous duct epithelium results in obstruction that contributes to ductal dilatation and could eventually lead to the formation of lactiferous duct fistulas (35,36). The mammographic abnormalities include calcifications, spiculated masses, and lobulated masses and can rarely simulate carcinoma (37).

The composition of the intraluminal contents in duct ectasia is variable, ranging from galactocele-like lesions (Fig. 2.8) to eosinophilic (granular or amorphous) proteinaceous material to an admixture of lipid-containing histiocytic cells and desquamated epithelial cells. Cholesterol crystals and calcifications may be found amid such debris. Histiocytes that contain a yellow-brown pigment, related to lipofuscin, have been termed *ochrocytes* by Davies (38). Foam cells, histiocytes with finely vacuolated cytoplasm, may be found within ductal lumina, between the epithelial and myoepithelial layers of ducts, and in periductal tissues (**Fig. 2.9**). The presence of neutrophils, lymphocytes, and plasma cells within the ducts indicates an intense inflammatory reaction (**Fig. 2.10**). Disruption of ectatic ducts leads to spillage of stasis material (including cholesterol crystals) into periductal tissue, leading to periductal inflammation. Deposition of cholesterol crystals is the predominant finding in NCB of mass-forming lesions related to duct ectasia ("cholesteroloma") (39,40). Plasma cells and granulomata are inconspicuous features of duct ectasia. Calcium oxalate crystals may be found when stasis occurs in a duct with apocrine epithelium (Fig. 2.10).

Histiocytes with clear or "foamy" cytoplasm positioned in ductal epithelia can be confused with pagetoid carcinoma cells. In most instances, the distinction is made with ease on the basis of bland nuclear cytology of these cells, and the associated characteristic reactive features, of duct ectasia. The histiocytic phenotype of foam cells can be confirmed by CD68 (KP-1) immunoreactivity. These cells are negative for cytoplasmic cytokeratin and actin but may

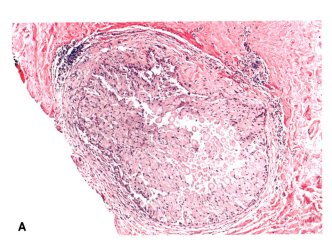
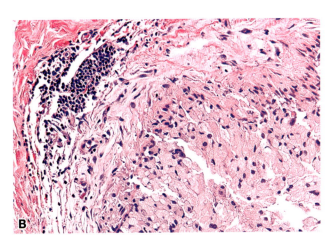

FIGURE 2.9 **Duct Ectasia. A, B:** Discovery of an ill-defined palpable lesion led to a needle core biopsy that demonstrated this dilated duct with a prominent (mainly) intraluminal accumulation of histiocytes.

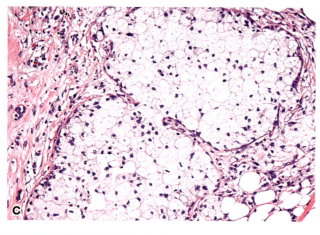
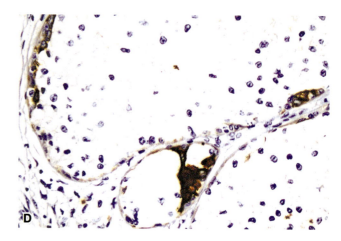
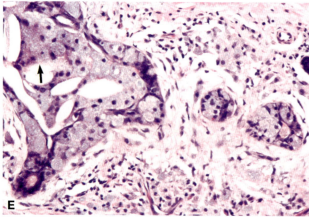

FIGURE 2.9 (*continued*) **C:** Histiocytes with vacuolated, granular cytoplasm are clustered in this dilated duct in another case. **D:** Ectasia of a duct with a solid accumulation of histiocytes mimics clear cell ductal carcinoma in situ. Residual ductal epithelial cells are highlighted by cytokeratin immunostain. The intraluminal histiocytes are cytokeratin-negative. **E:** Ochrocytes (ie, histiocytes with finely granular ceroid pigment) (arrow) are present in the lumen and in the lining epithelia of the duct and in periductal tissue.

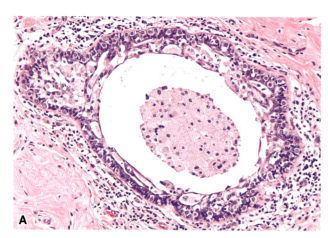
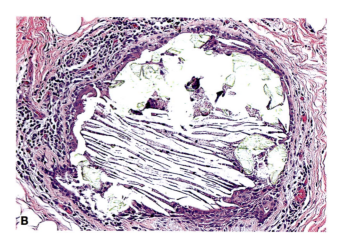
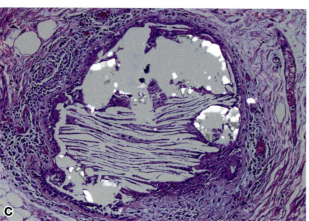

FIGURE 2.10 Duct Ectasia. Luminal Appearances. **A:** This dilated duct with intraluminal histiocytes is surrounded by lymphocytes. Note the histiocytes in the epithelial lining at the perimeter of the duct. **B, C:** A prominent inflammatory cell reaction composed of neutrophils, lymphocytes, and histiocytes involves this duct. Note loss of the native ductal epithelial lining. The intraductal "transparent" calcium oxalate crystals glow when viewed with polarized light **(C)**.

INFLAMMATORY AND REACTIVE LESIONS

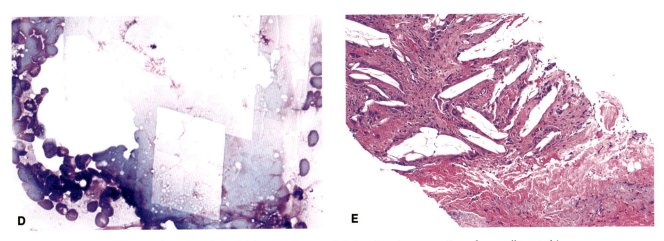

FIGURE 2.10 (*continued*) **D:** Calcium oxalate crystals in a touch preparation of a needle core biopsy. The latter mainly showed duct ectasia and focal cystic apocrine hyperplasia (Diff-Quik stain). **E:** Healed duct ectasia with intraductal deposition of cholesterol crystals associated with fibrosis. This pattern has been called a "cholesteroloma" when it is associated with a mass.

display misleading surface cytokeratin staining from the cell membranes of contiguous epithelial cells or weak reactivity for adsorbed antigens such as gross cystic disease fluid protein-15 (GCDFP-15) (41).

In advanced cases of duct ectasia, the development of periductal fibrosis and hyperelastosis, often with a lamellar distribution, leads to mural thickening. The inflammatory cell reaction is less conspicuous, and the ducts are encased in thickened laminated layers of fibrous and elastic tissue (42). The duct lumen can become widely dilated, or even partially obliterated with formation of secondary lumens at its perimeter, resulting in a distinctive "garland-like" pattern (a pattern that has been termed "mastitis obliterans") **(Fig. 2.11)**. In some instances, the periductal reactive process includes proliferating granulation tissue and hyperelastosis that can narrow, and even occlude, ducts (43,44). The affected ducts may eventually be reduced to a fibrous scar. Remnants of persisting epithelium may proliferate to form secondary glands within such sclerotic ducts.

The diagnosis of primary "histiocytoid" breast carcinoma should be considered in cases wherein minimally atypical histiocyte-like cells proliferate with neither admixed inflammatory cell infiltrate nor ductal disruption. Use of epithelial (cytokeratin) and histiocytic (CD68) immunostains can be helpful in confirming the diagnosis (45).

Occasionally, it may be difficult to distinguish duct ectasia from cystic change—particularly in NCB material **(Fig. 2.12)**. Typically, cysts are clustered, display a rounder outline, and lack periductal elastosis. Abundant intraluminal and periductal histiocytes are more common in duct ectasia.

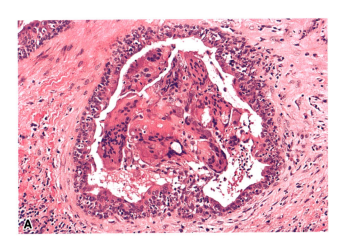
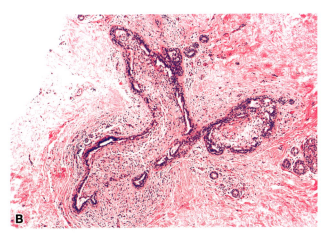

FIGURE 2.11 **Evolution of Ductitis Obliterans (Duct Ectasia, Later Phases). A:** Early duct ectasia with intraluminal multinucleated histiocytes. These are replaced by fibrosis. **B-D:** Duct ectasia showing phases in the development of mastitis obliterans, in three different cases. Healing fibrous "polyp" formation progressively "obliterates" most of the ductal lumen. The garland-like structure (best developed in **D**) is characteristic of healed duct ectasia (ie, ductitis obliterans).

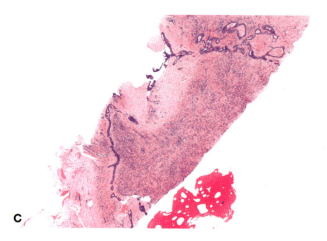
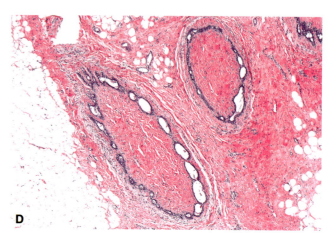

FIGURE 2.11 (continued)

SO-CALLED PLASMA CELL MASTITIS

The ill-defined disease process known as plasma cell mastitis (PCM) has been used for a form of periductal mastitis with a prominent plasma cell reaction. Lesions that have been diagnosed as PCM have shown marked diffuse plasma cell infiltrate surrounding ducts and lobules, typically in the vicinity of duct ectasia. **(Fig. 2.13)**. Lymphocytes and neutrophils have been variably present. The term PCM has been loosely used for a variety of lesions in which there is an overwhelming plasma cell infiltration. Plasmacytoma and myeloma should be considered in the differential diagnosis.

DIABETIC (LYMPHOCYTIC) MASTOPATHY

The occurrence of tumor-forming stromal proliferations in patients with diabetes mellitus is referred to as diabetic mastopathy (DM) (46). The initial clinical symptom is a palpable, firm-to-hard mass, which may suggest carcinoma. Most patients (~75%) have insulin-dependent diabetes mellitus (47-49); however, similar lesions have been reported in patients with another type of autoimmune disease (including autoimmune thyroiditis) and in patients without any autoimmune disease (50,51).

With rare exceptions (52), DM has been limited to females. In six series, the mean age of patients at the time of biopsy varied from 36 to 57 years, with a range of 20 to 77 years (48). Most patients with DM with type I insulin-dependent diabetes mellitus are younger than 30 years, and the interval between the onset of DM and detection of the breast lesion is about 20 years. Bilateral lesions have been present in nearly 50% of the cases. Most of the patients with DM have had complications of juvenile-onset diabetes, with diabetic retinopathy being reported in many instances.

The mammogram in DM often reveals localized, increased density or a heterogeneous parenchymal pattern, but no specific features have been identified (53,54). The mammographic appearance of the mass can resemble a fibroadenoma or carcinoma (50,55). An irregular hypoechoic mass

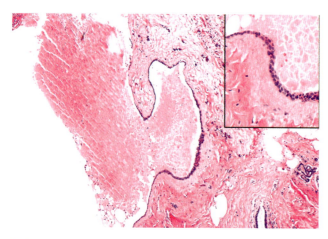

FIGURE 2.12 **Duct Ectasia, Without Inflammation.** The dilated duct is lined by flat epithelium. There is no inflammation. A cellular proteinaceous material fills the duct lumen. Inset shows detail of the epithelial cells lining the dilated duct.

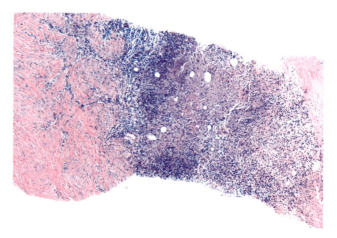

FIGURE 2.13 **So-called "Plasma Cell Mastitis."** A needle core biopsy specimen from a patient with a breast mass clinically suspected to be carcinoma. Plasma cells are a prominent element in the cellular infiltrate—possibly related to duct ectasia in the vicinity.

INFLAMMATORY AND REACTIVE LESIONS 23

with variable acoustic shadowing is found on ultrasonography (53). Breast density associated with DM could obscure a coexistent lesion such as carcinoma, a setting in which MRI may be useful (56,57). Spontaneous regression and clinical disappearance of DM have been described (58).

The lesional tissue of DM is "pink" (owing to the predominance of eosin, rather than hematoxylin, staining tissues), consisting of collagenized "glassy" stroma with keloidal features and variably prominent stromal cells. Polygonal epithelioid cells are found dispersed in the collagen among the spindly stromal cells in most, but not all, cases. The stromal cells are myofibroblasts with variable fibroblastic and myoid differentiation **(Fig. 2.14)** and are immunoreactive for actin, CD34, and desmin. The breast glands are typically atrophic. Multinucleated stromal giant cells and mitotic activity are not part of this proliferative process. Rarely, CD10-positive *atypical* myofibroblastic cells may be present (59). Mature perivascular, periductal, and perilobular lymphocytes are clustered throughout the lesion. Few, if any, plasma cells or neutrophils are present in the infiltrates. Lymphoid follicles with germinal centers are rare. When studied by immunohistochemistry, the lymphocytes have a B-cell phenotype. No Ig heavy-chain gene rearrangements was detected via polymerase chain reaction (PCR) in tissue samples from six patients with DM (60).

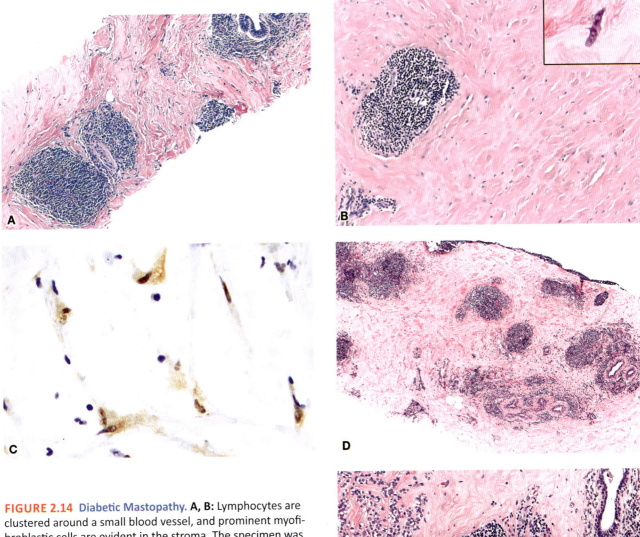

FIGURE 2.14 Diabetic Mastopathy. A, B: Lymphocytes are clustered around a small blood vessel, and prominent myofibroblastic cells are evident in the stroma. The specimen was obtained from a young woman with type 1 (autoimmune) diabetes mellitus who presented with a unilateral breast mass. Inset in **(B)** shows detail of an altered myofibroblast. **C:** The spindly myofibroblasts are CD34-positive. **D:** Another case of diabetic mastopathy with the characteristic prominent perivascular and periglandular lymphocytic response amid fibrotic stroma. **E:** A needle core biopsy showing invasive carcinoma (left) and changes characteristic of diabetic mastopathy in a 38-year-old patient with childhood-onset type 1 diabetes mellitus.

In one series of 20 patients with DM, 13 (65%) showed all 4 of its histopathologic characteristics (ie, keloid-like fibrosis, epithelioid fibroblasts, widespread periductal/lobular lymphocytic infiltration, and widespread perivascular lymphocytic infiltration), but one or more of these typical findings was absent in the remainder of the cases (61). Infarcts, fat necrosis, granulomas, duct stasis, arteritis, and other inflammatory lesions are not features of DM. Stromal collagen fibers are sometimes prominent. Proliferative epithelial changes may be present coincidentally but are not an integral component of DM. The differential diagnosis of DM includes nonspecific lymphocytic lobulitis (Fig. 2.15) and fibromatosis.

DM is generally regarded as a self-limited stromal abnormality. Recurrent tumors have occurred in the ipsilateral breast in a minority of cases, and these patients are prone to asynchronous, as well as synchronous, bilateral involvement. Excisional biopsy is adequate treatment. There is no evidence to suggest that DM predisposes to mammary carcinoma or stromal neoplastic diseases such as fibromatosis. Nonetheless, patients with DM can coincidentally harbor mammary carcinoma (62).

Lymphocytic Mastitis and Sclerosing Lymphocytic Mastitis

Lymphocytic mastitis and sclerosing lymphocytic mastitis are terms used for immune-mediated, nonspecific lymphocytic infiltrative lesions in the breast. The term lymphocytic mastitis is sometimes used as a synonym for DM. However, the latter term ought to be used only when the disease process forms a palpable mass and is associated with DM. *Lymphocytic mastitis* can be diagnosed when there is a dense intralobular, perilobular, and perivascular lymphocytic infiltrate associated with lobular atrophy and sclerosis. When the sclerotic process is intense, the term *sclerosing lymphocytic mastitis* can be used.

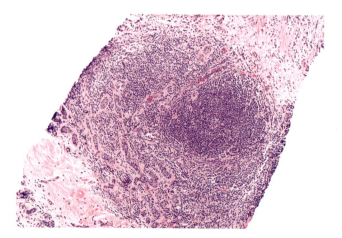

FIGURE 2.15 Lymphocytic Lobulitis. This needle core biopsy was performed to assess a nonpalpable mass on mammography. The patient had no known systemic illness. A lobule heavily infiltrated by lymphocytes is shown. The infiltrate was polyclonal by immunohistochemistry (not shown).

GRANULOMATOUS MASTITIS

Numerous pathogenetic processes responsible for granulomatous inflammation are included under the generic heading of *granulomatous mastitis* (GM) (63). The differential diagnosis of GM includes specific entities such as tuberculosis and other bacterial infections, as well as fungal and parasitic infestations (63-66). It is necessary to exclude the presence of acid-fast bacilli (AFB) or other bacteria and fungi with histochemical stains, cultures, PCR, and other appropriate tests (67). Reactive non-necrotizing epithelioid sarcoid-like granulomatous inflammation that develops in association with breast carcinomas is restricted to intratumoral and peritumoral tissue and ipsilateral axillary lymph nodes (68). Rheumatoid nodules, characterized by noncaseating and nonvasculitic granulomata with fibrinoid necrosis, have been diagnosed on NCB sampling in a case of mammary involvement with rheumatoid arthritis (69).

Granulomatous Lobular Mastitis

Granulomatous lobular mastitis is a clinicopathologic condition characterized by perilobular granulomatous inflammation (70,71). This pattern of distribution of the granulomata suggests a cell-mediated reaction to one or more substances in mammary secretions or in lobular epithelial cells; however, no specific antigen has been identified. The lesion usually appears approximately 2 years after a pregnancy. The age at diagnosis ranges from 17 to 42 years, with a mean of about 33 years (71). Virtually all patients are parous. The distinct, firm-to-hard mass may involve any portion of the breast, but it tends to spare the subareolar region. Granulomatous lobular mastitis can form a mass that can span as much as 8 cm, although it averages 6 cm. The clinical findings often suggest carcinoma, and mammography has been described as "suspicious" (63). In one report, sonograms were characterized by "multiple clustered, often contiguous tubular hypoechoic lesions" (72). The primary histopathologic finding is granulomatous lobulitis (Fig. 2.16). The granulomas are composed of epithelioid histiocytes and Langhans giant cells (giant cells with multiple nuclei, typically arranged at the perimeter of the cell) accompanied by lymphocytes, plasma cells, and occasional eosinophils. Fat necrosis and abscesses containing neutrophils are occasionally present, and these processes contribute to the effacement of the lobulocentric distribution in confluent lesions. Asteroid bodies and calcifications in the giant cells are rare. Spaces that develop in the centers of the abscesses contain no foreign material, demonstrable secretion, or bacteria. Squamous metaplasia of duct and lobular epithelium is unusual. Vasculitis is not present. Stains and cultures for bacteria, AFB, and fungi are negative. The management of nonspecific GM is generally difficult, unless a specific etiology for the process is determined. NCB, as the initial diagnostic procedure, can be useful in planning management (73,74). Steroids may be of use in appropriately selected cases, and surgical excision can alleviate chronic pain in cases refractory to medical management (75).

INFLAMMATORY AND REACTIVE LESIONS 25

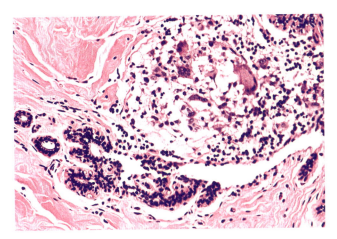

FIGURE 2.16 **Granulomatous Lobulitis, Nonspecific.** A non-necrotizing granuloma with epithelioid giant cells in a lobule in a needle core biopsy. No specific etiology could be established in this patient. Note similarity between this granuloma and those of sarcoidosis seen in **Figure 2.17**.

Cystic Neutrophilic Granulomatous Mastitis

Cystic neutrophilic granulomatous mastitis (CNGM) is a particular form of GM characterized by minute cystic spaces in the center of granulomata. A zone of neutrophils outlines the central space. The latter contains rare gram-positive bacilli (76,77). Culture studies have identified *Corynebacterium* spp., which are sensitive to the tetracycline group of antibiotics. Please see Chapter 3 for a detailed discussion.

SARCOIDOSIS

Sarcoidosis usually involves the breasts of women in their 20s and 30s, reflecting the overall age distribution of the disease (78-81). Mammary involvement is often detected after the diagnosis of sarcoidosis has been established in another organ. The primary manifestation of the disease in the breast is rare. In some patients, mammary sarcoidosis produces a firm-to-hard mass that may be clinically mistaken for carcinoma. Occasionally, mammary sarcoidosis is clinically inapparent, and the disease is incidentally discovered in a biopsy performed for an unrelated condition.

The mammographic, ultrasound, MRI, and positron emission tomography (PET) characteristics of mammary sarcoidosis are not specific and can be interpreted as "suggestive" of carcinoma (82,83), especially if a spiculated lesion is seen on mammography (84). Rarely, sarcoidosis produces multiple, bilateral mammographically detected lesions (80).

Microscopic examination of mammary sarcoidosis reveals non-necrotizing epithelioid granulomata in periductal and perilobular distribution **(Fig. 2.17)**. Multinucleated Langhans giant cells within the granulomata may contain

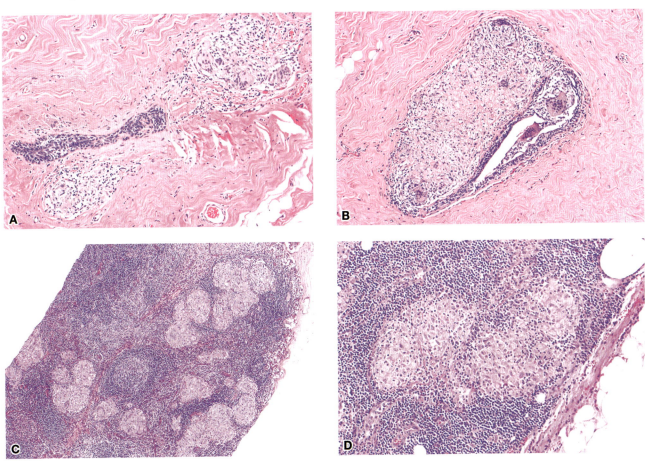

FIGURE 2.17 **Mammary and Axillary Nodal Sarcoidosis. A, B:** Epithelioid non-necrotizing granulomata, typical of sarcoidosis, lie adjacent to mammary ducts. **C, D:** Epithelioid non-necrotizing granulomata involve a palpable axillary lymph node in a 45-year-old woman with sarcoidosis.

cytoplasmic asteroid bodies (eosinophilic stellate forms) or intracellular Schaumann structures (proteinaceous calcified crystals). A variable lymphoplasmacytic and fibrotic reaction is present. Minute isolated sarcoid granulomata may be dispersed throughout the breast in some cases.

MASTITIS RELATED TO IMPLANT PLACEMENT

Some 5 million women in the United States have had mammary implants placed, two-thirds of which were for cosmetic (augmentation) purposes and the rest as part of breast reconstruction following mastectomy. The typical implant comprises a silicone shell filled with either silicone gel (most) or saline. Leakage of silicone from implants may or may not be a clinically subtle process; however, it can cause significant tissue reaction. Rupture of saline-filled implants results in immediate "deflation" with a much lesser degree of tissue reaction. Parenthetically, the term "tissue expander" is used for an implant placed temporarily after mastectomy, pending removal at a later date during definitive reconstructive surgery.

In the postimplant setting, the ability to detect carcinoma by mammography and ultrasound is usually impaired by GM caused by leakage of implant contents (eg, silicone) and/or an inflammatory reaction to the coating of the implant (85-87). Calcifications that deposit in the leaked contents of a mammary implant are generally irregular and coarse. Finer calcifications, resembling those of carcinoma, should be biopsied (88). Enhanced MRI is an important procedure for detecting carcinoma in a breast distorted by leakage of implant contents (89).

Mammary implants are usually filled with either foreign chemicals (silicone and other substances) or saline. Upon leakage, silicone and other fillers typically elicit a foreign body giant cell granulomatous reaction associated with fat necrosis **(Fig. 2.18)**. Occasionally, this process can mimic liposarcoma because of the presence of numerous enlarged multivacuolated histiocytes that are "disarming replicas of lipoblasts" (90). The accompanying chronic inflammatory reaction and fibrosis vary in intensity. Silicone and other fillers may also enter the lumina of ducts and lobules (91). Some of the foreign material is lost from the tissue during histologic processing, leaving clear spaces of varying size on hematoxylin and eosin (H&E) stained sections. The presence of silicone and other substances can be confirmed by electron microscopy, spectroscopy, spectrophotometry, and so on (92).

The most common etiology for a mass that forms in the postaugmentation setting is leakage-related GM; however, it should be noted that mammary implants have been associated with a variety of neoplasms, including anaplastic large cell lymphoma (93,94), fibromatosis, and other fibroblastic neoplasms (95).

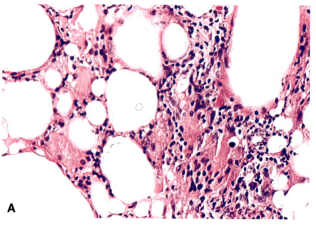

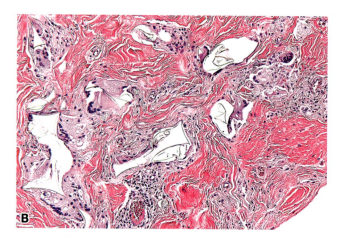

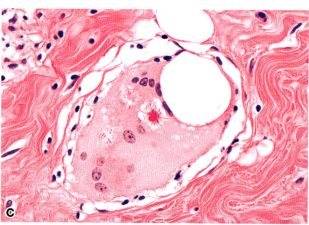

FIGURE 2.18 Implant-Associated Mastitis. A: This chronic inflammatory cell infiltrate surrounds vacuolar spaces that contain silicone material. **B:** Refractile fragments of polyurethane from the outer surface of a silicone cosmetic breast implant are present in this needle core biopsy sample from a 44-year-old woman who presented with a breast mass. **C:** An "asteroid" body (central) is present within a multinucleated giant cell in this granulomatous reaction to leaked implant material.

Lastly, cosmetic augmentation of the breasts can also be achieved by direct injection of silicone, other chemicals, and autologous adipose tissue. Direct injections invariably lead to intramammary granulomatous reaction of the foreign body type. The ipsilateral axillary lymph nodes can show a similar reaction owing to drainage of the foreign material. Injection of autologous fat tissue can result in the formation of intramammary *liponecrotic pseudocysts* (96).

INFLAMMATORY PSEUDOTUMOR

IPT is a poorly characterized entity. Indeed, it may not be an entity at all. The term has been loosely used for a variety of benign and malignant breast lesions. Localized nodular lesions with interlacing bundles of bland myofibroblastic cells with lymphocytes, plasma cells, histiocytes, and giant cells have been diagnosed as IPT (12,97-102). In most cases, lesions diagnosed as IPT have been the result of fat necrosis or duct ectasia associated with mastitis. Typically, NCB of lesions diagnosed as IPT has shown nonspecific "inflammatory" features (98). Please also see the section on fat necrosis for a discussion of the related *cellular spindled histiocytic pseudotumor*.

IgG4-RELATED DISEASE

IgG4-related disease is a relatively new entity characterized by mass-forming IgG4-dominant plasma cells associated with fibrosclerosis and phlebitis. The prototype of this disease is autoimmune (sclerosing) pancreatitis, and involvement of various organs, including the breast, has been described—either synchronously or metachronously. Most patients with IgG4 mastitis are premenopausal women who present with unilateral, palpable, painless mass. The histopathologic features of the disease are variable; however, a combination of prominent lymphocytic and plasma (pseudolymphomatous) cell infiltrate, obliterative phlebitis, dense storiform fibrosis, and glandular atrophy is usually present (103). Giant cells and granulomata are usually, but not always, absent (104). NCB sampling may show severe lymphoplasmacytic infiltration (105). Predictably, IgG4-immunoreactive plasma cells are prominent within the mass. The proportion of IgG4+ plasma cells to IgG+ plasma cells (>70%) and greater than 50 IgG4 plasma cells/hpf (in the area of highest infiltrate) are of diagnostic significance. Serum IgG4 levels are elevated. Immunosuppressive therapy and/or excision of the mass is usually curative.

INFLAMMATORY MYOFIBROBLASTIC TUMOR

Inflammatory myofibroblastic tumor (IMT), including its nomenclature, diagnostic criteria, and malignant potential, continues to be controversial. The entity is best regarded as a low-grade neoplasm with recurrent potential, rather than a reactive inflammatory condition. IMTs usually present as a solitary, circumscribed, solid, less than 5-cm mass in the abdominopelvic region in younger patients. A minority of patients present with systemic symptoms, including fever. IMT is rare in the breast (106,107). The histogenesis of IMT is uncertain, although a clonal origin is favored. Approximately two-thirds of IMTs harbor clonal rearrangements of the *ALK* gene at 2p23, and approximately one-half are immunoreactive for anaplastic lymphoma kinase (ALK).

IMT is histopathologically characterized by the proliferation of spindle (slender to plump) myofibroblastic spindle cells without overt cytologic atypia, interspersed by variably prominent lymphoplasmacytic and eosinophilic infiltrate **(Fig. 2.19)**. It is possible that some cases of IMT have been diagnosed as IPT or as "inflammatory myofibrohistiocytic proliferation" or "plasma cell granuloma." ALK immunohistochemistry is highly specific for IMT but lacks sensitivity. There is no histologic difference between IMTs harboring *ALK* gene abnormalities and those that do not. ALK reactivity is regarded as a favorable prognostic indicator.

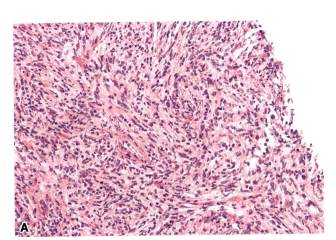 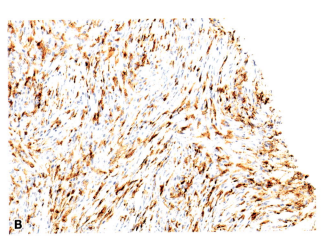

FIGURE 2.19 Inflammatory Myofibroblastic Tumor. A, B: This needle core biopsy specimen is from a circumscribed 1.5-cm tumor. The lesion is composed mainly of spindle cells with a lymphocytic and plasma cell infiltrate. The lesional cells are diffusely immunoreactive for ALK-1 (**B**).

Most mammary IMTs can be treated successfully by excision (although *ALK*-targeted therapy has potential in this regard). IMTs recur in about one-third of cases and rarely metastasize; thus, the entity is regarded as a low-grade malignant neoplasm. Be that as it may, surgical excision is usually curative (106,107).

ALK (+) Histiocytosis

ALK (+) histiocytosis usually presents as a systemic self-limiting disease in infants; however, the spectrum of the disease has expanded to include localized disease in the breast (with mainly spindle cell characteristics) in older children and young adults. The typical lesion is well circumscribed with monotonous spindled histiocytes cells arranged in storiform and fascicular patterns. There are more conventional (rather epithelioid) histiocytes, admixed with lymphocytes, and rare Touton giant cells. There is negligible atypia (108). The spindle and epithelioid cells are typically positive for ALK and CD163 and occasionally positive for S-100. Myofibroblasts within the tumor are positive for actin. The disease is defined by recurrent KIF5B-ALK fusion, and complete remission has been reported with ALK inhibitor therapy.

As could be ascertained from the aforementioned passages, IPT, IMT, ALK (+) histiocytosis, and even IgG4-related disease have some degree of histologic, if not etiologic, similarities. Clinical correlation is recommended before any of these diagnoses is rendered.

AMYLOID TUMOR (AMYLOIDOMA)

Amyloid tumor (AT), also referred to as amyloidoma, is a mass-forming amyloid deposition. AT in the breast has been described in patients with systemic diseases that predispose to amyloid deposition, including lymphoma, multiple myeloma, rheumatoid arthritis, and primary amyloidosis. More than one-half of patients with mammary amyloidosis have a concurrent hematologic disorder—most commonly, mucosa-associated lymphoid tissue (MALT) lymphoma, followed by plasma cell neoplasm.

AT limited to the breast is uncommon (109-111) and typically presents as a unilateral solitary mass in middle-aged or older women. Bilateral involvement has been described (112,113). ATs have been reported at the site of insulin injections (114). This is notable because the underside of the breast is a favored site for insulin injection in some diabetic women. Clinical examination reveals a discrete, hard mass that mimics carcinoma. Mammography of AT typically shows calcifications (115-118). MRI features of mammary amyloidosis have not been fully characterized; however, one case of bilateral mammary amyloidosis demonstrated a high signal on T2 imaging (generally, a low signal is indicative of a benign lesion) (119). Concurrent mammary carcinoma and amyloidosis have been described (120-122).

Histologically, AT is characterized by amorphous, faintly eosinophilic, homogeneous, "waxy," extracellular deposits of amyloid in adipose tissue, fibrous stroma, and in walls of blood vessels **(Fig. 2.20)**. Deposits of amyloid around ducts and lobules are associated with atrophy and obliteration of the affected structures. In adipose tissue, thin ribbons of amyloid ("rings") may be formed around individual adipocytes. These amyloid rings are accentuated when Congo red–stained sections are examined with polarized light (123). Lymphocytes, plasma cells, and multinucleated giant cells may be present in association with the amyloid deposits; however, the inflammatory cell reaction is seldom prominent. The latter can show punctate or irregular calcifications. Rarely, osseous metaplasia of AT is evident (116,124). Amyloid is periodic acid–Schiff (PAS)-positive, appears to be metachromatic with the crystal violet stain, and exhibits apple-green birefringence when the Congo red–stained section is examined under polarized light. Thicker (10 μm) sections may provide better staining. Most breast amyloid depositions are of the AL (usually kappa) type, although the deposits can be of AA, AL, and β2-microglobulin types. Mammary amyloidosis can be readily diagnosed on NCB (110,117,118); however, the findings can be mistaken for atrophy (or even as infarct).

The lesion can be treated by excision. The prognosis of patients with mammary lesions and systemic amyloidosis depends on the clinical course of the underlying disease. When limited to the breast, AT is an innocuous condition (in the limited follow-up reported so far). Notably, one woman who presented with bilateral mammary AT developed systemic amyloidosis 1 year later (125).

VASCULITIS

Inflammatory lesions of blood vessels (ie, vasculitis) are encountered in a variety of systemic disorders that are broadly grouped under the heading of collagen-vascular disease. Vasculitis in the breast may present as an isolated process or with multiorgan involvement. Although there are subtle differences in the pathologic features of the vasculitides associated with various collagen-vascular diseases, the diagnosis of a specific condition is more often rendered on the composite clinical and histopathologic findings. The clinical manifestations of mammary vasculitis sometimes resemble those of carcinoma (126).

Giant Cell and Other Types of Arteritis

Giant cell arteritis clinically limited to the breast has been reported in postmenopausal women who presented with one or more palpable breast tumors (127-130). The lesions can be bilateral. The firm tumors range from less than 1 to 4 cm, and carcinoma is clinically suspected in most patients (131). Axillary nodal enlargement has been noted in some cases (128). Systemic symptoms include headache, muscle and joint pain, fever, and night sweats. Mild anemia and an elevated erythrocyte sedimentation rate are found in most cases. Microscopically, transmural inflammation involves small- and medium-sized arteries throughout the affected tissue **(Fig. 2.21)**. Veins and arterioles are largely spared.

INFLAMMATORY AND REACTIVE LESIONS 29

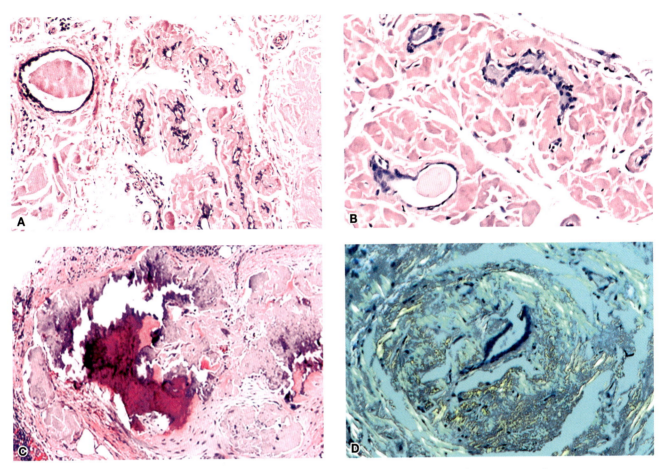

FIGURE 2.20 **Amyloidosis. A-C:** A thick layer of amyloid is deposited in the basement membranes of the glands. This palpable amyloid tumor is composed of masses of amyloid, fibrosis, and calcification with ossification. **D:** Apple-green birefringence of amyloid with Congo red stain (under polarized light) in periductal tissue in this case.

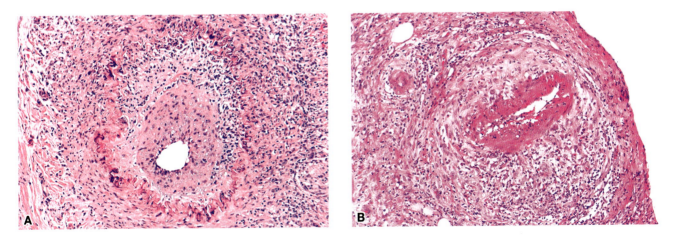

FIGURE 2.21 **Mammary Vasculitis. A:** The patient with long-standing history of giant cell (temporal) arteritis presented with a breast mass. Core biopsy revealed fat necrosis caused by arteritis. The artery is almost totally occluded by the inflammatory process. The elastic layer is fragmented. No giant cells are evident in this particular focus. **B:** This patient with systemic lupus erythematosus (SLE), presented with a painful breast mass. Needle core biopsy showed markedly active vasculitis with fibrinoid necrosis involving small-sized arteries.

Fibrinoid necrosis is not a consistent feature, but fragmentation of the intramural elastic fibers is demonstrable with an elastic stain. Multinucleated giant cells tend to be oriented around the disrupted elastic fibers. The vascular lumen may be narrowed or occluded. The differential diagnosis includes other types of arteritis, phlebitis, traumatic fat necrosis, and infarction related to pregnancy or lactation.

Breast involvement has also been reported in patients with Wegener granulomatosis (132,133), polyarteritis (134,135), scleroderma (136), dermatomyositis (137), lupus erythematosus (138-140), and Churg-Strauss syndrome (ie, allergic granulomatous angiitis) (141). NCB can reveal vasculitis involving various types and sizes of vessels and different kinds of inflammatory cell infiltrates, with or without granulomas or necrosis (142). The lesions in several of these vasculitides may be manifested by a mass with vascular calcifications or with irregular dystrophic calcifications (126). Fat necrosis is often present. Patients with one of these forms of systemic vasculitis may develop coincidental breast carcinoma in the absence of mammary vasculitis (143-145).

Lupus Mastitis

Lupus mastitis is a rare complication of lupus erythematosus (138,146) and is essentially a form of panniculitis (fat necrosis of subcutaneous tissue) and mastitis (necrosis of breast fat). The ischemia is presumably caused by vasculitis. (Fig. 2.21). The disease is characterized clinically by nodular lesions (147). There is a dense lymphoplasmacytic infiltrate around the affected fat lobules. Concentric perivascular fibrosis and hyalinized stromal fibrosis extending around ducts and lobules have been reported (139). NCB of lupus mastitis may show a "dense lymphoplasmacytic infiltrate with no normal breast ducts or lobules" (129). Advanced lesions may show calcification. Immunoglobulin deposits can be demonstrated around blood vessels, and serum antinuclear antibodies (ANAs) are present. Clinical findings in the skin may mimic inflammatory carcinoma (148).

OTHER INFLAMMATORY AND REACTIVE LESIONS

Several other inflammatory and reactive lesions in addition to those that have been described in this chapter, such as *Rosai-Dorfman disease, eosinophilic mastitis,* and *nephrogenic systemic fibrosis,* can be encountered in NCB (149-151). This possibility highlights the need to be constantly on the alert for unanticipated and novel diseases in the breast. A striking example of the latter is *pandemic (COVID-19)–related lesions.* COVID-19 is a multisystem disease, and manifestations of the disease have been reported in the breast—mainly in the form of abscesses and gangrene (152,153).

Lastly, a type of reactive process that follows the performance of NCB of breast (154) deserves mention. This type of lesion follows the deployment of various types of marking

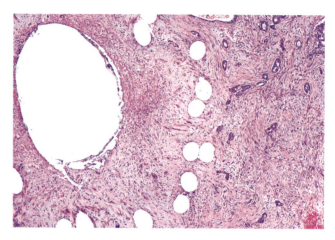

FIGURE 2.22 Excisional Biopsy With Healing Marker Clip Deployment Site Following Needle Core Biopsy. Dense fibrotic reaction around gel-polymer pellets (represented by nearly empty spaces, because polymer is dissolved in tissue processing). Note multinucleated giant cells. The various packing material (gel-polymer pellets, collagen plugs, or other substances) can resemble suture or amyloid.

devices ("clips") at the biopsied site. Placement of the clip at the time of NCB facilitates surgical and radiologic localization of the site later. The titanium clips are placed with some form of "plug" (either a resorbable chemical or bovine collagen). The "plug" minimizes the risk of "clip migration" as well as enhances hemostasis and invariably elicits a prominent nonspecific mixed inflammatory cell and granulation tissue response **(Fig. 2.22)**. Over time, there is fibrous scarring of the site. These findings are, of course, evident in excisional biopsies and mastectomies performed *after* NCB but can be encountered in NCB samples in cases wherein the biopsy is repeated at the same site for any reason.

REFERENCES

1. Layfield LJ, Frazier S, Schanzmeyer E. Histomorphologic features of biopsy sites following excisional and core needle biopsies of the breast. *Breast J.* 2015;21:370-376.
2. Tan PH, Lai LM, Carrington EV, et al. Fat necrosis of the breast—a review. *Breast.* 2006;15:313-318.
3. Akyol M, Kayali A, Yildirim N. Traumatic fat necrosis of male breast. *Clin Imaging.* 2013;37:954-956.
4. Hogge JP, Robinson RE, Magnant CM, Zuurbier RA. The mammographic spectrum of fat necrosis of the breast. *Radiographics.* 1995;15:1347-1356.
5. Martin BF, Phillips JD. Gangrene of the female breast with anticoagulant therapy: report of two cases. *Am J Clin Pathol.* 1970;53:622-626.
6. Clarke D, Curtis JL, Martinez A, Fajardo L, Goffinet D. Fat necrosis of the breast simulating recurrent carcinoma after primary radiotherapy in the management of early stage breast carcinoma. *Cancer.* 1983;52:442-445.
7. Rostom AY, el-Sayed ME. Fat necrosis of the breast: an unusual complication of lumpectomy and radiotherapy in breast cancer. *Clin Radiol.* 1987;38:31.
8. Girling AC, Hanby AM, Millis RR. Radiation and other pathological changes in breast tissue after conservation treatment for carcinoma. *J Clin Pathol.* 1990;43:152-156.
9. Isenberg JS, Tu Q, Rainey W. Mammary gangrene associated with warfarin ingestion. *Ann Plast Surg.* 1996;37:553-555.
10. Taboada JL, Stephens TW, Krishnamurthy S, Brandt KR, Whitman GJ. The many faces of fat necrosis in the breast. *AJR Am J Roentgenol.* 2009;192:815-825.
11. Bargum K, Nielsen SM. Case report: fat necrosis of the breast appearing as oil cysts with fat-fluid levels. *Br J Radiol.* 1993;66:718-720.
12. Sciallis AP, Chen B, Folpe AL. Cellular spindled histiocytic pseudotumor complicating mammary fat necrosis: a potential diagnostic pitfall. *Am J Surg Pathol.* 2012;36:1571-1578.
13. Chang MC, Eslami Z, Ennis M, Goodwin PJ. Crown-like structures in breast adipose tissue of breast cancer patients: associations with CD68 expression,

obesity, metabolic factors and prognosis. *NPJ Breast Cancer*. 2021;7:97. doi:10.1038/s41523-021-00304-x

14. Provenzano E, Barter SJ, Wright PA, Forouhi P, Allibone R, Ellis IO. Erdheim-Chester disease presenting as bilateral clinically malignant breast masses. *Am J Surg Pathol*. 2010;34:584-588.

15. Guo S, Yan Q, Rohr J, Wang Y, Fan L, Wang Z. Erdheim-Chester disease involving the breast—a rare but important differential diagnosis. *Hum Pathol*. 2015;46:159-164.

16. Aggon AA, Eakin LO, Desimone N, Snyder JA. Extensive multifocal mammary infarction—a case report. *Breast Care (Basel)*. 2013;8:143-145.

17. Oh YJ, Choi SH, Chung SY, Yang I, Woo JY, Lee MJ. Spontaneously infarcted fibroadenoma mimicking breast cancer. *J Ultrasound Med*. 2009;28:1421-1423.

18. Toy H, Esen HH, Sonmez FC, Kucukkartallar T. Spontaneous infarction in a fibroadenoma of the breast. *Breast Care (Basel)*. 2011;6:54-55.

19. Skenderi F, Krakonja F, Vranic S. Infarcted fibroadenoma of the breast: report of two new cases with review of the literature. *Diagn Pathol*. 2013;8:38.

20. Kavdia R, Kini U. WCAFTI: worrisome cytologic alterations following tissue infarction; a mimicker of malignancy in breast cytology. *Diagn Cytopathol*. 2008;36:586-588.

21. Agnihotri M, Naik L, Kothari K, Fernandes G, Ojha S. Fine-needle aspiration cytology of breast lesions with spontaneous infarction: a five-year study. *Acta Cytol*. 2013;57:413-417.

22. Flint A, Oberman HA. Infarction and squamous metaplasia of intraductal papilloma: a benign breast lesion that may simulate carcinoma. *Hum Pathol*. 1984;15:764-767.

23. Ginter PS, Hoda SA, Ozerdem U. Exuberant squamous metaplasia in an intraductal papilloma of breast. *Int J Surg Pathol*. 2015;23:125-126.

24. Murad TM, Contesso G, Mouriesse H. Papillary tumors of large lactiferous ducts. *Cancer*. 1981;48:122-133.

25. Jones EL, Codling BW, Oates GD. Necrotic intraduct breast carcinomas simulating inflammatory lesions. *J Pathol*. 1973;110:101-103.

26. Yu L, Yang W, Cai X, Shi D, Fan Y, Lu H. Centrally necrotizing carcinoma of the breast: clinicopathological analysis of 33 cases indicating its basal-like phenotype and poor prognosis. *Histopathology*. 2010;57:193-201.

27. Zaman S, Gupta R, Gupta S. Crystallizing galactocele of the breast masquerading as a malignancy: report of a rare case with cytological diagnosis. *Diagn Cytopathol*. 2022;50:E236-E239.

28. Salvador R, Salvador M, Jimenez JA, Martinez M, Casas L. Galactocele of the breast: radiologic and ultrasonographic findings. *Br J Radiol*. 1990;63:140-142.

29. Novotny DB, Maygarden SJ, Shermer RW, Frable WJ. Fine needle aspiration of benign and malignant breast masses associated with pregnancy. *Acta Cytol*. 1991;35:676-686.

30. Heymann JJ, Halligan AM, Hoda SA, Facey KE, Hoda RS. Fine needle aspiration of breast masses in pregnant and lactating women: experience with 28 cases emphasizing Thinprep findings. *Diagn Cytopathol*. 2015;43:188-194.

31. Adams EG, Kemp JD, Holcomb KZ, Sperling LC. Xanthogranulomatous reaction to a ruptured galactocele. *J Cutan Pathol*. 2010;37:973-976.

32. Tung A, Carr N. Postaugmentation galactocele: a case report and review of literature. *Ann Plast Surg*. 2011;67:668-670.

33. Taylor D, Kulawansa ST, McCallum DD, Saunders C. Peri-implant galactocele following vacuum-assisted core biopsy of the breast: a cautionary tale. *BMJ Case Rep*. 2013;2013:bcr2012007127. doi:10.1136/bcr-2012-007127

34. Rahal RM, de Freitas-Júnior R, Carlos da Cunha L, Moreira MA, Rosa VD, Conde DM. Mammary duct ectasia: an overview. *Breast J*. 2011;17:694-695.

35. Habif DV, Perzin KH, Lipton R, Lattes R. Subareolar abscess associated with squamous metaplasia of lactiferous ducts. *Am J Surg*. 1970;119:523-526.

36. Passaro ME, Broughan TA, Sebek BA, Esselstyn CB Jr. Lactiferous fistula. *J Am Coll Surg*. 1994;178:29-32.

37. Sweeney DJ, Wylie EJ. Mammographic appearances of mammary duct ectasia that mimic carcinoma in a screening programme. *Australas Radiol*. 1995;39:18-23.

38. Davies JD. Pigmented periductal cells (ochrocytes) in mammary dysplasias: their nature and significance. *J Pathol*. 1974;114(4):205-216.

39. Seidman MA, Scognamiglio T, Hoda SA. "Cholesteroloma": a rare cause of "indeterminate" microcalcifications on mammography. *Breast J*. 2009;15:303-304.

40. Bezić J, Piljić-Burazer M. Breast cholesterol granuloma: a report of two cases with discussion on potential pathogenesis. *Pathologica*. 2013;105:349-352.

41. Tashiro T, Hirokawa M, Sano T. Are mammary pagetoid foam cells histiocytic or epithelial? *Virchows Arch*. 2001;439:102-104.

42. Davies JD. Inflammatory damage to ducts in mammary dysplasia: a cause of duct obliteration. *J Pathol*. 1975;117:47-54.

43. Davies JD. Hyperelastosis, obliteration and fibrous plaques in major ducts of the human breast. *J Pathol*. 1973;110:13-26.

44. Wang Z, Leonard MH Jr, Khamapirad T, Castro CY. Bilateral extensive ductitis obliterans manifested by bloody nipple discharge in a patient with long-term diabetes mellitus. *Breast J*. 2007;13:599-602.

45. Tan PH, Harada O, Thike AA, Tse GM. Histiocytoid breast carcinoma: an enigmatic lobular entity. *J Clin Pathol*. 2011;64:654-659.

46. Tomaszewski JE, Brooks JS, Hicks D, Livolsi VA. Diabetic mastopathy: a distinctive clinicopathologic entity. *Hum Pathol*. 1992;23:780-786.

47. Chan CL, Ho RS, Shek TW, Kwong A. Diabetic mastopathy. *Breast J*. 2013;19:533-538.

48. Dorokhova O, Fineberg S, Koenigsberg T, Wang Y. Diabetic mastopathy, a clinicopathological correlation of 34 cases. *Pathol Int*. 2012;62:660-664.

49. Seidman JD, Schnaper LA, Phillips LE. Mastopathy in insulin-requiring diabetes mellitus. *Hum Pathol*. 1994;25:819-824.

50. Ashton MA, Lefkowitz M, Tavassoli FA. Epithelioid stromal cells in lymphocytic mastitis—a source of confusion with invasive carcinoma. *Mod Pathol*. 1994;7:49-54.

51. Love JE, Lawton TJ. Diabetic mastopathy in patients with non-diabetic autoimmune disease. *Mod Pathol*. 2005;18(suppl 1):41A.

52. Weinstein SP, Conant EF, Orel SG, Lawton TJ, Acs G. Diabetic mastopathy in men: imaging findings in two patients. *Radiology*. 2001;219:797-799.

53. Andrews-Tang D, Diamond AB, Rogers L, Butler D. Diabetic mastopathy: adjunctive use of ultrasound and utility of core biopsy in diagnosis. *Breast J*. 2000;6:183-188.

54. Camuto PM, Zetrenne E, Ponn T. Diabetic mastopathy: a report of 5 cases and a review of the literature. *Arch Surg*. 2000;135:1190-1193.

55. Byrd BF Jr, Hartmann WH, Graham LS, Hogle HH. Mastopathy in insulin-dependent diabetics. *Ann Surg*. 1987;205:529-532.

56. Gabriel HA, Feng C, Mendelson EB, Benjamin S. Breast MRI for cancer detection in a patient with diabetic mastopathy. *AJR Am J Roentgenol*. 2004;182:1081-1083.

57. Tuncbilek N, Karakas HM, Okten O. Diabetic fibrous mastopathy: dynamic contrast-enhanced magnetic resonance imaging findings. *Breast J*. 2004;10:359-362.

58. Bayer U, Horn LC, Schulz HG. Bilateral, tumorlike diabetic mastopathy-progression and regression of the disease during 5-year follow up. *Eur J Radiol*. 1998;26:248-253.

59. Shousha S. Diabetic mastopathy: strong CD10+ immunoreactivity of the atypical stromal cells. *Histopathology*. 2008;52:648-650.

60. Valdez R, Thorson J, Finn WG, Schnitzer B, Kleer CG. Lymphocytic mastitis and diabetic mastopathy: a molecular, immunophenotypic, and clinicopathologic evaluation of 11 cases. *Mod Pathol*. 2003;16:223-228.

61. Morgan MC, Weaver MG, Crowe JP, Abdul-Karim FW. Diabetic mastopathy: a clinicopathologic study in palpable and nonpalpable breast lesions. *Mod Pathol*. 1995;8:349-354.

62. Alkhudairi SS, Abdullah MM, Alselais AG. Diabetic mastopathy in a patient with high risk of breast carcinoma: a management dilemma. *Cureus*. 2020;12:e7003.

63. Fitzgibbons PL. Granulomatous mastitis. *N Y State J Med*. 1990;90:287.

64. Cooper NE. Rheumatoid nodule in the breast. *Histopathology*. 1991;19:193-194.

65. Lacambra M, Thai TA, Lam CC, et al. Granulomatous mastitis: the histological differentials. *J Clin Pathol*. 2011;64:405-411.

66. Pandhi D, Verma P, Sharma S, Dhawan AK. Borderline-lepromatous leprosy manifesting as granulomatous mastitis. *Lepr Rev*. 2012;83:202-204.

67. Nalini G, Kusum S, Barwad A, Gurpreet S, Arvind R. Role of polymerase chain reaction in breast tuberculosis. *Breast Dis*. 2015;35:129-132.

68. Bässler R, Birke F. Histopathology of tumour associated sarcoid-like stromal reaction in breast cancer. An analysis of 5 cases with immunohistochemical investigations. *Virchows Arch A Pathol Anat Histopathol*. 1988;412:231-239.

69. Iqbal FM, Ali H, Vidya R. Breast lumps: a rare site for rheumatoid nodules. *BMJ Case Rep*. 2015;2015:bcr2014208586. doi:10.1136/bcr-2014-208586

70. Fletcher A, Magrath IM, Riddell AR, Talbot IC. Granulomatous mastitis: a report of seven cases. *J Clin Pathol*. 1982;35:941-945.

71. Going JJ, Anderson TJ, Wilkinson S, Chetty U. Granulomatous lobular mastitis. *J Clin Pathol*. 1987;40:535-540.

72. Han BK, Choe YH, Park JM, et al. Granulomatous mastitis: mammographic and sonographic appearances. *AJR Am J Roentgenol*. 1999;173:317-320.

73. Oran EŞ, Gürdal SÖ, Yankol Y, et al. Management of idiopathic granulomatous mastitis diagnosed by core biopsy: a retrospective multicenter study. *Breast J*. 2013;19:411-418.

74. Joseph KA, Luu X, Mor A. Granulomatous mastitis: a New York public hospital experience. *Ann Surg Oncol*. 2014;21:4159-4163.

75. Hovanessian Larsen LJ, Peyvandi B, Klipfel N, Grant E, Iyengar G. Granulomatous lobular mastitis: imaging, diagnosis, and treatment. *AJR Am J Roentgenol*. 2009;193:574-581.

76. Renshaw AA, Derhagopian RP, Gould EW. Cystic neutrophilic granulomatous mastitis: an underappreciated pattern strongly associated with gram-positive bacilli. *Am J Clin Pathol*. 2011;136:424-427.

77. D'Alfonso TM, Moo TA, Arleo EK, Cheng E, Antonio LB, Hoda SA. Cystic neutrophilic granulomatous mastitis: further characterization of a distinctive histopathologic entity not always demonstrably attributable to Corynebacterium infection. *Am J Surg Pathol*. 2015;39:1440-1447.

78. Fitzgibbons PL, Smiley DF, Kern WH. Sarcoidosis presenting initially as breast mass: report of two cases. *Hum Pathol*. 1985;16:851-852.

79. Reis J, Boavida J, Bahrami N, Lyngra M, Geitung JT. Breast sarcoidosis: clinical features, imaging, and histological findings. *Breast J*. 2021;27:44-47.

80. Nicholson BT, Mills SE. Sarcoidosis of the breast: an unusual presentation of a systemic disease. *Breast J*. 2007;13:99-100.

81. Zujić PV, Grebić D, Valenčić L. Chronic granulomatous inflammation of the breast as a first clinical manifestation of primary sarcoidosis. *Breast Care (Basel)*. 2015;10:51-53.

82. Kenzel PP, Hadijuana J, Hosten N, et al. Boeck sarcoidosis of the breast: mammographic, ultrasound, and MR findings. *J Comput Assist Tomogr.* 1997;21:439-441.

83. Ito T, Okada T, Murayama K, et al. Two cases of sarcoidosis discovered accidentally by positron emission tomography in patients with breast cancer. *Breast J.* 2010;16:561-563.

84. Kirshy D, Gluck B, Brancaccio W. Sarcoidosis of the breast presenting as a spiculated lesion. *AJR Am J Roentgenol.* 1999;172:554-555.

85. Venkataraman S, Hines N, Slanetz PJ. Challenges in mammography: part 2, multimodality review of breast augmentation—imaging findings and complications. *AJR Am J Roentgenol.* 2011;197:W1031-W1045.

86. Destouet JM, Monsees BS, Oser RF, Nemecek JR, Young VL, Pilgram TK. Screening mammography in 350 women with breast implants: prevalence and findings of implant complications. *AJR Am J Roentgenol.* 1992;159:973-978.

87. Cheung YC, Su MY, Ng SH, Lee KF, Chen SC, Lo YF. Lumpy silicone-injected breasts: enhanced MRI and microscopic correlation. *Clin Imaging.* 2002;26:397-404.

88. Morgenstern L, Gleischman SH, Michel SL, Rosenberg JE, Knight I, Goodman D. Relation of free silicone to human breast carcinoma. *Arch Surg.* 1985;120:573-577.

89. Maijers MC, Niessen FB, Veldhuizen JF, Ritt MJ, Manoliu RA. MRI screening for silicone breast implant rupture: accuracy, inter- and intraobserver variability using explantation results as reference standard. *Eur Radiol.* 2014;24:1167-1175.

90. Goldblum JR, Weiss SW, Folpe AL, eds. *Enzinger and Weiss's Soft Tissue Tumors.* 7th ed. Elsevier; 2020.

91. Leibman AJ, Kossoff MB, Kruse BD. Intraductal extension of silicone from a ruptured breast implant. *Plast Reconstr Surg.* 1992;89:546-547.

92. Travis WD, Balogh K, Abraham JL. Silicone granulomas: report of three cases and review of the literature. *Hum Pathol.* 1985;16:19-27.

93. Taylor CR, Siddiqi IN, Brody GS. Anaplastic large cell lymphoma occurring in association with breast implants: review of pathologic and immunohistochemical features in 103 cases. *Appl Immunohistochem Mol Morphol.* 2013;21:13-20.

94. Hoda S, Rao R, Hoda RS. Breast implant-associated anaplastic large cell lymphoma. *Int J Surg Pathol.* 2015;23:209-210.

95. Balzer BL, Weiss SW. Do biomaterials cause implant-associated mesenchymal tumors of the breast? Analysis of 8 new cases and review of the literature. *Hum Pathol.* 2009;40:1564-1570.

96. Kim H, Yang EJ, Bang SI. Bilateral liponecrotic pseudocysts after breast augmentation by fat injection: a case report. *Aesthetic Plast Surg.* 2012;36:359-362.

97. Yip CH, Wong KT, Samuel D. Bilateral plasma cell granuloma (inflammatory pseudotumour) of the breast. *Aust N Z J Surg.* 1997;67:300-303.

98. Pettinato G, Manivel JC, Insabato L, De Chiara A, Petrella G. Plasma cell granuloma (inflammatory pseudotumor) of the breast. *Am J Clin Pathol.* 1988;90:627-632.

99. Haj M, Weiss M, Loberant N, Cohen I. Inflammatory pseudotumor of the breast: case report and literature review. *Breast J.* 2003;9:423-425.

100. Hill PA. Inflammatory pseudotumor of the breast: a mimic of breast carcinoma. *Breast J.* 2010;16:549-550.

101. Sari A, Yigit S, Peker Y, Morgul Y, Coskun G, Cin N. Inflammatory pseudotumor of the breast. *Breast J.* 2011;17:312-314.

102. Shin SJ, Scamman W, Gopalan A, Rosen PP. Mammary presentation of adult-type "juvenile" xanthogranuloma. *Am J Surg Pathol.* 2005;29:827-831.

103. Wallace ZS, Naden RP, Chari S, et al. The 2019 American College of Rheumatology/European League Against Rheumatism classification criteria for IgG4-related disease. *Ann Rheum Dis.* 2020;79:77-87.

104. Ogura G, Matsumoto T, Aoki Y, Kitabatake T, Fujisawa M, Kojima K. IgG4-related tumour-forming mastitis with histological appearances of granulomatous lobular mastitis: comparison with other types of tumour-forming mastitis. *Histopathology.* 2010;57:39-45.

105. Ogiya A, Tanaka K, Tadokoro Y, et al. IgG4-related sclerosing disease of the breast successfully treated by steroid therapy. *Breast Cancer.* 2014;21:231-235.

106. Coffin CM, Hornick JL, Fletcher CD. Inflammatory myofibroblastic tumor: comparison of clinicopathologic, histologic, and immunohistochemical features including ALK expression in atypical and aggressive cases. *Am J Surg Pathol.* 2007;31:509-520.

107. Kovács A, Máthé G, Mattsson J, Stenman G, Kindblom LG. ALK-positive inflammatory myofibroblastic tumor of the nipple during pregnancy—an unusual presentation of a rare disease. *Breast J.* 2015;21:297-302.

108. Kashima J, Yoshida M, Jimbo K, et al. ALK-positive histiocytosis of the breast: a clinicopathologic study highlighting spindle cell histology. *Am J Surg Pathol.* 2021;45:347-355.

109. Charlot M, Seldin DC, O'hara C, Skinner M, Sanchorawala V. Localized amyloidosis of the breast: a case series. *Amyloid.* 2011;18:72-75.

110. Huerter ME, Hammadeh R, Zhou Q, Weisberg A, Riker AI. Primary amyloidosis of the breast presenting as a solitary nodule: case report and review of the literature. *Ochsner J.* 2014;14:282-286.

111. Duckworth LA, Cotta CV, Rowe JJ, Downs-Kelly E, Komforti MK. Amyloid in the breast: retrospective review with clinicopathological and radiological correlation of 32 cases from a single institution. *Histopathology.* 2021;79:57-66.

112. Silverman JF, Dabbs DJ, Norris HT, Pories WJ, Legier J, Kay S. Localized primary (AL) amyloid tumor of the breast. Cytologic, histologic, immunocytochemical and ultrastructural observations. *Am J Surg Pathol.* 1986;10:539-545.

113. Fleury AM, Buetens OW, Campassi C, Argani P. Pathologic quiz case: a 77-year-old woman with bilateral breast masses. Amyloidosis involving the breast. *Arch Pathol Lab Med.* 2004;128:e67-e69.

114. Yumlu S, Barany R, Eriksson M, Röcken C. Localized insulin-derived amyloidosis in patients with diabetes mellitus: a case report. *Hum Pathol.* 2009;40:1655-1660.

115. Liaw YS, Kuo SH, Yang PC, Chen CL, Luh KT. Nodular amyloidosis of the lung and the breast mimicking breast carcinoma with pulmonary metastasis. *Eur Respir J.* 1995;8:871-873.

116. Lynch LA, Moriarty AT. Localized primary amyloid tumor associated with osseous metaplasia presenting as bilateral breast masses: cytologic and radiologic features. *Diagn Cytopathol.* 1993;9:570-575.

117. Eghtedari M, Dogan BE, Gilcrease M, Roberts J, Cook ED, Yang WT. Imaging and pathologic characteristics of breast amyloidosis. *Breast J.* 2015;21:197-199.

118. Ngendahayo P, Faverly D, Hérin M. Primary breast amyloidosis presenting solely as nonpalpable microcalcifications: a case report with review of the literature. *Int J Surg Pathol.* 2013;21:177-180.

119. O'Brien J, Aherne S, McCormack O, Jeffers M, McInerney D. MRI features of bilateral amyloidosis of breast. *Breast J.* 2013;19:338-339.

120. Sabate JM, Clotet M, Torrubia S, et al. Localized amyloidosis of the breast associated with invasive lobular carcinoma. *Br J Radiol.* 2008;81:e252-e254.

121. Rocken C, Kronsbein H, Sletten K, Roessner A, Bässler R. Amyloidosis of the breast. *Virchows Arch.* 2002;440:527-535.

122. Munson-Bernardi BD, DePersia LA. Amyloidosis of the breast coexisting with ductal carcinoma in situ. *AJR Am J Roentgenol.* 2006;186:54-55.

123. Libbey CA, Skinner M, Cohen AS. Use of abdominal fat tissue aspirate in the diagnosis of systemic amyloidosis. *Arch Intern Med.* 1983;143:1549-1552.

124. Yokoo H, Nakazato Y. Primary localized amyloid tumor of the breast with osseous metaplasia. *Pathol Int.* 1998;48:545-548.

125. Hecht AH, Tan A, Shen JF. Case report: primary systemic amyloidosis presenting as breast masses, mammographically simulating carcinoma. *Clin Radiol.* 1991;44:123-124.

126. Kim SM, Park JM, Moon WK. Dystrophic breast calcifications in patients with collagen diseases. *Clin Imaging.* 2004;28:6-9.

127. Clement PB, Senges H, How AR. Giant cell arteritis of the breast: case report and literature review. *Hum Pathol.* 1987;18:1186-1189.

128. Lau Y, Mak YF, Hui PK, Ahchong AK. Giant cell arteritis of the breast. *Aust N Z J Surg.* 1996;66:259-261.

129. Kadotani Y, Enoki Y, Itoi N, Kojima F, Kato G, Lee CJ. Giant cell arteritis of the breast: a case report with a review of literatures. *Breast Cancer.* 2010;17:225-232.

130. Marie I, Audeguy P, François A, DE Kergal F, Richard C. Giant cell arteritis presenting as a breast lesion: report of a case and review of the literature. *Am J Med Sci.* 2008;335:489-491.

131. Pappo I, Beglaibter N, Amir G. Mammary arteritis mimicking cancer. Case report. *Eur J Surg.* 1992;158:191-193.

132. Jordan JM, Rowe WT, Allen NB. Wegener's granulomatosis involving the breast. Report of three cases and review of the literature. *Am J Med.* 1987;83:159-164.

133. Allende DS, Booth CN. Wegener's granulomatosis of the breast: a rare entity with daily clinical relevance. *Ann Diagn Pathol.* 2009;13:351-357.

134. Yamashina M, Wilson TK. A mammographic finding in focal polyarteritis nodosa. *Br J Radiol.* 1985;58:91-92.

135. Dhaon P, Bansal N, Das SK, Wakhlu A, Tandon V. Cutaneous polyarteritis nodosa presenting with digital gangrene and breast ulcer. *Int J Rheum Dis.* 2013;16:774-776.

136. Harrison GO, Elliott RL. Scleroderma of the breast: light and electron microscopy study. *Am Surg.* 1987;53:526-531.

137. Gyves-Ray KM, Adler DD. Dermatomyositis. An unusual cause of breast calcifications. *Breast Dis.* 1989;2:195-201.

138. Cernea SS, Kihara SM, Sotto MN, Vilela MA. Lupus mastitis. *J Am Acad Dermatol.* 1993;29:343-346.

139. Nigar E, Contractor K, Singhal H, Matin RN. Lupus mastitis—a cause of recurrent breast lumps. *Histopathology.* 2007;51:847-849.

140. Kinonen C, Gattuso P, Reddy VB. Lupus mastitis: an uncommon complication of systemic or discoid lupus. *Am J Surg Pathol.* 2010;34:901-906.

141. Visentin MS, Salmaso R, Modesti V, et al. Parotid, breast, and fascial involvement in a patient who fulfilled the ACR criteria for Churg-Strauss syndrome. *Scand J Rheumatol.* 2012;41:319-321.

142. Hernández-Rodríguez J, Tan CD, Molloy ES, Khasnis A, Rodríguez ER, Hoffman GS. Vasculitis involving the breast: a clinical and histopathologic analysis of 34 patients. *Medicine (Baltimore).* 2008;87:61-69.

143. Bonnetblanc JM, Bernard P, Fayol J. Dermatomyositis and malignancy. A multicenter cooperative study. *Dermatologica.* 1990;180:212-216.

144. Sigurgeirsson B, Lindelöf B, Edhag O, Allander E. Risk of cancer in patients with dermatomyositis or polymyositis. A population-based study. *N Engl J Med.* 1992;326:363-367.

145. Kontos M, Fentiman IS. Systemic lupus erythematosus and breast cancer. *Breast J.* 2008;14:81-86.

146. Chen X, Hoda SA, Delellis RA, Seshan SV. Lupus mastitis. *Breast J.* 2005;11:283-284.
147. Holland NW, McKnight K, Challa VR, Agudelo CA. Lupus panniculitis (profundus) involving the breast: report of 2 cases and review of the literature. *J Rheumatol.* 1995;22:344-346.
148. Fernandez-Flores A, Crespo LG, Alonso S, Montero MG. Lupus mastitis in the male breast mimicking inflammatory carcinoma. *Breast J.* 2006;12:272-273.
149. Adejolu M, Huo L, Rohren E, Santiago L, Yang WT. False-positive lesions mimicking breast cancer on FDG PET and PET/CT. *AJR Am J Roentgenol.* 2012;198:W304-W314.
150. Singh A, Kaur P, Sood N, Puri H, Garg B. Bilateral eosinophilic mastitis: an uncommon unheard entity. *Breast Dis.* 2015;35:33-36.
151. Solomon GJ, Wu E, Rosen PP. Nephrogenic systemic fibrosis mimicking inflammatory breast carcinoma. *Arch Pathol Lab Med.* 2007;131:145-148.
152. Van Wert M, Ghio M, Graham C, Smetherman D, Sanders R, Corsetti R. Multicentric breast abscesses in a patient who had COVID-19. *Ochsner J.* 2021;21:402-405.
153. Abbas A, Turner N, MacNeill F. Managing breast gangrene during the COVID-19 pandemic. *Ann R Coll Surg Engl.* 2021;103:e141-e143.
154. Guarda LA, Tran TA. The pathology of breast biopsy site marking devices. *Am J Surg Pathol.* 2005;29:814-819.

3

Specific Infections and Infestations

RAZA S. HODA AND SYED A. HODA

INTRODUCTION

A wide variety of microbial infections caused by bacteria, fungi, parasites, and viruses can afflict the breast. Most forms of infectious mastitis are a manifestation of a systemic infection. It is rare for the breast to be the only organ involved in an infectious disease process outside of the settings of pregnancy and lactation or in the absence of a compromised immune status.

The presence of most specific infectious processes in needle core biopsy specimens is unexpected. Often, the only clinical information available in such cases is either a mass or an imaging abnormality. The pathologist is typically unaware of any concurrent systemic or local infection. Thus, pathologists ought to be alert to the possibility of encountering infectious disease processes in needle core biopsies.

BACTERIAL INFECTION

Abscess

Bacterial infections are the commonest cause of mastitis and are most frequent during lactation and pregnancy. *Staphylococcus aureus* is the usual cause of bacterial abscesses, including those that occur during lactation **(Fig. 3.1)**. A minor (~10%) proportion of *S. aureus* that cause mammary abscess result from the methicillin-resistant variety (1), and antibiotic use ought to be guided by results of bacterial cultures.

Rare instances of mammary abscesses caused by *Nocardia* (2), *Salmonella* (3-5), *Pseudomonas* (6), and brucellosis (7) have been reported. Mammary lesions resulting from cat-scratch disease caused by *Bartonella* present as a mass with inflammatory signs, often accompanied by axillary nodal enlargement that may mimic inflammatory carcinoma (8). The mammary lesion of bartonellosis is typically either in an axillary or in an intramammary lymph node rather than in mammary parenchyma.

The existence of an immunodeficiency or immunocompromised state (including HIV/AIDS) can predispose to infections, including those caused by *Salmonella* and *Pseudomonas aeruginosa* (9). Mammary gangrene has been reported in patients with HIV infection in the absence of prior trauma or other injury to the breast (10). Among other predisposing factors for mammary bacterial infections are the performance of needle core biopsy (11) and insertion of nipple rings purportedly for adornment purposes (12).

Actinomycotic infection of the breast typically presents as an abscess near the nipple and areola. Predisposing factors include lactation, diabetes, nipple piercing, and immunosuppressive therapy (13-15). Sinus tracts can develop following incision and drainage of an actinomycotic abscess or with progression of the untreated lesion. A chronic abscess may form, creating a firm mass that can simulate carcinoma (13). Axillary lymph node enlargement generally reflects reaction to the mammary inflammatory process rather than spread of actinomycosis to lymph nodes; however, primary actinomycotic axillary lymphadenitis has been reported (14,15). In advanced cases, the infection can spread to the chest wall. Extension of pulmonary actinomycosis to the breast has also been described (16). The diagnosis of actinomycosis is rendered by the demonstration of the gram-positive organism in filaments or colonies ("sulfur" granules). Isolates from mammary actinomycosis include *Actinomyces meyeri* (17), *A. viscosus* (18), *A. radingae, A. turicensis* (15), and *A. israelii* (19). Treatment with penicillin has reportedly been effective (14), but recurrent or advanced infections may require multiple antibiotics (15) and rarely wide local excision or mastectomy.

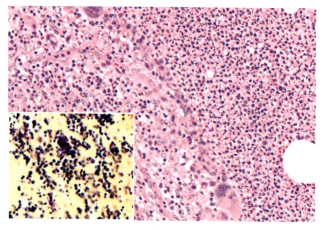

FIGURE 3.1 Staphylococcal Abscess. Purulent mastitis in a 35-year-old woman who had been nursing until a few weeks prior to the biopsy. The abscess contained gram-positive cocci (inset). *S. aureus* was cultured.

Mycobacterial Infections

Mycobacterium tuberculosis infection of the breast, in immunosuppressed as well as immunocompetent men and women, is not an uncommon condition in many regions of the world (20-23). Tuberculous mastitis has been reported as a manifestation of AIDS, and this presentation is encountered with increasing frequency in HIV-positive individuals (9,24).

Mammary tuberculosis unassociated with HIV infection is primarily a disease of premenopausal women with a predilection for the lactating breast, but it can also affect postmenopausal women. Infection of the breast may be the primary manifestation of tuberculosis, but the breasts are probably infected secondarily in most patients even when the primary nonmammary focus remains clinically inapparent.

It is difficult to make a clinical diagnosis of tuberculous mastitis because the disease can present variably. The most common presentation is with a slow-growing mass. The mammographic presentation of such masses may resemble carcinoma (25,26). Calcifications are typically absent. Advanced masses become fixed to the skin and may develop draining sinuses. An acute and diffuse type of tuberculous mastitis is characterized by the development of multiple painful nodules throughout the breast, producing a pattern that can mimic inflammatory carcinoma (26). A third, sclerosing variety of infection occurs predominantly in elderly women, resulting in diffuse induration of the breast and diffusely increased density on mammography. The clinical distinction between tuberculous mastitis and mammary carcinoma can be complicated by the occasional coexistence of both conditions (27). Rarely, tuberculosis of the chest wall can present as a breast lump (20).

Microscopically, granulomatous lesions in tuberculous mastitis usually, but not always, feature granulomata with "caseous" necrosis **(Fig. 3.2)**. Associated fibrosis may be prominent in chronic cases. The granulomas are associated with ducts and lobules. Acid-fast bacteria are detected in a minority of cases **(Fig. 3.3)**. Neutrophils can obscure the

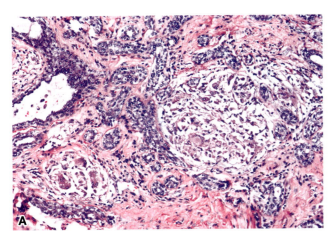 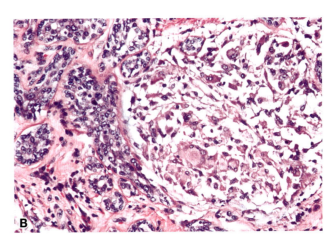

FIGURE 3.2 Tuberculous Mastitis. A, B: Granulomatous inflammation in sclerosing adenosis in a patient with active pulmonary tuberculosis. The needle core biopsy was performed to evaluate a breast mass. No acid-fast bacteria were found with the acid-fast (Ziehl–Neelsen) stain.

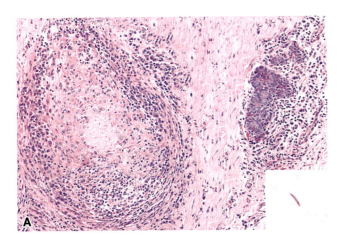 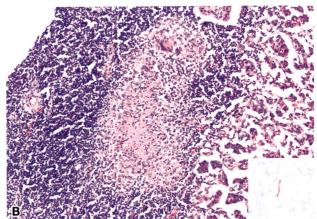

FIGURE 3.3 Tuberculous Mastitis. A: A granuloma with central "caseous" necrosis is present in the vicinity of inactive mammary glands. Inset shows an acid-fast bacillus on a Ziehl–Neelsen preparation. **B:** Needle core biopsy of axillary lymph node with a caseating granuloma present in the vicinity of metastatic mammary micropapillary carcinoma. Inset shows acid-fast bacilli on a Ziehl–Neelsen preparation.

granulomatous character of the process in specimens from patients with necrotizing abscesses. The finding of caseous necrosis in granulomata in a needle core biopsy of the breast may be considered presumptive evidence of tuberculosis in the appropriate clinical setting. If mycobacterial infection is clinically suspected, samples obtained via a fine needle aspirate or needle core biopsy should be submitted for microbiologic culture or polymerase chain reaction (PCR) study.

A wide variety of *atypical (nontuberculous) mycobacteria* can infect breast tissue in acute, subacute, and chronic forms (28) and can simulate a neoplasm (29). Breast abscess formation attributable to atypical mycobacterial infection such as *Mycobacterium fortuitum* (12,30) and *M. abscessus* (31) has been observed following nipple piercing. *M. fortuitum* infections have also complicated prosthetic breast implants (32).

The precise diagnosis of mammary mycobacterial and atypical (nontuberculous) mycobacterial infection and other granulomatous conditions is facilitated by the PCR technique (21,28,33).

Cystic Neutrophilic Granulomatous Mastitis

A particular type of granulomatous mastitis associated with cystic degeneration and marked neutrophilic infiltrate has been associated with *Corynebacterium*, a gram-positive bacterial organism (34-38) **(Fig. 3.4)**. Cystic neutrophilic granulomatous mastitis (CNGM) usually presents as a mass. The disease is characterized by lobulocentric granulomata with mixed inflammatory cell infiltrate and clear vacuoles. The latter are lined by neutrophils within the granulomas. Gram-positive bacilli are identified in approximately one-half of the cases. Examination of thicker, that is, 6 μm, sections of Gram stain preparations from representative tissue blocks of CNGM has been shown to improve the detection rate of the responsible bacilli. Molecular techniques utilizing broad-range bacterial 16S ribosomal DNA PCR on formalin-fixed paraffin-embedded tissue can facilitate the diagnosis of CNGM (39,40). In general, tuberculous granulomata (a potential consideration in the differential diagnosis) show frankly caseous necrosis and a lesser extent (if any) of cystic change. Other forms of granulomatous mastitis are discussed in detail in Chapter 2.

FUNGAL INFECTIONS

Infection with *Histoplasma capsulatum* is endemic in the Ohio and Mississippi river valleys of the United States and in many geographic zones on all continents. Calcified granulomata have not been described in the breast, but there have been rare instances of localized mammary *Histoplasma* infection. The latter can present as a solitary unilateral mass that may clinically simulate a neoplasm (41,42). Histologically, the lesions consist of confluent necrotizing

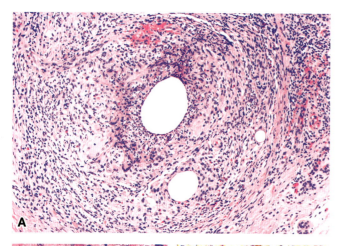

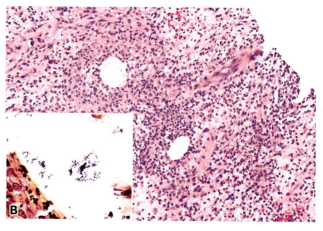

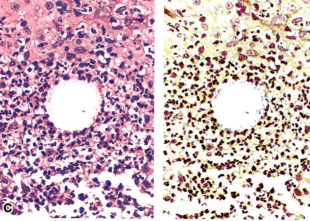

FIGURE 3.4 Cystic Neutrophilic Granulomatous Mastitis.
A: The archetypal lesion of this disease shows granulomatous mastitis with cyst lined by neutrophils. Note multinucleated giant cells. Bacilli were evident within the cysts on deeper sections. **B:** Mammary glandular and stromal tissue has been destroyed by abscess formation with the characteristic central cystic structure. Neutrophils are dominant amid the inflammatory cell infiltrate. Inset shows gram-positive rods. *Corynebacterium* sp. was cultured. **C:** Bacilli at the rim of the central cystic structure in this example of cystic neutrophilic granulomatous mastitis (CNGM) (left). The slide was de-stained and then re-stained by Gram method (right). The latter stain showed the bacilli to be gram-positive.

granulomas in which *H. capsulatum* is demonstrated by a methenamine silver reaction. The granulomatous reaction is essentially similar to that of nonspecific granulomatous lobular mastitis (42,43).

Rare instances of other fungal infections of the breast have also been reported. These include *Cryptococcus* **(Fig. 3.5)** (44,45), *Aspergillus* (46), *Coccidioides* (47), *Paracoccidioides* (48), and *Blastomyces* (49). *Aspergillus* infection has been reported at the site of breast augmentation implants (50). Notably, and inexplicably, coccidioidomycosis can "flare up" during pregnancy—occasionally with breast involvement (51,52).

PARASITIC INFESTATION

A variety of parasites can infest female and male breast tissue. In almost all instances, the mammary involvement is part of a systemic disease process.

Mammary filariasis is caused most frequently by *Wuchereria bancrofti* and has been reported from tropical and semitropical regions in South America, China, and South Asia, where infection with this organism is endemic. Involvement of the breast occurs in the chronic phase of the disease, sometimes more than a decade after last exposure to infection.

The patient with mammary filariasis usually presents with a solitary, nontender, painless unilateral breast mass. Multiple lesions occur in a minority of cases. Many lesions involve subcutaneous tissue, and they may be fixed to the skin. The resultant hard mass with cutaneous attachment, sometimes accompanied by inflammatory changes including edema, appears to be clinically indistinguishable from carcinoma (53). In this setting, axillary lymph nodal enlargement caused by filarial lymphadenitis further complicates the differential diagnosis. Viable microfilariae can be detected in the breast by ultrasound examination if they produce a distinctive pattern of movement referred to as the "filaria dance" sign (54). Mammographically detected calcifications attributed to *W. bancrofti* and *Loa loa* infection have been described as having a spiral or serpiginous configuration (55). Microscopic examination of fine needle aspiration or tissue biopsy samples reveals adult filarial worms that may be well preserved or in different stages of degeneration (56) **(Fig. 3.6)**. Granulomatous reaction with eosinophilia is present in tissues around the parasites. Fully degenerated worms are likely to become calcified. Microfilariae are not always detected in the peripheral blood (57). Adult worms and microfilariae may also be found in axillary lymph nodes (58).

Several cases of mammary *cysticercosis*, an infection caused by larvae of tapeworms, that have been described have mimicked a neoplasm (59-61). Most instances of mammary cysticercosis are caused by *Taenia solium*, and such a case diagnosed by needle core biopsy in a *male* breast has been reported (62). *T. solium* is typically acquired by ingesting undercooked pork; however, mammary infection has been reported in a vegetarian presumably by ingestion of *T. solium* eggs in contaminated food (61).

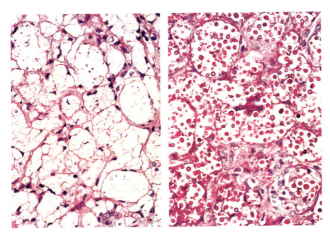

FIGURE 3.5 A needle core biopsy of a breast mass shows encapsulated yeast form diagnostic of *Cryptococcus neoformans*. Hematoxylin and eosin (H&E) stain (left) and mucicarmine stain (right). Culture studies were confirmatory. (Courtesy of Dr Dam Thuy Trang, Hanoi, Vietnam.)

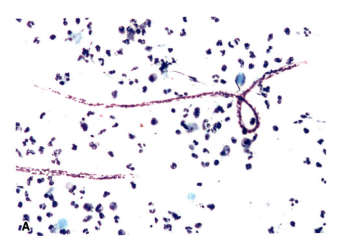
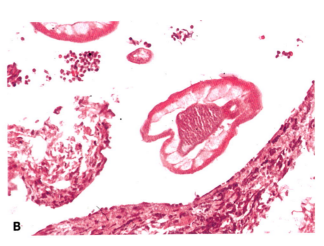

FIGURE 3.6 **Mammary Filariasis. A:** Microfilariae in a fine needle aspiration specimen with *W. bancrofti* infection. **B:** Biopsy specimen from a mammary filarial abscess showing a microfilaria in cross section and fragments of the surrounding tissue. (Courtesy of Dr Kusum Kapila, Kuwait.)

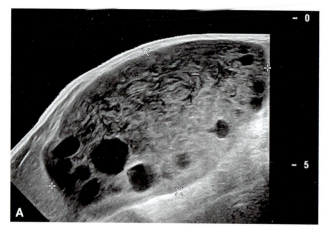
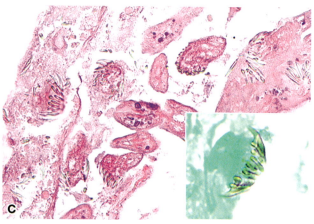
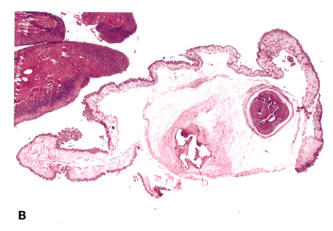

FIGURE 3.7 **Echinococcal (Hydatid) Diseases. A:** Ultrasound image of a breast showing a mass with multiple internal anechoic cysts. (Courtesy of Dr Abdulmohsen Alkushi, Riyadh, Kingdom of Saudi Arabia.) **B:** Part of an echinococcal cyst wall and a cross section of the larval tapeworm in another breast specimen. (Courtesy of Dr Kusum Kapila, Kuwait.) **C:** A portion of yet another mammary hydatid (echinococcal) cyst wall with numerous echinococcal scolices. Inset shows the detail of a scolex.

The breast can also be the site of hydatid cyst formation caused by *Echinococcus granulosus*. The lesion typically presents as a firm, discrete mobile mass. Mammography reveals a dense, well-circumscribed tumor within which internal ring structures representing air fluid levels may be seen. Ultrasound evaluation displays air fluid levels and multiple cysts to better advantage (63,64) **(Fig. 3.7)**. Rarely, mammographically detected calcifications in clinically inapparent cysts have been the first evidence of mammary cysticercosis (65,66). Mammary hydatid disease can be recognized by finding fragments of the adult worm, the hydatid membranes, and hooklets in aspirated cyst contents or a needle core biopsy (67).

The diagnosis of mammary *sparganosis* by needle core biopsy caused by the tapeworm *Spirometra* has been described (68) **(Fig. 3.8)**. Complete excision is the treatment of choice (69,70).

Calcified ova of *schistosomiasis* can simulate a carcinoma on mammograms (71) **(Fig. 3.9),** or the inflammatory nodule may be mistaken for a fibroadenoma (72).

Microcalcifications attributed to *trichinellosis*, that is, *Trichinella* infection, have been found in the pectoral muscles by mammography (73).

Cutaneous *myiasis* caused by larvae of the botfly *Dermatobia hominis* results in a mass lesion accompanied by local inflammation. The mammographic and ultrasound findings in five patients with mammary lesions were reported by de Barros et al (74). The mammographically ill-defined tumors measured 0.7 to 2.0 cm. Paired linear microcalcifications were visualized in three lesions. Oval larvae outlined by a hypoechoic zone were demonstrated by ultrasound examination. Although the diagnosis of myiasis could be suggested by a history of origin from or a visit to an endemic area, the clinical signs, the ultrasound findings, the presence of an ill-defined mass with calcification, and inflammation may

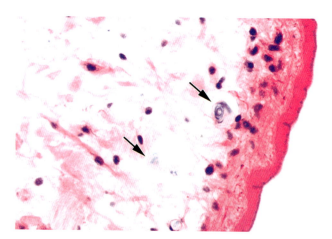

FIGURE 3.8 **Mammary Sparganosis.** Portion of a sparganum larva obtained by needle core biopsy of the breast. Note the presence of whorled calcifications in the larva (arrows). (Courtesy of Dr Amy Bik-Wan Chan, Hong Kong.)

SPECIFIC INFECTIONS AND INFESTATIONS 39

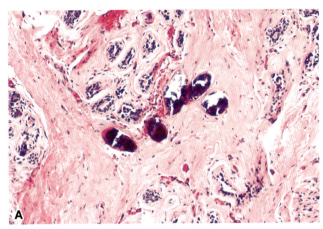
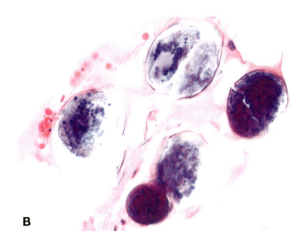
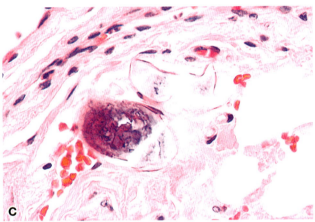
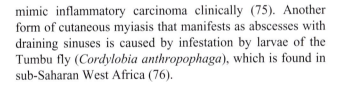

FIGURE 3.9 Mammary Schistosomiasis. This young woman with gastrointestinal symptoms was found to have numerous calcifications in the breast by mammography. **A:** The needle core biopsy sample shown here has five calcified ova of *Schistosoma mansoni* in the stroma next to a lobule. **B:** Five calcified ova in fat from the same specimen. **C:** Magnified view showing the characteristic spine. (Courtesy of Dr Rhonda Yantiss, Miami, FL.)

mimic inflammatory carcinoma clinically (75). Another form of cutaneous myiasis that manifests as abscesses with draining sinuses is caused by infestation by larvae of the Tumbu fly (*Cordylobia anthropophaga*), which is found in sub-Saharan West Africa (76).

VIRAL INFECTION

Although a variety of secondary infections can involve the breast in patients with HIV infection (vide supra), the disease can manifest itself in an intramammary lymph node (77). The characteristic findings in this setting are florid follicular hyperplasia with "follicle-lysis."

Infection of the mammary skin, and rarely of the nipple, with a variety of viruses, including *Human papillomavirus* (causing verruca vulgaris), *Herpes simplex*, and *Herpes zoster*, has been reported (78); however, these infectious processes are unlikely to be encountered in needle core biopsy specimens.

REFERENCES

1. Dabbas N, Chand M, Pallett A, Royle GT, Sainsbury R. Have the organisms that cause breast abscess changed with time? Implications for appropriate antibiotic usage in primary and secondary care. *Breast J.* 2010;16:412-415.
2. Simpson AJH, Jumaa PA, Das SS. Breast abscess caused by *Nocardia asteroides*. *J Infect.* 1995;30:266-267.
3. Banu A, Hassan MM, Anand M. Breast abscess: sole manifestation of *Salmonella typhi* infection. *Indian J Med Microbiol.* 2013;31:94-95.
4. Vattipally V, Thatigotla B, Nagpal K, et al. *Salmonella typhi* breast abscess: an uncommon manifestation of an uncommon disease in the United States. *Am Surg.* 2011;77:E133-E135.
5. Singh S, Pandya Y, Rathod J, Trivedi S. Bilateral breast abscess: a rare complication of enteric fever. *Indian J Med Microbiol.* 2009;27:69-70.
6. Harji DP, Rastall S, Catchpole C, Bright-Thomas R, Thrush S. Pseudomonal breast infection. *Ann R Coll Surg Engl.* 2010;92:W20-W22.
7. Gurleyik E. Breast abscess as a complication of human brucellosis. *Breast J.* 2006;12:375-376.
8. Povoski SP, Spigos DG, March WL. An unusual case of cat-scratch disease from *Bartonella quintana* mimicking inflammatory breast cancer in a 50-year old woman. *Breast J.* 2003;9:497-500.
9. Pantanowitz L, Connolly JL. Pathology of the breast associated with HIV/AIDS. *Breast J.* 2002;8:234-243.
10. Venkatramani V, Pillai S, Marathe S, Rege SA, Hardikar JV. Breast gangrene in an HIV-positive patient. *Ann R Coll Surg Engl.* 2009;91:W13-W14.
11. Roque DR, MacLaughlan S, Tejada-Berges T. Necrotizing infection of the breast after core needle biopsy. *Breast J.* 2013;19:201-202.
12. Bengualid V, Singh V, Singh H, Berger J. *Mycobacterium fortuitum* and anaerobic breast abscess following nipple piercing: case presentation and review of the literature. *J Adolesc Health.* 2008;42:530-532.
13. Thambi R, Devi L, Sheeja S, Poothiode U. Primary breast actinomyces simulating malignancy: a case diagnosed by fine-needle aspiration cytology. *J Cytol.* 2012;29:197-199.
14. Jain BK, Sehgal VN, Jagdish S, Ratnakar C, Smile SR. Primary actinomycosis of the breast: a clinical review and a case report. *J Dermatol.* 1994;21:497-500.
15. Attar KH, Waghorn D, Lyons M, Cunnick G. Rare species of actinomyces as causative pathogens in breast abscess. *Breast J.* 2007;13:501-505.
16. Pinto MM, Longstreth GB, Khoury GM. Fine needle aspiration of Actinomyces infection of the breast: a novel presentation of thoracopleural actinomycosis. *Acta Cytol.* 1991;35:409-411.
17. Allen JN. *Actinomyces meyeri* breast abscess. *Am J Med.* 1987;83:186-187.
18. Capobianco G, Dessole S, Becchere MP, et al. A rare case of primary actinomycosis of the breast caused by *Actinomyces viscosus*: diagnosis by fine needle aspiration cytology under ultrasound guidance. *Breast J.* 2005;11:57-59.
19. Akhlaghi M, Ghazvini RD. Clinical presentation of primary actinomycosis of the breast. *Breast J.* 2009;15:102-103.
20. Teo TH, Ho GH, Chaturverdi A, Khoo BKJ. Tuberculosis of the chest wall: unusual presentation as a breast lump. *Singapore Med J.* 2009;50:e97-e99.
21. Miller K, Harrington SM, Propcop GW. Acid-fast smear and histopathology results provide guidance for the appropriate use of broad-range polymerase chain reaction and sequencing for mycobacteria. *Arch Pathol Lab Med.* 2015;139:1020-1023.
22. Kumar M, Chand G, Nag VL, et al. Breast tuberculosis in immunocompetent patients at tertiary care center: a case series. *J Res Med Sci.* 2012;17:199-202.

23. Hale JA, Peters GN, Cheek JH. Tuberculosis of the breast: rare but still extant. *Am J Surg.* 1985;150:620-624.
24. Hartstein M, Leaf HL. Tuberculosis of the breast as a presenting manifestation of AIDS. *Clin Infect Dis.* 1992;15:692-693.
25. Makanjuola D, Murshid K, Sulaimani A, Al Saleh M. Mammographic features of breast tuberculosis: the skin bulge and sinus tract sign. *Clin Radiol.* 1996;51: 354-358.
26. Sopeña B, Arnillas E, Garcia-Vila LM, Climent A, Miramontes S. Tuberculosis of the breast: unusual clinical presentation of extrapulmonary tuberculosis. *Infection.* 1996;24:57-58.
27. Rothman GM, Meroz A, Kolkov Z, Lewinski UH. Breast tuberculosis and carcinoma. *Isr J Med Sci.* 1989;25:339-340.
28. Yoo H, Choi SH, Kim YJ, Kim SJ, Cho YU, Choi SJ. Recurrent bilateral breast abscess due to nontuberculous mycobacterial infection. *J Breast Cancer.* 2014;17:295-298.
29. Mohamad B, Iqbal MN, Gopal KV, Arshad SN, Daw HA. MAI infection simulating metastatic breast cancer. *BMJ Case Rep.* 2012;2012:bcr0120125640. doi:10.1136/bcr-01-2012-5640
30. Lewis CG, Wells MK, Jennings WC. *Mycobacterium fortuitum* breast infection following nipple-piercing, mimicking carcinoma. *Breast J.* 2004;10:363-365.
31. Trupiano JK, Sebek BA, Goldfarb J, Levy LR, Hall GS, Procop GW. Mastitis due to *Mycobacterium abscessus* after body piercing. *Clin Infect Dis.* 2001;33: 131-134.
32. Haiavy J, Tobin H. *Mycobacterium fortuitum* infection in prosthetic breast implants. *Plast Reconstr Surg.* 2002;109:2124-2128.
33. Wolfrum A, Kümmel S, Theuerkauf I, Pelz E, Reinisch M. Granulomatous mastitis: a therapeutic and diagnostic challenge. *Breast Care (Basel).* 2018;13: 413-418.
34. Renshaw AA, Derhagopian RP, Gould EW. Cystic neutrophilic granulomatous mastitis: an underappreciated pattern strongly associated with gram-positive bacilli. *Am J Clin Pathol.* 2011;136:424-427.
35. Gautham I, Radford DM, Kovacs CS, et al. Cystic neutrophilic granulomatous mastitis: the Cleveland Clinic experience with diagnosis and management. *Breast J.* 2019;25:80-85.
36. D'Alfonso TM, Moo TA, Arleo EK, Cheng E, Antonio LB, Hoda SA. Cystic neutrophilic granulomatous mastitis: further characterization of a distinctive histopathologic entity not always demonstrably attributable to *Corynebacterium* infection. *Am J Surg Pathol.* 2015;39:1440-1447.
37. Wu JM, Turashvili G. Cystic neutrophilic granulomatous mastitis: an update. *J Clin Pathol.* 2020;73:445-453.
38. Sangoi AR. "Thick section" Gram stain yields improved detection of organisms in tissue sections of cystic neutrophilic granulomatous mastitis. *Am J Clin Pathol.* 2020;153:593-597.
39. Naik MA, Korlimarla A, Shetty ST, Fernandes AM, Pai SA. Cystic neutrophilic granulomatous mastitis: a clinicopathological study with 16s rRNA sequencing for the detection of *Corynebacteria* in formalin-fixed paraffin-embedded tissue. *Int J Surg Pathol.* 2020;28:371-381.
40. Tariq H, Menon PD, Fan H, et al. Detection of *Corynebacterium kroppenstedtii* in granulomatous lobular mastitis using real-time polymerase chain reaction and Sanger sequencing on formalin-fixed, paraffin-embedded tissues. *Arch Pathol Lab Med.* 2022;146:749-754.
41. Salfelder K, Schwarz J. Mycotic "pseudotumors" of the breast. *Arch Surg.* 1975; 110:751-754.
42. Johnston KT, Dang PA, Specht MC, Letourneau AR, Gudewicz TM. Case records of the Massachusetts General Hospital. Case 29-2016. A 53-year-old woman with pain and a mass in the breast. *N Engl J Med.* 2016;375:1172-1180.
43. Payne S, Kim S, Das K, Mirani N. A 36-year-old woman with a unilateral breast mass: necrotizing granulomatous mastitis secondary to budding yeast forms morphologically consistent with *Histoplasma capsulatum. Arch Pathol Lab Med.* 2006;130:e1-e2.
44. Ramos-Barbosa S, Guazzelli LS, Severo LC. Cryptococcal mastitis after corticosteroid therapy. *Rev Soc Bras Med Trop.* 2004;37:65-66.
45. Haddow LJ, Sahid F, Moosa MY. Cryptococcal breast abscess in an HIV-positive patient: arguments for reviewing the definition of immune reconstitution inflammatory syndrome. *J Infect.* 2008;57:82-84.
46. Giovindarajan M, Verghese S, Kuruvilla S. Primary aspergillosis of the breast: report of a case with fine needle aspiration cytology. *Acta Cytol.* 1993;37: 234-236.
47. Bocian JJ, Fahmy RN, Michas CA. A rare case of "coccidioidoma" of the breast. *Arch Pathol Lab Med.* 1991;115:1064-1067.

48. de Oliveira DCL, Guarachi GIY, Marinho JES, Vianna JAS, de Melo ASA, Rêgo SJF. Systemic paracoccidioidomycosis involving breast. *Breast J.* 2018;24:831-832.
49. Propeck PA, Scanlan KA. Blastomycosis of the breast. *AJR Am J Roentgenol.* 1996;166:726.
50. Williams K, Walton RL, Bunkis I. Aspergillus colonization associated with bilateral silicone mammary implants. *J Surg Pathol.* 1982;71:260-261.
51. Hooper JE, Lu Q, Pepkowitz SH. Disseminated coccidioidomycosis in pregnancy. *Arch Pathol Lab Med.* 2007;131:652-655.
52. Babycos PB, Hoda SA. A fatal case of disseminated coccidioidomycosis in Louisiana. *J La State Med Soc.* 1990;142:24-27.
53. Choudhury M. Bancroftian microfilaria in the breast clinically mimicking malignancy. *Cytopathology.* 1995;6:132-133.
54. Dreyer G, Brandão AC, Amaral F, Medeiros Z, Addiss D. Detection by ultrasound of living adult *Wuchereria bancrofti* in the female breast. *Mem Inst Oswaldo Cruz.* 1996;91:95-96.
55. Chow CK, McCarthy JS, Neafie R, et al. Mammography of lymphatic filariasis. *AJR Am J Roentgenol.* 1996;167:1425-1426.
56. Mondal SK. Incidental detection of filaria in fine-needle aspirates: a cytologic study of 14 clinically unsuspected cases at different sites. *Diagn Cytopathol.* 2012;40:292-296.
57. Parida G, Rout N, Samantaray S, Devi P, Pattanayak L, Kakkar S. Filariasis of breast simulating carcinoma. *Breast J.* 2008;14:598-599.
58. Chen YH, Qun X. Filarial granuloma of the female breast: a histopathologic study of 131 cases. *Am J Trop Med Hyg.* 1981;30:1206-1210.
59. Conde DM, Kashimoto E, Carvalho LE, Hidalgo SR, Torresan RZ. Cysticercosis of the breast: an uncommon cause of lumps. *Breast J.* 2006;12:179.
60. Karthikeyan TM, Manimaran D, Mrinalini VR. Cysticercus of the breast which mimicked a fibroadenoma: a rare presentation. *J Clin Diagn Res.* 2012;6:1555-1556.
61. Bhattacharjee HK, Ramman TR, Agarwal L, Nain M, Thomas S. Isolated cysticercosis of the breast masquerading as a breast tumor: report of a case and review of literature. *Ann Trop Med Parasitol.* 2011;105:455-461.
62. Lobaz J, Millican-Slater R, Rengabashyam B, Turton P. Parasitic infection of the male breast. *BMJ Case Rep.* 2014;2014:bcr2013202493.
63. Alamer A, Aldhilan A, Makanjuola D, Alkushi A. Preoperative diagnosis of hydatid cyst of the breast: a case report. *Pan Afr Med J.* 2013;14:99.
64. Vega A, Ortega E, Cavada A, et al. Hydatid cyst of the breast: mammographic findings. *AJR Am J Roentgenol.* 1994;162:825-826.
65. Lucarelli AP, Martins MM, de Oliviera VM, et al. A short report: cysticercosis of the breast. *Am J Trop Med Hyg.* 2008;279:864-865.
66. Haholy A, Sonmez G, Karaman M, Demirbilek O, Baloglu H. Unilocular cystic hydatidosis in breast. *Breast J.* 2008;14:393-394.
67. Sagin HB, Kiroglu Y, Aksoy F. Hydatid cyst of the breast diagnosed by fine needle aspiration biopsy: a case report. *Acta Cytol.* 1994;38:965-967.
68. Chan ABW, Wan SK, Leung S.L, et al. Sparganosis of the breast. *Histopathology.* 2004;44:510-511.
69. Koo M, Kim JH, Kim JS, et al. Cases and literature review of breast sparganosis. *World J Surg.* 2011;35:573-579.
70. Min KW, Kim DY, Kim HJ, Kang HJ, Song JS, Gong G. Sparganosis infection presenting as a palpable mass in male breast. *Int J Infect Dis.* 2013;17:e663-e664.
71. Sloan BS, Rickman LS, Blau EM, Davis CE. Schistosomiasis masquerading as carcinoma of the breast. *South Med J.* 1996;89:345-347.
72. Elma CA, Cavalcanti AC, Lima MM, Piva N. Pseudoneoplastic lesion of the breast caused by *Schistosoma mansoni. Rev Soc Bras Med Trop.* 2004;37:63-64.
73. Valdes PV, Prieto A, Diaz A, Calleja M, Gomez JL. Microcalcifications of pectoral muscle in trichinosis. *Breast J.* 2005;11:150.
74. de Barros N, D'Avila MS, de Pace Bauab S, et al. Cutaneous myiasis of the breast: mammographic and US features—report of five cases. *Radiology.* 2001; 218:517-520.
75. Ugwu BT, Nwadiaro PO. *Cordylobia anthropophaga* mastitis mimicking breast cancer: a case report. *East Afr Med J.* 1999;76:115-116.
76. Adisa CA, Mbanaso A. Furuncular myiasis of the breast caused by the larvae of the Tumbu fly (*Cordylobia anthropophaga*). *BMC Surg.* 2004;4:5.
77. Konstantinopoulos PA, Dezube BJ, March D, Pantanowitz L. HIV-associated intramammary lymphadenopathy. *Breast J.* 2007;13:192-195.
78. Das DK, Rifaat AA, George SS, Grover VK, Mathew TC, Mirza K. Morphologic changes in fibroadenoma of breast due to chickenpox: a case report with suspicious cytology in fine needle aspiration smears. *Acta Cytol.* 2008;52:337-343.

4

Benign Papillary Tumors

ELAINE W. ZHONG AND SYED A. HODA

INTRADUCTAL PAPILLOMA

A papilloma is a discrete benign neoplasm consisting of branching fibrovascular cores lined by ductal epithelium and myoepithelium. Papillomas most often arise from lactiferous ducts in the central part of the breast but can occur peripherally and in any quadrant. *Intracystic papilloma* is the descriptor applied to a papilloma protruding into a large, cystic cavity. An *adenomyoepithelioma* is biphasic neoplasm related to papilloma (see Chapter 5).

A *solitary papilloma* is a single discrete papillary tumor in one duct, typically central or subareolar, whereas *multiple papillomas* grow as independent tumors and often occupy contiguous branches of the ductal system. Solitary papillomas are more commonly diagnosed than multiple papillomas, because they are more frequently symptomatic (1). The term *papillomatosis* refers to the presence of multiple papillomas as well as to various papillary-like epithelial proliferations. Because of the possibility of confusion, it is best to avoid the diagnosis of papillomatosis in most circumstances. Juvenile papillomatosis and florid papillomatosis of the nipple are distinctive clinicopathologic entities.

Of note, papilloma-like features are seen on a more limited scale in *papillary hyperplasia*, a proliferative process that is a component of fibrocystic change (2). Papillary hyperplasia is characterized by epithelial proliferation on a vascular stalk (as opposed to a *fibro*vascular core), and tiered or branching architecture is usually not evident. In general, papillary hyperplasia is a purely microscopic lesion, whereas bona fide papilloma ought to be manifested macroscopically and/or radiologically (3). Indiscriminate application of the term "papilloma" to a minuscule, incidental, nonneoplastic lesion in a needle core biopsy (NCB) sample may raise management issues (4).

Clinical Features

Solitary papillomas occur at any age from infancy to the ninth decade but are most frequent in the sixth and seventh decades of life. Women with multiple papillomas tend to be younger than women with solitary papillomas, and the former most often present in their 40s and early 50s. Males with papillomas span the same age range as women (5). Papillomas may occur more frequently in African-American women than in those of other ethnicities (6).

Papillomas have developed in unusual settings. One report (7) documented the growth of a papilloma in residual breast tissue status-post mastectomy following a transverse rectus abdominis myocutaneous (TRAM) flap reconstruction. At least three publications (8-10) describe the presence of papillomas in ectopic breast tissue in axillary lymph nodes of women with intramammary papillomas.

Central papillomas often induce a discharge from the nipple. A profusely bloody discharge occurs more commonly with papillary carcinomas than with papillomas, but degenerative changes in a papilloma can give rise to bleeding and sporadic blood-stained discharge. A subareolar mass may be palpable. A papilloma in a 44-year-old man produced a hard, lobulated mass fixed to the chest wall (11). Multiple papillomas develop peripherally more often than centrally and typically present as palpable masses.

Imaging Studies

Cystic, solitary papillary tumors may appear well circumscribed on mammography (12). The presence of a cystic component is best appreciated on ultrasonography. The latter technique appears to be more sensitive than mammography for the detection of papillomas (12). Ductography may demonstrate the presence of a central papilloma, and magnetic resonance imaging (MRI) typically reveals duct dilation and small, oval, smoothly contoured, enhancing intraductal masses. After a detailed mammographic and sonographic study of 40 papillary tumors, Lam et al (13) concluded that "radiologic features are not sufficiently sensitive or specific to differentiate benign from malignant papillary lesions." By using a combination of both imaging modalities, the authors achieved a sensitivity of 61%, a specificity of 33%, a positive predictive value of 85%, and a negative predictive value of 13%.

Histologic Evaluation

The basic microscopic structure of a papilloma consists of a layer of benign mammary epithelium supported by branching stromal fronds, which are attached to the duct wall at one or more points **(Figs. 4.1 and 4.2)**. Epithelium lining the nonpapillary portion of the duct may be unremarkable or hyperplastic **(Fig. 4.3)**.

Superimposed secondary processes such as epithelial hyperplasia and stromal overgrowth can mask the underlying papillary architecture of a papilloma and thereby hinder

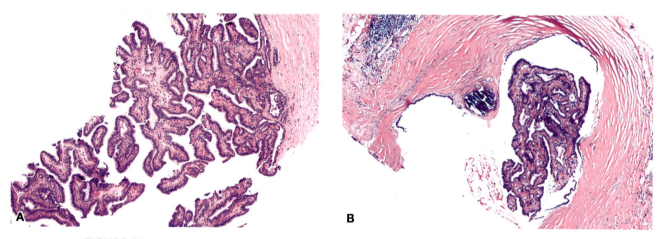

FIGURE 4.1 Intracystic Papilloma. A: Arborizing fronds float within a cystic space in this needle core biopsy. **B:** The sample displays a portion of an intracystic papilloma and the surrounding cyst wall. Note the calcification in the cyst wall at the center of the image.

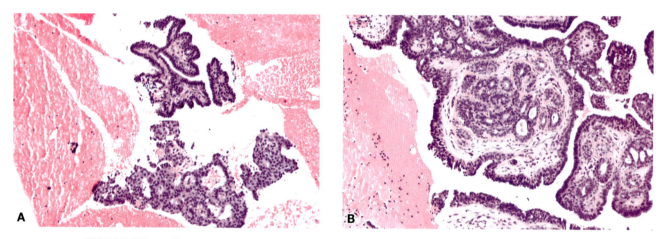

FIGURE 4.2 Papilloma. A, B: One can see detached papillary epithelial fragments in this needle core biopsy specimen. Note the simple surface epithelium showing minimal hyperplasia and the distinct fibrovascular stroma.

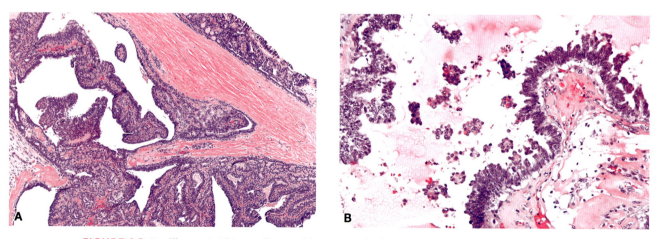

FIGURE 4.3 Papilloma. A: This needle core biopsy sample shows a cyst wall and papillary fronds extending into the lumen. The epithelium lining the cyst between the papillary fronds is minimally hyperplastic. **B:** The epithelium of this papilloma demonstrates slight micropapillary hyperplasia. The stroma of the papilloma contains histiocytes with clear cytoplasm.

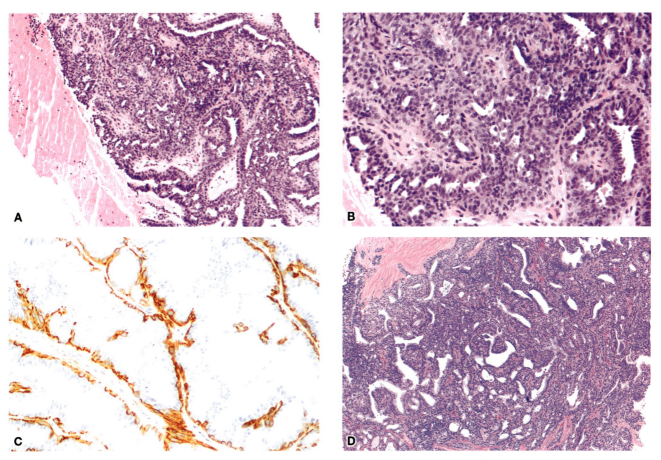

FIGURE 4.4 Papilloma With Ductal Hyperplasia. A, B: Hyperplasia in a needle core biopsy sample is manifested by increased thickness of the epithelial layer and bridging of the epithelium across the spaces between fronds, resulting in the formation of microlumina. **C:** Myoepithelium is demonstrated by reactivity for SMA. **D:** Hyperplasia in this papilloma contributes to a low-power impression of a complex, hypercellular tumor.

its recognition. Secondary microlumina can develop within the hyperplastic epithelium, and micropapillary ductal hyperplasia may be present **(Fig. 4.4)**. Proliferation of glands within the papilloma results in a pattern resembling sclerosing adenosis **(Figs. 4.5-4.7)**. When glandular proliferation and ductal hyperplasia occur together, the hyperplastic ductal cells fill virtually all the space between stromal stalks, and the papilloma takes on a solid appearance **(Fig. 4.8)**.

The epithelium of the typical papilloma consists of both luminal and myoepithelial cells. The luminal cells are

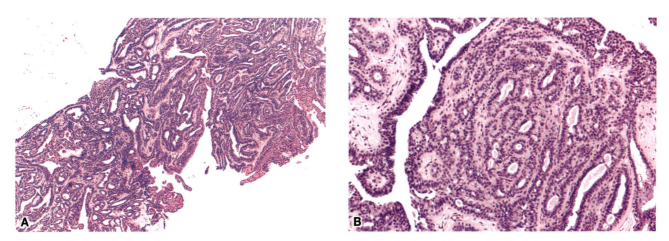

FIGURE 4.5 Papilloma With Adenosis. A, B: Hyperplasia in these needle core samples takes the form of nodular adenosis within the fibrovascular stroma. The surface epithelium is focally hyperplastic.

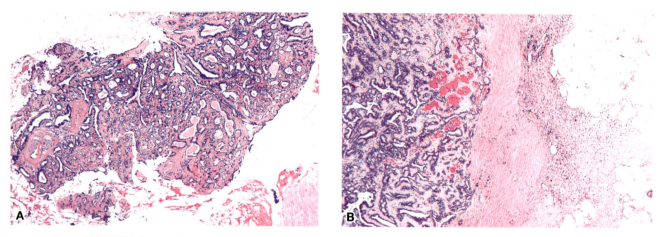

FIGURE 4.6 Papilloma With Adenosis. A: This needle core biopsy sample was obtained from a mammographically detected circumscribed papillary tumor. The mass consists almost entirely of small adenosis-type glands embedded in stroma. **B:** The excision specimen is shown. The scarring around the papilloma is attributable to the needle core biopsy.

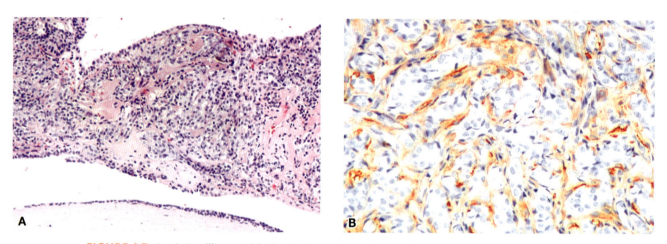

FIGURE 4.7 Cystic Papilloma With Florid Adenosis. A: This needle core biopsy sample contains a compact proliferation of adenosis in which the glands lack lumina. Part of the cyst wall is shown at the lower border. **B:** The immunostain for smooth muscle actin (SMA) highlights myoepithelial cells around the glands.

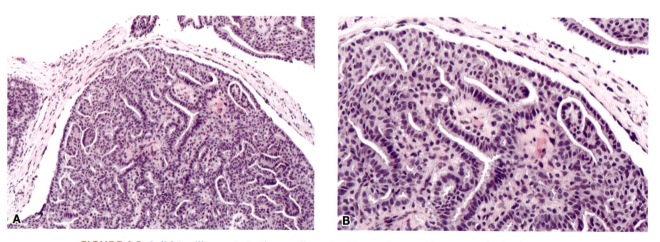

FIGURE 4.8 Solid Papilloma. A, B: The papilloma in this needle core biopsy sample displays a multinodular circumscribed architecture. Epithelial hyperplasia fills the spaces between the fibrovascular cores.

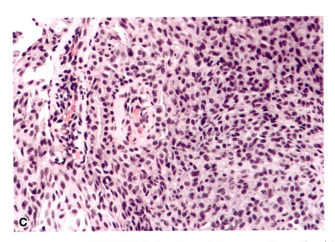
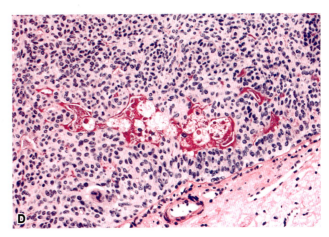

FIGURE 4.8 (*continued*) **C:** An area in another biopsy sample shows solid epithelial hyperplasia and inconspicuous fibrovascular cores. **D:** Florid epithelial hyperplasia masks the underlying papillary architecture of this solid papilloma. Histiocytes help to identify the fibrovascular stromal cores.

cuboidal to columnar, and they display minimal pleomorphism, nuclear hyperchromasia, or mitotic activity. Apocrine metaplasia occurs in many papillomas (**Fig. 4.9**), and rarely nearly all or all the epithelium is of the apocrine type (14). In most papillomas, the apocrine cells appear bland, but occasionally atypical apocrine cells can be seen with nuclear pleomorphism or cytoplasmic clearing. The presence of cytologically bland or mildly atypical apocrine epithelium almost always indicates that a papillary tumor is benign. Sebaceous metaplasia of the luminal cells of a papilloma has been reported (15).

The myoepithelial cells vary in their appearance and their distribution. Quiescent myoepithelial cells appear flattened along the basement membrane, whereas hyperplastic myoepithelial cells form a prominent layer of cuboidal cells occasionally exhibiting clear cytoplasm (**Fig. 4.10**). Some papillomas have markedly hyperplastic myoepithelial cells that assume an epithelioid appearance (**Fig. 4.11**). In this

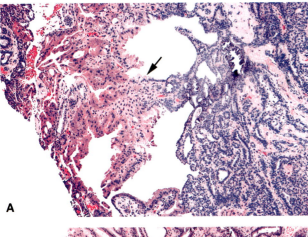
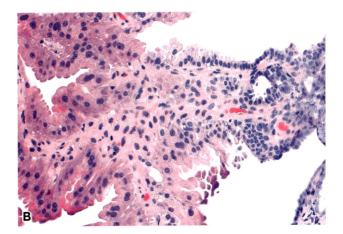
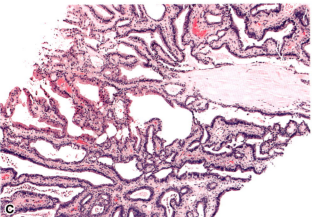

FIGURE 4.9 **Papilloma With Apocrine Metaplasia. A, B:** Metaplastic apocrine cells mingle with hyperplastic ductal cells in this needle core biopsy sample of a papilloma. The junction of the two types of epithelium is shown by the arrow in (**A**) and at higher magnification in (**B**). **C:** Another biopsied papilloma with focal apocrine metaplasia. The presence of these bland apocrine cells suggests that the tumor is benign.

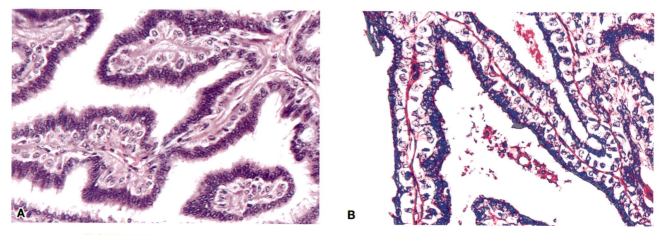

FIGURE 4.10 Papillomas With Prominent Myoepithelial Cells. A: A layer of prominent myoepithelial cells lies beneath the columnar luminal cells in this papilloma. **B:** Myoepithelial cells with clear cytoplasm outline glands in another needle core biopsy sample.

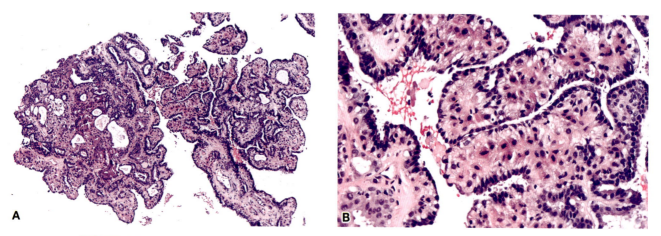

FIGURE 4.11 Papilloma With Hyperplastic Myoepithelial Cells. A, B: Clusters of myoepithelial cells with epithelioid and myoid appearances fill the subepithelial space in this needle core biopsy sample.

setting, the differential diagnosis includes adenomyoepithelioma. Myoepithelial cells are not equally apparent in all portions of a papilloma. They may become noticeably attenuated and focally undetectable even with the use of immunostains in sclerotic regions of a papilloma. The focal absence of myoepithelium does not, by itself, establish the diagnosis of carcinoma.

The appearance of the fibrovascular stroma varies considerably among papillomas. In some lesions, slender inconspicuous strands consisting of capillaries, fibroblasts, and collagen form the stromal network. The architecture and distribution of the stroma stands out clearly in sections stained for reticulin, vimentin, basement membrane proteins, or vascular markers such as CD34 and CD31. Expansion of the fibrovascular stroma by histiocytes occurs commonly in papillomas but only rarely in papillary carcinomas (see Figs. 4.3B and 4.8D).

In some papillomas, dense collagenization of the fibrovascular stroma occurs. The papillary architecture is accentuated when this process is limited to the intrinsic papillary structure. If myofibroblastic proliferation accompanies collagenization of the stroma, the papillary arrangement can become distorted **(Fig. 4.12)**. Epithelial elements entrapped in this stroma within or at the periphery of the lesion may simulate invasive carcinoma **(Fig. 4.13)**. In extreme situations, fibrous sclerosis is so severe as to virtually obliterate the papilloma, reducing it to a nodular scar containing sparse benign glandular elements. Such a lesion may be difficult to distinguish from a fibroadenoma.

Infarction, that is, ischemic necrosis, occurs in both solitary and multiple papillomas **(Fig. 4.14)**. It can occur as a result of vascular injury occurring in the course of antecedent NCB; however, in most cases, one cannot identify a specific cause for the phenomenon. The presence of chronic inflammatory cells and hemosiderin in and around many papillomas suggests that these lesions are prone to transient bleeding. Spontaneous infarction usually involves superficial portions of a papilloma. Extensively infarcted or sclerotic papillomas are occasionally mistaken for fibroepithelial lesions, or vice versa **(Fig. 4.15)**. Rarely, the entire lesion is infarcted. The underlying structure of a fully infarcted papilloma can be demonstrated with reticulin stain, cytokeratin, or p63 stains (16). There is no procedure for reliably distinguishing a completely infarcted papilloma from a papillary carcinoma;

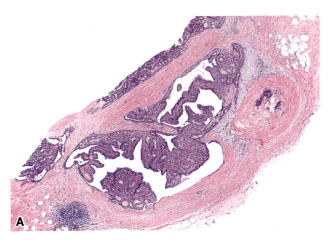 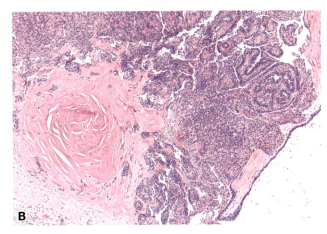

FIGURE 4.12 Papilloma With Sclerosis. A: This needle core biopsy sample of a mammographically detected circumscribed mass shows a papilloma with a dense calcifying nodule of sclerosis at the periphery. **B:** Another sclerosing papilloma, with pseudoangiomatous stromal hyperplasia (PASH)–like slits and entrapped epithelium within the sclerotic focus.

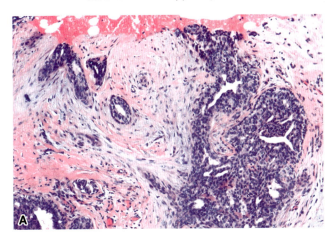 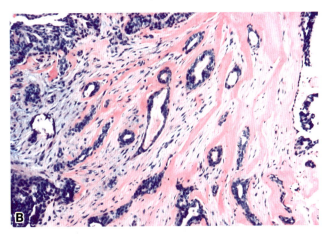

FIGURE 4.13 Papilloma With Sclerosis. A: This needle core biopsy has an area of papillary hyperplasia in sclerotic stroma. Note the epithelium cut tangentially as it protrudes into the stroma. This appearance should not be interpreted as invasive carcinoma. **B:** The cords of cells mostly appear distributed in parallel arrays between bands of collagenized stroma. The glands with angular contours resemble tubular carcinoma. Myoepithelial cells are inconspicuous.

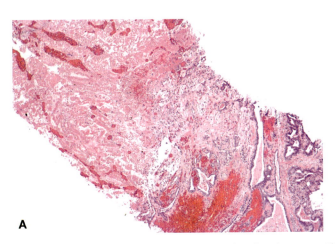 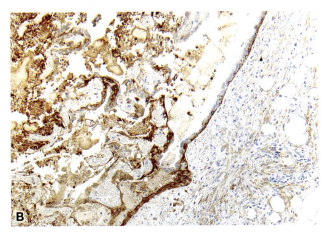

FIGURE 4.14 Papilloma With Infarction. A, B: This needle core biopsy sample was obtained from a patient with bloody nipple discharge and a mammographically detected nonpalpable mass. A needling procedure was not performed before the needle core biopsy. The ghost architecture of a papillary lesion is evident in this almost completely infarcted sample. A stain for CD10 **(B)** reveals myoepithelial cells abutting the fibrovascular stroma of the papillary tumor and along the wall of the dilated duct.

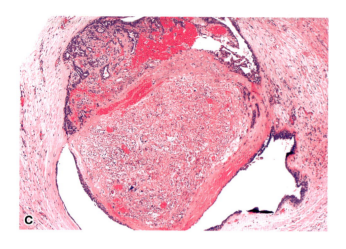

FIGURE 4.14 (*continued*) **C:** A partially infarcted papilloma with relative preservation in the top center of the field.

however, if one can demonstrate myoepithelium in the infarcted tissue, the tumor is more likely to be a papilloma than a papillary carcinoma. Cytologic atypia manifested by nuclear hyperchromasia and pleomorphism in the degenerated epithelium adjacent to infarcts can be commonly observed. These cytologic abnormalities may lead to an erroneous diagnosis of carcinoma in a fine needle aspiration (FNA) sample or an NCB specimen.

Squamous metaplasia can occur in the epithelium of a papilloma **(Fig. 4.16)** and is more likely to be found when there is infarction. In this setting, the phenomenon represents a reactive or reparative process (17). Rarely, squamous metaplasia constitutes a conspicuous component of the papilloma or of the epithelium lining the cystic portion of the lesion. Extension of squamous metaplasia to the epithelium of adjacent ducts is uncommon. Metaplastic epithelium entrapped in the stromal reaction may simulate metaplastic squamous carcinoma, and the distinction between metaplastic and neoplastic lesions can be difficult.

Like mammary epithelial cells in other lesions, those within papillomas can give rise to atypical or malignant populations. The diagnostic criteria for ductal and lobular proliferations arising in the usual settings apply when evaluating those involving a papilloma. The diagnosis of atypical ductal hyperplasia ("atypical papilloma") is appropriate for a limited focus of low-grade atypical ductal cells, <3 mm according to the WHO (4) **(Fig. 4.17)**. An expansive (>3 mm) collection of atypical ductal cells and those with marked cytologic atypia merit the diagnosis of ductal carcinoma in situ (DCIS) **(Fig. 4.18A and B)**. Chapter 11 discusses the diagnosis of ductal carcinoma involving a papilloma. The presence of atypical, dyscohesive, nonpolarized epithelial cells establishes the diagnosis of atypical lobular hyperplasia (ALH) or lobular carcinoma in situ **(Fig. 4.18C and D)**, which can be confirmed by E-cadherin.

Immunohistochemistry

Immunohistochemical staining of papillomas reveals the presence of epithelial, myoepithelial, and stromal cells therein. The epithelial cells exhibit scattered reactivity for estrogen receptor (ER), whereas it is typically diffuse in papillary carcinoma. Stains for actin, calponin, smooth muscle myosin heavy chain, CD10, and CK5/6 highlight

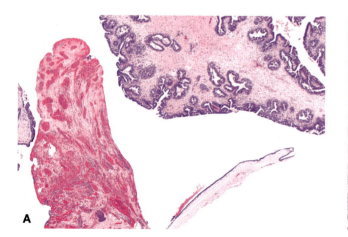 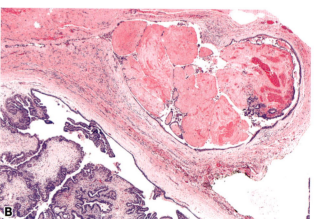

FIGURE 4.15 **Fibroepithelial Lesion Simulating Papilloma. A:** This infarcted lesion with branching epithelial and stromal elements was interpreted as papilloma on needle core biopsy. **B:** In the excision of the lesion in **A**, the preserved lesion in the adjacent tissue resolves the diagnosis as a partially infarcted phyllodes tumor.

BENIGN PAPILLARY TUMORS 49

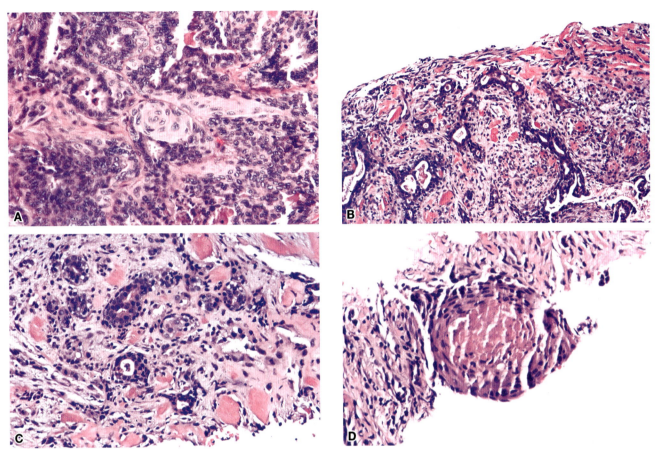

FIGURE 4.16 Papilloma With Squamous Metaplasia. A: A nest of squamous cells is present among the hyperplastic cells of the papillary glandular epithelium. **B-D:** This needle core biopsy sample from a sclerosing papilloma has focal squamous metaplasia **(D)**. The biopsy was misinterpreted as infiltrating carcinoma with squamous differentiation.

myoepithelial cells in most circumstances, but the staining reactions differ somewhat depending on the antibody. Because these cytoplasmic proteins also occur in stromal and vascular cells to varying degrees, one could have difficulty distinguishing such cells from myoepithelial cells. To minimize this problem, it is advisable to include a nuclear stain, p63 or p40, among those chosen to detect myoepithelial cells. One must remember that the p63 and p40 immunostains can stain the nuclei in neoplastic cells in some papillary carcinomas (17) and the nuclei of squamous cells.

Several panels of immunostains to aid in the distinction of papillomas from papillary carcinomas have been proposed.

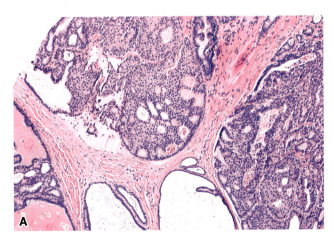
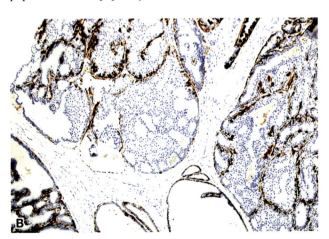

FIGURE 4.17 Papillomas With Atypical Ductal Hyperplasia. A, B: The papillary fronds of this tumor are partially populated by a low-grade cribriform proliferation. Residual benign epithelium is seen on the right. CK 5/6 **(B)** highlights the myoepithelium of the underlying papilloma and shows absence of expression in the cribriform area, supporting the atypical nature.

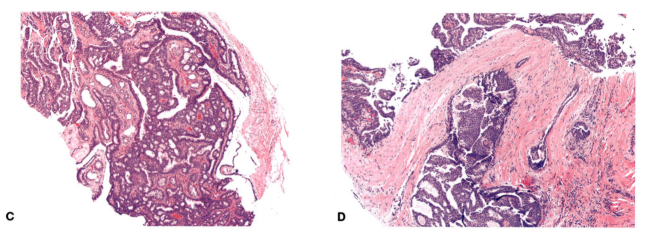

FIGURE 4.17 (*continued*) **C:** Papillary fronds fuse and form complex cribriform structures in this biopsied focus. Discontinuous and limited involvement make atypical ductal hyperplasia (ADH) the most appropriate diagnosis. **D:** Needle core biopsy of a papilloma with a focus of solid and cribriform ADH.

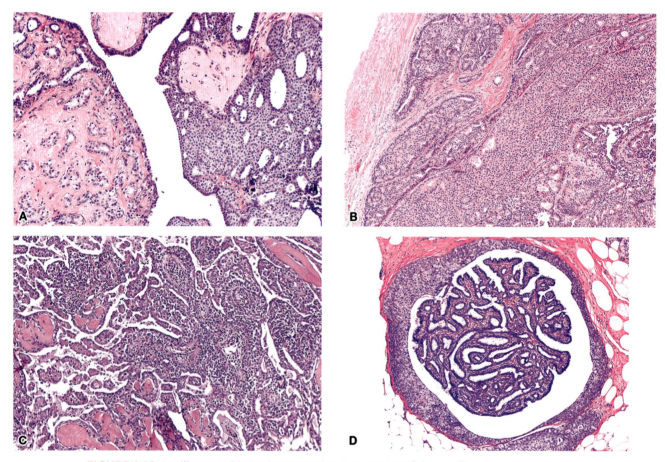

FIGURE 4.18 Papillomas With Carcinoma In Situ. A: A portion of the papilloma remains in the left of the field. Ductal carcinoma in situ covers fronds in the right of the field. **B:** Solid pattern ductal carcinoma in situ distends the space between fibrovascular cores. **C:** Neoplastic lobular cells mingle with the preexisting normal and hyperplastic ductal cells of this papilloma. **D:** Lobular carcinoma in situ rings this intraductal papilloma.

These panels are summarized in Chapter 11. When using staining for CK5/6 to identify a neoplastic population in the setting of a papillary tumor, one must remember that conventional apocrine cells do not express this cytokeratin. The lack of CK5/6 staining can lead observers to misclassify benign apocrine cells as neoplastic ductal cells (14,18).

Correlation Between Findings in Needle Core and Excision Specimens

The correlation between the findings in NCB and excisions of papillary tumors has been the subject of extensive investigation (19-21). A meta-analysis (22) using 34 studies published between 1999 and 2012 revealed that 36.9% of papillomas with atypia demonstrated carcinoma (most commonly DCIS) in an excision specimen, whereas only 7.0% of papillomas lacking atypical cells did. Series that included only radiology-pathology concordant cases have reported lower upgrade rates between 0% and 6.6% (23-25). Moreover, many carcinomas in the excisions were spatially apart from the biopsied papillomas and were likely coincidental (23,26).

Researchers have attempted to improve the predictive values of the findings in NCB by incorporating ancillary clinical, radiologic, or histologic features in their analyses. Some reports have identified findings such as older age, larger size, and peripheral location of the lesion, which seem to indicate an increased risk of atypical cells in subsequent excisions. However, other investigations have not borne out the predictive value of such findings. In the meta-analysis by Wen and Cheng (22), the presence of two findings, a palpable mass and suspicious mammographic features, indicated a heightened risk for carcinoma in subsequent excision.

Pathologists have searched for ways to improve their diagnostic abilities, and the use of immunostains and expertise of pathologists have come under study. Shah et al (27) reported that the use of immunostaining for calponin, CK5/6, and p63 allowed the recognition of atypical ductal hyperplasia (ADH) associated with papillomas. This technique improved the accuracy of all four participating pathologists to the point that the authors concluded that papillomas lacking atypia "do not require excision in the absence of suspicious clinical/radiological findings." Using a mixture of antibodies to CK5, p63, and CK8/18 to stain NCBs and comparing the diagnoses with those rendered on corresponding excision specimens, Reisenbichler et al (18) correctly identified all 19 papillary carcinomas in their study group of 58 papillary tumors. Grin et al (28) employed staining for CK5 and ER to identify the presence of atypical cells in NCBs of papillary tumors. This approach allowed the authors to classify NCBs of 15 of 15 papillomas and 14 of 15 papillary tumors containing atypical or malignant cells correctly when compared with the findings on excisions. Tse et al (29) stained for ER, CK14, and p63 to resolve discrepancies encountered in 15 NCBs. Although the use of these stains reduced the rate of discordance by 69%, the staining results did not completely eliminate either false-positive or false-negative cases.

Prognosis

Papillomas do not recur when completely excised. The development of subsequent papillomas is thought to represent the formation of de novo tumors.

Follow-up studies of patients with excised papillomas show that their presence indicates a slightly increased risk for the development of breast carcinoma. Moon et al (30) found that 4.3% of women with papillomas lacking atypia developed breast carcinoma. The relative risk (compared with women lacking suspicious findings on ultrasonography) was 4.8. When stratified by age, the relative risk for women >40 years was 5.1, whereas in women <40 years the presence of a papilloma without atypia did not increase the risk for breast carcinoma. The carcinomas arose in both breasts with equal frequency. MacGrogan and Tavassoli (31) studied the follow-up of 119 patients who underwent excisions of papillomas. Approximately 5% of women with benign papillomas or papillomas with "focal atypia" developed breast carcinoma at intervals between 3 and 14 years. Approximately 10% of women whose papillomas showed significant atypia developed breast carcinoma during the same span. The authors noted that the atypical cells in most cases were confined to the papilloma and that the excision seemed to have removed the entire lesional population. Cuneo et al (32) demonstrated similar outcomes: the 5-year risk for the development of noninvasive or invasive carcinoma in either breast was 4.6% for patients with a papilloma without atypia and 13% for patients with a papilloma with atypia.

It is important to note that in the foregoing studies, the carcinomas arose in the breasts contralateral to the ones harboring the papillomas as frequently as they did in the ipsilateral breasts. These findings would seem to indicate that the presence of a solitary papilloma poses a low risk for the development of an ipsilateral carcinoma and that papillomas do not often give rise to carcinomas. The presence of a solitary papilloma may foretell a slightly heightened propensity for the entirety of the mammary tissue to develop neoplastic proliferations, but the papilloma itself does not represent a clinically significant premalignant lesion.

A greater risk for concurrent (33) or subsequent carcinoma has been demonstrated in women with multiple papillomas compared with women with solitary papillomas (1), and women with multiple papillomas are at greater risk of developing carcinoma in the contralateral breast (33). Lewis et al (1) examined the follow-up of patients with solitary and multiple papillomas treated at the Mayo Clinic and determined the risk for developing breast carcinoma by comparison with an age- and calendar-period–matched cohort from the Surveillance, Epidemiology and End Results (SEER) database. The authors reported standardized incidence rates for breast carcinoma for women with solitary or multiple papillomas without atypia of 2.04 and 3.01, respectively. For women with solitary or multiple papillomas with atypia, the corresponding values were 5.11 and 7.01, respectively. In the study by Moon et al (30), the relative risks posed by central and peripheral papillomas (4.8 and 5.2, respectively) did not differ across the entire cohort, but they did differ in younger women. In women <40 years of age, the presence of a peripheral papilloma indicated a relative risk for developing breast carcinoma of 13.2 compared with a relative risk of 2.1 associated with a central papilloma. The corresponding relative risks for women >40 years of age are 4.0 and 5.8.

Treatment

Based on data from the foregoing studies, surveillance can substitute for excision for many patients with benign papilloma on NCB. The American Society of Breast Surgeons (34) does not recommend routine excision of papillomas without atypia and advises that those not excised should be followed by imaging. The decision to excise should be "individualized based on risk, including such criteria as size; symptomatology, including palpability and presence of nipple discharge; and breast cancer risk factors." It has also been suggested that vacuum-assisted NCB provides sufficient sampling of a lesion or even complete excision, such that surgical excision may not be necessary (35-40).

Many published reports include follow-up data of patients who underwent radiologic follow-up in lieu of surgery following the diagnosis of benign papilloma on NCB. Most studies involved relatively small numbers of patients, but in several recent ones (20,38,39,41-43) the study groups contain 50 or more patients. Among this aggregate of more than 1,000 women, approximately 2% developed carcinoma. Follow-up periods ranged from 2 to 5 years, and the nature of the follow-up varied. In Corbin et al's study (41), of 238 nonexcised papillomas followed for a mean of 60 months, there were no subsequent breast carcinomas diagnosed at the sites of the antecedent papilloma.

Among women recommended for follow-up without initial excision, some will require subsequent excision. In a series studied by Sexton et al (44), 59 of 78 (75%) patients with a papilloma diagnosed by NCB did not undergo excision and were followed for 3 to 5 years. Subsequent interval mammographic changes necessitated surgical excision in 10 of the 59 (17%), and 2 (3%) had a subsequent NCB. All subsequent cores and excisions were reportedly "benign." This study suggests that up to 20% of patients enrolled in follow-up after NCB diagnosis of papilloma will undergo another procedure within 5 years of the initial NCB.

RADIAL SCLEROSING LESION

Radial sclerosing lesions (RSLs) are proliferative abnormalities that have a stellate configuration radiologically and histologically. Clinical interest in RSLs derives from the realization that these abnormalities may be difficult to distinguish from invasive carcinoma by mammography and the concern that they are precursors to the development of carcinoma.

RSLs have been referred to by a variety of names introduced since the 1970s. Sclerosing papillary proliferation, complex sclerosing lesion, nonencapsulated sclerosing lesion, infiltrating epitheliosis, and indurative mastopathy represent just a few of the terms. *Radial scar*, a widely used designation for this lesion, is a translation of "strahlige Narben," the term Hamperl (45) introduced in 1975. This term refers to the stellate shape of the typical example; it is short and avoids terminology that suggests an association with a specific proliferative ductal lesion. However, inclusion of the word "scar" in the diagnosis implies that the changes represent a reparative process. Although the stellate configuration has a cicatrix-like appearance, it is possible that the stromal change is an integral part of the proliferative lesion rather than a reparative process. The term used here, *radial sclerosing lesion*, is preferable because it describes the mammographic and histologic appearance of the process without implying a histogenesis; furthermore, this designation is sufficiently generic to encompass the many histologic variants included in this category. The term *complex sclerosing lesion* is used to refer to an RSL over 1 cm in extent. RSLs are discussed in this chapter devoted to benign papillary tumors because many include a papillary component.

Clinical Features

Most RSLs are microscopic lesions not detectable by palpation or mammography. They are usually discovered during examination of specimens resected for unrelated indications. Consequently, the distribution of the ages of women with RSLs parallels that of women undergoing breast surgery. RSLs are uncommon before the age of 30 and most frequent between the ages of 40 and 60. The reported frequency of incidental lesions varies by study and diagnostic criteria. RSLs have been detected in 0.8% of image-guided NCBs (46), in 1.7% (47) to 7.1% (48) of benign breast excisions, and in 4% (49) to 26% (50) of mastectomies from patients with carcinomas. These data suggest that RSLs occur in women without carcinoma as frequently as in women with carcinomas. Multiple microscopic RSLs are not uncommon, and both breasts can be affected. Anderson and Battersby (51) described a woman with 80 RSLs in her right breast and 46 in her left breast. RSLs almost never affect men. One report (52) mentions in passing the presence of an RSL in the breast of a man with breast carcinoma.

Imaging Studies

Most RSLs are smaller than 2 cm when detected radiologically. Typical lesions are characterized by a lucent or dense center, radiating slender strands of tissue, and changes in appearance in different imaging projections. Calcifications are detected in some RSLs. When evident using sonography, RSLs form an irregular hypoechoic mass with ill-defined borders and diminished posterior acoustic transmission. Tomosynthesis may offer a more sensitive technique for the detection of RSLs (53). Certain radiologic features favor the diagnosis of an RSL over a stellate carcinoma, but these are not sufficiently distinctive to render specific diagnosis. MRI findings may help to differentiate RSLs from invasive carcinomas (54).

Histologic Evaluation

Andersen et al (55) described the histologic appearance of the RSL as "a distinct histologic structure, characterized by a sclerotic center with a central core containing obliterated duct(s), elastin deposits, and mostly infiltrating tubules and the center is surrounded by a corona of contracted ducts and lobules, which may show different types of proliferative lesions." Dense collagen, elastic tissue, and sparse stromal cells make up the *nidus* of the well-established "scar" **(Fig. 4.19)**. The elastic tissue, which one can highlight with an elastin stain, consists of dense, sometimes granular, weakly eosinophilic material in the walls of ducts and the stroma. The fibroelastotic stroma typically entraps distorted glands. A *corona* of ducts, terminal duct lobular units, and cysts arrayed in a radial orientation around the nidus is created by incorporation of these structures. The glandular tissue displays varying degrees of *proliferation,* including usual ductal hyperplasia, sclerosing adenosis, and cyst formation, and minute papillomas are frequently present **(Fig. 4.20)**. The peripheral zone can also include nonproliferative ducts and lobules, and cysts occasionally make up most or all of the corona. The proliferative zone sometimes appears asymmetric because of off-center planes of sectioning or intrinsic differences among lesions **(Fig. 4.21)**.

The epithelium within an RSL can exhibit a range of changes. Apocrine metaplasia frequently occurs in the cysts of RSLs, and occasionally it may be present in the proliferative component, especially in areas of sclerosing adenosis. Clear cell change and nuclear atypia are common in apocrine epithelium. Squamous metaplasia occurs infrequently in RSLs. Examples with squamous metaplasia may resemble low-grade adenosquamous carcinoma.

The fibrous reaction associated with RSLs typically entraps ductules. Similar to nests of epithelium trapped in the stroma at the peripheries of sclerosing papillomas, those in an RSL may simulate invasive carcinoma. This is an important consideration when examining NCB. The presence of a myoepithelial cell layer characterizes epithelial entrapment within an RSL. Ductules in the center of an RSL may appear to lack myoepithelial cells on routine hematoxylin and eosin (H&E) stain; consequently, this finding does not establish the diagnosis of invasive carcinoma. Less than 5% of RSLs demonstrate entrapment of small nerves (56).

Sections of an RSL in a relatively early phase of development reveal branching and budding ductal structures in

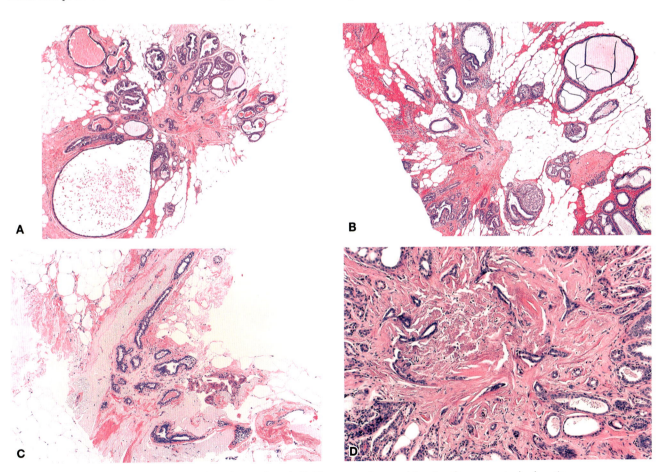

FIGURE 4.19 Radial Sclerosing Lesion. A, B: These needle core biopsies show a central sclerotic zone surrounded by radiating ducts with varying degrees of epithelial proliferation. The lesions are nearly entirely removed in the cores. **C:** Elastosis is prominent in this core needle sample of a radial sclerosing lesion. **D:** The small glands trapped in the nidus of this lesion resemble those of a tubular carcinoma.

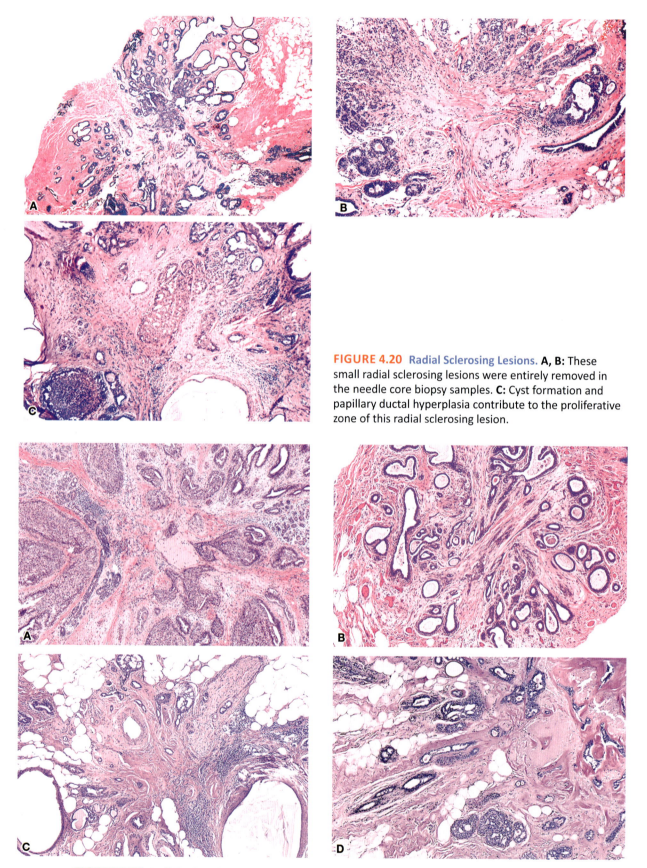

FIGURE 4.20 **Radial Sclerosing Lesions. A, B:** These small radial sclerosing lesions were entirely removed in the needle core biopsy samples. **C:** Cyst formation and papillary ductal hyperplasia contribute to the proliferative zone of this radial sclerosing lesion.

FIGURE 4.21 **Radial Sclerosing Lesions. A:** Florid ductal hyperplasia distends several ducts in the corona of this radial sclerosing lesion (RSL). **B:** Another RSL features adenosis with microcystic dilation of glands in the corona. **C:** The corona of a third RSL contains apocrine cysts and an entrapped nerve (upper right). **D:** In this RSL, the elastotic center is in the upper right corner. Mild ductal hyperplasia is present at the periphery.

the core. The ductal epithelial proliferation can appear especially florid and display necrosis. The stroma appears cellular, and the extracellular matrix appears myxoid rather than collagenous. Many of the stromal cells are myofibroblasts, surrounding the ductal structures and extending in radiating bands toward the periphery. Lymphocytes and plasma cells often sit at the junction of fat and fibrous tissue.

RSLs usually occur as isolated, separate lesions, but occasionally, contiguous foci may become confluent to form a larger complex and palpable mass in a fashion analogous to the formation of adenosis tumor.

Ductal Hyperplasia and Carcinoma in Radial Sclerosing Lesions

Ductal proliferations in RSLs can take the form of florid and atypical hyperplasia as well as DCIS. Duct hyperplasia in an RSL may be solid, cribriform, micropapillary, or a combination thereof **(Fig. 4.22)**. Focal necrosis occurs in the hyperplastic duct epithelium in about 10% of RSLs. The epithelial cells within these comedo-like foci are usually indistinguishable from those in hyperplastic foci lacking necrosis in the same RSL. Foci of ADH or atypical lobular hyperplasia (ALH) have been observed in 21% (57) to 51% (58) of RSLs. Often, the atypical foci are distributed in multiple tissue fragments in NCB. This disruption of the architecture of the lesion makes it difficult to determine the distribution and characteristics of the atypical population, and caution is warranted when considering a diagnosis of DCIS or invasive carcinoma in this setting **(Fig. 4.23)**.

The association of carcinomas, including tubular carcinomas, with RSLs has been well documented (59), but the literature does not provide a coherent estimate of its frequency. Values as high as 32% have been reported (57), and in one series 28% of mammographically detected RSLs >1 cm had foci of carcinoma (60). Mammographically occult RSLs, on the other hand, rarely contain carcinoma (61). One finds carcinoma most frequently in RSLs larger than 0.6 cm (62) and in women older than 50 years (62,63). Both ductal and lobular carcinomas **(Fig. 4.24)** occur in RSLs, and the frequency of noninvasive carcinomas exceeds that of invasive carcinomas (56,57,62,63). The carcinomas usually involve only a minor proportion of the RSL, sometimes as little as 5%, and they more frequently occupy the periphery rather than the center of the lesion (56,62,63). Typical ductal and lobular carcinomas account for most malignancies seen in RSLs, but low-grade adenosquamous carcinoma and metaplastic carcinoma sometimes develop in the setting of an RSL (64,65).

Immunohistochemistry

Myoepithelial cells can be demonstrated around the perimeter of most hyperplastic ducts in RSLs by immunostaining for p63, CD10, smooth muscle myosin heavy chain, or actin; however, in the central part of the lesion, myoepithelium may be substantially attenuated and even undetectable. The epithelial cells within RSLs display the staining characteristics seen in mammary epithelial cells in other locations. Stains for CK5/6, ER, and E-cadherin will usually allow one to classify epithelial proliferations involving RSLs.

Differential Diagnosis

NCB is usually sufficient to establish the diagnosis of RSL, but the distorted small glands or foci of sclerosing adenosis trapped in the stroma of an RSL can be misinterpreted. The major consideration in the differential diagnosis is tubular carcinoma. The glands in tubular carcinoma have round or distinctive angular shapes not ordinarily found in RSLs, and myoepithelium is absent. Since benign glands entrapped within the nidus of an RSL sometimes lack myoepithelial cells, one cannot rely solely on the absence of myoepithelium to distinguish an RSL from an invasive carcinoma. Permeation of the lesional glands beyond the confines of the nidus and into fat and the presence of cytologic atypia are evidence of malignancy. The overtly cystic and apocrine components of RSLs are absent from tubular carcinomas.

Correlation With Excision Specimens

Many studies have compared the pathologic findings of RSLs in NCB specimens with those in subsequent excisions, and several recent publications have compiled the results (66-68). Although these investigations vary in details, three conclusions seem appropriate. First, approximately 4% of excisions from women with RSLs lacking atypia on NCB contain either DCIS or invasive carcinoma. Second, approximately 20% of these excisions contain atypia (ADH, ALH, lobular carcinoma in situ [LCIS], and other rare types of epithelial atypia) in the absence of DCIS and invasive carcinoma. Third, approximately 20% of excisions from women whose RSLs display atypia on NCB contain either DCIS or invasive carcinoma. Rakha et al (69) published the largest study centering on RSLs harboring atypia detected in NCB. Excisions from 157 such cases disclosed carcinoma in 39 cases (24.8%). In this study, the upgrade rate for RSL with ADH was 35%; those of RSL with lobular neoplasia or apocrine atypia were 12% and 8%, respectively; and that for RSL with flat epithelial atypia (FEA) was 0%. These generalizations mirror the findings of literature reviews reported by Bianchi et al (70) and Conlon et al (71), and a meta-analysis by Farshid and Buckley (68).

It seems that most upgrades occur because of incomplete sampling of the radiologic target or the presence of unrelated lesions. A study by Douglas-Jones et al (72) included six cases in which NCB revealed RSL but failed to detect coexisting carcinomas. In each case, the needle track left by the NCB missed the carcinoma, usually by several millimeters. The use of the vacuum-assisted technique for NCB sampling, the practice of obtaining multiple samples (58,73), and correlation of radiologic and pathologic findings help to minimize the problem of unrepresentative sampling.

RSLs can occur as incidental, microscopic lesions seemingly entirely removed on NCB or in specimens sampled for unrelated indications. Data from multiple studies suggest that

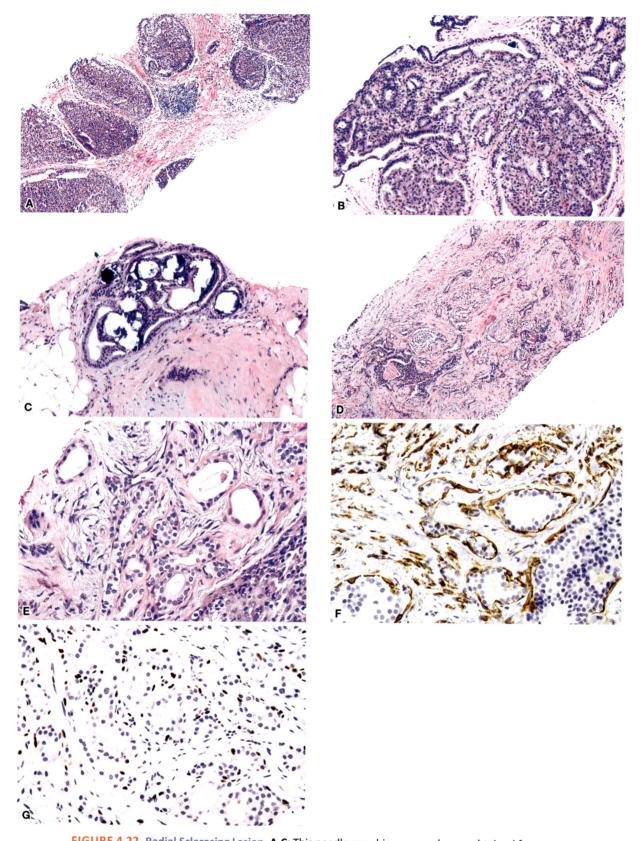

FIGURE 4.22 **Radial Sclerosing Lesion. A-C:** This needle core biopsy sample was obtained from a patient with a nonpalpable, mammographically detected stellate lesion containing calcifications. Florid ductal hyperplasia is shown in **(A, B)**. Calcifications are present in a hyperplastic duct next to a sclerotic stromal nodule in **(C)**. **D-G:** This needle core biopsy sample, mistakenly interpreted as invasive ductal carcinoma, was obtained from a radial sclerosing lesion with duct hyperplasia and adenosis. The adenosis architecture simulates the appearance of invasive ductal carcinoma **(D, E)**. Myoepithelial cells highlighted by myosin **(F)** and p63 **(G)** immunostains surround the benign glands.

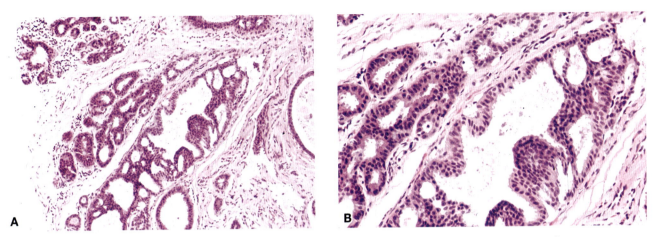

FIGURE 4.23 Radial Sclerosing Lesion With Atypical Duct Hyperplasia. **A, B:** A focus of atypical micropapillary hyperplasia in the periphery of a radial sclerosing lesion is seen in this needle core biopsy. Note the radiating arrangement of the glands and the microcyst at the right border in **(A)**. These findings suggest the presence of an underlying radial sclerosing lesion. An excision showed only reactive changes at the biopsy site.

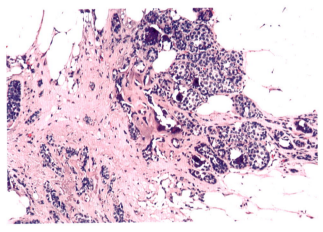

FIGURE 4.24 Radial Sclerosing Lesion With Carcinoma In Situ. A mammographically detected stellate mass with calcifications led to a needle core biopsy. Lobular carcinoma in situ fills glands with an adenosis pattern in sclerotic tissue in the right portion of the image.

RSLs discovered in these situations do not require excision. In one study (74) of 18 patients with microscopic RSLs without atypia mostly detected using a vacuum-assisted method, the subsequent excisions did not disclose carcinoma in any; however, the excisions did contain ADH in 6 patients (33%) and atypical apocrine adenosis in another 6%. The study of Conlon et al (71) included 18 RSLs not believed to represent the abnormalities targeted by imaging. The investigators identified epithelial atypia in 4 (22%) of the NCB. The excisions did not disclose carcinoma in any of the 18 cases, nor did any of the patients develop carcinoma at the sites of RSLs.

Treatment

Citing the infrequent detection of carcinomas in excisions subsequent to a diagnosis of RSL lacking atypia, several investigators suggest that radiologic follow-up can replace excision provided that the radiologic target is adequately sampled, pathologic findings correlate with imaging findings, and other clinical features do not indicate the advisability of an excision (71,75-77). Thus, incidental RSLs and those seemingly entirely removed via NCB may not need excision. Some authors recommend that at least 12 needle core samples be obtained (58,73). Several publications (46,53,71,73,75-79) report follow-up data of 425 such patients followed for mean periods of 26 months (46) to 84 months (71). Six women (1.5%) developed carcinoma (two invasive ductal carcinoma [IDC], four DCIS), but five of them were located apart from the RSL site and therefore considered incidental (71,75,76,78). Radiologists have used the vacuum-assisted technique to completely remove RSLs without atypia (80,81). This approach may prove a satisfactory alternative to surgical excision, but extended clinical follow-up and study of a large number of patients are required before reaching this conclusion.

Based on available data, excision would be prudent for RSLs displaying epithelial atypia. If the RSL does not have an atypical component and there are no coexisting atypical proliferative lesions, the decision whether to excise or follow up should be made on a case-by-case basis. Factors to consider include prior biopsy findings, other risk factors such as family history, ease of clinical or radiologic follow-up, and extent of removal of the targeted lesion via the NCB.

Prognosis

The preneoplastic nature of RSLs has been a source of controversy. For example, RSLs are no more common in the breasts of women with carcinoma than in those of women without carcinoma, and the morphologic features of RSLs are the same whether or not they are associated with carcinoma (51).

Some investigators have suggested that the presence of an RSL indicates a generalized heightened risk for the development of breast carcinoma, but the data relating to this notion are conflicting. One prospective investigation of 1,396 women with "radial scars" in excision specimens followed for a median of 12 years discovered a relative risk of 1.8 for subsequent carcinoma for women with a "radial scar" compared with those not having a "radial scar" (48). The carcinomas arose in both breasts with equal frequency; thus, the authors concluded that "scars" constitute indicators of an increased risk for breast carcinoma rather than direct precursors to carcinomas in most cases. An update of this study reaffirmed these findings (82). Several other studies (47,52,83-85), including one (83) involving 439 women followed up for a mean interval of 17 years, did not detect an increased risk for carcinoma for women with RSLs, nor did a meta-analysis (86) conducted using eligible studies published since 2000. RSLs frequently coexist with proliferative breast disease, including atypical hyperplasia. The presence of ADH increases the risk for carcinoma, but the presence of a coexisting RSL does not seem to confer any additional risk (82,83,85,86). Data regarding the risk posed by RSL in the setting of proliferative disease without atypia are conflicting. Two studies (82,86) suggest that the presence of an RSL indicates a heightened risk in this circumstance, whereas two others do not (83,85).

SUBAREOLAR SCLEROSING DUCTAL HYPERPLASIA

Subareolar sclerosing duct hyperplasia (SSDH) is a form of RSL that occurs beneath the nipple (87). The lesion forms a tumor of the central or subareolar breast parenchyma without involving the nipple parenchyma. The latter feature, among others, distinguishes SSDH from florid papillomatosis of the nipple (or "nipple adenoma").

Clinical Features

The age at diagnosis ranges from 26 to 73 years, averaging about 50 years. The left and right breasts are equally affected. The literature does not contain reports of bilateral SSDH.

The presenting symptom is a breast mass beneath the nipple or the areola, or both, or close to the areola. None of the lesions has been within the nipple. Erosion or ulceration of the nipple is absent. Nipple retraction or bloody nipple discharge may occur. The mammographic findings are nonspecific and may suggest carcinoma.

Histologic Evaluation

The histologic structure of SSDH is similar to that of RSLs in other parts of the breast. Sclerosis and elastosis are more marked toward the center of the tumor, whereas ductal hyperplasia is most prominent at the periphery **(Fig. 4.25)**. Cartilaginous metaplasia, a rare occurrence in these lesions, typically occurs in the sclerotic center. In some cases, hyperplastic ducts are seen at the edge, resulting in irregular borders. More often, much of the tumor has a rounded border created by the nodular expansion of confluent large ducts. Scattered mitotic figures may be encountered in the florid hyperplastic epithelium or in hyperplastic myoepithelial cells, which are found throughout much of the lesion. Rarely, focal necrosis is found in the hyperplastic epithelium. In contrast to RSLs that occur elsewhere in the breast, SSDH generally lacks cysts, cystic and papillary apocrine change, and squamous metaplasia. Carcinoma rarely arises in SSDH.

Treatment and Prognosis

The tumors should be treated by excision, which can usually be performed through a circumareolar incision and spares the nipple. Recurrences following complete excision have not developed during follow-up periods as long as 15.75 years (88). However, DCIS (two cases), ADH (two cases), and ALH (one case) subsequently developed in the ipsilateral breasts of 35 women in one study. One woman developed DCIS in the contralateral breast (88). Total mastectomy has been performed when DCIS was present in SSDH or when the lesion was mistakenly diagnosed as carcinoma.

CYSTIC APOCRINE METAPLASIA

The breasts develop from anlage that give rise to apocrine glands, but apocrine cells do not constitute a component of the "normal" mammary gland. Any benign proliferative

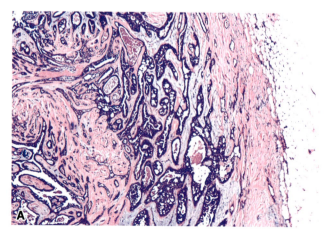
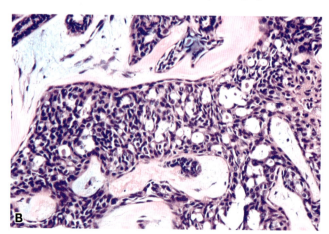

FIGURE 4.25 **Subareolar Sclerosing Duct Hyperplasia.** **A:** The border of the lesion is well circumscribed. **B:** Florid duct hyperplasia with a fenestrated pattern is evident.

lesion, including sclerosing adenosis, complex fibroadenomas, papillomas, RSLs, and gynecomastia (to name just a few), may contain apocrine cells. In their most banal form, metaplastic apocrine cells are similar to the cells that comprise cutaneous apocrine glands. Apocrine cells possess abundant, pink, finely granular cytoplasm, which forms apical tufts or blebs at the luminal surface. Round, regular nuclei containing small- to medium-size nucleoli are situated near the bases of the cells.

Parenthetically, the term "molecular apocrine" refers to the subset of triple-negative carcinomas that have a high rate of androgen receptor (AR) signaling based on gene expression analysis (see Chapter 15), unrelated to the benign histologic finding described in this section.

Clinical Features

There are no clinical features attributable to cystic apocrine metaplasia. Apocrine metaplasia is a common finding in the epithelial lining of cysts in gross cystic disease. Haagensen et al (89) reported finding apocrine metaplasia in 78% of 1,169 biopsies performed for gross cystic disease. The lesion was detected in 39% of 155 of MR-guided biopsies of women aged 30 to 76 years (90). One group of investigators reported that apocrine cysts were significantly more numerous in the lower quadrants of the breasts than in the upper quadrants (91).

Microscopic foci of apocrine metaplasia are common in the female breast after 25 years of age (92). The frequency of apocrine change plateaus in the fifth decade, possibly reflecting physiologic alterations associated with menopause. Apocrine cysts and apocrine hyperplasia are more common in the breasts of American women in New York than in Japanese women in Tokyo (93).

Histologic Evaluation

Cystic apocrine metaplasia consists of flat and cuboidal cells, which form either a single layer or isolated blunt papillae **(Fig. 4.26)**. The cells are usually evenly spaced and contain round nuclei with homogeneous, moderately dense chromatin. The nuclei typically have a single, central nucleolus of modest size. Metaplastic apocrine epithelium in cysts is prone to regressive changes that may lead to complete disappearance of these cells. This phenomenon is marked by conversion of columnar and cuboidal apocrine epithelium to a layer of flattened cells. The latter may ultimately be shed into the cyst, leaving only a fibrous shell. Mitotic figures are almost never seen in ordinary apocrine metaplasia.

A myoepithelial cell layer is usually apparent beneath the apocrine luminal cells; however, the myoepithelial cells may be inconspicuous, and large gaps between them may be observed. Rarely, the myoepithelium may be focally absent in otherwise ordinary, benign apocrine cysts (94). A network of congested capillaries typically underlies the basement membrane in foci of apocrine metaplasia.

Proliferation of apocrine cells can produce elaborate patterns of hyperplasia with either micropapillary or papillary architectures. In regions of proliferation, cellular crowding first gives rise to stratification of the apocrine epithelial cells. Exuberant growth can create a nodule composed of confluent glands lined by proliferative apocrine epithelium **(Fig. 4.27)**. The apocrine cells have cuboidal to tall columnar shapes, and tufts or snouts of epithelium protrude from the apical surfaces of the cells into the glandular lumen. The cytoplasm typically is finely granular and uniformly stained, but in rare instances coarse granules are conspicuous.

Micropapillary and papillary apocrine change most frequently occurs alongside other proliferative fibrocystic changes. The apocrine epithelium is usually arranged in a micropapillary pattern composed of regularly spaced, cytologically benign cells. Fibrovascular stroma appears scant or is entirely absent from these fronds. Foci of papillary apocrine metaplasia sometimes coexist with columnar cell lesions (95).

Calcifications associated with cystic and papillary apocrine metaplasia may be coarse, basophilic, easily fractured particles of calcium hydroxyapatite (phosphate) or birefringent crystals of calcium oxalate **(Fig. 4.28)**.

Atypical changes can be encountered in apocrine metaplasia in virtually any proliferative configuration (96).

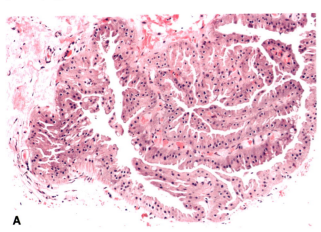
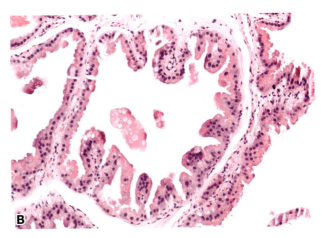

FIGURE 4.26 Cystic Apocrine Metaplasia. A, B: Note the evenly spaced, basally oriented nuclei and blunt papillae.

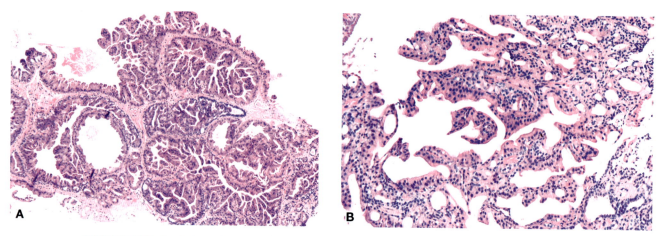

FIGURE 4.27 Cystic Apocrine Metaplasia. A, B: Apocrine metaplasia is present throughout this complex cystic and papillary lesion. The hyperplastic epithelium has micropapillae and cribriform areas. Complex branching papillary fronds and cysts with hyperplastic apocrine epithelium are shown in this needle core biopsy sample.

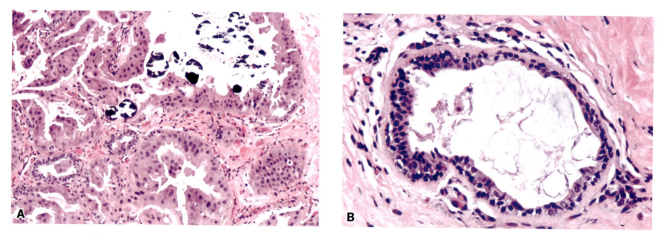

FIGURE 4.28 Cystic Apocrine Metaplasia With Calcifications. A: Round basophilic calcifications can be seen in a lesion composed of papillary apocrine epithelium. **B:** Plate-like, transparent calcium oxalate crystals occupy the lumen of a small apocrine cyst.

Architectural atypia consists of irregular fronds with little or no stromal support in which the apocrine cells are distributed in a rigid manner **(Fig. 4.29)**. Epithelial bridges and cribriform areas may be present.

Apocrine cells with mild cytologic atypia retain abundant granular eosinophilic cytoplasm and exhibit characteristic decapitation secretion. Minute cytoplasmic vacuoles may be found, especially in the suprabasal region of the cell.

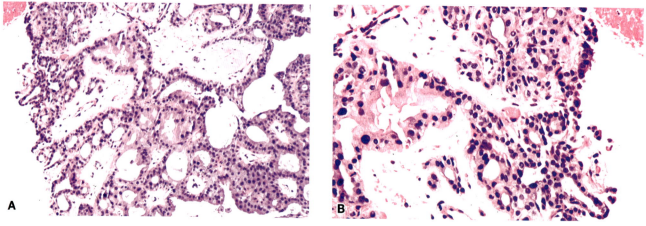

FIGURE 4.29 Cystic Apocrine Metaplasia With Atypia. A, B: The epithelium has focal cribriform microlumina and isolated hyperchromatic enlarged nuclei in these needle core biopsy specimens.

In comparison with conventional apocrine metaplasia, the nuclei in mild apocrine atypia appear irregularly placed and may not be basally oriented. Nucleoli appear slightly pleomorphic, and occasionally a nucleus has more than one nucleolus. With the development of more severe atypia, the cytoplasm of individual cells becomes increasingly vacuolated or clear, and the decapitation of cytoplasm at the luminal border becomes inapparent. Nuclear pleomorphism, with at least 3-fold variation in nuclear size, and hyperchromasia may be striking (97,98). The nuclear-to-cytoplasmic ratio increases as apocrine metaplasia becomes more atypical, but the cells generally retain relatively abundant cytoplasm.

Cytologic atypia tends to be more severe in the apocrine epithelium of sclerosing lesions such as sclerosing adenosis and RSLs, but it may be found in apocrine foci in fibroadenomas, cysts, and papillomas. Atypical cytologic features were present in 71% of adenosis tumors with apocrine metaplasia reported by Nielsen (99). Apocrine atypia can be particularly pronounced after radiation therapy.

When atypical apocrine metaplasia is present, the severity of the change is usually not homogeneous in a given lesion. Bland metaplastic apocrine change is usually found in the vicinity. The distinction between atypical apocrine metaplasia and apocrine carcinoma is usually not difficult, but it may be a challenge in NCB. In this situation, cytologic features may be less important than the growth pattern, especially in sclerosing lesions. A diagnosis of carcinoma is warranted in a sclerosing lesion when the atypical apocrine proliferation has the configuration of one of the conventional forms of DCIS (96). Prominent mitoses, intraluminal or single-cell necrosis, strong HER2 expression, and extent >2 mm may push the diagnosis to apocrine DCIS (92,98). Because myoepithelial cells may not always be detectable in benign apocrine lesions, the diagnosis of in situ or invasive apocrine carcinoma depends primarily on the cytologic and architectural characteristics of the proliferative cells. The results of myoepithelial stains can provide confirmatory evidence.

Immunohistochemistry

The apical cytoplasm of apocrine cells is immunoreactive for epithelial membrane antigen (EMA). The cytoplasm shows diffuse reactivity for GCDFP-15. A proportion of normal mammary cells and cutaneous adnexal cells also stain for this protein, so a positive reaction for GCDFP-15 does not establish the apocrine nature of a cell.

Apocrine cells typically do not stain for ER or PR (progesterone receptor), but they consistently stain for AR. Two reports (100,101) described staining for human epidermal growth factor receptor 2 (HER2) along the basal and lateral cell membranes. The cytoplasmic granules in apocrine cells sometimes stain for HER2. One must not misinterpret this finding as evidence of HER2 overexpression.

The myoepithelial cells in apocrine lesions vary in their reactivity for myoepithelial markers such as calponin, smooth muscle myosin heavy chain, CD10, and p63. Tramm et al (94) observed a substantial number of cases showing large gaps between p63-positive myoepithelial cells, although staining for calponin demonstrated a continuous layer of myoepithelium. The authors also observed rare instances in which large gaps were evident between calponin-immunoreactive myoepithelial cells but not between p63-immunoreactive myoepithelial cells. These data indicate that any effort to investigate the extent of myoepithelium in apocrine lesions must include not only p63 but also at least one cytoplasmic maker, an admonition that applies equally to all breast lesions.

Prognosis

The relationship of apocrine metaplasia to the development of mammary carcinoma is uncertain. In most instances, apocrine metaplasia appears to be part of the fibrocystic complex manifested by cysts with simple or papillary epithelium or ductal hyperplasia with intermingled apocrine change. Although anatomic studies of apocrine metaplasia have not shown an association between apocrine metaplasia and concurrent carcinoma (99,102,103), the findings of certain follow-up studies suggest that apocrine metaplasia may be a predictor for carcinoma. Haagensen et al (89) reported a 10-fold greater frequency of carcinoma in women who had apocrine metaplasia in a prior biopsy when compared with those in whom apocrine change was absent. Most of the subsequent carcinomas had "apocrine features," but origin in apocrine metaplasia was rarely traceable. When compared with Connecticut state incidence figures, patients with apocrine metaplasia had 3.5 times the expected frequency of carcinoma, whereas the risk was only 0.3 times expected when apocrine metaplasia was absent. Page et al (104) observed a slight overall increase in the number of subsequent carcinomas in women with papillary apocrine change in an antecedent biopsy when compared with the expected number of carcinomas based on an age-matched comparison with the Third National Cancer survey. The difference was statistically significant only in women who were older than 45 when the apocrine lesion was detected.

Histologic evidence of transitions from apocrine metaplasia to apocrine carcinoma has been reported. Yates and Ahmed (105) recounted a case in which a biopsy that disclosed "florid apocrine metaplasia intermingled with atypical apocrine cells" was followed by the detection of a 2.5-cm apocrine carcinoma 19 months later. Haagensen et al (89) reported that they had "traced the transformation of benign apocrine metaplasia into apocrine carcinoma in a considerable number of cases." Florid apocrine metaplasia with atypia often coexists with apocrine carcinoma (106), but few examples of apocrine carcinoma have been traced to atypical apocrine lesions. A recent study of 17 atypical apocrine lesions diagnosed on NCB reported a 25% upgrade rate to malignancy on excision, including one apocrine DCIS and one apocrine IDC (107). When carcinoma arises in the opposite breast of a patient with apocrine atypia or apocrine carcinoma, the contralateral carcinoma is not necessarily apocrine.

Treatment

Specific treatment is not indicated for proliferative lesions with apocrine metaplasia. Most cysts with metaplastic apocrine epithelium collapse and do not re-form after aspiration. Surgical excision of apocrine cysts is not indicated unless atypia is present. The need for follow-up of women with apocrine metaplasia on NCB depends on the overall findings in the specimen and the clinical circumstances. Patients with atypical apocrine metaplasia require clinical evaluation comparable to that of women with other atypical proliferative lesions.

FLORID PAPILLOMATOSIS AND SYRINGOMATOUS ADENOMA OF THE NIPPLE

Owing to their superficial location in the nipple, these lesions are ordinarily not subjected to NCB; nevertheless, pathologists do receive specimens from this location obtained by punch biopsy or incisional biopsy.

Florid Papillomatosis

Florid papillomatosis, also known as *nipple adenoma*, refers to a proliferative lesion of the nipple producing a constellation of clinicopathologic findings, which can include erosion of the nipple with replacement of the epidermis by glandular epithelium, inflammation, and enlargement of the nipple by a firm mass—hence the other term for the lesion: "erosive papillomatosis." The dominant histologic finding in most cases is florid ductal hyperplasia (once called papillomatosis).

Clinical Features

Approximately one-third of patients with florid papillomatosis present in the fifth decade, but the reported ages at diagnosis range from birth to 89 years (108). Approximately 15% of patients are <35 years, and an equal proportion are >65 years. Adolescents and infants account for a small percentage of the cases. Fewer than 5% of the reported examples of florid papillomatosis have involved men (109). Bilateral florid papillomatosis is extremely uncommon (110). Several examples of florid papillomatosis involving ectopic breast tissue have been reported (111,112).

In most cases of florid papillomatosis, the nodules have been present for a few months before the patients seek medical attention. The most frequent presenting symptom is nipple discharge, often described as bloody. Pain, itching, or burning sensations are not unusual. In many instances, the nipple appears enlarged, and a mass can be palpated. The surface of the nipple may appear granular, ulcerated, reddened, warty, or crusted. Often, these symptoms and clinical findings are mistaken for Paget disease or a papilloma.

Imaging Studies

Radiologic studies usually reveal the presence of a mass, although its small size and location within the nipple often make it difficult to detect by mammography. The nodules typically appear well defined and smoothly contoured. Unusual cases can present mammographic or sonographic features that suggest malignancy (113). Increased flow associated with the nodule can be seen with Doppler studies (114).

Histologic Evaluation

The lesions can be grouped into four categories according to histologic growth pattern. In three subtypes, one structural feature dominates or is present exclusively, whereas the fourth group consists of tumors with mixed patterns. No prognostic significance can be attached to these subtypes, and there is no evidence that they differ in pathogenesis. Some clinicopathologic correlations have been noted with these categories.

Florid papillomatosis with the *sclerosing papillomatosis pattern* typically presents as a discrete tumor. Scaling of the nipple skin may occur, but redness, ulceration, and inflammation are rarely present. The nipple contains a firm tumor, although the edges of the lesion may not seem well defined. The histologic features resemble those of a sclerosing papilloma. Exuberant papillary hyperplasia of ductal epithelium is distorted by a stromal proliferation within and around the affected ducts **(Fig. 4.30)**. The complex proliferative process is arranged in papillary, solid, tubular, and glandular structures. Squamous cysts are commonly formed in the terminal portions of lactiferous ducts. Focal necrosis may be found in the hyperplastic duct epithelium, sometimes associated with infrequent mitoses in epithelial cells. Apocrine metaplasia and extension of glandular epithelium to the nipple surface are uncommon.

Lesions with the *papillomatosis pattern* usually present with induration rather than a mass. Microscopic examination reveals florid papillary hyperplasia of ductal epithelium, causing expansion and crowding of the affected ducts **(Fig. 4.31)**. Focal necrosis and scattered mitotic figures may be found. These tumors lack the stromal proliferation that characterizes the sclerosing papillomatosis type of lesion. Hyperplastic glandular tissue may replace the overlying squamous epithelium over a part or the entire skin of the nipple. Squamous-lined cysts and apocrine metaplasia are not prominent in this variety.

Florid papillomatosis with the *adenosis pattern* forms a discrete nodule in the nipple. Microscopically, the lesion consists of crowded, orderly glands arranged in a pattern indistinguishable from that of florid sclerosing adenosis or an adenosis tumor. Myoepithelial hyperplasia accompanies the epithelial proliferation. Prominent apocrine metaplasia, hyperplasia of the squamous epithelium, and the formation of squamous cysts may be encountered. Mitotic figures and focal necrosis are uncommon.

Examples showing the *mixed proliferative pattern* contain different combinations of the other three patterns. Prominent features present in most cases include squamous metaplasia of ducts with cyst formation, apocrine metaplasia, and hyperplasia of the overlying epithelium. Hyperplastic duct epithelium may ulcerate the nipple surface. Adenosis occurs in about one-third of these lesions, and a syringomatous pattern may be found at the edges.

BENIGN PAPILLARY TUMORS

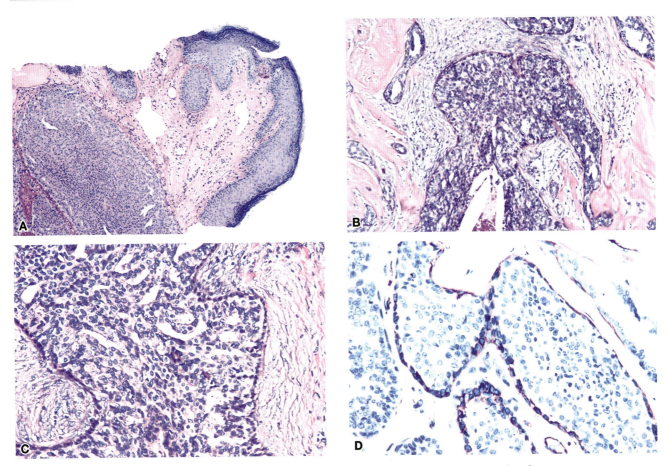

FIGURE 4.30 Florid Papillomatosis of Nipple. A: This needle core biopsy sample taken from a nodule in the nipple shows florid ductal hyperplasia just beneath the epidermis. **B:** Hyperplastic epithelium with a fenestrated pattern in sclerotic stroma is commonly present in the sclerosing type of florid papillomatosis. **C:** Myoepithelial cells outline the hyperplastic epithelium. **D:** Myoepithelial cells are accentuated by the immunostain for actin.

Immunohistochemistry

The cells lining the glands stain for "luminal" markers such as EMA, CK18 (CAM5.2), and MUC1, whereas the cells at the periphery of the glands stain for myoepithelial markers such as smooth muscle actin (SMA), calponin, and p63. One may not detect myoepithelial cells around glands within the center of a benign sclerosing lesion. Staining for CK7, keratin AE1/3, S-100, GCDFP-15, and CEA has yielded variable results.

Differential Diagnosis

On rare occasions, carcinoma can arise within a focus of florid papillomatosis (108). Such carcinomas can be difficult

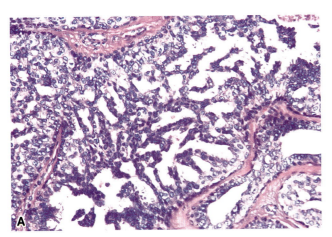 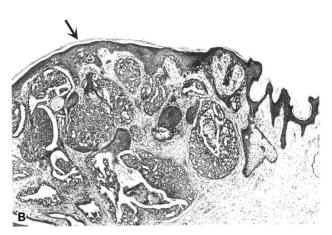

FIGURE 4.31 Florid Papillomatosis of Nipple. A: Micropapillary hyperplasia occupies this duct in a papillomatosis-type lesion. **B:** Ducts in this region of a nodule of florid papillomatosis harbor DCIS. The arrow marks carcinoma cells in the epidermis (Paget disease).

to detect because the hyperplastic areas in many examples of florid papillomatosis exhibit atypical features such as necrosis, cribriform and micropapillary growth patterns, mitotic figures, and cytologic atypia. In the absence of definitive evidence of invasion, Paget disease of nipple is the most reliable evidence of DCIS arising in florid papillomatosis. CAM5.2 and CK7 immunostains are helpful for detecting Paget cells. When Paget disease is found, underlying areas of DCIS, which differ in their pattern of growth from the rest of the tumor, are usually readily identifiable. A conservative approach to the diagnosis of florid papillomatosis is recommended.

Prognosis and Treatment

Incisional biopsy and NCB may not yield sufficient tissue to exclude the presence of carcinoma arising in the lesion. Complete excision, which is recommended as definitive treatment, may require removal of the nipple. Local recurrence of florid papillomatosis may occur following incomplete excision, but some patients have reportedly remained asymptomatic after a minimal amount of lesional tissue was left, and the margins of the excision specimen were only focally involved.

Syringomatous Adenoma of Nipple

Syringomatous adenoma of nipple is a benign, locally infiltrating neoplasm that has a close histopathologic resemblance to syringomatous tumors found in the facial skin and at other sites (115). The anatomic origin of the breast lesion is uncertain. The absence of epithelial proliferation in the mammary ducts and the lack of connection with the epidermis in most cases suggest an origin from other structures, possibly sweat ducts.

Clinical Features

The patients range in age from 11 to 76 at diagnosis. The median and mean ages at diagnosis are approximately 40 years (115,116). Isolated cases in men have been reported (115,117).

Typical syringomatous adenomas are unilateral lesions that affect either breast with approximately equal frequency. In one case, tumors appeared in both breasts synchronously (118), and another woman presented with a 4.2-cm fungating syringomatous adenoma in the left breast and a mammographically detected syringomatous adenoma in the right breast (119). Most patients report that signs and symptoms began within the year prior to diagnosis, but durations of symptoms of several years have been recorded. The initial symptom is a mass in the nipple or subareolar region. A few patients have described pain, tenderness, redness, itching, discharge, or nipple inversion. Crusting of the nipple caused by hyperkeratosis has been reported, but ulceration and erosion are not features of syringomatous adenoma. The occurrence of syringomatous adenoma in supernumerary nipples has been reported (120,121).

Imaging Studies

Mammography can demonstrate a dense stellate tumor, calcifications, or both (118,122,123). Sonography sometimes shows an irregular mass that may be accompanied by dilated ducts or calcifications (116,118,124).

Microscopic Pathology

The lesion consists of tubules, ductules, and strands composed of small, uniform cells that infiltrate the dermis and the stroma of the nipple. The neoplastic glands sometimes seem to connect with the basal layer of the epidermis. Hyperplasia of the epidermis is slight in most cases, but occasionally pseudoepitheliomatous hyperplasia may be encountered.

The ducts, lined by one or more layers of cells, have teardrop or comma-like shapes; with lumina that appear either open and round or filled with small uniform cells (**Fig. 4.32**). Some cells may exhibit cytoplasmic clearing. Mitoses are virtually absent, and the nuclei lack prominent nucleoli and pleomorphism. Flattening of cells around the lumina

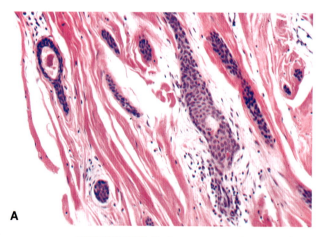
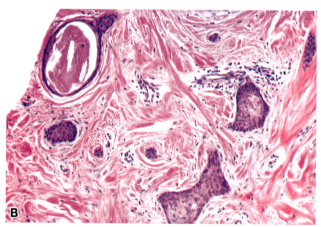

FIGURE 4.32 **Syringomatous Adenoma of Nipple. A:** This area from a needle core biopsy specimen shows elongated duct-like structures, one of which has an open lumen containing secretion. Squamous differentiation can be seen in the center. **B:** An area with cystic dilatation and prominent squamous differentiation is evident.

constitutes evidence of early squamous differentiation, which in a fully developed form results in keratotic cysts. A foreign body giant cell reaction may be elicited in the vicinity of ruptured squamous cysts. Calcification is rarely seen in the keratinized epithelium. The lumina of the ducts either appear empty or contain deeply eosinophilic, retracted secretion. The secretion is periodic acid–Schiff (PAS)-positive and sometimes weakly mucicarmine-positive (115).

The adenomatous tubules diffusely infiltrate the periductal stroma of nipple and may extend into the subareolar breast parenchyma in larger lesions. Invasion into the smooth muscle bundles of the nipple is common, and occasionally perineural invasion is observed. The stroma appears minimally altered in the vicinity of the infiltrating tubules. The collagen and fibroblasts tend to be concentrically oriented around the epithelial structures, albeit to a lesser degree than that observed in low-grade adenosquamous carcinoma.

Syringomatous glands may be found in proximity to and, rarely, in direct contact with the epithelium of nipple ducts, mammary lobules, and nipple epidermis. This continuity probably results from infiltrative growth of the neoplasm, and one should not misinterpret the finding as evidence of origin from any of these structures. Coincidental epithelial hyperplasia of lactiferous ducts or underlying breast tissue may occasionally be seen, but this is not an intrinsic component of syringomatous adenoma. Paget disease is not a feature of syringomatous adenoma.

Immunohistochemistry

The literature contains limited information regarding the immunohistochemical characteristics of syringomatous adenoma. The inner cells express keratin. In one report (119), the outer cells stained strongly for smooth muscle myosin heavy chain, 34βE12, and CK5/6. The outer cells and others showing squamous features stained for p63. ER is generally partial, weak, or negative (118,119,124).

Differential Diagnosis

Several lesions should be considered in the differential diagnosis of syringomatous adenoma of nipple. Florid papillomatosis is a hyperplastic epithelial proliferation of the major lactiferous ducts. Patients with florid papillomatosis tend to be older and are more likely to have erosion of the nipple with bleeding. Syringomatous foci are occasionally encountered as a minor component of florid papillomatosis.

Tubular carcinoma sometimes arises in the subareolar region and nipple, where it displays an infiltrative growth pattern that may be difficult to distinguish from syringomatous adenoma. Both invade smooth muscle and nerves. Features of tubular carcinoma in the nipple that are not seen in syringomatous adenoma include DCIS and angular glands. Squamous metaplasia and the formation of round glands, findings seen in syringomatous adenoma, are not features of tubular carcinoma.

Syringomatous adenoma and low-grade adenosquamous carcinoma share certain structural characteristics (125); however, the two lesions are not differing appearances of a single type of neoplasm. Syringomatous adenoma arises in the nipple and secondarily involves the breast parenchyma underlying the nipple in almost all cases. Low-grade adenosquamous carcinoma usually develops peripherally, sparing the nipple, although infrequently it can arise in the subareolar region and involve the nipple.

Treatment and Prognosis

Most patients have been treated by local excision, which required removing the entire nipple in some instances. Local recurrence, sometimes with invasive growth, after incomplete excision has occurred in approximately 30% of cases reported (115,116,126). Reexcision should be considered if the tumor involves the margin of the specimen. The time to recurrence has varied from <1 year to 8 years. In one case (115), the lesion slowly enlarged for 22 years after initial biopsy, at which time a partial mastectomy was performed for a 3-cm tumor that invaded the breast parenchyma. One patient experienced three recurrences over a 4-year period (127). None of the patients with lesions correctly diagnosed as syringomatous adenoma have developed metastases in regional lymph nodes or at distant sites. There is no evidence of association with mammary carcinoma.

COLLAGENOUS SPHERULOSIS

This nonneoplastic structural alteration represents a clinically insignificant incidental microscopic finding; and it occurs as a component of another benign breast lesion such as a papilloma (most commonly), adenomyoepithelioma, fibroadenoma, or sclerosing adenosis (128-131). Rarely, the collagenous spherulosis constitutes the dominant alteration (132).

First described by Clement et al in 1987 (133), this lesion features nodules of eosinophilic or basophilic basement membrane material enclosed in rounded spaces, superficially resembling adenoid cystic carcinoma (134). In 2006, Resetkova et al (131) summarized the clinical and morphologic features of 59 cases identified at a single institution and tabulated data from 61 reported cases.

Clinical Features

It is difficult to determine the incidence of collagenous spherulosis because the lesion often goes unrecognized or is misinterpreted. Estimates place the frequency of the lesion at <1% of excision specimens (135). Collagenous spherulosis affects women throughout adulthood; the ages of patients in reported cases range from 19 years (136) to 90 years (131). The literature does not contain reports of collagenous spherulosis in men.

The clinical presentation of collagenous spherulosis depends on the nature of the underlying lesion. Patients may complain of a mass, but more often the underlying lesion is detected by imaging studies. Radiologic imaging of collagenous spherulosis may demonstrate either calcifications or a mass, but the images do not have distinctive features.

Histologic Evaluation

Spherules composed of acellular material surrounded by epithelial cells constitute the defining features of collagenous spherulosis (**Figs. 4.33** and **4.34**). The spherules, which measure 20 to 100 μm, may be eosinophilic, amphophilic, or nearly transparent. Certain spherules appear as dense as the cylindromatous deposits in adenoid cystic carcinoma. In other instances, the centers of the spherules look nearly transparent, and stellate fibrils may be seen radiating from a central nidus to the periphery. Degenerative changes in the spherules can result in the loss of the radial structure and create a lumen-like space; however, at least a thin rim of basement membrane material encompassed by a ring of myoepithelial cells remains. At times, this layer collapses into the cystic spherule (**Fig. 4.35**). Constituents of the spherules include components of basement membranes: elastin, PAS-positive polysaccharides, type IV collagen, and laminin (135,137).

Myoepithelial and luminal cells contribute to the formation of collagenous spherulosis, and these cells give rise to two types of spaces. Myoepithelial cells constitute the dominant population, and they have long spindly shapes, flattened oval hyperchromatic nuclei, and attenuated eosinophilic cytoplasm, which is sometimes referred to as a "cuticle." The myoepithelial cells create the rounded spaces that enclose the spherules. The attenuated myoepithelial cells may be difficult to identify in H&E sections, but immunostains will highlight them. Collections of cuboidal luminal cells containing bland nuclei, inconspicuous nucleoli, and dense eosinophilic cytoplasm form glands interspersed among the myoepithelial cells and spherules. These glands sometimes contain eosinophilic secretory material. This pattern of growth creates an adenoid cystic–like arrangement; however, the glandular spaces tend to have relatively more irregular shapes than those of adenoid cystic carcinoma.

Collagenous spherulosis usually occurs as a multifocal process. Atypical epithelial proliferations and carcinomas

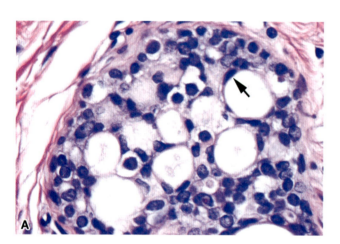
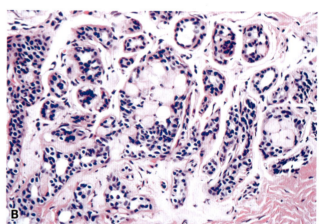

FIGURE 4.33 Collagenous Spherulosis. A: Each of the spherules in this duct is outlined by a membrane-like border surrounded by myoepithelial cells with elongated nuclei (*arrows*). Fibrillar material is present in some spherules. **B:** Solid eosinophilic nodules of basement membrane material are present in sclerosing adenosis in a needle core biopsy sample obtained for calcifications.

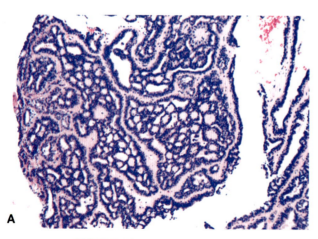
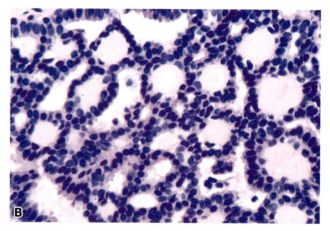

FIGURE 4.34 Collagenous Spherulosis in a Papilloma. A, B: The spherules are round, weakly eosinophilic bodies in the epithelium. Myoepithelial cells are inconspicuous, but they can be seen rimming spherules in the lower right corner of **(B)**. The true empty glandular lumina have irregular contours.

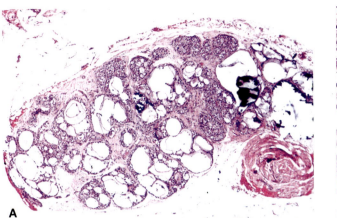 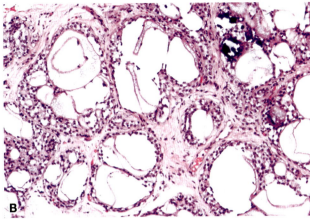

FIGURE 4.35 **Collagenous Spherulosis With Degenerative Changes. A, B:** The spherules in this case of collagenous spherulosis have undergone cystic degeneration. Detached strips of basement membrane material have collapsed into the cystic spherules. The biopsy was performed for mammographically detected calcifications, some of which are shown.

can supervene in foci of collagenous spherulosis, but coexisting neoplastic proliferations represent independent, unrelated processes. Resetkova et al (131) observed ADH in 3 of 59 (5%) cases and lobular carcinoma in situ (LCIS) in 15 of 59 (25%) cases. When LCIS colonizes collagenous spherulosis and replaces the luminal cells, an appearance similar to that of low-grade DCIS results (131,138) **(Fig. 4.36)**.

Immunohistochemistry

The two types of cells stain in the expected ways. The myoepithelial cells stain for proteins such as SMA, p63, and CD10, and the latter antibody sometimes stains the spherules. Luminal cells stain for low-molecular-weight CK, ER, and PR. By using a panel of these and other markers, collagenous spherulosis can be distinguished from adenoid cystic carcinoma. Cabibi et al (139) found that the cells of collagenous spherulosis stained intensely for CD10, HHF35 actin, ER, and PR, whereas those of adenoid cystic carcinoma did not. Conversely, the cells of adenoid cystic carcinoma stained intensely for c-Kit (CD117), but the cells of collagenous spherulosis did so only weakly. Rabban et al (140) pointed out that both lesions can express SMA, S-100, and p63 and suggested the use of other myoepithelial markers. These authors found that the cells of collagenous spherulosis stain intensely for calponin and smooth muscle myosin heavy chain and that those of adenoid cystic carcinoma do not.

Prognosis and Treatment

There is no evidence to indicate that collagenous spherulosis is precancerous (132,133) or that it is associated with adenoid cystic carcinoma. The prognosis and treatment of a patient with collagenous spherulosis depends on the nature of the associated lesion.

REFERENCES

1. Lewis JT, Hartmann LC, Vierkant RA, et al. An analysis of breast cancer risk in women with single, multiple, and atypical papilloma. *Am J Surg Pathol*. 2006;30:665-672.
2. Rakha EA, Ellis IO. Diagnostic challenges in papillary lesions of the breast. *Pathology*. 2018;50:100-110.
3. Patel A, Hoda RS, Hoda SA. Papillary breast tumors: continuing controversies and commentary on WHO's 2019 criteria and classification. *Int J Surg Pathol*. 2022;30:124-137.
4. Allison KH, Brogi E, Ellis IO, et al. *WHO Classification of Breast Tumours*. 5th ed. IARC; 2019.
5. Yamamoto H, Okada Y, Taniguchi H, et al. Intracystic papilloma in the breast of a male given long-term phenothiazine therapy: a case report. *Breast Cancer*. 2006;13:84-88.
6. Rizzo M, Lund MJ, Oprea G, Schniederjan M, Wood WC, Mosunjac M. Surgical follow-up and clinical presentation of 142 breast papillary lesions diagnosed by ultrasound-guided core-needle biopsy. *Ann Surg Oncol*. 2008;15:1040-1047.
7. Mesurolle B, Kethani K, El-Khoury M, Meterissian S. Intraductal papilloma in a reconstructed breast: mammographic and sonographic appearance with pathologic correlation. *Breast*. 2006;15:680-682.
8. Cottom H, Rengabashyam B, Turton PE, Shaaban AM. Intraductal papilloma in an axillary lymph node of a patient with human immunodeficiency virus: a case report and review of the literature. *J Med Case Rep*. 2014;8:162.
9. Dzodic R, Stanojevic B, Saenko V, et al. Intraductal papilloma of ectopic breast tissue in axillary lymph node of a patient with a previous intraductal papilloma of ipsilateral breast: a case report and review of the literature. *Diagn Pathol*. 2010;5:17.

FIGURE 4.36 **Collagenous Spherulosis With In Situ Carcinoma.** Lobular carcinoma in situ has filled and expanded the epithelium between spherules. Note the loss of cohesion between the neoplastic cells and the fine filamentous material in some spherules.

10. Ichihara S, Ikeda T, Kimura K, et al. Coincidence of mammary and sentinel lymph node papilloma. *Am J Surg Pathol.* 2008;32:784-792.
11. Shim JH, Son EJ, Kim EK, Kwak JY, Jeong J, Hong SW. Benign intracystic papilloma of the male breast. *J Ultrasound Med.* 2008;27:1397-1400.
12. Francis A, England D, Rowlands D, Bradley S. Breast papilloma: mammogram, ultrasound and MRI appearances. *Breast.* 2002;11:394-397.
13. Lam WW, Chu WC, Tang AP, Tse G, Ma TK. Role of radiologic features in the management of papillary lesions of the breast. *AJR Am J Roentgenol.* 2006;186:1322-1327.
14. Hayashi H, Ohtani H, Yamaguchi J, Shimokawa I. A case of intracystic apocrine papillary tumor: diagnostic pitfalls for malignancy. *Pathol Res Pract.* 2013; 209:808-811.
15. Jiao YF, Nakamura S, Oikawa T, Sugai T, Uesugi N. Sebaceous gland metaplasia in intraductal papilloma of the breast. *Virchows Arch.* 2001;438:505-508.
16. Judkins AR, Montone KT, LiVolsi VA, van de Rijn M. Sensitivity and specificity of antibodies on necrotic tumor tissue. *Am J Clin Pathol.* 1998;110:641-646.
17. Stefanou D, Batistatou A, Nonni A, Arkoumani E, Agnantis NJ. p63 expression in benign and malignant breast lesions. *Histol Histopathol.* 2004;19:465-471.
18. Reisenbichler ES, Adams AL, Hameed O. The predictive ability of a CK5/p63/CK8/18 antibody cocktail in stratifying breast papillary lesions on needle biopsy: an algorithmic approach works best. *Am J Clin Pathol.* 2013; 140:767-779.
19. Brennan SB, Corben A, Liberman L, et al. Papilloma diagnosed at MRI-guided vacuum-assisted breast biopsy: is surgical excision still warranted? *AJR Am J Roentgenol.* 2012;199:W512-W519.
20. Hawley JR, Lawther H, Erdal BS, Yildiz VO, Carkaci S. Outcomes of benign breast papillomas diagnosed at image-guided vacuum-assisted core needle biopsy. *Clin Imaging.* 2015;39:576-581.
21. Nayak A, Carkaci S, Gilcrease MZ, et al. Benign papillomas without atypia diagnosed on core needle biopsy: experience from a single institution and proposed criteria for excision. *Clin Breast Cancer.* 2013;13:439-449.
22. Wen X, Cheng W. Nonmalignant breast papillary lesions at core-needle biopsy: a meta-analysis of underestimation and influencing factors. *Ann Surg Oncol.* 2013;20:94-101.
23. Grimm LJ, Bookhout CE, Bentley RC, Jordan SG, Lawton TJ. Concordant, non-atypical breast papillomas do not require surgical excision: a 10-year multi-institution study and review of the literature. *Clin Imaging.* 2018;51:180-185.
24. Jaffer S, Bleiweiss IJ, Nagi C. Incidental intraductal papillomas (<2 mm) of the breast diagnosed on needle core biopsy do not need to be excised. *Breast J.* 2013;19:130-133.
25. Pareja F, Corben AD, Brennan SB, et al. Breast intraductal papillomas without atypia in radiologic-pathologic concordant core-needle biopsies: rate of upgrade to carcinoma at excision. *Cancer.* 2016;122:2819-2827.
26. Asirvatham JR, Jorns JM, Zhao L, Jeffries DO, Wu AJ. Outcomes of benign intraductal papillomas diagnosed on core biopsy: a review of 104 cases with subsequent excision from a single institution. *Virchows Arch.* 2018;473:679-686.
27. Shah VI, Flowers CI, Douglas-Jones AG, Dallimore NS, Rashid M. Immunohistochemistry increases the accuracy of diagnosis of benign papillary lesions in breast core needle biopsy specimens. *Histopathology.* 2006;48:683-691.
28. Grin A, O'Malley FP, Mulligan AM. Cytokeratin 5 and estrogen receptor immunohistochemistry as a useful adjunct in identifying atypical papillary lesions on breast needle core biopsy. *Am J Surg Pathol.* 2009;33:1615-1623.
29. Tse GM, Tan PH, Lacambra MD, et al. Papillary lesions of the breast—accuracy of core biopsy. *Histopathology.* 2010;56:481-488.
30. Moon HJ, Jung I, Kim MJ, Kim EK. Breast papilloma without atypia and risk of breast carcinoma. *Breast J.* 2014;20:525-533.
31. MacGrogan G, Tavassoli FA. Central atypical papillomas of the breast: a clinicopathological study of 119 cases. *Virchows Arch.* 2003;443:609-617.
32. Cuneo KC, Dash RC, Wilke LG, Horton JK, Koontz BF. Risk of invasive breast cancer and ductal carcinoma in situ in women with atypical papillary lesions of the breast. *Breast J.* 2012;18:475-478.
33. Ali-Fehmi R, Carolin K, Wallis T, Visscher DW. Clinicopathologic analysis of breast lesions associated with multiple papillomas. *Hum Pathol.* 2003;34:234-239.
34. The American Society of Breast Surgeons. *Consensus guideline on concordance assessment of image-guided breast biopsies and management of borderline or high-risk lesions.* https://www.breastsurgeons.org/docs/statements/Consensus-Guideline-on-Concordance-Assessment-of-Image-Guided-Breast-Biopsies.pdf
35. Carder PJ, Khan T, Burrows P, Sharma N. Large volume "mammotome" biopsy may reduce the need for diagnostic surgery in papillary lesions of the breast. *J Clin Pathol.* 2008;61:928-933.
36. Choi HY, Kim SM, Jang M, et al. Benign breast papilloma without atypia: outcomes of surgical excision versus US-guided directional vacuum-assisted removal or US follow-up. *Radiology.* 2019;293:72-80.
37. Kibil W, Hodorowicz-Zaniewska D, Popiela TJ, Kulig J. Vacuum-assisted core biopsy in diagnosis and treatment of intraductal papillomas. *Clin Breast Cancer.* 2013;13:129-132.
38. Mosier AD, Keylock J, Smith DV. Benign papillomas diagnosed on large-gauge vacuum-assisted core needle biopsy which span <1.5 cm do not need surgical excision. *Breast J.* 2013;19:611-617.
39. Yamaguchi R, Tanaka M, Tse GM, et al. Management of breast papillary lesions diagnosed in ultrasound-guided vacuum-assisted and core needle biopsies. *Histopathology.* 2015;66:565-576.
40. Youk JH, Kim MJ, Son EJ, Kwak JY, Kim EK. US-guided vacuum-assisted percutaneous excision for management of benign papilloma without atypia

diagnosed at US-guided 14-gauge core needle biopsy. *Ann Surg Oncol.* 2012;19:922-928.
41. Corbin H, Bomeisl P, Amin AL, Marshall HN, Gilmore H, Harbhajanka A. Upgrade rates of intraductal papilloma with and without atypia diagnosed on core needle biopsy and clinicopathologic predictors. *Hum Pathol.* 2022;128:90-100.
42. Swapp RE, Glazebrook KN, Jones KN, et al. Management of benign intraductal solitary papilloma diagnosed on core needle biopsy. *Ann Surg Oncol.* 2013;20:1900-1905.
43. Wyss P, Varga Z, Rossle M, Rageth CJ. Papillary lesions of the breast: outcomes of 156 patients managed without excisional biopsy. *Breast J.* 2014;20:394-401.
44. Sexton K, Brill YM, Atkins L, et al. Outcome of benign papillary lesions of the breast diagnosed by needle core and mammotome biopsies with 3 to 5 year follow up. *Mod Pathol.* 2006;19:42a.
45. Hamperl H. Radial scars (scarring) and obliterating mastopathy (author's transl) [in German]. *Virchows Arch A Pathol Anat Histol.* 1975;369:55-68.
46. Kim EM, Hankins A, Cassity J, et al. Isolated radial scar diagnosis by core-needle biopsy: is surgical excision necessary? *Springerplus.* 2016;5:398.
47. Andersen JA, Gram JB. Radial scar in the female breast. A long-term follow-up study of 32 cases. *Cancer.* 1984;53:2557-2560.
48. Jacobs TW, Byrne C, Colditz G, Connolly JL, Schnitt SJ. Radial scars in benign breast-biopsy specimens and the risk of breast cancer. *N Engl J Med.* 1999;340:430-436.
49. Fisher ER, Palekar AS, Kotwal N, Lipana N. A nonencapsulated sclerosing lesion of the breast. *Am J Clin Pathol.* 1979;71:240-246.
50. Wellings SR, Alpers CE. Subgross pathologic features and incidence of radial scars in the breast. *Hum Pathol.* 1984;15:475-479.
51. Anderson TJ, Battersby S. Radial scars of benign and malignant breasts: comparative features and significance. *J Pathol.* 1985;147:23-32.
52. Patterson JA, Scott M, Anderson N, Kirk SJ. Radial scar, complex sclerosing lesion and risk of breast cancer. Analysis of 175 cases in Northern Ireland. *Eur J Surg Oncol.* 2004;30:1065-1068.
53. Dominguez A, Durando M, Mariscotti G, et al. Breast cancer risk associated with the diagnosis of a microhistological radial scar (RS): retrospective analysis in 10 years of experience. *Radiol Med.* 2015;120:377-385.
54. Linda A, Zuiani C, Londero V, Cedolini C, Girometti R, Bazzocchi M. Magnetic resonance imaging of radial sclerosing lesions (radial scars) of the breast. *Eur J Radiol.* 2012;81:3201-3207.
55. Andersen JA, Carter D, Linell F. A symposium on sclerosing duct lesions of the breast. *Pathol Annu.* 1986;21(pt 2):145-179.
56. Doyle EM, Banville N, Quinn CM, et al. Radial scars/complex sclerosing lesions and malignancy in a screening programme: incidence and histological features revisited. *Histopathology.* 2007;50:607-614.
57. Manfrin E, Remo A, Falsirollo F, Reghellin D, Bonetti F. Risk of neoplastic transformation in asymptomatic radial scar. Analysis of 117 cases. *Breast Cancer Res Treat.* 2008;107:371-377.
58. Cawson JN, Malara F, Kavanagh A, Hill P, Balasubramanium G, Henderson M. Fourteen-gauge needle core biopsy of mammographically evident radial scars: is excision necessary? *Cancer.* 2003;97:345-351.
59. Alvarado-Cabrero I, Tavassoli FA. Neoplastic and malignant lesions involving or arising in a radial scar: a clinicopathologic analysis of 17 cases. *Breast J.* 2000;6:96-102.
60. Caneva A, Bonetti F, Manfrin E, et al. Is radial scar of the breast a premalignant lesion? *Lab Invest.* 1997;76:77.
61. Park VY, Kim EK, Kim MJ, Yoon JH, Moon HJ. Mammographically occult asymptomatic radial scars/complex sclerosing lesions at ultrasonography-guided core needle biopsy: follow-up can be recommended. *Ultrasound Med Biol.* 2016;42:2367-2371.
62. Sloane JP, Mayers MM. Carcinoma and atypical hyperplasia in radial scars and complex sclerosing lesions: importance of lesion size and patient age. *Histopathology.* 1993;23:225-231.
63. Farshid G, Rush G. Assessment of 142 stellate lesions with imaging features suggestive of radial scar discovered during population-based screening for breast cancer. *Am J Surg Pathol.* 2004;28:1626-1631.
64. Denley H, Pinder SE, Tan PH, et al. Metaplastic carcinoma of the breast arising within complex sclerosing lesion: a report of five cases. *Histopathology.* 2000;36:203-209.
65. Gobbi H, Simpson JF, Jensen RA, Olson SJ, Page DL. Metaplastic spindle cell breast tumors arising within papillomas, complex sclerosing lesions, and nipple adenomas. *Mod Pathol.* 2003;16:893-901.
66. Chou WYY, Veis DJ, Aft R. Radial scar on image-guided breast biopsy: is surgical excision necessary? *Breast Cancer Res Treat.* 2018;170:313-320.
67. Cohen MA, Newell MS. Radial scars of the breast encountered at core biopsy: review of histologic, imaging, and management considerations. *AJR Am J Roentgenol.* 2017;209:1168-1177.
68. Farshid G, Buckley E. Meta-analysis of upgrade rates in 3163 radial scars excised after needle core biopsy diagnosis. *Breast Cancer Res Treat.* 2019;174:165-177.
69. Rakha E, Beca F, D'Andrea M, et al. Outcome of radial scar/complex sclerosing lesion associated with epithelial proliferations with atypia diagnosed on breast core biopsy: results from a multicentric UK-based study. *J Clin Pathol.* 2019;72:800-804.
70. Bianchi S, Giannotti E, Vanzi E, et al. Radial scar without associated atypical epithelial proliferation on image-guided 14-gauge needle core biopsy: analysis of 49 cases from a single-centre and review of the literature. *Breast.* 2012;21:159-164.

71. Conlon N, D'Arcy C, Kaplan JB, et al. Radial scar at image-guided needle biopsy: is excision necessary? *Am J Surg Pathol*. 2015;39:779-785.
72. Douglas-Jones AG, Denson JL, Cox AC, Harries IB, Stevens G. Radial scar lesions of the breast diagnosed by needle core biopsy: analysis of cases containing occult malignancy. *J Clin Pathol*. 2007;60:295-298.
73. Brenner RJ, Jackman RJ, Parker SH, et al. Percutaneous core needle biopsy of radial scars of the breast: when is excision necessary? *AJR Am J Roentgenol*. 2002;179:1179-1184.
74. Lee KA, Zuley ML, Chivukula M, Choksi ND, Ganott MA, Sumkin JH. Risk of malignancy when microscopic radial scars and microscopic papillomas are found at percutaneous biopsy. *AJR Am J Roentgenol*. 2012;198:W141-W145.
75. Donaldson AR, Sieck L, Booth CN, Calhoun BC. Radial scars diagnosed on breast core biopsy: frequency of atypia and carcinoma on excision and implications for management. *Breast*. 2016;30:201-207.
76. Nakhlis F, Lester S, Denison C, Wong SM, Mongiu A, Golshan M. Complex sclerosing lesions and radial sclerosing lesions on core needle biopsy: low risk of carcinoma on excision in cases with clinical and imaging concordance. *Breast J*. 2018;24:133-138.
77. Resetkova E, Edelweiss M, Albarracin CT, Yang WT. Management of radial sclerosing lesions of the breast diagnosed using percutaneous vacuum-assisted core needle biopsy: recommendations for excision based on seven years' experience at a single institution. *Breast Cancer Res Treat*. 2011;127:335-343.
78. Mesa-Quesada J, Romero-Martin S, Cara-Garcia M, Martínez-López A, Medina-Pérez M, Raya-Povedano JL. Cicatriz radial sin atipia en biopsia percutánea. ¿Puede evitarse la biopsia quirúrgica? [Radial scars without atypia in percutaneous biopsy specimens: can they obviate surgical biopsy?] *Radiologia*. 2017;59:523-530.
79. Sohn VY, Causey MW, Steele SR, Keylock JB, Brown TA. The treatment of radial scars in the modern era—surgical excision is not required. *Am Surg*. 2010;76:522-525.
80. Rajan S, Wason AM, Carder PJ. Conservative management of screen-detected radial scars: role of mammotome excision. *J Clin Pathol*. 2011;64:65-68.
81. Tennant SL, Evans A, Hamilton LJ, et al. Vacuum-assisted excision of breast lesions of uncertain malignant potential (B3)—an alternative to surgery in selected cases. *Breast*. 2008;17:546-549.
82. Aroner SA, Collins LC, Connolly JL, et al. Radial scars and subsequent breast cancer risk: results from the nurses' health studies. *Breast Cancer Res Treat*. 2013;139:277-285.
83. Berg JC, Visscher DW, Vierkant RA, et al. Breast cancer risk in women with radial scars in benign breast biopsies. *Breast Cancer Res Treat*. 2008;108:167-174.
84. Bunting DM, Steel JR, Holgate CS, Watkins RM. Long term follow-up and risk of breast cancer after a radial scar or complex sclerosing lesion has been identified in a benign open breast biopsy. *Eur J Surg Oncol*. 2011;37:709-713.
85. Sanders ME, Page DL, Simpson JF, Schuyler PA, Dale Plummer W, Dupont WD. Interdependence of radial scar and proliferative disease with respect to invasive breast carcinoma risk in patients with benign breast biopsies. *Cancer*. 2006;106:1453-1461.
86. Lv M, Zhu X, Zhong S, et al. Radial scars and subsequent breast cancer risk: a meta-analysis. *PLoS One*. 2014;9:e102503.
87. Rosen PP. Subareolar sclerosing duct hyperplasia of the breast. *Cancer*. 1987;59:1927-1930.
88. Cheng E, D'Alfonso TM, Arafah M, Marrero Rolon R, Ginter PS, Hoda SA. Subareolar sclerosing ductal hyperplasia. *Int J Surg Pathol*. 2017;25:4-11.
89. Haagensen CD, Bodian C, Haagensen DE. Apocrine epithelium. In: *Breast Carcinoma: Risk and Detection*. W.B. Saunders; 1981:83-105.
90. Gao Y, Dialani V, DeBenedectis C, Johnson N, Brachtel E, Slanetz P. Apocrine metaplasia found at MR biopsy: is there something to be learned? *Breast J*. 2017;23:429-435.
91. Benigni G, Squartini F. Uneven distribution and significant concentration of apocrine metaplasia in lower breast quadrants. *Tumori*. 1986;72:179-182.
92. Wells CA, El-Ayat GA. Non-operative breast pathology: apocrine lesions. *J Clin Pathol*. 2007;60:1313-1320.
93. Schuerch C 3rd, Rosen PP, Hirota T, et al. A pathologic study of benign breast diseases in Tokyo and New York. *Cancer*. 1982;50:1899-1903.
94. Tramm T, Kim JY, Tavassoli FA. Diminished number or complete loss of myoepithelial cells associated with metaplastic and neoplastic apocrine lesions of the breast. *Am J Surg Pathol*. 2011;35:202-211.
95. Kosemehmetoglu K, Guler G. Papillary apocrine metaplasia and columnar cell lesion with atypia: is there a shared common pathway? *Ann Diagn Pathol*. 2010;14:425-431.
96. Carter DJ, Rosen PP. Atypical apocrine metaplasia in sclerosing lesions of the breast: a study of 51 patients. *Mod Pathol*. 1991;4:1-5.
97. Asirvatham JR, Falcone MM, Kleer CG. Atypical apocrine adenosis: diagnostic challenges and pitfalls. *Arch Pathol Lab Med*. 2016;140:1045-1051.
98. Tavassoli FA, Norris HJ. Intraductal apocrine carcinoma: a clinicopathologic study of 37 cases. *Mod Pathol*. 1994;7:813-818.
99. Nielsen BB. Adenosis tumour of the breast—a clinicopathological investigation of 27 cases. *Histopathology*. 1987;11:1259-1275.
100. Feuerhake F, Unterberger P, Hofter EA. Cell turnover in apocrine metaplasia of the human mammary gland epithelium: apoptosis, proliferation, and immunohistochemical detection of Bcl-2, Bax, EGFR, and c-erbB2 gene products. *Acta Histochem*. 2001;103:53-65.
101. Selim AG, El-Ayat G, Wells CA. Expression of c-erbB2, p53, Bcl-2, Bax, c-myc and Ki-67 in apocrine metaplasia and apocrine change within sclerosing adenosis of the breast. *Virchows Arch*. 2002;441:449-455.

102. Foote FW, Stewart FW. Comparative studies of cancerous versus noncancerous breasts. *Ann Surg*. 1945;121:6-53.
103. McCarty KS Jr, Kesterson GH, Wilkinson WE, Georgiade N. Histopathologic study of subcutaneous mastectomy specimens from patients with carcinoma of the contralateral breast. *Surg Gynecol Obstet*. 1978;147:682-688.
104. Page DL, Vander Zwaag R, Rogers LW, Williams LT, Walker WE, Hartmann WH. Relation between component parts of fibrocystic disease complex and breast cancer. *J Natl Cancer Inst*. 1978;61:1055-1063.
105. Yates AJ, Ahmed A. Apocrine carcinoma and apocrine metaplasia. *Histopathology*. 1988;13:228-231.
106. Abati AD, Kimmel M, Rosen PP. Apocrine mammary carcinoma. A clinicopathologic study of 72 cases. *Am J Clin Pathol*. 1990;94:371-377.
107. Jung HK, Kim SJ, Kim W, et al. Ultrasound features and rate of upgrade to malignancy in atypical apocrine lesions of the breast. *J Ultrasound Med*. 2020;39:1517-1524.
108. Rosen PP, Caicco JA. Florid papillomatosis of the nipple. A study of 51 patients, including nine with mammary carcinoma. *Am J Surg Pathol*. 1986;10: 87-101.
109. Fernandez-Flores A, Suarez-Penaranda JM. Immunophenotype of nipple adenoma in a male patient. *Appl Immunohistochem Mol Morphol*. 2011;19:190-194.
110. Sasi W, Banerjee D, Mokbel K, Sharma AK. Bilateral florid papillomatosis of the nipple: an unusual indicator for metachronous breast cancer development-a case report. *Case Rep Oncol Med*. 2014;2014:432609.
111. Shinn L, Woodward C, Boddu S, Jha P, Fouroutan H, Péley G. Nipple adenoma arising in a supernumerary mammary gland: a case report. *Tumori*. 2011;97: 812-814.
112. Shioi Y, Nakamura S, Kawamura S, Kasami M. Nipple adenoma arising from axillary accessory breast: a case report. *Diagn Pathol*. 2012;7:162.
113. Fornage BD, Faroux MJ, Pluot M, Bogomoletz W. Nipple adenoma simulating carcinoma. Misleading clinical, mammographic, sonographic, and cytologic findings. *J Ultrasound Med*. 1991;10:55-57.
114. Parajuly SS, Peng YL, Zhu M, Gang YZ, Gyawali S. Nipple adenoma of the breast: sonographic imaging findings. *South Med J*. 2010;103:1280-1281.
115. Rosen PP. Syringomatous adenoma of the nipple. *Am J Surg Pathol*. 1983;7:739-745.
116. Kubo M, Tsuji H, Kunitomo T, Taguchi K. Syringomatous adenoma of the nipple: a case report. *Breast Cancer*. 2004;11:214-216.
117. Paramaguru R, Ramkumar S. Syringomatous adenoma of the nipple in a male breast: a case report with a brief review of literature and histomorphological approach to diagnosis. *Cureus*. 2021;13:e19586.
118. Mrklic I, Bezic J, Pogorelic Z, et al. Synchronous bilateral infiltrating syringomatous adenoma of the breast. *Scott Med J*. 2012;57:121.
119. Montgomery ND, Bianchi GD, Klauber-Demore N, Budwit DA. Bilateral syringomatous adenomas of the nipple: case report with immunohistochemical characterization of a rare tumor mimicking malignancy. *Am J Clin Pathol*. 2014;141: 727-731.
120. Owall L, Mygind H, Rosenborg A, Lænkholm AV. Syringomatous tumour presenting as inversion of a supernumerary nipple. *Case Rep Pathol*. 2019;2019: 9461815.
121. Page RN, Dittrich L, King R, Boulos F, Page DL. Syringomatous adenoma of the nipple occurring within a supernumerary breast: a case report. *J Cutan Pathol*. 2009;36:1206-1209.
122. AlSharif S, Tremblay F, Omeroglu A, Altinel G, Sun S, Mesurolle B. Infiltrating syringomatous adenoma of the nipple: sonographic and mammographic features with pathologic correlation. *J Clin Ultrasound*. 2014;42:427-429.
123. Kim HM, Park BW, Han SH, et al. Infiltrating syringomatous adenoma presenting as microcalcification in the nipple on screening mammogram: case report and review of the literature of radiologic features. *Clin Imaging*. 2010;34: 462-465.
124. Odashiro M, Lima MG, Miiji LN, et al. Infiltrating syringomatous adenoma of the nipple. *Breast J*. 2009;15:414-416.
125. Rosen PP, Ernsberger D. Low-grade adenosquamous carcinoma. A variant of metaplastic mammary carcinoma. *Am J Surg Pathol*. 1987;11:351-358.
126. Carter E, Dyess DL. Infiltrating syringomatous adenoma of the nipple: a case report and 20-year retrospective review. *Breast J*. 2004;10:443-447.
127. Jones MW, Norris HJ, Snyder RC. Infiltrating syringomatous adenoma of the nipple. A clinical and pathological study of 11 cases. *Am J Surg Pathol*. 1989;13:197-201.
128. Gangane N, Joshi D, Anshu, Shivkumar VB. Cytological diagnosis of collagenous spherulosis of breast associated with fibroadenoma: report of a case with review of literature. *Diagn Cytopathol*. 2007;35:366-369.
129. Ohta M, Mori M, Kawada T, Maegawa H, Yamamoto S, Imamura Y. Collagenous spherulosis associated with adenomyoepithelioma of the breast: a case report. *Acta Cytol*. 2010;54:314-318.
130. Reis-Filho JS, Fulford LG, Crebassa B, Carpentier S, Lakhani SR. Collagenous spherulosis in an adenomyoepithelioma of the breast. *J Clin Pathol*. 2004;57:83-86.
131. Resetkova E, Albarracin C, Sneige N. Collagenous spherulosis of breast: morphologic study of 59 cases and review of the literature. *Am J Surg Pathol*. 2006; 30:20-27.
132. Hill P, Cawson J. Collagenous spherulosis presenting as a mass lesion on imaging. *Breast J*. 2008;14:301-303.
133. Clement PB, Young RH, Azzopardi JG. Collagenous spherulosis of the breast. *Am J Surg Pathol*. 1987;11:411-417.

134. Rosen PP. Adenoid cystic carcinoma of the breast. A morphologically heterogeneous neoplasm. *Pathol Annu*. 1989;24 Pt 2:237-254.
135. Wells CA, Wells CW, Yeomans P, Viña M, Jordan S, d'Ardenne AJ. Spherical connective tissue inclusions in epithelial hyperplasia of the breast ("collagenous spherulosis"). *J Clin Pathol*. 1990;43:905-908.
136. Highland KE, Finley JL, Neill JS, Silverman JF. Collagenous spherulosis. Report of a case with diagnosis by fine needle aspiration biopsy with immunocytochemical and ultrastructural observations. *Acta Cytol*. 1993;37:3-9.
137. Grignon DJ, Ro JY, Mackay BN, Ordóñez NG, Ayala AG. Collagenous spherulosis of the breast. Immunohistochemical and ultrastructural studies. *Am J Clin Pathol*. 1989;91:386-392.
138. Hill P, Cawson J. Collagenous spherulosis with lobular carcinoma in situ: a potential diagnostic pitfall. *Pathology*. 2007;39:361-363.
139. Cabibi D, Giannone AG, Belmonte B, Aragona F, Aragona F. CD10 and HHF35 actin in the differential diagnosis between collagenous spherulosis and adenoid-cystic carcinoma of the breast. *Pathol Res Pract*. 2012;208: 405-409.
140. Rabban JT, Swain RS, Zaloudek CJ, Chase DR, Chen YY. Immunophenotypic overlap between adenoid cystic carcinoma and collagenous spherulosis of the breast: potential diagnostic pitfalls using myoepithelial markers. *Mod Pathol*. 2006;19:1351-1357.

Adenomyoepithelial and Myoepithelial Neoplasms

RAZA S. HODA AND SYED A. HODA

Myoepithelial cells (MECs) are located between the glandular epithelium and the basement membrane of normal mammary ducts and lobules. These cells are under hormonal influence and have contractile properties (1). It ought to be recognized that MECs are integral to almost all proliferative lesions of the breast (including sclerosing adenosis, and usual as well as papillary ductal hyperplasia). MECs may be reduced or absent around ducts involved in ductal carcinoma in situ (DCIS). Most MECs have spindle cell morphology. MECs with globoid morphology and abundant clear cytoplasm occur physiologically during the luteal phase of the menstrual cycle and are also common as an incidental finding and in sclerosing lesions and in adenomyoepithelial and myoepithelial tumors **(Figs. 5.1-5.3)**. Relative prominence, clear cell change, and hyperplasia of the MECs are also common after radiation. Rarely, myoid transformation of MECs ("myoid metaplasia") can occur, especially in sclerosing lesions. The immunoprofile of MECs is summarized in **Table 5.1**.

Hyperplastic MECs may occasionally mimic atypical lobular hyperplasia (ALH) and classic lobular carcinoma in

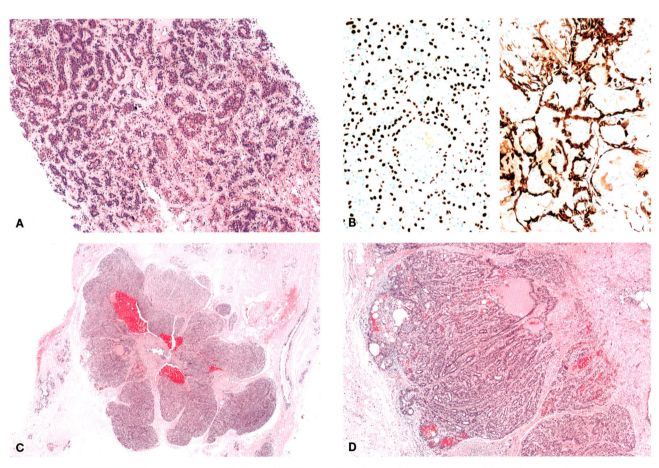

FIGURE 5.1 **Adenomyoepithelioma (AME). A, B:** Needle core biopsy shows an AME. The biphasic appearance of the neoplasm is evident at low-power microscopy. **B:** The myoepithelial cells of this AME are immunoreactive for p63 (left) and smooth muscle myosin heavy chain and calponin (right). **C, D:** The excised AME shows its characteristic circumscription and multinodularity.

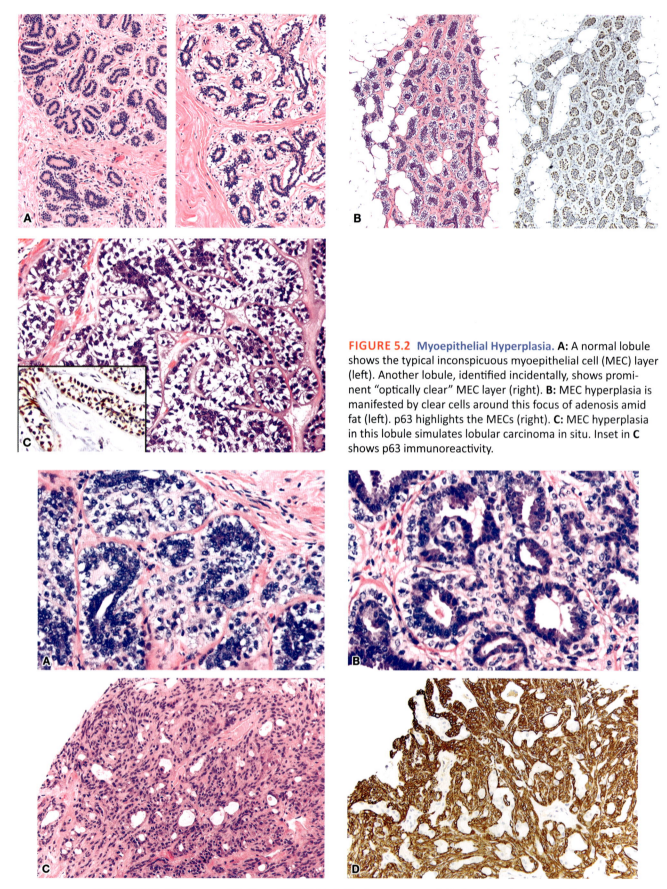

FIGURE 5.2 Myoepithelial Hyperplasia. A: A normal lobule shows the typical inconspicuous myoepithelial cell (MEC) layer (left). Another lobule, identified incidentally, shows prominent "optically clear" MEC layer (right). B: MEC hyperplasia is manifested by clear cells around this focus of adenosis amid fat (left). p63 highlights the MECs (right). C: MEC hyperplasia in this lobule simulates lobular carcinoma in situ. Inset in C shows p63 immunoreactivity.

FIGURE 5.3 Adenomyoepithelioma (AME), Variable Appearances. A, B: Prominent myoepithelial cells (MECs) with clear cytoplasm provide contrast to the darker staining epithelial cells. C, D: Spindled MECs surround lesional glands. Smooth muscle myosin heavy chain (SMMHC) (D) highlights the former.

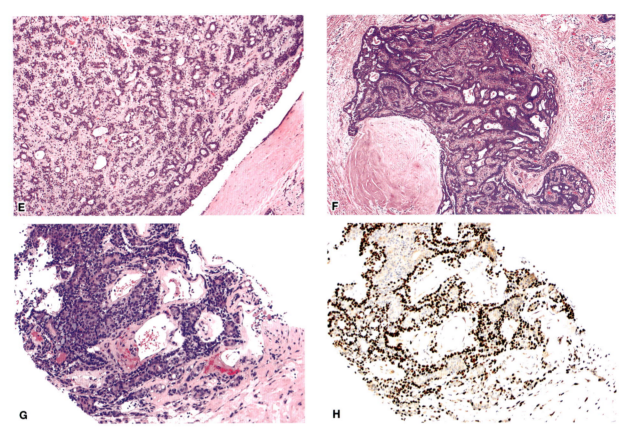

FIGURE 5.3 (*continued*) **E:** This "intraductal" AME was mistaken for a conventional intraductal papilloma. Note the fibrous inactive ductal wall (right). **F:** A densely sclerotic AME mistaken for sclerosing papilloma. **G, H:** A well-vascularized AME shows inconspicuous "biphasic" growth. p63 highlights the MECs **(H)**.

situ (LCIS). The circumferential distribution along the periphery of the acini is usually sufficient for the identification of MECs. E-cadherin staining of MECs yields either negative or weak membranous reactivity. The latter pattern of E-cadherin staining in MECs should not be misdiagnosed as aberrant expression of E-cadherin in ALH or classic LCIS. Immunohistochemical stains for MEC markers can be used to resolve problematic cases.

Neoplasms associated with MECs include adenomyoepithelioma (and malignancies associated with it), pleomorphic adenoma (MT), myoepithelioma, and myoepithelial carcinoma.

ADENOMYOEPITHELIOMA

Adenomyoepithelioma (AME) is a rare benign biphasic mammary neoplasm composed of epithelial ("luminal") and myoepithelial ("basal") cells (2). Other than a few relatively small series (3-6), most reports of AME are case studies. Some AME have atypical features (atypical AME). Rarely, carcinoma can arise in an AME.

AMEs tend to occur in postmenopausal women and are uncommon in young women (3,4). Rare examples of AME have been described in men (7,8).

AME has no documented familial association. A 41-year-old woman with neurofibromatosis type 1 and multiple gastrointestinal stromal tumors had a "malignant myoepithelioma" (ie, myoepithelial carcinoma) arising in an AME, but no other family member was affected (9).

AME typically presents as a solitary and painless mass. The tumor can arise in the center or at the periphery of the breast. Nipple discharge is uncommon. Patients with carcinoma (epithelial and/or myoepithelial) in an AME may describe recent rapid growth of a long-standing lesion.

Mammographically, AME usually appears as a single mass with well circumscribed to lobulated borders. The mammographic appearance often suggests a fibroadenoma (10-13). Mammographic calcifications are rare (12,14-16). On ultrasound examination, AME appears as a solid, round, or oval mass with hypo- or complex echogenic texture (10,14). The edge of the tumor is typically smooth or lobulated and rarely irregular (10,14). Posterior acoustic enhancement may be present (10,14). Hypervascularity in the vicinity of an AME has been reported (17). Associated duct ectasia is common. Mammographically inapparent AMEs can be detected by sonography (11,14). Information on the MRI features of AME is limited. Homogeneous to heterogeneous enhancement with a delayed washout pattern is reported (10,14).

AME has a mean and median size of about 2.5 cm (range: 0.5-8.0), although recently reported cases tend to be smaller. Most AMEs are solid, well circumscribed, and firm. Some AMEs are intracystic (4,5,14,18,19).

TABLE 5.1
Immunohistochemical Markers for Myoepithelial Cells

Marker	Cytoplasm	Nucleus
Calponin[a]	Positive	Negative
CD10[a]	Positive	Negative
Caldesmon	Positive	Negative
Cytokeratin, basal[b]	Positive	Negative
D2-40	Positive	Negative
DOG-1	Positive	Negative
MSA[a]	Positive	Negative
p40	Negative	Positive
p63	Negative	Positive
SMA[a]	Positive	Negative
SMM-HC[a]	Positive	Negative
SOX-10	Negative	Positive
WT-1	Negative	Positive

Less commonly utilized myoepithelial immunostains include maspin, caveolin, nestin, stratifin (14-3-3 sigma), and P-cadherin. E-cadherin can show weak immunoreactivity in myoepithelial cells. Estrogen receptor, progesterone receptor, HER2, androgen receptor, GCDFP-15 are typically negative in myoepithelial cells. CD, cluster designation; DOG-1, discovered on GIST 1; EMA, epithelial membrane antigen; MSA, muscle-specific actin; SMA, smooth muscle actin; SMMHC, smooth muscle myosin heavy chain; SOX-10, SRY-Box transcription factor 10; WT, Wilms tumor.
[a]May be immunoreactive in myofibroblasts.
[b]Cytokeratins 5, 5/6, 14, 17, 34BE12. These cytokeratins can be expressed in some normal and hyperplastic epithelial cells.

AME is a circumscribed tumor, related to intraductal papilloma, devoid of a fibrous capsule. Most lesions consist of an aggregate of solid or papillary nodules (Fig. 5.1). AME bears some morphologic resemblance to papilloma and "ductal adenoma" (18,20,21). The latter neoplasm (a circumscribed biphasic tumor) refers to a densely sclerotic intraductal papilloma. A few AMEs appear to arise from a lobular proliferation or areas of adenomyoepithelial hyperplasia in adenosis (Fig. 5.2). An AME consists of closely juxtaposed small glands and tubules composed of cuboidal epithelial cells and MECs. The MECs of an AME are often polygonal or spindle shaped with strikingly clear or eosinophilic cytoplasm. The juxtaposition of the darker staining cytoplasm of the epithelial cells and the pale ("optically clear") cytoplasm of MECs is a helpful clue to the diagnosis (Fig. 5.3). Rarely, the lesional MECs can show plasmacytoid features—with eccentrically placed nuclei. Apocrine metaplasia of the glandular epithelium is common, particularly in papillary areas. Squamous metaplasia can be florid, especially in foci of infarction, and can raise the differential diagnosis of squamous cell carcinoma **(Fig. 5.4)**. Sebaceous **(Fig. 5.5)** or mucoepidermoid metaplasia can also occur. In some AMEs, MECs with clear cytoplasm are numerous and compress the tubular lumina, resulting in zones virtually devoid of glandular lumina **(Fig. 5.6)**. MECs can undergo myoid metaplasia **(Fig. 5.7)**. Palisading of spindle cells and alveolar clustering of polygonal MECs are common myoid patterns. The glandular elements may be intermixed with myoid areas or overgrown by myoepithelial proliferation. Myoid hyperplasia may give rise to areas with leiomyomatous cytologic features or a storiform ("star-like" or "cartwheel-like") architectural pattern (17). Stromal and myoepithelial elements may have an adenoid cystic pattern. Collagenous spherulosis (22) **(Fig. 5.8)** and cartilaginous metaplasia are rarely encountered. Occasional calcifications are present **(Fig. 5.9)**. Foci of stromal fibrosis or infarct (ie, ischemic necrosis) are rarely associated with coarse calcification.

Immunostains for myoepithelial (Table 5.1) and epithelial cells can be helpful in highlighting the proportion of the two types of cells in AMEs. Of note, the characteristic biphasic pattern of staining is not always evident. There may be considerable intratumoral and intertumoral variation in immunoreactivity with various markers.

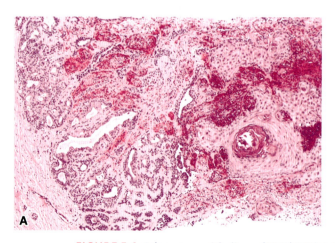 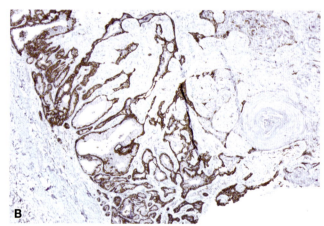

FIGURE 5.4 **Adenomyoepithelioma (AME) With Infarction and Squamous Metaplasia. A, B:** Most of the tumor in this needle core biopsy (NCB) is infarcted. Myoepithelium is highlighted in non-infarcted areas by CD10 immunoreactivity **(B)**.

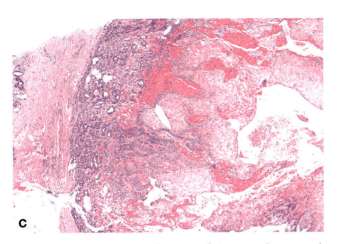
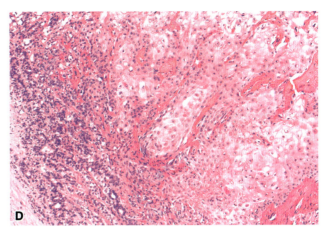

FIGURE 5.4 (*continued*) **C, D:** Another example of a partially infarcted AME with squamous metaplasia in the infarcted area. This NCB had been misinterpreted as a metaplastic squamous cell carcinoma.

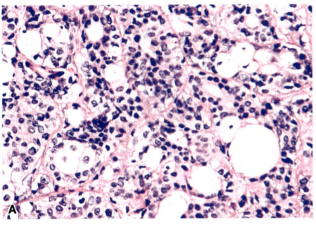
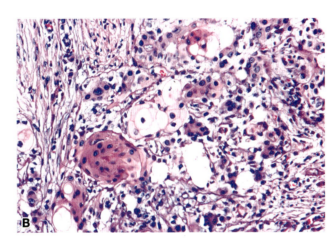
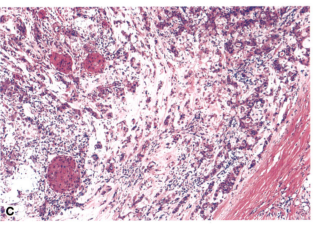

FIGURE 5.5 **Adenomyoepithelial Tumors With Sebaceous and Squamous Differentiation. A, B:** The myoepithelial cells with vacuolated cytoplasm have largely overgrown the epithelial cells in a benign adenomyoepithelioma (AME). Sebaceous **(A, B)** and squamous **(B)** differentiation is evident. **C:** Squamous metaplasia is seen in this malignant AME.

Mixed Tumor (Pleomorphic Adenoma)

Mixed tumor (MT) (pleomorphic adenoma) of the breast (23-27) is a variant of AME. It occurs more frequently in the subareolar region (25,26). Most MTs are solid and circumscribed. The matrix of a mammary MT can be loosely myxoid **(Fig. 5.10)** or collagenized and occasionally shows chondroid or osseous metaplasia. Calcification and ossification can occur. Foci resembling hypercellular MT of the salivary glands and a distinct papillary component can occur. Squamous and/or sebaceous metaplasia may be encountered. Although MT is rare in human breasts, it is a relatively common neoplasm in those of female dogs.

Atypical Adenomyoepithelioma

Atypical features in an AME include mitotic activity (~5 mitoses/10 high-power fields) in the epithelium and/or myoepithelium (6), focal nuclear pleomorphism, nuclear hyperchromasia, and occasional multinucleated cells. Apocrine

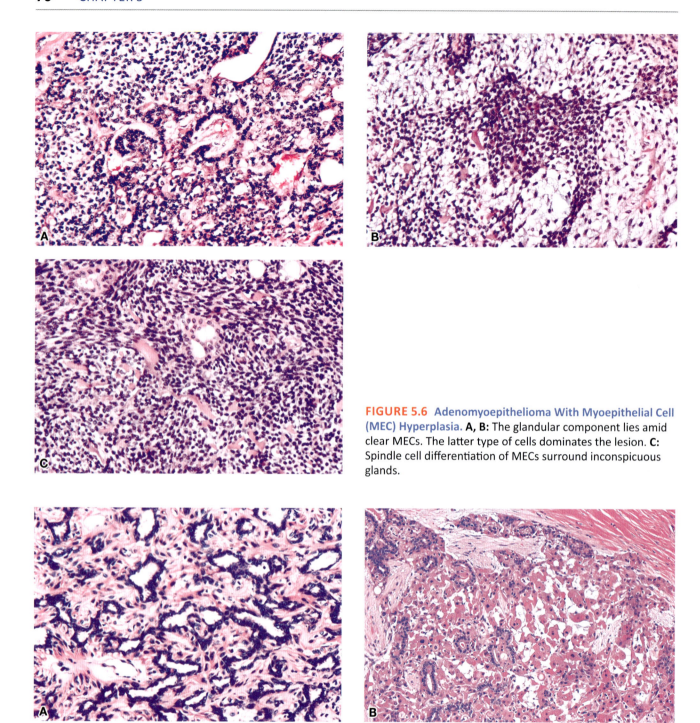

FIGURE 5.6 Adenomyoepithelioma With Myoepithelial Cell (MEC) Hyperplasia. A, B: The glandular component lies amid clear MECs. The latter type of cells dominates the lesion. C: Spindle cell differentiation of MECs surround inconspicuous glands.

FIGURE 5.7 Adenomyoepithelioma (AME) With Myoid Differentiation. A: The spindly myoepithelial cells (MECs) in this lesion have a myoid phenotype with *subtle* eosinophilic cytoplasm. B: The polygonal MECs in another AME have *prominent* eosinophilic cytoplasm.

atypia is a common finding in an atypical AME. Cytologic atypia is more common in AMEs in which MECs have spindle cell, myoid, or clear appearance.

Carcinoma (Epithelial and/or Myoepithelial) Arising in AME

Carcinomatous transformation in an AME can be limited to either the epithelial or the myoepithelial component or can involve both elements **(Figs. 5.11 and 5.12)**. The diagnosis of (adeno)carcinoma arising in an AME applies when only the epithelium is malignant. When only the myoepithelium is malignant, the diagnosis of myoepithelial carcinoma in an AME is appropriate. *A malignant neoplasm with myoepithelial differentiation not arising in an AME is classified as metaplastic carcinoma* (see Chapter 13). The term malignant AME ought to be reserved for exceedingly rare biphasic neoplasms in which both epithelial and myoepithelial components are carcinomatous.

High mitotic activity, necrosis, cellular pleomorphism, overgrowth of myoepithelium or epithelium, and invasion at

ADENOMYOEPITHELIAL AND MYOEPITHELIAL NEOPLASMS

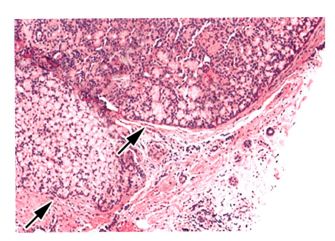

FIGURE 5.8 Adenomyoepithelioma (AME) With Collagenous Spherulosis. AME in this needle core biopsy shows prominent collagenous spherulosis (arrows).

the periphery of the tumor are features of a malignant AME. Carcinomatous AMEs with a biphasic growth pattern in the breast, and at their metastatic sites, have been reported (28-32).

Various histologic types of carcinoma associated with AME have been described, including adenoid cystic carcinoma (33), low-grade adenosquamous carcinoma (34,35), squamous carcinoma (35), sarcomatoid carcinoma (35), undifferentiated carcinoma (36), invasive ductal carcinoma (37), undifferentiated carcinoma with heterologous (osteogenic and spindle cell) differentiation (38), and myoepithelial carcinoma (39-41).

Myoepithelial carcinoma (**Fig. 5.11**) is the result of malignant overgrowth of the myoepithelial component of an AME. It consists of spindle and/or epithelioid cells with high mitotic activity and cytologic atypia (39-42). Necrosis is common.

The immunophenotype of malignant MECs is sometimes different from that of benign MECs. Malignant MECs are not necessarily reactive for all MEC markers. Therefore, a panel of immunostains should be used to maximize the detection of MECs. Inclusion of calponin and p63 stains is recommended in this regard.

The epithelium of a benign AME usually displays some nuclear reactivity for estrogen receptor (ER), whereas progesterone receptor (PR) is typically absent. The MECs of an AME do not express ER and PR. Carcinomas arising in AMEs, whether consisting of only epithelial or

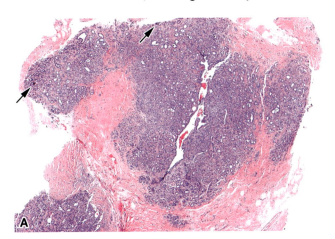
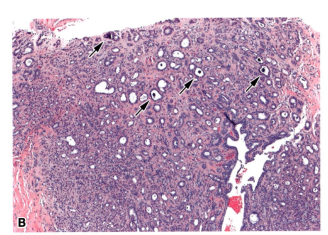

FIGURE 5.9 Adenomyoepithelioma (AME) With Calcifications. A, B: The AME in this needle core biopsy harbors deposits of calcifications (arrows).

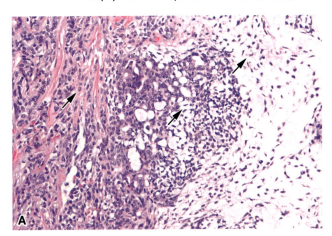
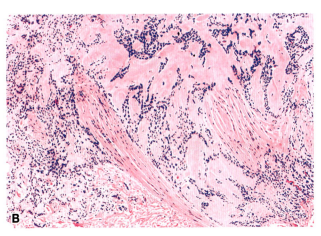

FIGURE 5.10 Mixed Tumor (MT, Pleomorphic Adenoma) and Myoepithelioma. A: This MT (pleomorphic adenoma) of the breast consists of epithelial and myoepithelial cells (MECs) without evidence of atypia. The MECs are mainly spindly (arrows) and lie amid a myxoid matrix. **B:** This myoepithelioma shows uniform spindled MECs infiltrating fibrous stroma. The lesional cells were immunoreactive with p63 and calponin (neither shown here).

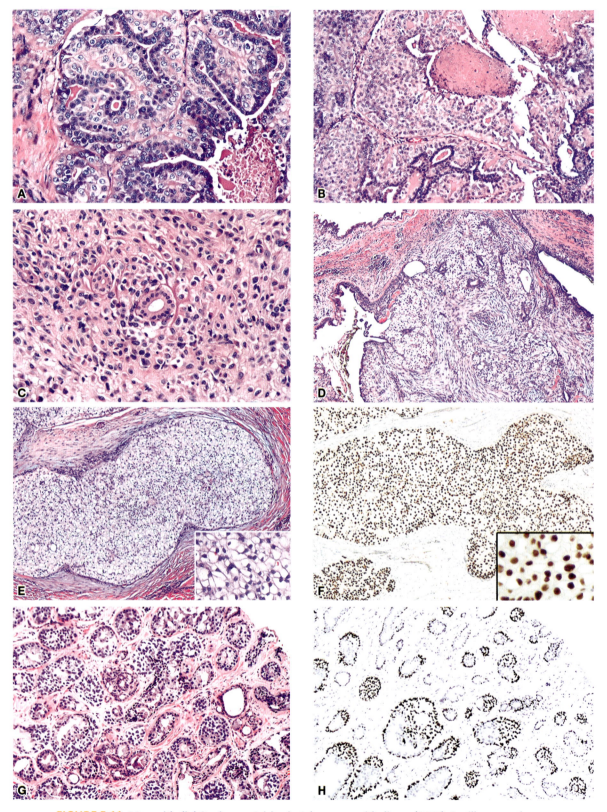

FIGURE 5.11 Myoepithelial Carcinoma Arising in Adenomyoepithelioma (AME), Papilloma, and Adenosis. A-D: Proliferating epithelioid myoepithelial cells (MECs) with large vesicular nuclei are indicative of malignancy in this AME. **A:** Note focal necrosis in lower right corner. **B:** Sheets of neoplastic MECs surround another necrotic focus. Residual glands are evident. **C:** Invasive myoepithelial carcinoma surrounds benign glands (center). The tumor cells have eosinophilic cytoplasm. **D, E:** Intraductal myoepithelial carcinoma in a sclerosing papilloma **(D)** and in adjacent ducts **(E)**. Inset in **E** shows the clear cytoplasm in the cells of myoepithelial carcinoma. **F:** Nuclear immunoreactivity for p63 in the intraductal myoepithelial carcinoma. Inset in **F** shows detail. **G-H:** Intraductal myoepithelial carcinoma arising in adenosis. Nuclear p63 immunoreactivity in the neoplastic MECs **(H)**.

myoepithelial carcinoma or of the combination of the two, are usually negative for both ER and PR (31,32,43), and for HER2 (32,43).

Prognosis and Management of Benign and Atypical Myoepithelial Lesions

Most AMEs are benign tumors that can be treated by local excision (4). Local recurrence has been reported, usually more than 2 years after the initial excision (3,5,44). In some cases, recurrence of AME (4,44) could be attributed to incomplete excision, possibly related to multinodularity and peripheral intraductal extension (4). There is no evidence that cytologic atypia or the proportions of spindle or clear or polygonal MECs are related to local recurrence. Carcinoma may be detected as a separate lesion coincidentally or subsequent to excision of an AME (5). Mastectomy, radiation, and axillary dissection are not appropriate treatments for benign or atypical AME.

Nadelman et al (45) reported two morphologically "benign" AMEs that developed lung metastases with the same histologic appearance as the primary tumors. These two cases are most unusual. One of the mammary AMEs had been sampled by needle core biopsy (NCB), and the possibility of tumor dissemination secondary to this needling procedure cannot be entirely ruled out in this case.

Wiens et al studied the outcome in 24 patients with adenomyoepithelial neoplasms (12 of which were histologically confirmed to be benign in 6, atypical in 3, and malignant in 3) (46). Eleven lesions were excised. Mean follow-up was 44 months (range 1-138 months) during which no case recurred. Notably, two patients with benign AME had concurrent contralateral breast carcinoma. One patient with malignant AME died with metastatic disease.

Moritz et al reported follow-up in 13 cases of AME and one malignant AME (47). Clinical follow-up (mean: 75 months) was obtained for all but one case. Five patients underwent mastectomy. No recurrences were noted. Three benign AME were associated with breast carcinoma. The case of malignant AME had a synchronous malignant phyllodes tumor. The authors concluded that conservative excision with attainment of negative margins seems appropriate treatment for AME.

Carcinoma (Epithelial and/or Myoepithelial) Arising in AME

Carcinoma arising in AMEs is treated as any other type of breast carcinoma of similar grade and stage. Some such carcinomatous tumors have recurred locally (3,29,36-38,43,48) or resulted in distant metastases and fatal outcome (30-32,36-40). Metastatic sites include lung (31,38), liver (40), bone (39), thyroid gland (30), brain (37), and kidney (32). Some patients developed distant metastases a few months after primary diagnosis (31,36,39), whereas others developed metastatic disease 12 years (30) and 15 years (37) after diagnosis of the primary tumor.

Differential Diagnosis of Adenomyoepithelial and Myoepithelial Lesions

Myoepitheliosis refers to an incidental, focal, minute (non–mass forming) finding with a relative increase in the number of MECs vis-à-vis epithelial cells in normal lobules or in foci of sclerosing adenosis. **Adenomyoepitheliosis** is another incidental, focal, non–mass forming lesion with increased numbers of *both* myoepithelial and epithelial cells. At higher power microscopic examination, adenomyoepitheliosis is similar to AME—and the relationship between these two lesions is unclear at this time.

In an NCB sample, clear cell epithelioid myoepithelial hyperplasia in an AME with an adenosis pattern could be mistaken for **invasive carcinoma** (Fig. 5.12). Benign AME in which glandular elements are dispersed amid spindled MECs can also be mistaken for invasive carcinoma (49). The differential diagnosis of a **mixed tumor** (pleomorphic adenoma) includes **metaplastic carcinoma** with myxoid/chondroid matrix (50). Metaplastic carcinoma shows cytologic atypia, hypercellularity, necrosis, mitotic activity, and relative overgrowth of the neoplastic epithelial component. The definitive diagnosis of mammary MT (pleomorphic adenoma) in an NCB sample is not possible, and excision of the lesion is essential to rule out metaplastic carcinoma. The myxoid matrix of a mammary MT (pleomorphic adenoma), especially when abundant, can occasionally simulate **mucinous carcinoma** (27,51). The spindle cell component of an AME or myoepithelial carcinoma arising in an AME can simulate a **phyllodes tumor**. AME lacks frond-like architecture.

Rarely, **syringomatous adenoma of the nipple with myxochondroid stroma** may raise the differential diagnosis of a mammary MT. Usually, syringomatous adenoma is based in the dermis and not in the breast parenchyma. Lastly, several MEC–associated tumors that are primary in the **salivary glands** can arise in the breast. Such tumors show similar histopathologic features in these two locations, although the clinical behavior thereof may differ. The latter is exemplified by adenoid cystic carcinoma, which usually has a relatively high proclivity to metastasize when it arises in salivary glands and typically has a better outcome in the breast (52).

Myoepithelioma is an extremely rare tumor comprising benign MECs. Tumors referred to as muscular (53) and myoid hamartomas (54) probably arise from myoepithelial hyperplasia with myoid transformation. Most myoepitheliomas (including myoid hamartomas) are reported in peri- and postmenopausal women (53-59). Men are not affected. A myoepithelioma consists of bundles of benign spindle cells sometimes arranged in a storiform pattern (Fig. 5.10). The cytoplasm tends to be eosinophilic or sometimes clear; however, it may also be inconspicuous. The lesional cells are immunoreactive for the usual MEC markers. Mitoses are exceedingly rare or absent.

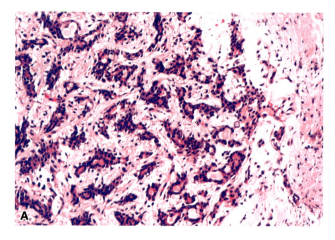
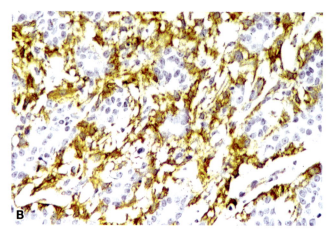
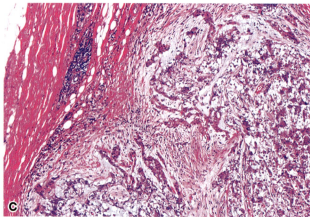

FIGURE 5.12 Adenomyoepithelioma (AME) Mistaken for Carcinoma (A) and Malignant AME (B). A: This needle core biopsy from an AME was misinterpreted as invasive ductal carcinoma. The markedly "optically clear" myoepithelial cells (MECs) are difficult to recognize between the somewhat unevenly shaped glands—resulting in an appearance that simulates invasive carcinoma. Please see **C** for comparison. **B:** The excisional biopsy of the lesion showed a circumscribed nodule richly endowed with CD10-positive MECs. **C:** An invasive malignant AME is shown for comparison, with stromal invasion by both components: epithelial (darker) and myoepithelial (clear) cells.

Pure spindle cell myoepithelial tumors may be difficult to distinguish by light microscopy from other spindle cell mammary neoplasms. The differential diagnosis includes myofibroblastoma, metaplastic carcinoma, and primary spindle cell sarcomas (especially leiomyosarcoma). Some lesions reported in the past as myoepithelioma with peripheral infiltration into the surrounding fat might have been unrecognized examples of low-grade metaplastic spindle cell carcinoma (also see Chapter 13). Excision is required for any neoplasm showing spindle cell proliferation with myoepithelial differentiation in NCB material.

Molecular Pathology Aspects

In molecular terms, epithelial/myoepithelial neoplasms have been studied more in the salivary glands than in the breast (60). Rakha et al have provided a brief overview of genetic alterations in this group of tumors (61).

In general, benign AMEs have a low mutation burden and a low number of copy number alterations. Most ER-negative AMEs show concurrent mutations affecting the *HRAS Q61* hotspot and *PI3K* pathway genes, and immunostains for RAS Q61R can be useful in the diagnostic workup of ER-negative mammary AMEs (62). Ginter et al studied the molecular pathology of seven mammary AMEs via Oncomine Comprehensive Assay v3 (63). These cases included one benign, two atypical, one in situ, and three invasive. Two atypical AMEs and the malignant in situ AME harbored the same gain-of-function phosphoinositide 3-kinase (*PI3K*) mutation. The malignant in situ AME also showed *EGFR* amplification. The same gain-of-function *HRAS* mutation was present in an atypical AME and in a malignant invasive AME. No fusion drivers were detected. The authors concluded that alterations in *PI3K/AKT* and other pathways could provide the option of targeted therapy in malignant mammary AMEs.

REFERENCES

1. Pandey PR, Saidou J, Watabe K. Role of myoepithelial cells in breast tumor progression. *Front Biosci.* 2010;15:226-236.
2. Hamperl H. The myothelia (myoepithelial cells): normal state; regressive changes; hyperplasia; tumors. *Curr Top Pathol.* 1970;53:161-220.
3. Loose JH, Patchefsky AS, Hollander IJ, Lavin LS, Cooper HS, Katz SM. Adenomyoepithelioma of the breast: a spectrum of biologic behavior. *Am J Surg Pathol.* 1992;16:868-876.
4. Rosen PP. Adenomyoepithelioma of the breast. *Hum Pathol.* 1987;18:1232-1237.
5. Tavassoli FA. Myoepithelial lesions of the breast: myoepitheliosis, adenomyoepithelioma, and myoepithelial carcinoma. *Am J Surg Pathol.* 1991;15:554-568.
6. McLaren BK, Smith J, Schuyler PA, Dupont WD, Page DL. Adenomyoepithelioma: clinical, histologic, and immunohistologic evaluation of a series of related lesions. *Am J Surg Pathol.* 2005;29:1294-1299.
7. Tamura G, Monma N, Suzuki Y, Satodate R, Abe H. Adenomyoepithelioma (myoepithelioma) of the breast in a male. *Hum Pathol.* 1993;24:678-681.
8. Berna JD, Arcas I, Ballester A, Bas A. Adenomyoepithelioma of the breast in a male. *AJR Am J Roentgenol.* 1997;169:917-918.
9. Hegyi L, Thway K, Newton R, et al. Malignant myoepithelioma arising in adenomyoepithelioma of the breast and coincident multiple gastrointestinal stromal tumours in a patient with neurofibromatosis type 1. *J Clin Pathol.* 2009;62:653-655.
10. Adejolu M, Wu Y, Santiago L, Yang WT. Adenomyoepithelial tumors of the breast: imaging findings with histopathologic correlation. *AJR Am J Roentgenol.* 2011;197:W184-W190.

11. Chang A, Bassett L, Bose S. Adenomyoepithelioma of the breast: a cytologic dilemma: report of a case and review of the literature. *Diagn Cytopathol.* 2002;26:191-196.
12. Iyengar P, Ali SZ, Brogi E. Fine-needle aspiration cytology of mammary adenomyoepithelioma: a study of 12 patients. *Cancer.* 2006;108:250-256.
13. Mercado CL, Toth HK, Axelrod D, Cangiarella J. Fine-needle aspiration biopsy of benign adenomyoepithelioma of the breast: radiologic and pathologic correlation in four cases. *Diagn Cytopathol.* 2007;35:690-694.
14. Lee JH, Kim SH, Kang BJ, Lee AW, Song BJ. Ultrasonographic features of benign adenomyoepithelioma of the breast. *Korean J Radiol.* 2010;11:522-527.
15. Han JS, Peng Y. Multicentric adenomyoepithelioma of the breast with atypia and associated ductal carcinoma in situ. *Breast J.* 2010;16:547-549.
16. Howlett DC, Mason CH, Biswas S, Sangle PD, Rubin G, Allan SM. Adenomyoepithelioma of the breast: spectrum of disease with associated imaging and pathology. *AJR Am J Roentgenol.* 2003;180:799-803.
17. Park YM, Park JS, Jung HS, Yoon HK, Yang WT. Imaging features of benign adenomyoepithelioma of the breast. *J Clin Ultrasound.* 2013;41:218-223.
18. Gusterson BA, Sloane JP, Middwood C, et al. Ductal adenoma of the breast—a lesion exhibiting a myoepithelial/epithelial phenotype. *Histopathology.* 1987;11:103-110.
19. Hikino H, Kodama K, Yasui K, Ozaki N, Nagaoka S, Miura H. Intracystic adenomyoepithelioma of the breast—case report and review. *Breast Cancer.* 2007;14:429-433.
20. Guarino M, Reale D, Squillaci S, Micoli G. Ductal adenoma of the breast: an immunohistochemical study of five cases. *Pathol Res Pract.* 1993;189:515-520.
21. Jensen ML, Johansen P, Noer H, Sørensen IM. Ductal adenoma of the breast: the cytological features of six cases. *Diagn Cytopathol.* 1994;10:143-145.
22. Reis-Filho JS, Fulford LG, Crebassa B, Carpentier S, Lakhani SR. Collagenous spherulosis in an adenomyoepithelioma of the breast. *J Clin Pathol.* 2004;57:83-86.
23. Chen KT. Pleomorphic adenoma of the breast. *Am J Clin Pathol.* 1990;93:792-794.
24. Diaz NM, McDivitt RW, Wick MR. Pleomorphic adenoma of the breast: a clinicopathologic and immunohistochemical study of 10 cases. *Hum Pathol.* 1991;22:1206-1214.
25. Narita T, Matsuda K. Pleomorphic adenoma of the breast: case report and review of the literature. *Pathol Int.* 1995;45:441-447.
26. Nevado M, Lopez JI, Dominguez MP, Ballestin C, Garcia H. Pleomorphic adenoma of the breast: case report. *APMIS.* 1991;99:866-868.
27. Reid-Nicholson M, Bleiweiss I, Pace B, Azueta V, Jaffer S. Pleomorphic adenoma of the breast: a case report and distinction from mucinous carcinoma. *Arch Pathol Lab Med.* 2003;127:474-477.
28. Trojani M, Guiu M, Trouette H, De Mascarel I, Cocquet M. Malignant adenomyoepithelioma of the breast: an immunohistochemical, cytophotometric, and ultrastructural study of a case with lung metastases. *Am J Clin Pathol.* 1992;98:598-602.
29. Qureshi A, Kayani N, Gulzar R. Malignant adenomyoepithelioma of the breast: a case report with review of literature. *BMJ Case Rep.* 2009;2009:bcr01.2009.1442.
30. Bult P, Verwiel JM, Wobbes T, Kooy-Smits MM, Biert J, Holland R. Malignant adenomyoepithelioma of the breast with metastasis in the thyroid gland 12 years after excision of the primary tumor: case report and review of the literature. *Virchows Arch.* 2000;436:158-166.
31. Kihara M, Yokomise H, Irie A, Kobayashi S, Kushida Y, Yamauchi A. Malignant adenomyoepithelioma of the breast with lung metastases: report of a case. *Surg Today.* 2001;31:899-903.
32. Honda Y, Iyama K. Malignant adenomyoepithelioma of the breast combined with invasive lobular carcinoma. *Pathol Int.* 2009;59:179-184.
33. Van Dorpe J, De Pauw A, Moerman P. Adenoid cystic carcinoma arising in an adenomyoepithelioma of the breast. *Virchows Arch.* 1998;432:119-122.
34. Van Hoeven KH, Drudis T, Cranor ML, Erlandson RA, Rosen PP. Low-grade adenosquamous carcinoma of the breast: a clinocopathologic study of 32 cases with ultrastructural analysis. *Am J Surg Pathol.* 1993;17:248-258.
35. Foschini MP, Pizzicannella G, Peterse JL, Eusebi V. Adenomyoepithelioma of the breast associated with low-grade adenosquamous and sarcomatoid carcinomas. *Virchows Arch.* 1995;427:243-250.
36. Michal M, Baumruk L, Burger J, Manhalová M. Adenomyoepithelioma of the breast with undifferentiated carcinoma component. *Histopathology.* 1994;24:274-276.
37. Rasbridge SA, Millis RR. Adenomyoepithelioma of the breast with malignant features. *Virchows Arch.* 1998;432:123-130.

38. Simpson RH, Cope N, Skálová A, Michal M. Malignant adenomyoepithelioma of the breast with mixed osteogenic, spindle cell, and carcinomatous differentiation. *Am J Surg Pathol.* 1998;22:631-636.
39. Chen PC, Chen CK, Nicastri AD, Wait RB. Myoepithelial carcinoma of the breast with distant metastasis and accompanied by adenomyoepitheliomas. *Histopathology.* 1994;24:543-548.
40. Jones C, Tooze R, Lakhani SR. Malignant adenomyoepithelioma of the breast metastasizing to the liver. *Virchows Arch.* 2003;442:504-506.
41. Buza N, Zekry N, Charpin C, Tavassoli FA. Myoepithelial carcinoma of the breast: a clinicopathological and immunohistochemical study of 15 diagnostically challenging cases. *Virchows Arch.* 2010;457:337-345.
42. Hungermann D, Buerger H, Oehlschlegel C, Herbst H, Boecker W. Adenomyoepithelial tumours and myoepithelial carcinomas of the breast—a spectrum of monophasic and biphasic tumours dominated by immature myoepithelial cells. *BMC Cancer.* 2005;5:92.
43. Oka K, Sando N, Moriya T, Yatabe Y. Malignant adenomyoepithelioma of the breast with matrix production may be compatible with one variant form of matrix-producing carcinoma: a case report. *Pathol Res Pract.* 2007;203:599-604.
44. Young RH, Clement PB. Adenomyoepithelioma of the breast: a report of three cases and review of the literature. *Am J Clin Pathol.* 1988;89:308-314.
45. Nadelman CM, Leslie KO, Fishbein MC. "Benign" metastasizing adenomyoepithelioma of the breast: a report of 2 cases. *Arch Pathol Lab Med.* 2006;130:1349-1353.
46. Wiens N, Hoffman DI, Huang CY, Nayak A, Tchou J. Clinical characteristics and outcomes of benign, atypical, and malignant breast adenomyoepithelioma: a single institution's experience. *Am J Surg.* 2020;219:651-654.
47. Moritz AW, Wiedenhoefer JF, Profit AP, Jagirdar J. Breast adenomyoepithelioma and adenomyoepithelioma with carcinoma (malignant adenomyoepithelioma) with associated breast malignancies: a case series emphasizing histologic, radiologic, and clinical correlation. *Breast.* 2016;29:132-139.
48. Pauwels C, De Potter C. Adenomyoepithelioma of the breast with features of malignancy. *Histopathology.* 1994;24:94-96.
49. Zhang C, Quddus MR, Sung CJ. Atypical adenomyoepithelioma of the breast: diagnostic problems and practical approaches in core needle biopsy. *Breast J.* 2004;10:154-155.
50. Djakovic A, Engel JB, Geisinger E, Honig A, Tschammler A, Dietl J. Pleomorphic adenoma of the breast initially misdiagnosed as metaplastic carcinoma in preoperative stereotactic biopsy: a case report and review of the literature. *Eur J Gynaecol Oncol.* 2011;32:427-430.
51. Iyengar P, Cody HS III, Brogi E. Pleomorphic adenoma of the breast: case report and review of the literature. *Diagn Cytopathol.* 2005;33:416-420.
52. Marchiò C, Weigelt B, Reis-Filho JS. Adenoid cystic carcinomas of the breast and salivary glands (or "The strange case of Dr Jekyll and Mr Hyde" of exocrine gland carcinomas). *J Clin Pathol.* 2010;63:220-228.
53. Eusebi V, Cunsolo A, Fedeli F, Severi B, Scarani P. Benign smooth muscle cell metaplasia in breast. *Tumori.* 1980;66:643-653.
54. Daroca PJ Jr, Reed RJ, Love GL, Kraus SD. Myoid hamartomas of the breast. *Hum Pathol.* 1985;16:212-219.
55. Erlandson RA, Rosen PP. Infiltrating myoepithelioma of the breast. *Am J Surg Pathol.* 1982;6:785-793.
56. Bigotti G, Di Giorgio CG. Myoepithelioma of the breast: histologic, immunologic, and electromicroscopic appearance. *J Surg Oncol.* 1986;32:58-64.
57. Rode L, Nesland JM, Johannessen JV. A spindle cell breast lesion in a 54-year-old woman. *Ultrastruct Pathol.* 1986;10:421-425.
58. Schurch W, Potvin C, Seemayer TA. Malignant myoepithelioma (myoepithelial carcinoma) of the breast: an ultrastructural and immunocytochemical study. *Ultrastruct Pathol.* 1985;8:1-11.
59. Thorner PS, Kahn HJ, Baumal R, Lee K, Moffatt W. Malignant myoepithelioma of the breast: an immunohistochemical study by light and electron microscopy. *Cancer.* 1986;57:745-750.
60. Foschini MP, Morandi L, Asioli S, Giove G, Corradini AG, Eusebi V. The morphological spectrum of salivary gland type tumours of the breast. *Pathology.* 2017;49:215-227.
61. Rakha E, Tan PH, Ellis I, Quinn C. Adenomyoepithelioma of the breast: a proposal for classification. *Histopathology.* 2021;79:465-479.
62. Pareja F, Toss MS, Geyer FC, et al. Immunohistochemical assessment of HRAS Q61R mutations in breast adenomyoepitheliomas. *Histopathology.* 2020;76:865-874.
63. Ginter PS, McIntire PJ, Kurtis B, et al. Adenomyoepithelial tumors of the breast: molecular underpinnings of a rare entity. *Mod Pathol.* 2020;33:1764-1772.

6

Adenosis and Microglandular Adenosis

RAZA S. HODA AND SYED A. HODA

ADENOSIS

Adenosis ("simple" adenosis) refers to an increase in the number of glands without any significant level of either architectural or cytologic alteration. All forms of adenosis, except microglandular adenosis (MGA), are nonneoplastic lobulocentric proliferations of terminal ducts and lobules lined by epithelium as well as myoepithelium—and are enveloped by basement membrane **(Table 6.1)**. Stromal sclerosis is commonly associated with adenosis, resulting in "sclerosing adenosis" (SA). Coalescent foci of adenosis can form a mass ("adenosis tumor" or "nodular adenosis") (1).

Age and Incidence

Adenosis is usually included in the spectrum of fibrocystic change. The mean age at diagnosis of adenosis tumor in a series of 15 cases (2) was 37 years (range, 21-68); 12 women were premenopausal. There were 88 cases with diagnosis of SA out of a total of 1,166 consecutive needle core biopsies (NCBs) (7.5%) performed over 5 years at one center (3). The mean age of women with NCB diagnosis of SA not associated with carcinoma or atypia was 48 years (range, 35-72); 23 (70%) women were younger than 50 years, and 19 (58%) were 45 to 54 years old. Taskin et al found SA to be present in 76 of 723 (10.5%) breast NCBs as either a major (41 cases) or minor (35 cases) finding (4). Adenosis is exceedingly rare in men.

Symptoms

Adenosis consisting of closely adjacent or merging lobules can form a palpable and/or radiographically detectable mass (2). The mean size of 15 adenosis tumors in one study (2) was 1.9 cm. Patients rarely report pain or tenderness (2,4,5). A 37-year-old woman with bilateral adenosis tumors had palpable and tender masses with indistinct margins in each breast (5). Calcifications are common in adenosis and tend to be minute and clustered, especially in SA.

Imaging

An adenosis tumor can appear as a lobulated solid mass mammographically and by ultrasound examination (2) and can mimic a fibroadenoma. A patient with bilateral adenosis tumors (5) had multiple oval masses with angulated margins, complex posterior acoustic shadowing, and orientation parallel to the skin by ultrasound examination. Mild vascularity was detected on color Doppler ultrasound. On magnetic resonance imaging (MRI), the masses were ovoid with indistinct borders, had intermediate enhancement on T1-weighted and T2-weighted images, and had a homogeneous signal.

Nonpalpable adenosis is usually detected mammographically because of associated calcifications. Gill et al (3) studied the radiologic findings of 44 lesions that yielded SA as the major component in an NCB sample, including 4/44 with ductal carcinoma in situ (DCIS), and 7/44 with atypical ductal hyperplasia (ADH). DCIS in SA was associated with pleomorphic calcifications, and ADH with amorphous calcifications. The 33 NCBs that yielded SA without carcinoma or atypia targeted clustered calcifications (16 cases), mass (15 cases), circumscribed mass with calcifications (1 case), and spiculated mass (1 case).

Microscopic Pathology

Sclerosing Adenosis

SA is the most common form of adenosis. An *adenosis tumor* (nodular adenosis) is a mass lesion formed by closely juxtaposed and/or coalescent foci of adenosis **(Figs. 6.1-6.3)**.

TABLE 6.1

Adenosis: Types and Variants

"Simple" adenosis
SA
Florid adenosis
Tubular adenosis
Blunt duct adenosis
Apocrine adenosis
Atypical apocrine adenosis
ALH and LCIS in SA
ADH and DCIS in SA
SA in fibroepithelial lesions
"Secretory" adenosis
MGA
Atypical MGA
In situ and/or invasive carcinoma associated with MGA

ADH, atypical ductal hyperplasia; ALH, atypical lobular hyperplasia; DCIS, ductal carcinoma in situ; LCIS, lobular carcinoma in situ; MGA, microglandular adenosis; SA, sclerosing adenosis.

ADENOSIS AND MICROGLANDULAR ADENOSIS 83

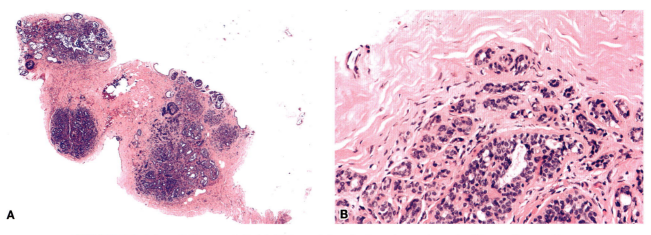

FIGURE 6.1 Adenosis Tumor. A, B: Multiple nodules of adenosis are shown in this needle core biopsy. Larger nodules represent coalescent lobules, such as the one shown in **B**.

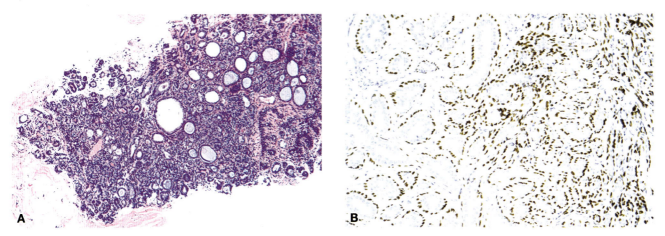

FIGURE 6.2 Adenosis Tumor. A, B: A dense proliferation of hyperplastic epithelial and myoepithelial cells characterizes this lesion. Note the distinct border on the left **(A)** and numerous microcysts. **B:** Myoepithelial hyperplasia is highlighted by nuclear reactivity for p63.

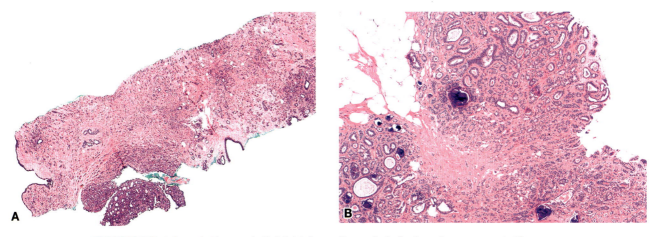

FIGURE 6.3 Adenosis Tumor. A, B: Multiple confluent foci of adenosis are present. Abundant calcifications are shown in **B**.

SA shows variable attenuation of the glandular epithelium, preservation of the myoepithelium, and lobular fibrosis. The glands are arranged in a swirling "organoid" lobulocentric pattern, and the glandular lumina are compressed and often inapparent **(Fig. 6.4)**. The myoepithelium can undergo myoid metaplasia **(Fig. 6.5)**. In some cases, fibrosis separates the glands, resulting in a dispersed pattern that can mimic tubular carcinoma **(Fig. 6.6)**. In general, early SA appears richer in glands and later lesions richer in stroma. It follows that SA tends to have a more glandular pattern in

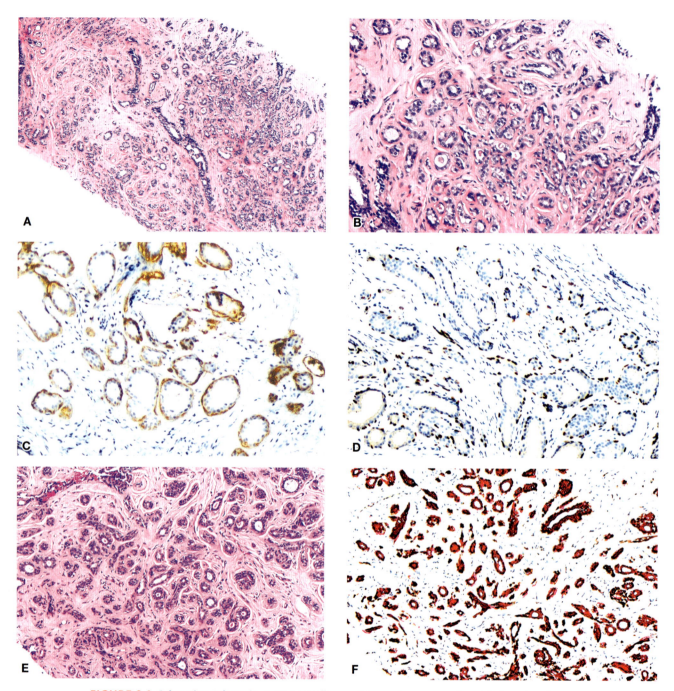

FIGURE 6.4 Sclerosing Adenosis. A, B: A needle core biopsy shows a confluent lesion showing stromal fibrosis, thickened periglandular basement membranes, and atrophy of some glands. **C:** Myoepithelium is highlighted by cytoplasmic reactivity for CD10. **D:** Myoepithelium around adenosis glands is identified by nuclear p63 reactivity. **E, F:** Sclerosing adenosis with features of tubular adenosis. Note relatively elongated tubules. ADH5 immunostain demonstrates presence of myoepithelial cells around each "tubule."

premenopausal women, but sclerosis and epithelial atrophy are common after menopause **(Fig. 6.7)**. Minute calcifications are common **(Fig. 6.8)**.

Florid Adenosis

Florid adenosis is the most cellular form of adenosis with hyperplasia of epithelial and myoepithelial cells **(Fig. 6.9)**. Pregnancy-associated mass-forming florid adenosis can sometimes exhibit apoptosis and mitotic activity **(Fig. 6.10)**. Calcifications are less common and extensive than in SA. Necrosis is rare.

Tubular Adenosis

Tubular adenosis (TA) consists of proliferating, elongated ductules. Most ductules are cut longitudinally and appear as tubules **(Fig. 6.11)**. TA lacks the lobulocentric distribution

ADENOSIS AND MICROGLANDULAR ADENOSIS   85

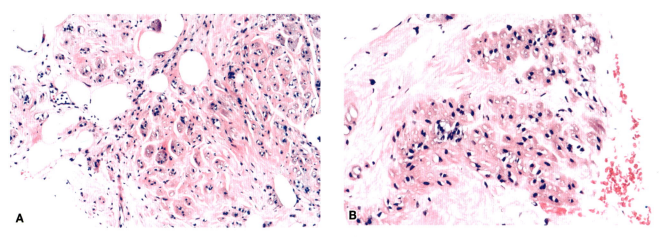

FIGURE 6.5 **Sclerosing Adenosis With Myoid Metaplasia. A, B:** Well-developed myoid metaplasia of myoepithelial cells is shown in this needle core biopsy. Epithelial cells are almost absent, and the myoepithelial cells have the eosinophilic cytoplasm of smooth muscle. **B:** Epithelioid myoid metaplasia of myoepithelium is shown in this sclerosing adenosis.

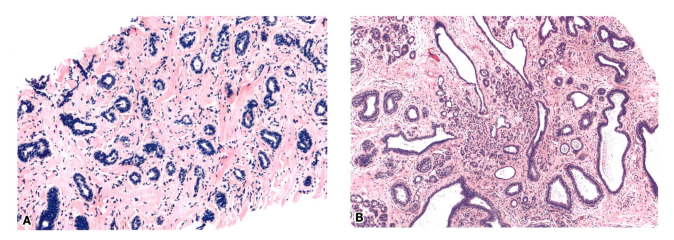

FIGURE 6.6 **Sclerosing Adenosis With Dispersed and Compact Patterns. A:** Glands with round, angular, and tubular shapes are dispersed in collagenous stroma that exhibits pseudoangiomatous hyperplasia. This type of adenosis resembles tubular carcinoma. **B:** Compact pattern of sclerosing adenosis amid dilated ducts with columnar cell change.

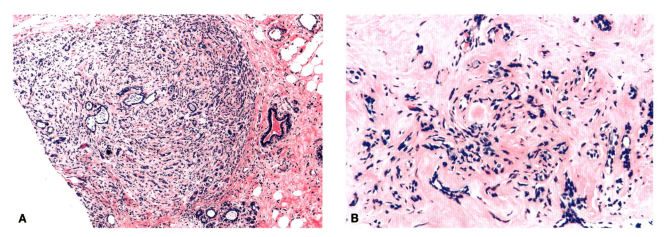

FIGURE 6.7 **Sclerosing Adenosis With Variable Appearances. A:** Atrophic sclerosing adenosis. This needle core biopsy shows nodular atrophic sclerosing adenosis that resembles invasive lobular carcinoma. **B:** Markedly atrophic sclerosing adenosis. There is atrophy of glandular cells, leaving swirling elongated myoepithelial cells.

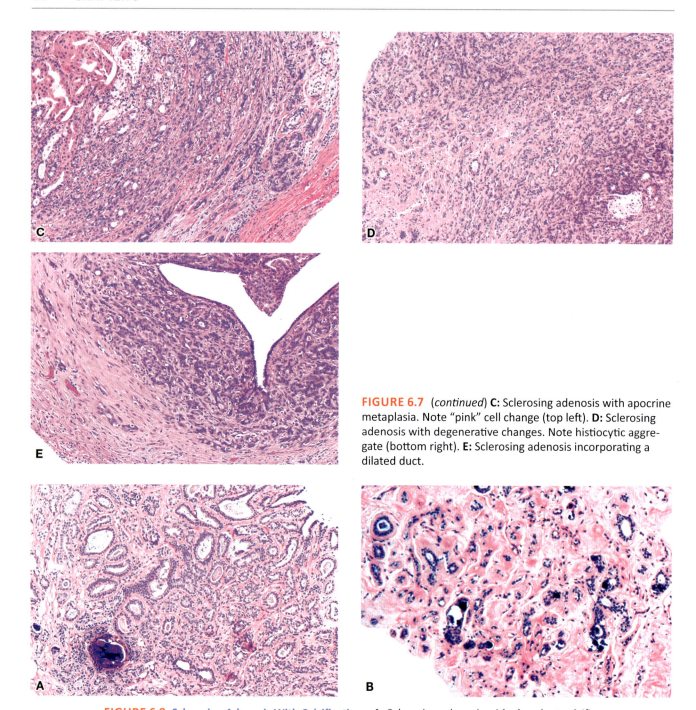

FIGURE 6.7 (*continued*) **C:** Sclerosing adenosis with apocrine metaplasia. Note "pink" cell change (top left). **D:** Sclerosing adenosis with degenerative changes. Note histiocytic aggregate (bottom right). **E:** Sclerosing adenosis incorporating a dilated duct.

FIGURE 6.8 Sclerosing Adenosis With Calcifications. A: Sclerosing adenosis with abundant calcifications. **B:** Sclerosing adenosis with epithelial atrophy and calcifications.

of florid adenosis or SA, and the ductules often extend in a seemingly haphazard pattern into fibrous mammary stroma **(Fig. 6.11)**. Infiltration into adipose tissue is less common. Intraluminal secretion may undergo calcification. The presence of basement membranes and an outer myoepithelial cell layer (6) is useful in separating TA and tubular carcinoma.

Distorted ductules and glands can closely mimic invasive carcinoma in all forms of adenosis. Cystic dilation of ductules or glands is uncommon, but TA tends to show relatively more open lumina. The epithelium lining the tubules and glands is usually inconspicuous, slightly columnar or flat. Signet ring cell morphology or intracytoplasmic vacuoles are exceedingly rare in adenosis. Apocrine metaplasia can involve all forms of adenosis (except MGA). Epithelial mitoses are rare to absent. The myoepithelial cells can be spindled or cuboidal, with conspicuous clear cytoplasm, or attenuated. Perineural invasion may occur **(Fig. 6.12)**. Invasion of the wall of blood vessels by florid adenosis was documented in 10% of cases in one study (7). Lesional necrosis (usually ischemic in origin) occasionally occurs in adenosis tumor, typically during either pregnancy or lactation.

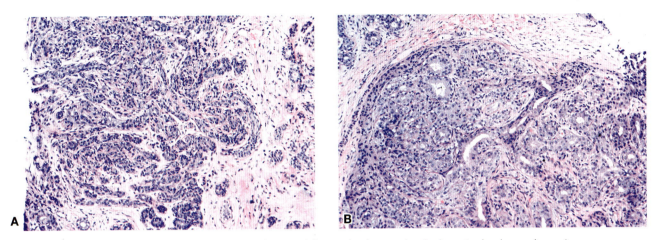

FIGURE 6.9 **Florid Adenosis. A, B:** Elongated, hyperplastic, entwined adenosis glands are shown in a needle core biopsy. The epithelium in the lesion in **B** shows apocrine features.

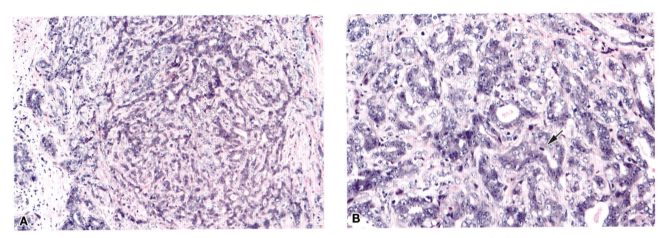

FIGURE 6.10 **Florid Adenosis in Pregnancy.** This needle core biopsy is from a palpable tumor in a 35-year-old woman who was 9 weeks pregnant. **A, B:** There is marked hyperplasia of epithelial and myoepithelial cells in florid adenosis. Note epithelial mitosis (arrow).

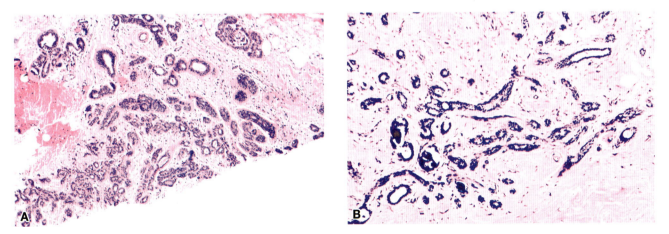

FIGURE 6.11 **Tubular Adenosis. A:** Elongated adenosis glands that resemble tubules with thick basement membranes are present in this needle core biopsy from a premenopausal woman. **B:** Epithelial atrophy, calcifications, and stromal fibrosis in a biopsy from a postmenopausal patient.

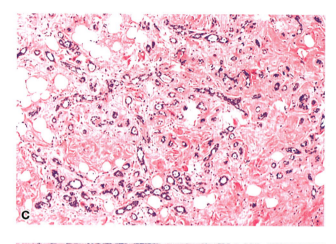

FIGURE 6.11 (*continued*) **C:** Tubular adenosis in an excision demonstrates the infiltrative nature of this lesion that closely mimics invasive carcinoma.

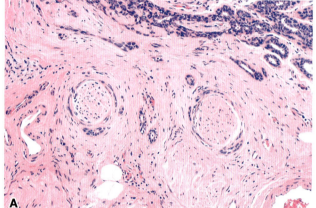
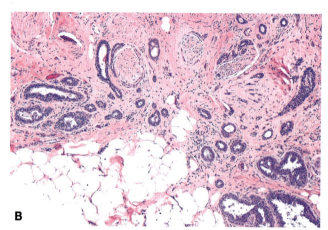

FIGURE 6.12 Adenosis With Perineural Invasion. A: Two nerves are surrounded circumferentially by adenosis glands. **B:** Adenosis glands encircle nerves at the perimeter of a sclerosing lesion in this needle core biopsy.

Blunt Duct Adenosis

Blunt duct adenosis (BDA) is a form of terminal duct change (both hyperplasia and hypertrophy) characterized by abortive lobule formation (1). The lesional glands typically form aggregates of rounded glands, with "blunt lateral outlines" and "blunt endings" **(Fig. 6.13)**. There is mild epithelial hyperplasia. The myoepithelium in cystic BDA also shows mild hypertrophy. The stroma surrounding BDA glands is expanded and relatively more cellular than usual intralobular stroma. BDA occasionally exhibits apocrine metaplasia.

Apocrine Adenosis and Atypical Apocrine Adenosis

Apocrine adenosis (AA) designates a focus of adenosis with apocrine metaplasia (8,9) **(Fig. 6.14)**. It is a common alteration, especially in the context of SA. It is readily detected at low-power examination because the apocrine cells have more abundant apocrine-type cytoplasm than the cuboidal to flat epithelium typically found in adenosis. The cytoplasm is finely granular and eosinophilic; however, it can be gray to amphophilic. The nuclei are round with prominent nucleoli and show no atypical features. No mitoses are present.

Atypical apocrine adenosis (AAA) consists of apocrine cells with cytoplasmic clearing or vacuolization and anisonucleosis. The nuclei have irregular nuclear membranes, as much as 3-fold variation in size, and nuclear pleomorphism **(Fig. 6.15)**. Nuclear hyperchromasia and prominent nucleoli are found in extreme examples of AAA. Mitotic figures are uncommon, and their identification raises the differential diagnosis of apocrine DCIS (10,11). The diagnosis of DCIS with apocrine morphology is reserved for cases with substantial cytologic atypia *and/or* mitotic activity *and/or* fully developed architectural patterns characteristic of DCIS, such as solid growth, cribriform or papillary architecture.

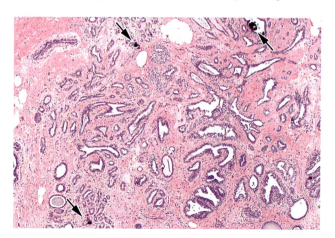

FIGURE 6.13 Blunt Duct Adenosis. An example of blunt duct adenosis in an excision. Calcifications are present (arrows).

ADENOSIS AND MICROGLANDULAR ADENOSIS 89

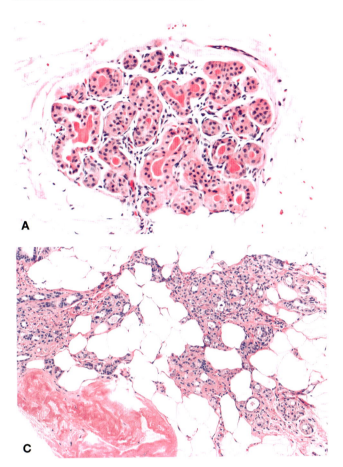

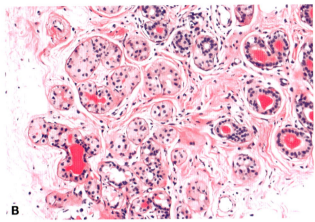

FIGURE 6.14 Apocrine Adenosis. A: Apocrine metaplasia in a lobule. **B:** Apocrine metaplasia in adenosis. **C:** Apocrine metaplasia involving atrophic sclerosing adenosis.

It is unclear whether AAA is a morphologic precursor of DCIS with apocrine features. One study (12) found that the median Ki-67 proliferation rate of AA was significantly higher than that of normal mammary epithelium but did not differ significantly from that of AAA (3.7% vs 4.8%). Calhoun and Booth (13) reported a retrospective series including 22 NCBs with diagnosis of AA and 12 with diagnosis of AAA. The mean and median age at diagnosis was 60 and 58 years, respectively. The NCBs sampled calcifications (11 cases), a mass or density (18 cases), and a mass or density with calcifications (3 cases). Two NCBs sampled a focus of MRI enhancement. Seven NCBs with AA also contained atypia and/or carcinoma (one invasive carcinoma, one DCIS, and five atypical hyperplasia). Five NCBs with AAA also contained other forms of atypia or carcinoma (two atypical hyperplasia and three DCIS). No carcinoma was found in subsequent excisional biopsies in patients who had only AA or AAA in the index NCB material. No long-term follow-up information was provided.

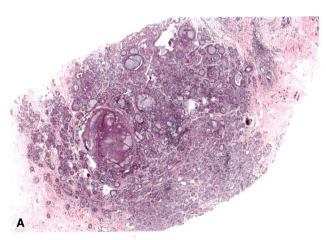

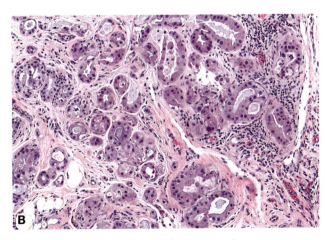

FIGURE 6.15 Atypical Apocrine Adenosis. A-D: A needle core biopsy with atypical apocrine adenosis. **A:** The epithelium in a focus of sclerosing adenosis is expanded. The apocrine epithelial cells have abundant cytoplasm. **B:** The apocrine cells are enlarged, and a few have hyperchromatic nuclei.

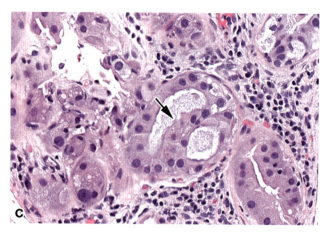
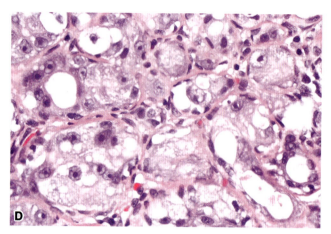

FIGURE 6.15 (*continued*) **C:** Nuclear hyperchromasia and anisonucleosis are evident. The epithelium in one gland forms a small arch (arrow). **D:** The cytoplasm of the atypical apocrine cells is vacuolated. The nuclei are enlarged, and nucleoli are prominent.

Atypical Lobular Hyperplasia and Lobular Carcinoma In Situ in Adenosis

Classic lobular carcinoma in situ (LCIS) is the most common form of carcinoma in situ (CIS) in adenosis **(Figs. 6.16-6.18)**. LCIS causes an expansion of the epithelium in a focus of adenosis, and intercellular dyscohesion is usually evident. Signet ring cell morphology can be identified in LCIS, but it is not a feature of benign epithelium in adenosis. Atypical lobular hyperplasia (ALH) involving adenosis can be a subtle finding **(Fig. 6.19)**. The diagnosis of LCIS and ALH in adenosis is supported

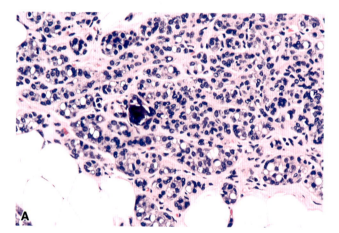
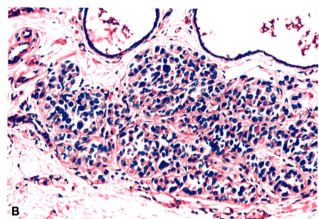

FIGURE 6.16 **Sclerosing Adenosis With Lobular Carcinoma In Situ. A, B:** Lobular carcinoma in situ with signet ring cells. Note intracytoplasmic mucin demonstrated with the mucicarmine stain **(B)**.

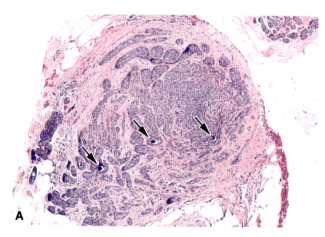
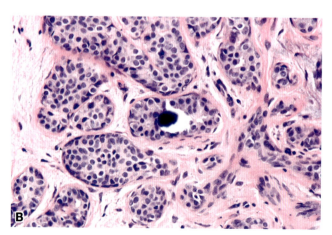

FIGURE 6.17 **Tubular Adenosis With Lobular Carcinoma In Situ (LCIS). A, B:** Swirling tubular adenosis glands are expanded by LCIS. The needle core biopsy was performed for calcifications that were detected on screening (arrows).

ADENOSIS AND MICROGLANDULAR ADENOSIS 91

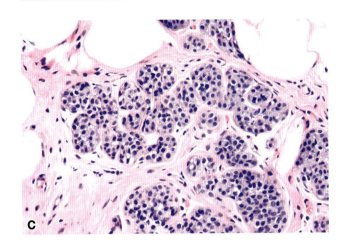

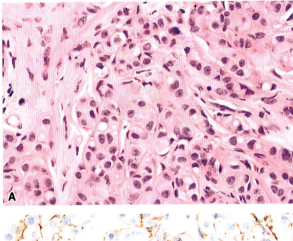

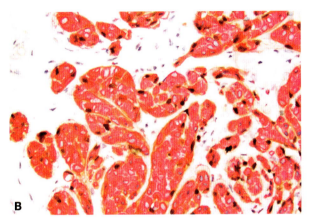

FIGURE 6.17 (*continued*) **C:** LCIS in adenosis from the same specimen with a lesser degree of architectural distortion.

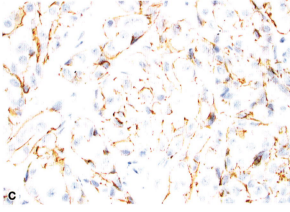

FIGURE 6.18 **Sclerosing Adenosis With Lobular Carcinoma In Situ (LCIS). A:** Sclerosing adenosis with LCIS mimics invasive carcinoma. LCIS cells have intracytoplasmic vacuoles. Basement membranes outline most lobules. **B:** Staining with ADH5 antibody cocktail highlights the myoepithelial layer (brown chromogen: nuclear p63 and cytoplasmic CK5 and CK14), ruling out stromal invasion. LCIS cells show cytoplasmic reactivity for luminal cytokeratins (red chromogen: cytoplasmic CK7 and CK18). **C:** Weak membranous E-cadherin reactivity highlights myoepithelial cells. There is no reactivity around LCIS cells.

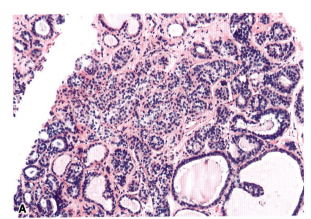

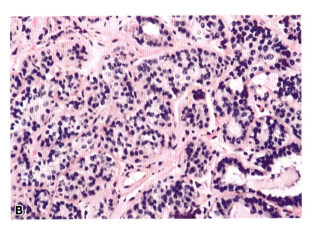

FIGURE 6.19 **Adenosis With Atypical Lobular Hyperplasia. A, B:** The monomorphic cells of atypical lobular hyperplasia are apparent in some adenosis glands. The biopsy was performed for screen-detected calcifications. Note the microcystic dilation of some glands and calcification right of center **(B)**.

by negative membranous reactivity for E-cadherin **(Fig. 6.18)** and diffuse cytoplasmic staining for p120.

Atypical Ductal Hyperplasia and Ductal Carcinoma In Situ in Adenosis

ADH and DCIS can be associated with adenosis. DCIS in adenosis is less common than LCIS. The diagnosis of DCIS in adenosis needs to fulfill the same criteria required for the diagnosis of DCIS outside of adenosis, and it is appropriate when an atypical epithelial proliferation shows solid, cribriform, or papillary architecture *and/or* substantial cytologic atypia, *and/or* prominent central ("comedo") necrosis *and/or* mitotic activity **(Fig. 6.20)**. The distinction between AAA and apocrine DCIS in adenosis can be especially difficult (10,11,14) **(Fig. 6.21)**. Cytoplasmic clearing or vacuolization can occur in atypical sclerosing apocrine lesions as well as in DCIS with apocrine features (see Chapter 15).

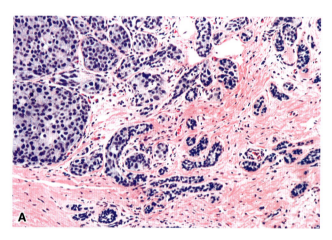
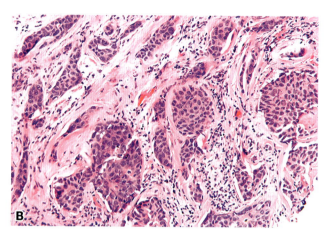
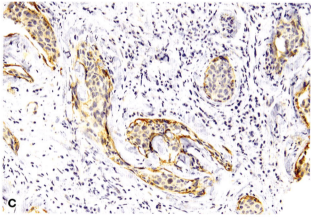

FIGURE 6.20 Sclerosing Adenosis With Ductal Carcinoma In Situ (DCIS). A, B: The glands are enlarged by solid DCIS. Sclerosing adenosis was mistaken for invasive carcinoma in these two cases. **C:** CD10 immunostain performed on the lesion in **B** demonstrates myoepithelial lining of the lesional glands.

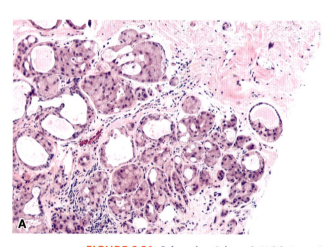
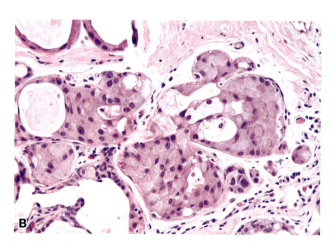

FIGURE 6.21 Sclerosing Adenosis With Apocrine Ductal Carcinoma In Situ. A, B: The adenosis glands in this needle core biopsy are expanded by apocrine carcinoma composed of cells with abundant eosinophilic cytoplasm and pleomorphic nuclei.

Adenosis in Fibroepithelial Neoplasms

A fibroadenoma with SA, cystic apocrine hyperplasia, macrocysts, and calcifications is a "complex fibroadenoma" (see Chapter 7). SA may be limited to a part of a fibroadenoma (**Fig. 6.22**), or it may be diffuse, obscuring the underlying fibroepithelial structure. An NCB sample of a complex fibroadenoma with confluent SA can simulate invasive carcinoma. Phyllodes tumors can also have foci of adenosis.

Immunohistochemistry

Adenosis can closely mimic invasive carcinoma, especially when the glands and tubules are compact, or appear to infiltrate the adjacent fatty breast parenchyma, or are markedly distorted by extensive sclerosis, and/or CIS is present. These scenarios may require immunostains using a panel of myoepithelial markers (6,15). In a study (16) evaluating the reactivity of myoepithelial markers in SA, calponin was negative in 1/22 (4.5%) cases, myosin in 3/21 (14.3%), and CK5/6 in 4/20 (20%), whereas SMA, CD10, and p63 stained the myoepithelium in all cases tested for these markers.

Differential Diagnosis

Adenosis can mimic invasive carcinoma, especially when the glands and tubules are compact, or appear to infiltrate the adjacent adipose tissue (**Figs. 6.23 and 6.24**) and breast parenchyma, or are markedly distorted by extensive sclerosis (**Fig. 6.25**), and/or involved by CIS. Conversely, it is difficult to diagnose stromal invasion within foci of adenosis. The most convincing evidence for a diagnosis of invasive carcinoma arising in adenosis is the presence of invasive foci extending *beyond* the adenosis lesion. Careful evaluation of the interface of the lesion with the surrounding uninvolved breast parenchyma is most informative, although the latter is often only minimally represented in an NCB sample. A focal mixed inflammatory cell infiltrate and reactive stromal changes often accompany stromal (micro)invasion (**Fig. 6.26**). TA and SA can mimic well-differentiated

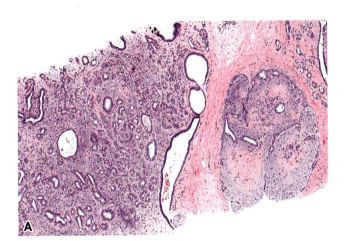
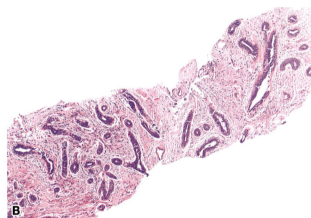

FIGURE 6.22 Sclerosing Adenosis in a Fibroadenoma. **A:** This needle core biopsy specimen of a fibroadenoma shows adenosis concentrated in one part of the lesion (left), whereas a few elongated ducts and lobules with fibroadenomatoid changes are seen in another part of the lesion (right). **B:** Adenosis with features of tubular adenosis is evident in this fibroadenoma.

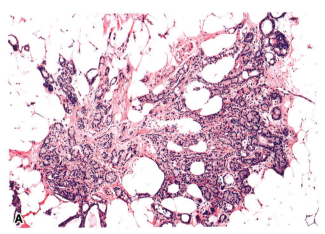
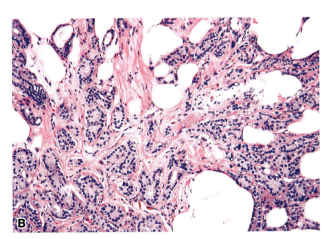

FIGURE 6.23 Adenosis Mimics Invasive Carcinoma. **A, B:** This needle core biopsy shows sclerosing adenosis invading adipose tissue, simulating invasive carcinoma.

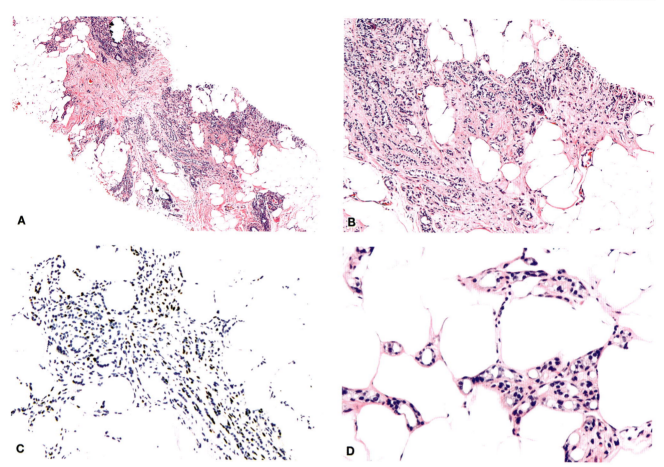

FIGURE 6.24 **Sclerosing Adenosis With an Invasive Pattern. A, B:** Sclerosing adenosis in this needle core biopsy extends into fat in a pattern resembling invasive carcinoma. Note the fibrous stroma that surrounds the adenosis glands. **C:** Nuclear p63 staining decorates myoepithelial cells. **D:** Another needle core biopsy in which sclerosing adenosis lies amid fat.

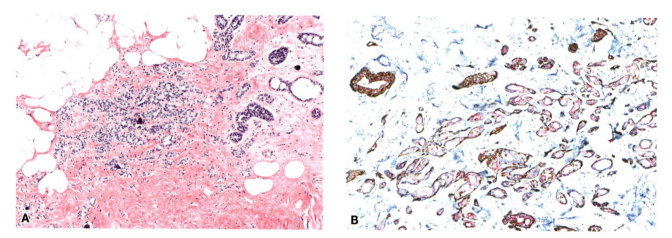

FIGURE 6.25 **Sclerosing Adenosis With an Invasive Pattern. A:** Sclerosing adenosis in this needle core biopsy simulates tubular carcinoma. **B:** Staining of the focus in **A** with the ADH5 antibody cocktail highlights the myoepithelial cells (brown chromogen: nuclear p63 and cytoplasmic CK5 and CK14). The cytoplasm of the epithelial cells is positive for luminal cytokeratins (red chromogen: CK7 and CK18).

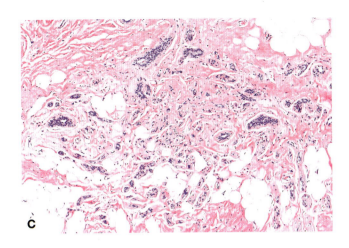

FIGURE 6.25 (*continued*) **C:** Another needle core biopsy sample in which sclerosing adenosis mimics invasive carcinoma.

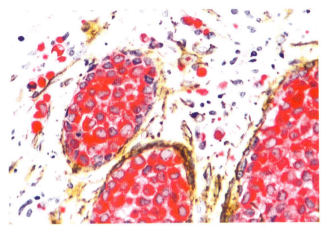

FIGURE 6.26 Sclerosing Adenosis With Microinvasive and In Situ Lobular Carcinoma. Double immunolabeling has been used to detect microinvasive carcinoma in which LCIS involves sclerosing adenosis. Scattered AE1:AE3-positive epithelial cells (red chromogen) devoid of myoepithelium are evident in the stroma outside glands. The latter are bounded by myoepithelial cells positive for smooth muscle actin (brown chromogen).

carcinoma **(Figs. 6.11, 6.24, 6.25, and 6.27)** and tubular carcinoma. LCIS or DCIS involving adenosis can mimic invasive carcinoma, but the underlying adenosis tends to retain a lobulocentric arrangement **(Fig. 6.17)**. A radial scar is distinguished from SA by its typical stellar configuration with glands radiating out from a central fibroelastotic nidus. Occasionally, foci of SA may be incorporated into a radial scar.

Treatment and Prognosis

Radiologic-pathologic correlation needs to be assessed whenever adenosis is present in an NCB specimen. Surgical excision is recommended if the lesion has a spiculated contour, harbors suspicious calcifications, is associated with a complex (radial) sclerosing lesion, or atypical epithelial hyperplasia is present (3). In the absence of one or more of the aforementioned features, clinical follow-up of a circumscribed tumor or of a "nonpalpable indistinctly marginated mass" that yields microscopic SA at NCB is a reasonable option (3) if the imaging and pathologic findings are concordant. Excisional biopsy is often pursued for adenosis tumor. Gill et al (3) reported follow-up information on a series of 33 NCBs with a major component of SA and no atypia and/or carcinoma. In one case, the radiologic target was a suspicious mass, and the NCB radiologic-pathologic findings were deemed discordant. Follow-up surgical excision yielded invasive carcinoma. The remaining 32 cases had concordant radiologic-pathologic findings: one lesion was excised as part of a mastectomy for ipsilateral invasive carcinoma, and 24 of the remaining 31 lesions were benign on radiologic follow-up.

Calhoun and Booth (13) reported the findings in the surgical excision specimens of patients with NCB diagnosis of AAA. Excision of seven lesions with NCB diagnosis of AAA yielded AAA (five cases), AA (one case), and atypical hyperplasia (one case).

The treatment of carcinoma arising in adenosis depends on the stage and extent of the lesion. In many of these cases, carcinoma is also present in breast tissue outside the area of adenosis (17–19).

Risk of Subsequent Carcinoma

Foote and Stewart (1) reported that adenosis was not a precursor lesion or risk factor for carcinoma. Page et al (20) did not detect a significantly increased risk of subsequent carcinoma associated with SA in a retrospective study of women with fibrocystic changes but reported increased relative risk (RR) in two subsequent studies (21,22), amounting to a 2.1 RR in women with SA with atypia, and 1.7 RR in women with SA without atypia (22). The RR was not significantly affected by a family history of breast carcinoma, but the risk was 6.7-fold when SA was accompanied by atypical hyperplasia, often of the lobular type. Others have also reported an increased risk of subsequent carcinoma after a diagnosis of SA (23–27). At a median follow-up of 15.7 years, the RR of carcinoma for 3,733 women with SA in the Mayo Clinic Benign Breast Disease Cohort (28) was 2.1 (95% confidence

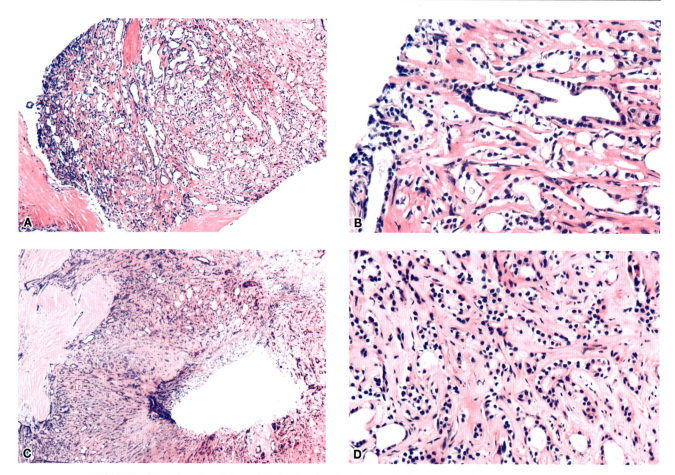

FIGURE 6.27 **Sclerosing Adenosis Mistaken for Carcinoma. A, B:** This needle core biopsy of a palpable adenosis tumor was interpreted as invasive, well-differentiated duct carcinoma. The lesion has a well-circumscribed border and lacks lobulocentric architecture. Myoepithelial cells with clear cytoplasm are evident at higher magnification. **C, D:** The subsequent excision revealed a circumscribed focus of sclerosing adenosis. The defect in the center represents the site of the antecedent needle core biopsy.

interval [CI], 1.9-2.3) versus 1.52 (95% CI, 1.42-1.63) in 9,701 women without SA. Overall, the RR associated with SA without atypia is so small that no intervention is required beyond clinical surveillance.

The precancerous significance of AAA has also been evaluated. In a study by Carter and Rosen (10), none of the 51 patients with sclerosing proliferative lesions with AAA developed carcinoma after a mean follow-up of 35 months. Seidman et al (11) reported that at a mean follow-up of 8.7 years, 4/37 (10.8%) patients with AAA developed invasive ductal carcinoma (three ipsilateral and one contralateral), but the authors did not mention whether the carcinoma had apocrine features. All carcinomas occurred more than 3 years after the index diagnosis of AAA, with a mean interval of 5.6 years. The RR of carcinoma was 5.5 (95% CI, 1.9-16) when compared to age-specific incidence rates. All patients who developed carcinoma were older than 60 years when AAA was diagnosed, and patients in this age group had an RR of 14 for carcinoma (95% CI, 4.1-48). AAA was present in only 37/9,340 excisional biopsy specimens from patients in the Mayo Clinic Benign Breast Disease Cohort (29). The

mean age at diagnosis of AAA was 59.3 years, versus 51.4 years for all women in the cohort. Only three women (8%) with AAA developed subsequent carcinoma, a rate comparable to that of 7.8% for all women in the cohort. Two ipsilateral invasive carcinomas developed 4 and 18 years after the index biopsy. The third patient developed contralateral DCIS 12 years after the index biopsy. None of the carcinomas had apocrine morphology, and no AAA was present in the background breast parenchyma.

All forms of adenosis **(Table 6.1)**, except MGA, vide infra, are regarded as nonneoplastic and have not been associated with any molecular or genetic abnormality.

MICROGLANDULAR ADENOSIS

MGA is a proliferative glandular lesion that mimics carcinoma, both clinically and pathologically. MGA differs substantially from all other forms of adenosis, as the glands thereof do not have a myoepithelial layer. MGA was characterized as a distinct clinicopathologic entity in 1983 (30-32), and there are only a few reports of MGA without atypia or associated carcinoma (33-35). MGA often has areas of atypia (atypical MGA). Carcinoma can arise in MGA, and either it retains the distribution of MGA ("CIS arising in MGA") or it can be frankly invasive.

Clinical Presentation

All reported patients with MGA have been women, ranging from 28 to 82 years of age; most patients are 45 to 55 years old. Atypical MGA and carcinoma arising in MGA have an age distribution rather akin to that of MGA (33,36-42). The median age of patients with MGA-associated carcinoma was 47 years (range, 26-68) in a series from Memorial Hospital in New York (42) and 46 years (range, 31-61) in a series from China (43).

In most instances, MGA is detected as a mass (33,35), but can be an incidental finding near another lesion (33). In two separate series, all patients with MGA-associated invasive carcinoma presented with a mass lesion (33,42,43).

In one series (42), six patients with MGA-associated carcinoma had a family history of breast carcinoma. A 22-year-old woman with MGA had a *BRCA1* germline mutation (5625G>T mutation in exon 24) (44). Another patient with MGA had neurofibromatosis (45).

Imaging

MGA and MGA-associated lesions typically present as breast masses. Mammography of MGA may reveal increased density and is sometimes reported as "suspicious" (46), but no specific radiologic changes have been described, and some lesions may not be apparent radiologically (44). None of the three cases of MGA reported by Khalifeh et al (33) was detected mammographically. One case appeared as an ill-defined hypoechoic mass by ultrasound examination, and a mammogram showed only dense breast tissue (35). Another case appeared as a hypoechoic mass with well-defined, but irregular borders, lobulations, and angular margins. The mass was wider than tall, had an antiparallel orientation, and was suspicious sonographically (44). On MRI, the lesion consisted of a noncircumscribed mass with moderate early and delayed enhancement, and hyperintense T2-weighted images. The radiologic differential diagnosis included fibroadenoma. Atypical MGA and carcinoma arising in MGA tend to appear mammographically as infiltrative masses (33), but no radiologic abnormality was detected in the breast of a 74-year-old woman with a palpable breast mass consisting of invasive carcinoma arising in MGA (40).

Microscopic Pathology

MGA is an infiltrative proliferation of small glands in fibrous or fatty mammary stroma **(Table 6.2)**. At low magnification, the glands lack the "organoid" growth pattern of SA and typically display a relatively random and disorganized distribution **(Fig. 6.28)**. Smaller lesions may show lobular arrangement **(Figs. 6.29 and 6.30)**. The glands of

---

TABLE 6.2

Microglandular Adenosis: Typical Histopathologic Features

Proliferation of uniform, relatively small, round glands amid fibrous and/or adipose tissue
Haphazard distribution of glands
Glandular epithelium is one cell layered, and the cells are flat-to-cuboidal.
Lesional glands lack myoepithelial layer, but are surrounded by basement membrane.
Small round nuclei, inconspicuous or absent nucleoli
Cytoplasm is clear or amphophilic; rarely eosinophilic
Intraluminal eosinophilic (PAS-positive) secretions common
Calcifications in luminal secretions occur.

PAS, periodic acid–Schiff.

MGA are small, and round to oval; tubule formation is rare. The glands can be crowded, but gland fusion is uncommon. The epithelium consists of a monolayer of flat-to-cuboidal cells **(Fig. 6.30)**, with small round nuclei and inconspicuous or absent nucleoli. The cytoplasm is clear or amphophilic; rarely, eosinophilic and granular cytoplasm can occur. Intraluminal homogeneous eosinophilic secretions are common, and they occasionally undergo calcification **(Fig. 6.30)**. The secretion is usually positive for periodic acid–Schiff (PAS) positive (diastase resistant), Alcian blue, and mucicarmine. The glands of MGA lack a myoepithelial layer but are surrounded by basement membrane. The latter can be highlighted using PAS and/or reticulin stain, or immunostains for laminin and collagen IV.

Atypical MGA **(Fig. 6.31)** is MGA with one or more of the following features: larger and/or merging glands, lesser secretions, focal solid growth, larger nuclei, nuclear hyperchromasia, and rare mitotic activity **(Table 6.3)**. The atypical epithelium has hyperchromatic and focally pleomorphic nuclei and varying amounts of clear-to-amphophilic cytoplasm. Cytoplasmic eosinophilic granules are uncommon.

Carcinoma arising in association with MGA is of major clinical and pathologic concern (32-34,36-42,46,47). The term "CIS in MGA" is used for a neoplastic epithelial proliferation that consists of basaloid epithelial cells with solid growth, cytologic atypia, and mitotic activity, but is surrounded by basement membrane, retains the growth pattern of MGA, and is neither associated with stromal desmoplasia nor with lymphoplasmacytic infiltrate **(Figs. 6.32 and 6.33; Table 6.3)**. Necrosis within the solid epithelial nests is common. Extensive sampling is often necessary to identify residual foci of MGA without atypia, and the latter may not be present in the limited samples obtained by NCB. In rare cases, ordinary DCIS or LCIS (31) coexists with MGA or atypical MGA. Ordinary DCIS surrounded by myoepithelium was present in a case of MGA and MGA-associated invasive carcinoma (34).

Invasive carcinoma arising in MGA usually forms microscopic solid tumor nodules substantially larger than the

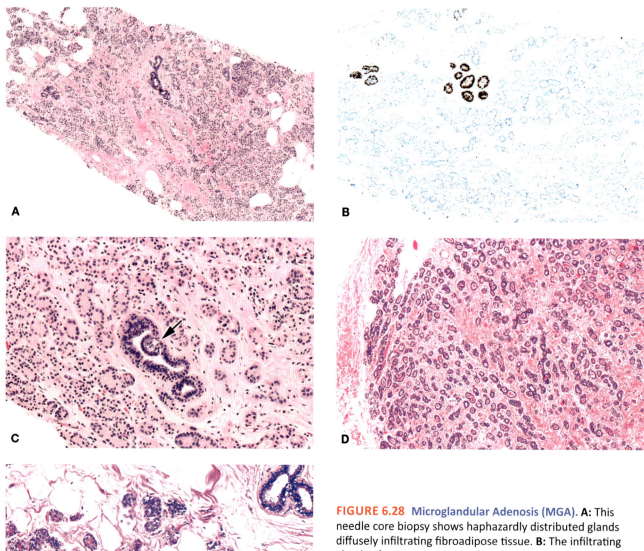

FIGURE 6.28 Microglandular Adenosis (MGA). **A:** This needle core biopsy shows haphazardly distributed glands diffusely infiltrating fibroadipose tissue. **B:** The infiltrating glands of MGA are negative for estrogen receptor. The normal epithelium in the few entrapped benign glands shows positivity for estrogen receptor. **C:** The "micro" glands are round and are lined by monostratified epithelium with no cytologic atypia. MGA surrounds a duct with calcification (arrow). This lesion was originally diagnosed as a well-differentiated "triple-negative" invasive ductal carcinoma. **D:** A compact, relatively circumscribed, focus of MGA lying amid fibrous tissue. **E:** MGA with minimal extension into adipose tissue.

MGA glands filled by CIS and are typically poorly differentiated, grade 3 (in ~75% of cases) and grade 2 (in ~25% of cases) (Table 6.3). The invasive foci are associated with stromal desmoplasia and enveloped by a conspicuous lymphocytic reaction. Necrosis may be present. Mitoses are readily apparent in these regions. Basement membranes are disrupted around invasive nests, but this finding can be difficult to evaluate, especially in limited NCB material. Poorly differentiated carcinoma with high-grade basaloid morphology is the most common form of MGA-associated invasive carcinoma. Other morphologies include invasive metaplastic matrix carcinoma (in one-third of cases) and those of the squamous and adenoid cystic variety (33,34,39,43). MGA-associated acinic cell ("serous" with zymogen-type granules) differentiation is uncommon (33,43,48,49). Invasive carcinomas arising in this setting are usually "triple-negative" (ie, negative for estrogen receptor [ER], progesterone receptor [PR], and human epidermal growth factor receptor 2 [HER2]) and are positive for S-100.

Immunohistochemistry

The glands of MGA are devoid of myoepithelium but are surrounded by basement membrane. The latter is not readily

ADENOSIS AND MICROGLANDULAR ADENOSIS

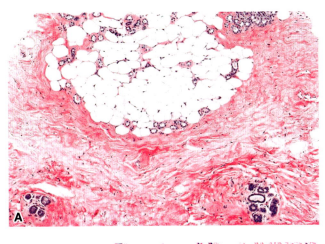
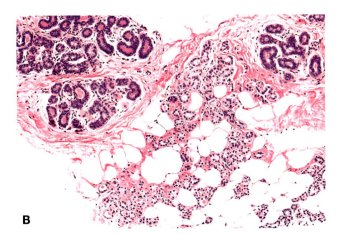
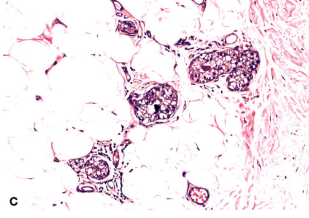

FIGURE 6.29 Microglandular Adenosis (MGA). **A:** This needle core biopsy shows "micro" glands haphazardly distributed in fat. **B:** Another needle core biopsy with pseudolobulated MGA. **C:** A minuscule focus of MGA amid adipose tissue.

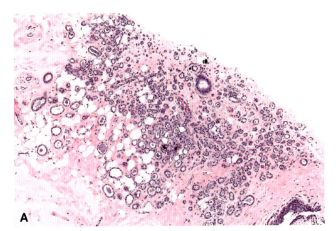
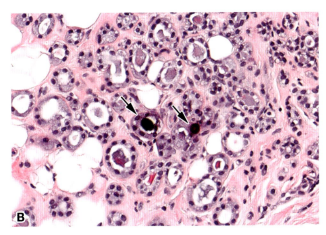
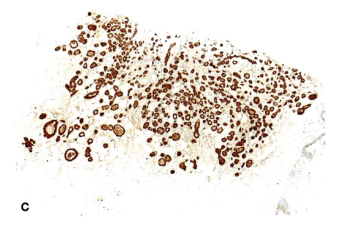

FIGURE 6.30 Microglandular Adenosis (MGA). **A:** This needle core biopsy shows MGA that resembles conventional adenosis. **B:** The glandular epithelium is cytologically bland. Basement membrane is evident around the glands. Minute intraluminal calcifications are present (arrows). **C:** The glandular proliferation is strongly and uniformly positive for S-100 but lacks myoepithelium (not shown).

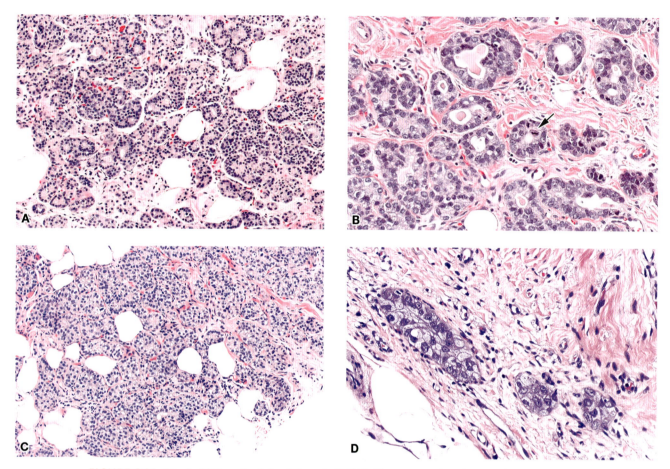

FIGURE 6.31 Atypical Microglandular Adenosis (MGA). Three examples of atypical MGA in needle core biopsies. **A:** In this case, a few glands appear to be interconnected. **B:** In another case, the glands have a more solid growth, nuclear hyperchromasia, and rare mitoses (arrow). **C, D:** Yet another case of atypical MGA with marked cellular crowding and overgrowth. Cytologic atypia is evident in each case.

evident on hematoxylin and eosin (H&E) stained sections and can be highlighted with immunostains for laminin and type IV collagen. Reticulin (silver impregnation) and PAS stains can highlight the basement membrane around MGA glands (42,50), but these stains can be difficult to interpret. Some low-grade invasive carcinomas can show focal basement membrane (51).

The cells forming MGA are strongly immunoreactive for S-100 (Fig. **6.30**) and negative for ER **(Fig. 6.28)**, PR, HER2 (42), gross cystic disease fluid protein 15 (GCDFP-15), and epithelial membrane antigen (EMA) (50). p53 is absent (42) or minimally expressed (<3% of cells) (33,37) in MGA. Ki-67 staining cells tend to be sparse (<3%) (33).

Atypical MGA and MGA-associated carcinoma are positive for S-100; however, the staining tends to be spotty and less intense with increasing atypia within the lesion (33,36,37). p53 was detected in 5% to 10% of atypical MGA cells and in more than 30% of the cells of MGA-associated carcinoma in one series (33), but another study found no difference in the percentage of p53-positive cells in MGA-associated lesions (37). Increase in the percentage of Ki67-positive cells with increasing severity of the lesions has been reported (33,36,37). Together with recent molecular evidence (34,37), these data suggest that MGA is a nonobligate morphologic precursor of MGA-associated invasive breast carcinoma (see later).

Although MGA is reported as EMA-negative in most series, 8/15 cases of atypical MGA, 3/9 of MGA-associated CIS, and 4/6 MGA-associated invasive carcinomas were EMA-positive in one study (36). All atypical MGA cases in one series were CK7-positive and CK20-negative (36). CK5/6 (33) and 34βE12 (36) were negative in all cases of atypical MGA, CIS in MGA, and MGA-associated invasive carcinoma in two separate studies. CK5/6 was negative in 3/3 cases of MGA in one series (33). The luminal keratins CK8/18 were positive in MGA and MGA-related lesions in two studies (33,34). Epidermal growth factor receptor (EGFR), another basal marker, decorated 11/11 MGA-related lesions in one series (33) and 13/14 cases in another (34). EGFR expression was also detected in an MGA-associated invasive carcinoma (41). Focal positivity for CD117 (c-kit) was detected in 3/6 cases of MGA-associated invasive carcinoma, two of which were matrix-producing and one with acinic-like features (33).

MGA-associated invasive carcinomas are consistently negative for ER, PR, and HER2 (33,34,36,43), but one case reportedly showed focal ER positivity (36).

ADENOSIS AND MICROGLANDULAR ADENOSIS

TABLE 6.3
Atypical MGA, Carcinoma In Situ, and Invasive Carcinoma Associated With MGA: Typical Histopathologic Features

Atypical MGA
Relatively larger glands
Glandular crowding, gland fusion, solid growth
Enlarged pleomorphic nuclei, nuclear hyperchromasia, and mitotic activity
Relatively uniform clear-to-amphophilic cytoplasm

Carcinoma In Situ Associated With MGA
Retains the usual architecture of MGA
Solid growth
Basaloid cells
Nuclear atypia
Readily evident mitotic activity
Rarely, necrosis in solid epithelial nests
No stromal desmoplasia
No lymphoplasmacytic infiltrate

Invasive Carcinoma Arising in MGA
Higher-grade carcinoma (basaloid morphology is most common)
Relatively larger, more solid nodules
Nuclear atypia
Mitoses readily apparent
Basement membrane disrupted
Stromal desmoplasia and lymphocytic reaction
Necrosis variable
May show matrix production, squamous differentiation, acinic cell change

MGA, microglandular adenosis.

Differential Diagnosis of Microglandular Adenosis at Needle Core Biopsy

Tubular carcinoma is composed of angular glands of varying size, arranged in a stellate or radial configuration. The neoplastic glands are lined by predominantly columnar-to-cuboidal epithelium, which tends to have amphophilic cytoplasm. Desmoplasia and stromal elastosis are common. The glands composing well-differentiated invasive ductal carcinoma and tubular carcinoma are devoid of myoepithelium and basement membrane, and are usually strongly and diffusely positive for ER and PR but negative for S-100. Tubular carcinoma is positive for EMA, whereas MGA is usually regarded as EMA-negative (50), although few cases of MGA and MGA-associated lesions were reported as EMA-positive in one series (36). In general, one or more lesions of the morphologic spectrum of low-grade mammary neoplasia (low-grade DCIS, ADH, columnar cell change with atypia/flat epithelial atypia, classical LCIS, and ALH) are present near well-differentiated invasive ductal carcinoma and tubular carcinoma, at least focally (also see Chapter 10).

Areas that resemble MGA can be found in adenosis. SA is usually distinctly lobulocentric, and the compressed glands tend to be arranged in a whorled or laminated fashion within the lobular nodules. TA consists predominantly of elongated glands and tubules, whereas most MGA glands are round to oval. Immunostains for p63, calponin, and other myoepithelial markers highlight the myoepithelial cells in all forms of adenosis, except MGA. Khalifeh et al (33) reported the histologic findings in 54 cases that had initially been misdiagnosed as MGA. The revised diagnosis included 48 cases of adenosis (21 ordinary adenosis, 17 infiltrating

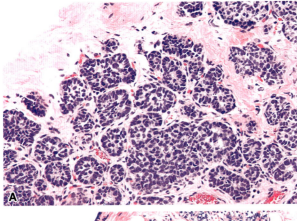

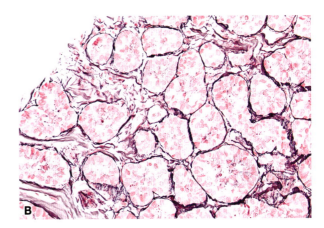

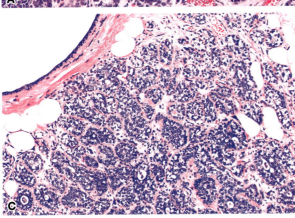

FIGURE 6.32 Ductal Carcinoma In Situ (DCIS) in Microglandular Adenosis (MGA). **A, B:** A needle core biopsy with DCIS in MGA. Basement membranes are highlighted by reticulin stain **(B)**. **C:** Glandular crowding is evident in this example of DCIS in MGA.

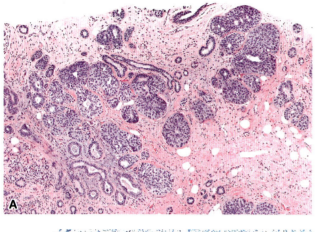
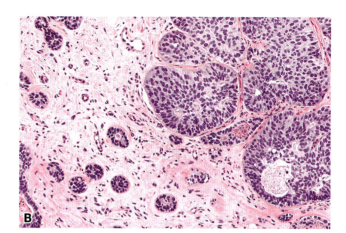
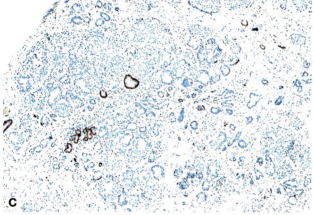

FIGURE 6.33 Ductal Carcinoma In Situ (DCIS) in Microglandular Adenosis (MGA). A, B: A needle core biopsy with DCIS in MGA. **C:** Calponin immunostain shows the absence of myoepithelium around DCIS in MGA and around MGA. Reactivity for calponin is present around entrapped normal glands.

adenosis, 9 adenosis with clear cell changes, and 1 BDA), 2 cases of AAA, and 4 cases with no obvious pathologic abnormality. All glands present in these cases had a complete myoepithelial cell layer, as demonstrated by myoepithelial immunostains.

The differential diagnosis of atypical MGA and CIS in MGA includes invasive carcinoma. In the absence of the usual form of MGA, it is difficult to separate atypical MGA and CIS arising in MGA from invasive carcinoma—especially on NCB material. The absence of stromal desmoplasia and of a stromal inflammatory cell infiltrate associated with a high-grade infiltrative epithelial proliferation with triple-*negative* profile should raise the possibility of atypical MGA and CIS in MGA. In these cases, positivity for S-100 further increases the suspicion of MGA-associated carcinoma, but it is insufficient for an unequivocal diagnosis. Excision of the lesion is required for its definitive classification.

MGA-associated acinic cell differentiation (with zymogen-like granules) is uncommon (33,43,48,49) **(Fig. 6.34).** MGA and atypical MGA can show some histopathologic features that overlap with so-called acinic cell carcinoma (52).

"Secretory adenosis" refers to a lesion that resembles MGA, but the glands therein possess myoepithelial cell layer (the term "secretory" in this context refers to the intraluminal eosinophilic secretions in the lesional glands).

Prognosis and Treatment

Even though MGA is regarded as a benign lesion, excisional biopsy is *always* recommended when an NCB sample contains MGA. MGA is typically treated by local excision. Reexcision should be considered if MGA involves the surgical margins microscopically because little is known about the long-term course of incompletely excised MGA. In one case, MGA involved the final margins of a lumpectomy specimen with MGA-associated in situ and invasive carcinoma (41). No radiotherapy was administered, and the patient did not undergo chemotherapy. Ten years later, a mass lesion consisting of MGA-associated CIS developed in the same region of the breast.

Patients with atypical MGA should undergo wide excision of the lesion to achieve negative margins. Further excision is strongly recommended if the margins are involved. Carcinoma is reported in association with MGA and atypical MGA in most published series (33,34,36,37,42,46), and in almost all cases the carcinoma arose within the MGA lesion. One unusual patient had concurrent but separate foci of MGA and carcinoma in one breast (32). A patient with MGA in one breast developed invasive ductal carcinoma not associated with MGA in the contralateral breast (42).

In one study (42), lymph node metastases were documented in 3 of 11 patients with MGA-associated invasive carcinoma who underwent axillary dissection. Ten patients treated by mastectomy were recurrence-free with a median

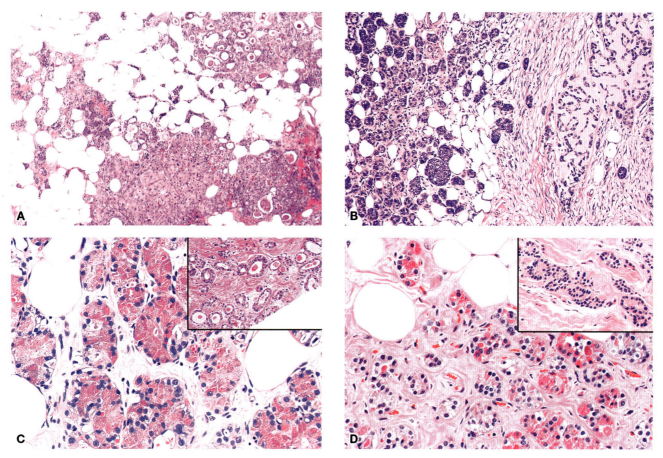

FIGURE 6.34 **Invasive Carcinoma Associated With Microglandular Adenosis (MGA).** A case of invasive carcinoma with basaloid features associated with MGA **(A)**, another with metaplastic matrix-producing features associated with MGA **(B)**, and two others with acinic-type differentiation (with intracytoplasmic zymogen-like granules in lesional cells) in invasive carcinomas associated with MGA **(C, D)**. Insets show associated MGA **(C, D)**.

follow-up of 57 months (range, 3-108). Two of three patients treated by excisional surgery were recurrence-free 12 and 105 months later. The third woman developed bone metastases at 51 months and was alive at 98 months posttreatment. Khalifeh et al (33) reported that two of six patients with MGA-associated carcinoma presented with distant metastases. One patient had only bone metastases, whereas the other had widespread systemic disease, including metastases to lymph nodes, brain, bone, and spinal cord. The metastases were morphologically similar to the primary carcinoma. In a recent series (43), 7 of 11 women with MGA-associated carcinoma (1 DCIS and 10 invasive carcinomas) underwent mastectomy, and 4 were treated with lumpectomy and adjuvant radiotherapy. None of the patients had lymph node metastases at presentation. One patient received neoadjuvant chemotherapy, and all others received adjuvant chemotherapy, including the patient with MGA-associated DCIS. A patient developed lung metastases 24 months after initial diagnosis and was alive with disease at 34 months' follow-up.

Based on published reports with limited data and a median follow-up of nearly 5 years, patients with MGA-associated carcinomas appear to have a relatively favorable outcome, even though MGA-associated carcinoma has histopathologic and immunohistochemical features of basal-like carcinoma that is usually associated with a poor prognosis. The treatment of MGA-associated carcinoma should be based on the stage of disease in the individual patient. In cases of MGA-associated DCIS and MGA-associated invasive carcinoma, breast-conserving surgery should always be combined with radiotherapy. Adjuvant chemotherapy is recommended for patients with axillary lymph node metastases or with invasive tumors larger than 1 cm in the absence of nodal metastases.

Caution is recommended in the diagnostic evaluation of NCB material that contains a triple-negative small glandular proliferation devoid of myoepithelium, and immunostaining for S-100 should be performed to rule out the possibility of MGA. In the current era of neoadjuvant treatment, it is imperative to remember that well-differentiated invasive ductal carcinoma with triple-negative profile is *exceedingly* rare and can be confidently diagnosed only upon review of the morphology of the entire tumor.

Molecular Pathology of Microglandular Adenosis

MGA with neither associated atypia nor carcinoma is heterogeneous at the molecular level. MGA with atypia and/or carcinoma shows complex copy number alterations (with gains of 1q, 2q, 7p, and 8q; and losses of 1p, 3p, 5q, 6q, 8p, 14q, 16q, 17p, and 17q) (34,37,53-55) and *TP53* and *PIK3CA* mutations (in >75% and ~10% of such cases, respectively).

Molecular studies investigating MGA and its associated lesions suggest that the entity is a nonobligate precursor of triple-negative breast carcinoma. Comparative genomic and array-based hybridization studies demonstrate similar copy number alterations across MGA, atypical MGA, and carcinoma associated with MGA (34,37). Additional alterations have been found in the invasive carcinoma component. Most cases of MGA with neither atypia nor associated carcinoma show no significant chromosomal abnormality. Next-generation sequencing (NGS) studies reveal similar findings (53,54). Cases of MGA with associated invasive carcinoma most frequently harbor somatic mutations in *TP53* and canonical cancer-associated pathways, such as *PIK3*-related genes. MGA with neither atypia nor invasive carcinoma typically lacks such genomic changes.

REFERENCES

1. Foote FW, Stewart FW. Comparative studies of cancerous versus noncancerous breasts. *Ann Surg*. 1945;121:197-222.
2. Markopoulos C, Kouskos E, Phillipidis T, et al. Adenosis tumor of the breast. *Breast J*. 2003;9:255-256.
3. Gill HK, Ioffe OB, Berg WA. When is a diagnosis of sclerosing adenosis acceptable at core biopsy? *Radiology*. 2003;228:50-57.
4. Taşkın F, Köseoğlu K, Unsal A, Erkuş M, Ozbaş S, Karaman C. Sclerosing adenosis of the breast: radiologic appearance and efficiency of core needle biopsy. *Diagn Interv Radiol*. 2011;17:311-316.
5. Oztekin PS, Tuncbilek I, Kosar P, Gültekin S, Oztürk FK. Nodular sclerosing adenosis mimicking malignancy in the breast: magnetic resonance imaging findings. *Breast J*. 2011;17:95-97.
6. Lee KC, Chan JK, Gwi E. Tubular adenosis of the breast: a distinctive benign lesion mimicking invasive carcinoma. *Am J Surg Pathol*. 1996;20:46-54.
7. Eusebi V, Azzopardi JG. Vascular infiltration in benign breast disease. *J Pathol*. 1976;118:9-16.
8. Nielsen BB. Adenosis tumour of the breast—a clinicopathological investigation of 27 cases. *Histopathology*. 1987;11:1259-1275.
9. Simpson JF, Page DL, Dupont WD. Apocrine adenosis—a mimic of mammary carcinoma. *Surg Pathol*. 1990;3:289-299.
10. Carter DJ, Rosen PP. Atypical apocrine metaplasia in sclerosing lesions of the breast: a study of 51 patients. *Mod Pathol*. 1991;4:1-5.
11. Seidman JD, Ashton M, Lefkowitz M. Atypical apocrine adenosis of the breast: a clinicopathologic study of 37 patients with 8.7-year follow-up. *Cancer*. 1996;77:2529-2537.
12. Elayat G, Selim AG, Wells CA. Cell cycle alterations and their relationship to proliferation in apocrine adenosis of the breast. *Histopathology*. 2009;54:348-354.
13. Calhoun BC, Booth CN. Atypical apocrine adenosis diagnosed on breast core biopsy: implications for management. *Hum Pathol*. 2014;45:2130-2135.
14. Abati AD, Kimmel M, Rosen PP. Apocrine mammary carcinoma: a clinicopathologic study of 72 cases. *Am J Clin Pathol*. 1990;94:371-377.
15. Eusebi V, Collina G, Bussolati G. Carcinoma in situ in sclerosing adenosis of the breast: an immunocytochemical study. *Semin Diagn Pathol*. 1989;6:146-152.
16. Hilson JB, Schnitt SJ, Collins LC. Phenotypic alterations in myoepithelial cells associated with benign sclerosing lesions of the breast. *Am J Surg Pathol*. 2010;34:896-900.
17. Moritani S, Ichihara S, Hasegawa M, et al. Topographical, morphological and immunohistochemical characteristics of carcinoma in situ of the breast involving sclerosing adenosis: two distinct topographical patterns and histological types of carcinoma in situ. *Histopathology*. 2011;58:835-846.
18. Oberman HA, Markey BA. Noninvasive carcinoma of the breast presenting in adenosis. *Mod Pathol*. 1991;4:31-35.
19. Fechner RE. Lobular carcinoma in situ in sclerosing adenosis: a potential source of confusion with invasive carcinoma. *Am J Surg Pathol*. 1981;5:233-239.
20. Page DL, Vander Zwaag R, Rogers LW, Williams LT, Walker WE, Hartmann WH. Relation between component parts of fibrocystic disease complex and breast cancer. *J Natl Cancer Inst*. 1978;61:1055-1063.
21. Dupont WD, Page DL. Risk factors for breast cancer in women with proliferative breast disease. *N Engl J Med*. 1985;312:146-151.
22. Jensen RA, Page DL, Dupont WD, Rogers LW. Invasive breast cancer risk in women with sclerosing adenosis. *Cancer*. 1989;64:1977-1983.
23. Bodian CA, Perzin KH, Lattes R, Hoffmann P, Abernathy TG. Prognostic significance of benign proliferative breast disease. *Cancer*. 1993;71:3896-3907.
24. Carter CL, Corle DK, Micozzi MS, Schatzkin A, Taylor PR. A prospective study of the development of breast cancer in 16,692 women with benign breast disease. *Am J Epidemiol*. 1988;128:467-477.
25. Hutchinson WB, Thomas DB, Hamlin WB, Roth GJ, Peterson AV, Williams B. Risk of breast cancer in women with benign breast disease. *J Natl Cancer Inst*. 1980;65:13-20.
26. Kodlin D, Winger EE, Morgenstern NL, Chen U. Chronic mastopathy and breast cancer: a follow-up study. *Cancer*. 1977;39:2603-2607.
27. Krieger N, Hiatt RA. Risk of breast cancer after benign breast diseases: variation by histologic type, degree of atypia, age at biopsy, and length of follow-up. *Am J Epidemiol*. 1992;135:619-631.
28. Visscher DW, Nassar A, Degnim AC, et al. Sclerosing adenosis and risk of breast cancer. *Breast Cancer Res Treat*. 2014;144:205-212.
29. Fuehrer N, Hartmann L, Degnim A, et al. Atypical apocrine adenosis of the breast: long-term follow-up in 37 patients. *Arch Pathol Lab Med*. 2012;136:179-182.
30. Clement PB, Azzopardi JG. Microglandular adenosis of the breast—a lesion simulating tubular carcinoma. *Histopathology*. 1983;7:169-180.
31. Rosen PP. Microglandular adenosis: a benign lesion simulating invasive mammary carcinoma. *Am J Surg Pathol*. 1983;7:137-144.
32. Tavassoli FA, Norris HJ. Microglandular adenosis of the breast: a clinicopathologic study of 11 cases with ultrastructural observations. *Am J Surg Pathol*. 1983;7:731-737.
33. Khalifeh IM, Albarracin C, Diaz LK, et al. Clinical, histopathologic, and immunohistochemical features of microglandular adenosis and transition into in situ and invasive carcinoma. *Am J Surg Pathol*. 2008;32:544-552.
34. Geyer FC, Lacroix-Triki M, Colombo PE, et al. Molecular evidence in support of the neoplastic and precursor nature of microglandular adenosis. *Histopathology*. 2012;60:E115-E130.
35. Kim DJ, Sun WY, Ryu DH, et al. Microglandular adenosis. *J Breast Cancer*. 2011;14:72-75.
36. Koenig C, Dadmanesh F, Bratthauer GL, Tavassoli FA. Carcinoma arising in microglandular adenosis: an immunohistochemical analysis of 20 intraepithelial and invasive neoplasms. *Int J Surg Pathol*. 2000;8:303-315.
37. Shin SJ, Simpson PT, Da Silva L, et al. Molecular evidence for progression of microglandular adenosis (MGA) to invasive carcinoma. *Am J Surg Pathol*. 2009;33:496-504.
38. Shui R, Yang W. Invasive breast carcinoma arising in microglandular adenosis: a case report and review of the literature. *Breast J*. 2009;15:653-656.
39. Shui R, Bi R, Cheng Y, Lu H, Wang J, Yang W. Matrix-producing carcinoma of the breast in the Chinese population: a clinicopathological study of 13 cases. *Pathol Int*. 2011;61:415-422.
40. Geyer FC, Kushner YB, Lambros MB, et al. Microglandular adenosis or microglandular adenoma? A molecular genetic analysis of a case associated with atypia and invasive carcinoma. *Histopathology*. 2009;55:732-743.
41. Resetkova E, Flanders DJ, Rosen PP. Ten-year follow-up of mammary carcinoma arising in microglandular adenosis treated with breast conservation. *Arch Pathol Lab Med*. 2003;127:77-80.
42. James BA, Cranor ML, Rosen PP. Carcinoma of the breast arising in microglandular adenosis. *Am J Clin Pathol*. 1993;100:507-513.
43. Zhong F, Bi R, Yu B, et al. Carcinoma arising in microglandular adenosis of the breast: triple negative phenotype with variable morphology. *Int J Clin Exp Pathol*. 2014;7:6149-6156.
44. Sabate JM, Gomez A, Torrubia S, et al. Microglandular adenosis of the breast in a BRCA1 mutation carrier: radiological features. *Eur Radiol*. 2002;12:1479-1482.
45. Kay S. Microglandular adenosis of the female mammary gland: study of a case with ultrastructural observations. *Hum Pathol*. 1985;16:637-641.
46. Rosenblum MK, Purrazzella R, Rosen PP. Is microglandular adenosis a precancerous disease? A study of carcinoma arising therein. *Am J Surg Pathol*. 1986;10:237-245.
47. Lin L, Pathmanathan N. Microglandular adenosis with transition to breast carcinoma: a series of three cases. *Pathology*. 2011;43:498-503.
48. Damiani S, Pasquinelli G, Lamovec J, Peterse JL, Eusebi V. Acinic cell carcinoma of the breast: an immunohistochemical and ultrastructural study. *Virchows Arch*. 2000;437:74-81.
49. Coyne JD, Dervan PA. Primary acinic cell carcinoma of the breast. *J Clin Pathol*. 2002;55:545-547.
50. Eusebi V, Foschini MP, Betts CM, et al. Microglandular adenosis, apocrine adenosis, and tubular carcinoma of the breast: an immunohistochemical comparison. *Am J Surg Pathol*. 1993;17:99-109.
51. Cserni G. Presence of basement membrane material around the tubules of tubulolobular carcinoma. *Breast Care (Basel)*. 2008;3:423-425.
52. Rosen PP. So-called acinic cell carcinoma of the breast arises from microgladular adenosis and is not a distinct entity. *Mod Pathol*. 2017;30:1504.
53. Guerini-Rocco E, Piscuoglio S, Ng CK, et al. Microglandular adenosis associated with triple-negative breast cancer is a neoplastic lesion of triple-negative phenotype harbouring TP53 somatic mutations. *J Pathol*. 2016;238:677-688.
54. Schwartz CJ, Dolgalev I, Yoon E, et al. Microglandular adenosis is an advanced precursor breast lesion with evidence of molecular progression to matrix-producing metaplastic carcinoma. *Hum Pathol*. 2019;85:65-71.
55. WHO Classification of Tumours Editorial Board. *WHO Classification of Tumours: Breast Tumours*. 5th ed. International Agency for Research on Cancer; 2019.

7

Fibroepithelial Neoplasms

RAZA S. HODA AND SYED A. HODA

Fibroepithelial tumors encompass a wide spectrum of proliferative lesions as well as neoplasms—both benign and malignant. Definitions of fibroadenoma (FA) and of phyllodes tumors (PTs) as well as variants thereof and related lesions appear in **Tables 7.1 and 7.2**. The distinction between the specific "fibroepithelial" entities may be difficult to make in many cases, particularly on needle core biopsy (NCB) sampling.

SCLEROSING LOBULAR HYPERPLASIA (FIBROADENOMATOID CHANGE)

Sclerosing lobular hyperplasia (SLH) is a benign fibroepithelial alteration that can form a palpable mass (1,2). SLH may be associated with tenderness. Patient age ranges from 12 (3) to 46 (4) years, with a mean age of about 30 years. There is no known predisposing factor. Imaging findings closely resemble those of FA.

TABLE 7.1

Definitions of Fibroadenoma (FA) and Related Benign Biphasic Tumors

Fibroadenoma: A biphasic (fibrous and epithelial) circumscribed mass composed of fibrous and glandular elements. The growth pattern is either intracanalicular or pericanalicular. The *intracanalicular pattern* shows elongated and compressed epithelial-lined clefts. The *pericanalicular pattern* displays stromal cells in a circumferential manner around open (noncompressed) glands.

Cellular Fibroadenoma: A FA with modest homogeneous increase in stromal cellularity, pericanalicular pattern, and some stromal cell mitotic activity (<2/10 hpf or 1/mm^2). There is negligible stromal cell atypia. There is no periductal stromal hypercellularity ("condensation").

Complex Fibroadenoma: An FA with some (or all) of the following features: cysts (>3 mm), sclerosing adenosis, cystic apocrine hyperplasia, and glandular-based calcifications. Approximately 20% of FAs show complex features. There is a slightly increased relative risk (<3×) of developing subsequent breast carcinoma.

Fibroadenomatoid Change (Sclerosing Lobular Hyperplasia): A multinodular, yet circumscribed, mass in younger women. There is compact proliferation of ducts and lobules (without epithelial hyperplasia). The glands show normal architecture. The intralobular stroma, and to a lesser degree, the interlobular parenchyma, is fibrotic.

"Giant" Fibroadenoma: An FA that spans >5 cm or weighs >500 g. Such tumors typically occur in younger women (age: <30)

Hamartoma: An uncommon, circumscribed, round or lenticular mass composed of (otherwise unremarkable) nonhyperplastic components of breast tissue (ducts and lobules, fibrous and adipose tissues). The proportion of the three ("fibro," "adeno," and "lipo") components vary. Imaging is considered characteristic: "breast within a breast." The lesion has also been described as "encapsulated fat."

"Juvenile" Fibroadenoma: Typically, a large rapidly growing FA in an adolescent. There is pericanalicular (rather than intracanalicular) growth pattern. The stroma is usually not prominent and is relatively homogeneous. Stromal cell mitoses are readily evident (~2/10 hpf). The epithelial component displays variable degrees of hyperplasia. More common in Americans of African descent.

"Lactating/Lactational Adenoma": This seemingly biphasic "tumor" occurs in pregnant (or nursing) women and is best regarded as *nodular lactational hyperplasia*. The glandular component shows diffuse secretory change. The latter is characterized by "hobnailing," vacuolated cytoplasm, and luminal secretions.

Myxoid Fibroadenoma: An FA with prominent myxoid change in stroma. Myxoid fibroadenomas have been reported in the Carney complex.

Nodular Pseudoangiomatous Stromal Hyperplasia (PASH): Myofibroblastic cells form a mass with uniformly distributed otherwise unremarkable glands. The glands are not compressed, i.e., the stroma surrounds the native glands—without distortion. The nodule can appear to be "fibroadenomatoid." Glands may be absent ("fibrous tumor") or inconspicuous within the nodule.

Tubular Adenoma: A biphasic fibroepithelial tumor with well-defined borders and scanty stroma. The glandular component is tightly packed with bland round to tubule-like glands. There is minimal stroma, and atypia is negligible. Glandular secretions are inconspicuous.

TABLE 7.2
Definitions of Phyllodes Tumor (PT) and Related Tumors

Benign Phyllodes Tumor: A circumscribed biphasic (fibrous and epithelial) neoplasm. The growth pattern is intracanalicular, with development of exaggerated "leaf-like" stromal fronds. The stroma is hypercellular. This is the most common type of PT.
Borderline (Low-Grade Malignant) Phyllodes Tumor: Histopathologic characteristics are intermediate between benign and malignant phyllodes tumor. See **Tables 7.4 and 7.5**.
Malignant Phyllodes Tumor: An infiltrative biphasic (fibrous and epithelial) neoplasm. The stroma is diffusely hypercellular, and the stromal cells exhibit nuclear atypia and mitotic activity. Stromal overgrowth (no glandular component on low-power microscopic examination, i.e., at 4× objective with a 10× ocular, or 22.9 mm^2) is evident. Least common type of PT
Periductal Stromal Tumor: This poorly characterized tumor may be best regarded as a variant of PT, and usually behaves as a low-grade malignancy. It shows an infiltrative biphasic growth pattern with proliferation of variably hypercellular atypical spindly stromal cells. The latter surround unremarkable or minimally hyperplastic mammary glands (mainly ducts). "Leaf-like" architecture is absent.
Carcinosarcoma: An uncommon biphasic neoplasm with concurrent carcinomatous and sarcomatous component

Nodular pseudoangiomatous stromal hyperplasia (PASH), infiltrative variant of myofibroblastoma, and metaplastic spindle cell carcinoma may mimic PT—particularly on needle core biopsy sampling.

In SLH, there is an increased number, and enlargement, of lobules. The intralobular stroma is collagenized, with variable sclerosis **(Fig. 7.1)**. The individual lobules appear to be minute FAs, albeit with a prominent glandular component. The acini are lined by single-layered epithelium. Secretory activity may be present. Calcifications are uncommon. SLH can occur in the vicinity of FAs, PTs and hamartomas **(Fig. 7.2)** (1,5).

SLH does not require treatment. Excision might be considered if the NCB of a mass-forming lesion yields SLH to rule out inadequate sampling of a PT. Clinical and imaging correlation is necessary.

FIBROADENOMA

Clinical Presentation

FA is the most common benign neoplasm of the breast. It can occur at any age; however, the median age at presentation ranges from 20 to 40, approximately 20 years lower than that of patients with PT. Juvenile FA tends to occur in girls younger than 20 and is the most common fibroepithelial lesion in pediatric patients (6,7). Fibroepithelial lesions with features of juvenile FA can occur in adult women (8). The mean age of complex FAs was 34.5 in one study (9). In another series (10), the median age of patients with complex FA was higher than that of patients with noncomplex FAs (47 vs 28.5, respectively).

A relationship of FA with hormonal treatment has been debated. Some FAs develop just after puberty (6). The familial occurrence of multiple synchronous and metachronous FAs has been observed. Rare examples of FAs are reported in men (11-15), usually in association with gynecomastia. Women treated with cyclosporin for immunosuppression may develop large, multiple, and bilateral FAs (16,17). The duration of cyclosporin treatment prior to the detection of an FA is generally greater than 1 year. Some, but not all, FAs have regressed after cyclosporin was discontinued. (18). Women with Carney syndrome may develop myxoid FAs (19). The percentage of women with myxoid FA who have Carney syndrome is unknown.

FA usually presents as a painless, firm or rubbery, well-circumscribed, solitary mass. Some patients have multiple,

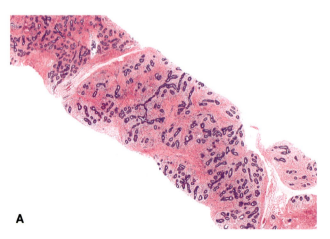
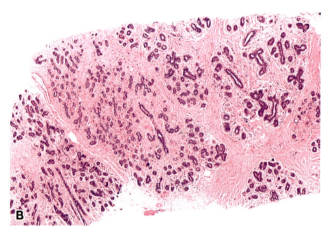

FIGURE 7.1 Sclerosing Lobular Hyperplasia (Fibroadenomatoid Change). A, B: These needle core biopsies were obtained from breast nodules in teenage girls. The biopsies show enlarged lobules with sclerotic stroma.

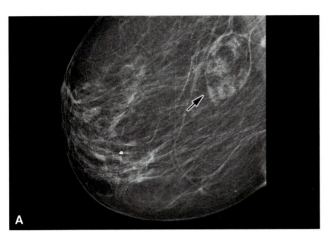
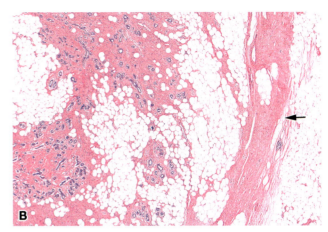

FIGURE 7.2 **Mammary Hamartoma. A:** Imaging is considered characteristic: "breast within a breast" (arrow). Image courtesy: Dr Serine Baydoun, Cleveland, OH. **B:** Circumscribed mass composed of nonhyperplastic components of breast tissue (ducts and lobules, fibrous and adipose tissues). Note fibrous band enclosing the lesion (arrows).

bilateral, synchronous or metachronous FAs. FAs can undergo infarction during pregnancy, either following trauma or de novo. An infarcted FA can be painful. FA in axillary breast tissue can mimic lymphadenopathy, clinically and on imaging.

Imaging

An increasing percentage of FAs are nonpalpable tumors detected on imaging as discrete nodular densities (19). Stromal calcifications in FAs are common in postmenopausal women. On ultrasonography, most FAs are nodular, iso- or hypo-echoic solid masses with circumscribed borders. In one study (20), myxoid FAs showed significantly greater depth-to-width ratio than usual FAs, and some were suspicious for mucinous carcinoma. Magnetic resonance imaging (MRI) appearance of FAs is variable and is influenced by the relative proportions of epithelial and stromal components. In an MRI study of 81 FAs (21), 70.4% had well-defined margins, 90.1% were round or lobulated, 49.4% had heterogeneous internal structures, and 27.2% displayed nonenhancing internal septations. After contrast injection, 22.2% of FAs had a suspicious signal intensity–time course.

Size

Most FAs span less than 3 cm. FAs that span more than 4 cm are more frequent in patients under 20 (22) and usually have the morphology of juvenile FA. The so-called "giant" FA (a term that we cannot condone) and juvenile FA (a term that we reluctantly accept—given its wide usage) are usually clinicopathologically similar. The mean size of 23 juvenile FAs in women 18 or younger studied by Ross et al (6) was 3.1 cm (range 0.5-7). In one series (10), the mean size of complex FAs (1.3 ± 0.57 cm) was about one-half the size of usual FAs (2.5 ± 1.44 cm).

Histopathology

FA is mainly a tumor of specialized mammary stroma—with secondary proliferation of glandular elements. The stroma shows either intra- or pericanalicular growth pattern **(Fig. 7.3)**. The *intracanalicular pattern* shows elongated and compressed epithelial-lined clefts. The *pericanalicular pattern* displays stromal cells in a circumferential manner around open glands. FAs with a prominent intracanalicular pattern can mimic benign phyllodes tumor (BnPT) and papilloma, especially in NCB. Within any given FA, the stroma has homogeneous cellularity, and the epithelium-to-stroma ratio is similar **(Fig. 7.3)**. In contrast, PTs have uneven distribution of glands and heterogeneous stromal cellularity. BnPT can harbor foci indistinguishable from FA. Adipocytic (lipomatous) differentiation is not encountered in FA but may occur in PT.

Multinucleated stromal giant cells can be found in FAs (23) and PTs (23), in some benign tumors (24), as well as in nonlesional stroma. The nuclei in the giant cells are typically pleomorphic and hyperchromatic and can show a florette-like pattern. Per se, the presence of such giant cells has no known prognostic significance. FAs with giant cells should not be misclassified as PTs, even if the cells are focally p53-positive and Ki-67-positive (24).

The usual (adult-type) is the most common type of FA **(Fig. 7.4)**. FAs in postmenopausal women tend to be hypocellular and hyalinized, and may harbor coarse dystrophic stromal-based calcifications **(Fig. 7.5)**. FAs in younger women have more cellular stroma. Epithelial hyperplasia is usually absent. Focal secretory change may be present **(Fig. 7.6)**. Mitoses are uncommon in FAs but may be observed in FAs in adolescent girls (6,7).

A **tubular adenoma** is a variant of pericanalicular FA. **(Fig. 7.7)**. There is adenosis with closely approximated round or oval glands lined by single-layered glandular epithelium and myoepithelium.

A FA with hypercellular stroma is often referred to as **cellular FA**, but this diagnosis has low interobserver reproducibility. The differential diagnosis between cellular FA and BnPT can be problematic, especially on NCB **(Figs. 7.8 and 7.9; Table 7.3)**; and excision is warranted for its definitive classification. Nevertheless, most FAs rarely pose a diagnostic challenge on NCB. A hyalinized FA with

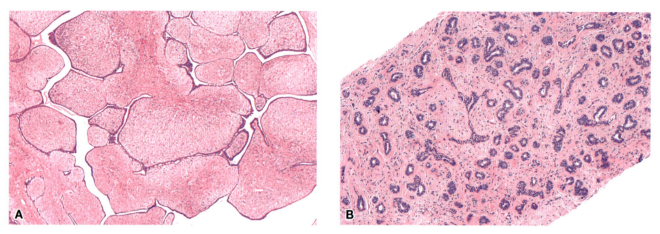

FIGURE 7.3 **Fibroadenoma, Growth Patterns. A:** The *intracanalicular* growth pattern is formed by compressed epithelial-lined clefts. **B:** A *pericanalicular* lesion in which the stroma is arranged in a circumferential nodular pattern around the epithelial-lined glands.

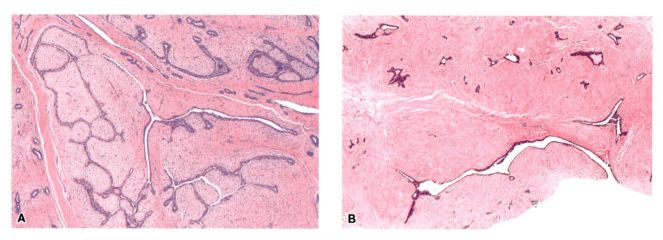

FIGURE 7.4 **Fibroadenoma, Usual Type. A:** Excisional biopsy of a usual fibroadenoma in a 26-year-old woman. **B:** Needle core biopsy of a usual fibroadenoma in a 55-year-old woman.

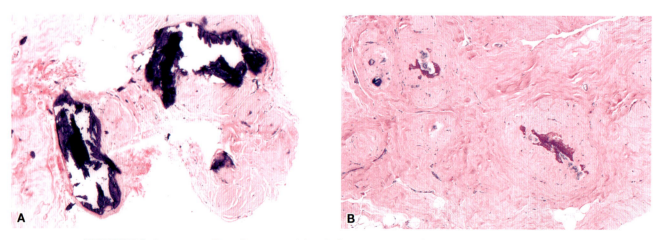

FIGURE 7.5 **Senescent Fibroadenoma, With Calcification and Ossification. A, B:** Two examples of nonpalpable atrophic fibroadenomas (both discovered on screening) in octogenarians. Note coarse calcifications in both, and ossification in **B**.

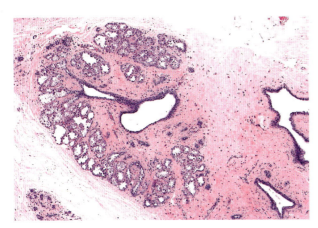

FIGURE 7.6 **Fibroadenoma, With Secretory Change.** This needle core biopsy is from a palpable lesion in a 32-year-old woman. The patient is a *BRCA1* germline mutation carrier, and the tumor was clinically suspicious for malignancy.

and eosin (H&E)-stained sections and can be highlighted with Masson trichrome and/or CK stains **(Fig. 7.10)**. FA (and lactational adenoma/nodular lactational hyperplasia) can undergo infarction during pregnancy as well as in the postpartum period.

Myxoid FAs are characterized by diffuse and homogenous myxoid stromal change **(Fig. 7.11)**. These FAs have uniformly hypocellular stroma, whereas myxoid change in a PT tends to be less homogeneous. The differential diagnosis of myxoid FA in NCB includes mucinous carcinoma **(Fig. 7.12)** and PT with myxoid stroma.

"Complex" FAs are those with at least one of the following findings: sclerosing adenosis (SA), papillary apocrine hyperplasia, macrocysts (≥3 mm), and epithelial-based calcifications **(Fig. 7.13)** (9,25). In a series of 63 complex FAs (10), 57% had SA, 8% had apocrine metaplasia, and 1.6% had cysts. Calcifications in SA were found in 9.5% of cases. Papillary hyperplasia and SA can mask the basic fibroepithelial nature of a complex FA, especially in an NCB, and raise the differential diagnosis of fibrocystic changes (FCCs) **(Fig. 7.13)**, juvenile papillomatosis, and papilloma **(Fig. 7.14)**. Differential diagnosis of complex FAs with confluent SA

conspicuous epithelium may raise the differential diagnosis of a sclerotic papilloma, but the pseudopapillary fronds in FA lack true fibrovascular cores. The underlying architecture of an **infarcted FA** can usually be identified in hematoxylin

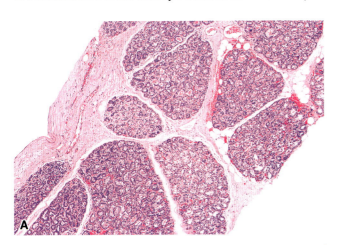
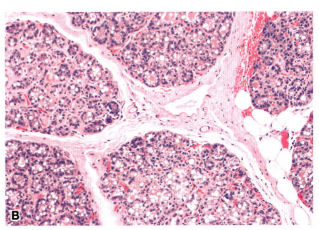

FIGURE 7.7 **Nodular Lactational Hyperplasia (So-called "Lactating Adenoma" or "Lactational Adenoma"). A, B:** Enlarged lobules with lactational/secretory hyperplasia in needle core biopsy from a breast tumor in a 37-year-old pregnant woman.

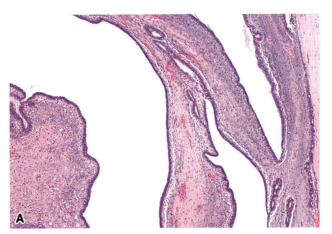
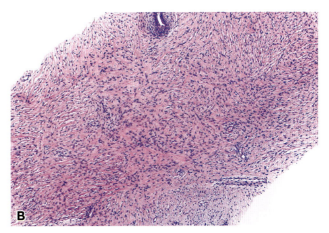

FIGURE 7.8 **"Fibroepithelial Lesions." A:** Wider (as opposed to narrower) epithelial-lined clefts suggest a phyllodes tumor (PT). **B.** Relative stromal prominence (or frank "overgrowth") also suggests PT.

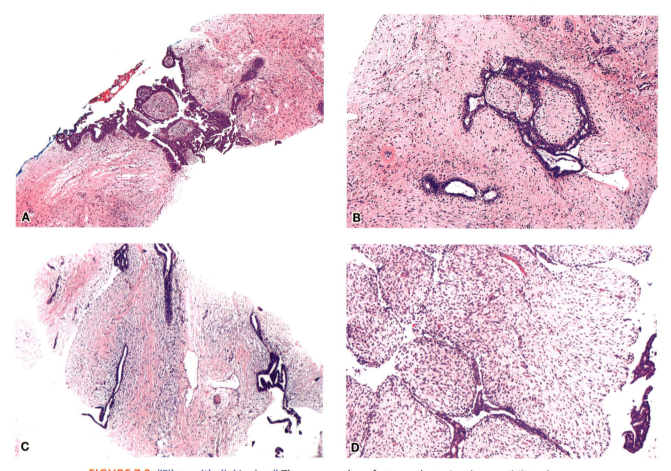

FIGURE 7.9 "Fibroepithelial Lesion." These cases show features that raise the possibility of benign phyllodes tumor. Excision is warranted in these cases. **A:** The stroma of the fibroepithelial lesion in this needle core biopsy (NCB) shows increased cellularity without cytologic atypia. A duct is lined by hyperplastic epithelium. Within the duct lumen are detached fragments of stroma lined by epithelium all around, in a frond-like arrangement. **B:** This NCB shows a fibroepithelial tumor with moderately cellular stroma. **C:** This NCB shows moderately cellular stroma and epithelial-lined clefts. **D:** This needle core shows apparent fragmentation of cores. Each fragment is epithelial-lined.

TABLE 7.3

Differential Diagnosis: Fibroepithelial Tumors on Needle Core Biopsy List of Factors Favoring Benign Phyllodes Tumor

Histopathologic Feature	Details
Stromal overgrowth	No glands in a 40× total microscopy field (or 22.9 mm^2)
Stromal heterogeneity	Regional variation in cellularity
Stromal cellularity	Higher (see **Table 7.6**)
Stromal cell mitoses	Readily evident
Condensation of stroma	In subepithelial location
Pleomorphism	Of stromal cell nuclei
Fragmentation of cores	Fragmented cores lined near-circumferentially by epithelium
Adipose tissue	Incorporation within the tumor
Edges (whenever evaluable)	Tumor infiltrative into adjacent fibroadipose tissue

No one factor, in isolation, is diagnostic.

FIBROEPITHELIAL NEOPLASMS 111

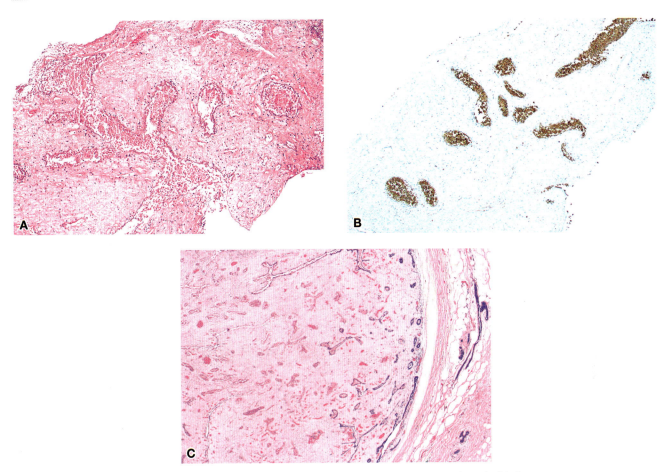

FIGURE 7.10 Fibroadenoma With Infarct. A-C: This needle core biopsy of a palpable breast mass in a 15-year-old girl had been initially interpreted as a vascular lesion, but the "ghostly" outline of the tissue is typical of an infarcted fibroadenoma. Cytokeratin 7 stain highlights the necrotic epithelium, confirming that the lesion is an infarcted fibroadenoma **(B). C:** A case of *de novo* acute infarct of the breast. Excision of a largely necrotic fibroadenoma in a 30-year-old nonpregnant woman who developed acute pain in the breast 2 days prior to excision. Note preservation of viable glandular elements at the perimeter of the tumor.

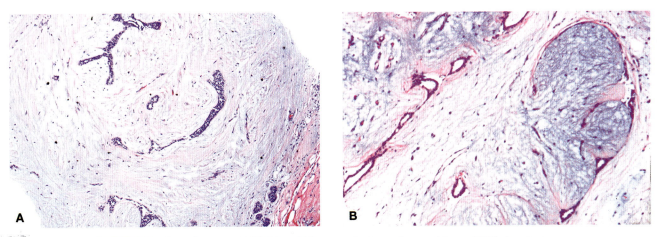

FIGURE 7.11 Fibroadenomas With Myxoid Stroma. A: A needle core biopsy (NCB) showing myxoid stroma in a fibroadenoma. **B:** NCB in which the epithelium is compressed into slender cords and minute glands by the myxoid stroma.

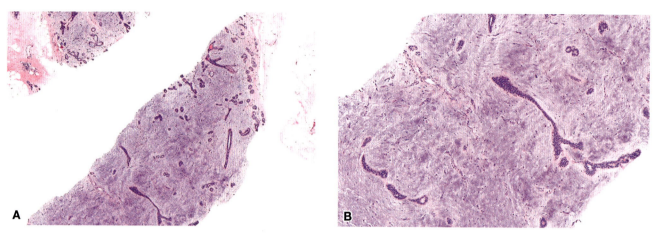

FIGURE 7.12 Fibroadenoma With Myxoid Stroma. A, B: A needle core biopsy showing myxoid stroma in a fibroadenoma. This lesion had been misinterpreted as mucinous carcinoma.

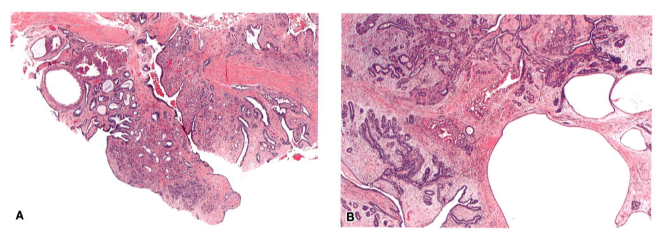

FIGURE 7.13 Complex Fibroadenoma. A, B: A needle core biopsy **(A)** and subsequent excision **(B)** showing a complex fibroadenoma with apocrine hyperplasia, macrocysts, and adenosis.

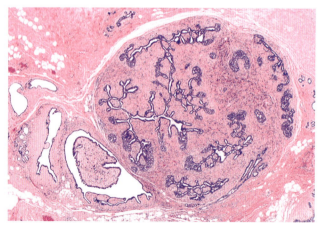

FIGURE 7.14 Partial Papillary Appearance of a Fibroadenoma. A needle core biopsy of the papillary portion of the tumor (lower left) could result in the mistaken diagnosis of a papilloma. A papilloma should have true fibrovascular cores.

also includes invasive carcinoma **(Fig. 7.15)**. Excision of a complex FA is not necessary, unless there is atypical ductal hyperplasia (ADH) or whenever the diagnosis is uncertain.

Juvenile fibroadenoma is characterized by increased stromal cellularity and epithelial hyperplasia. Pericanalicular architecture is more common than intracanalicular architecture (6,7). The tumor border is well-defined. The stroma tends to be uniformly cellular, with scant separation between intralobular/periglandular stroma and interlobular stroma (6). The glandular element tends to be uniformly distributed; however, some juvenile FAs can show stromal expansion as well as gland-rich areas (6), creating an impression of intratumoral heterogeneity, especially on NCB. The uniform quality of stromal proliferation and lack of stromal atypia are features that support the diagnosis of FA. Epithelial hyperplasia is typical in juvenile FAs and can be conspicuous. ADH or ductal carcinoma in situ (DCIS) are rare in this setting. Necrosis and/or calcifications are uncommon **(Fig. 7.16)**.

FIBROEPITHELIAL NEOPLASMS **113**

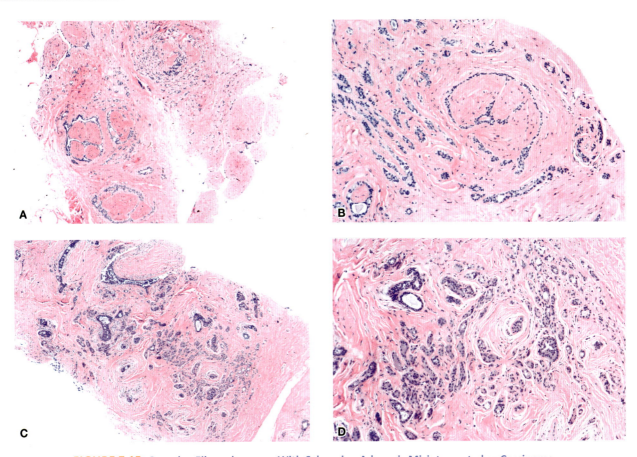

FIGURE 7.15 Complex Fibroadenomas With Sclerosing Adenosis Misinterpreted as Carcinoma.
A, B: A needle core biopsy (NCB) showing sclerosing adenosis in a fibroadenoma. This biopsy was erroneously interpreted as infiltrating lobular carcinoma. **C, D:** This NCB with sclerosing adenosis in a fibroadenoma was diagnosed as invasive tubular carcinoma.

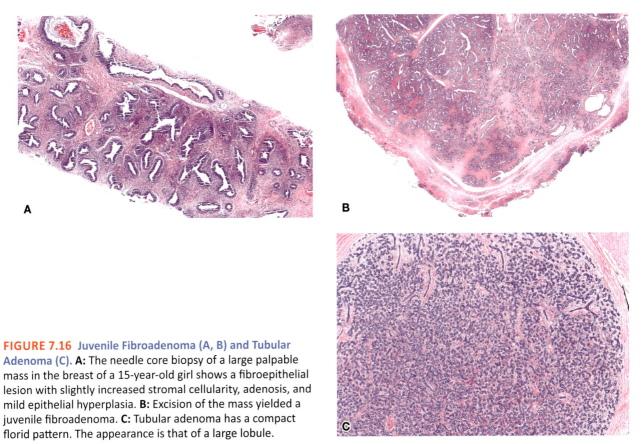

FIGURE 7.16 Juvenile Fibroadenoma (A, B) and Tubular Adenoma (C). A: The needle core biopsy of a large palpable mass in the breast of a 15-year-old girl shows a fibroepithelial lesion with slightly increased stromal cellularity, adenosis, and mild epithelial hyperplasia. **B:** Excision of the mass yielded a juvenile fibroadenoma. **C:** Tubular adenoma has a compact florid pattern. The appearance is that of a large lobule.

Fibroadenoma With ALH, LCIS, ADH, and DCIS

Lobular carcinoma in situ (LCIS) and DCIS can be associated with FAs. Atypical lobular hyperplasia (ALH) and classic LCIS **(Fig. 7.17)** are the most common atypical epithelial proliferations in this setting. Pleomorphic LCIS is rare in an FA. Rarely, ALH or LCIS are confined to the FA. Occasionally, ADH and DCIS **(Fig. 7.17)** are identified (26,27). The differential diagnosis of ADH in FA includes artifactual telescoping of the benign epithelium in the epithelial clefts **(Fig. 7.18)**. An FA may be secondarily involved by invasive carcinoma in its vicinity.

Immunohistochemistry

The epithelium and stroma of FAs show some degree of positivity for estrogen receptor (ER) and progesterone receptor (PR), but these findings have no clinical value. The stromal cells of FAs are CD34-positive and show immunoreactivity for actin and desmin in cases with myoid/myofibroblastic proliferation. Nuclear staining for β-catenin has been documented in the stromal cells of FAs (28). Significant differences are in Ki-67 indices of FAs and BnPTs in NCB (29,30), but substantial overlap exists, limiting the utility of this marker.

Treatment and Prognosis

Clinically symptomatic masses, for example, those causing pain or physical distortion, are typically excised. In the absence of symptoms and atypical histopathologic findings, excision is not warranted for radiologic–pathologic concordant lesions. Clinical, imaging, and pathologic correlations are of foremost importance. Molecular studies suggest that PTs could develop from FAs (31-33), but such occurrences are rare.

Percutaneous Forms of Treatment

Relatively small (≤1.5 cm) FAs can be completely excised via vacuum-assisted, ultrasound-guided *biopsy* (34,35). Vacuum-assisted *excision* for FAs that are less than 2 cm is particularly feasible, with minimal morbidity (34). In a series of 52 FAs (35) removed percutaneously under sonographic guidance, and followed-up with clinical and sonographic examination every 6 months, the recurrence rate was 15% at a median follow-up of 22 months (range 7-59), with an actuarial recurrence rate of 33% at 59 months. Only three of the recurrent lesions were palpable. All recurrences occurred in FAs that were 2 cm or more at initial diagnosis (range 2.1-2.8).

Cryoablation has been used for treating FAs (36-38). The mean pretreatment tumor diameter of 444 FAs treated with cryoablation was 1.8 cm (37). A palpable abnormality was present in 46% of patients at 6-month follow-up and in 35%

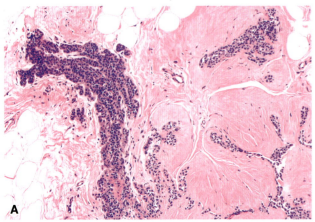

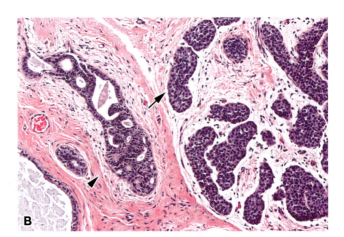

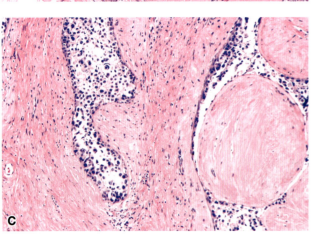

FIGURE 7.17 Fibroadenomas With Lobular Carcinoma In Situ (LCIS), Atypical Ductal Hyperplasia (ADH), and Ductal Carcinoma In Situ (DCIS). A: The fibroadenoma in this needle core biopsy from a 55-year-old woman shows LCIS of the classic type. **B:** This image shows a focus of ADH (arrowhead) and LCIS (arrows). **C:** DCIS is present in this sclerotic fibroadenoma.

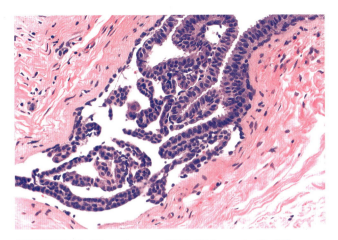

FIGURE 7.18 Fibroadenoma With "Telescoping" of the Epithelium Simulating Ductal Hyperplasia. The ductal epithelium in this fibroadenoma is detached from the duct wall and shows "telescoping" within the luminal space—in a pattern that simulates ductal hyperplasia. Occasionally, "telescoping" can mimic atypical ductal hyperplasia.

at 12 months. In two other series (37,38), a persistent palpable abnormality was more common if the index FA was 2 cm or more. The residual tumor consisted of shrunken hyaline matrix in two cases in which tissue evaluation was undertaken (38).

Excision

Most solitary FAs are treated by excision. Excision of juvenile FAs in adolescent patients should preserve as much of the native immature breast tissue as possible. The risk of upgrade to carcinoma (DCIS and/or invasive carcinoma) at excision following radiologic–pathologic concordant NCB diagnosis of FA (or any of its variants) is negligible.

Follow-Up Without Excision

Some patients with radiologic–pathologic concordant NCB diagnosis of FA do not undergo excision. Regular clinical and mammographic follow-up to document the stability of the lesion is recommended. Features that raise concern for PT include rapid increase in size, development of multilobulation, and cystic change in a previously solid mass.

Relative Risk of Subsequent Carcinoma

The relative risk (RR) of subsequent carcinoma in women with FA is minimal, even in those with proliferative epithelial changes in the FA or in its vicinity, or in those with a family history of breast carcinoma (25). Proliferative changes are more common within/near complex FAs than in noncomplex FAs. In one study (25), the RR of invasive carcinoma for women with any type of FAs was 1.6, but it was 2.4 for women with complex FA, and 3.72 for women with a complex FA and a family history of breast carcinoma. Follow-up information of patients with juvenile FAs is limited but does not reveal a predisposition to develop carcinoma (6,7). Some FAs may recur after excision, especially juvenile FAs with more than 2 mitoses/10 hpf (7).

"FIBROEPITHELIAL TUMOR" AND PHYLLODES TUMOR

PTs are rare fibroepithelial tumors characterized by increased cellularity and heterogeneity of the stromal component. The epithelium-to-stroma ratio varies within the tumor, and some foci in BnPT may resemble FA. PTs are further classified as *benign*, *borderline* (BoPT, *low-grade malignant*), or *malignant* (MPT) based on histopathologic characteristics. This grade-based classification is predictive of probable clinical course **(Tables 7.4 and 7.5)**.

The generic "diagnostic" term "*fibroepithelial tumor/lesion*" is used in NCB whenever the findings therein are equivocal, and in particular when the distinction between cellular FA and BnPT, as well as between BnPT and BoPT, cannot be made (39).

Clinical Presentation

PT usually presents as a discrete firm palpable mass. Larger tumors (>5 cm) may invade the skin or extend into the chest wall. PT can present with bloody nipple discharge (40). Clinically, a size of more than 4 cm and/or "rapid" growth favor PT over FA; however, no one clinical feature can reliably distinguish among the types of PTs (or between cellular FA and BnPT). Enlargement of an erstwhile stable fibroepithelial tumor suggests grade progression. There is emerging evidence that PTs rarely develop from FAs (32,33).

Multifocal ipsilateral or bilateral PTs are rare (5,41-44). There are reports of MPTs with para-neoplastic production of human chorionic gonadotropin (HCG) (45) and of insulin-like growth factor II (46-48). The latter event may result in hypoglycemia.

The median age at diagnosis of PT is about 45 to 50. PTs are rare in women younger than 30 and are exceedingly uncommon before menarche (40,49-51). Most PTs in girls younger than 18 years are benign (6,7). MPTs are rare in pediatric patients and during pregnancy (44,52-54). A BnPT that developed in a 31-week pregnant woman did not recur in a subsequent pregnancy (53), and another PT may have developed from a preexisting FA during endocrine modulating treatment for in vitro fertilization (55). The annual age-adjusted incidence of MPT in a population-based study was 2.1 per 1 million women (56). The risk of MPT was 3- to 4-folds higher for foreign-born than for US-born Latina. Another study (57) found a higher percentage of BoPT and MPTs in Hispanic patients. Asian ethnicity also appears to be associated with a higher risk of PTs. In a study conducted in Australia (58), 31% of 65 women with PTs and 6/9 (67%) women with recurrent PTs were of Asian descent. Furthermore, 32% of the Asian patients developed recurrent disease versus only 7% of non-Asian patients. Women with *TP53* germline mutation (Li-Fraumeni syndrome) have a significantly increased risk of developing MPT ($P = .0003$) (59). PTs are rare in men. A 70-year-old man with gynecomastia and a breast tumor growing over 5 decades had a focally MPT in a 30-cm FA (60).

116 CHAPTER 7

TABLE 7.4
Differential Diagnosis: Fibroadenoma and Benign Phyllodes Tumor

	Fibroadenoma	Phyllodes[a]
Pathologic and Clinical Features		
Stromal cellularity	Lower	Higher
Stromal overgrowth[b]	Absent	May be present
Stromal cell mitoses	Absent/lower	Higher
Edges of the lesion	Sharper	Ill-defined
Stromal atypia/pleomorphism	Uncommon	Common
Epithelial hyperplasia	(+/−)	(++)
Epithelial-lined clefts	Shorter	Elongated
Incorporation of adipocytes	Uncommon	More common
Subepithelial condensation of stroma	Less common	More common
Infarct	Uncommon	Less uncommon
Fragmentation of cores	Uncommon	More common
Clinical size	Typically smaller	Typically larger
Mutations		
MED12	Similar incidence (~60%)	Similar incidence
RARA	Less frequent	More frequent
TERT promotor	Less frequent	More frequent

[a]See **Table 7.5** also.
[b]No glands at 40× microscopy (10× eyepiece, 4× objective).

TABLE 7.5
Differential Diagnosis: Benign, Borderline and Malignant Phyllodes Tumor

	Benign	Borderline	Malignant
Proportion of phyllodes tumors (PTs)[c]	~75%	~15%	~10%
Stromal cellularity	Mild	(~)[a]	Marked
Stromal heterogeneity	Lower	(~)[a]	Higher
Stromal overgrowth	Absent	(~)[a]	Present
Stromal cell mitoses	≤4/10 hpf	5-9/10 hpf [a]	≥10/10 hpf
	2.5/mm^2	2.5-5/mm^2	5/mm^2
Stromal cell atypia	Minimal	(~)[a]	Maximal
Malignant heterologous elements[b]	Absent	(−)[a]	Rare
Fragmentation of cores	Minimal	(~)[a]	Maximal
Edges of the lesion	Circumscribed	(~)[a]	Infiltrative
CD34 immunostaining of stroma	(+)	(~)[a]	(−/+)
Cytokeratin/p63 immunostaining	(−)	(~)[a]	(−/+)
Local recurrence rate[c]	~10%	(~)[a]	~25%
Metastases[c]	(−)	~2%	~15%

[a]These three categories of PTs represent a spectrum, and "borderline" phyllodes tumor lies mid-spectrum, just as "cellular fibroadenoma" is a category between FA and benign phyllodes tumor.
[b]*Well-differentiated* liposarcoma does not represent a malignant heterologous element.
[c]Based on review of cumulative literature. *Note: Clinical size, epithelial-lined clefts, epithelial hyperplasia, and infarction are not relevant to grade stratification.*
hpf: high power field; total magnification: 400×: 40× objective, 10× eyepiece.

Size

The mean tumor size in a study of 605 PTs was 5.2 cm (range 0.3-25) (41). MPTs tend to be larger than BnPTs, but there are exceptions. In a study of 293 PTs (5), the size was 3 cm or less in 54% of cases: 66% of BnPTs measured 3 cm or less, whereas 67% of BoPTs and MPTs were more than 3 cm.

Imaging

Mammography reveals a rounded or lobulated, sharply defined opaque mass (61,62). Sonographically, most PTs appear well-circumscribed; however, some are structurally nonhomogeneous (61). Calcifications are uncommon. Neither mammography nor ultrasonography can reliably classify PT, or distinguish BnPT from cellular FA. MRI of BnPTs reveals an oval or lobulated shape with internal septations (21), but MRI characteristics do not permit separation from cellular FA. A study of 30 PTs (21,63) found no significant difference in MRI characteristics of BnPT and MPT; however, cystic change is suggestive of the latter.

Histopathology

PTs are fibroepithelial tumors characterized by increased cellularity and expansion of the stromal component. Further classification of PTs takes into account multiple parameters; including stromal cellularity, overgrowth, atypia, mitotic activity, edges of the tumor, and presence of heterologous elements. Cellularity and atypia of stromal cells are the more subjective elements among these criteria **(Table 7.6)**. It is usually not possible to definitively classify a fibroepithelial tumor based on evaluation of NCB alone because of intratumoral heterogeneity inherent in most PTs. Stromal cellularity, atypia, and mitotic activity in NCBs of a PT tend to be indicators of PT grade. Diagnostic interpretation should convey the possibility that the lesion may be of higher-grade than evident in the NCB.

Stromal cellularity within a PT tends to be heterogeneous, with more cellular regions in (either abrupt or gradual) juxtaposition to less cellular foci. Some of the latter might be indistinguishable from FA. Varied stromal cellularity in an NCB suggests a PT **(Fig. 7.19)**.

TABLE 7.6

Assessment of Stromal Cellularity and Stromal Cell Atypia in Fibroepithelial Tumors

Stromal Cellularity	
Mildly hypercellular	Slightly more cellular than uninvolved perilobular stroma
	Uniformly spaced cells
	No nuclear overlap
Markedly hypercellular	Tightly packed cells
	Considerable nuclear overlap
	Confluent appearance
	Considerably more cellular than uninvolved perilobular stroma
Moderately hypercellular	Cellularity between mildly and markedly hypercellular
Stromal cell atypia	
Mild atypia	Minimal nuclear pleomorphism
	Slightly more hyperchromatic
	Mildly irregular nuclear contour
	Inconspicuous nucleoli
Marked atypia	Minimal nuclear pleomorphism
	Much more hyperchromatic
	Markedly irregular nuclear contour
	Prominent nucleoli
Moderate atypia	Atypia between mild and marked atypia

Hematoxylin and eosin sections should be of routine (4-5) micron thickness for optimal assessment of stromal cellularity and stromal cell atypia. Atypia and mitotic rate may not be congruent.

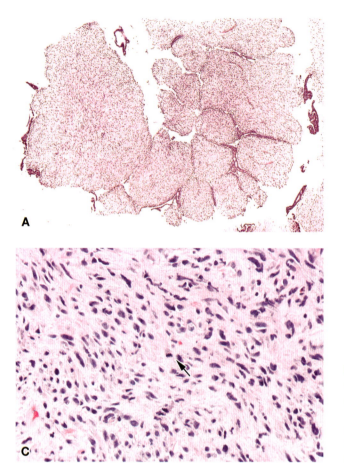
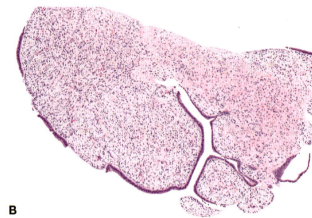

FIGURE 7.19 **Features of Phyllodes Tumors (PTs).** **A:** Fragmentation of tissue cores, relative paucity of epithelial components, expansion of stroma, and stromal hypercellularity are features of PTs. **B:** In this needle core biopsy of a benign phyllodes tumor, the stroma is cellular and forms small fronds lined by epithelium. **C:** A stromal mitosis (arrow) in the same tumor shown in **B**.

Elongated and dilated ducts with cleft-like appearance (resulting in a "cauliflower"-like gross appearance) are one of the characteristic features of PT. The stromal fronds protruding into the ducts usually do *not* tightly mold to one another. In NCB, the frond-like architecture of PTs correlates with fragmentation of cores, and the presence of detached, round-to-oval stromal fragments of different sizes which are lined by epithelium **(Fig. 7.19)**. FAs with an intracanalicular structure can superficially resemble BnPTs, but the fronds tend to completely fill the duct lumina and fit into one another like pieces of a jigsaw puzzle. The stroma of intracanalicular FAs also tends to be uniform and hypocellular. In NCBs of some BnPT or BoPTs, the intracanalicular pattern of clefts sometimes may be obscured by ductal epithelial hyperplasia or by a focally conspicuous glandular component.

Stromal myxoid change is common in PT, but it tends to be patchy. Pseudoangiomatous stromal hyperplasia (PASH) is more commonly identified than FA (64) **(Fig. 7.20)**. Multinucleated stromal giant cells **(Fig. 7.21)** occur in about

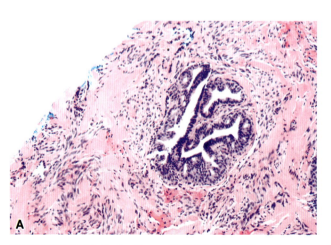
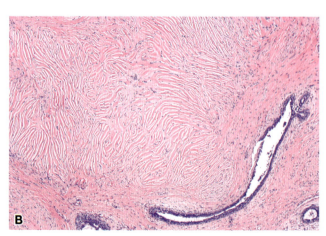

FIGURE 7.20 **Phyllodes Tumor (PT) With Pseudoangiomatous Stromal Hyperplasia (PASH).** **A:** This benign phyllodes tumor (BnPT) has a prominent fascicular stromal pattern composed of bundles of myofibroblasts. The patient was a 75-year-old woman with a recently detected 1.5-cm tumor. **B:** Fascicular PASH in a BnPT from a 45-year-old woman.

FIBROEPITHELIAL NEOPLASMS

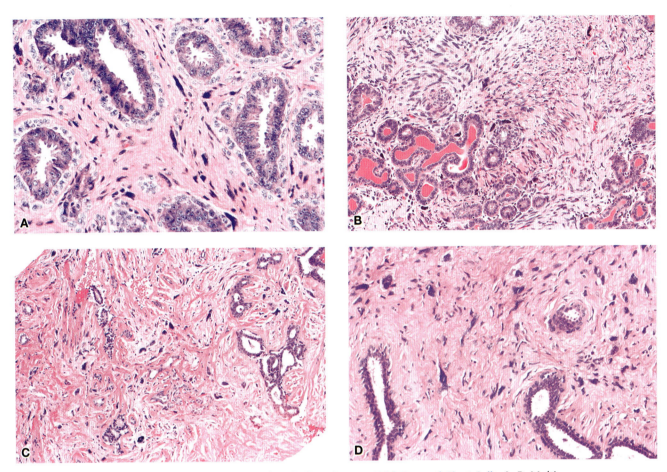

FIGURE 7.21 Phyllodes Tumor (PT) and Fibroadenoma With Stromal Giant Cells. **A, B:** Multinucleated giant cells are present in the stroma of this *benign phyllodes tumor*. **C, D:** A *fibroadenoma* with numerous multinucleated stromal cells.

10% of PTs (64), especially in higher-grade ones. Squamous metaplasia is not characteristic of FAs or BnPTs, but it can occur in BoPTs and in MPTs. The most frequent stromal change consists of atypical lipomatous or *well-differentiated* liposarcoma-like foci. Such lipomatous changes lack *MDM2* and *CDK4* amplifications, and their presence does *not* represent a malignant heterologous element. Rhabdomyosarcoma-, angiosarcoma-, and osteosarcoma-like foci can also occur.

Stromal overgrowth (65), defined as the absence of an epithelial component in at least one microscopic field at 40× total magnification, that is, 4× ocular and 10× eyepiece, or 22.9 mm^2) is associated with an increased risk of metastases. This feature is more common in MPTs, but it can also occur in BnPTs and BoPTs. Stromal overgrowth cannot be definitively assessed in NCB, but lack of epithelium at lesser, for example, 10× (29,68) *total* magnification in NCB material is regarded as an indicator thereof. Stromal mitotic activity is also an important parameter of grade of a PT.

BENIGN PHYLLODES TUMOR

A BnPT has minimal-to-mild stromal atypia, stromal cellularity, and mitotic activity. Stromal cellularity and mitoses are relatively more pronounced around the ducts. Epithelial hyperplasia can be prominent. The edges of the tumor show stromal infiltration **(Fig. 7.22)**, but this feature is not always evident on NCB. Multinucleated stromal giant cells with hyperchromatic nuclei may be present **(Fig. 7.21)**. Focal stromal myxoid change is not uncommon in a BnPT, but it is usually focal. Tumoral necrosis is infrequent. The most common differential diagnosis of a BnPT in NCB is with cellular FA **(Figs. 7.8, 7.9, 7.19, and 7.22)**. Many studies have tried to identify clinical and morphologic features predictive of PT in excisions, but no single morphologic feature, or any combination thereof, is reliable. Findings in NCB which correlate with the diagnosis of PT in the follow-up excision include at least two (29,30,66) or three (67) stromal mitoses/10 hpf, stromal hypercellularity (29,66), stromal overgrowth (defined as absence of epithelial elements in at least one final 40× field) (29,68), invasive margins (defined as microscopic extension of the tumor into the adjacent mammary fibroadipose tissue), fragmentation of the tissue cores (defined as detached stromal fragments mostly or even entirely surrounded by epithelium) (66,68), presence of adipose tissue admixed with stroma (68), and nuclear atypia. Patient aged higher than 50 to 55 years favors a diagnosis of PT in some studies (66,69) but not in others (67,68). In a study evaluating morphologic parameters predictive of PT versus cellular FA, 74% of PTs had at least three stromal mitoses/10 hpf in

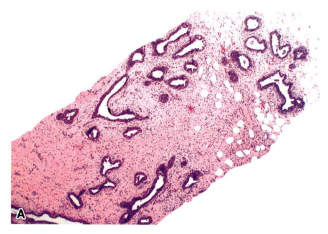
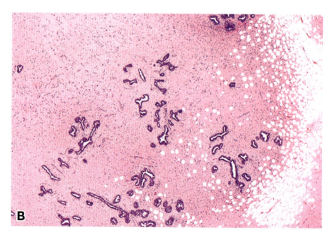

FIGURE 7.22 Benign Phyllodes Tumor, Edge. In this needle core biopsy (A) and excisional biopsy (B), the stroma is minimally hypercellular. Infiltration (permeation) into the adjacent fat at the edge of the lesion is evident in both specimens. There was stromal "overgrowth" (not shown).

NCB, and 11% had 1 to 2 mitoses/10 hpf, whereas the NCB of cellular FAs showed 3 or more stromal mitoses in 11% of cases, 1 to 2 mitoses/10 hpf in 30% of cases, and no mitotic activity in the remaining 60% (67). All of the aforementioned features can be difficult to assess in NCB. One study (70) found that despite training, interobserver agreement was poor for mitotic count and stromal cellularity, and it was fair for other features. In sum, if review of NCB raises the differential diagnosis of BnPT, excision is prudent. Excision should be aimed at attaining negative margins.

Borderline (Low-Grade Malignant) Phyllodes Tumor

A BoPT is best regarded as a low-grade MPT. BoPT has moderately cellular stroma with a heterogeneous distribution. Invasion of spindle cells into fibroadipose tissue is often observed. Focal atypical adipose metaplasia with lipoblast-like cells as well as chondroid and osseous metaplasia can be encountered (Fig. 7.23). Focal necrosis may be present. Stromal mitoses are readily evident (Fig. 7.23). In most cases, the epithelial component of a BoPT is at least focally present in NCB, enabling the diagnosis of a fibroepithelial tumor. However, the grade of the fibroepithelial tumor is difficult to assess because of intratumoral heterogeneity. Nuclear pleomorphism and 2 or more mitoses/10 hpf in an NCB usually correlate with the finding of at least BoPT upon excision.

The differential diagnosis of BnPT and BoPT in NCB includes MPT. In some cases, the differential diagnosis may also include PASH, myofibroblastoma, fibromatosis, and "low-grade" spindle cell carcinoma.

Malignant Phyllodes Tumor

A MPT is characterized by hypercellular stroma with high-grade nuclei and conspicuous mitotic activity (Fig. 7.24). The edges of the tumor are infiltrative. Tumoral degeneration and necrosis, with cystic change, are common. The relative paucity of the epithelial component within MPT correlates with limited and widely spaced epithelial elements in NCB. Lack of epithelium in a 40× *total* magnification is an indicator of stromal overgrowth. Areas of sarcomatous metaplasia are common. Notably, the presence of lipoblasts (associated with *well-differentiated* liposarcomatous-like change) does *not* represent a malignant heterologous element (vide supra). Squamous metaplasia can be present. Rarely, carcinomas develop in MPT (71).

NCB of MPT usually yields only a minimal amount of epithelium, often times limited to a single flat layer lining stretched-out ducts. In some cases, no duct/glandular elements are present in the NCB. In the latter scenario, the differential diagnosis of MPT includes metaplastic spindle cell carcinoma with high-grade morphology (Table 7.7), high-grade angiosarcoma, other sarcomas, either primary or metastatic, and melanoma with spindle cell morphology. In such cases, the use of an appropriate immunostain panel with CK34βE12, CK14, CK5/6, MNF116, p63, CD34, CD31, ERG, S100, and HMB45 may be helpful. In the event of equivocal results, the report should indicate diagnostic uncertainty and emphasize the need for excision to allow comprehensive evaluation.

Epithelial Component in Phyllodes Tumors

Many PTs exhibit epithelial hyperplasia, which tends to be more frequent and pronounced in BnPTs and BoPTs, and less common in MPTs. The latter usually have inconspicuous, flattened epithelium. Myoepithelial hyperplasia can occur. Squamous metaplasia of the ductal epithelium occurs in 3.6% (64) to 10% of PTs (72,73), whereas it is quite uncommon in FA. The presence of a cyst lined by squamous epithelium within a cellular fibroepithelial lesion favors the diagnosis of PT. Apocrine metaplasia can occur in PTs; however, it is also encountered in FAs, especially in complex FAs. Foci of adenosis can be present within a PT. In rare instances, adenosis and/or papillary hyperplasia can obscure the underlying architecture of a PT, mimicking nodular adenosis, adenomyoepithelioma, or papilloma.

FIBROEPITHELIAL NEOPLASMS

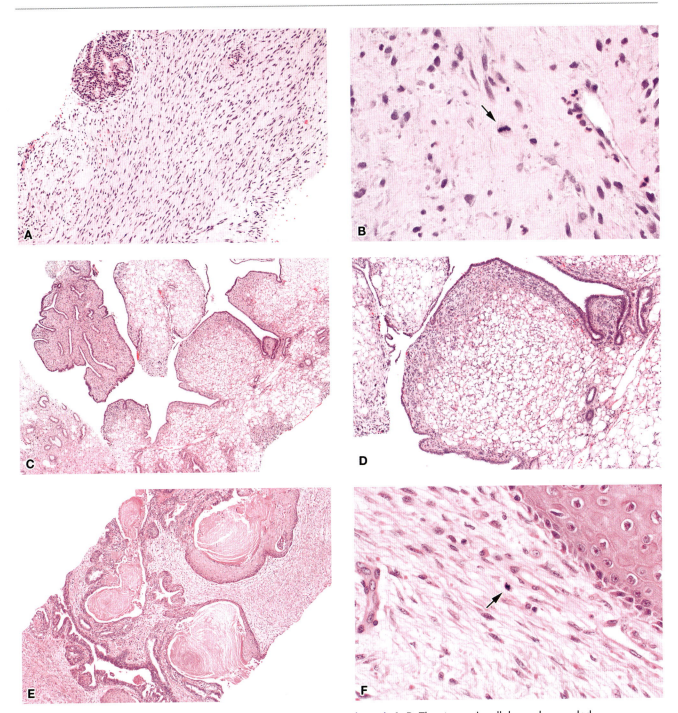

FIGURE 7.23 Borderline (Low-Grade) Phyllodes Tumor (BoPT). **A, B:** The stroma is cellular and expanded. A stromal cell mitosis is shown (arrow in **B**). Excision of the lesion yielded a BoPT. **C, D:** This needle core biopsy shows detached fragments of cellular stroma lined by epithelium. The stroma shows extensive atypical adipose differentiation, and the stromal cells tend to be denser in subepithelial location. **E, F:** Another BoPT with marked cystic squamous metaplasia. Note detail with stromal cell mitosis (arrow in **F**).

ALH, LCIS, ADH, and DCIS are uncommon in PTs (58,64). The diagnosis of DCIS should be rendered with extreme caution on NCB if an underlying fibroepithelial lesion is recognized because florid hyperplasia involving elongated compressed ducts can appear worrisome for in situ carcinoma. On the other hand, the unequivocal identification of DCIS amid a spindle cell tumor supports the diagnosis of metaplastic spindle cell carcinoma. Invasive carcinoma is rare in PTs (58,64,74-81). An invasive carcinoma with squamous differentiation arising in a high-grade MPT has been reported (82).

Recurrent and Metastatic Phyllodes Tumor

Ductal elements may or may not be present in locally recurrent PTs in the breast. The morphology of recurrent tumors is usually similar to that of primary PT. Occasionally, the recurrent PT differs from the primary and may be of higher-grade (5,64).

Metastatic PT at distant sites almost always consists entirely of the stromal component. At least one case with concomitant glandular component has been reported (83). The most common appearance in metastatic PT is that of a

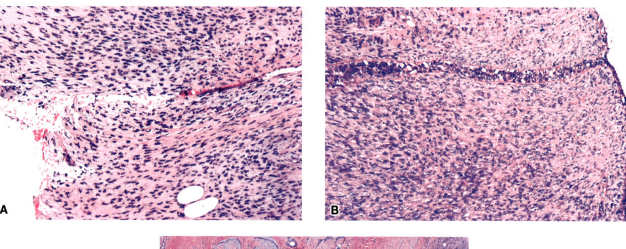

FIGURE 7.24 **Malignant Phyllodes Tumor (MPT).** **A:** This needle core biopsy (NCB) is from a fibrosarcomatous phyllodes tumor. **B:** The epithelial-lined cleft is virtually obliterated in this NCB from a tumor with leiomyosarcomatous differentiation. **C:** This MPT shows marked stromal heterogeneity. Fibroadenoma-like area (left) and the malignant (high-grade, right) phyllodes portion of the tumor are evident. This case highlights the importance of adequate sampling (particularly in larger tumors).

TABLE 7.7

Phyllodes Tumors and Metaplastic Carcinoma: Immunohistochemical and Molecular Features

	Phyllodes Tumors	Metaplastic Carcinoma
Immunohistochemistry		
Cytokeratin	(−) (rarely+, focal)	usually (+)
p63	(−) (rarely+, focal)	usually (+)
p40	(−) (rarely+, focal)	usually (+)
CD34	(+), in lower grade	(−) (rarely+, focal)
p53	(+)	(+)
Mutations		
RARA	(+)	(−)
MED12	(+)	(−)

EGFR, NF1, PIK4C, RB1, TERT, and *TP53* mutations observed in both.

high-grade spindle cell tumor with a fibrosarcomatous pattern. Rarely, locally recurrent or metastatic lesions exhibit heterologous differentiation which was not apparent in the primary MPT.

Immunohistochemistry

Immunohistochemical stains are not useful in the subclassification of PTs but play a role in their differential diagnosis.

CD34 is expressed in the stroma of most PTs (84-86). A study (87) reported CD34 staining in 72.5% of BnPTs, 66.7% of BoPTs, and 44.4% of (high-grade) MPTs. This finding suggests lesser expression of CD34 in higher-grade PTs.

Cytokeratins and p63 (and its isoform p40) are useful in the differential diagnosis of PTs, especially MPT and metaplastic spindle cell carcinoma, with the caveat that the latter may show only focal or even no staining for CKs. Furthermore, a study of 109 PTs (87) identified focal patchy stromal staining for CK7 in 28.4% of cases, for 34βE12 in 22%, for MNF116 in 11.9%, for AE1:AE3 in 8.3%, and for CAM5.2 and CK14 in 1.8% of cases each. MNF116 and 34βE12 staining in the stromal cells decreased significantly with increasing PT grade. In one series, no p63 staining was identified in the neoplastic stromal cells (87). Another group (88) reported p63 and p40 staining in the stromal cells of MPTs but not in BnPT and BoPTs. A subsequent study of six MPTs did not confirm these findings, although it documented focal p63 staining in a spindle cell sarcoma (89). Based on these observations, cautious interpretation of focal CK or p63 positivity in NCB of mammary spindle cell tumors is prudent (**Fig. 7.25**).

The expression of **ER and PR** in the epithelium of PTs appears inversely correlated with increasing grade of the PT. AR occurs in less than 5% of the epithelium and stroma of all PTs (90). Focal membranous reactivity for **HER2** is detected in the epithelium but not in the stroma of PTs, and does not correlate with prognosis (91). None of these biomarkers has prognostic or predictive utility in the evaluation of fibroepithelial lesions.

Nuclear β-catenin diffusely stains 80% to 100% of cases of primary mammary fibromatosis (92,93) and also decorates the stromal cells of approximately three-fourths of PTs (93-95), including 94% of stromal cells of BnPTs, mostly in periductal distribution. Staining for nuclear β-catenin is weaker in BoPTs and MPTs compared with BnPTs. Nuclear β-catenin is also detected in 23% of metaplastic mammary carcinomas (93). The finding of *focal*, rather than *diffuse*, nuclear β-catenin staining in an NCB should be interpreted cautiously.

A few studies (84,96-100) have reported staining for **CD117/c-kit** in PTs. One group (101) attributed the staining for c-kit to infiltrating mast cells and reported focal expression in the stromal cells of only two PTs.

p53 is present in the nucleus of the neoplastic stromal cells, and its expression correlates with higher-grade

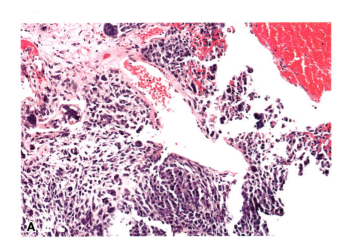
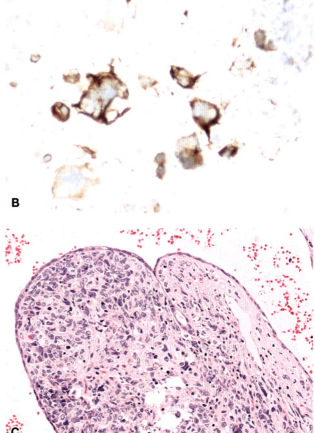

FIGURE 7.25 Malignant Phyllodes Tumor (MPT) With Focal Cytokeratin Staining. A: This needle core biopsy from a 3-cm solid and cystic mass showed a cluster of viable tumor cells. **B:** Focal CAM5.2 staining was identified. No reactivity for other epithelial markers, as well as for vascular and melanocytic antigens, was documented (not shown), and a diagnosis of poorly differentiated carcinoma was rendered. **C:** The tumor in the excision consisted of epithelial-lined fronds. CAM5.2 immunostain did not decorate the neoplastic spindle cells. The final interpretation was MPT with focal aberrant CAM5.2 staining.

(91,99,100,102-107), with the greatest reactivity in the periductal stroma of MPTs (108). p53 reactivity in PTs correlated with reduced survival (106,109), but it was not predictive of recurrence in other series (91,99,102).

Ki-67 immunoreactivity also correlates with tumor grade (102,104,105,107); however, the interpretation of Ki-67 staining is notorious for poor interobserver reproducibility—except at the extremes of the range that is, less than 5% and more than 30%. Immunohistochemical studies have been applied to the diagnosis of fibroepithelial tumors in NCB. **Ki-67** and **topoisomerase II** immunoreactivity showed a statistically significant correlation with PT diagnosis in two studies (29,30). However, some overlap exists between the results in FAs and PTs using both markers (Ki-67 index: 1.6, range 0.4-4 in FAs vs. 6.0, range 0-18 in PTs; topoisomerase II index: 2.8, range 0-10 in FAs vs. 7.0, range 1.2-29 in PTs), even though the results were statistically significant, especially for Ki-67 (P = .002) (30). In another study (29), Ki-67 and topoisomerase II indexes greater or equal to 5% and reduced or patchy CD34 staining in lesional stromal cells in NCB correlated with the diagnosis of PT in the excision. These stains are not used in routine practice.

CD10 is expressed in the stromal cells of fibroepithelial lesions, including FAs. Some studies (110,111) report higher CD10 expression in MPTs, including 6 of 10 PTs that developed distant metastases (111), but another group found no difference in the expression of CD10 in FAs and PTs (112).

Treatment and Prognosis

The treatment of PT primarily entails complete excision to prevent local recurrence (5,41,52,64,113-116). Most studies recommend a margin clearance of at least 1.0 cm (52,113,115,117,118), although the need for such a wide margin continues to be debated. Higher rates of local recurrence are reported if the final margin is diffusely (rather than focally) involved (64); however, local recurrences also occur in approximately 10% of patients with negative margins. Mastectomy might be indicated if a large MPT cannot be excised with cosmetically acceptable results. The risk of lymph node (LN) metastases is extremely low (52,115), and axillary nodal LN biopsy is not indicated in the absence of a coexisting ipsilateral invasive carcinoma or lymphadenopathy (see section on Survival).

Local Recurrence

BnPTs do not metastasize but locally recur in 11% to 17% of cases (5,41,64,119). The recurrent tumor has higher-grade morphology than the index PT in more than one-third of cases (5,41). Recently, some groups (113,120-124) have reported less than 10% rate of local recurrence for BnPTs and suggested a wait-and-see approach instead of re-excision of BnPTs with positive margins, particularly for smaller BnPTs. In recent series (123,124), most recurrent BnPT also had BnPT morphology, and none was morphologically malignant. Historically, BoPTs recur locally in 14% to 25% of cases (41,64,125); the recurrence may have malignant morphology. About one-third of patients with MPT (41) develop a local recurrence which tends to occur earlier than for BnPT or BoPTs.

Distant Metastases

Distant metastases of PTs are rare and occur almost exclusively with malignant tumors (5,41), usually within 3 years (5,52,64,117,126). In a study of 605 PT, 440 (72.7%) were benign, 111 (18.4%) borderline, and 54 (8.9%) malignant (41). Recurrences, mostly local, were recorded in 80 (13.2%) cases. Fatality due to PT occurred in 12 (2%) women. Multivariate analysis showed stromal cell atypia, stromal overgrowth, and status of margins to be independently predictive of clinical outcome. Stromal cell mitoses achieved "near significance." Stromal hypercellularity and tumor borders were not significant in this study. The authors developed a nomogram based on *a*typia, *m*itoses, *o*vergrowth, and *s*urgical margins ("AMOS") which predictive recurrence-free survival (RFS) at 1, 3, 5, and 10 years. This AMOS-based nomogram is yet to be fully validated (41).

Radiotherapy may be beneficial in preventing local recurrence of BoPTs and MPTs, but two studies evaluating this approach had limited numbers of cases and lacked study control groups, limiting the interpretation of the findings (118,127). At present, radiotherapy is not part of the standard treatment of PT managed with breast-conserving surgery. Radiotherapy is usually part of the management of a PT invading the chest wall. The RFS in patients with primary MPTs who received chemotherapy was not significantly improved (128).

Survival

Analysis of 821 patients with MPTs recorded in the Surveillance, Epidemiology, and End Results (SEER) program with median follow-up of 5.7 years revealed disease-free survival (DFS) of 91%, 89%, and 89% at 5, 10, and 15 years, respectively (129), with no statistically significant difference in disease-specific survival between patients treated with excision versus mastectomy. The most common sites of metastatic disease are the lungs and bone. Most deaths occur within 5 years of the initial diagnosis of PT (5,41,64,117). Nearly all fatalities occur in patients who presented with MPTs or developed malignant recurrences. Stromal overgrowth, invasive borders, pleomorphism, and mitoses are factors associated with distant metastases (5,64,65). In one of the largest series published to date, margin involvement, atypia, and stromal overgrowth were significant predictors of recurrence, and mitotic rate was nearly statistically significant (41).

Role of Molecular Pathology in Diagnosis of Fibroepithelial Tumors

Molecular pathology is assuming an ever-increasing role in the unequivocal establishment of diagnoses of mesenchymal (soft tissue) neoplasms—including those of the breast (130).

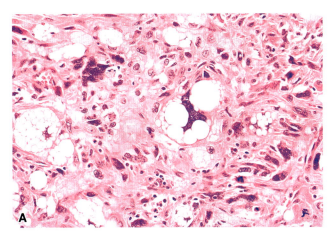
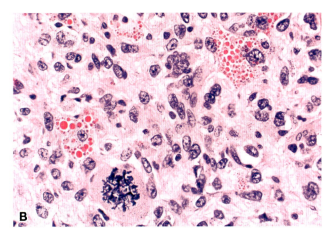

FIGURE 7.26 Malignant Phyllodes Tumor (MPT) With Unusual Findings: Sarcomatous Change With Lipoblasts and Thanatosomes. **A:** This needle core biopsy (NCB) from a 5-cm solid mass showed a MPT with high-grade "pleomorphic" lipoblasts. **B:** This NCB from a 7-cm solid tumor showed a MPT with thanatosomes (from *thanatos,* Greek: death). Thanatosomes are a form of degenerative intracellular hyaline globules and indicate a rare form of apoptosis. These structures have been described in high-grade malignancies in several organs.

The diagnosis of fibroepithelial tumors of the breast can also be facilitated via molecular testing.

The limited sampling of spindle cell and fibroepithelial tumors obtained in NCBs occasionally leads to diagnostic uncertainty on routine histopathologic evaluation (131). Such samplings are particularly suitable for molecular testing—especially in cases in which a firm diagnosis is critical in planning immediate management, for example, the use of neoadjuvant chemotherapy in a case in which the differential diagnosis includes metaplastic carcinoma or a large tumor in a young patient in whom mastectomy is being considered (132).

Several recent publications have reported on the molecular "landscape" of fibroepithelial tumors (130-133), and the key findings can be summarized as follows: Genetic mutations observed in fibroepithelial tumors include those in *MED12, RARA,* and *TERT* promoter (133). *MED12* mutations are found with similar frequency in FA and BnPTs (~60%); however, both *RARA* and *TERT* promoter mutations are relatively more frequent in PTs than in FAs. Of note, neither *RARA* nor *MED12* mutations are found in metaplastic carcinoma. *EGFR, NF1, PIK4C, RB1, TERT,* and *TP53* mutations can be present in both PTs and metaplastic carcinomas.

The molecular pathology of MPTs with high-grade ("true") liposarcomatous components and those with thanatosomes **(Fig. 7.26)** has yet to be elucidated. Thanatosomes are degenerative intracellular hyaline globules, which almost certainly indicate a form of apoptotic cell death (134).

REFERENCES

1. Kovi J, Chu HB, Leffall LD Jr. Sclerosing lobular hyperplasia manifesting as a palpable mass of the breast in young black women. *Hum Pathol.* 1984;15:336-340.
2. Poulton TB, de Paredes ES, Baldwin M. Sclerosing lobular hyperplasia of the breast: imaging features in 15 cases. *AJR Am J Roentgenol.* 1995;165:291-294.
3. Kapur P, Rakheja D, Cavuoti DC, et al. Sclerosing lobular hyperplasia of breast: cytomorphologic and histomorphologic features: a case report. *Cytojournal.* 2006;3:8.
4. Panikar N, Agarwal S. Sclerosing lobular hyperplasia of the breast: fine-needle aspiration cytology findings—a case report. *Diagn Cytopathol.* 2004;31:340-341.
5. Barrio AV, Clark BD, Goldberg JI, et al. Clinicopathologic features and long-term outcomes of 293 phyllodes tumors of the breast. *Ann Surg Oncol.* 2007;14:2961-2970.
6. Ross DS, Giri DD, Akram MM, et al. Fibroepithelial lesions in the breast of adolescent females: a clinicopathological study of 54 cases. *Breast J.* 2017;23:182-192.
7. Tay TK, Chang KT, Thike AA, et al. Paediatric fibroepithelial lesions revisited: pathological insights. *J Clin Pathol.* 2015;68:633-641.
8. Lerwill MF, Lee AHS, Tan PH. Fibroepithelial tumours of the breast—a review. *Virchows Arch.* 2022;480:45-63.
9. Kuijper A, Mommers EC, van der Wall E, et al. Histopathology of fibroadenoma of the breast. *Am J Clin Pathol.* 2001;115:736-742.
10. Sklair-Levy M, Sella T, Alweiss T, et al. Incidence and management of complex fibroadenomas. *AJR Am J Roentgenol.* 2008;190:214-218.
11. Ansah-Boateng Y, Tavassoli FA. Fibroadenoma and cystosarcoma phyllodes of the male breast. *Mod Pathol.* 1992;5:114-116.
12. Gupta P, Foshee S, Garcia-Morales F, et al. Fibroadenoma in male breast: case report and literature review. *Breast Dis.* 2011;33:45-48.
13. Uchida T, Ishii M, Motomiya Y. Fibroadenoma associated with gynaecomastia in an adult man: case report. *Scand J Plast Reconstr Surg Hand Surg.* 1993;27:327-329.
14. Kanhai RC, Hage JJ, Bloemena E, et al. Mammary fibroadenoma in a male-to-female transsexual. *Histopathology.* 1999;35:183-185.
15. Lemmo G, Garcea N, Corsello S, et al. Breast fibroadenoma in a male-to-female transsexual patient after hormonal treatment. *Eur J Surg Suppl.* 2003;(588):69-71.
16. Weinstein SP, Orel SG, Collazzo L, et al. Cyclosporin A-induced fibroadenomas of the breast: report of five cases. *Radiology.* 2001;220:465-468.
17. Son EJ, Oh KK, Kim EK, et al. Characteristic imaging features of breast fibroadenomas in women given cyclosporin A after renal transplantation. *J Clin Ultrasound.* 2004;32:69-77.
18. Iaria G, Pisani F, De Luca L, et al. Prospective study of switch from cyclosporine to tacrolimus for fibroadenomas of the breast in kidney transplantation. *Transplant Proc.* 2010;42:1169-1170.
19. Carney JA, Toorkey BC. Myxoid fibroadenoma and allied conditions (myxomatosis) of the breast: a heritable disorder with special associations including cardiac and cutaneous myxomas. *Am J Surg Pathol.* 1991;15:713-721.
20. Yamaguchi R, Tanaka M, Mizushima Y, et al. Myxomatous fibroadenoma of the breast: correlation with clinicopathologic and radiologic features. *Hum Pathol.* 2011;42:419-423.
21. Wurdinger S, Herzog AB, Fischer DR, et al. Differentiation of phyllodes breast tumors from fibroadenomas on MRI. *AJR Am J Roentgenol.* 2005;185:1317-1321.
22. Foster ME, Garrahan N, Williams S. Fibroadenoma of the breast: a clinical and pathological study. *J R Coll Surg Edinb.* 1988;33:16-19.
23. Powell CM, Cranor ML, Rosen PP. Multinucleated stromal giant cells in mammary fibroepithelial neoplasms: a study of 11 patients. *Arch Pathol Lab Med.* 1994;118:912-916.

24. Ryska A, Reynolds C, Keeney GL. Benign tumors of the breast with multinucleated stromal giant cells: immunohistochemical analysis of six cases and review of the literature. *Virchows Arch.* 2001;439:768-775.

25. Dupont WD, Page DL, Parl FF, et al. Long-term risk of breast cancer in women with fibroadenoma. *N Engl J Med.* 1994;331:10-15.

26. Ben Hassouna J, Damak T, Ben Slama A, et al. Breast carcinoma arising within fibroadenomas: report of four observations. *Tunis Med.* 2007;85:891-895.

27. Petersson F, Tan PH, Putti TC. Low-grade ductal carcinoma in situ and invasive mammary carcinoma with columnar cell morphology arising in a complex fibroadenoma in continuity with columnar cell change and flat epithelial atypia. *Int J Surg Pathol.* 2010;18:352-357.

28. Sawyer EJ, Hanby AM, Poulsom R, et al. Beta-catenin abnormalities and associated insulin-like growth factor overexpression are important in phyllodes tumours and fibroadenomas of the breast. *J Pathol.* 2003;200:627-632.

29. Jara-Lazaro AR, Akhilesh M, Thike AA, et al. Predictors of phyllodes tumours on core biopsy specimens of fibroepithelial neoplasms. *Histopathology.* 2010;57:220-232.

30. Jacobs TW, Chen YY, Guinee DG Jr, et al. Fibroepithelial lesions with cellular stroma on breast core needle biopsy: are there predictors of outcome on surgical excision? *Am J Clin Pathol.* 2005;124:342-354.

31. Piscuoglio S, Murray M, Fusco N, et al. MED12 somatic mutations in fibroadenomas and phyllodes tumours of the breast. *Histopathology.* 2015;67:719-729.

32. Yoshida M, Ogawa R, Yoshida H, et al. TERT promoter mutations are frequent and show association with MED12 mutations in phyllodes tumors of the breast. *Br J Cancer.* 2015;113:1244-1248.

33. Piscuoglio S, Ng CK, Murray M, et al. Massively parallel sequencing of phyllodes tumours of the breast reveals actionable mutations, and TERT promoter hotspot mutations and TERT gene amplification as likely drivers of progression. *J Pathol.* 2016;238:508-518.

34. Thurley P, Evans A, Hamilton L, James J, Wilson R. Patient satisfaction and efficacy of vacuum-assisted excision biopsy of fibroadenomas. *Clin Radiol.* 2009;64:381-385.

35. Grady I, Gorsuch H, Wilburn-Bailey S. Long-term outcome of benign fibroadenomas treated by ultrasound-guided percutaneous excision. *Breast J.* 2008;14:275-278.

36. Graña-López L, Pérez-Ramos T, Villares A, Vázquez-Caruncho M. Cryoablation of breast lesions: our experience. *Radiologia (Engl Ed).* 2022;64(suppl 1):49-53.

37. Nurko J, Mabry CD, Whitworth P, et al. Interim results from the FibroAdenoma Cryoablation Treatment Registry. *Am J Surg.* 2005;190:647-651.

38. Kaufman CS, Littrup PJ, Freeman-Gibb LA, et al. Office-based cryoablation of breast fibroadenomas with long-term follow-up. *Breast J.* 2005;11:344-350.

39. Jacklin RK, Ridgway PF, Ziprin P, et al. Optimising preoperative diagnosis in phyllodes tumour of the breast. *J Clin Pathol.* 2006;59:454-459.

40. Tagaya N, Kodaira H, Kogure H, et al. A case of phyllodes tumor with bloody nipple discharge in juvenile patient. *Breast Cancer.* 1999;6:207-210.

41. Tan PH, Thike AA, Tan WJ, et al. Predicting clinical behaviour of breast phyllodes tumours: a nomogram based on histological criteria and surgical margins. *J Clin Pathol.* 2012;65:69-76.

42. Mallory MA, Chikarmane SA, Raza S, et al. Bilateral synchronous benign phyllodes tumors. *Am Surg.* 2015:81:E192-E194.

43. Seal SK, Kuusk U, Lennox PA. Bilateral and multifocal phyllodes tumours of the breast: a case report. *Can J Plast Surg.* 2010;18:145-146.

44. Mrad K, Driss M, Maalej M, et al. Bilateral cystosarcoma phyllodes of the breast: a case report of malignant form with contralateral benign form. *Ann Diagn Pathol.* 2000;4:370-372.

45. Reisenbichler ES, Krontiras H, Hameed O. Beta-human chorionic gonadotropin production associated with phyllodes tumor of the breast: an unusual paraneoplastic phenomenon. *Breast J.* 2009;15:527-530.

46. Kataoka T, Haruta R, Goto T, et al. Malignant phyllodes tumor of the breast with hypoglycemia: report of a case. *Jpn J Clin Oncol.* 1998;28:276-280.

47. Hino N, Nakagawa Y, Ikushima Y, et al. A case of a giant phyllodes tumor of the breast with hypoglycemia caused by high-molecular-weight insulin-like growth factor II. *Breast Cancer.* 2010;17:142-145.

48. Aguiar Bujanda D, Rivero Vera JC, Cabrera Suarez MA, et al. Hypoglycemic coma secondary to big insulin-like growth factor II secretion by a giant phyllodes tumor of the breast. *Breast J.* 2007;13:189-191.

49. Selamzade M, Gidener C, Koyuncuoglu M, et al. Borderline phyllodes tumor in an 11-year-old girl. *Pediatr Surg Int.* 1999;15:427-428.

50. Inder M, Vaishnav K, Mathur DR. Benign breast lesions in prepubertal female children—a study of 20 years. *J Indian Med Assoc.* 2001;99:619-620.

51. Sorelli PG, Thomas D, Moore A, et al. Malignant phyllodes tumor in an 11-year-old premenarchal girl. *J Pediatr Surg.* 2010:45:e17-e20.

52. Guillot E, Couturaud B, Reyal F, et al. Management of phyllodes breast tumors. *Breast J.* 2011;17:129-137.

53. Way JC, Culham BA. Phyllodes tumour in pregnancy: a case report. *Can J Surg.* 1998;41:407-409.

54. Blaker KM, Sahoo S, Schweichler MR, et al. Malignant phylloides tumor in pregnancy. *Am Surg.* 2010;76:302-305.

55. Pacchiarotti A, Frati P, Caserta D, et al. First case of transformation for breast fibroadenoma to high-grade malignant cystosarcoma in an in vitro fertilization patient. *Fertil Steril.* 2011;96:1126-1127.

56. Bernstein L, Deapen D, Ross RK. The descriptive epidemiology of malignant cystosarcoma phyllodes tumors of the breast. *Cancer.* 1993;71:3020-3024.

57. Pimiento JM, Gadgil PV, Santillan AA, et al. Phyllodes tumors: race-related differences. *J Am Coll Surg.* 2011;213:537-542.

58. Karim RZ, Gerega SK, Yang YH, et al. Phyllodes tumours of the breast: a clinicopathological analysis of 65 cases from a single institution. *Breast.* 2009;18:165-170.

59. Birch JM, Alston RD, McNally RJ, et al. Relative frequency and morphology of cancers in carriers of germline TP53 mutations. *Oncogene.* 2001;20:4621-4628.

60. Pantoja E, Llobet RE, Lopez E. Gigantic cystosarcoma phyllodes in a man with gynecomastia. *Arch Surg.* 1976;111:611.

61. Buchberger W, Strasser K, Heim K, et al. Phylloides tumor: findings on mammography, sonography, and aspiration cytology in 10 cases. *AJR Am J Roentgenol.* 1991;157:715-719.

62. Cosmacini P, Zurrida S, Veronesi P, et al. Phyllode tumor of the breast: mammographic experience in 99 cases. *Eur J Radiol.* 1992;15:11-14.

63. Yabuuchi H, Soeda H, Matsuo Y, et al. Phyllodes tumor of the breast: correlation between MR findings and histologic grade. *Radiology.* 2006;241:702-709.

64. Tan PH, Jayabaskar T, Chuah KL, et al. Phyllodes tumors of the breast: the role of pathologic parameters. *Am J Clin Pathol.* 2005;123:529-540.

65. Hawkins RE, Schofield JB, Fisher C, et al. The clinical and histologic criteria that predict metastases from cystosarcoma phyllodes. *Cancer.* 1992;69:141-147.

66. Tsang AK, Chan SK, Lam CC, et al. Phyllodes tumours of the breast—differentiating features in core needle biopsy. *Histopathology.* 2011;59:600-608.

67. Yasir S, Gamez R, Jenkins S, et al. Significant histologic features differentiating cellular fibroadenoma from phyllodes tumor on core needle biopsy specimens. *Am J Clin Pathol.* 2014;142:362-369.

68. Lee AH, Hodi Z, Ellis IO, et al. Histological features useful in the distinction of phyllodes tumour and fibroadenoma on needle core biopsy of the breast. *Histopathology.* 2007;51:336-344.

69. Morgan JM, Douglas-Jones AG, Gupta SK. Analysis of histological features in needle core biopsy of breast useful in preoperative distinction between fibroadenoma and phyllodes tumour. *Histopathology.* 2010;56:489-500.

70. Bandyopadhyay S, Barak S, Hayek K, et al. Can problematic fibroepithelial lesions be accurately classified on core needle biopsies? *Hum Pathol.* 2016;47:38-44.

71. Sin EI, Wong CY, Yong WS, et al. Breast carcinoma and phyllodes tumour: a case series. *J Clin Pathol.* 2016;69:364-369.

72. Grimes MM. Cystosarcoma phyllodes of the breast: histologic features, flow cytometric analysis, and clinical correlations. *Mod Pathol.* 1992;5:232-239.

73. Norris HJ, Taylor HB. Relationship of histologic features to behavior of cystosarcoma phyllodes: analysis of ninety-four cases. *Cancer.* 1967;20:2090-2099.

74. Grove A, Deibjerg Kristensen L. Intraductal carcinoma within a phyllodes tumor of the breast: a case report. *Tumori.* 1986;72:187-190.

75. Knudsen PJ, Ostergaard J. Cystosarcoma phylloides with lobular and ductal carcinoma in situ. *Arch Pathol Lab Med.* 1987;111:873-875.

76. Yamaguchi R, Tanaka M, Kishimoto Y, et al. Ductal carcinoma in situ arising in a benign phyllodes tumor: report of a case. *Surg Today.* 2008;38:42-45.

77. Korula A, Varghese J, Thomas M, et al. Malignant phyllodes tumour with intraductal and invasive carcinoma and lymph node metastasis. *Singapore Med J.* 2008;49:e318-e321.

78. Nomura M, Inoue Y, Fujita S, et al. A case of noninvasive ductal carcinoma arising in malignant phyllodes tumor. *Breast Cancer.* 2006;13:89-94.

79. Kodama T, Kameyama K, Mukai M, et al. Invasive lobular carcinoma arising in phyllodes tumor of the breast. *Virchows Arch.* 2003;442:614-616.

80. Quinlan-Davidson S, Hodgson N, Elavathil L, et al. Borderline phyllodes tumor with an incidental invasive tubular carcinoma and lobular carcinoma in situ component: a case report. *J Breast Cancer.* 2011;14:237-240.

81. Choi Y, Lee KY, Jang MH, et al. Invasive cribriform carcinoma arising in malignant phyllodes tumor of breast: a case report. *Korean J Pathol.* 2012;46:205-209.

82. Sugie T, Takeuchi E, Kunishima F, et al. A case of ductal carcinoma with squamous differentiation in malignant phyllodes tumor. *Breast Cancer.* 2007;14:327-332.

83. Kracht J, Sapino A, Bussolati G. Malignant phyllodes tumor of breast with lung metastases mimicking the primary. *Am J Surg Pathol.* 1998;22:1284-1290.

84. Noronha Y, Raza A, Hutchins B, et al. CD34, CD117, and Ki-67 expression in phyllodes tumor of the breast: an immunohistochemical study of 33 cases. *Int J Surg Pathol.* 2011;19:152-158.

85. Chen CM, Chen CJ, Chang CL, et al. CD34, CD117, and actin expression in phyllodes tumor of the breast. *J Surg Res.* 2000;94:84-91.

86. Moore T, Lee AH. Expression of CD34 and bcl-2 in phyllodes tumours, fibroadenomas and spindle cell lesions of the breast. *Histopathology.* 2001;38:62-67.

87. Chia Y, Thike AA, Cheok PY, et al. Stromal keratin expression in phyllodes tumours of the breast: a comparison with other spindle cell breast lesions. *J Clin Pathol.* 2012;65:339-347.

88. Cimino-Mathews A, Sharma R, Illei PB, et al. A subset of malignant phyllodes tumors express p63 and p40: a diagnostic pitfall in breast core needle biopsies. *Am J Surg Pathol.* 2014;38(12):1689-1696.

89. D'Alfonso TM, Ross DS, Liu YF, et al. Expression of p40 and laminin 332 in metaplastic spindle cell carcinoma of the breast compared with other malignant spindle cell tumours. *J Clin Pathol.* 2015;68:516-521.

90. Tse GM, Lee CS, Kung FY, et al. Hormonal receptors expression in epithelial cells of mammary phyllodes tumors correlates with pathologic grade of the tumor: a multicenter study of 143 cases. *Am J Clin Pathol.* 2002;118:522-526.

91. Shpitz B, Bomstein Y, Sternberg A, et al. Immunoreactivity of p53, Ki-67, and c-erbB-2 in phyllodes tumors of the breast in correlation with clinical and morphologic features. *J Surg Oncol.* 2002;79:86-92.

92. Abraham SC, Reynolds C, Lee JH, et al. Fibromatosis of the breast and mutations involving the APC/beta-catenin pathway. *Hum Pathol.* 2002;33:39-46.

93. Lacroix-Triki M, Geyer FC, Lambros MB, et al. beta-catenin/Wnt signalling pathway in fibromatosis, metaplastic carcinomas and phyllodes tumours of the breast. *Mod Pathol.* 2010;23:1438-1448.

94. Sawyer EJ, Hanby AM, Rowan AJ, et al. The Wnt pathway, epithelial-stromal interactions, and malignant progression in phyllodes tumours. *J Pathol.* 2002;196:437-444.

95. Karim RZ, Gerega SK, Yang YH, et al. Proteins from the Wnt pathway are involved in the pathogenesis and progression of mammary phyllodes tumours. *J Clin Pathol.* 2009;62:1016-1020.

96. Tse GM, Putti TC, Lui PC, et al. Increased c-kit (CD117) expression in malignant mammary phyllodes tumors. *Mod Pathol.* 2004;17:827-831.

97. Carvalho S, de Silva AO, Milanezi F, et al. c-KIT and PDGFRA in breast phyllodes tumours: overexpression without mutations? *J Clin Pathol.* 2004;57:1075-1079.

98. Sawyer EJ, Poulsom R, Hunt FT, et al. Malignant phyllodes tumours show stromal overexpression of c-myc and c-kit. *J Pathol.* 2003;200:59-64.

99. Tan PH, Jayabaskar T, Yip G, et al. p53 and c-kit (CD117) protein expression as prognostic indicators in breast phyllodes tumors: a tissue microarray study. *Mod Pathol.* 2005;18:1527-1534.

100. Korcheva VB, Levine J, Beadling C, et al. Immunohistochemical and molecular markers in breast phyllodes tumors. *Appl Immunohistochem Mol Morphol.* 2011;19:119-125.

101. Djordjevic B, Hanna WM. Expression of c-kit in fibroepithelial lesions of the breast is a mast cell phenomenon. *Mod Pathol.* 2008;21:1238-1245.

102. Kleer CG, Giordano TJ, Braun T, et al. Pathologic, immunohistochemical, and molecular features of benign and malignant phyllodes tumors of the breast. *Mod Pathol.* 2001;14:185-190.

103. Tse GM, Lui PC, Scolyer RA, et al. Tumour angiogenesis and p53 protein expression in mammary phyllodes tumors. *Mod Pathol.* 2003;16:1007-1013.

104. Erhan Y, Zekioglu O, Ersoy O, et al. p53 and Ki-67 expression as prognostic factors in cystosarcoma phyllodes. *Breast J.* 2002;8:38-44.

105. Esposito NN, Mohan D, Brufsky A, et al. Phyllodes tumor: a clinicopathologic and immunohistochemical study of 30 cases. *Arch Pathol Lab Med.* 2006;130:1516-1521.

106. Kuijper A, de Vos RA, Lagendijk JH, et al. Progressive deregulation of the cell cycle with higher tumor grade in the stroma of breast phyllodes tumors. *Am J Clin Pathol.* 2005;123:690-698.

107. Gatalica Z, Finkelstein S, Lucio E, et al. p53 protein expression and gene mutation in phyllodes tumors of the breast. *Pathol Res Pract.* 2001;197:183-187.

108. Millar EK, Beretov J, Marr P, et al. Malignant phyllodes tumours of the breast display increased stromal p53 protein expression. *Histopathology.* 1999;34:491-496.

109. Yonemori K, Hasegawa T, Shimizu C, et al. Correlation of p53 and MIB-1 expression with both the systemic recurrence and survival in cases of phyllodes tumors of the breast. *Pathol Res Pract.* 2006;202:705-712.

110. Tse GM, Tsang AK, Putti TC, et al. Stromal CD10 expression in mammary fibroadenomas and phyllodes tumours. *J Clin Pathol.* 2005;58:185-189.

111. Al-Masri M, Darwazeh G, Sawalhi S, et al. Phyllodes tumor of the breast: role of CD10 in predicting metastasis. *Ann Surg Oncol.* 2012;19(4):1181-1184.

112. Zamecnik M, Kinkor Z, Chlumska A. CD10+ stromal cells in fibroadenomas and phyllodes tumors of the breast. *Virchows Arch.* 2006;448:871-872.

113. Bartoli C, Zurrida S, Veronesi P, et al. Small sized phyllodes tumor of the breast. *Eur J Surg Oncol.* 1990;16:215-219.

114. Toussaint A, Piaget-Rossel R, Stormacq C, et al. Width of margins in phyllodes tumors of the breast: the controversy drags on? A systematic review and meta-analysis. *Breast Cancer Res Treat.* 2021;185:21-37.

115. Ben Hassouna J, Damak T, Gamoudi A, et al. Phyllodes tumors of the breast: a case series of 106 patients. *Am J Surg.* 2006;192:141-147.

116. Asoglu O, Ugurlu MM, Blanchard K, et al. Risk factors for recurrence after primary surgical treatment of malignant phyllodes tumors. *Ann Surg Oncol.* 2004;11:1011-1017.

117. Chaney AW, Pollack A, McNeese MD, et al. Primary treatment of cystosarcoma phyllodes of the breast. *Cancer.* 2000;89:1502-1511.

118. Belkacemi Y, Bousquet G, Marsiglia H, et al. Phyllodes tumor of the breast. *Int J Radiat Oncol Biol Phys.* 2008;70:492-500.

119. Barth RJ Jr. Histologic features predict local recurrence after breast conserving therapy of phyllodes tumors. *Breast Cancer Res Treat.* 1999;57:291-295.

120. Zurrida S, Bartoli C, Galimberti V, et al. Which therapy for unexpected phyllode tumour of the breast? *Eur J Cancer.* 1992;28:654-657.

121. Teo JY, Cheong CS, Wong CY. Low local recurrence rates in young Asian patients with phyllodes tumours: less is more. *ANZ J Surg.* 2012;82:325-328.

122. Park HL, Kwon SH, Chang SY, et al. Long-term follow-up result of benign phyllodes tumor of the breast diagnosed and excised by ultrasound-guided vacuum-assisted breast biopsy. *J Breast Cancer.* 2012;15:224-229.

123. Borhani-Khomani K, Talman ML, Kroman N, et al. Risk of local recurrence of benign and borderline phyllodes tumors: a Danish population-based retrospective study. *Ann Surg Oncol.* 2016;23:1543-1548.

124. Kim S, Kim JY, Kim do H, et al. Analysis of phyllodes tumor recurrence according to the histologic grade. *Breast Cancer Res Treat.* 2013;141:353-363.

125. Reinfuss M, Mitus J, Duda K, et al. The treatment and prognosis of patients with phyllodes tumor of the breast: an analysis of 170 cases. *Cancer.* 1996;77:910-916.

126. Tan EY, Tan PH, Yong WS, et al. Recurrent phyllodes tumours of the breast: pathological features and clinical implications. *ANZ J Surg.* 2006;76:476-480.

127. Barth RJ Jr, Wells WA, Mitchell SE, et al. A prospective, multi-institutional study of adjuvant radiotherapy after resection of malignant phyllodes tumors. *Ann Surg Oncol.* 2009;16:2288-2294.

128. Morales-Vasquez F, Gonzalez-Angulo AM, Broglio K, et al. Adjuvant chemotherapy with doxorubicin and dacarbazine has no effect in recurrence-free survival of malignant phyllodes tumors of the breast. *Breast J.* 2007;13:551-556.

129. Macdonald OK, Lee CM, Tward JD, et al. Malignant phyllodes tumor of the female breast: association of primary therapy with cause-specific survival from the Surveillance, Epidemiology, and End Results (SEER) program. *Cancer.* 2006;107:2127-2133.

130. Anderson WJ, Fletcher CDM. Mesenchymal lesions of the breast. *Histopathology.* 2023;82:83-94.

131. Li JJX, Tse GM. Core needle biopsy diagnosis of fibroepithelial lesions of the breast: a diagnostic challenge. *Pathology.* 2020;52:627-634.

132. Mon KS, Tang P. Fibroepithelial lesions of the breast: update on molecular profile with focus on pediatric population. *Arch Pathol Lab Med.* 2023;147:38-45.

133. Chang HY, Koh VCY, Md Nasir ND, et al. *MED12, TERT* and *RARA* in fibroepithelial tumours of the breast. *J Clin Pathol.* 2020;73:51-56.

134. D'Alfonso TM, Ginter PS, Salvatore SP, Antonio LB, Hoda SA. Phylloides tumor with numerous thanatosomes ("death bodies"): a report of two cases and a study of thanatosomes in breast tumors. *Int J Surg Pathol.* 2014;22:337-342.

Ductal Hyperplasia, Atypical Ductal Hyperplasia, and Ductal Carcinoma In Situ

RAZA S. HODA AND SYED A. HODA

DUCTAL HYPERPLASIA AND ATYPICAL DUCTAL HYPERPLASIA

The distinction between ductal hyperplasia (DH), atypical ductal hyperplasia (ADH), and ductal carcinoma in situ (DCIS) is important for the appropriate management of patients because these lesions, particularly the latter two, are "associated with an increased risk, albeit of different magnitudes, for the development of invasive carcinoma" (1,2) **(Table 8.1)**. In most instances, ductal epithelial proliferations are readily classified by pathologists based on generally accepted definitions, including those offered by the World Health Organization (WHO) **(Table 8.2)**, and histopathologic features (3,4) **(Table 8.3)**, despite some differences in terminology **(Table 8.4)**. There exists a subset of lesions for which assignment to either of these categories is less certain. These "borderline" lesions may be diagnosed as either ADH or DCIS (synonym: intraductal carcinoma) or even DH by different pathologists depending on the criteria applied. Studies of interobserver differences in the interpretation of highly selected examples of these lesions with "blurry boundaries" (5) have focused attention on this troublesome diagnostic problem which, nonetheless, applies to a relatively minor proportion of proliferative epithelial lesions (6-9).

Microscopic examination of glass slides prepared from needle core biopsy (NCB) and surgical specimens is likely to remain the only means to diagnose DH, ADH, and DCIS—until the use of artificial intelligence (AI) applied to whole slide imaging (WSI) becomes prevalent. Diagnoses with AI may eventually become more consistent and reproducible than human visual grading. Key issues that need to be resolved before adoption of AI on WSI for objectively resolving the differential diagnosis of DH, ADH, and DCIS include dealing with intra- and interlaboratory variations in tissue fixation and processing, as well as slide sectioning and staining (9). In this regard, obtaining standardization of, and consistency in, H&E staining (and establishment of firmer diagnostic criteria) may be the more significant impediments.

Clinical Features

There are no clinical features specifically associated with DH. The alterations caused by epithelial proliferation in individual ducts or in groups of ducts are almost always "microscopic" in extent. DH of various degrees is a common constituent of "fibrocystic changes." The latter may be detected via imaging studies or form a palpable mass. The lesion complex can include sclerosing adenosis, cystic apocrine hyperplasia, duct ectasia, and fibrosis.

An important corollary to the lack of clinical indicators of DH is the inability to determine the duration of these lesions. The date on which DH was first diagnosed is customarily used as if it were the date of "onset." This practice, which is a consequence of the inability to determine the preclinical duration of hyperplastic ductal lesions, is almost certainly a significant source of bias in assessing the precancerous significance of proliferative lesions.

TABLE 8.1

Clinical Implications of Various Degrees of Intraductal Epithelial Proliferation

	UDH	ADH	DCIS
Risk of breast carcinoma	1.5-2×	2-5×[a]	~10×
Risk of ipsilateral breast carcinoma	(+)	×2	Higher
Risk of contralateral breast carcinoma	(+)	(+)	(−/+)
Typical long-term management	Screening	Surveillance	Multidisciplinary

Based on review of literature.

ADH, atypical ductal hyperplasia; DCIS, ductal carcinoma in situ; UDH, usual ductal hyperplasia.

[a]Approximately 5% are expected to develop breast carcinoma in lifetime; risk is higher in those with family history.

TABLE 8.2

World Health Organization (WHO) Definitions of Various Intraductal Lesions

Usual Ductal Hyperplasia (UDH)
Usual ductal hyperplasia is an architecturally, cytologically, and molecularly heterogeneous benign epithelial proliferation primarily involving terminal duct lobular units.

Columnar Cell Lesions
Columnar cell lesions are clonal alterations of the terminal duct lobular units characterized by enlarged, variably dilated acini lined by columnar epithelial cells.

Flat Epithelial Atypia/Atypical Columnar Cell Hyperplasia (FEA/ACCH)
Atypical columnar cell hyperplasia/flat epithelial atypia is characterized by low-grade (monomorphic) cytologic atypia.

Atypical Ductal Hyperplasia (ADH)
Atypical ductal hyperplasia is an epithelial proliferative lesion with cytologic and architectural features similar to those of low-grade ductal carcinoma in situ but less developed in architecture, degree of terminal duct lobular unit involvement, and contiguous extent.

Ductal Carcinoma In Situ (DCIS)
Ductal carcinoma in situ is a noninvasive proliferation of cohesive neoplastic epithelial cells confined to the mammary ductal-lobular system, exhibiting a range of architectural patterns and nuclear grades.

Modified from World Health Organization. *Breast Tumours. WHO Classification of Tumours*. Vol 2. 5th ed. International Agency for Research on Cancer; 2019.

TABLE 8.3

Distinguishing Between Lower-Grade Intraductal Lesions

	UDH	ADH	LG-DCIS
Lesional cells	Heterogeneous	Homogeneous	Homogeneous
Cell arrangement	Overlapping, cell borders: ill-defined	No overlapping, cell borders: well-defined	No overlapping, cell borders: well-defined
Growth pattern	Cribriform, micropapillary, solid	Cribriform, micropapillary, solid	Cribriform, micropapillary, solid
Luminal Spaces	Irregular, variable, slit-like	Mixed pattern	Rounded, rigid, punched-out
Cell polarization around spaces	Nonpolarized	Variably polarized	Polarized
Cellular arcades and bridges	Variable: stretched and attenuated	Variable thickness	Uniform thickness

ADH, atypical ductal hyperplasia; LG-DCIS, low-grade ductal carcinoma in situ; UDH, usual ductal hyperplasia.

TABLE 8.4

Synonyms of Various Intraductal Epithelial Proliferative Lesions

Usual Ductal Hyperplasia (UDH)
Epithelial hyperplasia, epitheliosis, intraductal hyperplasia

Atypical Columnar Cell Hyperplasia/Flat Epithelial Atypia (ACCH/FEA)
Flat epithelial atypia
Columnar cell hyperplasia (with atypia)

Atypical Ductal Hyperplasia (ADH)
Atypical intraductal hyperplasia

Ductal Carcinoma In Situ (DCIS)
Intraductal carcinoma
Noninvasive carcinoma

Imaging

The imaging manifestations of DH, usually in the context of fibrocystic changes, include density, distortion, nonpalpable mass formation, and calcifications. The latter are the most frequent mammographic indications of DH, ADH, and DCIS—in the absence of a palpable abnormality (10-12). Lesions described on mammography as radial scars (ie, radial sclerosing lesions) often have a component of DH. Some, but not all, radial scars contain calcifications. Before the widespread use of mammography, DH was found in about 25% of biopsies performed for a palpable abnormality (13,14). No more than around 5% of these biopsies showed ADH. The frequency of these atypical abnormalities is higher (~15%) among mammographically directed biopsies and excisional biopsies (15-19). The yield of ADH in MRI-directed vacuum-assisted NCB ranged from 3% to 8% in several earlier studies (20-22).

CHAPTER 8

DH can be found in adult women at any age. In younger patients (age <30 years), most examples of DH occur either as juvenile papillomatosis (23) or as one of the group of lesions referred to as papillary DH in teenage girls and young women (24). Most women with DH are between 35 and 60 years of age (mean age of ~55, ~5 years younger than patients with ADH). After age 60, DH becomes relatively infrequent, and when present it is relatively less florid than in younger women. Occasionally, an older woman (age >60 years) may have extensive proliferative changes with florid DH. Use of exogenous estrogens can be documented in some, but not all, of these cases. Of note, the risk for breast carcinoma with usual ductal hyperplasia (UDH) alone, albeit minimal, is conferred on both breasts and is higher in women with strong family history of breast carcinoma.

Histopathology of Ductal Hyperplasia

DH describes a proliferative epithelial process that is manifested by an increase in the number of epithelial cells within ducts and terminal duct lobular units (TDLUs). DH with neither cytologic nor architectural atypia is typically termed *usual ductal hyperplasia* (UDH) **(Table 8.5)**. The normal

resting ductal epithelium consists of a continuous monolayer of cuboidal-to-columnar epithelial cells supported by a layer of myoepithelial cells. An increase in cellularity of the epithelial cells typically constitutes hyperplasia and may result in partial or complete obstruction of the ductal lumen. If DH is traced in serial sections, it is often possible to observe its discontinuous and multifocal nature. Various distortions of the basic ductal architecture occur when hyperplastic ducts become serpiginous or are incorporated into complex proliferative lesions, such as papillomata or radial sclerosing lesions. DH can extend into smaller ducts. The lesion may rarely extend into lobules.

The histologic criteria for DH are the same for NCB and excisional biopsies. However, fragmented portions of the lesion often appear in NCB. This lesional disintegration disrupts the helpful topographical information provided by the larger intact samples of an excisional biopsy. This circumstance can lead to either overinterpretation of individual isolated ductal proliferative processes in NCB or failure to recognize the presence of a significant abnormality.

Usual Ductal Hyperplasia

When individual cell borders are inconspicuous, the epithelial proliferation in DH (also referred to as *usual ductal hyperplasia*) often has a syncytial appearance. The proliferative epithelial process appears to be polymorphous and haphazard, with cellular heterogeneity. Intracytoplasmic (and intranuclear) vacuolization may occur. True cytoplasmic microlumina that contain secretions (positive for mucicarmine or alcian blue–PAS stains) are uncommon in hyperplastic ductal epithelia (25). The presence of intracytoplasmic, mucin-containing microlumina is an atypical feature that should result in careful consideration of the diagnosis of DCIS or of "pagetoid" extension of lobular carcinoma in situ (LCIS) into ducts. In DH, nuclear spacing is uneven so that in some foci the cells are crowded, with overlapping of nuclei. Depending upon the plane of section, nuclei in DH are round, ovoid, elliptical, or kidney shaped. Nucleoli are typically inconspicuous—unless there is apocrine metaplasia. Nuclei are variable in size. In a minority of cases, nuclear grooves and intranuclear "acidophilic" inclusions may be prominent (26). Despite the obviously proliferative nature of DH, mitotic activity is typically infrequent, and no abnormal mitotic figures are evident. Apocrine metaplastic cells are a common component of UDH. Cells with clear cell cytoplasmic change (usually admixed with apocrine metaplasia) are encountered less commonly.

UDH is identified in approximately 20% to 25% of benign NCB of the breast. DH has been subdivided based on qualitative and quantitative criteria, into the categories of mild, moderate, and florid (or marked). The application of this classification is limited by the fact that disordered epithelial growth with varied structural patterns is a characteristic feature of DH. Consequently, hyperplastic epithelium is not uniformly distributed in a stratified fashion, which permits ready determination of the in vivo number of cell

TABLE 8.5

UDH: Pathologic Features

Degree	Features
Mild	<3 cell layers
Moderate	~3-4
Florid	>4 cell layers

Architectural	Features
Cribriform	Irregular lumina, slit-like, nonpolarization of cells lining spaces, spaces are preferentially located at the perimeter of the duct, epithelial bridges are partly attenuated.
Micropapillary	Arcades and bridges are nonrigid, stretched, and partly attenuated.
Solid	Usually nondistended, with heterogeneous cell population
Gynecomastoid	Mimics low-grade micropapillary ductal carcinoma in situ

Cytologic
Heterogeneous epithelial component
Variation in cell size and shape
Ill-defined cell borders
Overlapping cells
Nuclei may have grooves and intranuclear inclusions.
May incorporate apocrine and squamous metaplastic cells
Necrosis is rare (most common amid hyperplastic cells of florid papillomatosis of the nipple)

UDH, usual ductal hyperplasia.

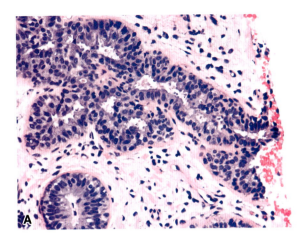
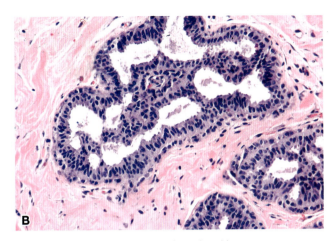

FIGURE 8.1 **Ductal Hyperplasia, Mild. A:** The ducts in this needle core biopsy (NCB) are lined by epithelium that is up to two cell layers in thickness. **B:** Mild hyperplasia is shown in another NCB. Hyperplasia of myoepithelial cells is also evident.

layers. Also, epithelial thickness is difficult to appraise in tangentially sectioned glands. Furthermore, the criteria for making these distinctions based on the number of epithelial layers are difficult to apply to smaller ducts and TDLUs. In these structures, the lumen is minuscule, and it can be filled even when there is a minimal increase in epithelial layers. Degrees of hyperplasia based on epithelial layers are meaningful only when applied to selected nontangential sections of glandular structures of sufficient dimension to manifest diagnostic features. In sum, the classification of DH based on epithelial thickness alone has significant limitations.

Mild hyperplasia may affect the entire epithelium circumferentially in a ductal cross section or only a segment of the duct **(Fig. 8.1)**. It occurs as an increase in the amount of epithelium, which rarely exceeds three cell layers in thickness, and may assume a papillary configuration.

In **moderate hyperplasia,** the epithelia tend to be more than three cell layers in thickness. Epithelial proliferation is more pronounced relative to that in mild hyperplasia, and secondary glandular lumina may form **(Fig. 8.2)**. Parts of the ductal lumen may persist as crescentic spaces at the perimeter of the duct or as intraductal cribriform spaces **(Fig. 8.3)**. Micropapillary hyperplasia is part of the spectrum of mild and moderate DH **(Fig. 8.4)**. The papillae appear as slender, irregular fronds of hyperplastic epithelium, in which the apical cells are relatively smaller and may assume a pyramidal structure. The cells in the latter structure are more condensed with seemingly pinched nuclei. The nuclei in moderate hyperplasia are often irregularly spaced, frequently overlap, and may be distributed in a "streaming" manner **(Fig. 8.5)**. Streaming refers to a growth pattern in which the nuclei of hyperplastic epithelial cells are oriented parallel to the long axes of cells **(Fig. 8.6)**. Because the cytoplasmic borders of these cells are often indistinct, streaming is usually detected as parallel orientation of oval- or spindle-shaped nuclei (ie, resembling a "school of fish"). Streaming occurs in most structural patterns of DH (and less commonly in ADH). The association of streaming pattern with DH has been confirmed by computerized morphometric analysis of the orientation of nuclei in proliferative ductal lesions (27).

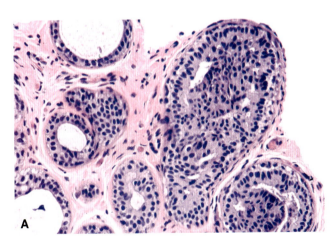
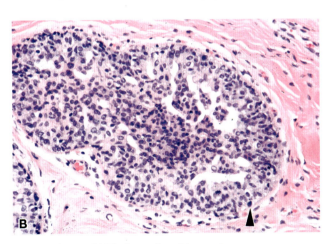

FIGURE 8.2 **Ductal Hyperplasia, Moderate. A:** This needle core biopsy (NCB) shows ductal hyperplasia in an enlarged duct. Note the persistent columnar duct epithelium at the periphery of hyperplastic ducts. **B:** This duct from another specimen is nearly filled with hyperplastic epithelium. Note condensation of the cells with diminished cytoplasm in the center of the duct and a mitotic figure (arrowhead).

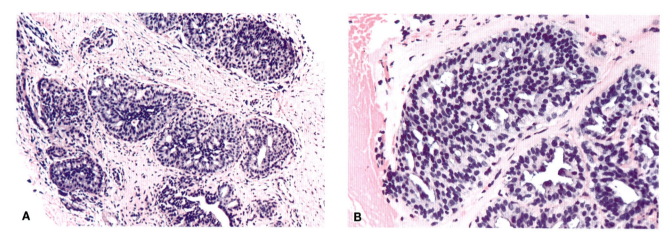

FIGURE 8.3 Ductal Hyperplasia, Moderate. A, B: Hyperplastic epithelium fills the ducts in this needle core biopsy (NCB) forming a cribriform pattern. Cells in the center of the duct have relatively smaller condensed nuclei and scant cytoplasm. Columnar epithelium is present at the perimeter of the affected duct **(B)**.

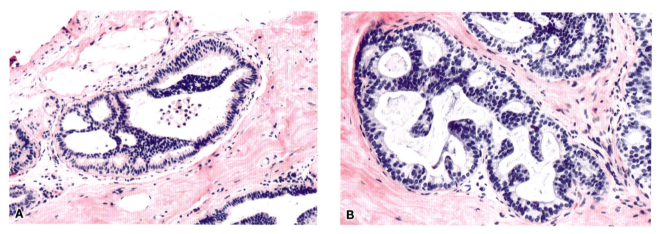

FIGURE 8.4 Ductal Hyperplasia, Micropapillary. A: Well-preserved columnar ductal epithelium is present at the periphery of this duct, with a more complex micropapillary proliferation in the lumen. There is mild architectural atypia. **B:** Micropapillary hyperplasia. There is mild architectural atypia.

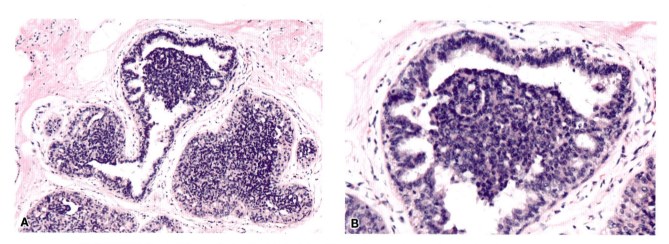

FIGURE 8.5 Ductal Hyperplasia, Florid. A, B: In this needle core biopsy (NCB), the dense overlapping cellular proliferation has solid and papillary patterns. Columnar cell and micropapillary hyperplasia are shown in **(B)** at the periphery of the duct.

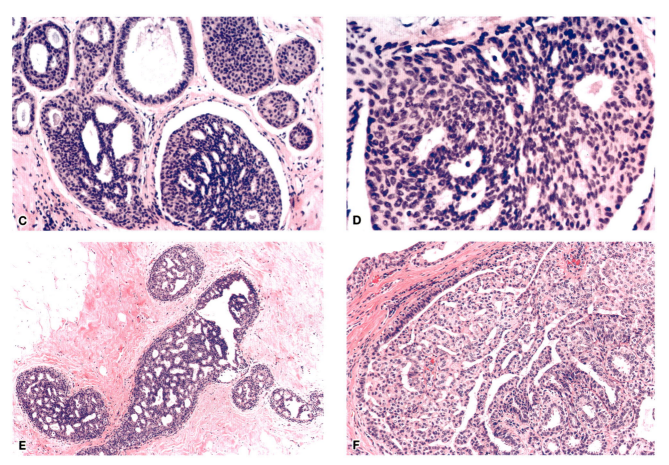

FIGURE 8.5 (*continued*) **C, D:** Solid and cribriform florid hyperplasia is seen in these lesions. The epithelium in the duct in (**D**) has a streaming pattern. Note the loss of cytoplasm and nuclear condensation in cells in the centers of ducts. **E:** Cribriform florid hyperplasia, involving multiple duct profiles, is seen in this biopsy. **F:** The cribriform florid hyperplasia in this biopsy involves an intraductal papilloma.

The distinction between moderate and **florid hyperplasia** is not sharp, but lesions are generally placed in the latter category when the affected ducts are appreciably expanded and filled with proliferative epithelium in comparison with their nonhyperplastic counterparts. Florid hyperplasia has the papillary and bridging growth patterns that are encountered in moderate hyperplasia, but the overall proliferative process tends to be more cellular and complex than in moderate hyperplasia (**Fig. 8.7**). Foci of florid hyperplasia are more likely to fill the entire ductal lumen in a solid or cribriform (fenestrated) manner.

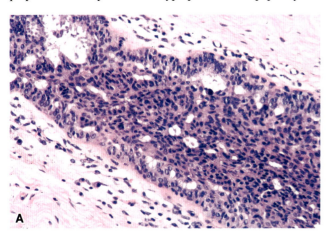
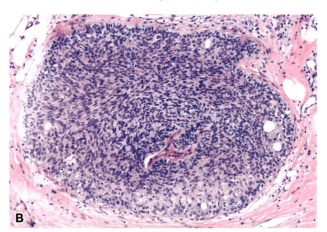

FIGURE 8.6 **Ductal Hyperplasia, Florid With Streaming. A:** The hyperplastic epithelium in the lumen of this duct is composed of cells with a streaming pattern. Note the persistent columnar ductal epithelium and microlumina at the border of the duct. **B:** This solid papillary ductal hyperplasia, with fibrovascular stroma, is composed of spindle cells with a streaming pattern. Microlumina are present at the perimeter of the duct.

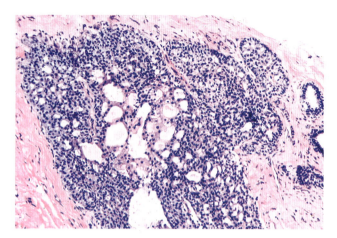

FIGURE 8.7 Ductal Hyperplasia, Florid. The hyperplastic duct in this needle core biopsy (NCB) is enlarged and filled by epithelium with solid and cribriform areas. Apocrine metaplasia is present in the center of the duct.

ducts with hyperplastic epithelium without necrosis. Histiocytes ("foam" cells) are relatively common in the lumina of hyperplastic ducts. Degenerating histiocytes should not be mistaken for necrotic debris. In sum, per se, necrosis is not diagnostic of DCIS, and it is the architectural and cytologic features of a proliferative lesion which determine the diagnosis.

The **cribriform (fenestrated) growth pattern** that occurs in moderate and florid DH results from the formation of epithelial bridges which traverse the ductal lumen. The cribriform spaces represent portions of original ductal lumen which have been subdivided by the complex arborizing epithelial proliferation. Using a serial section-3D reconstruction method, Ohuchi et al (28) demonstrated that the lumina which appear separate in a two-dimensional histologic section of a hyperplastic focus were part of a network of channels representing the original ductal lumen surrounded by hyperplastic epithelium. By contrast, 3D reconstruction of DCIS revealed that the fenestrations in these lesions were newly formed disconnected spaces bounded by polarized neoplastic cells.

Features that facilitate the distinction between UDH and low-grade DCIS include cellular (especially nuclear) heterogeneity in UDH. The nuclei of the cells surrounding the secondary lumina tend to run parallel to the lumina. Cellular polarization around spaces within the duct and/or at the periphery of the afflicted duct supports the diagnosis of DCIS.

Necrotic cellular debris is rarely present in hyperplastic ducts. Necrosis may be present in association with florid papillary hyperplasia **(Fig. 8.8)**, sclerosing papillary lesions, subareolar sclerosing DH, and florid papillomatosis of the nipple (so-called nipple adenoma). The latter lesion is notorious for harboring necrosis—not only most commonly but also most prominently. When necrosis occurs in UDH, the hyperplastic ducts with necrosis are cytologically and architecturally indistinguishable from adjacent

The spaces that are found in cribriform DH have distinctive features. The secondary lumina tend to be larger and relatively more numerous at the perimeter of the duct (rather than centrally), but the reverse distribution may be encountered. Cells outlining these spaces are distributed in a haphazard fashion except at the edge of the duct, where residual columnar or cuboidal epithelium composed of cells with more regularly oriented nuclei may persist. The spaces in a hyperplastic duct may have varied shapes (ovoid, crescentic, irregular, or serpiginous) rather than being rounded as in cribriform DCIS **(Fig. 8.9)**. The spaces in DH may be empty or may contain secretions and histiocytes. Calcifications can develop in the glandular lumina of DH. The rare gynecomastoid type of UDH may mimic low-grade micropapillary DCIS.

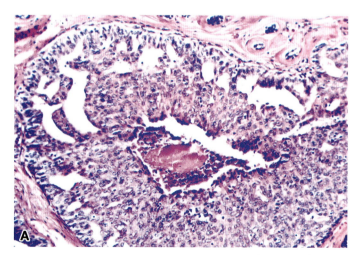 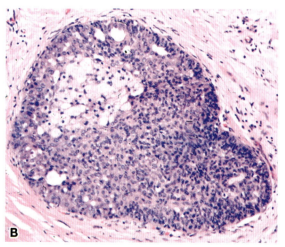

FIGURE 8.8 Ductal Hyperplasia, Florid With Necrosis and Histiocytes. A: Necrosis is present in the center of this hyperplastic duct that was part of sclerosing papillary duct hyperplasia. Columnar epithelium can be seen at the periphery of the duct, where there are microlumina of various sizes and shapes. **B:** The epithelial proliferation in this enlarged duct is relatively solid with peripheral fenestrations. Histiocytes are present in the duct.

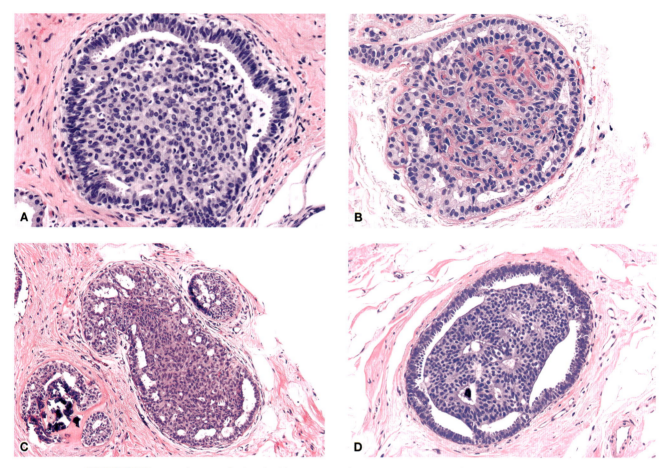

FIGURE 8.9 Ductal Hyperplasia, Florid. A-D: Microlumina are present at the periphery of multiple ducts in different needle core biopsies. Polypoid florid duct hyperplasia is focally anchored to the persisting columnar cell epithelium at the perimeter of the duct.

A monolayer of myoepithelial cells, or variably hyperplastic myoepithelial cells, may be evident at the edge of a duct with DH **(Fig. 8.10)**. These cells may accompany the proliferative process into the ductal lumen when the fibrovascular stromal framework of papillary hyperplasia is present. Immunostains readily highlight the myoepithelial contribution to DH, ADH, and DCIS. Experience has led to the conclusion that the reactivity of individual markers is unpredictable in an individual case. Thus, it is prudent to employ multiple myoepithelial markers. p63 and p40 (also SOX10 and WT1) are localized in the nuclei of myoepithelial cells (29,30). These nuclear markers are not reactive in myofibroblasts and blood vessels. Nuclear staining with p63 and p40 produces a "string of dots" between the epithelium and the basement membrane in benign ducts and lobules. Rarely, p63 and p40 may be positive in epithelial cell nuclei

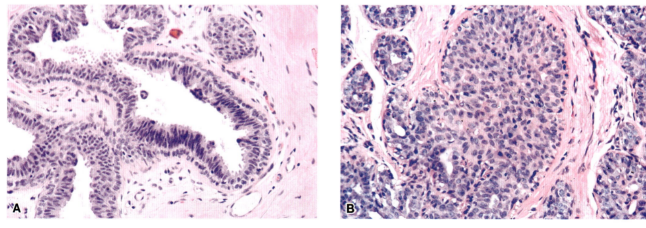

FIGURE 8.10 Ductal Hyperplasia With Myoepithelial Cells. A: Columnar cell hyperplasia with prominent myoepithelium. **B:** Solid hyperplasia with inconspicuous myoepithelium.

in papillary lesions and in high-grade DCIS, and much less often in DH. These epithelial cells can be distinguished from myoepithelial cells by their cytologic appearance and position thereof. SOX10 and WT1 can also be used as a myoepithelial (nuclear) marker (31).

Several cytoplasmic markers are available for highlighting the myoepithelium including smooth muscle actin (SMA), smooth muscle myosin-heavy chain (SMM-HC), calponin, and CD10. These markers exhibit variable degrees and extent of cross-reactivity with myofibroblasts and blood vessels (30,32-34). Due to the variable reactivity of these reagents with myoepithelial cells, it is prudent to employ one or more cytoplasmic and nuclear markers for the evaluation of myoepithelia.

Myoepithelium is usually uniformly present in ducts with proliferative fibrocystic changes, such as in adenosis and in various degrees of DH. Attenuation of myoepithelial cells, which occurs in some forms of epithelial hyperplasia, especially sclerosing papillary lesions and ADH, results in increased space between p63/p40/SOX-10/WT1 reactive nuclei relative to the staining pattern observed in inactive glands. In this situation, myoepithelial integrity can usually be demonstrated with one of the immunostains that show cytoplasmic reactivity. Because stromal proliferation accompanies many of these proliferative lesions, care must be taken not to mistake myofibroblastic reactivity for myoepithelial positivity. The demonstration of a myoepithelial cell layer is useful in demonstrating the presence of myoepithelial cells at the perimeter of most ducts with DH, ADH, and DCIS. An intraductal proliferative lesion that is devoid of myoepithelium both within the duct and at its perimeter is almost certainly DCIS—except for some densely sclerosing papillary proliferations and certain types of apocrine lesions (35).

The cells of DH show variable positivity, often in a "mosaic pattern," for high-molecular-weight cytokeratin (HMW-CK: eg, CK 5/6 and CK-K903) and variable reactivity for estrogen receptor (ER). In contrast, the epithelial cells that comprise ADH (and DCIS) are negative for HMW-CK and are typically diffusely positive for ER (**Fig. 8.11**). Notably, some high-grade DCIS can be positive for HMW-CK

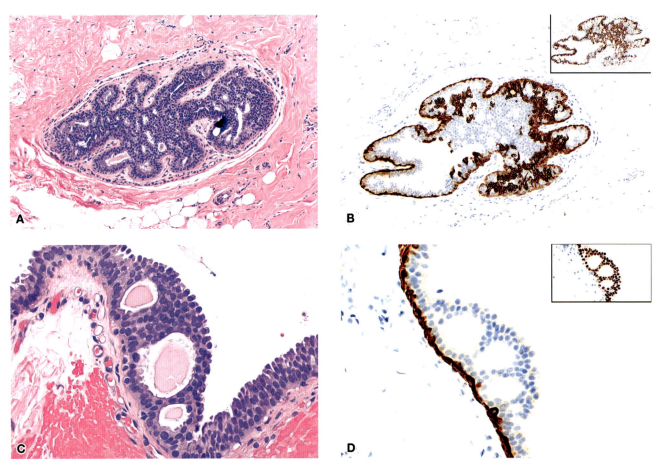

FIGURE 8.11 Differential Diagnosis of Florid Ductal Hyperplasia, Atypical Ductal Hyperplasia (ADH) and Low-Grade Ductal Carcinoma In Situ (DCIS), Role of Cytokeratin (CK) 5/6 and Estrogen Receptor (ER). **A, B:** Florid ductal hyperplasia. **B,** shows CK5/6 staining with "mosaic" pattern. ER (*inset*) shows heterogeneous staining. **C, D:** Atypical ductal hyperplasia. **D,** shows no staining of the lesional cells with CK5/6. ER (*inset*) shows strong homogeneous staining.

DUCTAL HYPERPLASIA, ATYPICAL DUCTAL HYPERPLASIA, AND DUCTAL CARCINOMA IN SITU 137

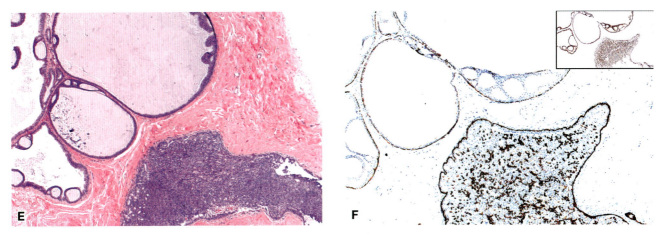

FIGURE 8.11 (*continued*) **E, F:** ADH and florid ductal hyperplasia. **E:** ADH (top) and florid ductal hyperplasia (bottom). **F:** ADH (top) shows no staining of the lesional cells with CK5/6, and ER shows strong homogeneous staining. Florid ductal hyperplasia (bottom) shows CK5/6 staining with "mosaic" pattern. ER (inset) shows heterogeneous staining.

(and also for p63 and p40). It must also be remembered that *columnar cell lesions* (CCLs, including flat epithelial atypia [FEA]) and apocrine metaplastic cells are generally negative for HMW-CK (36,37). A commercially available immunohistochemical cocktail (ADH5, Biocare) that combines low-molecular-weight CK (CK7/CK18, using Fast Red chromogen), HMW-CK (CK5/CK14 utilizing brown DAB chromogen), and p63 (also using DAB) is of use in distinguishing DH from ADH/DCIS—although the interpretation of ADH5 immunostaining can be difficult (38). Both ER and PR are variably reactive in DH. Please see **Table 8.6** for use of immunostains in the differential diagnosis of lower-grade intraductal epithelial proliferative and neoplastic lesions.

Collagenous Spherulosis

Collagenous spherulosis (CS) is a special form of hyperplasia wherein myoepithelial cells contribute to the formation of nodular subepithelial deposits of acellular basement membrane material (usually <100 μm) akin to those encountered in adenoid cystic carcinoma (**Fig. 8.12**). CS can develop in papillomata and in other proliferative lesions, as well as in LCIS. The myoepithelial cells in CS are compressed, elongated, and bland. The interspersed luminal cells are characteristically cuboidal. The center of the spherule can resemble a glandular lumen (with or without calcifications). The PAS-positive and laminin-positive basement membrane material is usually eosinophilic (on H&E stain), fibrillary, and wispy; however, the material may also be either basophilic and condensed or even mucoid. This material can undergo degeneration and may be present as thin fibrils or amorphous myxoid-like material.

Immunostains (especially calponin and myosin) can demonstrate myoepithelial cells around these spherules and distinguish these structures from true glandular lumina in cribriform spaces that form in DH and cribriform type of DCIS. In cribriform DCIS, the myoepithelium is usually present only at the perimeter of the duct. The epithelial cells in CS may be patchily CD117-positive and ER-positive. Histochemical stains for basement membrane (eg, PAS and

TABLE 8.6
Immunostains in the Differential Diagnosis of Lower-Grade Intraductal Lesions

Immunostains	UDH	ADH	LG-DCIS[a]
HMW-CK[b]	Variably positive: Heterogeneous "Mosaic-like"	Negative	Negative
ER	Variably heterogeneous, weak-strong	Less heterogeneous, moderate-strong	Homogeneous, strong

Based on review of literature.
ADH, atypical ductal hyperplasia; ER, estrogen receptor; HMW-CK, high-molecular-weight cytokeratin (typically CK5/6, also: CK5, CK14, and CK17); LG-DCIS, low-grade ductal carcinoma in situ; UDH, usual ductal hyperplasia;
[a]Some high-grade DCIS, particularly those of the "basal-like" subtype will be CK5/6-positive.
[b]HMW-CK: CK5, CK5/6, CK14, and CK17 are most suitable in this regard. Exceptions include some cases of intraductal proliferations with apocrine, columnar cell, papillary, and high-grade features. Of note, some normal cells may be negative for HMW-CK. Columnar cell lesions are strongly and diffusely ER-positive. Low-molecular-weight CKs (eg, CK8, CK 18, CK19) are generally expressed in ADH and LG-DCIS.

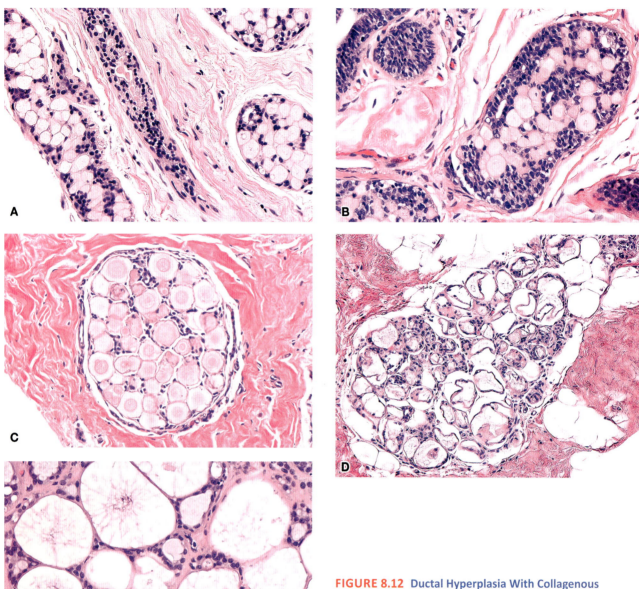

FIGURE 8.12 **Ductal Hyperplasia With Collagenous Spherulosis Which Mimics Cribriform Architecture.** Patterns of hyperplasia with collagenous spherulosis. **A-E:** Cribriform hyperplasia where microspherules are present amid the microlumina in these cases. The collagenous spherules are well formed. Degenerative changes are present in the collagenous spherules (in **D** and **E**).

reticulin) and stains for basement membrane (eg, reticulin and laminin) may be used to highlight the luminal contents. MYB RNA ISH testing can be useful to support the diagnosis of adenoid cystic carcinoma (39).

Atypical Ductal Hyperplasia

There is broad agreement on the general definition of atypical ductal hyperplasia (ADH) as a proliferative epithelial lesion that fulfills some, but not all, criteria for the diagnosis of DCIS. The 2012 WHO classification of breast tumors defined ADH, in part, as "proliferation of monomorphic, evenly placed epithelial cells involving TDLUs" (2). This definition could also easily have been applied to low-grade DCIS. The subsequent, and latest, 2019 WHO classification of breast tumors redefined ADH as "an epithelial proliferative lesion with cytological and architectural features similar to those of low-grade DCIS but less developed in architecture, degree of terminal duct lobular unit involvement and contiguous extent" (3).

The difficulty in arriving at a crisper definition of ADH lies in the specifics of the atypical hyperplastic process. In general, these specifics can be considered under two headings: quantitative and qualitative. The former refers to the amount and extent of the proliferative abnormality whereas the latter is concerned with architectural and cytologic details.

Quantitative criteria for distinguishing between DH and DCIS based on the number of duct cross sections that exhibit the abnormality, or the dimension of the affected area, have been proposed. Some investigators have classified proliferative lesions limited to a single duct as ADH, even if the abnormality is qualitatively consistent with DCIS (14). Based on a criterion requiring at least two fully involved duct cross sections for a diagnosis of DCIS, cases are arbitrarily assigned to the category of ADH when only one qualitatively diagnostic duct is present.

Another scheme emphasizes the histologic extent of a lesion as the basis for the diagnosis of ADH (40). According to this criterion, foci spanning less than 2 mm are diagnosed as ADH, regardless of the number of duct cross sections, even if the individual ducts qualify as DCIS. The 2-mm criterion was selected because ". . . it was at the level of one or more small ducts or ductules measuring around 2 mm in aggregate cross-sectional diameter that most pathologists felt hesitant in diagnosing a lesion as intraductal carcinoma" (41). Another explanation offered by the proponents of this criterion was that "questions about quantity are raised generally when dispersed lesions add up to from 1.6 to 2.7 mm in aggregate size. Therefore, we arbitrarily chose 2 mm as a cutoff point" (40).

No scientific study has compared the clinical significance of different quantitative criteria for diagnosing ADH. There is no a priori reason for choosing two duct cross sections or 2 mm as the critical "tipping points" in relation to risk stratification. For example, no data exist for the risk to develop subsequent carcinoma in patients whose biopsies contained epithelial proliferative lesions qualitatively consistent with DCIS limited to one, two, or three duct cross sections, respectively. Regarding the dimensions of these lesions, no analysis comparing foci measuring 1.5, 2.0, 2.5 mm, or larger has been reported.

Several technical issues hinder the application of quantitative criteria, especially in the diagnosis of findings in NCB. What appear to be two contiguous cross sections may prove in serial sections to be part of a single duct, or deeper sections of what appears to be a single duct lesion may uncover additional involved cross sections of the duct. How close must two duct cross sections be to be considered contiguous? Is the stroma between duct cross sections included in the measurement? Quantitative criteria assume that the ducts in question have been sectioned perpendicular to their long axis. How to assess ducts cut longitudinally has not been adequately addressed. If the longitudinal dimension of a duct in a section exceeds 2 mm but the transverse span is 1 mm, should this focus be considered DCIS when using the 2-mm criterion?

Others have also rejected utilizing quantitative factors in the diagnosis of ADH. This position was elaborated by Fisher et al (42) who stated that "our definition of ADH consists of a ductal epithelial alteration approximating but not unequivocally satisfying the criteria for a diagnosis of DCIS. It does not include arbitrarily established quantities of unequivocal DCIS (less than 2.0 mm or 2 'spaces')." In their study of the prognostic significance of proliferative breast "disease," Bodian et al (13) reported that "during the course of many years, intraductal carcinoma has been diagnosed if the characteristic features are present in only one ductal space."

The role of quantitative factors in the diagnosis of proliferative ductal lesions seems to lie between these extremes. The use of rigid criteria such as two ductal cross sections or 2 mm can be justified in research settings to ensure a homogeneous study group or to assess a particular criterion, but the strict application of these arbitrary rules in a clinical setting is difficult for the technical reasons stated earlier and is poorly substantiated by existing data. Given the limitations of current methods for diagnosing ductal lesions, quantitative factors sometimes play a role in the assessment of a particular lesion in material obtained in an NCB. This situation arises when the biopsy contains detached fragments of cytologically atypical epithelium (**Fig. 8.13**) or when only part of one duct with changes suggestive of DCIS is represented (**Figs. 8.14-8.17**). The same issue arises when a process suggests lobular extension of DCIS (**Fig. 8.18**).

It is notable that the 2 mm and two duct thresholds (or more appropriately "guidelines") were originally developed for excisional biopsies. These thresholds were developed for ducts uniformly involved by a monotonous process with well-developed architecture and low-grade cytology. As stated earlier, it is hard to imagine any significant level of pathobiologic difference between ducts that either span a few microns less or more than 2 mm or involve one or three duct profile (which may be the same duct coming in and out of the plane of section).

In many instances, the diagnosis of ADH depends on the presence of structural elements of DCIS mingling with hyperplasia. Architecturally, this may be manifested by a cribriform pattern partially involving a duct (**Figs. 8.19 and 8.20**). These foci feature sharply defined round-to-ovoid spaces outlined by cells with distinct borders and a rigid arrangement. Rarely, ADH can display a solid growth pattern. Cribriform, micropapillary and papillary foci involving hyperplastic ducts constitute other architectural manifestations

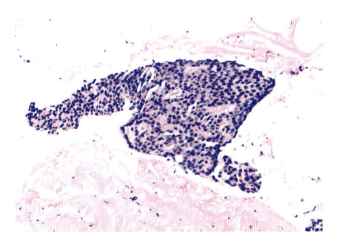

FIGURE 8.13 Atypical Ductal Hyperplasia. This needle core biopsy (NCB) included a detached fragment of nearly solid proliferative duct epithelium.

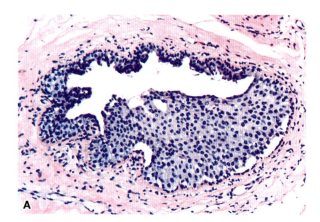
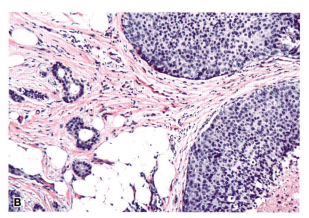

FIGURE 8.14 **Atypical Ductal Hyperplasia. A:** The needle core biopsy (NCB) from this patient contained this duct that is partly occupied by a solid epithelial proliferation of monomorphic cells. This partially involved duct provides insufficient evidence for the diagnosis of ductal carcinoma in situ (DCIS). **B:** The excisional biopsy revealed in situ and invasive carcinoma. The area of DCIS shown here has a relatively denser and cytologically more atypical cell population than does the duct in **(A)**.

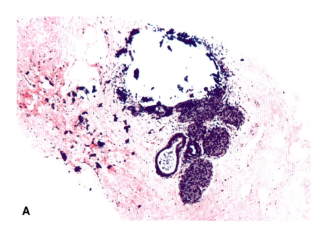
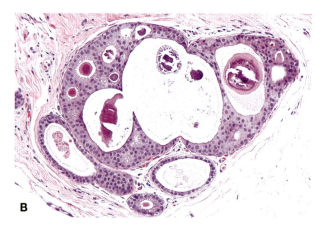

FIGURE 8.15 **Atypical Ductal Hyperplasia. A:** This needle core biopsy (NCB) of mammographically detected calcifications shows solid atypical duct hyperplasia with calcification. Intraductal calcification was fractured in preparing the slide. **B:** Cribriform atypical duct hyperplasia with concentrically laminated calcifications. The hyperplastic epithelial cells display apocrine cytoplasmic traits. Note the orderly distribution of nuclei at the perimeter of the duct.

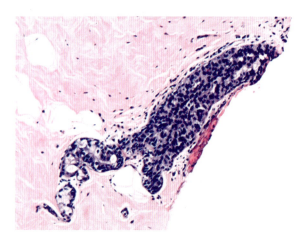

FIGURE 8.16 **Atypical Ductal Hyperplasia.** The duct at the edge of this specimen was the only significant abnormality in this needle core biopsy (NCB). Note the overlapping, hyperchromatic, pleomorphic nuclei. Excisional biopsy yielded a 3-mm focus of atypical duct hyperplasia similar to this duct.

of ADH **(Fig. 8.21)**. The latter can be rarely encountered in ducts exhibiting apocrine metaplasia **(Figs. 8.21 and 8.22)**. Cytologic atypia may involve individual cells, groups of cells, or the entire population of a proliferative epithelial lesion. Atypical features include nuclear enlargement with increased nuclear-to-cytoplasmic ratio, nuclear hyperchromasia, irregular chromatin pattern, mitoses, and macronucleoli **(Fig. 8.23)**.

Most cases of ADH and low-grade DCIS can be readily differentiated; however, some ADH lesions are at the cusp of DCIS (ie, "borderline" for DCIS). These cases are diagnostically challenging. Most of these foci retain a minor characteristic of hyperplasia, such as epithelial overlapping, with a structure that is otherwise typical of DCIS **(Figs. 8.23-8.25)**. These slight variations will be disregarded by observers who classify the lesions as DCIS, whereas others may diagnose ADH. Similarly, those who place credence in quantitative criteria will diagnose ADH because the extent of a lesion is not sufficient, whereas others, not adhering

DUCTAL HYPERPLASIA, ATYPICAL DUCTAL HYPERPLASIA, AND DUCTAL CARCINOMA IN SITU 141

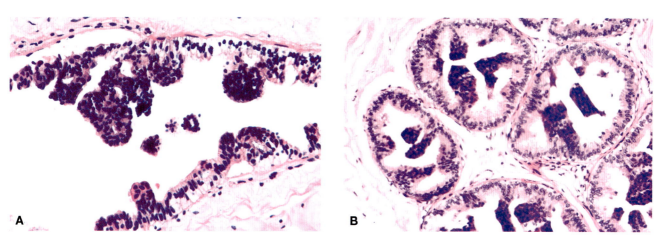

FIGURE 8.17 Atypical Ductal Hyperplasia, Micropapillary. A: Mammographically detected calcifications led to this needle core biopsy (NCB). The micropapillae are composed of cells with overlapping, hyperchromatic nuclei. **B:** Atypical micropapillary hyperplasia with condensation of nuclei in the micropapillae.

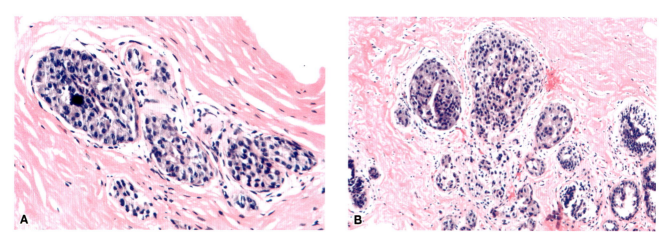

FIGURE 8.18 Atypical Ductal Hyperplasia, Lobular Extension. A: A thin layer of persistent glandular epithelium outlines a narrow, slit-shaped lumen next to calcification. Solid ductal carcinoma in situ (DCIS) was found in the excisional biopsy. **B:** An irregular proliferation of cells fills lobular glands in this needle core biopsy (NCB).

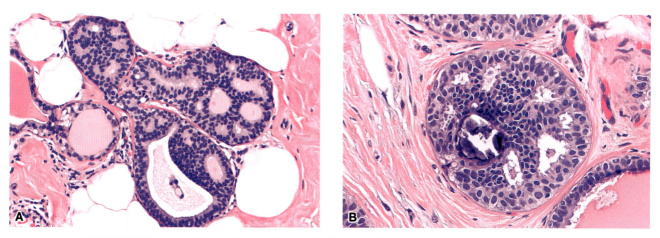

FIGURE 8.19 Atypical Ductal Hyperplasia, Cribriform. A: The only proliferative abnormality in the needle core biopsy (NCB) in this case was one focus of cribriform proliferation in a duct. **B:** Atypical cribriform hyperplasia in another case.

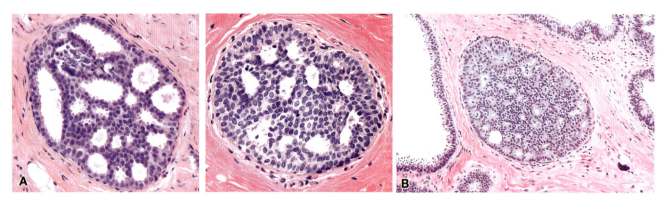

FIGURE 8.20 Atypical Ductal Hyperplasia, Cribriform. A, B: The atypical hyperplasia in multiple ducts show cribriform microlumen formation.

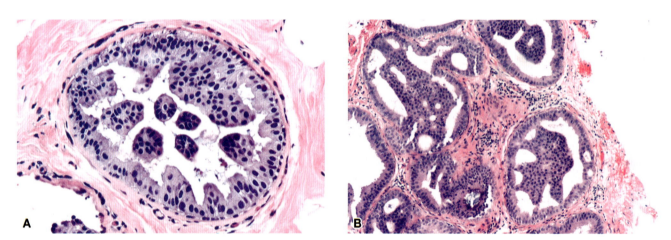

FIGURE 8.21 Atypical Ductal Hyperplasia, Micropapillary. A: Crowded multilayered cells in atypical hyperplasia. Crowding and hyperchromasia of shrunken nuclei at the tips of some micropapillae is apparent in this duct. There is a ring of evenly spaced ductal cell nuclei at the periphery of the duct. **B:** A monomorphic population of cells forms bridges across these ducts, creating irregularly shaped microlumina. Epithelium at the perimeter of each duct consists of cuboidal or low columnar cells with evenly spaced, basally oriented nuclei.

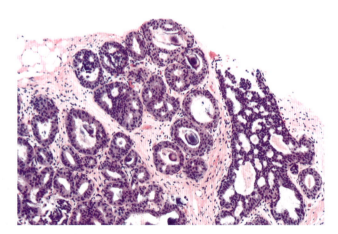

FIGURE 8.22 Atypical Columnar Cell Hyperplasia. Note cytologic (columnar cells with hyperchromatic nuclei) and architectural (cribriform and micropapillary) atypia.

to these rules, will diagnose DCIS. It has been shown that reproducible categorization as ADH or DCIS in "borderline" lesions cannot be achieved, and "borderline" may even be an entity per se (43). We would recommend exercising diagnostic restraint in diagnosing DCIS whenever the evidence is scant—particularly in NCB samplings.

Insufficient emphasis has been placed on diagnosing specific proliferative lesions in the context of the overall spectrum of histologic changes in NCB material. In a research setting, a pathologist can be required to make a diagnosis that is based only on one focus or selected foci on a single slide. This situation, duplicated to a large extent in assessing NCB, is different from the circumstances under which the various diagnostic criteria were originally developed: by review of multiple histologic sections (14,40,42).

When faced with an atypical ductal proliferative lesion in an NCB, slides from previous biopsies diagnosed as ADH

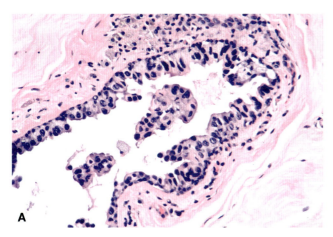
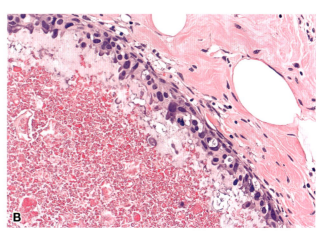

FIGURE 8.23 Atypical Micropapillary Hyperplasia With Marked Cytologic Atypia Compared to "Clinging" Ductal Carcinoma In Situ. A: The only proliferative abnormality in this needle core biopsy (NCB) was this duct at the edge of one core. The epithelial layer is thickened and composed of cells distributed in a disordered pattern. Many nuclei are hyperchromatic, especially at the luminal border, and there is some nuclear overlap. This minuscule atypical proliferative process has micropapillary traits. **B:** Flat micropapillary ("clinging") carcinoma. The cytologic atypia is more pronounced than that observed in **A**.

or DCIS should be reviewed whenever possible. A focus of concern in an NCB may be found to be substantially more atypical than the previously diagnosed ADH, or it may be as atypical, or it may be less so. The first situation would tend to support a diagnosis of DCIS, whereas the second would suggest ADH, and the third should prompt reevaluation of the diagnosis of ADH.

Obtaining H&E-stained "serial" sections, "levels," or "deepers" from the corresponding tissue block can be useful in most, if not all, cases (please see Chapter 26). Immunohistochemical evaluation, with either various cytokeratins or hormonal receptors, is seldom helpful in this regard—as these stains may be able to separate UDH (heterogeneous in intensity and proportion) from ADH (diffusely strong), but cannot separate ADH from DCIS (both diffusely strong). It must also be remembered that the "highest level of accuracy" of diagnosis in NCB material is achieved "using the triple approach, combining imaging and clinical examination assessment with pathological results" and that pathologic findings "should not be reported in isolation" (44). In dealing with ADH and "borderline" lesions, it is our practice to review the case in a peer review session—preferably after multiple (serials, levels, or deepers) and/or appropriate immunostains are available.

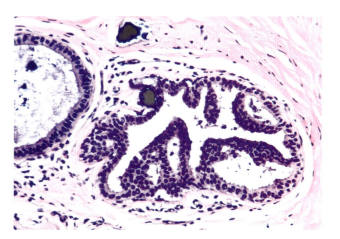

FIGURE 8.25 Atypical Ductal Hyperplasia, Borderline. The needle core biopsy (NCB) that yielded this lesion was performed for clustered microcalcifications. Calcifications are present in microcysts and stroma. The proliferation has a micropapillary structure and is composed of cells with condensed, hyperchromatic nuclei. The non-papillary peripheral epithelium consists of regular cuboidal cells that are indistinguishable from cells lining the adjacent nonproliferative cyst. The micropapillary abnormality was limited to this site.

FIGURE 8.24 Atypical Ductal Hyperplasia, Borderline. The ducts in this needle core biopsy (NCB) have a solid central population of small, monomorphic cells. Microlumina outlined by cells oriented around the rounded fenestrations are present at the periphery of some ducts.

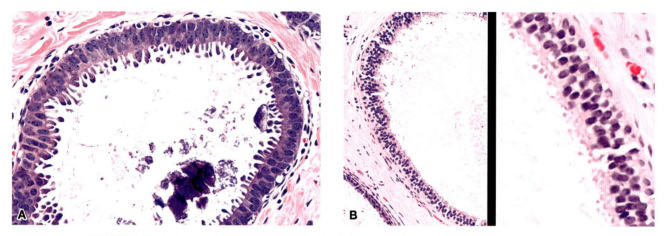

FIGURE 8.26 **Columnar Cell Change. A, B:** Cystic dilatation of ducts lined by cuboidal and columnar cells with closely approximated, basally oriented nuclei. Luminal cytoplasmic tufts ("snouts") are evident in **A**. The cystic columnar cell change in **B** shows less prominent cytoplasmic snouts and epithelial hyperplasia with stratification. Right panel in **B** shows detail.

ADH can involve proliferative lesions such as sclerosing adenosis and radial scars and may also be associated with benign neoplasms (most often fibroadenomas and papillomas). In the latter instance, the term atypical papilloma (ie, papilloma with ADH) is used. ADH can, of course, accompany DCIS and invasive carcinoma.

Columnar Cell Lesions

Columnar cell lesions (CCLs), often considered to be part of the spectrum of DH, have come under enhanced scrutiny as a result of being increasingly detected on mammography and sampled via NCB. Lubelsky et al (45) reported that 21% of NCB obtained for calcifications in mammographically screened women had CCLs. These abnormalities have also been known as *columnar cell change* (CCC) *or columnar cell hyperplasia* (CCH) (46,47) and *flat epithelial atypia* (FEA) (48). Other more cumbersome names that have been offered include *atypical cystic lobules* (49), *cancerization of lobules and ADH adjacent to DCIS* (50), and *columnar alteration with prominent apical snouts and secretions* (CAPSS) (51).

The fundamental lesion, **columnar cell change (CCC)**, is localized in a TDLU, which becomes variably enlarged due to cystic dilatation. The latter is due to accumulation of distinctly eosinophilic secretions. The simplest form of this process features a thin, single, epithelial layer composed of cuboidal-to-tall columnar cells distributed in a relatively uniform pattern. Of note, in some cases, CCC mainly comprises *cuboidal* (rather than the namesake columnar) cells. Because the nuclei in CCC tend to be relatively large, the cells appear crowded and dark. The apical cell surface usually has an apocrine-type of cytoplasmic protrusion ("snout"), and in some cases, this is an unusually prominent feature. In the plainest form of CCL, the epithelium is one to two cells deep, and there is minimal nuclear pleomorphism **(Fig. 8.26)**. Nucleoli are uncommon, and mitotic figures are rare. When present, calcification is in the form of amorphous granular material or discrete basophilic deposits **(Fig. 8.27)**. Notably, the lesional cells in CCC (typically tall with apical snouts) can resemble those of tubular carcinoma. The cytologic features of CCLs can suggest apocrine differentiation. The cells often express GCDFP-15 (BRST-2), an apocrine marker. The proliferation rate is relatively low, even in hyperplastic foci (52). The epithelium in CCL is almost always strongly and diffusely ER-positive, whereas cells with apocrine change are typically ER-negative (52) and androgen receptor (AR)-positive.

Columnar cell hyperplasia (CCH) is a multifocal process that may also be bilateral. CCH is most often encountered in women aged 35 to 50 years; however, it can also be present after menopause. CCH rarely produces a palpable abnormality, and it is typically detected on mammogram because calcifications are frequently formed. CCH is present when the epithelium is more than two cells deep. This is most readily apparent when cellular crowding becomes pronounced, and nuclei are not distributed in a single plane relative to the basement membrane. This tendency toward "stacking" of nuclei is usually accompanied by nuclear hyperchromasia. Diminutive epithelial mounds may be formed

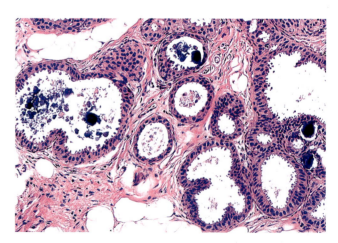

FIGURE 8.27 **Columnar Cell Change, With Calcifications.** Granular and punctate basophilic calcifications are shown.

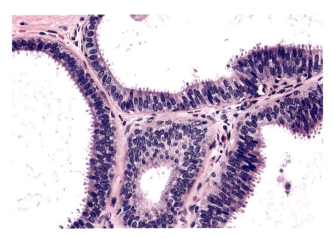

FIGURE 8.28 **Columnar Cell Hyperplasia.** The thickened epithelium is composed of crowded, columnar cells with overlapping nuclei.

in the hypercellular regions **(Fig. 8.28)**. Notably, CCLs may not show the mosaic-like heterogeneity with HMW-CKs (so characteristic of UDH), and most CCH lesions are strongly and diffusely ER-positive.

More involved columnar cell proliferative foci comprise lesions described as **atypical columnar cell hyperplasia (ACCH)/flat epithelia atypia (FEA) (Table 8.7)**. The term flat epithelial atypia (FEA) has been used as a synonym for the lesion described as ACCH. Mild ACCH is usually manifested by the presence of minute (and often isolated) foci of micropapillary growth in a background of otherwise usual CCH **(Fig. 8.29)**. The presence of more elaborate growth patterns as well as cytologic atypia characterizes CCH with moderate-to-marked atypia, which in its most severe form approaches DCIS **(Figs. 8.30 and 8.31)**. In most instances of ACCH/FEA, the cytologic atypia is more pronounced than the architectural abnormality **(Fig. 8.32)**. When carcinoma arises in the setting of CCH, the growth pattern is usually one of the characteristic forms of DCIS **(Figs. 8.33 and 8.34)**. Flat micropapillary (so-called clinging) DCIS with minimal epithelial complexity can be encountered in this setting **(Fig. 8.35)**. Atypical lobular hyperplasia (ALH) and LCIS frequently accompany CCL, and tubular carcinoma may also be present **(Fig. 8.36)**. CCLs are part of a triad that includes LCIS and tubular carcinoma (ie, "The Rosen Triad") (53-55) **(Table 8.8)**.

The term **flat epithelial atypia (FEA)** has been used as a synonym for the lesion described as ACCH (please see the foregoing section also). The term "flat" implies simple (ie, noncomplex) architecture, mainly represented by epithelium of a single layer or at most a few layers (hence the term "flat"). "Flat" refers to the architectural pattern, that is, an even luminal surface of the epithelium—and does not refer to the cytologic shape of the lesional cells, which are either columnar or cuboidal (and almost never flattened).

TABLE 8.7

Histopathologic Features of Columnar Cell Change, Columnar Cell Hyperplasia, Atypical Columnar Cell Hyperplasia/Flat Epithelial Atypia and Flat Micropapillary ("Clinging") Carcinoma In Situ

	CCC	CCH	ACCH/FEA[a]	Clinging DCIS
TDLU	Variably dilated, irregular	Variably dilated, irregular	Dilated, smooth inner contour	May be dilated, variable contour
Cell layer	1-2	>2	>1	>1
Cells	Columnar	Columnar	Cuboidal-columnar	Columnar
N:C ratio	Normal	Slightly higher	Increased	Markedly increased
Nuclei	Ovoid, even chromatin	Ovoid, even chromatin	Rounded-ovoid, low-grade "atypia"	Irregular, hyperchromatic
Nucleoli	Not prominent	Inconspicuous	Usually prominent	Prominent
Cell polarization	++	++	−/+	−/+
Mitoses	−	+/−	+/−	+
Secretions	+/−	+	+	+/−
Necrosis	−	−	−	+/−
Calcifications	+	++	++	+

Based on review of literature.
ACCH, atypical columnar cell hyperplasia; CCC, columnar cell change; CCH, columnar cell hyperplasia; DCIS, ductal carcinoma in situ; FEA, flat epithelial atypia; N:C ratio, nuclear-to-cytoplasmic ratio; TDLU, terminal duct lobular unit.
[a]The term "flat" implies simple (or noncomplex) architecture. Of note, "flat" in this context does *not* refer to the shapes of the lesional cells, which are either columnar or cuboidal (and almost never flattened), rather "flat" refers to the architectural pattern of the lesion, that is, flat luminal surface.

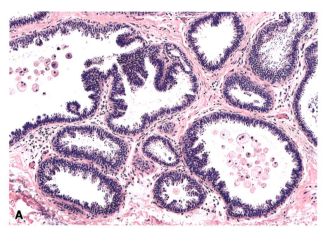
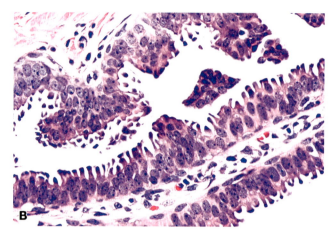

FIGURE 8.29 **Columnar Cell Hyperplasia, With Atypia. A:** Minute epithelial mounds are formed in the epithelium, and there is mild cytologic atypia. Histiocytes are present in some lumina. **B:** Focal blunt micropapillary proliferation of the hyperplastic columnar cell epithelium. Note apical snouts of the lesional cells.

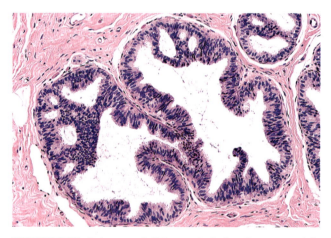

FIGURE 8.30 **Columnar Cell Hyperplasia (Moderate Atypia).** Atypical micropapillary hyperplasia, with the formation of epithelial arcades and bridges.

The proliferating ductal epithelium in ACCH/FEA shows "low-grade" atypia. The recognition of "low-grade" atypia is challenging—not only because of "inherent subjectivity in the interpretation of atypia, which presents as a morphologic continuum reflecting a biological spectrum." Also, "the lack of standardization in defining 'atypia' augments diagnostic discordance in breast pathology with potential implications for patient management" (9).

Be that as it may, cytologic atypia is generally assessed based on cellular pleomorphism, nuclear hyperchromasia, rate of mitoses, presence and size of nucleoli, and type of apoptosis/necrosis. Low-grade atypia (such as that encountered in ACCH/FEA) is characterized by monomorphic cells with uniform rounded nuclei that measure up to 2 times the size of red blood cells. The chromatin appears even, nucleoli are inconspicuous, and mitoses are rare. Minor degrees of architectural atypia including cellular tufts and mounds may

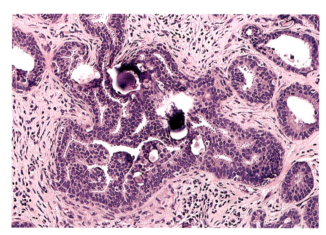

FIGURE 8.31 **Columnar Cell Hyperplasia (Moderate Atypia).** Micropapillary hyperplasia in a duct with calcifications.

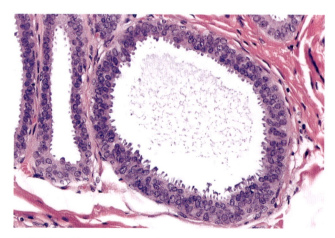

FIGURE 8.32 **Columnar Cell Hyperplasia With Atypia.** The epithelial cells display cytologic atypia. There are no structural abnormalities. No mitoses are evident.

DUCTAL HYPERPLASIA, ATYPICAL DUCTAL HYPERPLASIA, AND DUCTAL CARCINOMA IN SITU

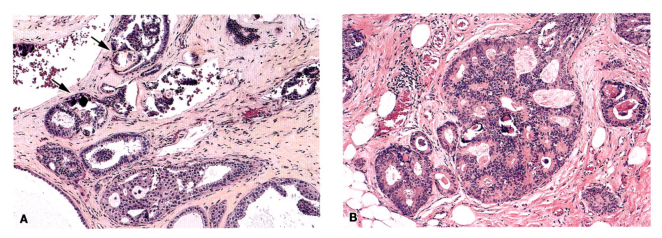

FIGURE 8.33 Ductal Carcinoma In Situ (DCIS), Atypical Columnar Cell Hyperplasia, and Columnar Cell Change With Ossifying-Type Calcifications. This needle core biopsy (NCB) was obtained from a focus of nonpalpable mammographically detected calcifications. **A:** Basophilic and ossifying-type calcifications (arrows) are associated with atypical hyperplasia. **B:** Cribriform DCIS with calcifications was present in the subsequent excisional biopsy.

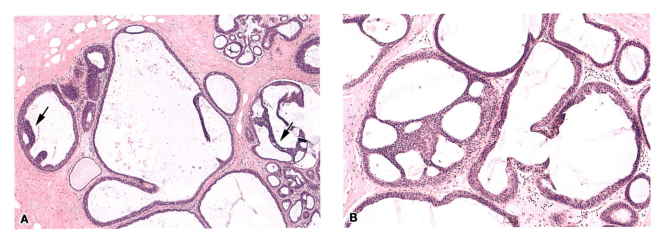

FIGURE 8.34 Ductal Carcinoma In Situ (DCIS) Following Atypical Columnar Cell Hyperplasia.
A: An excisional biopsy revealed multifocal, predominantly cystic columnar cell hyperplasia with focal atypia, shown here with micropapillary architecture (arrows). **B:** Four years later, needle core biopsy (NCB) at the same location (performed for calcifications) revealed cribriform DCIS (one duct thereof shown on left) associated with atypical columnar cell hyperplasia.

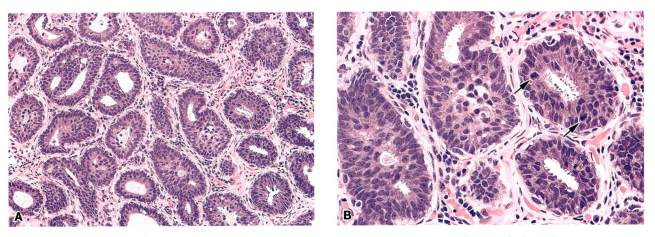

FIGURE 8.35 Ductal Carcinoma In Situ (DCIS) Associated With Columnar Cell Hyperplasia. A, B: Flat micropapillary and cribriform DCIS with mitoses (arrows).

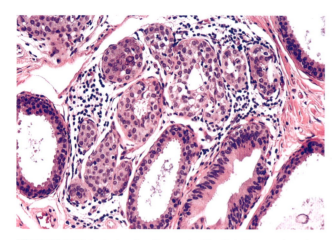

FIGURE 8.36 Lobular Carcinoma In Situ (LCIS) Associated With Columnar Cell Change. LCIS is surrounded by cystic columnar cell change.

TABLE 8.8
"Rosen Triad"

Columnar cell group of lesions
Lobular carcinoma in situ, classic type
Tubular carcinoma

From Brandt SM, Young GQ, Hoda SA. The "Rosen Triad": tubular carcinoma, lobular carcinoma in situ, and columnar cell lesions. *Adv Anat Pathol.* 2008;15:140-146.

be seen in ACCH/FEA. High-grade cytologic atypia of epithelial cells in an ACCH/FEA-type lesion is categorized as DCIS with flat micropapillary ("clinging") pattern.

By contrast, the term **atypical duct hyperplasia (ADH)** should be restricted to lesions that show *complex architecture*. It is not uncommon to find ACCH/FEA and ADH to be concurrent in an NCB. The two lesions can occasionally merge. Whether or not ACCH/FEA and ADH are biologically equivalent remains rather uncertain. Nevertheless, the rate of upgrade of ACCH/FEA found on NCB to either DCIS or invasive carcinoma on subsequent excision has been reported to be 3.2% in two series (56,57), and 5% (58), 9.5% (59), 9.6% (60), 15% (61), 19% (62), and 33% (63) in others. This extremely wide range (3.2%-33%) in the upgrade rate is most likely attributable to variations in the diagnostic threshold of "atypia," degree of sampling, and radiology-pathology concordance.

At presentation, CCLs can harbor *calcifications*. Two types of calcifications are encountered: crystalline and ossifying. The crystalline type, usually associated with lesions with less atypia, is deeply basophilic, opaque, round, or angular and is prone to fragmentation in the process of histologic sectioning. The ossifying type of calcification usually has a rounded, well-defined contour and an internal structure that resembles a "bony" nodule in which basophilic granular calcific deposits are embedded in spaces within an eosinophilic matrix **(Fig. 8.37)**. Ossifying type of calcifications occur throughout the range of CCLs and may also develop in UDH. Both types of calcifications can coexist.

The proliferative activity of CCLs was evaluated by Ki-67 immunoreactivity and was found to be significantly lower in CCC (mean 0.1%) and CCH without atypia (mean 0.76%) than in normal TDLU (mean 2.4%) (64). Ki-67 indices in ACCH/FEA (mean 8.2%) and low-grade DCIS (8.9%) have not been found to be significantly different. The highest Ki-67 index was found in intermediate- to high-grade DCIS (mean 25.5%).

Dabbs et al (65) studied molecular changes in selected microdissected CCLs and found "a gradient of progressive mutational change" between CCC and invasive carcinoma arising in the background of CCLs. Mutational changes manifested as loss of heterozygosity (LOH) at selected loci were absent from CCC and only rarely found in CCH. Increasing LOH was detected across the spectrum of ACCH/FEA, DCIS, and invasive carcinoma. These results parallel those obtained in non-columnar cell proliferative lesions (66) and appear to support the concept that ADH may, in situations yet to be fully defined, be a precursor to carcinoma.

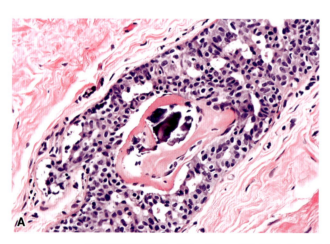 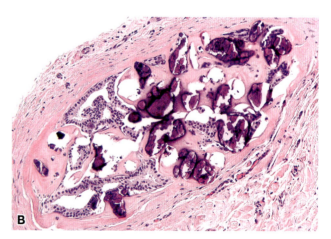

FIGURE 8.37 Ossifying Type of Calcifications in Columnar Cell Lesions. A: Ossifying calcification in cribriform ductal hyperplasia. **B:** In this needle core biopsy (NCB), ossifying-type calcifications nearly obliterate the luminal space in a duct with columnar cell change.

Although there is cumulative evidence to support the position that follow-up with imaging is a "reasonable" option for non-atypical CCLs diagnosed on NCB (67) and that patients with a diagnosis of ACCH/FEA on NCB should undergo excision of the lesional area (68), the management of CCLs found in NCB obtained for mammographically detected calcifications remains contentious (69). In this regard, two issues need to be considered.

The *first* concern is the likelihood that the NCB is not fully representative of abnormalities present. Guerra-Wallace et al (70) evaluated patients who underwent excisional biopsy after a CCL was found in NCB. They reported finding carcinoma in 10 of 135 (7.4%) women with CCH without atypia and in 11 of 60 (18.3%) with coexisting ADH. Chivukula et al (71) reported that ACH/FEA was detected in 301 of 8,054 (3.7%) of NCB obtained in a 2-year period. Excisional biopsies performed in 270 (90%) of the cases revealed invasive carcinoma in 18 patients (7%) and DCIS in 23 (8.5%) patients. Piubello et al (72) reported that 2 of 10 (20%) excisional biopsies from patients with ACCH/FEA and ADH in an NCB obtained for calcifications yielded DCIS and that invasive carcinoma was found in 3 of 10 (30%) of patients. In this study, no carcinoma was detected in excisional biopsies from 20 women who had ACCH/FEA without ADH in a prior NCB. DCIS was found in 1 of 51 (2%) of excisional biopsies performed after NCB diagnosis of CCH or ACCH/FEA without ADH reported by Senetta et al (73). DCIS associated with CCH and ACCH tends to have low-grade nuclei, micropapillary, and cribriform architecture, and no necrosis (74). ACCH/FEA is significantly related to ALH and LCIS (46,74), and it has been associated with invasive lobular carcinoma (75) as well as tubular carcinoma (46,53-55,75,76). The upgrade rate in a recent large follow-up study of ACCH/FEA, conducted at Memorial Sloan-Kettering Cancer Center in New York City, was extremely low. This study included 40 NCB cases (drawn from ~15,700 consecutive ones, from as many patients, over a 78-month period ending mid-2018). The target was calcifications in 36 (90%) cases, MRI enhancement in 3 (8%), and sonographic mass in 1 (2%). All NCBs were considered radiologic-pathologic concordant. ACCH/FEA was coexistent with ALH/LCIS in six cases. Subsequent excision yielded two low-grade invasive carcinomas, each spanning less than 2 mm, identified in sections without biopsy-site changes. About 38 cases had no upgrade. The presence of ALH/LCIS did not affect upgrade. *The upgrade rate of ACCH/FEA was 5%.* The study suggested that nonsurgical management may be considered in patients with radiology-pathology concordant NCB diagnosis of ACCH/FEA (58).

The *second* issue is the long-term risk for CCL to evolve into carcinoma. The role of CCL as precursors to carcinoma was reviewed by Turashvili et al (77), who concluded that "the natural history of CCLs is currently uncertain in any given patient." In a long-term follow-up study of a large series of patients with CCL, Boulos et al (78) reported a slight, statistically significant increased relative risk (RR) for developing breast carcinoma (1.47) when compared with controls with neither proliferative fibrocystic changes nor CCLs. In this study, the RR was not significantly affected by the presence or absence of ACCH/FEA.

With respect to immediate clinical management, some of the foregoing data support the recommendation to perform an excisional biopsy in a patient found to have ACCH/FEA in an NCB. An excisional biopsy would also be prudent if NCB reveals LCIS or ALH or ADH coexisting with CCL without ADH. Clinical circumstances such as the extent and character of the mammographically detected calcifications, the presence of a palpable lesion, or a family history of breast carcinoma may also play a role in deciding whether an excisional biopsy should follow the diagnosis of CCL without ADH on NCB.

The long-term significance of CCLs with or without ADH for the later development of DCIS or invasive carcinoma remains to be determined. Unfortunately, most studies of the cancer risk attributable to ADH discussed later in this chapter did not distinguish between ADH with and without CCLs. Hence, it is not certain that the elevated risk of carcinoma associated with ADH generally applies equally to CCLs with and without atypical hyperplasia. If the results presented by Boulos et al (78), *vide supra*, are confirmed by other investigators, CCLs may prove to be in a relatively low-risk category.

Presently, clinical follow-up with no other intervention is appropriate for the patient whose only abnormality is a non-atypical CCL or even ACCH/FEA diagnosed on NCB—if there is no other indication to perform an excisional biopsy. If the NCB shows ADH or LCIS in conjunction with CCL, treatment with excision *and* endocrine treatment may be appropriate.

Cumulative evidence, to date, suggests that whereas CCLs may be an early precursor lesion, UDH does not confer a substantial risk for the development of breast carcinoma (3). Furthermore, ACCH/FEA is associated with an exceedingly low risk of progression to carcinoma—lower than that associated with either ADH or ALH (3). Parenthetically, ADH is thought to be an early neoplastic step in the pathway to low-grade DCIS and invasive low-grade ER-positive ductal carcinoma.

Diagnosis of Atypical Ductal Hyperplasia by Needle Core Biopsy

It is often, and wisely, stated that the diagnosis of ADH should not be rendered until that of low-grade DCIS has been considered and rejected **(Tables 8.9 and 8.10)**. The histopathologic and cytopathologic features of ADH are well characterized, yet it suffers from a relatively low (as low as 40%) rate of diagnostic agreement. The rate is higher when a consensus diagnosis is obtained or appropriate immunostains are available. Notably, the results of immunostains can be similar in ACCH/FEA, ADH, and low-grade DCIS.

ADH typically involves TDLUs, and pagetoid extension of ADH along ducts (toward the nipple) is uncommon. More common is the extension of the process into lobules. Cells

TABLE 8.9

ADH: Pathologic Features

Architectural Patterns

Cribriform	Regular, round lumina with polarization of cells lining spaces
Micropapillary	Arcades and bridges are rigid, uniformly thick.
Flat micropapillary	Bulbous tips (club shaped), "clinging"
Solid	Cohesive cells, nondistended ducts

Cytologic Features

Uniform cells

Evenly spaced cells

Well-defined cell borders

Rounded nuclei

Expanse

Rule of thumb	<2 mm, <2 ducts/terminal duct lobular units; please see text.

10%-15% of cases of ADH diagnosed on needle core biopsy (NCB) show carcinoma; most commonly ductal carcinoma in situ on excision.

ADH, atypical ductal hyperplasia.

TABLE 8.10

Differential Diagnosis of ADH Versus LG-DCIS

Features	ADH	DCIS
Cytology		
Uniform	(+)	(++)
Cells evenly spaced	(+)	(++)
Distinct cell borders	(+)	(++)
Histology		
Cribriform		
Round, punched-out spaces	(+)	(++)
Micropapillary		
Bulbous micropapillae	(+)	(++)
Rigid arches/bridges/trabeculae	(+)	(++)
Solid		
Expansile, with cohesive cells	(+)	(++)
E-cadherin	(+)	(+)

Rule of thumb: Involvement of either >2 mm or >2 ducts/terminal duct lobular units supports the diagnosis of DCIS; please see text also.

ADH, atypical ductal hyperplasia; LG-DCIS, low-grade ductal carcinoma in situ.

with high-grade nuclei should not be encountered in ADH. Also, ADH associated with a mucocele-like lesion is uncommon. ADH is a microfocal disease, and its *extent* does not (counterintuitively) significantly contribute to breast cancer risk (79). Thus, the extent should not always influence *long-term* management.

In most clinical settings, *ADH is diagnosed in 10% to 15% of patients subjected to NCB* (11,12,80-83). In four studies consisting of 323 to 900 patients who underwent NCB of mammographically detected lesions, the frequencies of ADH were 6.7%, 4.7%, 4.5%, and 4.3% (84-87). Follow-up excisional biopsies were performed on most women with ADH in these reports. Among women who underwent excisional biopsy, the reported frequencies of DCIS in the excisional specimen were 27%, 12.5%, 33%, and 36%, respectively. Invasive carcinoma was found in 14%, 12.5%, 0%, and 11% of patients, respectively. In these reports, approximately 25% of excisional biopsies revealed additional foci of ADH. The yield of significant lesions in the excisional biopsy may be somewhat lower after NCB diagnosis of ADH if the entire radiologically detected lesion was removed by NCB (88). The relative high frequency of carcinoma reported after a diagnosis of ADH in an NCB has, over the years, dictated that excisional biopsy should be performed in this setting (12,89). Please see page 152 for further discussion of the trend of de-escalation of management.

The reported frequency of ADH in vacuum-assisted MRI-directed NCB ranges from 3% to 8% (20-22). Among patients with ADH detected in vacuum-assisted NCB who undergo excisional biopsy, the yield of carcinoma has averaged 34% (22). The higher yield of subsequent carcinoma, sometimes termed *underestimation of ADH*, found in MRI-detected lesions than in mammographically directed biopsies, probably reflects the tendency to employ MRI predominantly in women at higher risk for carcinoma. Most carcinomas found after the detection of ADH by MRI-directed NCB have been DCIS.

Due to the limited and often-fragmented nature of NCB, added consideration is given to quantitative issues in assessing these specimens. Pathologists should avoid overinterpretation of findings in an NCB because of the expectation that residual lesion tissue remains at the biopsy site. In the evaluation of NCB of breast lesions, especially those that are only evident by mammography, *it must be anticipated that the material seen in NCB may be the most extreme and potentially the only abnormality present*. ADH may be diagnosed if detached fragments of abnormal epithelium suggest carcinoma, or if only part of a duct with features of carcinoma is contained in the sample. The importance of quantitative issues and adequate sampling was documented by Jackman et al (11) who "progressively increased the average number of NCB obtained per lesion and have found a decrease in both the number of ADH lesions and the discordance of ADH lesion." The greater success in diagnosis was attributable to more lesions being diagnosed as DCIS rather than as ADH due to a more complete sampling (11). Wagoner et al (89) reported that the following features of ADH in NCB

TABLE 8.11

Features Predictive of DCIS on Excision Following Diagnosis of ADH on NCB

Extent of ADH on NCB	Multiple foci
Calcifications	Residual "suspicious"
Clinical	Palpable mass
Presentation	Mass
Age	Postmenopausal
Architecture	Micropapillary pattern of ADH

Based on review of literature.
ADH, atypical ductal hyperplasia; DCIS, ductal carcinoma in situ; NCB, needle core biopsy.

were predictive of finding DCIS in the subsequent excision: micropapillary ADH, greater than 2 foci of ADH, ADH in multiple samples, and residual calcifications (Please see **Table 8.11**).

Usual Ductal Hyperplasia/Atypical Ductal Hyperplasia and Breast Carcinoma Risk

Most women diagnosed with either UDH or ADH will develop neither DCIS nor invasive carcinoma. The major clinical concern related to UDH and ADH is the risk for the subsequent development of carcinoma. In a minority of women with biopsy findings classified as nonproliferative or proliferative, carcinoma subsequently develops in either breast. The overall proportion of women in whom carcinoma later develops rarely exceeds 10%, even with follow-up of two decades or more. Bodian et al (13) detected subsequent breast carcinoma in 139 of 1,521 patients (9.1%) with biopsy-proven proliferative changes, and in 18 of 278 (6.5%) with nonproliferative biopsies within a follow-up period of 21 years. Overall, 8.7% of the patients developed breast carcinoma. In other reports involving at least 1,000 patients, the proportions of women in whom carcinoma developed were 2.2% (90), 4.1% (91), and 4.9% (92). The proportion of patients with subsequent carcinoma tends to increase with the length of follow-up, being highest after a follow-up of more than a decade (91,92). This observation is consistent with the rising risk for developing breast carcinoma with advancing age. The incidence of ADH peaks in women in their 40s.

The risk for the development of carcinoma after the diagnosis of unilateral biopsy-proven proliferative changes affects both breasts. The bilaterality of risk was noted by Davis et al (93) in a review of 297 patients with "cystic disease." These authors also tabulated data from 11 articles with at least 100 patients, to show that carcinoma subsequently developed in 0.7% to 4.9% of patients, with 50% of carcinomas occurring in the contralateral breast. Krieger and Hiatt found that only 56% of subsequent carcinomas occurred in the previously sampled breast with benign proliferative changes (92). Laterality of subsequent carcinoma

was not significantly influenced by the type of antecedent proliferative change or age at biopsy. The mean interval to subsequent ipsilateral carcinomas (11.2 years) was less than that for contralateral carcinomas (14 years). Page et al (94) reported that 8/18 (44%) carcinomas after ADH occurred in the contralateral breast. Involvement of the contralateral breast in a similar proportion of patients was also described by Connolly et al (95).

The chances for the development of breast carcinoma are influenced by factors that can modify the level of risk associated with benign proliferative changes. Age at diagnosis is inversely related to subsequent risk. Carter et al (96) found that the rate of subsequent breast carcinoma, when compared with that of normal women, was increased 3.7-fold in women with ADH who were 46 to 55 years of age, and 2.3-fold in women older than 55 years. London et al (97) also observed an inverse relationship of age and risk, in which the RR increased 2.6-fold among premenopausal women who had biopsy-proven atypia in comparison with postmenopausal subjects.

A history of breast carcinoma among first-degree female relatives is a particularly strong additive factor in women who have ADH. Page et al (94) and Dupont and Page (98) found that the risk associated with ADH in women with a positive family history was more than double that of women without this factor. London et al (97) also reported that the increased risk associated with family history was strongest in patients with ADH.

Among women who have had a benign result on breast biopsy, the risk for developing subsequent carcinoma is related to the histologic components of the antecedent biopsy. When assessed independently, sclerosing adenosis has been associated with an increased risk in several studies (90,98,99). ADH coexisting with sclerosing adenosis may confer a greater increase in risk (98,100). The proportion of patients who develop carcinoma is highest in women with ADH, intermediate in those with proliferative ductal changes without atypia, and least when there are no proliferative changes. Proliferative changes were identified in 152 (85%) of 1,799 biopsies studied by Bodian et al (13). Moderate-to-severe atypia was present in 70 specimens, representing 3.8% of all cases and 4.6% of specimens with proliferative changes. Follow-up revealed that the RR for the development of carcinoma (in comparison with the general population) was higher in women with any proliferative changes (RR of 2.2) than in those with nonproliferative findings on biopsy (RR of 1.6). The RR associated with severe ductal atypia was 3.9. Page et al (94) found the RR to be 4.7 for women with ADH in comparison with women who had nonproliferative biopsy results. The RR for women with ADH and a family history of breast carcinoma was increased further in comparison with women with nonproliferative biopsies and a positive family history (94). Ma and Boyd (99) undertook a meta-analysis of studies that investigated the association between ADH and breast cancer risk. Fifteen reports between 1960 and 1992 fulfilled the authors' requirements for inclusion in the study, resulting in a total sample size of 182,980 women. The overall odds ratio in comparison with controls for the development of carcinoma in women with ADH was 3.67 (95% CI, 3.16-4.26).

In sum, the results of several major studies, which included more than 17,000 women, have established ADH as a risk factor for the subsequent development of breast carcinoma (98,101-105). The first such study by Dupont and Page in 1985 related breast cancer risk to histologic findings in benign biopsies (94). The main findings in that study were that women who had proliferative lesions without atypia had about a two-fold increase in the risk of subsequent breast cancer, and those with ADH had about a five-fold increase in breast cancer. Multiple other studies have yielded largely similar findings, despite obvious differences in materials and methods employed in each study.

Excision for Atypical Ductal Hyperplasia Diagnosed on Needle Core Biopsy

ADH, rarely encountered in the pre-mammographic period, was reportedly present in about 4% of benign biopsies in that era. This lesion has become relatively more common in the current mammographic era and is diagnosed in 10% to 20% of benign biopsies (94,106). Until recently, the need for an excisional biopsy following the diagnosis of ADH was unquestioned. Such automatic triggering of excision was based on the reportedly high rate of "upgrade"—ranging from 11.5% to 62% (17,107-109). The term "upgrade" implies the finding of a more significant lesion, DCIS, or invasive carcinoma, in the subsequent excision, and has varied somewhat with the radiologic method used to guide NCBs. For instance, ADH diagnosed on sonographically guided NCB shows a higher underestimation rate, which was as high as 56% in one series (110). Notably, no significant difference has been reported in upgrade rate of stereotactic vacuum-assisted NCB using 11-gauge (11.9%) versus 8-gauge (14.3%) needles (108).

When the number of foci of involvement by ADH on NCB (based on a mean of about 12 cores per case) was correlated with excisional biopsy results by Ely et al (111), all cases of ADH in less than or equal to 2 foci had no worse lesion on excision, whereas ADH present in greater than or equal to 4 foci was found to be statistically predictive of a worse lesion on excision.

It should be realized that some, if not all, "upgraded" lesions either represent cases of ADH associated with DCIS which were either minimally sampled or represent underdiagnosed cases of DCIS.

Recent reports have indicated that correlation of the histologic findings in an NCB with pre- and postprocedure mammograms could spare excision in some patients. Studies by de Mascarel et al (112) and Villa et al (17) showed that patients without residual calcification after a diagnosis of ADH on a vacuum-assisted breast biopsy could possibly be managed with follow-up alone. McGhan et al (107) reported that patients younger than 50 years of age with only focal atypia and no residual calcifications post-NCB may

represent a low-risk group and could potentially avoid excision. Nguyen et al (18) concluded that ADH without "significant cytologic atypia and/or necrosis," regardless of extent, and with more than 95% removal of the targeted calcifications, is associated with a minimal risk (<3%) of carcinoma and may undergo follow-up only.

Nomograms devised to calculate the likelihood of upgrade for ADH may facilitate decision-making in selected cases. A nomogram developed by Khoury et al (113) includes age, menopausal status, hormonal receptor status, personal history of breast carcinoma, number of involved cores, solid growth pattern, extent of largest focus, and presentation (mass vs calcification). Of note, palpability at the time of ADH diagnosis has been shown to be significantly associated with the development of breast carcinoma (114).

De-Escalation of Surgery in Atypical Ductal Hyperplasia

Ever since the practice of NCB has become commonplace, the diagnosis of ADH on NCB has routinely triggered an excision of the lesional area. The occasional, often anecdotal, upgrade of ADH to invasive carcinoma has reinforced this argument. Much more importantly, this practice has been supported by multiple "upgrade" studies (89,107,110,113,115-132). These studies have indicated an overall upgrade rate ranging from 10.5% to 56%, with a mean rate of around 15% to 30%. The upgrade rate has been shown to be lower in studies in which imaging was correlated and higher in cases in which smaller gauge needles were used. In studies in which complete excision of the target lesion has been achieved, the upgrade rate is much lower (~15%). One other factor that must be considered in management decisions is the extent of ADH. The upgrade rate of focal ADH, defined as one less than 2 mm focus, has recently been shown to be much lower (7%) (133) and that of multifocal ADH (16.5%) (134).

The National Cancer Comprehensive Network (NCCN) guidelines for 2022 recommend excision whenever ADH is diagnosed on NCB (135). The American Society of Breast Surgeons (ASBS) guidelines recommend offering excision in such cases—with the caveat that selected patients in whom the "target lesion" has been excised via NCB can be observed—without resorting to excision (136).

Although the cumulative historical data indicate that the upgrade rate on excision of ADH diagnosed on NCB to DCIS is approximately 15% to 20% and to invasive carcinoma is approximately 5%, at the present time, the need for excisional biopsy following the diagnosis of ADH on NCB should ideally be determined on an individual basis after clinical and radiologic correlation is undertaken. In particular, imaging may help in determining the *extent* of excision.

It can be hypothesized that the "upgrade" rate of ADH may not be the best measure of outcome. The evidence suggests that *most* cases of ADH do not progress to invasive carcinoma, and when they do, are of lower grade. However, "de-escalation" of the management of ADH has been challenged by emerging data that indicate that ADH can progress to either lower-grade or higher-grade carcinoma—suggesting that some cases of ADH could be more clinically significant than lower-grade DCIS (137).

Chemoprevention of Atypical Ductal Hyperplasia

ER is strongly expressed in more than 90% of breast carcinomas that develop in women with ADH (115). This finding provides a rationale for the use of selective estrogen receptor modulators (SERMs) and aromatase inhibitors to prevent breast carcinoma in women with ADH. Results of several chemoprevention trials, as well as subgroup analyses, have shown RR reductions ranging from 41% to 79% (116). Chemoprevention should be considered in at least a proportion of women with ADH and who are otherwise considered to be at higher risk. However, in most settings, such chemoprevention is "infrequently prescribed and infrequently used" (116).

DUCTAL CARCINOMA IN SITU

Frequency of Ductal Carcinoma In Situ

The introduction of mammographic screening in the early 1980s led to a dramatic increase in the detection of DCIS (138). Currently, approximately 19% of breast carcinomas are DCIS—**it is estimated that 55,720 women in the United States will be diagnosed to have DCIS in 2023 (out of 297,790 cases of all breast carcinomas)** (139). DCIS is uncommon in women younger than 30 years of age, and the risk of DCIS increases with age. The rate of DCIS increases with age from 0.6/1,000 screening examinations in women aged 40 to 49 years to 1.3/1,000 screening examinations in women aged 70 to 84 years (140). Risk of development of metastases and/or death in a patient diagnosed with pure DCIS is rare (<1%) (141). The beneficial effects of mammography as a diagnostic or screening modality and of improved systemic therapy are reflected in these trends (10).

Imaging in Ductal Carcinoma In Situ

The most common imaging correlates of DCIS include calcifications and architectural distortion on mammogram, mass-forming lesion on ultrasound, and nonmass enhancement on MRI evaluation.

Currently, DCIS is mostly detected on screening mammography. Mammography is a sensitive diagnostic procedure for detecting DCIS (142). Among nonpalpable carcinomas detected by mammography, approximately 25% were DCIS (143-145). Mammographically detected calcifications are found in 80% to 85% of DCIS (144,145). Other radiologic findings that lead to the "incidental" detection of a lesser proportion (about 5%) of DCIS are densities and asymmetric changes. Calcifications alone are more likely to be the mammographic indicator of DCIS in women younger than 50 years, whereas coexistent abnormalities are evident more often in women older than 50 years—a distinction that possibly results from differences in breast density between the age groups (145).

Mammographic calcifications associated with DCIS are generally large and pleomorphic, and either linear and cast-like or vermicular (worm-like) and branching (ie, follow the distribution of the disease in the ductal system) (146). Round or oval, well-circumscribed calcifications are less common in DCIS. Most DCIS have five or more calcifications (146). Mammographic calcifications have been used as a guide to assess the extent of DCIS. However, these measurements may underestimate the extent of the lesion (147). When the extent of lesions was measured both mammographically and histopathologically, discrepancies were found more often between the interpretations for cases that are mainly cribriform or micropapillary than for high-grade solid DCIS with necrosis. A discrepancy of more than 20 mm was found in 44% of pure cribriform-micropapillary lesions, in 12% of high-grade solid carcinomas, and in 50% of cases with both patterns (147). The likelihood of detecting multifocal DCIS (ie, multiple foci of DCIS in one quadrant) radiologically and pathologically is related to the size of the lesion as determined by either procedure. Multifocality is appreciably more frequent in lesions greater than 2.0 to 2.5 cm than in smaller foci of DCIS (148).

The mammographic appearance of calcifications bears some relationship to the histologic type of DCIS. In general, mammographic calcifications that are "highly suspicious for malignancy" are associated with high-grade DCIS (149); however, as noted by Stomper and Connolly (150), "there is considerable overlap, and the predominant histological subtype cannot be predicted on the basis of the microcalcification type with a high degree of accuracy." Predominantly linear or "casting-type" calcifications are found more often in "comedo" carcinomas than in "granular" calcification of cribriform, papillary, or solid types (147,150). Nonetheless, 22% of linear calcifications were associated with non-"comedo" carcinomas, and 47% of granular calcifications occurred in "comedo" DCIS in one series (150). The presence of casting-type calcifications occupying more than one quadrant in a mammogram was associated with high-grade DCIS, multifocal invasive carcinoma, and axillary nodal metastases (151). Abnormal mammographic findings without calcifications are more likely to call attention to DCIS of the *small cell type* than of the *large cell type*, regardless of the growth pattern (152). DCIS cases that overexpress human epidermal growth factor receptor 2 (HER2) are more likely to have calcifications than are HER2-negative DCIS (153).

Although DCIS can occur in adult women of any age, the mean age of patients at diagnosis in multiple studies is between 50 and 59 years. The age factor assumes considerable significance in determining screening guidelines. There are no significant differences in the age distribution of structural subtypes of DCIS (154). Extreme "density" of breast on mammography has been reported to be a risk factor for multicentricity (155).

Sonography is of limited value in the detection, or determination of extent, of DCIS. Scoggins et al (156) reported sonographic visibility in 362/691 (52%) of pure DCIS lesions. Lesion visibility was commonly due to the presence of a "mass." MRI is an effective method for detecting DCIS of all grades (157). The technique is relatively more sensitive for the diagnosis of invasive carcinoma, and the rate of false-negatives is higher for DCIS (158). Menell et al (159) found that MRI was overall more sensitive than mammography for detecting DCIS and for detecting multifocal DCIS. Manion et al (160) found that the most common types of carcinoma identified by MRI screening were ER-positive invasive carcinomas (mean size 0.7 cm) and high-grade DCIS. Detection of lesions is based on the finding of contrast enhancement in breast parenchyma after injection of a gadolinium contrast agent (161-163). Orel et al (164) described three patterns of enhancement associated with DCIS: ductal, regional, and a peripherally enhancing mass. The mean size of MRI-detected DCIS was 10 mm. It has been suggested that tumor angiogenesis contributes to MRI enhancement (161). Contrast-enhanced MRI has proven to be an effective method for the detection of concurrent, unsuspected contralateral carcinoma in women with ipsilateral DCIS (165).

Intraoperative Consultation (Frozen Section) Diagnosis of Ductal Carcinoma In Situ

DCIS can be recognized in frozen sections (FS) prepared from an excisional biopsy, but if any difficulty is encountered, the decision should be immediately deferred to permanent sections because there is a significant risk of trimming away the lesional area as FS are prepared **(Fig. 8.38)**. In one study of DCIS, 50% of the lesions were diagnosed at the time of FS, 36% were reported to be benign, 8% were deferred, 5% were diagnosed as ADH, and one case was diagnosed as invasive carcinoma (166). Approximately 3% of biopsies reported to be benign at FS examination prove to contain carcinoma when permanent sections are examined (167). Because of the limited amount of tissue that can be examined by FS during an intraoperative consultation, approximately 20% of patients with an FS diagnosis of DCIS eventually prove to have invasive carcinoma (168). FS is not recommended for the diagnosis of NCB unless there are exceptional clinical circumstances.

Histopathology of Ductal Carcinoma In Situ

The anatomic site of origin of most DCIS appears to be in the TDLU. Evidence for this conclusion originally came from the classic subgross microdissection studies of Wellings et al (169). Recently characterized CCLs, described earlier in this chapter, lend support to this conclusion with respect to low-grade micropapillary DCIS but not high-grade DCIS. However, a substantial but undetermined proportion of DCIS lesions possibly arise from primary or segmental ducts or their branches. Both sites of origin are compatible with the presence of DCIS involving the epithelium of lobules, which is referred to as "lobular cancerization" **(Fig. 8.39)**.

Tables 8.12 to 8.14 provide the classification, architectural patterns, cytologic features, and typical results of biomarkers in DCIS. The typical DCIS lesion is a unifocal disease and is characteristically limited to single duct system. DCIS which seemingly "skips" (up to 1 cm) on histologic sections may represent the solitary lesion coming in and out of the plane of section.

In standard histology sections, DCIS appears confined within the lumina of ducts and lobules involved in the process. When studied by immunohistochemistry, basement membranes in DCIS are intact or only focally discontinuous (and even occasionally reduplicated in high-grade DCIS) (170).

The presence or absence of mitotic figures is not a definitive feature in the diagnosis of DCIS because mitoses may also be found in normal lobules and in DH or ADH, albeit infrequently. The finding of numerous mitoses, such as greater than or equal to 1 per high-power field, strongly suggests DCIS. Myoepithelial cells are variably retained,

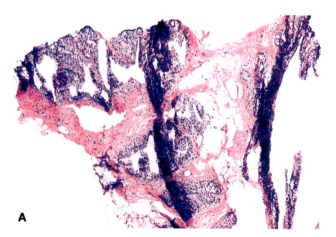 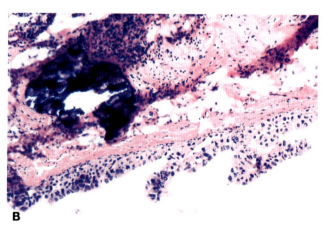

FIGURE 8.38 **Ductal Carcinoma In Situ (DCIS), Frozen Section.** The patient had a needle core biopsy (NCB) procedure for calcifications, and the NCB was submitted for frozen section. **A:** The frozen section slide has folds and tears. **B:** A displaced calcification is present near the center, and a band of atypical cells is present at the lower border of the tissue in the frozen section. The "frozen" diagnosis was deferred.

DUCTAL HYPERPLASIA, ATYPICAL DUCTAL HYPERPLASIA, AND DUCTAL CARCINOMA IN SITU 155

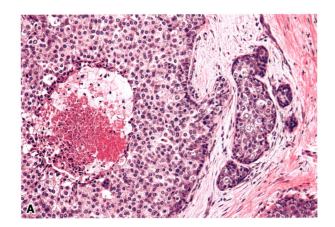
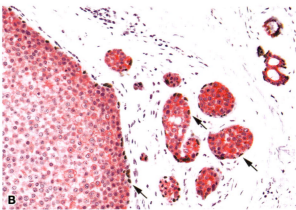

FIGURE 8.39 Ductal Carcinoma In Situ (DCIS), Lobular Extension ("Lobular Cancerization"). **A, B:** DCIS with central necrosis extending into a lobule in periductal fibrosis. This pattern can be mistaken for microinvasion. Myoepithelial cells at the perimeter of the lobular glands are highlighted via p63 (brown nuclear immunostain, arrows). Epithelial cells are decorated by cytokeratin (red cytoplasmic immunostain). **C:** In another case, the enlarged lobular complex is involved by DCIS with high-grade nuclei. There is prominent intralobular lymphocytic infiltrate.

TABLE 8.12
Classification of DCIS by Architectural Patterns and Cytologic Features

Architectural Patterns
Cribriform
Cystic hypersecretory
Flat micropapillary ("clinging")
Micropapillary
Paget disease
Papillary, various subtypes
Mucinous
Solid, low-grade
Solid, high-grade with necrosis ("comedo")

Cytologic Features
Apocrine (typically ER-negative and AR-positive)
Clear, usually admixed with apocrine features
Neuroendocrine (usually with solid papillary architecture)
Signet ring (mostly with solid papillary architecture)
Small (usually with neuroendocrine cytologic/immunohistochemical features)
Spindle (usually with neuroendocrine cytologic/immunohistochemical features)
Squamous

Most DCIS are unicentric (focal) and segmental in distribution. Multicentric/multifocal DCIS is uncommon. Multicentricity/multifocality of DCIS is most common in micropapillary DCIS. AR, androgen receptor; DCIS, ductal carcinoma in situ; ER, estrogen receptor.

TABLE 8.13
DCIS: Architectural and Cytologic Features[a]

Architectural	Description
Cribriform	Regular and round lumina with polarization of cells lining the spaces
Micropapillary	Arcades and bridges are rigid and uniformly thick.
Flat micropapillary	Bulbous tips, with "clinging" appearance
Solid	Cohesive cells in distended ducts
Cytologic	
Uniform, evenly spaced cells	
Well-defined cell borders	
Nonoverlapping cells	
Rounded nuclei	
Apoptosis and punctate necrosis	
Expanse	
Rule of thumb[b]	Involvement: >2 mm or >2 ducts/terminal duct lobular units—neither approach is preferred; please see text also.

DCIS, ductal carcinoma in situ.
[a]A more cautious approach to the diagnosis of DCIS in needle core biopsy (NCB) is recommended.
[b]Could be useful; however, only in low-grade DCIS.

TABLE 8.14
Typical Biomarker Results in Low-Grade Versus High-Grade DCIS

Biomarker	LG-DCIS	HG-DCIS
ER	(+)	(+/−)
PR	(+)	(+/−)
HER2	(−)	(−/+)
Ki-67 index	low	high

Based on review of literature.
ER, estrogen receptor; LG/HG-DCIS, low-grade/high-grade ductal carcinoma in situ; HER2, human epidermal growth factor receptor 2; Ki-67, proliferation marker; PR, progesterone receptor.

but attenuated, and occasionally hyperplastic at the periphery of a duct involved by DCIS **(Fig. 8.40)**. Carcinoma cells at the periphery of the duct exhibit loss of polarity as a manifestation of cellular crowding. Rarely, remnants of nonneoplastic duct epithelium persist in ducts involved by DCIS **(Fig. 8.41)**.

A range of cell types are found in DCIS. *Signet ring cells*, usually associated with lobular carcinoma, also occur in DCIS, most often in the papillary and cribriform types **(Fig. 8.42)**. Signet ring cells have eccentric nuclei that may be often indented by a cytoplasmic mucin vacuole. A minute droplet of secretion may be apparent in the vacuole. Intracytoplasmic mucin sometimes imparts a diffuse pale blue color to the cytoplasm without forming distinct vacuoles **(Fig. 8.43)**. Clear holes in the cytoplasm can be mistaken for signet ring vacuoles. These cytoplasmic defects, sometimes the site of glycogen accumulation, are not reactive with the mucicarmine stain, they do not indent the nucleus, and there is ordinarily no secretion evident in the lumen.

Clear cell DCIS is a poorly defined variant typically encountered with solid and "comedo" patterns. Some clear cell DCIS are composed of cells with an arrangement described as *mosaic* because of the appearance created by sharply defined cell borders **(Fig. 8.44)**. A large subset of lesions that are classified under this heading are a form of apocrine carcinoma. Occasionally, clear cell DCIS has strongly mucicarmine-positive cytoplasm. The presence of a monomorphic clear cell population in a ductal proliferative lesion is highly suggestive of DCIS. Other clear cell lesions are the in situ forms of lipid-rich or glycogen-rich carcinomas. Apocrine cytology is encountered in all architectural types of DCIS **(Fig. 8.45)**. These cells have abundant cytoplasm, which ranges from granular and eosinophilic to vacuolated or clear. There is variable nuclear pleomorphism, sometimes manifested by prominent nucleoli.

Spindle cell DCIS may express neuroendocrine markers such as chromogranin, synaptophysin, CD56, and neuron-specific enolase (171) **(Fig. 8.46)**. The swirling growth pattern of cells in spindle cell DCIS mimics "streaming" that is characteristically found in UDH. Spindle cell DCIS often coexists with cribriform DCIS.

The expression of *neuroendocrine markers* can be found in DCIS with non–spindle cell cytology and with various growth patterns. Kawasaki et al (172) found neuroendocrine marker expression in 20 of 294 (6.8%) DCIS. The diagnosis of neuroendocrine DCIS was made when at least 50% of the tumor cells expressed chromogranin A and/or synaptophysin. Neuroendocrine DCIS had a significantly higher frequency of presentation with bloody nipple discharge (72%) than non-neuroendocrine DCIS (5%). Most of the lesions had solid papillary or papillary architecture with low nuclear grade in 90% and an absence of calcifications in 75%. Neuroendocrine DCIS tended to express ER and PR and not to overexpress HER2.

Primary neuroendocrine carcinomas of the gastrointestinal tract and lung metastatic to the breast can mimic primary in situ carcinoma of the breast, and in this context, "clinical history is paramount for optimal diagnosis" (173).

Small cell DCIS is extremely uncommon **(Fig. 8.47)**. The growth patterns are typically cribriform and solid or a

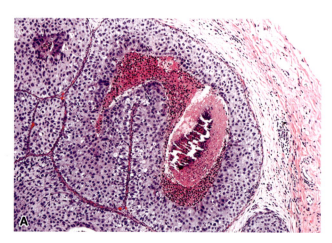
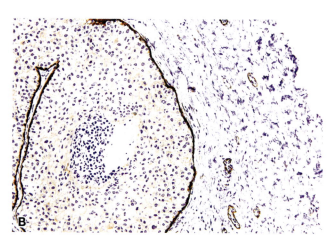

FIGURE 8.40 Ductal Carcinoma In Situ (DCIS). A: A duct involved by solid DCIS with necrosis and calcifications. **B:** DCIS is encircled by myosin-positive myoepithelial cells.

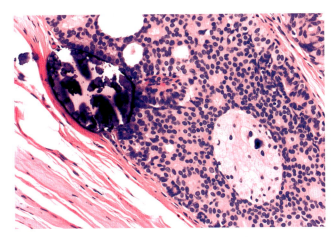

FIGURE 8.41 **Ductal Carcinoma In Situ (DCIS).** Microlumina are present in this cribriform DCIS with punctate necrosis, histiocytes, and calcifications.

mixture of these forms. When present by itself, the solid pattern can be distinguished from LCIS with E-cadherin immunostain. Membrane reactivity will be present in DCIS, and absent or fragmented and weak in LCIS.

Structure of DCIS: The cellular composition of low-grade DCIS is usually described as *monomorphic*, a term applied especially to cribriform, solid, and micropapillary carcinomas. In this context, monomorphic means that there is overall homogeneity in the cytologic appearance of the lesion, although the cells are not always similar in such features as the amount of cytoplasm or nuclear size. Cell and nuclear shape may be altered by the presence or absence of crowding in one or another part of the duct. The presence of a myoepithelial cell layer is not a consideration in judging whether a ductal proliferation is monomorphic. Dimorphic variants of DCIS, consisting of two distinctly different populations of cells, are unusual **(Fig. 8.47)**.

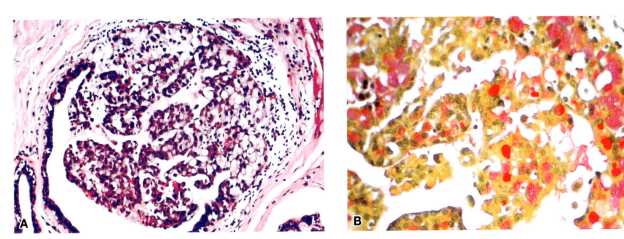

FIGURE 8.42 **Ductal Carcinoma In Situ (DCIS), Signet Ring Cells. A:** Papillary DCIS with signet ring cells. **B:** The intracytoplasmic mucin is stained magenta with the mucicarmine stain.

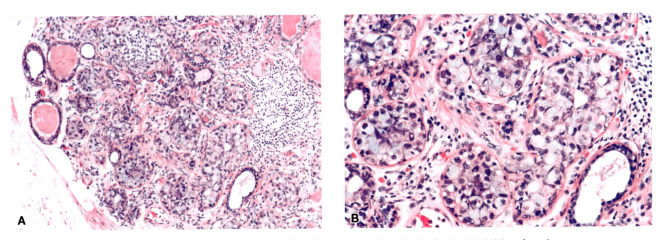

FIGURE 8.43 **Ductal Carcinoma In Situ (DCIS), Intracytoplasmic Mucin. A, B:** DCIS in sclerosing adenosis in a needle core biopsy (NCB). The carcinoma cells have pale blue mucin in the cytoplasm which was reactive with mucicarmine stain.

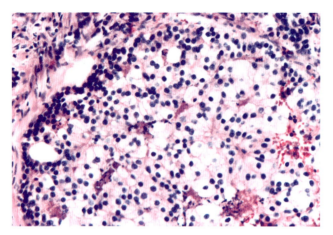

FIGURE 8.44 Ductal Carcinoma In Situ, Clear Cell Type. The cells have sharply defined borders and lower-grade nuclei.

DCIS in a particular case can have multiple cytologic, structural, or immunohistochemical phenotypes (154). Mixed histologic patterns are found in 30% to 40% of cases. Although some structural combinations such as micropapillary-cribriform and papillary-cribriform occur relatively more often than others, there is considerable heterogeneity with respect to growth patterns (174). The probability of structural variability increases with the extent of the lesion, a phenomenon that must be considered in using NCB for the subclassification of a mammographically detected DCIS.

Cytologic features, especially at the nuclear level, tend to be more homogeneous than the growth pattern in a given case. Some combinations of growth patterns and cytologic appearances occur more frequently, such as classic "comedo" DCIS, composed of pleomorphic cells with high-grade nuclei and necrosis, or the low nuclear grade typically present

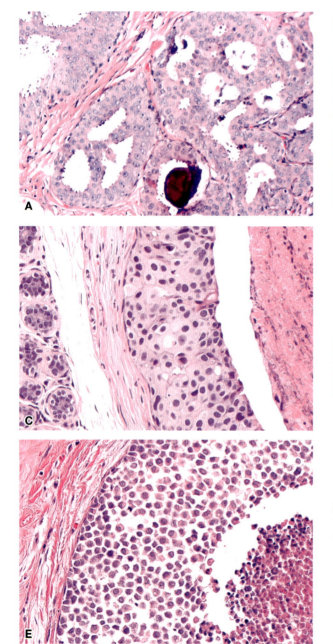

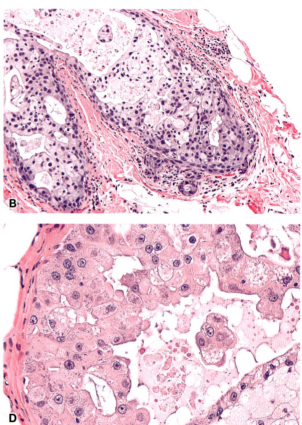

FIGURE 8.45 Ductal Carcinoma In Situ (DCIS), Apocrine Type (and Apocrine Pleomorphic Lobular Carcinoma In Situ [LCIS]). A: Cribriform DCIS with apocrine cytology. **B:** Micropapillary apocrine DCIS with intermediate nuclear grade. with clear cell change. **C, D:** Two additional cases of apocrine DCIS are shown. Note solid architecture and luminal necrosis in **(C)**. Pink granular cytoplasm of the apocrine type is shown in **(D)**. **E:** Apocrine pleomorphic LCIS is shown here for comparison. Note noncohesion of LCIS cells.

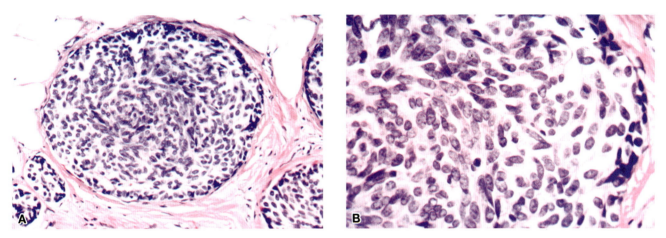

FIGURE 8.46 Ductal Carcinoma In Situ, Spindle Cell Type. A, B: The swirling spindle cell proliferation mimics the streaming pattern of ductal hyperplasia. The monomorphic spindle cells extend to the perimeter of the duct in this needle core biopsy (NCB).

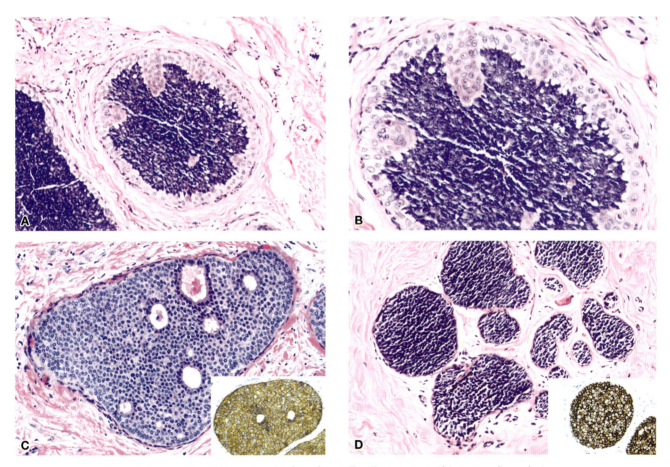

FIGURE 8.47 Ductal Carcinoma In Situ (DCIS), Small Cell Type. A, B: This extraordinary lesion consists of a central nearly syncytial mass of relatively small undifferentiated carcinoma cells and an outer zone of larger polygonal cells. Two protruding mounds of large cells show traces of squamous differentiation, a feature that was even more pronounced in other ducts. Persistent myoepithelial cells that were immunoreactive for actin are represented by the small dark elongated nuclei at the outer border of the duct. **C:** Solid, small cell DCIS with cribriform microlumina. This architectural and cytologic appearance of the lesion could be mistaken for pagetoid spread of LCIS in a duct. All cells were strongly E-cadherin positive (inset). **D:** Small cell DCIS in a lobule. The in situ carcinoma is E-cadherin positive (inset).

in cribriform and micropapillary DCIS. However, the considerable range of heterogeneity is illustrated by lesions composed of cytologically low-grade nuclei growing in a solid pattern with central "comedo" necrosis, and others having a micropapillary pattern composed of cells with high-grade nuclei found in some examples of flat micropapillary DCIS.

Micropapillary DCIS consists of ducts lined by a layer of neoplastic cells, which intermittently give rise to slender papillary fronds or arcuate formations that protrude into the ductal lumen (**Fig. 8.48**). The papillae are variable in appearance, ranging from blunt bumps or mounds to pronounced, slender, elongated processes. The latter almost always lacks a fibrovascular core and is lined by cytologically homogenous carcinoma cells. Arcuate structures, commonly referred to as "Roman bridge arches," occur when microlumina are formed beneath adjacent coalescent fronds or within a mound of neoplastic cells. These fenestrations resemble the lumina formed in cribriform DCIS. In conjunction with micropapillae, these are a feature of micropapillary DCIS.

The appearance of the micropapillary fronds varies somewhat with the plane of individual histologic sections. Whereas some micropapillae are cut perpendicular to their long axis, others are seen sectioned tangentially or transversely, resulting in irregular nests of seemingly detached cell clusters in the ductal lumen. Apart from epithelial proliferation, ducts with low nuclear-grade micropapillary DCIS are usually relatively free of cellular debris or inflammatory cells, but may contain calcifications.

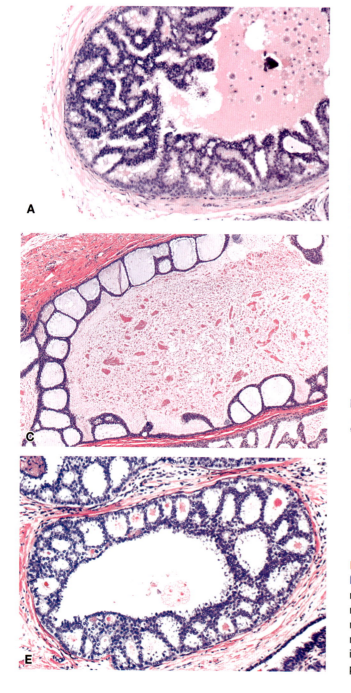
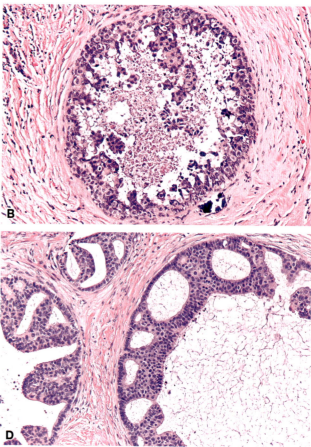

FIGURE 8.48 Ductal Carcinoma In Situ (DCIS), Micropapillary Type. A: Slender fronds of micropapillary DCIS with low nuclear grade form an irregular network of arches at the periphery of this duct in a needle core biopsy (NCB). **B:** Delicate micropapillary bands of monomorphic cells with lower-grade nuclei outline microlumina in this duct. **C:** Micropapillary DCIS in an NCB. **D, E:** Relatively "rigid" arches characterize micropapillary DCIS.

Micropapillary DCIS is usually composed of cytologically low-grade, relatively small homogeneous cells with a high nuclear-to-cytoplasmic ratio and dark nuclei **(Fig. 8.48)**. The nuclei typically vary little in size, and chromatin density between cells at the base and tip of micropapillae may be slightly smaller and darker at the surface (but marked disparity in these characteristics is a feature of micropapillary hyperplasia). At the margin of the duct, between papillary and arcuate structures, the neoplastic cells typically form a thin layer one to not more than three or four cells deep. Persistent nonneoplastic epithelium between micropapillae is a feature of micropapillary hyperplasia rather than micropapillary carcinoma. Mitoses are rarely evident in low-grade micropapillary DCIS. In most instances, the cells are so crowded that their individual borders and cytoplasm cannot be identified. Occasionally, the cells have slightly more abundant cytoplasm, with apocrine-type protrusions at the luminal border. In one variant of this cell type, the nuclei of the tumor cells are contained in cytoplasmic blebs that are extruded into the ductal lumen. Clear cell change and squamous metaplasia are rarely seen in micropapillary DCIS.

A minority of DCIS with a micropapillary structural phenotype are composed of cells with intermediate- or high-grade nuclei. This type of micropapillary carcinoma tends to occur in women between 35 and 50 years of age and is multifocal and sometimes bilateral. Cells forming this type of carcinoma, which is mainly localized in TDLU, differ from those in conventional micropapillary lesions in that they are larger, with more abundant cytoplasm. Nuclei are also correspondingly larger, and nucleoli are usually apparent. Mitoses can be seen in this epithelium, and the cells often have a distinctly apocrine appearance. This cytologically high-grade form of micropapillary DCIS is more likely to have calcifications than the low-grade variant, and necrotic cellular debris may be found in the ductal lumen. Florid micropapillary proliferation tends to result in fusion of the epithelial fronds and the formation of cribriform spaces. It is not unusual to find DCIS with a combination of micropapillary and cribriform features.

The term **flat micropapillary (clinging) carcinoma** refers to DCIS with the cytologic appearance of the micropapillary lesion that is lacking in fully developed epithelial fronds **(Fig. 8.48)**. Lesions composed entirely of flat micropapillary DCIS are uncommon, and more often one or more epithelial fronds or bridges are present. In the absence of calcification or necrosis, flat micropapillary DCIS is easily overlooked. This type of DCIS is most often found in the background of CCH. The lesions are typically multifocal or multicentric and can be bilateral. Calcifications with distinctive crystalline, ossifying, and laminated appearances tend to occur in CCH, leading to mammographic detection. Patients with CCH may have tubular carcinoma and LCIS ("the Rosen triad"), as well as invasive lobular carcinoma, and micropapillary DCIS.

Cribriform DCIS is a fenestrated epithelial proliferation in which microlumina are formed in the malignant epithelium that bridges most, or all, of the ductal lumen **(Fig. 8.49)**.

Extension into lobular epithelium (so-called lobular cancerization) or into the lactiferous ducts of the nipple is uncommon. Dilated ducts with cribriform DCIS can be mistaken for adenoid cystic carcinoma or complex papilloma.

The differential diagnosis of cribriform DCIS (positive for myoepithelial cells at the perimeter, via immunostains) includes invasive cribriform carcinoma (completely negative for myoepithelial cells) and adenoid cystic carcinoma (positive for myoepithelial cells, with cytoplasmic and nuclear c-Kit positivity of epithelial cells), not to mention UDH and ADH.

Collagenous spherulosis can be associated with LCIS, and this combined lesion can be mistaken for cribriform DCIS. The presence of CS can be confirmed with myoepithelial immunostains. The latter will highlight myoepithelial cells at the perimeter of spherules. Laminin and collagen IV immunostains can highlight the basement membrane components in the "spherules." The distinction between DCIS and LCIS with CS depends on cytologic features of the lesion and can be confirmed with E-cadherin or p120 immunostains. The appearance of coexisting in situ carcinoma in the immediate vicinity of CS can also be helpful.

The *secondary lumina* in cribriform DCIS tend to be round or oval, with smooth edges bordered by cuboidal cells. The distribution of microlumina is variable. In some instances, the spaces are spread across the entire duct, but in others they are concentrated toward the center or rarely in a zone largely at the periphery of the duct. Microlumina surrounded by homogeneous cells, uniformly distributed throughout the duct, are the hallmark of cribriform DCIS. The microlumina may contain secretions, degenerated or necrotic cells, and punctate calcifications.

Bands of neoplastic cells between and around the microlumina are described as rigid, a term that refers to the uniform, not overlapping distribution of polygonal cells, in contrast to the streaming pattern of overlapping oval cells in DH. Polarization of the cells in a radial fashion around the microlumina contributes to the rigid appearance. The most orderly type of low-grade cribriform DCIS is composed of monomorphic cuboidal-to-low columnar cells. Nucleoli are inconspicuous or absent, and mitoses are rarely encountered. The cells usually have sparse cytoplasm. Cribriform DCIS can be composed of cells with intermediate- to high-grade nuclei. Necrosis may be present in such foci.

Solid DCIS is formed by neoplastic cells that fill most or all of the duct space **(Fig. 8.50)**. Microlumina and papillary structures are absent, but calcifications may be present. Patients with "comedo" DCIS often have coexistent foci of non-necrotic solid DCIS. The polygonal cells are typically of a single type with low-to-intermediate nuclear grade. The cytoplasm has a spectrum of appearances including amphophilic, apocrine, clear, and granular.

"Comedo" DCIS should *not* be regarded as an architectural type of DCIS. The term "comedo" refers to expansive central necrosis occurring in certain forms of DCIS (including solid and micropapillary). "Comedo" DCIS is typically composed of carcinoma cells with mitotically

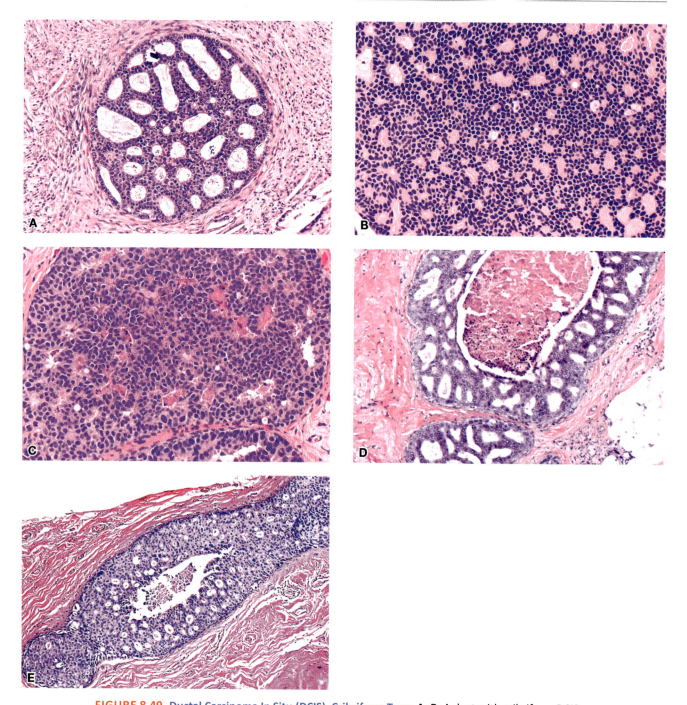

FIGURE 8.49 Ductal Carcinoma In Situ (DCIS), Cribriform Type. **A, B:** A duct with cribriform DCIS is shown. Note uniform microlumina. **C:** Cribriform DCIS, with punctate necrosis. **D:** Cribriform DCIS (showing micropapillary features) with necrosis. **E:** A longitudinal section of cribriform DCIS with necrosis.

active high-grade nuclei associated with its namesake type of necrosis **(Fig. 8.51)**. The term "comedo" necrosis could possibly be used only when there is DCIS (of any architectural type) with high-grade nuclei and *prominent* necrotic debris—a finding that is typically associated with degenerating cells characterized by karyorrhectic or pyknotic nuclei with variable degrees of loss in nuclear detail.

In a 1997 consensus report (175), **nuclear grade** was stratified into three categories **(Table 8.15)**. Pleomorphic nuclei of similar size were not consistent with low nuclear grade. The pathology report should reflect the overall highest nuclear grade but may indicate the relative proportions of grade when there is heterogeneity **(Fig. 8.52)**. *Necrosis* refers to karyorrhectic debris and dead cells and has been classified as "comedo" and "punctate" **(Table 8.16)**. Five architectural patterns were identified as follows: micropapillary, cribriform, solid, "comedo," and papillary. It was specified that "comedo" referred "to solid intraepithelial growth within the

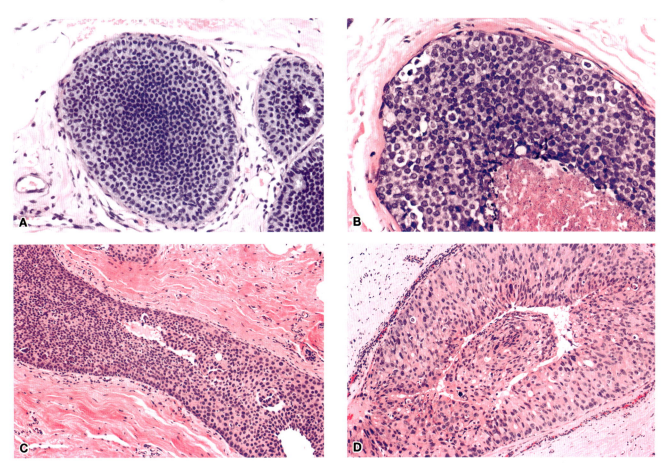

FIGURE 8.50 **Ductal Carcinoma In Situ (DCIS), Solid Type. A-D:** Multiple examples of solid type of DCIS. Periductal angiogenesis is prominent in **D**.

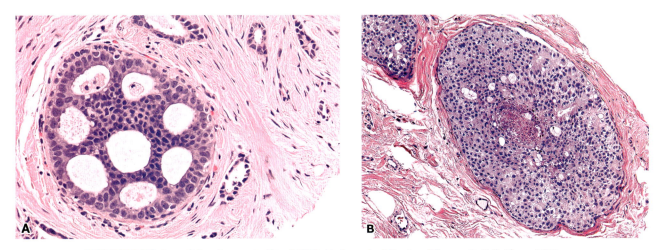

FIGURE 8.51 **Ductal Carcinoma In Situ (DCIS), Various Architectural Types. A:** Cribriform DCIS, without necrosis associated with tubular carcinoma. **B:** Cribriform DCIS, with punctate necrosis.

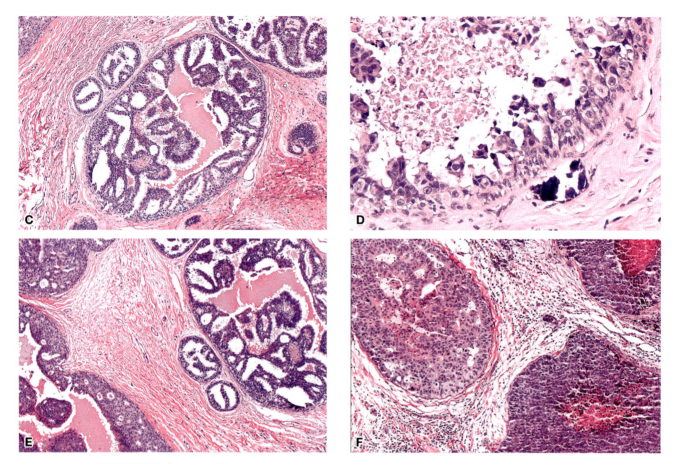

FIGURE 8.51 (*continued*) **C:** Micropapillary DCIS with luminal secretions (without necrosis). **D:** Flat micropapillary ("clinging") DCIS with high-grade nuclei and central necrosis. Note calcification. **E, F:** Two examples of "colliding" architectural types with differing cytology are shown. DCIS of cribriform and micropapillary types **(E)**. Cribriform DCIS and small cell DCIS with necrosis **(F)**.

TABLE 8.15
Grading of Nuclei in DCIS

Low-grade nuclei
Monomorphic (monotonous) appearance
Size of ductal epithelial nuclei or 1.5-2.0× normal red blood cells
Nuclear chromatin is diffuse and finely dispersed.
"Occasional nucleoli and mitoses"
Cells usually polarized
High-grade nuclei
"Markedly pleomorphic"
Size: usually more than 2.5× that of ductal epithelial nuclei
Chromatin: vesicular with irregular distribution
"Prominent, often multiple, nucleoli"
"Mitoses may be conspicuous"
Intermediate-grade nuclei
"Nuclei that are neither low grade nor high grade"

Cytologic monotony is characteristic of atypical columnar cell hyperplasia/flat epithelial atypia, atypical ductal hyperplasia, and low-grade DCIS—all of which demonstrate "low-grade" nuclear atypia. Cytologic heterogeneity is a feature of usual ductal hyperplasia (and, paradoxically, also of high-grade DCIS). Most usual ductal hyperplasia cells show negligible nuclear atypia.
DCIS, ductal carcinoma in situ
Based on the Consensus Conference on the classification of ductal carcinoma in situ. Consensus Conference Committee. *Cancer.* 1997;80:1798-1802.

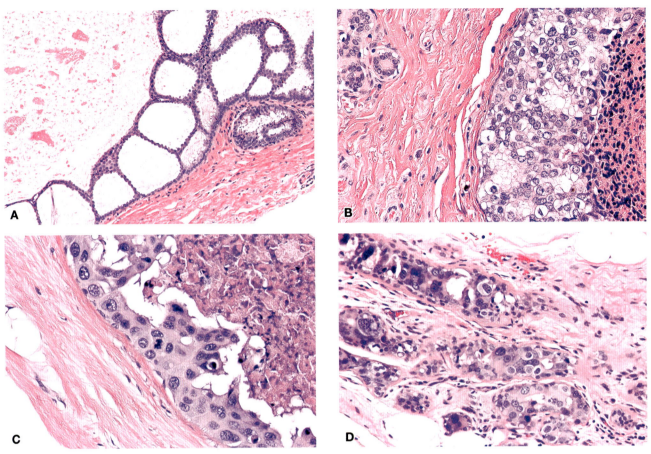

FIGURE 8.52 Ductal Carcinoma In Situ (DCIS), Various Nuclear Grades. **A:** DCIS, with low-grade nuclei. **B:** DCIS, cribriform type with intermediate-grade nuclei. **C:** DCIS, flat micropapillary ("clinging") type with high-grade nuclei. **D:** DCIS in terminal ducts, status-post chemotherapy. Note highly pleomorphic cells with scattered high-grade nuclei.

basement membrane with central (zonal) necrosis. Such lesions are often but not invariably high nuclear grade."

The **myoepithelial cell layer** is sometimes obscured in DCIS and only rarely eliminated (exhibiting "necrosis to the wall" pattern) by the carcinomatous proliferation, but in other instances, it may be hyperplastic and produce a distinct ring around the afflicted gland. The latter configuration is usually accompanied by accentuation of the basement membrane itself, as well as a circumferential periductal collar of desmoplastic stroma. A "cocktail" of antibodies to SMM-HC and p63 is especially sensitive for detecting myoepithelium in high-grade DCIS (176). The stroma immediately around high-grade DCIS is occasionally markedly desmoplastic with a mixed inflammatory cell infiltrate and capillary proliferation (ie, neoangiogenesis). Neovascularity in many instances is represented by proliferation of capillaries immediately external to the basement membrane (177). Occasionally, actin and other myoepithelial markers can highlight the smooth muscle in the walls of these new vessels—in a pattern that can mimic staining of myoepithelial cells. A variable inflammatory infiltrate is present in the periductal stroma, with a granulomatous reaction in foci where the ductal wall is partially disrupted, and it appears that necrotic contents of the duct have been discharged into the stroma.

It is important to distinguish between **"comedo" necrosis** and the accumulation of secretions accompanied by an inflammatory reaction that occurs in ductal stasis. Both conditions are prone to the formation of calcifications. Cellular necrosis is rarely seen in ductal stasis, and when present, the degenerated cells are usually histiocytes. The ductal contents in "comedo" DCIS consist of necrotic carcinoma cells represented by "ghost" outlines thereof and karyorrhectic debris

---

TABLE 8.16

Types of Necrosis in DCIS

"Comedo" necrosis
"Central zone necrosis within a duct, usually exhibiting a linear pattern within ducts if sectioned longitudinally"
Punctate necrosis
"Nonzonal-type necrosis (foci of necrosis that do not exhibit a linear pattern if longitudinally sectioned)"

DCIS, ductal carcinoma in situ.
Based on the Consensus Conference on the classification of ductal carcinoma in situ. Consensus Conference Committee. *Cancer.* 1997;80:1798-1802.

associated with minimal, if any, inflammation (**Fig. 8.53**). There is typically a sharp demarcation between viable carcinoma cells and the necrotic center. A space may be formed between the viable and necrotic elements. Dying cells at the inner edge of the viable zone have pyknotic nuclei and frayed cytoplasmic borders. The outlines of necrotic ("ghost") cells may be visible in the center of the duct.

Calcifications can develop in the necrotic center when there is "comedo" necrosis. The calcification can be finely granular and mixed with cellular debris in some instances, or it can form more solid irregular masses that correspond to casting calcifications on mammography. Calcifications in "comedo" DCIS almost always consist of calcium salts, mainly calcium phosphate, rather than crystalline calcium oxalate. The latter is typically found in benign apocrine lesions. In routine H&E-stained sections, calcium phosphate calcifications are magenta to purple. Calcifications and necrotic debris may become dislodged in an NCB, and rarely this material is the only component of the lesion found in the specimen. When dislodged calcifications are present in an NCB, serial sections of the biopsy should be prepared. An excisional biopsy may be indicated in such cases, even after radiologic correlation, when no epithelial elements are found in the NCB (**Fig. 8.54**).

If a dislodged fragment of carcinoma becomes embedded in stroma or fat in an NCB, the resulting appearance can be mistaken for invasive carcinoma (**Fig. 8.55**).

Occasionally, marked periductal **fibrosis** can be associated with extensive sclerotic obliteration of ducts that contain "comedo" DCIS, a process referred to as "healing" by Muir and Aitkenhead (178) or as "regressive change" by Wasserman and Parra-Herran (179). Prominent necrosis can contribute to this process. The residual structures typically consist of round-to-oval scars composed of circumferential layers of collagen and elastic tissue (**Fig. 8.56**). The center of the scar, representing the remnants of the duct, is often less dense, and it may contain a few residual carcinoma cells, histiocytes, and calcification. End-stage scars of periductal mastitis can be indistinguishable from those of obliterated DCIS (180). When this type of scar is found in an NCB, serial sections should be obtained because minute foci of atypical/carcinoma cells may be detected in the scar. "Distorting" periductal sclerosis around DCIS in an NCB, defined as "irregular angulation of gland" which "may be related to regressive change," has been shown to be predictive of upstaging to invasive carcinoma on subsequent excisional biopsy (181).

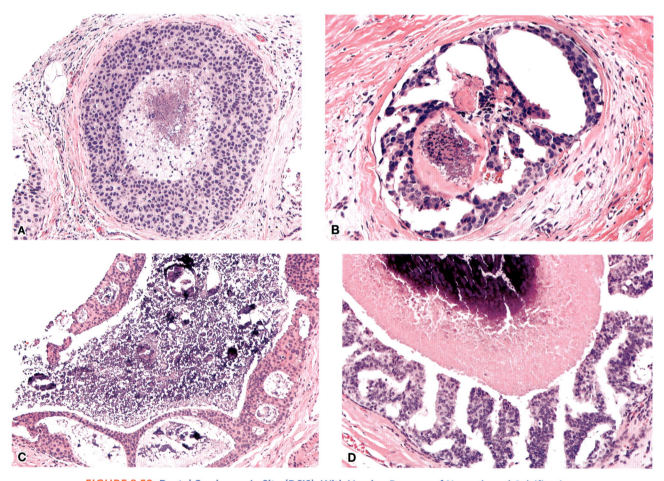

FIGURE 8.53 Ductal Carcinoma In Situ (DCIS), With Varying Degrees of Necrosis and Calcification.
A: Cribriform DCIS with punctate necrosis and minuscule deposits of calcifications. **B:** Micropapillary DCIS with punctate necrosis. **C:** Micropapillary DCIS with mainly granular calcifications obscuring necrosis. **D:** Micropapillary DCIS with necrosis and calcification.

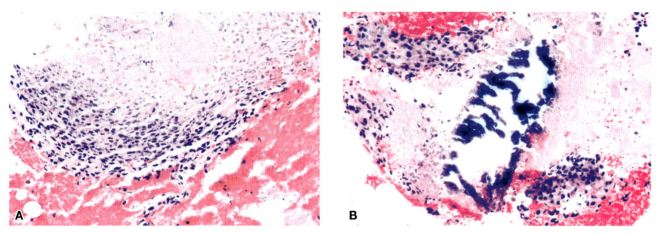

FIGURE 8.54 **Detached Probable Intraductal Carcinoma, Solid "Comedo" Type. A, B:** The needle core biopsy (NCB) had these fragments of calcification, "comedo"-type necrosis, and atypical cells. An NCB such as this is an indication for excisional biopsy to determine if carcinoma is present.

Triple-negative basal-like DCIS, which can show central necrosis, has a basal-like immunophenotype (negative for ER, PR, and HER2). This form of DCIS is the putative precursor to invasive basal-like ductal carcinoma (182-184). Bryan et al (183) found the basal-like immunophenotype in 4/55 (6%) DCIS with high-grade nuclei. This form of DCIS typically expresses basal cytokeratins and epidermal growth factor receptor (EGFR) significantly more often than high-grade DCIS, which did not have basal-like immunophenotype and may display solid, flat, or micropapillary architectural features (184).

Papillary DCIS is distinguished by the presence of prominent papillary fibrovascular stromal architecture and is discussed in Chapter 11. Spindle cell DCIS is sometimes a variant of papillary DCIS, but spindle cells also occur in non-papillary types of DCIS.

DCIS in sclerosing lesions assumes the structural configuration of the underlying lesion and may be mistaken for

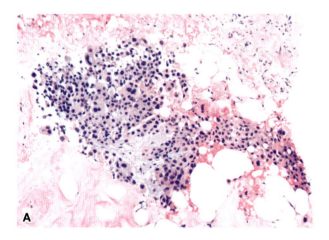
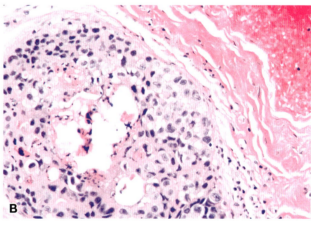
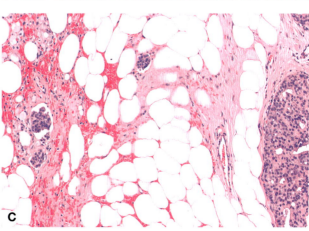

FIGURE 8.55 **Displaced Epithelium Mistaken for Invasive Carcinoma in a Needle Core Biopsy (NCB). A:** This fragment of carcinoma displaced in fibrofatty tissue was interpreted as invasive carcinoma. **B:** The excisional biopsy contained intraductal "comedo" carcinoma with no unequivocal invasion. Note hemorrhage caused by the NCB procedure in the upper right corner. **C:** Excisional biopsy with ductal carcinoma in situ (DCIS) in a case in which the antecedent NCB also showed DCIS. A focus of artifactually displaced tumor cells simulating lymphovascular involvement is present (left, center) along the healing biopsy tract.

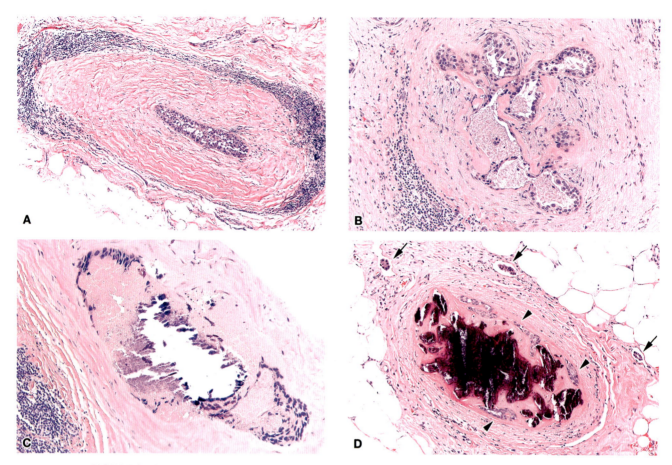

FIGURE 8.56 Intraductal Carcinoma, With Obliterative Sclerosis. A-D: Four different biopsies arranged in a sequence, which suggests progressive replacement of degenerating and necrotic ductal carcinoma in situ (DCIS) by circumferential sclerosis of the ducts and calcifications. In **(D)**, there is minimal evidence of DCIS (arrowheads); however, foci of lymphovascular involvement by carcinoma cells (arrows) are evident around the sclerotic duct.

invasive carcinoma (185-187). Because sclerosing adenosis is fundamentally a lesion formed by altered lobules, this presentation can be viewed as either DCIS which arose in TDLUs or as a form of intralobular extension of the ductal lesion **(Fig. 8.57)**. DCIS in sclerosing adenosis usually occurs focally, but it can be diffuse. The growth patterns of DCIS are usually solid and cribriform. An organoid appearance can be formed when there is alveolar expansion of lobular structures in adenosis. Calcifications may be present in the underlying adenosis or as part of the DCIS. DCIS can be limited to sclerosing adenosis, or there may be additional foci thereof in the vicinity (186). *Atypical apocrine adenosis*

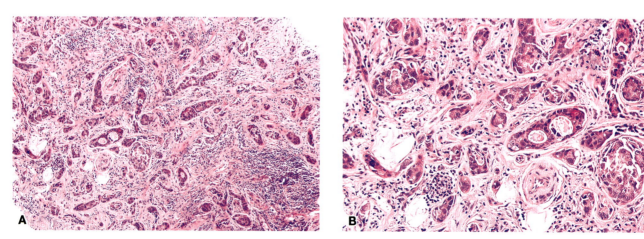

FIGURE 8.57 Ductal Carcinoma In Situ (DCIS) in Sclerosing Adenosis. A, B: Needle core biopsy (NCB) showing sclerosing adenosis involved by DCIS.

(ie, sclerosing adenosis with atypical apocrine metaplasia) can mimic invasive apocrine carcinoma (188). The underlying architecture of sclerosing adenosis can be appreciated with stains for myoepithelial cells (eg, myosin, calponin, etc) (186). Invasive carcinoma arising in sclerosing adenosis may be difficult to detect unless the invasive component has grown beyond adenosis and has an architectural pattern that differs from that of adenosis.

Features that distinguish apocrine ADH from **apocrine DCIS** include presence of the following in the latter: marked variation in nuclear size, prominence of nucleoli, mitoses, and necrosis. DCIS with apocrine cytoplasmic features can inhabit any architectural pattern of DCIS—most commonly of the solid and micropapillary types. The differential diagnosis of solid high-grade apocrine DCIS includes pleomorphic LCIS **(Table 8.17)**. Features that could assist in the diagnosis of the latter include relative dyscohesion of the neoplastic cells and presence of classic LCIS in its vicinity. Cytoplasmic localization of E-cadherin and p120 (as well as AR-positivity) can be further supportive of the diagnosis of apocrine variant of LCIS (189).

DCIS in radial sclerosing lesions may be difficult to diagnose. The presence of an underlying radial scar is indicated by the overall configuration of the lesion and association with cysts, sclerosing adenosis, and apocrine metaplasia **(Fig. 8.58)**. Fragmented portions of radial scars obtained in an NCB are difficult to assess for the presence of DCIS. *Neural entrapment* occurs when nerves are incorporated in sclerosing lesions when no carcinoma is present (190). The presence of this unusual finding coexisting with DCIS in sclerotic lesions is not indicative of invasion. Neural entrapment has also been observed in areas of sclerosing papillary DCIS not associated with sclerosing adenosis (191).

Concurrent DCIS and LCIS are present when there are separate foci of in situ carcinoma with the characteristic histologic features of each lesion. This is illustrated by instances in which the lobular lesion with the classic small cell phenotype of lobular carcinoma is limited to TDLUs that are separate from ducts with the classic features of "comedo," cribriform,

or micropapillary DCIS. In some instances, the distinction is less clear, especially when the proliferation in the ducts and lobules is composed of uniform cells with low- to intermediate-grade nuclei. The difficulty presented by these lesions is whether these should be classified as DCIS with "lobular cancerization" or as LCIS with "pagetoid type" of ductal extension. The E-cadherin and p120 stains will display strong membrane reactivity if the lesion is DCIS. E-cadherin staining will be attenuated, fragmented, or absent, and p120 reactivity will be localized in the cytoplasm, in LCIS. The presence of the cribriform pattern is suggestive, but not diagnostic, of DCIS with lobular extension. Cells with apocrine differentiation are more consistent with DCIS, although apocrine variant of pleomorphic LCIS is in the differential diagnosis. Ultimately, some cases defy classification even after careful consideration of all features. The definitive classification of in situ carcinoma in such cases should be deferred to examination of the excisional biopsy.

Coexistent DCIS and LCIS in a single duct lobular unit constitute one of the most unusual microscopic patterns of noninvasive carcinoma (192). This diagnosis depends on finding carcinoma with two distinctly different cytologic and architectural patterns in a single duct **(Fig. 8.59)**. In these combined lesions, LCIS with conventional cytology is typically present within lobular glands as well as in a pagetoid distribution in the ductal epithelium. The ductal lumen contains a cribriform, micropapillary, or solid proliferation composed of relatively more pleomorphic cells in DCIS. Coexistent DCIS and LCIS have been found in association with invasive ductal and invasive lobular carcinomas. With lobular extension of DCIS, so-called lobular cancerization, the nonneoplastic lobular epithelium is displaced by carcinoma cells with the same cytologic appearance as the DCIS. E-cadherin and p120 stains can be used to identify LCIS and DCIS in combined lesions.

Some types of DCIS, including **cystic hypersecretory carcinoma in situ** (discussed elsewhere) and **noninvasive adenoid cystic carcinoma** (193,194), are exceptionally uncommon.

TABLE 8.17

Differential Diagnosis of HG-DCIS Versus P-LCIS

Features	HG-DCIS	P-LCIS
Intracellular cohesion	Cohesive	Less cohesive/ noncohesive
Association with ADH	Common	Less common
Association with ALH/LCIS	Less common	Common
E-cadherin	Cytoplasmic membrane-positive	Cytoplasmic membrane-negative
p120	Cytoplasmic membrane-positive	Cytoplasm positive
β-catenin	Cytoplasmic membrane-positive	Negative

Based on review of literature.
HG-DCIS, high-grade ductal carcinoma in situ; P-LCIS, pleomorphic lobular carcinoma in situ.

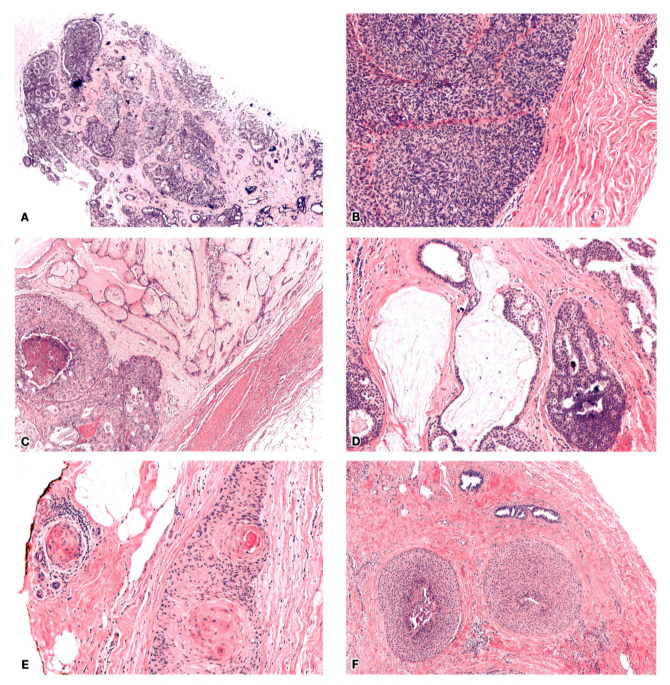

FIGURE 8.58 Ductal Carcinoma In Situ (DCIS) in Various Settings. **A:** Cribriform DCIS is present in a complex sclerosing lesion in the upper left portion of this needle core biopsy (NCB). Atypical ductal hyperplasia (ADH) occupies the midportion, and sclerosing adenosis is present on the lower right. **B:** DCIS with solid papillary features. **C:** DCIS abuts fibroadenoma. **D:** DCIS associated with extravasated mucin (mucocele-like lesion). **E:** A rare type of DCIS, squamous type. **F:** DCIS of the solid type in a male.

Distinct **genetic abnormalities** have been documented in DCIS (195). In general, loss of 16q occurs almost exclusively in lower-grade DCIS. Intermediate-grade DCIS shows frequent gains of 1q and loss of 11q. High-grade DCIS shows high frequency of amplifications at 17q12 and 11q13 and a higher rate of genetic imbalances. The key molecular characteristics of various intraductal proliferative and neoplastic lesions are listed in **Table 8.18**.

Grading of Ductal Carcinoma In Situ

The purpose of grading DCIS is to predict its biologic behavior. Over the years, multiple grading systems for DCIS have been proposed; however, no system has found universal acceptance.

At this time, DCIS is traditionally graded as low, intermediate, and high grade. Low-grade DCIS should be diagnosed

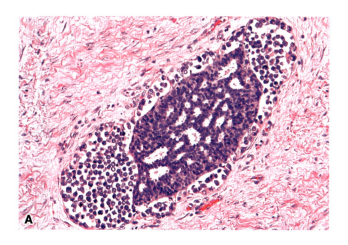
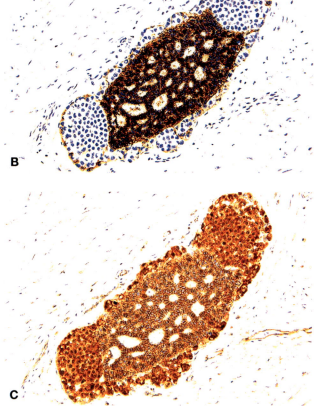

FIGURE 8.59 Coexistent Ductal Carcinoma In Situ (DCIS) and Lobular Carcinoma In Situ (LCIS) in a Single Duct Lobular Unit. **A:** DCIS of the cribriform type is present centrally, and LCIS of classic type is present at either end of the duct. Note the uniform cell population that inhabits the cribriform structure of DCIS. The LCIS is represented by uniform but noncohesive cells (which are cytologically different from the DCIS cells). **B:** An E-cadherin immunostain shows negative reaction in LCIS and strong cytoplasmic membrane staining in DCIS cells. Note weaker staining of myoepithelial cells at the perimeter of the duct. **C:** A p120 immunostain shows *cytoplasmic staining* in LCIS cells and strong *cytoplasmic membrane staining* in DCIS cells (similar to that seen with E-cadherin, in **B**). The difference in staining of E-cadherin ad p120 can be subtle and may be difficult to appreciate at low-power examination.

TABLE 8.18
Key Molecular Pathologic Characteristics of Various Intraductal Lesions

Usual Ductal Hyperplasia (UDH)
PIK3CA (~50%) point mutations
AKT1 (uncommon, ~15%) point mutations
Loss of heterozygosity (uncommon, ~15%)
Genetic abnormalities in UDH are generally not in common with those in ADH and DCIS.
Columnar Cell Lesions, and Atypical Columnar Cell Hyperplasia (ACCH)/Flat Epithelial Atypia (FEA)
Loss at 16q
Rosen Triad
Loss at 16q, 8p, 3p, 1p, 11q, and gain at 1q and 16p
Atypical Ductal Hyperplasia (ADH)[a]
Several recurrent alterations:
Loss of 16q and 17p, and gain at 1q
Low-Grade Ductal Carcinoma In Situ (LG-DCIS)
Several recurrent alterations:
Losses at 16q and 17p, and gains at 1q
High-Grade Ductal Carcinoma In Situ (HG-DCIS)
Genomic instability
Complex karyotypes:
Loss of 8p, 11q, 13q, and 14q; gains of 1q, 5p, 8q, and 17q; and amplification of 17q12 and 11q13

Based on review of literature.
[a]ADH is considered a nonobligate precursor of invasive carcinoma; however, its molecular taxonomy remains largely unclear.

with caution whenever the lesional material is minimally represented on the limited sampling of NCB. Notably, bland nuclear features that warrant a cytologic pleomorphism score of 1 are encountered only uncommonly in DCIS. In a study of almost 5,000 DCIS cases in the Netherlands, in which 48% had been reported as grade 3, 39.5% as grade 2, and 12.5% as grade 1, the proportion of low-grade DCIS varied between 6% and 24%, "by departments" participating (196).

Whenever an invasive carcinoma is associated with DCIS, both components tend to have similar nuclear grades (197). Also, there is a high degree of genomic concordance between synchronously occurring DCIS and invasive carcinoma.

Grading schemes consisting of two categories (high-grade and other grades) have been devised. The determination of grade is based largely upon nuclear cytology (175); however, the minimum proportion of cells with higher-grade nuclei in a DCIS case that warrants assignment to an overall higher grade has not been established. The finding of rare occasional giant nucleus should not be used to confer an overall nuclear grade of 3. Nuclear grade tends to be relatively constant in an individual case, even when substantial variation in architectural pattern is noted (198). Necrosis and architecture of DCIS are also considerations in grading.

The current College of American Pathologists (CAP) synoptic reporting form includes "comedo" pattern among the five main *architectural types* of DCIS: "comedo," solid, cribriform, micropapillary, and papillary—not including Paget disease of the nipple (199). Vide supra, it is imprecise to consider "comedo" as an "architectural" type of DCIS (200). However, the term "comedo" implies high-grade DCIS (197). Parenthetically, the CAP template classifies necrosis as focal (small foci or single cell) or central (expansive "comedo").

There is a significant correlation between the grade of DCIS and that of the corresponding invasive carcinoma (198). The grading categories also have significant associations with biologic characteristics of DCIS, especially lesions classified as high- and low grade. High-grade DCIS typically exhibits the following features: negativity for ER and for PR, HER2 expression, p53-positivity, high proliferation rate, and increased periductal angiogenesis. Low-grade DCIS is characterized by the following: positivity for ER and for PR, negativity for HER2 and for p53, low proliferation rate, and minimal periductal angiogenesis. Intermediate-grade DCIS tends to have mixed patterns of biologic marker expression.

The *Holland* classification system of DCIS is three-tiered (201). The system primarily utilizes nuclear grading and secondarily uses cellular polarization. The term "comedonecrosis" is not a criterion in this system. The *Lagios* system (202) stratifies DCIS into high grade (high-grade nuclei and extensive necrosis), intermediate grade (intermediate-grade nuclei with focal or absent necrosis), and low grade (low-grade nuclei without necrosis). The *Van Nuys* scale of DCIS (203) uses nuclear grade and necrosis to classify DCIS into three groups. Group 3 includes DCIS cases with high-grade nuclei (with or without necrosis). Group 2 DCIS cases are represented by those that are not high grade but show necrosis. Group 1 DCIS are not high grade and show no necrosis. The Van Nuys system has been shown to be the most reproducible vis-à-vis Holland and Lagios systems (204). An image analysis-based "automated proliferation index" utilizing nuclear grade and proliferation index (using Ki-67 immunostain) offers the promise of a less-subjective approach to grading DCIS (205).

No single grading system for DCIS has been demonstrated to be superior for anticipating successful breast conservation, and none has gained universal acceptance. A consensus conference convened in 1997 did not endorse any single system of classification but recommended that a pathology report for DCIS provides information about the descriptive characteristics considered to be necessary in most grading schemes (175). The three essential elements noted were *nuclear grade, necrosis, and architectural pattern(s)*. It was observed that the pathology report should reflect the highest nuclear grade but may indicate the relative proportions of grade when there is heterogeneity. Necrosis was defined as the "presence of ghost cells and karyorrhectic debris." Five architectural patterns were identified— "comedo," cribriform, papillary, micropapillary, and solid. It was specified that "comedo" referred "to solid intraepithelial growth within the basement membrane with central (zonal) necrosis. Such lesions are often but not invariably of high nuclear grade." Other elements recommended for inclusion in the diagnosis were lesion "size (extent, distribution)" and margin status. No method for assessing size or margins was suggested.

NCBs are commonly performed to assess imaging abnormalities detected in patients treated for DCIS. Radiation therapy can result in *scattered* markedly atypical cells in ducts and lobules. The markedly atypical cells are *diffusely* present in residual high-grade DCIS.

In the postchemotherapy setting, residual-treated DCIS can manifest itself as rare markedly atypical monster cells in ducts with intraluminal necrosis and histiocytes. The atypical cells rather resemble the pretreatment DCIS. Comparative review of pre- and posttreatment DCIS is helpful in assessment of residual disease.

Extent of Ductal Carcinoma In Situ

Extent of DCIS is difficult to determine in most cases. This difficulty is because of the (a) complex three-dimensional nature of the disease, (b) multifocality and multicentricity in some cases, (c) compressibility of breast tissue, (d) inherent limitations of sampling on NCB, and (e) the presence of DCIS in the initial NCB and in the subsequent excisional biopsy (206,207).

It may be possible to obtain an accurate measurement of DCIS size when DCIS is limited to a single core biopsy. Determination of size of DCIS when it is distributed in multiple, widely separated foci within an NCB or when it involves multiple foci in more than one NCB is imprecise.

Kestin et al (208) were unable to determine tumor size in 58% of the cases they analyzed. For this and other reasons summarized by Schnitt et al (209), classifications for assessing the prognosis of DCIS which depend on, and offer, size categories may be viewed, at best, as general guidelines rather than as strict criteria for making therapeutic decisions.

It is exceedingly unusual for DCIS to be limited to NCB. This material is not optimal for determining the size of DCIS even if the procedure is performed for calcifications alone and calcifications are no longer present in a follow-up mammogram. NCB cannot, in most cases, provide a single intact sample of DCIS. Lastly, it is not feasible to reassemble the foci from multiple NCBs to obtain a single measurement.

Biomarkers in Ductal Carcinoma In Situ

Approximately 75% of DCIS lesions express ER **(Fig. 8.60)**. The threshold for ER-positivity is the same as that for invasive carcinoma (>1% of staining in DCIS cells, even if it is weak in intensity, is regarded as ER-positive). A somewhat lower proportion of DCIS cases are PR-positive. Almost all low-grade DCIS are ER-positive. Any low-grade DCIS that is ER-negative should be reviewed not only for confirmation of diagnosis of DCIS but also for reliability of ER results (particularly with regard to pre-analytical handling of tissue). Of note, around one-half of even *high-grade* DCIS are ER-positive.

PR is frequently tested and reported in DCIS cases although there is no evidence that PR expression in DCIS is clinically relevant. The threshold for PR-positivity is the same as that for ER (ie, positivity in 1% of DCIS cells, even with weak intensity, is a positive result). Overall, PR expression in DCIS is "somewhat lower" than for ER (2).

Tamoxifen has been used in receptor-positive disease because NSABP-17 and B-24 trials demonstrated reduced ipsilateral breast tumor recurrence as well as reduced development of contralateral primary tumors. It is likely that other SERMs, including anastrozole, will replace tamoxifen for adjuvant endocrine therapy in postmenopausal women with DCIS (210,211).

Approximately 2/3 of high-grade DCIS are HER2-positive, and 40% of all DCIS demonstrate HER2 positivity—a finding that may have promise as a treatment option in this subset of DCIS, which is typically high grade and hormone receptor–negative (210,212).

A high rate of concordance in the status of ER, PR, and HER2 between DCIS and subsequent invasive carcinoma (213,214) likely demonstrates the importance of chemoprevention in patients with hormone-positive and HER2-positive cases of DCIS. Please see Chapter 27 for details of biomarker testing.

DUCTAL CARCINOMA IN SITU AND INVASIVE CARCINOMA

The diagnosis of DCIS by NCB cannot be relied upon to exclude the concurrent presence of invasive carcinoma in the affected breast. Several studies have reported the frequency of invasive carcinoma detected by excisional biopsy after an NCB diagnosis of DCIS to be in the range of 15% to 27% (11,87,215-217). In one study, the diagnosis of DCIS was reported to be more reliable with a directional vacuum-assisted biopsy procedure than with an automated NCB system (87).

Ultrastructural studies have detected foci of discontinuity in the basement membranes of ducts with DCIS (218), and similar observations have been reported in tissues studied by immunohistochemistry (219). Breaks in the basement membrane are common when DCIS is of a higher grade with central necrosis. In such foci, the neoplastic epithelium appears to protrude from the duct while it remains connected to the DCIS (220). This finding often elicits diagnostic uncertainty, reflected in such caveats as "microinvasive carcinoma is suspected" or "microinvasion cannot be ruled out."

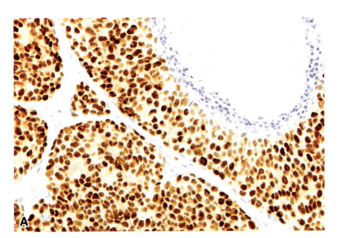
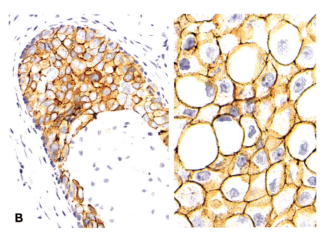

FIGURE 8.60 Ductal Carcinoma In Situ (DCIS), Biomarkers. **A:** Nuclear immunoreactivity for estrogen receptor (ER) in cribriform DCIS with intermediate-grade nuclei. Note absence of immunoreactivity in degenerating and necrotic cells. **B:** Strong complete-circumferential membrane immunoreactivity for human epidermal growth factor receptor 2 (HER2) in DCIS with necrosis and high-grade nuclei.

Microinvasive Ductal Carcinoma

Microinvasive ductal carcinoma (MiCa) is mostly encountered in association with DCIS and is only rarely detected in the absence of ADH or DCIS in its vicinity (221). In general, MiCa cells are cytologically similar to those of the associated "parent" DCIS—with similar nuclear grade. When MiCa is present, the carcinoma cells are distributed singly or in small cell groups with irregular shapes, without orientation relative to the DCIS, in the periductal stroma. The stroma at the sites of MiCa sometimes appears relatively less dense and occasionally edematous. The detection of MiCa can be difficult when there is a marked inflammatory cell reaction in the periductal region (as in most cases); however, MiCa of the lobular type is typically not associated with an inflammatory cell reaction. Granulomatous reaction may even be elicited at foci of MiCa (222). In this setting, tumor cells can resemble histiocytes, and it may require immunostains for cytokeratin to confirm their presence outside of the ducts **(Fig. 8.61)**. Carcinomatous epithelium displaced by needling procedures should not be misinterpreted as intrinsic invasive carcinoma. Hemorrhage, granulation tissue, reactive fibrosis, and hemosiderin deposition typically accompany artifactually displaced epithelia.

MiCa is more often associated with high-grade DCIS, but it may occur in other types as well (154). Assignation of overall grade of MiCa is not always possible; however, nuclear grade can be routinely assessed and should be assigned.

There have been several studies that have identified features of DCIS in NCB, which were predictive of detecting invasive carcinoma in the subsequent lumpectomy. Renshaw (216) reported that invasive carcinoma in the excisional biopsy was significantly associated with cribriform/papillary architecture and necrosis in DCIS and more than 4 mm of lobular extension. Hou et al (223) also found lobular extension to be predictive of invasion. Other features of DCIS in an NCB which have been cited as predictive of invasion include the presence of a mass lesion on imaging studies (223-225), high-grade nuclei (226-228), extensive calcifications (226,227), and palpability of lesion (228). In general, the diagnosis of MiCa carries an excellent prognosis (229-231). It is staged as T1*mic* in the TNM/UICC/AJCC classification system.

Lee et al (229) developed a nomogram to predict invasive carcinoma in the subsequent excision for DCIS cases diagnosed on NCB. The nomogram included five factors: hormone receptor expression, nuclear grade, extent, structure (cribriform or not), and type of biopsy (vacuum assisted or not). This nomogram could be useful in deciding on axillary sampling.

In view of the foregoing discussion, it is evident that there are instances in which the presence or absence of MiCa can be difficult to determine with certainty, even with immunohistochemistry. Some guidelines can be suggested.

1. The presence of myoepithelial cells at the perimeter of the lesional glands is the most convincing evidence of noninvasive carcinoma, especially if demonstrated with p63 or p40 immunostain. It is essential to use more than one immunostain because immunoreactivity is not equally evident with all reagents (232).
2. Absence of demonstrable immunoreactivity with an appropriate marker implies that myoepithelial cells are not present, although they can be severely attenuated and difficult to recognize in some cases. Loss of the myoepithelial cell layer can occur in some DCIS cases. By itself, the absence of myoepithelial cells is not indicative of invasive carcinoma, and the interpretation of this finding depends on the histologic appearance of the lesion in the corresponding H&E section(s).
3. A new "contemporaneous" H&E-stained section must be prepared whenever immunostains are performed for suspected MiCa (233). This is necessary because the structure of the lesional tissue may change as additional "levels" or "deeper" slides are prepared (234).
4. Cytokeratin immunostains are essential for the evaluation of any focus suspected to be the site of MiCa. Cytokeratin highlights the distribution of epithelial cells, helps in

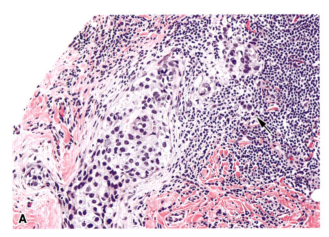 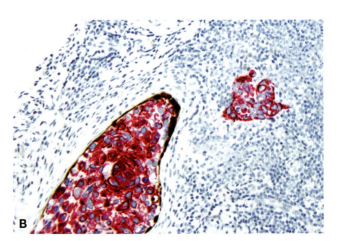

FIGURE 8.61 Ductal Carcinoma In Situ (DCIS) With Microinvasion. A, B: Microinvasive carcinoma surrounded by lymphocytes next to DCIS in a needle core biopsy (NCB) **(A)**. Myoepithelium around the DCIS stains brown and the carcinoma cells are red (cytokeratin-myosin/p63 immunostain) **(B)**.

determining the extent of invasive carcinoma, and prevents misinterpretation of histiocytes and endothelial cells.
5. Immunostains for basement membrane components laminin and collagen type IV are occasionally helpful (but can be difficult to interpret). Absence of reactivity for myoepithelial cells and basement membrane indicates a strong likelihood of invasive carcinoma.
6. The immunohistochemical demonstration of basal lamina in the absence of myoepithelial cells can rarely present a difficult diagnostic situation. The presence of laminin and collagen type IV favors a diagnosis of in situ carcinoma. However, consideration must be given to the possibility of MGA (a lesion in which myoepithelial cells are absent but basement membrane is present) and of the prospect that basal lamina is rarely formed by certain invasive carcinomas (including adenoid cystic carcinoma).

When multiple foci of microinvasive carcinoma are present, there is no precise method for estimating their aggregate dimension, and these cases qualify as multifocal MiCa (and staged as mT1mi). Invasive foci greater than 1 mm are diagnosed as invasive ductal carcinoma and reported on the basis of their measured extent (Figs. 8.61 and 8.62).

de Mascarel et al (235) subclassified MiCa into type 1 (single tumor cells) and type 2 (clusters of tumor cells). None of the 59 type 1 patients who had axillary lymph nodes removed had nodal metastases. On the other hand, there were nodal metastases in 14 (10%) of the 139 patients with type 2 MiCa who had axillary lymph nodes examined. Distant metastases were reported in 2 (3%) of the 72 patients with type 1 microinvasion and in 12 (7%) of 171 with type 2 microinvasion. The survival of patients with type 1 microinvasive carcinoma was similar to that of women with pure DCIS and significantly better than that of patients with type 2 M1Ca.

Occasionally, multiple foci of MiCa are identified in an NCB. The minimum expanse between such foci of MiCa may be significant in designating the lesion as MiCa ×2 or as a larger invasive carcinoma (incorporating the distance between the two foci of MiCa). Criteria to choose one or the other are not subject to any current guidelines. Be that as it may, in our opinion, each focus of MiCa unequivocally associated with a duct with DCIS should be considered a separate focus.

Epithelial Displacement of Ductal Carcinoma In Situ Cells into Lymphovascular Spaces in Needle Core Biopsy

The finding of (apparently displaced) neoplastic cells into lymphovascular spaces in pure DCIS cases in NCB specimens is an uncommon (yet challenging) event. Koo et al reported seven such cases in a study of 218 DCIS cases diagnosed on NCB (236). This rate of 3.2% is lower than the rate of 16% to 28% reported for such a finding in excision specimens (237,238). Obviously, such a finding in surgical excisions is accompanied by reactive changes (eg, granulation tissue, fat necrosis, inflammatory cells, etc) whenever there has been an antecedent NCB procedure.

The first step in the workup of such cases is to carefully review all cores from the case to exclude the possibility of any (micro)invasive carcinoma. Second, the possibility of retraction artifact in DCIS via myoepithelial immunostains should be excluded (concomitantly, it would be prudent to confirm the finding of true lymphovascular involvement, via endothelial immunostains). If no invasive carcinoma is identified and the finding of involvement of lymphovascular space is confirmed, then prompt excision of the lesional area is prudent to exclude invasive carcinoma in the immediate vicinity. If no invasive carcinoma is identified in the excision, then the possibility of invasive carcinoma elsewhere in the breast must be entertained (and investigated via imaging studies). If no invasive carcinoma is found in such a case, then the original finding of epithelial cells in lymphovascular spaces can reasonably be regarded as being artifactual (as per Koo et al) (236). The latter is likelier when spring-loaded, rather than vacuum-assisted, NCB tools are used to obtain the biopsy. Such artifacts are also more common in DCIS of the various papillary subtypes (including papillary DCIS, solid papillary DCIS, and intracystic [so-called encapsulated] papillary DCIS).

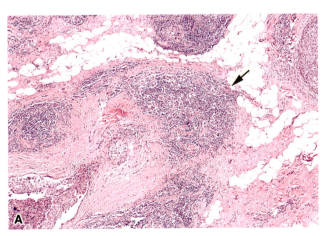
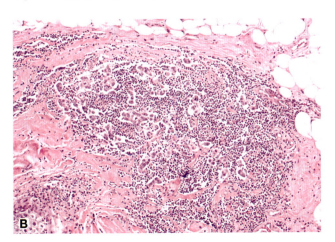

FIGURE 8.62 Ductal Carcinoma In Situ With Microinvasive Carcinoma. A: Focus of microinvasive carcinoma amid marked lymphocytic reaction (arrow). B: Magnified view of microinvasive carcinoma.

Reporting of Ductal Carcinoma In Situ on Needle Core Biopsy

DCIS is the stage of carcinoma at its most curable stage. The NCB pathology report of DCIS should include the following: nuclear grade (ie, low, intermediate, or high), architectural pattern (ie, cribriform, micropapillary, flat micropapillary/clinging, papillary, or solid), necrosis (ie, incipient/punctate or "comedo"), estimation of extent (239), and status of ER.

Given the increasing body of evidence indicating a therapeutic benefit for chemoprevention, biomarker testing of DCIS (at least for ER) in NCB has assumed considerable clinical importance (240). Results of ER and PR testing should record the proportion (between <1% and 100%) and intensity (weak, moderate, or strong) of reactivity. Immunohistochemical testing for HER2, if tested, should be reported on a scale of 0 to 3+, as per ASCO-CAP guidelines (241). The results of other biologic markers including those related to cell cycle regulation, apoptosis, and angiogenesis are novel in the context of DCIS and are currently of investigational interest (242).

Features predictive of local recurrence of DCIS are listed in **Table 8.19**.

Genetic Alterations

Consistent chromosomal aberrations have not been found in UDH. The characteristic genetic alterations in ADH and low-grade DCIS have not been detected in UDH. Thus, at least from the molecular level perspective, UDH could be regarded as a "dead end" process—or a marker, but not a direct precursor, of more significant lesions (243). Cumulative evidence suggests that the spectrum of CCLs (including FEA) are putative precursors of ADH and low-grade DCIS because loss of 16q is common in CCLs as well as in ADH in low-grade DCIS (244). DCIS and the associated invasive carcinomas, of all grades, can be similar in their respective genetic makeups, although considerable intratumoral genetic heterogeneity is present in some DCIS. It has been speculated that "the process of progression to invasive disease may constitute an 'evolutionary bottleneck,' resulting in the selection of subsets of tumor cells with specific genetic and/or epigenetic aberrations" (245).

TABLE 8.19
Features Predictive of Local Recurrence of DCIS

Age	Premenopausal
Nuclear grade	3 (of 3)
Necrosis	Expansive ("comedo")
Expanse	Larger
Margins	Positive

Based on review of literature. Nuclear grade and margin status are more significant factors.
DCIS, ductal carcinoma in situ.

A comprehensive description of the cytogenetic and molecular genetic aspects of DCIS appears in *Rosen's Breast Pathology,* 5th edition (246), and elsewhere (195).

Principles of Management of Ductal Carcinoma In Situ

In current clinical practice, most DCIS cases are diagnosed on NCB performed to evaluate mammographically detected abnormalities, and its management is optimally planned after an excision of the lesional area is performed. The management options are optimally offered by a team of specialists, and final decision is rendered after consultation with the patient. The management team includes the medical oncologist, surgeon, radiation oncologist, and pathologist. In some cases, reconstructive surgeons and genetic counselors are included in the team. The treatment plan is ideally "personalized," that is, based on specific clinical and pathologic findings. Important considerations include the manner of clinical presentation (eg, palpable mass or imaging abnormality), extent on imaging as measured macroscopically or microscopically (when possible), margin status, and histologic features including nuclear grade, growth pattern (eg, solid, cribriform, micropapillary, solid papillary, etc), and the presence or absence of necrosis. Ancillary studies, ranging from ER testing to genomic assays, play an increasingly important role in customizing management.

Numerous studies indicate that margin status and pathobiologic characteristics of DCIS including nuclear grade are the most important predictors of local recurrence after breast conservation with or without radiotherapy. Although the definitions of "negative" or "close" margins have evolved over time, most would agree that the goal of a lumpectomy is to resect all DCIS (ie, evident either clinically or on imaging) with no overt involvement of the margin ("no tumor at ink"). Other biologic characteristics, at least partially reflected in the histologic appearance of DCIS, have a complex influence on the success of treatment by affecting the rate of growth (and to some extent the time to detection of clinical recurrences) and radiosensitivity of residual DCIS after lumpectomy. Consequently, it is possible for patients with comparable amounts of incompletely excised residual high-grade and low-grade DCIS who receive the same treatment to have similar absolute risks for breast recurrence, but these two lesions may differ in time to clinical detection of recurrence, especially of invasive carcinoma, and in responsiveness to radiotherapy or to estrogen-modulating treatment.

Risk factors for noninvasive and invasive local recurrence may differ. The former has been associated with symptomatic presentation, and the latter has been shown to be associated with larger extent, margin status, among other factors (247).

Retrospective and prospective randomized studies have demonstrated that radiotherapy after excisional surgery reduces the risk of local recurrence by about 50%. The degree to which a reduced frequency of breast recurrence contributes to overall survival remains to be determined. The possibility that there could be a survival advantage conferred by reducing breast recurrences is suggested by a meta-analysis of randomized studies of radiotherapy and breast conservation in women with invasive breast carcinoma, which detected this beneficial effect. The addition of estrogen-modulating treatment to breast conservation therapy reduces breast recurrences in women with ER-positive DCIS.

Radiotherapy is usually indicated for any of the following circumstances: high-grade DCIS, positive margin, or close but free margin (described as <2 mm or less), and younger (<50 years) patients. SERM therapy can be considered for ER-positive DCIS. Omitting radiotherapy is an option for some women older than 50 years of age with clear margins (clearance >2 mm) and with low-grade histology.

Various imaging techniques, including MRI, are an essential component in the clinical follow-up of women treated by breast conservation with or without radiotherapy and/or SERMs. Attention should be paid to the follow-up of the contralateral breast, especially in women with ADH or LCIS coexisting with DCIS.

Some patients with DCIS may choose mastectomy even if they are candidates for breast conservation. Typically, a mastectomy is preferable for patients with such widespread DCIS that negative margins cannot be achieved with cosmetically acceptable results. Many of these patients have widely dispersed "suspicious" calcifications on mammography. Bilateral mastectomy is an option that is being increasingly exercised in younger women who have high-grade DCIS (248) or bilateral widespread (multifocal or multicentric) disease or those who are regarded as "high risk" (genetically predisposed to breast carcinoma or have a strong family history).

In general, a lumpectomy with or without radiation will suffice for most women with DCIS limited to a single focus, and if the margins are negative, and if the lesion is not of the "comedo" type (with high-grade nuclei and necrosis), and it is small (variously defined as <1.0 or <2.5 cm). Radiation after lumpectomy is recommended regardless of size when the DCIS is of high-grade nuclei with necrosis, is widespread (multifocal or multicentric), or is margin-positive.

As discussed earlier in this chapter, the management of ADH and low-grade DCIS is evolving. Although most authorities would continue to recommend excision for ADH (249), some have questioned the "necessity and benefit" of surgery for low-grade DCIS (250).

Axillary lymph node dissection is not indicated in most patients with DCIS. A sentinel lymph node biopsy or "low" axillary lymph node dissection may be performed in the course of a lumpectomy or mastectomy for high-grade and/or palpable DCIS (251).

Primary surgical treatment for most patients with MiCa is lumpectomy (or mastectomy in certain cases). In most published series of MiCa, the overall outcome was relatively favorable, but the studies were not directly comparable

because of differing criteria for defining microinvasion. Patients treated by breast conservation were described in several reports with results indicating that this was equally effective as mastectomy. These and other published reports indicate that the presence of MiCa, as variously defined in the past or as currently described in the TNM staging system (<1 mm), probably has minimal independent impact on the effectiveness of conservation therapy for local control. The characteristics of the DCIS which are associated with MiCa, such as formation of a palpable mass, high-grade nuclei, and necrosis, are crucial determinants for appropriate treatment. The significance of multiple foci of MiCa is yet to be determined. The finding of MiCa usually leads to sentinel lymph node biopsy prior to consideration of systemic therapy.

The University of Southern California/Van Nuys Prognostic Index

The University of Southern California/Van Nuys Prognostic Index (USC/VNPI) is a theoretically simple scoring method that can be used to stratify patients with regard to risk of local recurrence. The USC/VNPI uses age, grade, extent, margin width, and necrosis—as evaluated in *lumpectomies* (252,253). It should be noted that the scheme now referred to as the USC/NPI Index has undergone revisions involving inclusions and/or exclusions of various parameters or combinations of parameters since its initial presentation more than 20 years ago as the Van Nuys Prognostic Index (254,255). Consequently, the validity and usefulness of various versions of this scheme, including that currently proposed (253) for recommending treatment, is questionable, as evidenced by the authors' 2010 admonition that the recommendations in this article "represent substantial changes from those previously published" (252). The authors also noted more recently that "there is no difference in mortality rate regardless of which treatment is chosen" (253).

Memorial Sloan-Kettering Cancer Center's Ductal Carcinoma In Situ Nomogram

Rudloff et al (256) developed the Memorial Sloan-Kettering Cancer Center's (MSKCC) Nomogram to predict ipsilateral local recurrence in DCIS cases. Ten independent factors in *lumpectomies* were identified: age, personal/family history, presentation (clinical vs imaging), nuclear grade, necrosis, margins, adjuvant endocrine treatment, adjuvant radiotherapy, number of excisions, and duration of treatment period. The nomogram was internally validated, but Yi et al (257) evaluated Rudloff et al's nomogram in a cohort of 794 patients with DCIS at M.D. Anderson Cancer Center and found that the 5- and 10-year prediction for recurrence was "imperfect" and "limited." Another study published in 2023, using data from 296 patients from Barcelona, found that the MSKCC nomogram "did not accurately predict" local relapse (258).

Oncotype Ductal Carcinoma In Situ Score

The quest to reliably identify a subgroup of patients with DCIS who could benefit from less-aggressive management has brought about the development of the molecular-based *Oncotype DCIS score*. Using a validated technique, the 12-gene signature score independently predicts the risk of ipsilateral recurrence of DCIS or invasive carcinoma. The 12 genes include 5 that are related to proliferation: Ki-67, STK15, survivin, cyclin B1, and MYBL2. The other seven include PR and GSTM1 genes as well as five reference genes. Solin (259) reported that for patients with a low, intermediate, and high DCIS score, the 10-year risk of developing an ipsilateral carcinoma (DCIS or invasive carcinoma) were 10.6%, 26.7%, and 25.9%, respectively; and for invasive carcinoma were 3.7%, 12.3%, and 19.2%, respectively. The Oncotype DCIS score provides additional "personalized" information on DCIS which can affect management (260), and it has also been shown to provide independent information on the risk of local recurrence beyond those clinicopathologic variables that are usually assessed, such as size, age, grade, necrosis, multifocality, and subtype (261).

Declining Rate of Recurrence of Ductal Carcinoma In Situ

The declining rate of recurrence of DCIS after breast-conserving surgery over the last 30 years can be attributed not only to earlier detection, attainment of negative margins, and use of adjuvant therapies but also to improved pathologic assessment (262). Notwithstanding the foregoing, the management of DCIS ought to be guided by the following: high-grade DCIS has a more immediate risk of invasion (within 5 years in many cases), whereas low-grade DCIS has a much longer time course to invasive carcinoma (which may span many years). The risk is to the *ipsilateral* breast. Notably, with ADH, the risk is *bilateral*. Of note, approximately 20% of women with DCIS also develop either invasive or in situ carcinoma in the contralateral breast.

Clinical Trials of Nonsurgical Management of Ductal Carcinoma In Situ

An estimated 20% of untreated DCIS progresses to invasive carcinoma. At this time, almost all patients diagnosed with DCIS are managed essentially in a manner to those diagnosed with lower-grade invasive carcinoma, that is, with surgery aimed at attaining negative margins, radiation, and endocrine therapy. Currently, three phase III randomized controlled clinical trials are examining nonsurgical treatment options for patients with DCIS: COMET (Comparison of Operative to Monitoring and Endocrine Therapy) (263), LORD (LOw Risk DCIS) (264), and LORIS (LOw RISk) (265). These trials vary in enrollment criteria; however, all exclude patients with high-grade DCIS. The LORD and LORIS trials compare active surveillance and surgical arms, whereas endocrine therapy is a choice in the COMET trial.

REFERENCES

1. Connolly JL, Schnitt SJ. Benign breast disease. Resolved and unresolved issues. *Cancer.* 1993;71:1187-1189.
2. Lakhani SR, Ellis IO, Schnitt SR, et al, eds. *WHO/IARC Classification of Tumours of the Breast.* Vol 4. 4th ed. World Health Organization; 2012.
3. World Health Organization. *Breast Tumours. WHO Classification of Tumours.* Vol 2. 5th ed. International Agency for Research on Cancer; 2019.
4. Bodian CA, Perzin KH, Lattes R, et al. Reproducibility and validity of pathologic classifications of benign breast disease and implications for clinical applications. *Cancer.* 1993;71:3908-3913.
5. Choi DX, Eaton AA, Olcese C, et al. Blurry boundaries: do epithelial borderline lesions of the breast and ductal carcinoma in situ have similar rates of subsequent invasive cancer? *Ann Surg Oncol.* 2013;20:1302-1310.
6. Rosai J. Borderline epithelial lesions of the breast. *Am J Surg Pathol.* 1991;15:209-221.
7. Schnitt SJ, Connolly JL, Tavassoli FA, et al. Interobserver reproducibility in the diagnosis of ductal proliferative breast lesions using standardized criteria. *Am J Surg Pathol.* 1992;16:1133-1143.
8. Palli D, Galli M, Bianchi S, et al. Reproducibility of histological diagnosis of breast lesions: results of a panel in Italy. *Eur J Cancer.* 1996;32A:603-607.
9. Katayama A, Toss MS, Parkin M, et al. Atypia in breast pathology: what pathologists need to know. *Pathology.* 2022;54:20-31.
10. Helvie MA, Hessler C, Frank TS, et al. Atypical hyperplasia of the breast: mammographic appearance and histologic correlation. *Radiology.* 1991;179:759-764.
11. Jackman RJ, Nowels KW, Shepard MJ, et al. Stereotaxic large-core needle biopsy of 450 nonpalpable breast lesions with surgical correlation in lesions with cancer or atypical hyperplasia. *Radiology.* 1994;193:91-95.
12. Liberman L, Cohen MA, Abramson AF, et al. Atypical ductal hyperplasia diagnosed at stereotaxic core biopsy of breast lesions: an indication for surgical biopsy. *AJR Am J Roentgenol.* 1995;164:1111-1113.
13. Bodian CA, Perzin KH, Lattes R, et al. Prognostic significance of benign proliferative breast disease. *Cancer.* 1993;71:3896-3907.
14. Page DL, Rogers LW. Combined histologic and cytologic criteria for the diagnosis of mammary atypical ductal hyperplasia. *Hum Pathol.* 1992;23:1095-1097.
15. Rubin E, Visscher DW, Alexander RW, et al. Proliferative disease and atypia in biopsies performed for nonpalpable lesions detected mammographically. *Cancer.* 1988;61:2077-2082.
16. Stomper PC, Cholewinski SP, Penetrante RB, et al. Atypical hyperplasia: frequency and mammographic and pathologic relationships in excisional biopsies guided with mammography and clinical examination. *Radiology.* 1993;189:667-671.
17. Villa A, Tagliafico A, Chiesa F, et al. Atypical ductal hyperplasia diagnosed at 11-gauge vacuum-assisted breast biopsy performed on suspicious clustered microcalcifications: could patients without residual microcalcifications be managed conservatively? *AJR Am J Roentgenol.* 2011;197:1012-1018.
18. Nguyen CV, Albarracin CT, Whitman GJ, et al. Atypical ductal hyperplasia in directional vacuum-assisted biopsy of breast microcalcifications: considerations for surgical excision. *Ann Surg Oncol.* 2011;18:752-761.
19. Calhoun BC, Collins LC. Recommendations for excision following core needle biopsy of the breast: a contemporary evaluation of the literature. *Histopathology.* 2016;68:138-151.
20. Orel SG, Rosen M, Miles C, et al. MR imaging-guided 9-gauge vacuum-assisted core-needle breast biopsy: initial experience. *Radiology.* 2006;238:54-61.
21. Perlet C, Heywang-Kobrunner SH, Heinig A, et al. Magnetic resonance-guided, vacuum-assisted breast biopsy: results from a European multicenter study of 538 lesions. *Cancer.* 2006;106:982-990.
22. Liberman L, Holland AE, Marjan D, et al. Underestimation of atypical ductal hyperplasia at MRI-guided 9-gauge vacuum-assisted breast biopsy. *AJR Am J Roentgenol.* 2007;188:684-690.
23. Rosen PP, Cantrell B, Mullen DL, et al. Juvenile papillomatosis (Swiss cheese disease) of the breast. *Am J Surg Pathol.* 1980;4:3-12.
24. Wilson M, Cranor ML, Rosen PP. Papillary duct hyperplasia of the breast in children and young women. *Mod Pathol.* 1993;6:570-574.
25. Arapantoni-Dadioti P, Panayiotides J, Georgakila H, et al. Significance of intracytoplasmic lumina in the differential diagnosis between epithelial hyperplasia and carcinoma in situ of the breast. *Breast Dis.* 1996;9:277-282.
26. Lauer S, Oprea-Ilies G, Cohen C, et al. Acidophilic nuclear inclusions are specific for florid ductal hyperplasia among proliferative breast lesions. *Arch Pathol Lab Med.* 2011;135:766-769.
27. Ozaki D, Kondo Y. Comparative morphometric studies of benign and malignant intraductal proliferative lesions of the breast by computerized image analysis. *Hum Pathol.* 1995;26:1109-1113.
28. Ohuchi N, Abe R, Takahashi T, et al. Three-dimensional atypical structure in intraductal carcinoma differentiating from papilloma and papillomatosis of the breast. *Breast Cancer Res Treat.* 1985;5:57-65.
29. Kővári B, Szász AM, Kulka J, et al. Evaluation of p40 as a myoepithelial marker in different breast lesions. *Pathobiology.* 2015;82:166-171.
30. Barbareschi M, Pecciarini L, Cangi MG, et al. p63, a p53 homologue, is a selective nuclear marker of myoepithelial cells of the human breast. *Am J Surg Pathol.* 2001;25:1054-1060.
31. Rammal R, Goel K, Elishaev E, et al. The utility of SOX10 immunohistochemical staining in breast pathology. *Am J Clin Pathol.* 2022;158:616-625.

32. Kalof AN, Tam D, Beatty B, et al. Immunostaining patterns of myoepithelial cells in breast lesions: a comparison of CD10 and smooth muscle myosin heavy chain. *J Clin Pathol.* 2004;57:625-629.
33. Moritani S, Kushima R, Sugihara H, et al. Availability of CD10 immunohistochemistry as a marker of breast myoepithelial cells on paraffin sections. *Mod Pathol.* 2002;15:397-405.
34. Lerwill M. Current practical applications of diagnostic immunohistochemistry in breast pathology. *Am J Surg Pathol.* 2004;28:1076-1091.
35. Tramm T, Kim JY, Tavassoli FA. Diminished number or complete loss of myoepithelial cells associated with metaplastic and neoplastic apocrine lesions of the breast. *Am J Surg Pathol.* 2011;35:202-211.
36. Liu H. Application of immunohistochemistry in breast pathology: a review and update. *Arch Pathol Lab Med.* 2014;138:1629-1642.
37. Lee AH. Use of immunohistochemistry in the diagnosis of problematic breast lesions. *J Clin Pathol.* 2013;66:471-477.
38. Reisenbichler ES, Ross JR, Hameed O. The clinical use of a p63/cytokeratin7/18/cytokeratin5/14 antibody cocktail in diagnostic breast pathology. *Ann Diagn Pathol.* 2014;18:313-318.
39. Butcher MR, White MJ, Rooper LM, et al. MYB RNA in situ hybridization is a useful diagnostic tool to distinguish breast adenoid cystic carcinoma from other triple-negative breast carcinomas. *Am J Surg Pathol.* 2022;46:878-888.
40. Tavassoli FA, Norris HJ. A comparison of the results of long-term follow-up for atypical intraductal hyperplasia and intraductal hyperplasia of the breast. *Cancer.* 1990;65:518-529.
41. Tavassoli FA. Intraductal hyperplasias, ordinary and atypical. In: Tavassoli FA, ed. *Pathology of the Breast.* Elsevier Science Publishing; 1992:155-191.
42. Fisher ER, Costantino J, Fisher B, et al. Pathologic findings from the National Surgical Adjuvant Breast Project (NSABP) Protocol B-17. Intraductal carcinoma (ductal carcinoma in situ). *Cancer.* 1995;75:1310-1319.
43. Tozbikian G, Brogi E, Vallejo CE, et al. Atypical ductal hyperplasia bordering on ductal carcinoma in situ. *Int J Surg Pathol.* 2017;25:100-107.
44. Pinder SE, Reis-Filho JS. Non-operative breast pathology. *J Clin Pathol.* 2007;60:1297-1299.
45. Lubelsky SM, Bane AL, Shin V, et al. Columnar cell lesions and flat epithelial atypia: incidence and significance in a mammographically screened population. *Mod Pathol.* 2005;18(suppl):41A.
46. Rosen PP. Columnar cell hyperplasia is associated with lobular carcinoma in situ and tubular carcinoma. *Am J Surg Pathol.* 1999;23:1561.
47. Rosen PP. Ductal hyperplasia: ordinary and atypical. In: Rosen PP, ed. *Breast Pathology.* 2nd ed. Lippincott Williams & Wilkins; 2001:215-223.
48. Tavassoli FA, Hoefler H, Rosai J, et al. Intraductal proliferative lesions. In: Tavassoli FA, Devilee P, eds. *Pathology and Genetics of Tumours of the Breast and Female Genital Organs.* IARC Press; 2003:63-67.
49. Oyama T, Maluf H, Koerner F. Atypical cystic lobules: an early stage in the formation of low-grade ductal carcinoma in situ. *Virchows Arch.* 1999;435:413-421.
50. Goldstein NS, Lacerna M, Vicini F. Cancerization of lobules and atypical ductal hyperplasia adjacent to ductal carcinoma in situ of the breast. *Am J Clin Pathol.* 1998;110:357-367.
51. Fraser JL, Raza S, Chorny K, et al. Columnar alteration with prominent apical snouts and secretions: a spectrum of changes frequently present in breast biopsies performed for microcalcifications. *Am J Surg Pathol.* 1998;22:1521-1527.
52. Fraser JL, Pliss N, Connolly JL, et al. Immunophenotype of columnar alteration with prominent apical snouts and secretions (CAPSS). *Mod Pathol.* 2000;13:21A.
53. Brandt SM, Young GQ, Hoda SA. The "Rosen Triad": tubular carcinoma, lobular carcinoma in situ, and columnar cell lesions. *Adv Anat Pathol.* 2008;15:140-146.
54. Bezic J, Gugic D. Signet ring lobular carcinoma in situ as a part of the "Rosen Triad" (tubular carcinoma, columnar cell hyperplasia, and lobular carcinoma in situ). *Turk Patoloji Derg.* 2013;29:134-137.
55. Wang J, Liu Y, Zhang GL, et al. Breast Rosen triad: a clinicopathologic analysis of 5 cases. *Zhonghua Bing Li Xue Za Zhi.* 2017;46:49-50.
56. Prowler VL, Joh JE, Acs G, et al. Surgical excision of pure flat epithelial atypia identified on core needle breast biopsy. *Breast.* 2014;23:352-356.
57. Uzoaru I, Morgan BR, Liu ZG, et al. Flat epithelial atypia with and without atypical ductal hyperplasia: to re-excise or not. Results of a 5-year prospective study. *Virchows Arch.* 2012;461:419-423.
58. Grabenstetter A, Brennan S, Salagean ED, et al. Flat epithelial atypia in breast core needle biopsies with radiologic-pathologic concordance: is excision necessary? *Am J Surg Pathol.* 2020;44:182-190.
59. Bianchi S, Bendinelli B, Castellano I, et al. Morphological parameters of flat epithelial atypia (FEA) in stereotactic vacuum-assisted needle core biopsies do not predict the presence of malignancy on subsequent surgical excision. *Virchows Arch.* 2012;461:405-417.
60. Khoumais NA, Scaranelo AM, Moshonov H, et al. Incidence of breast cancer in patients with pure flat epithelial atypia diagnosed at core-needle biopsy of the breast. *Ann Surg Oncol.* 2013;20:133-138.
61. Peres A, Barranger E, Becette V, et al. Rates of upgrade to malignancy for 271 cases of flat epithelial atypia (FEA) diagnosed by breast core biopsy. *Breast Cancer Res Treat.* 2012;133:659-666.
62. Rajan S, Sharma N, Dall BJ, et al. What is the significance of flat epithelial atypia and what are the management implications? *J Clin Pathol.* 2011;64:1001-1004.
63. Biggar MA, Kerr KM, Erzetich LM, et al. Columnar cell change with atypia (flat epithelial atypia) on breast core biopsy-outcomes following open excision. *Breast J.* 2012;18:578-581.
64. Noel J-C, Fayt I, Fernandes-Aguillar S, et al. Proliferating activity in columnar cell lesions of the breast. *Virchows Arch.* 2006;449:617-621.
65. Dabbs DJ, Carter G, Fudge M, et al. Molecular alterations in columnar cell lesions of the breast. *Mod Pathol.* 2006;19:344-349.
66. Kaneko M, Arihiro K, Takeshima Y, et al. Loss of heterozygosity and microsatellite instability in epithelial hyperplasia of the breast. *J Exp Ther Oncol.* 2002;2:9-18.
67. Seo M, Chang JM, Kim WH, et al. Columnar cell lesions without atypia initially diagnosed on breast needle biopsies: is imaging follow-up enough? *AJR Am J Roentgenol.* 2013;201:928-934.
68. Verschuur-Maes AH, van Deurzen CH, Monninkhof EM, et al. Columnar cell lesions on breast needle biopsies: is surgical excision necessary? A systematic review. *Ann Surg.* 2012;255:259-265.
69. Schnitt SJ, Vincent-Salomon A. Columnar cell lesions of the breast. *Adv Anat Pathol.* 2003;10:113-124.
70. Guerra-Wallace MM, Christensen WN, White RL. A retrospective study of columnar alteration with prominent apical snouts and secretions and the association with cancer. *Am J Surg.* 2004;188:395-398.
71. Chivukula M, Bhargava R, Tseng G, et al. Clinicopathologic implications of "flat epithelial atypia" in core needle biopsy specimens of the breast. *Am J Clin Pathol.* 2009;131:802-808.
72. Piubello Q, Parisi A, Eccher A, et al. Flat epithelial atypia on core needle biopsy: which is the right management? *Am J Surg Pathol.* 2009;33:1078-1084.
73. Senetta R, Campanino PP, Mariscotti G, et al. Columnar cell lesions associated with breast calcifications on vacuum-assisted core biopsies: clinical, radiographic, and histological correlations. *Mod Pathol.* 2009;22:762-769.
74. Collins LC, Achacoso NA, Nekhlyudov L, et al. Clinical and pathologic features of ductal carcinoma in situ associated with the presence of flat epithelial atypia: an analysis of 543 patients. *Mod Pathol.* 2007;20:1149-1155.
75. Abdel-Fatah TM, Powe DG, Hodi Z, et al. High frequency of coexistence of columnar cell lesions, lobular neoplasia, and low grade ductal carcinoma in situ with invasive tubular carcinoma and invasive lobular carcinoma. *Am J Surg Pathol.* 2007;31:416-426.
76. Sahoo S, Recant WM. Triad of columnar cell alteration, lobular carcinoma in situ, and tubular carcinoma of the breast. *Breast J.* 2005;11:140-142.
77. Turashvili G, Hayes M, Gilks B, et al. Are columnar cell lesions the earliest histologically detectable non-obligate precursor of breast cancer? *Virchows Arch.* 2008;452:589-598.
78. Boulos FI, Dupont WD, Simpson JF, et al. Histologic associations and long-term cancer risk in columnar cell lesions of the breast: a retrospective cohort and a nested case-control study. *Cancer.* 2008;113:2415-2421.
79. Collins LC, Aroner SA, Connolly JL, et al. Breast cancer risk by extent and type of atypical hyperplasia: an update from the Nurses' Health Studies. *Cancer.* 2016;122:515-520.
80. Tocino I, Garcia BM, Carter D. Surgical biopsy findings in patients with atypical hyperplasia diagnosed by stereotaxic core needle biopsy. *Ann Surg Oncol.* 1996;3:483-488.
81. Jackman RJ, Birdwell RL, Ikeda DM. Atypical ductal hyperplasia: can some lesions be defined as probably benign after stereotactic 11-gauge vacuum-assisted biopsy, eliminating the recommendation for surgical excision? *Radiology.* 2002;224:548-554.
82. Maganini RO, Klem DA, Huston BJ, et al. Upgrade rate of core biopsy-determined atypical ductal hyperplasia by open excisional biopsy. *Am J Surg.* 2001;182:355-358.
83. Winchester DJ, Bernstein JR, Jeske JM, et al. Upstaging of atypical ductal hyperplasia after vacuum-assisted 11-gauge stereotactic core needle biopsy. *Arch Surg.* 2003;138:619-623.
84. Brem RF, Behrndt VS, Sanow L, et al. Atypical ductal hyperplasia: histologic underestimation of carcinoma in tissue harvested from impalpable breast lesions using 11-gauge stereotactically guided directional vacuum-assisted biopsy. *AJR Am J Roentgenol.* 1999;172:1405-1407.
85. Moore MM, Hargett CW, Hanks JB, et al. Association of breast cancer with the finding of atypical ductal hyperplasia at core breast biopsy. *Ann Surg.* 1997;225:726-733.
86. Gadzala DE, Cederbom GJ, Bolton JS, et al. Appropriate management of atypical ductal hyperplasia diagnosed by stereotactic core needle breast biopsy. *Ann Surg Oncol.* 1997;4:283-286.
87. Burbank F. Stereotactic breast biopsy of atypical ductal hyperplasia and ductal carcinoma in situ lesions: improved accuracy with directional, vacuum-assisted biopsy. *Radiology.* 1997;202:843-847.
88. Renshaw AA, Cartagena N, Schenkman RH, et al. Atypical ductal hyperplasia in breast core needle biopsies. Correlation of size of the lesion, complete removal of the lesion, and the incidence of carcinoma in follow-up biopsies. *Am J Clin Pathol.* 2001;116:92-96.
89. Wagoner MJ, Laronga C, Acs G. Extent and histologic pattern of atypical ductal hyperplasia present on core needle biopsy specimens of the breast can predict ductal carcinoma in situ in subsequent excision. *Am J Clin Pathol.* 2009;131:112-121.
90. Kodlin D, Winger EE, Morgenstern NL, et al. Chronic mastopathy and breast cancer. A follow-up study. *Cancer.* 1977;39:2603-2607.
91. Dupont WD, Page DL. Breast cancer risk associated with proliferative disease, age at first birth, and a family history of breast cancer. *Am J Epidemiol.* 1987;125:769-779.

92. Krieger N, Hiatt RA. Risk of breast cancer after benign breast diseases. Variation by histologic type, degree of atypia, age at biopsy, and length of follow-up. *Am J Epidemiol.* 1992;135:619-631.
93. Davis HH, Simons M, Davis JB. Cystic disease of the breast: relationship to carcinoma. *Cancer.* 1964;17:957-978.
94. Page DL, DuPont WD, Rogers LW, et al. Atypical hyperplastic lesions of the female breast. A long-term follow-up study. *Cancer.* 1985;55:2698-2708.
95. Connolly J, Schnitt S, London S, et al. Both atypical lobular hyperplasia (ALH) and atypical ductal hyperplasia (ADH) predict for bilateral breast cancer risk. *Lab Invest.* 1992;66:13A.
96. Carter CL, Corle DK, Micozzi MS, et al. A prospective study of the development of breast cancer in 16,692 women with benign breast disease. *Am J Epidemiol.* 1988;128:467-477.
97. London SJ, Connolly JL, Schnitt SJ, et al. A prospective study of benign breast disease and the risk of breast cancer. *JAMA.* 1992;267:941-944.
98. Dupont WD, Page DL. Risk factors for breast cancer in women with proliferative breast disease. *N Engl J Med.* 1985;312:146-151.
99. Ma L, Boyd NF. Atypical hyperplasia and breast cancer risk: a critique. *Cancer Causes Control.* 1992;3:517-525.
100. Jensen RA, Page DL, Dupont WD, et al. Invasive breast cancer risk in women with sclerosing adenosis. *Cancer.* 1989;64:1977-1983.
101. Schnitt SJ, Morrow M, Tung NM. Refining risk assessment in women with benign breast disease: an ongoing dilemma. *J Natl Cancer Inst.* 2017;109(10). doi:10.1093/jnci/djx036
102. Beca F, Oh H, Collins LC, et al. The impact of mammographic screening on the subsequent breast cancer risk associated with biopsy-proven benign breast disease. *NPJ Breast Cancer.* 2021;7:23.
103. Kabat GC, Jones JG, Olson N, et al. A multi-center prospective cohort study of benign breast disease and risk of subsequent breast cancer. *Cancer Causes Control.* 2010;21:821-828.
104. Hartmann LC, Sellers TA, Frost MH, et al. Benign breast disease and the risk of breast cancer. *N Engl J Med.* 2005;353:229-237.
105. Dupont WD, Parl FF, Hartmann WH, et al. Breast cancer risk associated with proliferative breast disease and atypical hyperplasia. *Cancer.* 1993;71: 1258-1265.
106. Bernstein L, Patel AV, Ursin G, et al. Lifetime recreational exercise activity and breast cancer risk among black women and white women. *J Natl Cancer Inst.* 2005;97:1671-1679.
107. McGhan LJ, Pockaj BA, Wasif N, et al. Atypical ductal hyperplasia on core biopsy: an automatic trigger for excisional biopsy? *Ann Surg Oncol.* 2012;19: 3264-3269.
108. McLaughlin CT, Neal CH, Helvie MA. Is the upgrade rate of atypical ductal hyperplasia diagnosed by core needle biopsy of calcifications different for digital and film-screen mammography? *AJR Am J Roentgenol.* 2014;203: 917-922.
109. Neal L, Sandhu NP, Hieken TJ, et al. Diagnosis and management of benign, atypical, and indeterminate breast lesions detected on core needle biopsy. *Mayo Clin Proc.* 2014;89:536-547.
110. Mesurolle B, Perez JCH, Azzumea F, et al. Atypical ductal hyperplasia diagnosed at sonographically guided core needle biopsy: frequency, final surgical outcome, and factors associated with underestimation. *AJR Am J Roentgenol.* 2014;202:1389-1394.
111. Ely KA, Carter BA, Jensen RA, et al. Core biopsy of the breast with atypical ductal hyperplasia: a probabilistic approach to reporting. *Am J Surg Pathol.* 2001;25:1017-1021.
112. de Mascarel I, Brouste V, Asad-Syed M, et al. All atypia diagnosed at stereotactic vacuum-assisted breast biopsy do not need surgical excision. *Mod Pathol.* 2011;24:1198-1206.
113. Khoury T, Chen X, Wang D, et al. Nomogram to predict the likelihood of upgrade of atypical ductal hyperplasia diagnosed on a core needle biopsy in mammographically detected lesions. *Histopathology.* 2015;67:106-120.
114. Yoon JH, Koo JS, Lee HS, et al. Factors predicting breast cancer development in women during surveillance after surgery for atypical ductal hyperplasia of the breast: analysis of clinical, radiologic, and histopathologic features. *Ann Surg Oncol.* 2020;27:3614-3622.
115. Visscher DW, Frost MH, Hartmann LC, et al. Clinicopathologic features of breast cancers that develop in women with previous benign breast disease. *Cancer.* 2016;122:378-385.
116. Hartmann LC, Degnim AC, Santen RJ, et al. Atypical hyperplasia of the breast—risk assessment and management options. *N Engl J Med.* 2015;372:78-89.
117. Liberman L, Smolkin JH, Dershaw DD, et al. Calcification retrieval at stereotactic, 11-gauge, directional, vacuum-assisted breast biopsy. *Radiology.* 1998; 208:251-260.
118. Philpotts LE, Lee CH, Horvath LJ, et al. Underestimation of breast cancer with II-gauge vacuum suction biopsy. *AJR Am J Roentgenol.* 2000;175:1047-1050.
119. Adrales G, Turk P, Wallace T, et al. Is surgical excision necessary for atypical ductal hyperplasia of the breast diagnosed by Mammotome? *Am J Surg.* 2000; 180:313-315.
120. Eby PR, Ochsner JE, DeMartini WB, et al. Frequency and upgrade rates of atypical ductal hyperplasia diagnosed at stereotactic vacuum-assisted breast biopsy: 9-versus 11-gauge. *AJR Am J Roentgenol.* 2009;192:229-234.
121. Kohr JR, Eby PR, Allison KH, et al. Risk of upgrade of atypical ductal hyperplasia after stereotactic breast biopsy: effects of number of foci and complete removal of calcifications. *Radiology.* 2010;255:723-730.

122. Allison KH, Eby PR, Kohr J, et al. Atypical ductal hyperplasia on vacuum-assisted breast biopsy: suspicion for ductal carcinoma in situ can stratify patients at high risk for upgrade. *Hum Pathol.* 2011;42:41-50.
123. Lacambra MD, Lam CC, Mendoza P, et al. Biopsy sampling of breast lesions: comparison of core needle- and vacuum-assisted breast biopsies. *Breast Cancer Res Treat.* 2012;132:917-923.
124. Youn I, Kim MJ, Moon HJ, Kim EK. Absence of residual microcalcifications in atypical ductal hyperplasia diagnosed via stereotactic vacuum-assisted breast biopsy: Is surgical excision obviated? *J Breast Cancer.* 2014;17:265-269.
125. Caplain A, Drouet Y, Peyron M, et al. Management of patients diagnosed with atypical ductal hyperplasia by vacuum-assisted core biopsy: a prospective assessment of the guidelines used at our institution. *Am J Surg.* 2014;208: 260-267.
126. Menes TS, Rosenberg R, Balch S, et al. Upgrade of high-risk breast lesions detected on mammography in the breast cancer surveillance consortium. *Am J Surg.* 2014;207:24-31.
127. Mooney KL, Bassett LW, Apple SK. Upgrade rates of high-risk breast lesions diagnosed on core needle biopsy: a single-institution experience and literature review. *Mod Pathol.* 2016;29:1471-1484.
128. Farshid G, Gill PG. Contemporary indications for diagnostic open biopsy in women assessed for screen-detected breast lesions: a ten-year, single institution series of consecutive cases. *Breast Cancer Res Treat.* 2017;162:49-58.
129. Schiaffino S, Calabrese M, Melani EF, et al. Upgrade rate of percutaneously diagnosed pure atypical ductal hyperplasia: systematic review and meta-analysis of 6458 lesions. *Radiology.* 2020;294:76-86.
130. Lewin AA, Mercado CL. Atypical ductal hyperplasia and lobular neoplasia: update and easing of guidelines. *AJR Am J Roentgenol.* 2020;214:265-275.
131. Karwowski P, Lumley D, Stokes D, et al. Atypical ductal hyperplasia on core needle biopsy: surgical outcomes of 200 consecutive cases from a high-volume breast program. *Breast J.* 2021;27:287-290.
132. Gagnon N, Martel E, Cadrin-Chênevert A, et al. Upgrade rate of atypical ductal hyperplasia: ten years experience and predictive factors. *J Surg Res.* 2021;266:311-318.
133. Miller-Ocuin JL, Fowler BB, Coldren DL, et al. Is excisional biopsy needed for pure FEA diagnosed on a core biopsy? *Am Surg.* 2020;86:1088-1090.
134. Rageth CJ, Rubenov R, Bronz C, et al. Atypical ductal hyperplasia and the risk of underestimation: tissue sampling method, multifocality, and associated calcification significantly influence the diagnostic upgrade rate based on subsequent surgical specimens. *Breast Cancer.* 2019;26:452-458.
135. National Comprehensive Cancer Network. *Breast cancer screening and diagnosis.* Guidelines Version 1.2021. Accessed June 28, 2023. https://www.nccn .org/professionals/physician_gls/pdf/breast-screening.pdf
136. American Society of Breast Surgeons. *Official Statement: consensus guideline on concordance assessment of image-guided breast biopsies and management of borderline or high-risk lesions.* 2017. Accessed June 28, 2023. https://www .breastsurgeons.org/docs/statements/Consensus-Guideline-on-Concordance-Assessment-of-Image-Guided-Breast-Biopsies.pdf?v2
137. Kader T, Hill P, Zethoven M, et al. Atypical ductal hyperplasia is a multipotent precursor of breast carcinoma. *J Pathol.* 2019;248:326-338.
138. Ryser MD, Hendrix LH, Worni M, et al. Incidence of ductal carcinoma in situ in the United States, 2000-2014. *Cancer Epidemiol Biomarkers Prev.* 2019;28: 1316-1323.
139. Siegel RL, Miller KD, Wagle NS, Jemal A. Cancer statistics, 2023. *CA Cancer J Clin.* 2023;73:17-48.
140. Kerlikowske K. Epidemiology of ductal carcinoma in situ. *J Natl Cancer Inst Monogr.* 2010;2010(41):139-141.
141. Roses RE, Arun BK, Lari SA, et al. Ductal carcinoma-in-situ of the breast with subsequent distant metastasis and death. *Ann Surg Oncol.* 2011;18: 2873-2878.
142. Verbeek ALM, Hendriks JHCL, Holland R, et al. Reduction of breast cancer mortality through mass screening with modern mammography: first results of the Nijmegen project 1975-1981. *Lancet.* 1984;1:1222-1224.
143. Ciatto S, Cataliotti L, Distante V. Nonpalpable lesions detected with mammography: review of 512 consecutive cases. *Radiology.* 1987;165:99-102.
144. Dershaw DD, Abramson A, Kinne DW. Ductal carcinoma in situ: mammographic findings and clinical implications. *Radiology.* 1989;170:411-415.
145. Stomper PC, Connolly JL, Meyer JE, et al. Clinically occult ductal carcinoma in situ detected with mammography: analysis of 100 cases with radiologic-pathologic correlation. *Radiology.* 1989;172:235-241.
146. Tse GM, Tan PH, Pang AL, et al. Calcification in breast lesions: pathologists' perspective. *J Clin Pathol.* 2008;61:145-151.
147. Holland R, Hendriks JHCL, Verbeek ALM, et al. Extent, distribution, and mammographic- histological correlations of breast ductal carcinoma in situ. *Lancet.* 1990;335:519-522.
148. Lagios MD. Multicentricity of breast carcinoma demonstrated by routine correlated subgross and radiographic examination. *Cancer.* 1977;40:1726-1734.
149. Hayes BD, Brodie C, O'Doherty A, et al. High-grade histologic features of DCIS are associated with R5 rather than R3 calcifications in breast screening mammography. *Breast J.* 2013;19:319-324.
150. Stomper PC, Connolly JL. Ductal carcinoma in situ of the breast: correlation between mammographic calcification and tumor subtype. *AJR Am J Roentgenol.* 1992;159:483-485.
151. Zunzunegui R, Chung MA, Oruwari J, et al. Casting-type calcifications with invasion and high-grade ductal carcinoma in situ: a more aggressive disease? *Arch Surg.* 2003;138:537-540.

152. Evans A, Pinder S, Wilson R, et al. Ductal carcinoma in situ of the breast: correlation between mammographic and pathologic findings. *AJR Am J Roentgenol.* 1994;162:1307-1311.

153. Evans AJ, Pinder SE, Ellis IO, et al. Correlations between the mammo-graphic features of ductal carcinoma in situ (DCIS) and C-erbB-2 oncogene expression. Nottingham Breast Team. *Clin Radiol.* 1994;49:559-562.

154. Patchefsky AS, Schwartz GF, Finkelstein SD, et al. Heterogeneity of intraductal carcinoma of the breast. *Cancer.* 1989;63:731-741.

155. Rauch GM, Kuerer HM, Scoggins ME, et al. Clinicopathologic, mammographic, and sonographic features in 1,187 patients with pure ductal carcinoma in situ of the breast by estrogen receptor status. *Breast Cancer Res Treat.* 2013;139:639-647.

156. Scoggins ME, Fox PS, Kuerer HM, et al. Correlation between sonographic findings and clinicopathologic and biologic features of pure ductal carcinoma in situ in 691 patients. *AJR Am J Roentgenol.* 2015;204:878-888.

157. Baur A, Bahrs SD, Speck S, et al. Breast MRI of pure ductal carcinoma in situ: sensitivity of diagnosis and influence of lesion characteristics. *Eur J Radiol.* 2013;82:1731-1737.

158. Pilewskie M, Morrow M. Applications for breast magnetic resonance imaging. *Surg Oncol Clin N Am.* 2014;23:431-449.

159. Menell JH, Morris EA, Dershaw DD, et al. Determination of the presence and extent of pure ductal carcinoma in situ by mammography and magnetic resonance imaging. *Breast J.* 2005;11:382-390.

160. Manion E, Brock JE, Raza S, et al. MRI-guided breast needle core biopsies: pathologic features of newly diagnosed malignancies. *Breast J.* 2014;20: 453-460.

161. Gilles R, Zafrani B, Guinebretiere J-M, et al. Ductal carcinoma in situ: MR imaging-histopathologic correlation. *Radiology.* 1995;196:415-419.

162. Orel S, Schnall M, Livolsi V, et al. Suspicious breast lesions: MR imaging with radiologic-pathologic correlation. *Radiology.* 1994;190:485-493.

163. Heywang-Kobrunner S. Contrast-enhanced magnetic resonance imaging of the breast. *Invest Radiol.* 1994;29:94-104.

164. Orel SG, Mendonca MH, Reynolds C, et al. MR imaging of ductal carcinoma in situ. *Radiology.* 1997;202:413-420.

165. Pediconi F, Catalano C, Roselli A, et al. Contrast-enhanced MR mammography for evaluation of the contralateral breast in patients with diagnosed unilateral breast cancer or high risk lesions. *Radiology.* 2007;243:670-680.

166. Cheng L, Al-Kaisi NK, Liu AY, et al. The results of intraoperative consultations in 181 ductal carcinomas in situ of the breast. *Cancer.* 1997;80:75-79.

167. Rosen PP. Frozen section diagnosis of breast lesions: recent experience with 556 consecutive biopsies. *Ann Surg.* 1978;187:17-19.

168. Rosen PP, Senie R, Schottenfeld D, et al. Noninvasive breast carcinoma: frequency of unsuspected invasion and implication for treatment. *Ann Surg.* 1979;189:98-103.

169. Wellings SR, Jensen HM, Marcum RG. An atlas of subgross pathology of the human breast with special reference to possible precancerous lesions. *J Natl Cancer Inst.* 1975;55:231-273.

170. Barsky SH, Siegal GP, Jannotta F, et al. Loss of basement membrane components by invasive tumors but not by their benign counterparts. *Lab Invest.* 1983;49:140-147.

171. Farshid G, Moinfar F, Meredith DJ, et al. Spindle cell ductal carcinoma in situ: an unusual variant of ductal intraepithelial neoplasia that stimulates ductal hyperplasia or a myoepithelial proliferation. *Virchows Arch.* 2001;439:70-77.

172. Kawasaki, T, Nakamura S, Sakamoto G, et al. Neuroendocrine ductal carcinoma in situ (NE-DCIS) of the breast-comparative clinicopathologic study of 20 NE-DCIS cases and 274 non-NE-DCIS cases. *Histopathology.* 2008;53:288-298.

173. Perry KD, Reynolds C, Rosen DG, et al. Metastatic neuroendocrine tumour in the breast: a potential mimic of in-situ and invasive mammary carcinoma. *Histopathology.* 2011;59:619-630.

174. Lennington WJ, Jensen RA, Dalton LW, et al. Ductal carcinoma in situ of the breast: heterogeneity of individual lesions. *Cancer.* 1994;73:118-124.

175. Consensus Conference on the classification of ductal carcinoma in situ. Consensus Conference Committee. *Cancer.* 1997;80:1798-1802.

176. Wen P, Marsh WL. SMMHC-p63 cocktail improves detection of myoepithelial layer in high-grade ductal carcinoma in-situ. *Mod Pathol.* 2005;18(suppl): 54A-55A.

177. Bose S, Lesser ML, Norton L, et al. Immunophenotype of intraductal carcinoma. *Arch Pathol Lab Med.* 1996;100:81-85.

178. Muir R, Aitkenhead AC. The healing of intraduct carcinoma of the mamma. *J Pathol Bacteriol.* 1934;38:117-127.

179. Wasserman JK, Parra-Herran C. Regressive change in high-grade ductal carcinoma in situ of the breast: histopathologic spectrum and biologic importance. *Am J Clin Pathol.* 2015;144:503-510.

180. Davies JD. Hyperelastosis, obliteration and fibrous plaques in major ducts of the human breast. *J Pathol.* 1973;110:13-26.

181. Walters LL, Pang JC, Zhao L, et al. Ductal carcinoma in situ with distorting sclerosis on core biopsy may be predictive of upstaging on excision. *Histopathology.* 2015;66:577-586.

182. Thike AA, Iqbal J, Cheok PY, et al. Ductal carcinoma in situ associated with triple negative invasive breast cancer: evidence for a precursor-product relationship. *J Clin Pathol.* 2013;66:665-670.

183. Bryan BA, Schnitt SJ, Collins LC. Ductal carcinoma in situ with basal-like phenotype: a possible precursor to invasive basal-like breast cancer. *Mod Pathol.* 2006;19:617-621.

184. Dabbs DJ, Chivukula M, Carter G, et al. Basal phenotype of ductal carcinoma in situ: recognition and immunohistologic profile. *Mod Pathol.* 2006;19:1506-1511.

185. Chan JKC, Ng WF. Sclerosing adenosis cancerized by intraductal carcinoma. *Pathology.* 1987;19:425-428.

186. Eusebi V, Collina G, Bussolati G. Carinoma in situ in sclerosing adenosis of the breast: an immunocytochemical study. *Semin Diagn Pathol.* 1989;6:146-152.

187. Oberman HA, Markey BA. Non-invasive carcinoma of the breast presenting in adenosis. *Mod Pathol.* 1991;4:31-35.

188. Calhoun BC, Booth CN. Atypical apocrine adenosis diagnosed on breast core biopsy: implications for management. *Hum Pathol.* 2014;45:2130-2135.

189. Zhong E, Solomon JP, Cheng E, et al. Apocrine variant of pleomorphic lobular carcinoma in situ. Further clinical, histopathologic, immunohistochemical, and molecular characterization of an emerging entity. *Am J Surg Pathol.* 2020; 44:1092-1103.

190. Taylor HB, Norris HJ. Epithelial invasion of nerves in benign diseases of the breast. *Cancer.* 1967;20:2245-2249.

191. Tsang WYW, Chan JKC. Neural invasion in intraductal carcinoma of the breast. *Hum Pathol.* 1992;23:202-204.

192. Rosen PP. Coexistent lobular carcinoma in situ and intraductal carcinoma in a single lobular-duct unit. *Am J Surg Pathol.* 1980;4:241-246.

193. Wells J, Ozerdem U, Scognamiglio T, et al. Invasive mammary adenoid cystic carcinoma with an intraductal component. *Breast J.* 2016;22(2):233-234. doi:10.1111/tbj.12558

194. Fusco N, Guerini-Rocco E, Schultheis AM, et al. The birth of an adenoid cystic carcinoma. *Int J Surg Pathol.* 2015;23:26-27.

195. Ross DS, Wen YH, Brogi E. Ductal carcinoma in situ: morphology-based knowledge and molecular advances. *Adv Anat Pathol.* 2013;20:205-216.

196. Van Dooijeweert C, van Diest PJ, Willems SM, et al. Significant inter- and intra-laboratory variation in grading of ductal carcinoma in situ of the breast: a nationwide study of 4901 patients in the Netherlands. *Breast Cancer Res Treat.* 2019;174:479-488.

197. Goldstein NS, Murphy T. Intraductal carcinoma associated with invasive carcinoma of the breast: a comparison of the two lesions with implications for intraductal carcinoma classification systems. *Am J Clin Pathol.* 1996;106:312-318.

198. Douglas-Jones AG, Gupta SK, Attanoos RL, et al. A critical appraisal of six modern classifications of ductal carcinoma in situ of the breast (DCIS): correlation with grade of associated invasive carcinoma. *Histopathology.* 1996;29: 397-409.

199. College of American Pathologists. Protocol for the examination of specimens from patients with ductal carcinoma in situ (DCIS) of the breast. Accessed June 28, 2023. https://documents.cap.org/protocols/cp-breast-dcis-18protocol--4100.pdf

200. Cserni G, Sejben A. Grading ductal carcinoma in situ (DCIS) of the breast—what's wrong with it? *Pathol Oncol Res.* 2020;26:665-671.

201. Holland R, Peterse JL, Millis RR, et al. Ductal carcinoma in situ: a proposal for a new classification. *Semin Diagn Pathol.* 1994;11:167-180.

202. Scott MA, Lagios MD, Axelsson K, et al. Ductal carcinoma in situ of the breast: reproducibility of histological subtype analysis. *Hum Pathol.* 1997;28: 967-973.

203. Consensus conference on the classification of ductal carcinoma in situ. *Hum Pathol.* 1997;28:1221-1225.

204. Schuh F, Biazús JV, Resetkova E, et al. Reproducibility of three classification systems of ductal carcinoma in situ of the breast using a web-based survey. *Pathol Res Pract.* 2010;206:705-711.

205. Stasik CJ, Davis M, Kimler BF, et al. Grading ductal carcinoma in situ of the breast using an automated proliferation index. *Ann Clin Lab Sci.* 2011;41: 122-130.

206. Saqi A, Osborne MP, Rosenblatt R, et al. Quantifying mammary duct carcinoma in situ: a wild-goose chase? *Am J Clin Pathol.* 2000;113(5 suppl 1): S30-S537.

207. Lester SC, Bose S, Chen YY, et al. Protocol for the examination of specimens from patients with ductal carcinoma in situ of the breast. *Arch Pathol Lab Med.* 2009;133:15-25.

208. Kestin I, Goldstein NS, Lacerna MD, et al. Factors associated with local recurrence of mammographically detected ductal carcinoma in situ in patients given breast conserving therapy. *Cancer.* 2000;88:596-607.

209. Schnitt SJ, Connolly JL. Classification of ductal carcinoma in situ: striving for clinical relevance in the era of breast conserving therapy. *Hum Pathol.* 1997;28:887-880.

210. Mitchell KB, Kuerer H. Ductal carcinoma in situ: treatment update and current trends. *Curr Oncol Rep.* 2015;17:48.

211. Wapnir IL, Dignam JJ, Fisher B, et al. Long-term outcomes of invasive ipsilateral breast tumor recurrences after lumpectomy in NSABP B-17 and B-24 randomized clinical trials for DCIS. *J Natl Cancer Inst.* 2011;103(6):478-488.

212. Siziopikou KP, Anderson SJ, Cobleigh MA, et al. Preliminary results of centralized HER2 testing in ductal carcinoma in situ (DCIS): NSABP B-43. *Breast Cancer Res Treat.* 2013;142:415-421.

213. King TA, Sakr RA, Muhsen S, et al. Is there a low-grade precursor pathway in breast cancer? *Ann Surg Oncol.* 2012;19:1115-1121.

214. Arvold ND, Punglia RS, Hughes ME, et al. Pathologic characteristics of second breast cancers after breast conservation for ductal carcinoma in situ. *Cancer.* 2012;118:6022-6030.

215. Liberman L, Dershaw DD, Rosen PP, et al. Stereotaxic core biopsy of breast carcinoma: accuracy at predicting invasion. *Radiology.* 1995;194:379-381.

216. Renshaw AA. Predicting invasion in the excision specimen from breast core needle biopsy specimens with only ductal carcinoma in situ. *Arch Pathol Lab Med.* 2002;126:39-41.

217. Mendez I, Andreu FJ, Saez E, et al. Ductal carcinoma in situ and atypical ductal hyperplasia of the breast diagnosed at stereotactic core biopsy. *Breast J.* 2001;7:14-18.

218. Ozzello L. Ultrastructure of intraepithelial carcinomas of the breast. *Cancer.* 1971;28:1508-1515.

219. Rajan PB, Perry RH. A quantitative study of patterns of basement membrane in ductal carcinoma in situ (DCIS) of the breast. *Breast J.* 1995;1:315-321.

220. Ozzello L. The behaviour of basement membranes in intraductal carcinoma of the breast. *Am J Pathol.* 1959;35:887-899.

221. Prasad ML, Osborne MP, Giri DD, et al. Microinvasive carcinoma (T1mic) of the breast: clinicopathologic profile of 21 cases. *Am J Surg Pathol.* 2000;24:422-428.

222. Coyne J, Haboubi NY. Microinvasive breast carcinoma with granulomatous stromal response. *Histopathology.* 1992;20:184-185.

223. Hou L, Sneige N, Hunt KK, et al. Predictors of invasion in patients with core-needle biopsy-diagnosed ductal carcinoma in situ and recommendations for a selective approach to sentinel lymph node biopsy in ductal carcinoma in situ. *Cancer.* 2006;107:1760-1768.

224. Jackman RJ, Burbank F, Parker SH, et al. Stereotactic breast biopsy of non-palpable lesions: determinants of ductal carcinoma in situ underestimation rates. *Radiology.* 2001;218:497-502.

225. King TA, Farr GH Jr, Cederblom GI, et al. A mass on breast imaging predicts coexisting invasive carcinoma in patients with a core biopsy diagnosis of ductal carcinoma in situ. *Am Surg.* 2001;67:907-912.

226. Bagnall MJ, Evans AJ, Wilson AR, et al. Predicting invasion in mammographically detected microcalcification. *Clin Radiol.* 2001;56:828-832.

227. Hoorntje LE, Schipper ME, Peeters PH, et al. The finding of invasive cancer after a preoperative diagnosis of ductal carcinoma in situ: causes of ductal carcinoma in situ underestimates with stereotactic 14-gauge needle biopsy. *Ann Surg Oncol.* 2003;10:748-753.

228. Yen TW, Hunt KK, Rose MI, et al. Predictors of invasive breast cancer in patients with an initial diagnosis of ductal carcinoma in situ: a guide to selective use of sentinel lymph node biopsy in management of ductal carcinoma in situ. *J Am Coll Surg.* 2005;200:516-526.

229. Lee SK, Yang JH, Woo SY, et al. Nomogram for predicting invasion in patients with a preoperative diagnosis of ductal carcinoma in situ of the breast. *Br J Surg.* 2013;100:1756-1763.

230. Matsen CB, Hirsch A, Eaton A, et al. Extent of microinvasion in ductal carcinoma in situ is not associated with sentinel lymph node metastases. *Ann Surg Oncol.* 2014;21:3330-3335.

231. Shatat L, Gloyeske N, Madan R, et al. Microinvasive breast carcinoma carries an excellent prognosis regardless of the tumor characteristics. *Hum Pathol.* 2013;44:2684-2689.

232. Hilson JB, Schnitt SJ, Collins LC. Phenotypic alterations in ductal carcinoma in situ-associated myoepithelial cells: biologic and diagnostic implication. *Am J Surg Pathol.* 2009;33:227-232.

233. Hoda SA, Rosen PP. Contemporaneous H&E sections should be standard practice in diagnostic immunopathology. *Am J Surg Pathol.* 2007;31:1627.

234. Lee AH, Villena Salinas NM, Hodi Z, et al. The value of examination of multiple levels of mammary needle core biopsy specimens taken for investigation of lesions other than calcification. *J Clin Pathol.* 2012;65:1097-1099.

235. de Mascarel I, MacGrogan G, Mathoulin-Pelissier S, et al. Breast ductal carcinoma in situ with microinvasion: a definition supported by a long-term study of 1248 serially sectioned ductal carcinomas. *Cancer.* 2002;94:2134-2142.

236. Koo JS, Jung W-H, Kim H. Epithelial displacement into the lymphovascular space can be seen in breast core needle biopsy specimens. *Am J Clin Pathol.* 2010;133:781-787.

237. Youngson BJ, Cranor M, Rosen PP. Epithelial displacement in surgical breast specimens following needling procedures. *Am J Surg Pathol.* 1994;18:896-903.

238. Bonneau C, Lebas P, Michener P. Histologic changes after stereotactic 11-gauge directional vacuum assisted breast biopsy for mammary calcifications: experience in 31 surgical specimens. *Ann Pathol.* 2002;22:441-447.

239. Provenzano E, Brown JP, Pinder SE. Pathological controversies in breast cancer: classification of ductal carcinoma in situ, sentinel lymph nodes and low volume metastatic disease and reporting of neoadjuvant chemotherapy specimens. *Clin Oncol (R Coll Radiol).* 2013;25:80-92.

240. Walker RA, Hanby A, Pinder SE, et al. Current issues in diagnostic breast pathology. *J Clin Pathol.* 2012;65:771-785.

241. Wolff AC, Hammond ME, Hicks DG, et al. Recommendations for human epidermal growth factor receptor 2 testing in breast cancer: American Society of Clinical Oncology/College of American Pathologists clinical practice guideline update. *J Clin Oncol.* 2013;31:3997-4013.

242. Lari SA, Kuerer HM. Biological markers in DCIS and risk of breast recurrence: a systematic review. *J Cancer.* 2011;2:232-261.

243. Boecker W, Moll R, Dervan P, et al. Usual ductal hyperplasia of the breast is a committed stem (progenitor) cell lesion distinct from atypical ductal hyperplasia and ductal carcinoma in situ. *J Pathol.* 2002;198:458-467.

244. Simpson PT, Gale T, Reis-Filho JS, et al. Columnar cell lesions of the breast: the missing link in breast cancer progression? A morphological and molecular analysis. *Am J Surg Pathol.* 2005;29:734-746.

245. Cowell CF, Weigelt B, Sakr RA, et al. Progression from ductal carcinoma in situ to invasive breast cancer: revisited. *Mol Oncol.* 2013;7:859-869.

246. Hoda SA. In: Hoda SA, Brogi E, Koerner F, et al, eds. *Rosen's Breast Pathology.* 5th ed. Ductal carcinoma in situ. Wolters Kluwer/Lippincott Williams Wilkins; 2020:363-450.

247. Collins LC, Achacoso N, Haque R, et al. Risk factors for non-invasive and invasive local recurrence in patients with ductal carcinoma in situ. *Breast Cancer Res Treat.* 2013;139:453-460.

248. Sue GR, Lannin DR, Au AF, et al. Factors associated with decision to pursue mastectomy and breast reconstruction for treatment of ductal carcinoma in situ of the breast. *Am J Surg.* 2013;206:682-685.

249. Vanden Bussche CJ, Khouri N, Sbaity E, et al. Borderline atypical ductal hyperplasia/low-grade ductal carcinoma in situ on breast needle core biopsy should be managed conservatively. *Am J Surg Pathol.* 2013;37:913-923.

250. Sagara Y, Mallory MA, Wong S, et al. Survival benefit of breast surgery for low-grade ductal carcinoma in situ: a population-based cohort study. *JAMA Surg.* 2015;150:739-745.

251. Shah DR, Canter RJ, Khatri VP, et al. Utilization of sentinel lymph node biopsy in patients with ductal carcinoma in situ undergoing mastectomy. *Ann Surg Oncol.* 2013;20:24-30.

252. Silverstein MJ, Lagios MD. Choosing treatment for patients with ductal carcinoma in situ: fine tuning the University of Southern California/Van Nuys Prognostic Index. *J Natl Cancer Inst Monogr.* 2010;2010(41):193-196.

253. Silverstein MJ, Lagios MD. Treatment selection for patients with ductal carcinoma in situ (DCIS) of the breast using the University of Southern California/Van Nuys (USC/VNPI) prognostic index. *Breast J.* 2015;21:127-132.

254. Silverstein MJ, Poller DN, Waisman JR, et al. Prognostic classification of breast ductal carcinoma-in-situ. *Lancet.* 1995;345:1154-1157.

255. Silverstein MJ, Lagios MD, Craig PH, et al. A prognostic index for ductal carcinoma in situ of the breast. *Cancer.* 1996;77:2267-2274.

256. Rudloff U, Jacks LM, Goldberg JI, et al. Nomogram for predicting the risk of local recurrence after breast-conserving surgery for ductal carcinoma in situ. *J Clin Oncol.* 2010;28:3762-3769.

257. Yi M, Meric-Bernstam F, Kuerer HM, et al. Evaluation of a breast cancer nomogram for predicting risk of ipsilateral breast tumor recurrences in patients with ductal carcinoma in situ after local excision. *J Clin Oncol.* 2012;30:600-607.

258. Oses G, Mension E, Pumarola C, et al. Analysis of local recurrence risk in ductal carcinoma in situ and external validation of the Memorial Sloan Kettering Cancer Center nomogram. *Cancers (Basel).* 2023;15:2392.

259. Solin LJ, Gray R, Baehner FL, et al. A multigene expression assay to predict local recurrence risk for ductal carcinoma in situ of the breast. *J Natl Cancer Inst.* 2013;105:701-710.

260. Alvarado M, Carter DL, Guenther JM, et al. The impact of genomic testing on the recommendation for radiation therapy in patients with ductal carcinoma in situ: a prospective clinical utility assessment of the 12-gene DCIS score™ result. *J Surg Oncol.* 2015;111:935-940.

261. Rakovitch E, Nofech-Mozes S, Hanna W, et al. A population-based validation study of the DCIS score predicting recurrence risk in individuals treated by breast-conserving surgery alone. *Breast Cancer Res Treat.* 2015;152:389-398.

262. Subhedar P, Olcese C, Patil S, et al. Decreasing recurrence rates for ductal carcinoma in situ: analysis of 2996 women treated with breast-conserving surgery over 30 years. *Ann Surg Oncol.* 2015;22:3273-3281.

263. Hwang ES, Hyslop T, Lynch T, et al. The COMET (comparison of operative versus monitoring and endocrine therapy) trial: a phase III randomised controlled clinical trial for low-risk ductal carcinoma in situ (DCIS). *BMJ Open.* 2019;9:e026797.

264. Elshof LE, Tryfonidis K, Slaets L, et al. Feasibility of a prospective, randomized, open-label, international multicentre, phase III, non-inferiority trial to assess the safety of active surveillance for low risk ductal carcinoma in situ-The LORD study. *Eur J Cancer.* 2015;51:1497-510.

265. Francis A, Thomas J, Fallowfield L, et al. Addressing overtreatment of screen detected DCIS; the LORIS trial. *Eur J Cancer.* 2015;51:2296-2303.

9

Invasive Ductal Carcinoma

RAZA S. HODA AND SYED A. HODA

NOMENCLATURE

Invasive ductal carcinoma (IDC) constitutes approximately 75% of mammary carcinomas. IDC, not otherwise specified (NOS), is a term employed by some for this type of neoplasm. This is a useful designation that recognizes the distinction between this, the most common, type of invasive mammary carcinoma and other specific forms of invasive carcinoma, such as tubular, medullary, mucinous, and papillary carcinoma.

Invasive *ductal* carcinoma was rebranded as "invasive carcinoma of no special type" in the 2012 WHO Classification System (1). It was the opinion of the authors of the WHO Classification that "the use of the term 'ductal' perpetuates the traditional but incorrect concept that these tumors are derived exclusively from mammary ductal epithelium in distinction from lobular carcinomas, which were deemed to have arisen from within lobules, for which there is also no evidence." This change is a meaningless amendment to a well-established term, for which no convincing data were presented. The inappropriate nature of this nomenclature is highlighted by the fact that the WHO Classification System has retained terms such as atypical *ductal* hyperplasia and *ductal* carcinoma in situ. Until a sound basis for the change in nomenclature is provided, we recommend the continued use of the term "invasive ductal carcinoma" where appropriate. Regrettably, the 2019 WHO Classification System retained the term "invasive carcinoma of no special type" (2).

IDC includes a subset of tumors that express, at least in part, characteristics of one of the specific types of breast carcinoma but that do not constitute pure examples of the latter. One example of this phenomenon is IDC with architectural and cytologic features of invasive lobular carcinoma (**Figs. 9.1 and 9.2**). Invasive "biphasic" carcinomas, that is,

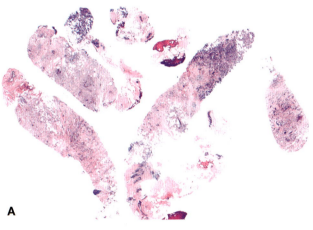

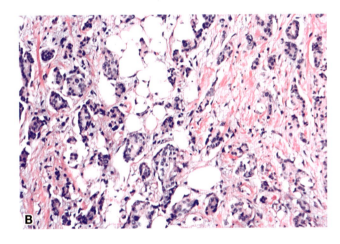

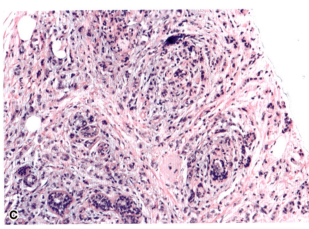

FIGURE 9.1 Concurrent Invasive Ductal and Lobular Carcinoma. A: Multiple needle cores from a single biopsy procedure are shown. **B:** A focus of invasive ductal carcinoma (moderately differentiated). **C:** A focus of invasive lobular carcinoma (classic type), with concentric ("target-like") and single (so-called "Indian") file growth patterns around native benign lobules and terminal ducts.

183

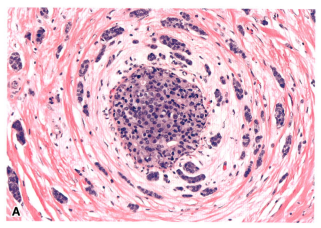 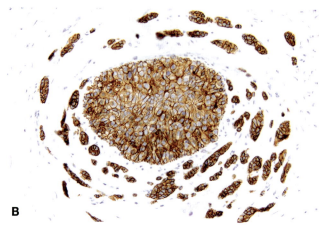

FIGURE 9.2 Ductal Carcinoma Simulating Lobular Carcinoma. A: An invasive ductal carcinoma with circumferential ("target-like" or "bull's eye") growth pattern around solid type of DCIS (center). The growth pattern mimics invasive and in situ lobular carcinoma. **B:** An E-cadherin immunostain shows the characteristic "chicken-wire" type of membrane reactivity in the invasive and in situ carcinoma—a finding that supports ductal differentiation of both.

those composed, in part, of definite ductal as well as unequivocally lobular features, are uncommon. Such tumors should be distinguished from those carcinomas in which two morphologically distinctive ductal and lobular carcinomas are concurrent in the same breast. These tumors may occasionally result in a pile-up of the two tumors ("collision tumors"). Foci of tubular, mucinous, or papillary differentiation can be present in IDCs. The presence of a mixed growth pattern in needle core biopsy (NCB) should be reported, with final classification deferred until the excisional biopsy is examined. The relatively favorable prognosis associated with certain specific histologic types of invasive carcinoma (eg, tubular) has been found to apply to those tumors that are composed entirely, or largely (approximately 90%), of the designated pattern.

Invasive tubulolobular carcinoma, a relatively uncommon type of carcinoma that displays features of tubular carcinoma as well as invasive lobular carcinoma, should be regarded as a variant of IDC—a categorization supported by immunoreactivity for E-cadherin in both components (tubular and "lobular") of the neoplasm (3).

An NCB specimen typically includes multiple samples of neoplastic tissue. The pathology report thereof ought to include all the key findings in these samplings **(Table 9.1)**. Occasionally, only a minuscule portion of the neoplasm may be present **(Fig. 9.3)**. All tissue on each slide must be examined to ensure that no material is overlooked. In extreme circumstances, the evidence for carcinoma is so scant that a definitive diagnosis cannot be rendered with confidence. In such cases, excisional biopsy is necessary to confirm carcinoma.

TABLE 9.1

Elements of Pathologic Reporting of Invasive Carcinoma in Needle Core Biopsy Specimen

Type	Ductal, lobular, etc.
Grade	1-3: gland formation, nuclear grade, and mitotic score
Maximum extent	in mm/cm
Number of cores involved	n
In situ carcinoma	Architectural type, nuclear grade, necrosis
Lymphovascular involvement	Present/absent/equivocal
Tumor-infiltrating lymphocytes	Score[a]
Calcifications	In invasive and/or in situ carcinoma, and/or in benign tissue
Biomarkers	ER, PR, HER2, Ki-67[b]

n, number. Relevant antecedent breast specimens on file should be reviewed and mentioned.

[a]TILs are defined as mononuclear immune cells that infiltrate tumor tissue and constitute a continuous variable quantified as a percentage of area occupied by TILs per total stromal area.

[b]Ki-67 of ≤5% or ≥30% can be used to estimate prognosis, particularly grade 2 and "luminal" tumors (*Appl Immunohistochem Mol Morphol.* 2022;30:237-245).

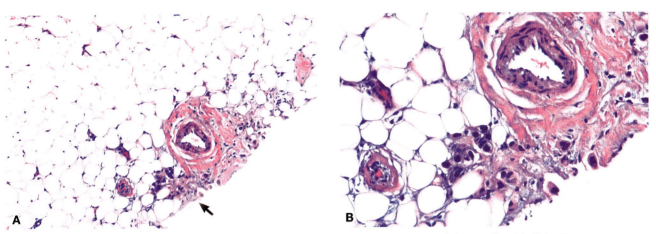

FIGURE 9.3 Invasive Ductal Carcinoma (IDC). A, B: A minuscule group of "atypical" epithelial cells amid adipose tissue (arrow) around a blood vessel in this needle core biopsy was the only evidence of invasive carcinoma. The material was not considered to be adequate for an unequivocal diagnosis of invasive carcinoma. Excisional biopsy of the 8-mm mass revealed IDC (not shown).

FROZEN SECTION AND RAPID CYTOLOGIC EVALUATION

In a series of 59 ultrasound-guided NCBs subjected to frozen section evaluation, Brunner et al (4) reported no false-positive case, a false-negative rate of 3.3% (n:2), and an unsatisfactory rate of 3.3% (n:2). Despite the technical feasibility of this procedure, the evaluation of NCBs by frozen section is not standard practice and should only be performed in *exceptional* situations—such as when there is strong clinical evidence of carcinoma and immediate intervention is planned in the event that a malignant diagnosis is rendered **(Fig. 9.4)**. Major reasons for avoiding frozen section diagnosis of NCBs include the inevitable loss of tissue from these limited specimens during slide preparation, as well as the potential for misinterpretation of benign pseudo-infiltrative lesions (sclerosing adenosis, radial scar, etc.), which can mimic IDC. Interpretive problems that apply to such deceptive lesions when they are examined in toto are compounded in the disrupted NCB material—especially when examined by frozen section.

Touch imprint cytology of NCBs can be a useful option to provide on-site assessment of adequacy and diagnosis in appropriate clinical settings (5). The technique of core wash cytology also has the potential for rapid diagnosis (6).

CLINICAL PRESENTATION

There are no specific clinical or imaging features that distinguish IDC from other types of invasive carcinoma and other benign mass-forming lesions such as radial sclerosing lesions. IDCs typically occur throughout the age range of adult women, either form a palpable mass or produce an imaging abnormality. Most IDC detected in the first four decades of life present as a palpable mass, whereas those occurring later are typically screen-detected. Various imaging

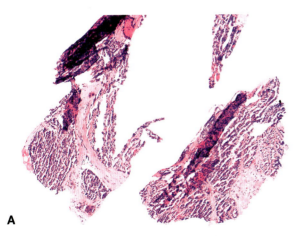
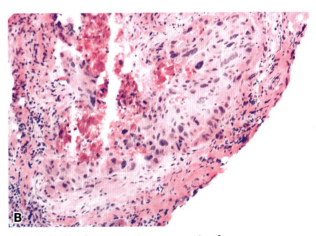

FIGURE 9.4 Invasive Ductal Carcinoma, Frozen Section. A, B: The frozen section preparation from a needle core biopsy shows ductal carcinoma with high-grade nuclei and necrosis. The presence of invasive carcinoma could not be firmly established in this preparation.

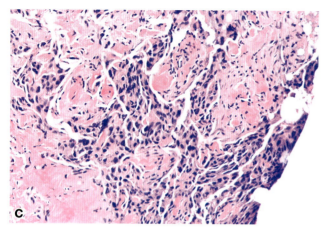 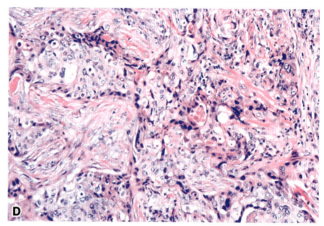

FIGURE 9.4 (*continued*) **C:** An invasive ductal carcinoma (poorly differentiated) was evident in the corresponding permanent section. The frozen section shows artifacts typical of the preparation. **D:** The artifact-free section from the subsequently performed excision is shown here for comparison.

techniques, including digital mammography, ultrasonography, magnetic resonance imaging (MRI), and positron emission tomography (PET), can detect nonpalpable IDCs early in their evolution.

MRI is a highly sensitive screening tool in women—especially for those who are considered "high risk" or those who have dense breasts. It is a rare IDC that is occult on MRI, and the technique detects up to 3 times as many breast carcinomas as mammography in high-risk patients. Be that as it may, MRI is not particularly specific, and most breast lesions (up to 79%) detected by MRI are benign (7). The most common benign lesion detected on MRI is cystic apocrine hyperplasia (8). Carcinomas detected by MRI screening are typically better differentiated IDC that span <1 cm and are positive for estrogen receptor (ER) and negative for human epidermal growth factor receptor 2 (HER2) (7).

It is uncommon for IDCs to present as a cyst—typically, a manifestation of central necrosis in a high-grade carcinoma. The uncommon presence of central fibrosis, that is, scarring following degeneration, is also usually indicative of a poorly differentiated carcinoma—and about one-quarter of the latter carcinomas are found to be "triple-negative," that is, negative for ER, PR (progesterone receptor), and HER2. Carcinomas with large central acellular zones (LCAZ) can be identified on imaging studies, including ultrasonography and MRI scans, owing to their characteristic appearance (9,10).

EXTENT/SIZE

Tumor volume rather than its one-dimensional extent (size) equates with tumor burden; however, at the present time, practical limitations inherent in pathologic evaluation preclude the reliable calculation of tumor volume owing to the asymmetric shapes of most IDC. It must also be realized that although breast tumors can be well visualized via various three-dimensional radiologic techniques, these methods cannot reliably differentiate between malignant and nonmalignant tissues, much less between IDC and ductal carcinoma in situ (DCIS). Thus, currently the size, that is, *greatest dimension*, of an invasive carcinoma is used to record its extent. The size of an invasive carcinoma, the "T" in the TNM (tumor-node-metastasis) staging system, is one of its most significant prognostic variables. The term "diameter" (defined as a straight line passing through the center of a circle or sphere) should not be used as a synonym for dimension (or extent)—because most IDCs are neither circular in two dimensions nor spherical in three dimensions.

The *gross* measurement of the size of a carcinoma is only an approximation of the actual amount of invasive tumor present (11,12). In some tumors, a considerable part of the gross mass is composed of invasive carcinoma, whereas other lesions of comparable size may have a substantial component of intraductal carcinoma, resulting in a lesser volume of invasive carcinoma. Histopathologic measurement of the invasive component, exclusive of peripheral extensions of intraductal carcinoma, is utilized for "T" staging of tumors that span <2 cm.

Survival decreases with increasing size of IDC and most other subtypes of breast carcinoma, and there is a coincidental increase in the frequency of axillary nodal metastases (13-15). This phenomenon applies not only to the overall spectrum of primary tumor size but also to subsets within those defined by TNM staging. For example, among T_1 breast carcinomas (≤2 cm), there is a significant relationship between size, the frequency of nodal metastases, and prognosis when the tumors are stratified in 5 to 10 mm groups: T1a, T1b, and T1c (16,17).

Concerted breast screening efforts have resulted in a progressive increase in the proportion of smaller tumors over recent decades. This is best reflected in earlier Surveillance, Epidemiology, and End Results (SEER) registry data, which showed that the proportion of carcinomas that measured <1 cm rose from <10% in the period 1975 to 1979 to about 25% in 1995 to 1999 among node-negative patients (18).

EXTENT/SIZE AND NEEDLE CORE BIOPSY SAMPLES

It is only rarely possible to accurately measure the in vivo extent of an IDC in an NCB, because it is difficult to ensure that the sample represents its largest dimension (19). The only focus of a microinvasive ductal carcinoma in a case may be limited to one of multiple slides prepared from a case **(Fig. 9.5)**. It is quite likely that a larger invasive carcinoma will be found on excision in cases wherein an NCB shows a smaller tumor.

Charles et al (20) did not find that NCBs affected the final staging of IDC except in 1/61 cases wherein no residual carcinoma was identified on subsequent excision. In a much larger study, Rakha et al (21) reported that NCBs resulted in the complete removal of the tumor in 165/40,395 (0.43%) of malignant NCBs. The median mammographic size of the tumor in this set was 0.6 cm. Complete removal of the tumor by NCBs was associated with vacuum-assisted procedure using a wide-bore needle. Edwards et al (22) showed that the size of invasive carcinoma on NCBs was greater than the size of residual invasive carcinoma on excisional biopsy in 24/222 (12%) cases. In 15 of these 24 cases (7.5% of all cases), the "T" was upstaged because a larger invasive carcinoma was present in the initial NCB than on the subsequent excisional biopsy. These data suggest that correlation of the extent of invasive ductal or other type of carcinoma in the initial NCB with that in the subsequent excision is crucial in determining "T." The extent of the radiologically evident tumor must also be a consideration in this regard.

MULTIFOCALITY/MULTICENTRICITY

A minority of patients have multifocal IDC (multiple foci of invasive carcinoma in the *same* quadrant) or multicentric IDC (multiple foci of IDC in *more than one* quadrant). When clinically apparent, multiple nodules may be sampled by NCBs to confirm this impression. The latest edition of the *American Joint Committee on Cancer Staging Manual* (AJCC) (23) refers to tumor size (the "T" in the TNM

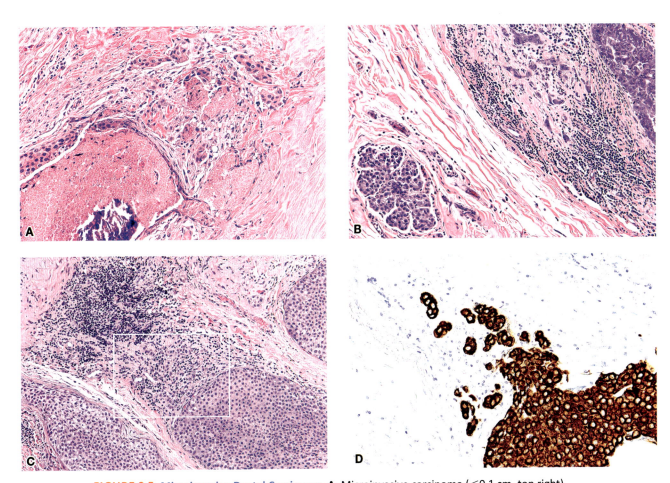

FIGURE 9.5 **Microinvasive Ductal Carcinoma. A:** Microinvasive carcinoma (<0.1 cm, top right) associated with high-grade ductal carcinoma in situ. The latter shows necrosis and calcification. **B:** Microinvasive carcinoma (top center) associated with high-grade DCIS (top right). Note lobular carcinoma in situ (LCIS) of classic type (lower left). **C, D:** Microinvasive carcinoma (box) associated with DCIS of solid type with intermediate-grade nuclei. The carcinoma has elicited a lymphocytic response that has obscured the microinvasive carcinoma. Cytokeratin AE1/AE3 immunostain highlights the microinvasive carcinoma **(D)**.

system) as the maximum dimension of the largest focus of invasive carcinoma—even when multiple separate invasive carcinomas are present with one caveat: macroscopic foci of "apparently distinct tumors" that lie "very close (eg, <5 mm)" should be regarded as a single mass, and in such cases the "T" should be reported with the combined dimension of such foci.

The pathology reports of excisions or mastectomies in cases of multifocal or multicentric invasive carcinoma should not only provide the maximum dimension of the single largest focus of invasive carcinoma but also the largest dimensions of each of the measurable foci of invasive carcinoma. This information can be provided separately for multiple grossly evident foci of invasive carcinoma and for additional foci that are only histologically identified. The data elements that could be used to compute the tumor volume in an NCB, if estimation of volume in such specimens ever assumes clinical significance, would be total aggregate length of invasive carcinoma in NCBs and the gauge (diameter) of the needles used in the procedure (24). As noted previously, NCBs are not a reliable basis for reporting maximum dimension of invasive carcinoma.

MRI offers an alternate method for determining the maximum dimension of a mammary tumor. Measurements of tumor extent obtained on MRI correlate more closely with pathologic tumor size than those obtained by mammography, ultrasound, or clinical examination (25,26). MRI has also proven to be an accurate method for measuring tumor size during, and after, neoadjuvant chemotherapy (27) and has been shown to correlate better than mammography in cases of IDC with an extensive intraductal component (EIC) (28); however, it must be realized that no imaging technique can reliably distinguish between invasive and noninvasive carcinoma.

The complexities and challenges in assessing the extent of invasive carcinoma have been detailed by Varma et al (12).

GRADING

Grading of IDCs provides an estimation of how closely an invasive carcinoma resembles normal breast glands and is regarded as one of its most important prognostic features. The most widely used histologic grading schema is the Nottingham Grading System (NGS), which is based on criteria established by Bloom and Richardson (29), as well as by Elston and Ellis (30). The parameters measured are the extent of gland formation, nuclear characteristics, and mitotic rate (31). Each of the three elements is assigned a score on a scale of 1 to 3, and the final grade is determined by the sum of the scores. Histologic grade is expressed in three categories: scores 3 to 5, well differentiated or grade 1; scores 6 to 7, intermediate or grade 2; scores 8 to 9, poorly differentiated or grade 3 **(Table 9.2)**. In IDCs that display morphologic heterogeneity, final grade of the tumor should be based on its most poorly differentiated portion.

Glandular differentiation assesses the formation of clear-cut glands by an invasive carcinoma. A true glandular structure is one with central luminal space lined by "polarized" tumor cells. This factor is best assessed on low-power examination of the entire tissue section (19). The proportion occupied by true glands is assessed **(Fig. 9.6)**.

Nuclear pleomorphism reflects grade at the cytopathologic level. The appearance of normal breast epithelial cells in the vicinity of an invasive carcinoma should be used as a standard for a nuclear score of 1 **(Fig. 9.7)**. Lymphocytes (and endothelial cells) can be used as a substitute in the event that normal breast tissue is absent in an NCB. Assignment of nuclear score of 1 is uncommon in IDC. The most

---

TABLE 9.2

Grading System for Invasive Carcinomas, Including Invasive Ductal Carcinoma

Gland formation in invasive carcinoma

Score 1:   >75%
Score 2:   10%-75%
Score 2:   <10%

The *overall* glandular differentiation of the invasive carcinoma should be taken into consideration. Specifically, the formation of those glands that exhibit open central lumina lined by polarized carcinoma cells over the entire tumor at low-power microscopy is assessed.

Nuclear features of invasive carcinoma cells

Score 1:   similar to nuclei of normal ductal cells ($\times 2$-$\times 3$ size of red blood cells [RBCs]) regular nuclear outlines and uniform chromatin
Score 2: $\times 1.5$-$\times 2$ nuclei of normal ductal cells open vesicular nuclei, visible nucleoli, moderate variability in size and shape
Score 3: $>\times 2$ nuclei of normal ductal cells, with prominent nucleoli, marked variation in both size and shape

Well-fixed foci with greatest atypia should be evaluated. Invasive carcinoma cells should be compared with nuclear size and shape of RBCs or benign "normal" ductal epithelial cells in the vicinity. Increasing size and number of nucleoli can contribute to assessment of pleomorphism.

TABLE 9.2
Grading System for Invasive Carcinomas, Including Invasive Ductal Carcinoma (*continued*)

Mitotic count of invasive carcinoma cells/10 high-power fields

- **Score 1:** 0-7 mitoses
- **Score 2:** 8-14 mitoses
- **Score 3:** >15 mitoses

Field area: 0.196 mm^2. The most mitotically active focus (typically at the periphery of the tumor) should be evaluated. Fields chosen should have as many tumor cells as possible and are selected by random meandering. Poorly preserved and necrotic foci should be avoided. Hyperchromatic, pyknotic nuclei are not counted. Cells in prophase should be disregarded. Delay in tissue fixation reduces mitotic count. Needle core biopsies (NCBs) should "fix" for several (~5) hours. Sections should be cut at 4-5 μm.

Histologic grading is an independent prognostic factor in estrogen receptor (ER)-positive invasive carcinomas. Grading on NCB material has quantitative limitations and can be imprecise. Grading on NCB is acceptable. Grade 1 and 3 tumors are seldom regraded on excision. In symptomatic invasive ductal carcinomas (IDCs), the distribution of grades 1, 2, and 3 is approximately 20%, 30%, and 50%, respectively. In asymptomatic (screen-detected) IDCs, the distribution of grades 1, 2, and 3 is approximately 30%, 40%, and 30%, respectively. Molecular studies indicate that most higher-grade invasive carcinomas are unlikely to progress from lower-grade ones, and that grade 1 and 3 invasive carcinomas have distinctive molecular profiles.

common type of invasive carcinoma cells with a nuclear score of 1 are those of classic invasive lobular carcinoma. Nuclear grading should be performed in the best-fixed and least-differentiated portion of the tumor (typically located at the advancing edge of an invasive carcinoma). Notably, nuclear grading is subject to a high degree of interobserver variation.

Mitotic count reflects the proliferation activity in an invasive carcinoma. Only cells that are unequivocally undergoing mitoses are counted. Most commonly, apoptotic cells or intratumoral lymphocytes are mistaken for a mitotic figure. Apoptotic cells commonly possess denser, more eosinophilic, cytoplasm. Absence of nuclear membrane and the presence of chromosomes support a mitotic (over an

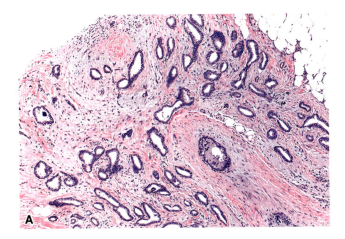
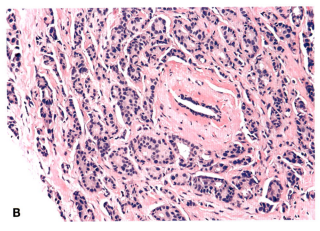
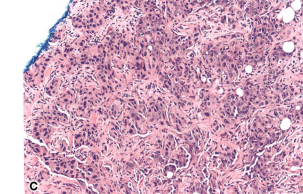

FIGURE 9.6 Invasive Ductal Carcinoma, Various Architectural Grades. A: Invasive well-differentiated ductal carcinoma characterized by glands with open lumina (gland score 1, with tubular features). **B:** Invasive moderately differentiated ductal carcinoma shows approximately one-half of glands with open lumina (gland score 2). **C:** Invasive poorly differentiated ductal carcinoma with no gland formation (gland score 3).

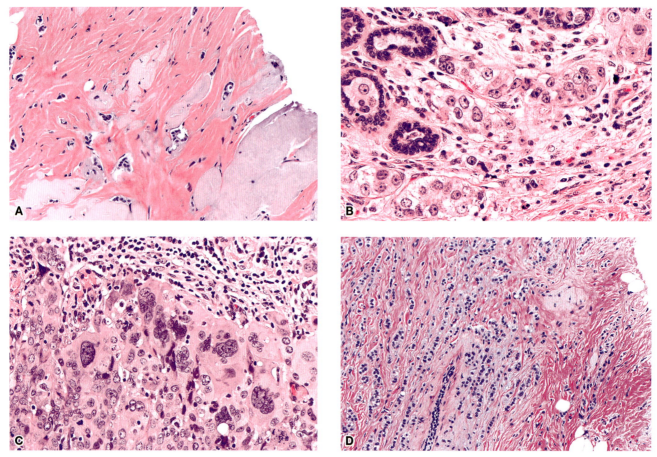

FIGURE 9.7 Invasive Carcinoma, Various Cytologic (Nuclear) Grades. A: An invasive carcinoma with tubulolobular architectural features and low-grade nuclei (nuclear score: 1). The myoepithelial cell layer was absent around the invasive carcinoma on p63 and ADH5 immunostains (not shown). **B:** Intermediate-grade nuclei (nuclear score: 2) in this invasive carcinoma are characterized by modest nuclear pleomorphism, moderate hyperchromasia, and enlargement. **C:** High-grade nuclei (nuclear score: 3) feature marked nuclear pleomorphism and hyperchromasia. **D:** The constituent cells of an invasive lobular carcinoma (classic type) with low-grade nuclei (nuclear score: 1) are shown here for comparison.

apoptotic) figure **(Fig. 9.8)**. As with nuclear grade, mitotic activity should be assessed at the advancing edge of an invasive carcinoma and/or its least differentiated (ie, most mitotically active) focus. Degenerated and necrotic foci should not be evaluated. Mitotic figures are scored on the number of mitoses per high-power field (hpf) used. The latter can vary between different microscopes, and this factor should be taken into consideration. The fields with the highest count should be recorded and the mean of 10/hpf calculated thereafter. Mitotic rates are being increasingly recorded as number of mitoses per mm^2 when digital image analysis is used.

Mitotic activity can be underassessed in NCBs owing to the limited nature of the specimen. In this regard, two studies seeking to (hypothetically) remedy this concern are notable. Firstly, it has been shown that the use of MIB-1 proliferation marker and PPH3 mitotic markers obtained on NCBs correlates better with mitotic count in the excisions (32). Secondly, it has been suggested that lowering the threshold for a mitotic score of 2 from 11 mitoses in 10 hpf to 6 mitoses in 10 hpf for invasive carcinomas in NCBs (particularly those with a gland formation score of 3 and nuclear grade score of 3) would improve agreement in the grading of IDC vis-a-vis excisional biopsy (33).

Several studies have investigated the accuracy of histologic grading based on NCBs when compared with the final grade determined from the excised tumor. The reported concordance rates ranged from 59% to 86% (34-39). In the same studies, concordance with respect to tumor type ranged from 66.6% to 81%. The data suggest that classification and grading of IDCs based on NCBs should be regarded as provisional. This consideration should be borne in mind when neoadjuvant chemotherapy is administered based on NCB diagnosis. Tumor heterogeneity is the most common source of discordant classification and grading; however, interobserver and intraobserver variation are also factors. Histologic grading is an independent prognostic factor in ER-positive invasive carcinomas.

Tumor grade is one of the key prognostic factors in IDC **(Table 9.3)**, especially in ER-positive and node-negative cases (40,41). Increasing tumor grade has been associated with several factors that are related to an increased risk

INVASIVE DUCTAL CARCINOMA **191**

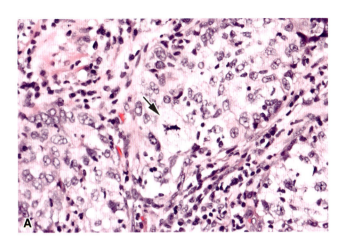
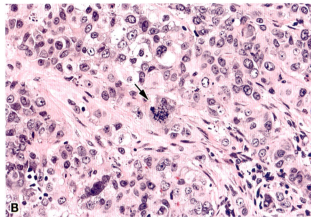
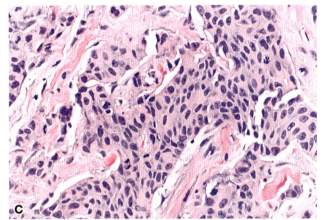

FIGURE 9.8 Invasive Ductal Carcinoma (IDC), Mitoses. Invasive carcinomas (poorly differentiated) with mitotic figures **(A)**. An abnormal mitotic figure in an IDC **(B)**. An IDC with intermediate-grade nuclei and brisk mitotic rate **(C)**. Arrows point to mitotic figures **(A and B)**.

TABLE 9.3
Prognostic and Predictive Factors of Invasive Ductal Carcinoma

	Prognostic Factor[a]	Predictive Factor[b]
Size	(+++)	(−)
Nodal status	(+++)	(−)
Metastasis	(+++)	(−)
Proliferation rate[c]	(+)	(+)
Grade[d]	(+)	(+)
Type of carcinoma	(++)	(+)
Lymphovascular involvement	(+)	(−)
Tumor-infiltrating lymphocytes	(+)	(+)
Age	(+)	(−)
Hormone (ER/PR) receptors	(+)	(++)
HER2	(+)	(++)
Oncotype (for ER+, HER2−)	(+)	(+)

The *AJCC TNM Staging Manual* (8th ed) combines anatomic prognostic factors with grade, ER, PR, HER, and Oncotype score (multigene assay) to identify groups of patients with similar survival at 5 years.

[a]A *prognostic factor* is a measurement associated with clinical outcome in the absence of therapy or with the application of a standard therapy likely to be received, ie, it is a measure of the natural history of the disease.

[b]A *predictive factor* is a measurement associated with response or no response to a particular therapy. Response is any of the clinical endpoints commonly used in clinical trials. A predictive factor implies a differential benefit from a treatment that depends on the status of the predictive biomarker.

[c]Per International Ki-67 in Breast Cancer Working Group "consensus": Ki-67 of ≤5% or ≥30% can be used to estimate prognosis in T1-2 N0-1 patients (*Appl Immunohistochem Mol Morphol*. 2022;30:237-245).

[d]Higher-grade carcinomas are typically more responsive to chemotherapy.

ER, estrogen receptor; HER2, human epidermal growth factor receptor 2; PR, progesterone receptor.

for breast recurrence after conservation therapy, including greater tumor size, diagnosis at a relatively young age, and absence of ER expression. Although some investigators have found a significant relationship between grade and local recurrence (42), others have concluded that grade is not a significant predictor of local recurrence (43).

Women with *BRCA1* mutations have a significantly higher frequency of invasive poorly differentiated ductal carcinomas when compared with individuals not carrying this mutation. *BRCA1* mutations occurring in sporadic and familial breast carcinomas have been associated with similar patterns of poorly differentiated growth. This is manifested by a higher nuclear grade, lower frequency of ER positivity, and high histologic grade (44). Women with *BRCA2* mutations generally develop IDCs of a higher grade than those that occur in sporadic age-matched controls but have a different histologic and immunohistochemical profile from that of *BRCA1* patients. Data from 4,325 *BRCA1* and 2,568 *BRCA2* mutation carriers showed strong evidence that the proportion of ER-negative breast tumors decreased with age at diagnosis among *BRCA1* but increased with age at diagnosis among *BRCA2* carriers. The proportion of "triple-negative" tumors decreased with age at diagnosis in *BRCA1* carriers but increased with age at diagnosis of *BRCA2* carriers (45).

LYMPHOVASCULAR INVOLVEMENT

Lymphatics are defined as vascular channels lined by endothelium without supporting smooth muscle or elastic tissue. Most lymphatics do not contain red blood cells, but, undoubtedly, some blood capillaries are included in this definition, and for *practical* purposes the terms lymphatic involvement (LI) and lymphovascular involvement (LVI) are synonymous.

LVI by tumor cells is identified in approximately 15% of IDC cases **(Figs. 9.9 and 9.10)**. LVI is an unfavorable prognostic finding and should be reported only when it is unequivocally identified **(Table 9.4)**. LVI can be simulated when artifactual spaces are formed around nests of invasive and in situ carcinoma owing to tissue retraction during tissue processing. It can be difficult to distinguish such retraction artifacts from true lymphatic spaces (46). Assessment for LVI is more reliably accomplished in breast tissue beyond the edges of the invasive carcinoma (47). An unusual pattern of invasive carcinoma associated with pseudoangiomatous stromal hyperplasia (PASH) can simulate LVI by carcinoma **(Fig. 9.11)**.

Retraction artifact is relatively more common in ductal than in lobular carcinomas. Carcinomas displaying such artifact tend to exhibit high histologic and nuclear grade.

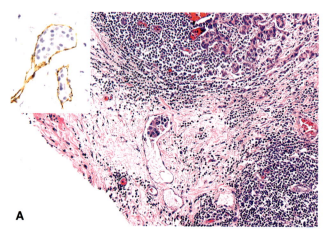

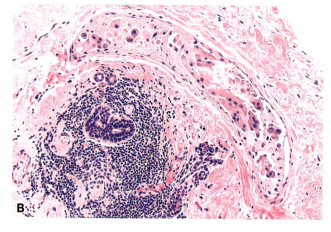

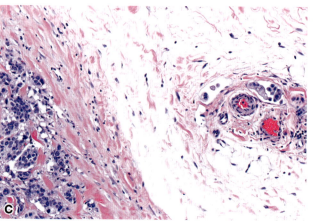

FIGURE 9.9 Invasive Ductal Carcinoma (IDC) With Lymphovascular Involvement (LVI). A: A cluster of carcinoma cells in a dilated lymphovascular channel adjacent to an IDC. Inset shows CD31 immunoreactivity in the endothelial cells. **B:** LVI in a case of invasive apocrine type of ductal carcinoma. This may be the only finding in a needle core biopsy in a case of an invasive apocrine carcinoma presenting with axillary nodal metastases ("occult primary"). **C:** Focus of lymphatic involvement (right) in an IDC (left). Note that this focus lies outside the limits of the invasive carcinoma. The lymphatic channel has an accompanying artery and vein.

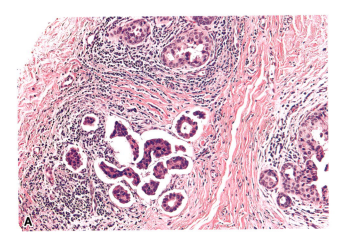
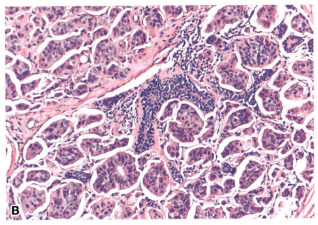
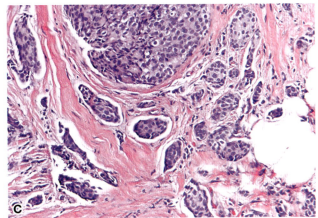

FIGURE 9.10 Artifacts Simulating Lymphovascular Involvement. A, B: Invasive micropapillary carcinoma in a needle core biopsy **(A)** and in an excisional biopsy **(B)**. **C:** An invasive ductal carcinoma with "retraction" artifact simulating invasive micropapillary carcinoma.

Acs et al (48) found a significant direct correlation between retraction artifact and LVI in patients with node-negative tumor. Furthermore, node-negative patients with retraction artifact had a significantly higher frequency of distant metastases than those without—suggesting that such artifact could possibly reflect an aspect of tumoral-stromal interaction related to the formation of lymphatic channels and not simply a passive phenomenon. The presence of foci of micropapillary features, possibly a special type of retraction artifact, also appears to predispose to axillary nodal metastases (49).

NCBs of breast can cause mechanically induced displacement of neoplastic and nonneoplastic epithelium—a finding that is commonly evident on the subsequently performed excisions. Rarely, epithelial displacement can be found in the initial NCB itself—a finding that can occasionally be diagnostically confounding. Koo et al (50) found epithelial displacement into lymphovascular channels in 7/218 (3.2%) NCBs with DCIS. There was no evidence of invasive carcinoma in the antecedent NCB or in the subsequent excision. This finding suggests that the presence of tumor cell clusters within lymphovascular channels in an NCB with DCIS may not always represent true LVI.

Immunostains for endothelial cells (including CD31, D2-40, ERG, FVIII, LYVE-1, VEGFR3, and WT1) can be confirmatory of LVI and can be useful to distinguish between retraction artifact and LVI (51-53). Thus far, ETS-related gene (ERG), a member of the erythroblast transformation-specific (ETS) family of transcription factors, is the only commercially available nuclear marker of endothelial cells (54). D2-40 is a monoclonal antibody directed at podoplanin with a high degree of specificity for lymphatic endothelia (*vide infra*). A vascular channel with endothelia that are

TABLE 9.4

Criteria for Unequivocal Lymphovascular Channel Involvement in Invasive Carcinomas

The focus should:

1. Be located outside the limits of the invasive carcinoma
2. *Should possess endothelial cells (endothelial and myoepithelial immunostains may confirm).*
   Lymphatic involvement is much more common than vascular involvement
1. Show lymphatics, arteries, and veins to be in close proximity ("travel together").[a]
2. *Have tumor cluster that is not of the same shape as the space in which it lies.*[a]

[a]May be helpful in distinguishing "retraction" artifact from true lymphovascular channel involvement. Rare instances of artifactual lymphovascular channel involvement have been reported in association with DCIS. Reference for latter: Koo JS, Jung WH, Kim H. Epithelial displacement into the lymphovascular space can be seen in breast core needle biopsy specimens. *Am J Clin Pathol.* 2010;133:781-787.

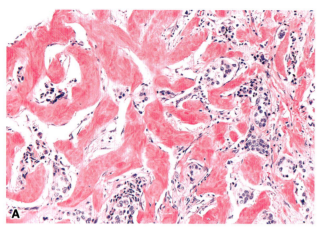 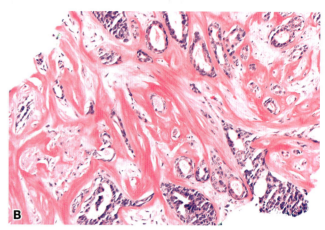

FIGURE 9.11 Invasive Ductal Carcinoma Amid Pseudoangiomatous Stromal Hyperplasia and Fibroelastotic Stroma. **A:** This invasive carcinoma infiltrates pseudoangiomatous stromal hyperplasia with dense collagenized stroma. **B:** This invasive carcinoma is associated with fibroelastotic stroma. The latter simulates pseudoangiomatous stromal hyperplasia.

D2-40 (+) and CD31 (−) is purportedly more likely to be a lymphatic space, whereas the reverse immunophenotype [D2-40 (−), CD31 (+)] is indicative of blood vessel channel. The presence of axillary nodal metastases was associated with peritumoral but not with intratumoral LVI detected by D2-40 immunostain by Van den Eynden et al (55) and de Mascarel et al (56). Periductal myoepithelial cells are sometimes immunoreactive for D2-40 (57), and this cross-reactivity is a potential source of misdiagnosis of LVI when DCIS cells become detached from the myoepithelial layer and are displaced into the ductal lumen.

Most patients with IDC associated with LVI also have axillary lymph node metastases; however, LVI is identified in 5% to 10% of patients with node-negative IDCs. Several studies have shown that LVI confers unfavorable prognosis on node-negative patients treated by either mastectomy (58-61) or breast conservation therapy (62). LVI does not predispose to local recurrence in patients treated by mastectomy (60), but they have been associated with an increased risk for recurrence in the breast after breast conservation therapy (62). Liljegren et al (63) reported that the relative risk for local recurrence after conservation therapy was 1.9% (95% CI: 1.1-3.5) in a comparison of women with or without LI.

The adverse effect of LVI is most pronounced in women with $T_1N_0M_0$ disease. In a 10-year follow-up study of 378 patients treated for $T_1N_0M_0$ carcinoma, 33% of 30 women with LI died of the disease. Death caused by breast carcinoma was observed in 20% of the 348 women who did not have LVI (47). Another study comparing similar subsets of $T_1N_0M_0$ patients found recurrences in 32% of those with LVI and in 10% of controls (64). In stage I patients with tumors larger than 2 cm ($T_2N_0M_0$), those with LVI also experienced a higher metastatic rate (61). Metastases that develop in node-negative patients who have LVI tend to occur in more than 5 years after diagnosis and are almost always systemic.

Blood vessel invasion, defined as the non-artifactual presence of carcinoma cells into the lumen of an artery or vein, is an uncommon finding in NCBs. Blood vessels are usually larger, with relatively thicker walls than lymphatics or capillaries, and can be identified by the presence of a smooth muscle wall supported by elastic fibers. Histochemical stains (eg, Verhoeff van Gieson stains) can highlight elastic tissue in arterial walls. Notably, elastic fibers may also be deposited or form around in situ and invasive carcinomas, and the resulting appearance of an elastic stain may be difficult to distinguish from blood vessel involvement. The independent prognostic significance of blood vessel involvement has not been established.

As stated earlier, various immunostains for endothelial cells can be employed in cases where there is uncertainty about the presence of LVI. Whenever such an investigation is undertaken, a contemporaneous hematoxylin and eosin (H&E)-stained slide should also be prepared to ensure correlation of the immunostained and routinely stained recut sections (65). A variety of diagnostic issues relating to LVI in breast carcinoma were reviewed by Hoda et al (66).

ANGIOGENESIS

Angiogenesis associated with breast carcinomas reflects the capacity of neoplastic tissue to induce vascular proliferation. Tumor growth is enhanced not only by increased perfusion associated with neovascularization **(Fig. 9.12)** but possibly also by growth factors produced by endothelial cells. Angiogenesis may have a significant role in progression of breast carcinoma (67), and antiangiogenic therapy may have a potential role in this regard (68). Studies of angiogenesis should take intratumoral variability into consideration (69). The limited tumor sampling obtained via NCBs is not ideal for estimating angiogenesis.

INVASIVE DUCTAL CARCINOMA

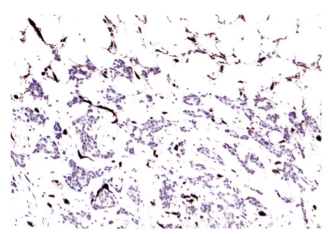

FIGURE 9.12 Invasive Ductal Carcinoma (IDC) With Angiogenesis. Capillary proliferation at the advancing edge of an IDC is highlighted via CD34 immunostain.

PERINEURAL INVASION

Perineural invasion can be identified in approximately 1% of IDCs **(Fig. 9.13)**; thus, it is about 10% less frequent than LVI (70). Perineural invasion tends to occur in higher-grade carcinomas and is frequently observed in association with LVI; however, it has not been proven as an independent prognostic factor.

Stromal Elastosis

Stromal elastosis refers to the presence of clumps of elastic fibers amid connective tissue and is *typically* observed in IDCs of lower grade **(Fig. 9.14)**. Some invasive carcinomas may show a radial scar–like appearance with central fibroelastotic core. Stromal elastosis has been significantly associated with ER positivity; however, it has not been proven to be an independent prognostic factor (71,72).

ABSENCE OF MYOEPITHELIUM

IDC lacks myoepithelium **(Figs. 9.15 and 9.16)**. This characteristic helps to distinguish it from benign proliferative lesions—with three notable exceptions: microglandular adenosis (discussed at length elsewhere), certain in situ carcinomas, and some apocrine lesions.

Per se the inability to *immunohistochemically* detect myoepithelium is not diagnostic of invasive carcinoma, because

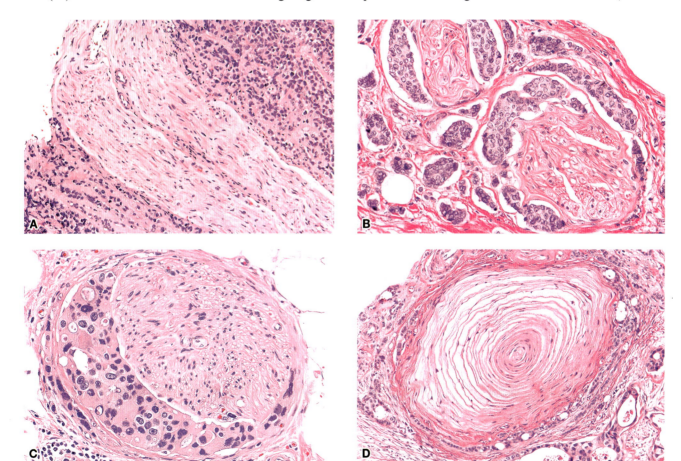

FIGURE 9.13 Invasive Ductal Carcinoma With Perineural Infiltration. A-D: Carcinoma cells are shown invading around nerves in different needle core biopsies. Illustrated here are perineural involvement of a major nerve trunk **(A)**, multiple peripheral nerves **(B)**, solitary peripheral nerve **(C)**, and Pacinian corpuscle **(D)**. The latter is a sensory neural receptor for pressure, vibration, and proprioception.

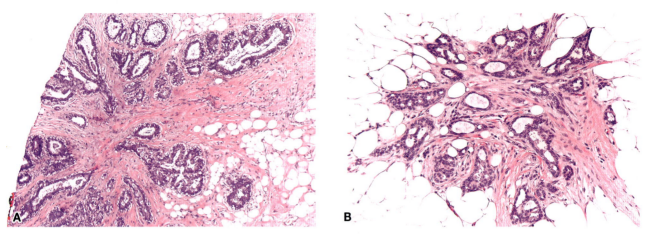

FIGURE 9.14 Radial Scar Versus Invasive Ductal Carcinomas (IDC). A: A radial scar with characteristic spoke-like glands radiating from a fibrotic nidus. Note symmetry of lesional glands. **B:** An IDC (well differentiated) with dense stroma. Note the relative asymmetry of lesional glands.

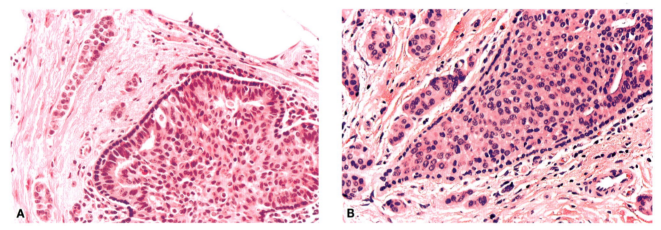

FIGURE 9.15 Invasive Ductal Carcinoma (IDC) without Myoepithelial Cell Layer on Routine hematoxylin and eosin Staining. A, B: Two examples of IDC in needle core biopsies. A hyperplastic myoepithelial cell layer (with dark staining nuclei) is evident in each case around the ducts with atypical hyperplasia but not around the invasive carcinoma.

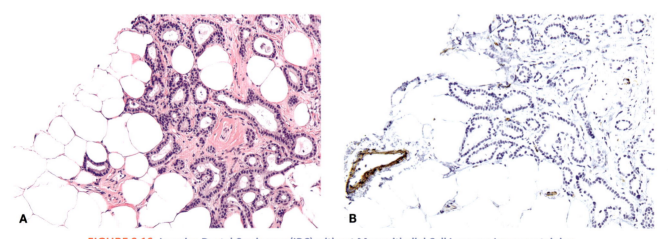

FIGURE 9.16 Invasive Ductal Carcinoma (IDC) without Myoepithelial Cell Layer on Immunostaining. A, B: IDC, well differentiated **(A)**. Heavy-chain myosin immunostain shows no staining around this invasive carcinoma, indicating absence of myoepithelial cell layer **(B)**. Myosin immunoreactivity is seen in a blood vessel wall.

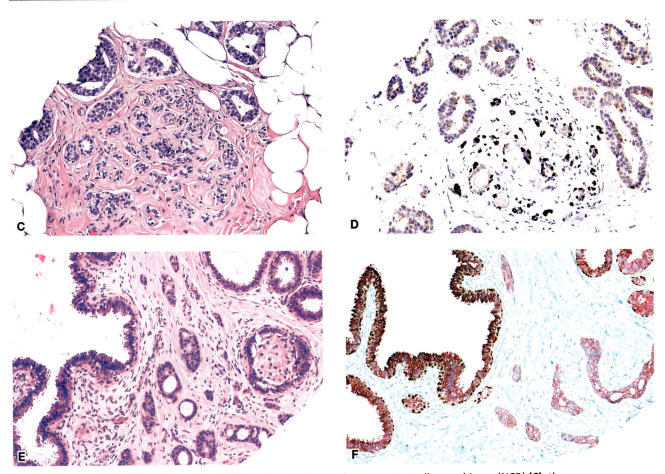

FIGURE 9.16 (*continued*) **C, D:** In this invasive carcinoma on a needle core biopsy (NCB) **(C)**, the p63 immunostain shows no staining around the invasive carcinoma **(D)**. Reactivity for p63 is seen in the associated adenosis **(D)**. **E, F:** An invasive ductal carcinoma in a NCB **(E)**. The corresponding ADH5 immunostain shows absence of myoepithelial cell staining (no brown staining) around the invasive carcinoma (red staining) cells.

myoepithelial cells can be diminished or completely lost in some in situ carcinomas—particularly those that are of the solid or apocrine types with high-grade nuclei. Myoepithelial cells can also be absent in certain forms of noninvasive papillary carcinoma (discussed at length elsewhere). The reduction and/or absence of myoepithelial cells, particularly as evident on p63 immunostain, in certain unequivocally benign apocrine lesions or in situ apocrine carcinomas is a well-documented (rather enigmatic) phenomenon (73,74). The latter finding emphasizes the need to utilize at least two myoepithelial markers and underlines the danger of interpreting immunohistochemical findings in isolation without regard to histopathologic features.

Cross-reactivity of stromal myofibrobasts with myoepithelial markers, particularly with smooth muscle actin, can be a confounding factor. This finding can create the false impression that myoepithelium is present in an IDC. For this reason, p63 or p40 immunostains are preferable—because reactivity thereof is limited to nuclei of myoepithelial cells (and cells of rare carcinomas, including those that are high grade or "basal" or those that populate low-grade adenosquamous carcinoma). It is also useful to employ a cytokeratin stain, or double or even triple immunostains (combining cytokeratin with various myoepithelial markers), to highlight foci of invasive carcinoma **(Fig. 9.17)**.

DUCTAL CARCINOMA IN SITU

DCIS is associated with IDC in approximately 75% of cases, and its presence in NCBs with IDC should be reported. Included in the diagnosis should be the architectural pattern and nuclear grade of DCIS, as well as the presence or absence of necrosis and calcifications.

IDC and its associated DCIS usually share similar nuclear grades, and the two components typically undergo similar molecular alterations (75). IDCs vary in the relative proportions of in situ and invasive components. As the proportion of DCIS increases, for any gross tumor size, there is a trend toward decreased nodal metastases and a more favorable prognosis. The distribution of DCIS in and around the primary tumor appears to correlate with the risk of local recurrence after breast conservation (76) but has no bearing on the risk of systemic recurrence in women treated by breast conservation or mastectomy (77). Local recurrence occurs more often after lumpectomy and radiation therapy in women who have high-grade DCIS or

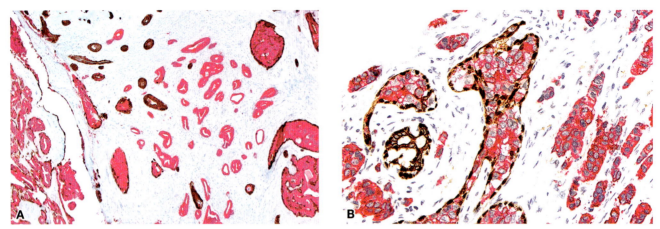

FIGURE 9.17 Invasive Ductal Carcinoma, ADH5 Triple Immunostain. A, B: Both of these ADH5 (triple) immunostained preparations facilitate the diagnosis of invasive carcinoma. The preparation uses a combination of cytokeratin AE1/3 (with red chromogen) and two myoepithelial markers: p63 to mark myoepithelial nuclei (with brown chromogen) and myosin (also with brown chromogen) to highlight myoepithelial cytoplasm. In this "cocktail," p63 and myosin stains decorate the entire myoepithelial cell (nucleus and cytoplasm) around the ductal carcinoma in situ in both cases.

an **extensive intraductal component** (EIC). The latter is defined as DCIS that comprises more than 25% of a tumor mass and extends beyond it. The increased risk of local recurrence after breast conservation attributable to EIC is probably a manifestation of a greater probability of there being carcinoma at margins of excision and beyond. In cases with negative margins, the presence of EIC may not increase the risk of local recurrence after breast conservation therapy (78,79).

An estimate of the proportion of DCIS associated with an invasive carcinoma and its extent beyond the invasive carcinoma cannot be reliably estimated in conventional NCBs.

BIOMARKERS

The practice of testing ER, PR, and HER2 on the initial NCB material rather than on the subsequent excision has been increasing in recent years **(Fig. 9.18)** (80). The

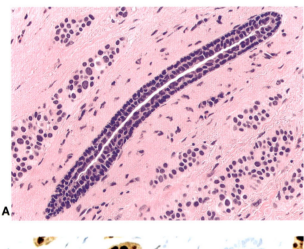

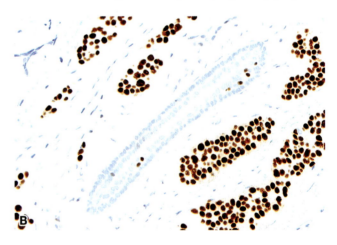

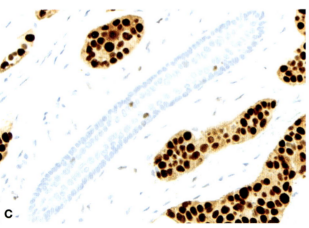

FIGURE 9.18 Invasive Ductal Carcinoma (IDC), Estrogen Receptor (ER) and Progesterone Receptor (PR) Immunostains. A: IDC around an inactive native duct. **B:** The ER stain shows strong and diffuse (>99%) staining in the invasive carcinoma. **C:** The PR stain, likewise, shows strong and diffuse (>99%) staining in the invasive carcinoma. The inactive epithelial cells in the native duct (center) show scattered reactivity. There is no reactivity for ER and PR in the abluminal myoepithelial cells **(B, C)**.

TABLE 9.5

Surrogate Immunohistochemical Classification, Frequency, and Associated Germline Mutations for Gene Expression Profile–Based Intrinsic Subtypes of Invasive Carcinomas

	Luminal A	Luminal B	HER2	Basal-Like
ER	(+)	(+)	(−)	(−)
PR	(+)	(+/weak)	(−)	(−)
HER2	(−)	(+/−)	(+)	(−)
Ki-67	Low	High	higher	highest
Proportion[a]	~40%	~15%	~15%	~15%
Association with germline mutations	(−)	BRCA2	TP53	BRCA1

[a]Proportion/frequency of cases in all invasive breast carcinomas. These four major types of invasive carcinoma based on ER, PR, HER2, and Ki-67 largely correlate with the four groups of carcinoma classified per mRNA expression (with ~75% overlap in each group).

use of NCB for this purpose offers the advantage of better tissue fixation and lesser ischemic time. The issue of tumor heterogeneity is a legitimate consideration; however, in one study, less than 3% of invasive carcinomas were heterogeneous enough to affect testing for predictive factors (81). Numerous studies comparing results of ER, PR, and HER2 testing on initial NCBs and on the subsequent excisions have shown excellent agreement between the two types of specimens (81-85). Results of biomarker testing can serve as a surrogate for gene expression profile–based intrinsic subtyping of invasive carcinomas **(Table 9.5)**.

Biomarker testing should be repeated on the excisional biopsy specimen in the following situations: (a) whenever there is a substantial time interval (ie, >6 months) between the NCB and the excision, (b) whenever there is intervening endocrine modulation therapy or chemotherapy, (c) whenever the grade of the invasive carcinoma is higher in the excision, and (d) whenever there is any reason to question the reliability of biomarker testing in the antecedent NCB (ie, poor fixation, questionable controls, etc.).

NCBs can also be used for genomic assays, including *Oncotype DX* (86). The latter test requires the presence of more than 1 mm of IDC in an NCB sample. The test not only provides prognostic information in terms of 10-year distant recurrence rate and predicts the likelihood of the benefit conferred by adjuvant chemotherapy in ER-positive invasive carcinomas but also provides the results of ER, PR, and HER2 results. The *Oncotype DX* results are based on the expression of a panel of 21 genes (including 16 cancer-related and 5 reference genes) on reverse transcription–polymerase chain reaction (RT-PCR) (and not on in situ hybridization). HER2 results based on RT-PCR testing, as reported by *Oncotype DX*, have generated controversy (87,88). *Mammaprint*, another genomic test, requires a minimum of 9 mm^2 of IDC in an NCB.

NEOADJUVANT CHEMOTHERAPY

Neoadjuvant chemotherapy has not been shown to improve overall survival compared with conventional adjuvant chemotherapy; however, the possibility of "downstaging" or elimination ("complete pathologic response") of the primary invasive carcinoma using this approach potentially reduces the need for mastectomy and axillary lymph node dissection. Thus, neoadjuvant chemotherapy can decrease the morbidity of extensive surgery, without compromising outcome. The objective of minimally invasive ablative techniques is to eradicate an invasive carcinoma by nonsurgical means. In the event that the carcinoma is entirely removed by these means, NCB may be the only diagnostic tissue that will ever be available to assess the histopathologic, immunohistochemical, and molecular pathologic characteristics of the invasive carcinoma.

At a minimum, pathologic information that must be available before the initiation of treatment includes diagnosis of IDC and its grade and type. ER, PR, and HER2 test results must also be available. In some cases, results of genomic assay (Oncotype DX, Mammaprint, etc.) obtained on NCB material could influence clinical decision-making. Every effort should be made to conserve as much tissue as possible in obtaining sections for these tests. In view of the foregoing, the practice of routinely obtaining multiple H&E-stained levels without saving intervening sections should be discontinued.

Selection of cases most likely to benefit from preoperative chemotherapy, and the development of personalized approaches based on the degree of response, is critical and is the subject of ongoing clinical trials. There is evidence suggesting that neoadjuvant endocrine and chemotherapy may not have a significant beneficial impact on the surgical treatment of invasive lobular carcinoma—usually a carcinoma with low proliferation rate; however, this subject also continues to be under investigation (89).

Of note, neoadjuvant chemotherapy as well as techniques of minimally invasive tumor ablation (such as radiofrequency ablation and cryoablation) rely on NCB for providing an unequivocal diagnosis of IDC.

TUMOR-INFILTRATING LYMPHOCYTES

Medullary carcinoma, characterized by prominent lymphocytic response as well as circumscription, syncytial growth, and high-grade nuclei, was first described in 1949 (90). Since then, the role of "tumor-infiltrating lymphocytes" (TIL) has been regarded as a major factor in influencing better prognosis of mammary carcinomas with an associated lymphocytic reaction (91). Pretherapy NCB provides an excellent substrate for the assay of predictive factors that could identify patients who would benefit most from several types of neoadjuvant chemotherapy. In this context, TIL has generated considerable interest and promise based on evidence that the likelihood and degree of response is directly related to the abundance of TIL **(Fig. 9.19)** (92-95).

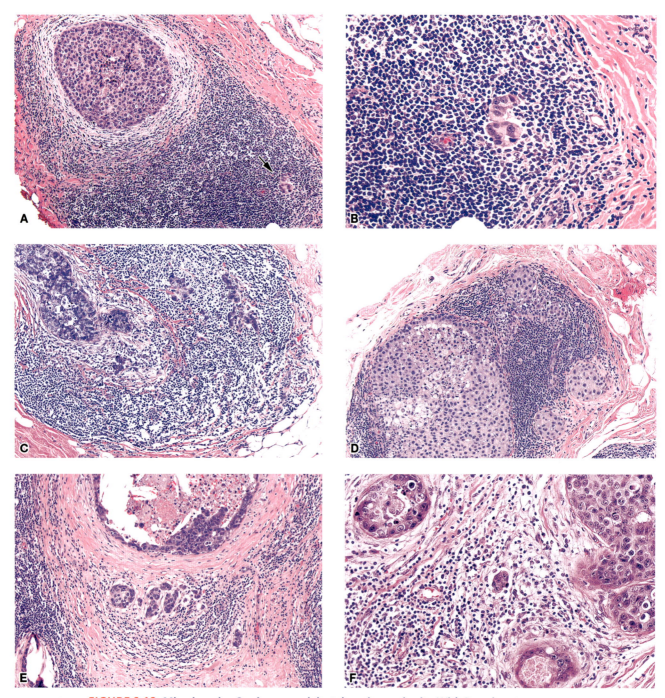

FIGURE 9.19 Microinvasive Carcinoma and ductal carcinoma in situ With Prominent Lymphoplasmacytic Infiltration. A-F: Needle core biopsies show five examples of microinvasive carcinomas (**A, B:** shows one lesion, **C-F:** each shows one lesion). Each microinvasive focus is associated with a marked peri- and intralesional lymphoplasmacytic inflammatory cell infiltrate.

Recommendations for a "pragmatic starting point" for the standardized evaluation of TIL in invasive breast carcinomas first appeared in 2014 and have continued unabated (92,96).

TIL may coexist with "tertiary lymphoid structures," which are peculiar lymph node–like structures characterized by lymphoid aggregates with venules lined by plump endothelial cells (94,97). Particularly abundant TILs are a feature of *BRCA* mutation–associated breast carcinomas—both carcinomas associated with better response to neoadjuvant chemotherapy (98). Given the potential significance of TIL, it has been suggested that "pathologists should perhaps get used to reporting this parameter as a part of the standard histological description of breast cancer" (99).

CHANGES AFTER NEOADJUVANT ENDOCRINE AND CHEMOTHERAPY

Neoadjuvant endocrine and chemotherapy are increasingly being utilized as treatment options for appropriately selected larger IDCs **(Table 9.6)**. In some clinical situations, sequential NCBs may be used to assess treatment response. The reporting of such specimens should include dimensions of "tumor bed," presence of residual invasive carcinoma, its histopathologic type, grade, cellularity (relative to that observed in preneoadjuvant chemotherapy sampling), presence or absence of LVI, DCIS, and so on (100). Of note, the tumor bed typically displays dense reparative-type stromal fibrosis rather than tumoral necrosis **(Fig. 9.20)**.

MOLECULAR CLASSIFICATION

"Intrinsic subtypes" of invasive breast carcinoma, including those of IDC, utilizing microarray-based gene expression profiling (101) were described in 2000. Four basic subtypes (ie, luminal, basal-like, HER2-positive, and normal-like) were initially described. Later, the luminal tumors were divided into A and B groups. The "normal-like" subtype is now considered to be the result of contamination of samples by nonneoplastic tissue rather than an authentic subtype.

Luminal A tumors are ER-positive, PR-positive, and HER2-negative and are of low grade. **Luminal B** tumors are ER-positive, PR-positive or -negative, and HER2-positive or -negative and are of a higher grade with a relatively higher proliferation rate based on Ki-67 **(Table 9.7)**.

TABLE 9.6
Histopathologic Changes in Invasive Ductal Carcinoma After Chemotherapy, Endocrine Therapy, and Radiation

Changes Post Chemotherapy

Vacuolization of tumor cells simulating histiocytes
Atrophy of terminal duct lobular units, with occasional atypia
The "tumor bed" is characterized by stromal fibrosis and hyalinization, lymphohistiocytic infiltrate, macrophages, hemosiderin deposits, and capillary proliferation

Changes Post Endocrine Therapy

Degenerative changes in tumor cells: nuclear aberrations, cytoplasmic vacuoles, cell membrane rupture, eventual necrosis. Changes can be patchy. Altered cells exist with non-altered cells.
Stromal fibrosis and hyalinization (scarring)
Downgrading of grade (in about a third of cases)
Change of hormone receptor (rare) and HER2 expression (rarer)

Changes Post Radiation Therapy
In breast carcinoma:

Giant tumor cells
Bizarre nuclear changes
"Naked" nuclei
Abnormal mitotic figures
Cytoplasmic vacuolization
Tumor necrosis and fibrosis post necrosis

In non-carcinomatous breast:

Lobular sclerosis and atrophy
Isolated nuclear atypia in epithelial cells of terminal ductules and in endothelial and stromal cells

Radiation-related changes persist for years.

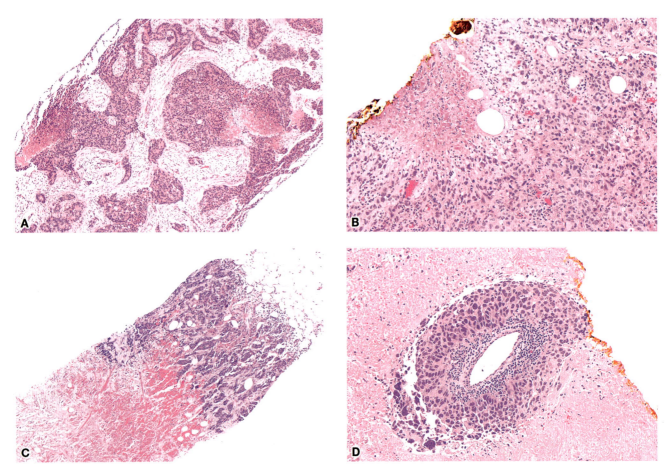

FIGURE 9.20 Invasive Ductal Carcinoma (IDC) With Necrosis. A-D: Needle core biopsies with varying degrees of necrosis. Tumoral necrosis is focally evident in **(A)** (and is increasingly prominent in **B-D**). **D:** The IDC is viable only around the blood vessel (center). The tumor shows a pseudopapillary appearance. None of these cases are status-post chemotherapy.

TABLE 9.7

Typical Treatment Response and Outcome in Major Molecular Categories of Breast Carcinoma

Luminal, A and B	
Typical treatment response	Variable response to endocrine therapy Variable response to chemotherapy, more to luminal B Pathologic complete response: <10%
Outcome	Type A: relapse rate low, but continuous <20 years Type B: relapse rate low (~4 years), higher late (~8 years) Late (>8 years) relapses uncommon Prognosis favorable for luminal A Prognosis less favorable for luminal B
HER2	
Typical treatment response	Responsive to anti-HER2 therapy Responsive to anthracycline-based chemotherapy Pathologic complete response: <60%
Outcome	Relapses peak early (~4 years) and peak late (~8 years) Poor prognosis

INVASIVE DUCTAL CARCINOMA **203**

TABLE 9.7

Typical Treatment Response and Outcome in Major Molecular Categories of Breast Carcinoma (*continued*)

Basal-like (including "triple-negative")[a]	
Typical treatment response	Not responsive to endocrine therapy Not responsive to anti-HER2 therapy May respond to platinum-based chemotherapy May respond to PARP inhibitors Pathologic complete response: 30%
Outcome	Relapses early (<4 years) Late (>8 years) relapses uncommon Poor prognosis

[a]Including some tumors with adenoid cystic carcinoma and secretory carcinoma: under investigation. PARP: Poly (ADP-ribose) polymerase is a group of proteins involved in DNA repair, genomic stability, and programmed cell death. References for latter: Bertucci F, Finetti P, Goncalves A, Birnbaum D. The therapeutic response of ER+/HER2− breast cancers differs according to the molecular basal or luminal subtype. *NPJ Breast Cancer.* 2020;6:8. 32195331, and Coleman WB, Anders CK. Discerning clinical responses in breast cancer based on molecular signatures. *Am J Pathol.* 2017;187:2199-2207.

A rare subset of luminal B tumors is "triple-positive" (ie, ER-positive, PR-positive, and HER2-positive). The minimum Ki-67 value required by most of the 2015 St. Gallen panel members for luminal B categorization was at least 20 (102). The two luminal subtypes differ in their genomic makeup, genetic alterations, and prognosis. Patients with luminal A tumors have better survival rates when compared with other groups (103).

The ER-negative groups include the basal-like and HER2-positive subtypes. The **basal-like** tumors are characterized by "triple-negativity" (ie, ER-negative, PR-negative, and HER2-negative) and immunoreactivity for high-molecular-weight cytokeratins as well as for epidermal growth factor receptor (EGFR). Attention has centered on CK5, CK5/6, CK14, and CK17, which have been referred to as "basal cytokeratins" owing to their localization mainly in the basal (myoepithelial) layer of the two-layered (ie, epithelial and myoepithelial) normal breast glands. Tumors that belong to this group have a high proliferation rate, are high grade, and, not surprisingly, display aggressive clinical behavior. The greatest molecular and clinical differences are between basal-like tumors and other subtypes (104,105). The **HER2** group is defined by high expression of HER2 and related genes. Several subtypes that are associated with different phenotypes as well as outcomes exist within the HER2 group. Tumors that are HER2-positive and ER-positive typically belong to the luminal B group.

Several additional subtypes (including claudin-low, molecular apocrine, and interferon-related) have been additionally described. **Claudin-low** tumors are usually also triple-negative and may show metaplastic or "medullary-like" differentiation (106). Survival rates for this group lie between those for luminal- and basal-like tumors.

Molecular apocrine group of tumors are ER-negative and androgen receptor (AR)-positive, and their constituent cells display apocrine cytologic features (107). These tumors may be HER2-positive or HER2-negative. The **interferon-related** group shows high expression of interferon-associated genes—including *STAT1* (103). The clinical significance of these more recently described subtypes remains to be established.

Gene expression profiling of breast carcinomas is used mainly in research settings. This sophisticated technique is of limited practical utility in clinical practice, because it is prohibitive in terms of time, effort, and cost. Some commercially available genomic tests—including the Blueprint 80-gene signature test—identify the intrinsic molecular subtypes of early-stage invasive carcinomas by assessing specific gene expression signatures of signaling pathways driving these molecular subtypes (basal-, luminal-, and HER2 type). Immunohistochemical surrogates for gene expression profile–based intrinsic subtypes have been developed. ER, PR, and HER2 are critical to these surrogate profiles. Ki-67 appears to be a useful discriminator between luminal A and B groups. The addition of CK5/6 and EGFR is helpful in identifying the basal-like type of tumors **(Fig. 9.21)** (104,105).

Surrogate immunohistochemical profiling overlaps, for the most part, with gene expression profiling; however, it does not replace it. The immunohistochemically characterized "triple-negative" carcinomas and gene expression–profiled "basal-like" carcinomas have some commonality; however, the two terms are not synonymous. A carcinoma cannot be identified as having the "basal-like" phenotype solely on the basis of "triple-negative" marker status. Not all triple-negative tumors express basal cytokeratins, and a subset of basal-like

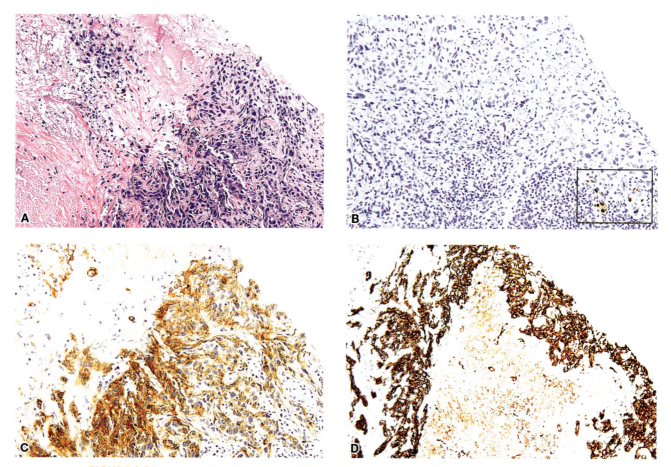

FIGURE 9.21 Invasive Ductal Carcinoma (IDC), Triple-Negative, and Basal-Like Immunophenotype. **A:** This needle core biopsy from a 30-year-old woman shows an IDC, poorly differentiated, associated with prominent lymphocytic infiltration and central necrosis. The latter two features are commonly found in triple-negative and basal-like carcinomas. The carcinoma expressed neither estrogen receptor (ER) nor progesterone receptor (PR). Human epidermal growth factor receptor 2 immunostain was negative (0, on a scale of 0 to 3+). **B:** ER reactivity is evident in the nuclei of nonneoplastic lobular cells (box). The carcinoma was immunoreactive for CK5/6 **(C)** and epidermal growth factor receptor **(D)**.

carcinomas are not triple-negative (108,109). In this respect, a discordance rate of up to 30% has been reported (110,111). Nevertheless, the role of "surrogate profiling," particularly with respect to "high" proliferation rate and "low-ER" status, continues to evolve with respect to implications for management (112).

MANAGEMENT OF INVASIVE DUCTAL CARCINOMA

The therapeutic options available for IDC, indeed of all invasive and noninvasive carcinomas, of the breast are "complex and varied" (113). Please visit the National Comprehensive Cancer Network's website, www.nccn.org (and other sources, eg, St. Gallen International Breast Cancer Conference) for the most current clinical practice guidelines—including those regarding endocrine, chemo-, radio-, and immune-therapies (113).

NOTE OF CAUTION

A variety of sclerosing lesions, including sclerosing adenosis, radial scar, subareolar sclerosing ductal hyperplasia, and sclerosing papilloma, can simulate IDC, particularly in NCB material. *It is prudent to establish the diagnosis of IDC via appropriate myoepithelial immunostains in all cases wherein the findings are equivocal* **(Fig. 9.22)**.

INVASIVE DUCTAL CARCINOMA 205

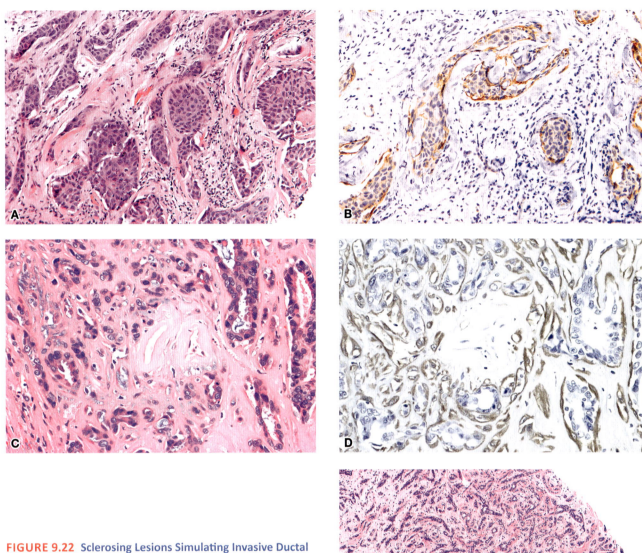

FIGURE 9.22 Sclerosing Lesions Simulating Invasive Ductal Carcinoma (IDC). A, B: A benign complex sclerosing lesion mimicking IDC in a needle core biopsy **(A)**. Smooth muscle actin immunostain highlights myoepithelial cells around the lesional glands **(B)**. **C, D:** Sclerosing adenosis mimicking IDC **(C)**. Smooth muscle myosin heavy chain immunostain highlights myoepithelial cells around the lesional glands **(D)**. **E:** Tubular adenosis simulating a well-differentiated IDC. Note proliferation of uniform appearing "tubules" with a relatively symmetric distribution.

REFERENCES

1. Lakhani SR, Ellis IO, Schnitt SJ, et al. *WHO Classification of Breast Tumors*. 4th ed. IARC Press; 2012.
2. Allison KH, Brogi E, Ellis IO, et al. *Microinvasive Carcinoma WHO Classification of Tumours of the Breast*. 5th ed. IARC Press; 2019.
3. Esposito NN, Chivukula M, Dabbs DJ. The ductal phenotypic expression of the E-cadherin/catenin complex in tubulolobular carcinoma of the breast: an immunohistochemical and clinicopathologic study. *Mod Pathol*. 2007;20:130-138.
4. Brunner AH, Sagmeister T, Kremer J, et al. The accuracy of frozen section analysis in ultrasound-guided core needle biopsy of breast lesions. *BMC Cancer*. 2009;9:341.
5. Kehl S, Mechler C, Menton S, et al. Touch imprint cytology of core needle biopsy specimens for the breast and quick stain procedure for immediate diagnosis. *Anticancer Res*. 2014;34:153-157.
6. Wauters CA, Sanders-Eras MC, de Kievit.van der Heijden IM, et al. Modified core wash cytology (CWC), an asset in the diagnostic work-up of breast lesions. *Eur J Surg Oncol*. 2010;36:957-962.
7. Manion E, Brock JE, Raza S, et al. MRI-guided breast needle core biopsies: pathologic features of newly diagnosed malignancies. *Breast J*. 2014;20:453-460.
8. Ginter PS, Winant AJ, Hoda SA. Cystic apocrine hyperplasia is the most common finding in MRI detected breast lesions. *J Clin Pathol*. 2014;67:182-186.
9. Sung JS, Jochelson MS, Brennan S, et al. MR imaging features of triple-negative breast cancers. *Breast J*. 2013;19:643-649.
10. Yamaguchi R, Tanaka M, Mizushima Y, et al. "High-grade" central acellular carcinoma and matrix-producing carcinoma of the breast: correlation between ultrasonographic findings and pathological features. *Med Mol Morphol*. 2011;44:151-157.

11. Seidman JD, Schnaper LA, Aisner SC. Relationship of the size of the invasive component of the primary breast carcinoma to axillary lymph node metastasis. *Cancer.* 1995;75:65-71.
12. Varma S, Ozerdem U, Hoda SA. Complexities and challenges in the pathologic assessment of size (T) of invasive breast carcinoma. *Adv Anat Pathol.* 2014;21:420-432.
13. Say CC, Donegan WL. Invasive carcinoma of the breast: prognostic significance of tumor size and involved axillary lymph nodes. *Cancer.* 1974;34:468-471.
14. Smart CR, Myers MH, Gloecker LA. Implications for SEER data on breast cancer management. *Cancer.* 1978;41:787-789.
15. Weaver DL, Rosenberg RD, Barlow WE. Pathologic findings from the breast cancer surveillance consortium: population-based outcomes in women undergoing biopsy after screening mammography. *Cancer.* 2006;106:732-742.
16. Rosen PP, Saigo PE, Braun DW Jr, et al. Predictors of recurrence in stage I ($T_1N_0M_0$) breast carcinoma. *Ann Surg.* 1981;193:15-25.
17. Rosen PP, Saigo PE, Braun DW Jr, et al. Prognosis in stage II ($T_1N_1M_0$) breast cancer. *Ann Surg.* 1981;194:576-584.
18. Elkin EB, Hudis C, Begg CB, et al. The effect of changes in tumor size on breast carcinoma survival in the U.S.: 1975-1999. *Cancer.* 2005;104;1149-1157.
19. Renshaw AA. Minimal (<0.1 cm) invasive carcinoma in breast core needle biopsies. *Arch Pathol Lab Med.* 2004;128:996-999.
20. Charles M, Edge SB, Winston JS, et al. Effect of stereotactic core needle biopsy on pathologic measurement of tumor size of T1 invasive breast carcinomas presenting as mammographic masses. *Cancer.* 2003;97:2137-2141.
21. Rakha EA, El-Sayed ME, Reed J, et al. Screen-detected breast lesions with malignant needle core biopsy diagnoses and no malignancy identified in subsequent surgical excision specimens (potential false-positive diagnosis). *Eur J Cancer.* 2009;45:1162-1167.
22. Edwards HD, Oakley F, Koyama T, et al. The impact of tumor size in breast needle biopsy material on final pathologic size and tumor stage: a detailed analysis of 222 consecutive cases. *Am J Surg Pathol.* 2013;37:739-744.
23. Edge SB, Byrd DR, Compton CC, et al, eds. *American Joint Committee on Cancer Staging Manual.* 7th ed. Springer-Verlag; 2010.
24. Ozerdem U, Hoda SA. Correlation of maximum breast carcinoma dimension on needle core biopsy and subsequent excisional biopsy: a retrospective study of 50 nonpalpable imaging-detected cases. *Pathol Res Pract.* 2014;210:603-605.
25. Berg WA, Gutierrez L, Ness-Aiver MS, et al. Diagnostic accuracy of mammography, clinical examination, US, and MR imaging in preoperative assessment of breast cancer. *Radiology.* 2004;233:830-849.
26. Thomassin-Naggara I, Siles P, Trop I, et al. How to measure breast cancer tumoral size at MR imaging? *Eur J Radiol.* 2013;82:e790-e800.
27. Yeh E, Slantez P, Kopans SB, et al. Prospective comparison of mammography, sonography, and MRI in patients undergoing neoadjuvant chemotherapy for palpable breast cancer. *AJR Am J Roentgenol.* 2005;184:868-877.
28. Schouten van der Velden AP, Boetes C, Bult P, et al. Magnetic resonance imaging in size assessment of invasive breast carcinoma with an extensive intraductal component. *BMC Med Imaging.* 2009;9:5.
29. Bloom HJ, Richardson WW. Histological grading and prognosis in breast cancer: a study of 1,049 cases, of which 359 have been followed 15 years. *Br J Cancer.* 1957;11:359-377.
30. Elston CW, Ellis IO. Pathological prognostic factors in breast cancer. I. The value of histological grade in breast cancer: experience from a large study with long-term follow-up. *Histopathology.* 1991;19:403-410.
31. Robbins P, Pinder S, de Klerk N, et al. Histological grading of breast carcinomas: a study of interobserver agreement. *Hum Pathol.* 1995;26:873-879.
32. Kwok TC, Rakha EA, Lee AH. Histological grading of breast cancer on needle core biopsy: the role of immunohistochemical assessment of proliferation. *Histopathology.* 2010;57:212-219.
33. O'Shea AM, Rakha EA, Hodi Z, et al. Histological grade of invasive carcinoma of the breast assessed on needle core biopsy—modifications to mitotic count assessment to improve agreement with surgical specimens. *Histopathology.* 2011;59:543-548.
34. Harris GC, Denley HE, Pinder SE, et al. Correlation of histologic prognostic factors in core biopsies and therapeutic excisions of invasive breast carcinoma. *Am J Surg Pathol.* 2003;27:11-15.
35. Sharifi S, Peterson MK, Baum JK, et al. Assessment of pathologic prognostic factors in breast core needle biopsies. *Mod Pathol.* 1999;12:941-945.
36. Andrade VP, Gobbi H. Accuracy of typing and grading invasive mammary carcinomas on core needle biopsy compared with the excisional specimen. *Virchows Arch.* 2004;445:597-602.
37. Ough M, Velasco J, Hieken TJ. A comparative analysis of core needle biopsy and final excision for breast cancer: histology and marker expression. *Am J Surg.* 2011;201:692-694.
38. Zheng J, Alsaadi T, Blaichman J, et al. Invasive ductal carcinoma of the breast: correlation between tumor grade determined by ultrasound-guided core biopsy and surgical pathology. *AJR Am J Roentgenol.* 2013;200:W71-W74.
39. Dhaliwal CA, Graham C, Loane J. Grading of breast cancer on needle core biopsy: does a reduction in mitotic count threshold improve agreement with grade on excised specimens? *J Clin Pathol.* 2014;67:1106-1108.
40. Dawson PJ, Ferguson DJ, Karrison T. The pathologic findings of breast cancer in patients surviving 25 years after radical mastectomy. *Cancer.* 1982;50:2131-2138.
41. LeDoussal V, Tubiana-Hulin M, Friedman S, et al. Prognostic value of histologic grade/nuclear components of Scarff-Bloom-Richardson (SBR): an improved score modification based on a multivariate analysis of 1262 invasive ductal carcinomas. *Cancer.* 1989;64:1914-1921.
42. Locker A, Ellis IO, Morgan DA, et al. Factors influencing local recurrence after excision and radiotherapy for primary breast cancer. *Br J Surg.* 1989;76:890-894.
43. Nixon AJ, Schnitt SJ, Gelman R, et al. Relationship of tumor grade to other pathologic features and to treatment outcome of patients with early stage breast carcinoma treated with breast-conserving therapy. *Cancer.* 1996;78:426-431.
44. Karp SE, Tonin PN, Begin LR, et al. Influence of BRCA1 mutations on nuclear grade and estrogen receptor status of breast carcinoma in Ashkenazi Jewish women. *Cancer.* 1997;80:435-441.
45. Mavaddat N, Barrowdale D, Andrulis IL, et al. Pathology of breast and ovarian cancers among BRCA1 and BRCA2 mutation carriers: results from the Consortium of Investigators of Modifiers of BRCA1/2 (CIMBA). *Cancer Epidemiol Biomarkers Prev.* 2012;21:134-147.
46. Gilchrist KW, Gould VE, Hirschl S, et al. Interobserver variation in the identification of breast carcinoma in intramammary lymphatics. *Hum Pathol.* 1982;13:170-172.
47. Rosen PP. Tumor emboli in intramammary lymphatics in breast carcinoma: pathologic criteria for diagnosis and clinical significance. *Pathol Annu.* 1983;18(pt 2):215-232.
48. Acs G, Dumoff KL, Solin LJ, et al. Extensive retraction artifact correlates with lymphatic invasion and nodal metastasis and predicts poor outcome in early stage breast carcinoma. *Am J Surg Pathol.* 2007;31:129-140.
49. Acs G, Paragh G, Chuang ST, et al. The presence of micropapillary features and retraction artifact in needle core biopsy material predicts lymph node metastasis in breast carcinoma. *Am J Surg Pathol.* 2009;33:202-210.
50. Koo JS, Jung WH, Kim H. Epithelial displacement into the lymphovascular space can be seen in breast core needle biopsy specimens. *Am J Clin Pathol.* 2010;133:781-787.
51. Saigo PE, Rosen PP. The application of immunohistochemical stains to identify endothelial-lined channels in breast carcinoma. *Cancer.* 1987;59:51-54.
52. Kahn HJ, Marks A. A new monoclonal antibody, D2-40, for detection of lymphatic invasion in primary tumors. *Lab Invest.* 2002;82:1255-1257.
53. Fukunaga M. Expression of D2-40 in lymphatic endothelium of normal tissues and in vascular tumors. *Histopathology.* 2005;46:396-402.
54. Miettinen M, Wang ZF, Paetau A, et al. ERG transcription factor as an immunohistochemical marker for vascular endothelial tumors and prostatic carcinoma. *Am J Surg Pathol.* 2011;35:432-441.
55. Van den Eynden GG, van der Auwera I, van Laere SJ, et al. Distinguishing blood and lymph vessel invasion in breast cancer: a prospective immunohistochemical study. *Br J Cancer.* 2006;94:1643-1649.
56. de Mascarel I, MacGrogan G, Debled M, et al. D2-40 in breast cancer: should we detect more vascular emboli? *Mod Pathol.* 2009;22:216-222.
57. Rabban JT, Chen Y-Y. D2-40 expression in breast myoepithelium: potential pitfalls in distinguishing intralymphatic carcinoma from in situ carcinoma. *Hum Pathol.* 2008;39:175-183.
58. Quiet CA, Ferguson DJ, Weichselbaum RR, et al. Natural history of node-positive breast cancer: the curability of small cancers with a limited number of positive nodes. *J Clin Oncol.* 1996;14:3105-3111.
59. Bettelheim R, Penman HG, Thornton-Jones H, et al. Prognostic significance of peritumoral vascular invasion in breast cancer. *Br J Cancer.* 1984;50:771-777.
60. Nime F, Rosen PP, Thaler H, et al. Prognostic significance of tumor emboli in intramammary lymphatics in patients with mammary carcinoma. *Am J Surg Pathol.* 1977;1:25-30.
61. Lauria R, Perrone F, Carlomagno C, et al. The prognostic value of lymphatic and blood vessel invasion in operable breast cancer. *Cancer.* 1995;76:1772-1778.
62. Clemente CG, Boracchi P, Andreola S, et al. Peritumoral lymphatic invasion in patients with node-negative mammary duct carcinoma. *Cancer.* 1992;69:1396-1403.
63. Liljegren G, Holmberg L, Bergh J, et al. 10-year results after sector resection with or without postoperative radiotherapy for stage I breast cancer: a randomized trial. *J Clin Oncol.* 1999;17:2326-2333.
64. Roses DF, Bell DA, Flotte TJ, et al. Pathologic predictors of recurrence in stage 1 ($T_1N_0M_0$) breast cancer. *Am J Clin Pathol.* 1982;78:817-820.
65. Hoda SA, Rosen PP. Contemporaneous H&E sections should be standard practice in diagnostic immunopathology. *Am J Surg Pathol.* 2007;31:1627.
66. Hoda SA, Hoda RS, Merlin S, et al. Issues relating to lymphovascular invasion in breast carcinoma. *Adv Anat Pathol.* 2006;13:308-315.
67. Rak JW, St Croix BD, Kerbel RS. Consequences of angiogenesis for tumor progression, metastasis and cancer therapy. *Anticancer Drugs.* 1995;6:3-18.
68. Vasudev NS, Reynolds AR. Anti-angiogenic therapy for cancer: current progress, unresolved questions and future directions. *Angiogenesis.* 2014;17:471-494.
69. de Jong JS, van Diest PJ, Baak JP. Methods in laboratory investigation: heterogeneity and reproducibility of microvessel counts in breast cancer. *Lab Invest.* 1995;73:922-926.
70. Karak SG, Quatrano N, Buckley J, et al. Prevalence and significance of perineural invasion in invasive breast carcinoma. *Conn Med.* 2010;74:17-21.
71. Tamura S, Enjoji M. Elastosis in neoplastic and non-neoplastic tissues from patients with mammary carcinoma. *Acta Pathol Jpn.* 1988;38:1537-1546.

72. Glaubitz LC, Bowen JH, Cox ED, et al. Elastosis in human breast cancer: correlation with sex steroid receptors and comparison with clinical outcome. *Arch Pathol Lab Med.* 1984;108:27-30.
73. Tramm T, Kim JY, Tavassoli FA. Diminished number or complete loss of myoepithelial cells associated with metaplastic and neoplastic apocrine lesions of the breast. *Am J Surg Pathol.* 2011;35:202-211.
74. Cserni G. Benign apocrine papillary lesions of the breast lacking or virtually lacking myoepithelial cells—potential pitfalls in diagnosing malignancy. *APMIS.* 2012;120:249-252.
75. Ross DS, Wen YH, Brogi E. Ductal carcinoma in situ: morphology-based knowledge and molecular advances. *Adv Anat Pathol.* 2013;20:205-216.
76. Schnitt SJ, Connolly JL, Harris JR, et al. Pathologic predictors of early local recurrences in stage I and II breast cancer treated by primary radiation therapy. *Cancer.* 1984;53:1049-1057.
77. Rosen PP, Kinne DW, Lesser ML, et al. Are prognostic factors for local control of breast cancer treated by primary radiotherapy significant for patients treated by mastectomy? *Cancer.* 1986;57:1415-1420.
78. Hurd TC, Sneige N, Allen PK, et al. Impact of extensive intraductal component on recurrence and survival in patients with stage I and II breast cancer treated with breast conservation therapy. *Ann Surg Oncol.* 1997;4:119-124.
79. Schnitt SJ, Abner A, Gelman R, et al. The relationship between microscopic margins of resection and the risk of local recurrence in patients with breast cancer treated with breast-conserving surgery and radiation therapy. *Cancer.* 1994;74:1746-1751.
80. Hicks DG, Fitzgibbons P, Hammond E. Core vs. breast resection specimen: does it make a difference for HER2 results? *Am J Clin Pathol.* 2015;144:533-535.
81. Arnould L, Roger P, Macgrogan G, et al. Accuracy of HER2 status determination on breast core-needle biopsies (immunohistochemistry, FISH, CISH and SISH vs FISH). *Mod Pathol.* 2012;25:675-682.
82. Petrau C, Clatot F, Cornic M, et al. Reliability of prognostic and predictive factors evaluated by needle core biopsies of large breast invasive tumors. *Am J Clin Pathol.* 2015;144:555-562.
83. Lee AH, Key HP, Bell JA, et al. Concordance of HER2 status assessed on needle core biopsy and surgical specimens of invasive carcinoma of the breast. *Histopathology.* 2012;60:880-884.
84. Chen X, Yuan Y, Gu Z, et al. Accuracy of estrogen receptor, progesterone receptor, and HER2 status between core needle and open excision biopsy in breast cancer: a meta-analysis. *Breast Cancer Res Treat.* 2012;134:957-967.
85. Hammond ME, Hicks DG. American Society of Clinical Oncology/College of American Pathologists HER2 testing clinical practice guideline upcoming modifications: proof that clinical practice guidelines are living documents. *Arch Pathol Lab Med.* 2015;139:970-971.
86. Markopoulos C. Overview of the use of Oncotype DX as an additional treatment decision tool in early breast cancer. *Expert Rev Anticancer Ther.* 2013;13:179-194.
87. Bartlett JM, Starczynski J. Quantitative reverse transcriptase polymerase chain reaction and the Oncotype DX test for assessment of human epidermal growth factor receptor 2 status: time to reflect again? *J Clin Oncol.* 2011;29:4219-4221.
88. Dabbs DJ, Klein ME, Mohsin SK, et al. High false-negative rate of HER2 quantitative reverse transcription polymerase chain reaction of the Oncotype DX test: an independent quality assurance study. *J Clin Oncol.* 2011;29:4279-4285.
89. Jakub JW, Zhang W, Solanki M, et al. Response rates of invasive lobular cancer in patients undergoing neoadjuvant endocrine or chemotherapy. *Am Surg.* 2023;89:230-237.
90. Moore OS Jr, Foote FW Jr. The relatively favorable prognosis of medullary carcinoma of the breast. *Cancer.* 1949;2:635-642.
91. Kuroda H, Tamaru J, Sakamoto G, et al. Immunophenotype of lymphocytic infiltration in medullary carcinoma of the breast. *Virchows Arch.* 2005;446:10-14.
92. Laenkholm AV, Callagy G, Balancin M, et al. Incorporation of TILs in daily breast cancer care: how much evidence can we bear? *Virchows Arch.* 2022;480:147-162.
93. Ocaña A, Diez-Gónzález L, Adrover E, et al. Tumor-infiltrating lymphocytes in breast cancer: ready for prime time? *J Clin Oncol.* 2015;33:1298-1299.
94. Lee HJ, Kim JY, Park IA, et al. Prognostic significance of tumor-infiltrating lymphocytes and the tertiary lymphoid structures in HER2-positive breast cancer treated with adjuvant trastuzumab. *Am J Clin Pathol.* 2015;144:278-288.
95. Ono M, Tsuda H, Shimizu C, et al. Tumor-infiltrating lymphocytes are correlated with response to neoadjuvant chemotherapy in triple-negative breast cancer. *Breast Cancer Res Treat.* 2012;132:793-805.
96. Salgado R, Denkert C, Demaria S, et al. The evaluation of tumor-infiltrating lymphocytes (TILs) in breast cancer: recommendations by an International TILs Working Group 2014. *Ann Oncol.* 2015;26:259-271.
97. Martinet L, Garrido I, Girard JP. Tumor high endothelial venules (HEVs) predict lymphocyte infiltration and favorable prognosis in breast cancer. *Oncoimmunology.* 2012;1:789-790.
98. Matsumoto H, Koo SL, Dent R, et al. Role of inflammatory infiltrates in triple negative breast cancer. *J Clin Pathol.* 2015;68:506-510.
99. Denkert C. Diagnostic and therapeutic implications of tumor-infiltrating lymphocytes in breast cancer. *J Clin Oncol.* 2013;31:836-837.
100. Provenzano E, Bossuyt V, Viale G, et al. Standardization of pathologic evaluation and reporting of postneoadjuvant specimens in clinical trials of breast cancer: recommendations from an international working group. *Mod Pathol.* 2015;28:1185-1201.
101. Perou CM, Søile T, Eisen MB, et al. Molecular portraits of human breast tumors. *Nature.* 2000;406:747-752.
102. Gnant M, Thomssen C, Harbeck N. St. Gallen/Vienna 2015: a brief summary of the consensus discussion. *Breast Care (Basel).* 2015;10:124-130.
103. Hu Z, Fan C, Oh DS, et al. The molecular portraits of breast tumors are conserved across microarray platforms. *BMC Genomics.* 2006;7:96.
104. Blows FM, Driver KE, Schmidt MK, et al. Subtyping of breast cancer by immunohistochemistry to investigate a relationship between subtype and short and long-term survival: a collaborative analysis of data for 10,159 cases from 12 studies. *PloS Med.* 2010;7:e1000279.
105. Green AR, Powe DG, Rakha EA, et al. Identification of key clinical phenotypes of breast cancer using a reduced panel of protein biomarkers. *Br J Cancer.* 2013;109:1886-1894.
106. Prat A, Parker JS, Karginova O, et al. Phenotypic and molecular characterization of the claudin-low intrinsic subtype of breast cancer. *Breast Cancer Res.* 2010;12:R68.
107. Farmer P, Bonnefoi H, Becette V, et al. Identification of molecular apocrine breast tumors by microarray analysis. *Oncogene.* 2005;24:4660-4671.
108. Reis-Filho JS, Tutt AN. Triple negative tumors: a critical review. *Histopathology.* 2008;52:108-118.
109. Rakha EA, Ellis IO. Triple negative/basal-like breast cancer: a review. *Pathology.* 2009;41:40-47.
110. Oakman C, Viale G, Di Leo A. Management of triple negative breast cancer. *Breast.* 2010;19:312-321.
111. Schmadeka R, Harmon BE, Singh M. Triple-negative breast carcinoma: current and emerging concepts. *Am J Clin Pathol.* 2014;141:462-477.
112. Coates AS, Winer EP, Goldhirsch A, et al. Tailoring therapies—improving the management of early breast cancer: St. Gallen International Expert Consensus on the Primary Therapy of Early Breast Cancer 2015. *Ann Oncol.* 2015;26:1533-1546.
113. National Comprehensive Cancer Network. Accessed March 22, 2023. www.nccn.org

Tubular Carcinoma

RAZA S. HODA AND SYED A. HODA

INTRODUCTION

Tubular carcinoma (TC) is a highly differentiated invasive ductal carcinoma (IDC) composed of at least 90% simple one-cell-layered neoplastic tubules with low-grade cytologic atypia (1). TC constitutes up to 2% of all breast carcinomas (2-6). It tends to have small size and is relatively more frequent among T1 tumors (5-15) and mammographically detected carcinomas (3,7,10,11,16,17). TC represents 3% to 4% of stage I and II breast carcinoma (9-11,15) and has an excellent prognosis (5-15).

CLINICAL PRESENTATION

TC usually occurs in peripheral portions of the breast. It rarely arises near the major lactiferous ducts of the nipple or in the subareolar region. Nipple discharge, Paget disease, and skin retraction are only rarely associated with TC.

Imaging

TC is frequently detected mammographically as a spiculated mass or an area of architectural distortion. In two recent series, TC constituted only 2% of interval carcinomas and of carcinomas found in women not participating in a mammographic screening program but constituted 8% of screen-detected carcinomas (3,16). In one study, the average radiographic size of nonpalpable TC was 0.8 cm and that of palpable lesions was 1.2 cm (18). TC often harbors calcifications. The main radiologic differential diagnosis of TC is radial sclerosing lesion (RSL, ie, "radial scar"). In particular, TC and RSL are indistinguishable radiologically, and TC can occasionally arise in a RSL (19,20). TC has no distinctive features by ultrasonography (5) or magnetic resonance imaging (21), compared with well-differentiated IDC. Because most TCs are detected by imaging studies, they are often the target of needle core biopsy (NCB) sampling.

Age, Ethnicity, and Gender

TC can occur at any age, but it is more common in postmenopausal women (5,6,8-15,17). A study based on SEER data for breast carcinomas diagnosed in the United States from 1992 to 2007 found that 73.6% of 4,477 TCs occurred in women 50 to 79 years old, 17.5% in women 40 to 49 years old, 6.9% in women older than 80 years, and only 2% in women 30 to 39 years old (4). Between 80% (22) and 90% (4) of TCs occur in non-Hispanic White women. TC constitutes less than 1% of male breast carcinomas (23).

Family History

A high frequency of breast carcinoma has been reported among first-degree relatives of women with TC. A study (10) found that 45% of patients with stage I or II TC had a family history of breast carcinoma, but this finding was not statistically significant compared with the 36% rate in a woman with IDC of similar stage. Rakha et al (11) reported a 20% rate of family history of breast carcinoma in women with TC. Family history of breast carcinoma in women with screen-detected carcinomas was associated with a relative risk of 1.71 for TC compared with 1.57 for any type of invasive carcinoma (24). A family history of breast carcinoma in a first-degree relative tripled the risk of TC in premenopausal women but was not significantly related to TC in postmenopausal patients (22). At least two studies have reported a 2- to 3-fold increase in the risk of TC in postmenopausal women who used hormone replacement therapy (22,25).

Size

Most TCs are 1 cm or smaller (7,9), but much larger tumors are also encountered. In one study (11), 59% of 102 TCs measured 1 cm or less, compared with only 30% of 212 IDC grade I; the median tumor size was also significantly smaller.

Multifocality

A few studies have documented multifocality in the setting of TC. In one study (26), 5% of 120 patients with TC treated by mastectomy had an additional and separate invasive carcinoma, and 3.3% had multifocal ductal carcinoma in situ (DCIS). In another study (27), invasive lobular carcinoma was identified in 7% of patients with TC. In a recent series (28), 9% of patients with TC had multifocal disease. A second invasive carcinoma of higher histologic grade was present in 15% of cases and consisted of moderately or poorly differentiated invasive ductal carcinoma in eight patients, an invasive lobular carcinoma in four patients, and a tubulolobular carcinoma in another patient. In another study (12), multifocal TC was identified in 9.7% of patients, including eight women with two foci each, one with four foci, and another patient with five foci. In general, it is not possible to comment on tumor multifocality when evaluating NCB material from a single radiologic target.

Contralateral Carcinoma

The reported frequency of contralateral carcinoma of any type in patients with TC ranges from 8% to 26% (5,10,29,30). Bilateral TC is uncommon (8,31-33). IDC is one of the most common types of contralateral carcinoma.

Histopathology

TC consists of a haphazard and infiltrative proliferation of small "tubule-like" glands lined by a single layer of neoplastic ductal epithelium with low-grade nuclear atypia **(Table 10.1)**. The diagnosis of TC applies only to lesions in which at least 90% of the tumor mass displays the aforementioned morphology **(Fig. 10.1)**. Multistratification of the neoplastic epithelium and/or complex glandular architecture is focal, if at all present **(Figs. 10.1 and 10.2)**. An IDC with low nuclear grade and tubular component representing less than 90% of the tumor is classified as a well-differentiated (grade I) IDC and does not carry the same excellent prognosis as a TC (11).

The tubules of TC have angular profile **(Fig. 10.1)**. Tear drop–shaped glands are common **(Fig. 10.2)**. The glandular lumen is usually widely patent, a feature best appreciated at low-power examination **(Figs. 10.1 and 10.2)**. The neoplastic epithelium lining the glands is either cuboidal or columnar. The neoplastic cells within a given lesion are usually homogeneous, but some variation in the height of the epithelium is often present, and nearly flat epithelium can be

found in continuity with columnar cells within an individual gland **(Fig. 10.2)**. The cytoplasm is relatively abundant and has amphophilic quality. Cytoplasmic snouts often protrude from the apical surface of the glandular epithelium of TC **(Fig. 10.2)**, but this finding is not exclusive to TC. Uncommon variants of TC feature mucin secretion **(Fig. 10.3)** or apocrine differentiation. Eosinophilic cytoplasm and apical intracytoplasmic granules characteristic of apocrine differentiation are usually not present in TC. The nuclei are basally located, round to oval, and show low-grade atypia, with even chromatin and a smooth nuclear membrane. Focally, intermediate-grade nuclei may be present. Nucleoli are inconspicuous or inapparent, and tend to be located adjacent to the nuclear membrane. Mitoses are rare, and necrosis is absent. Per Cserni, TCs "score 1+1+1 or at most 1+2+1 (3 or 4 overall) on the gland/tubule formation, nuclear pleomorphism, adjusted mitotic rate scheme" (34).

The stroma admixed with TC is rich in myofibroblasts and abundant elastic tissue, and myxoid matrix may also be encountered **(Figs. 10.1, 10.2, and 10.4)**. Stromal elements of TC tend to be more abundant than in well-differentiated IDC and separate the neoplastic glands more widely. Elastosis has been regarded as a histopathologic hallmark of TC **(Fig. 10.5)**, but it is not present in all cases, and it is often a prominent feature of RSL

Calcifications are detected microscopically in at least 50% of TC **(Fig. 10.6)**. They are present in the lumen of the neoplastic glands and in the tumoral stroma, or in the associated DCIS, atypical ductal hyperplasia (ADH), or columnar cell change (CCC). TC does not elicit a notable lymphocytic reaction. Lymphovascular involvement (LVI) is exceedingly rare (6,8,9,11), although artifactually displaced clusters of carcinoma can occasionally be identified in lymphovascular spaces in excision specimens after a needling procedure. Perineural invasion is extremely uncommon, especially in NCB samples.

Lesions Associated With Tubular Carcinoma

DCIS has been described in 21% to 41% of cases of TC (28,35,36). It usually has micropapillary, cribriform, or papillary architecture or a mixed pattern **(Fig. 10.7)**, and low- to intermediate-grade nuclei. TC is frequently associated with ADH and/or CCC (28,37) **(Figs. 10.8 and 10.9)**, a lesion previously designated informally as "pretubular" hyperplasia (38). The morphologic spectrum of columnar cell lesions ranges from CCC and columnar cell hyperplasia (CCH) without atypia through CCC and/or CCH with atypia, to ADH and low-grade DCIS. The term flat epithelial atypia (FEA) is also used to indicate atypical CCH (39). Apical snouts are present frequently at the luminal aspect of the epithelium showing CCC/CCH, but they are not exclusive to this alteration.

In CCH with atypia, the involved acini are cystically dilated and are lined by polarized cells showing slight nuclear enlargement, nuclear hyperchromasia, and increased

TABLE 10.1

Histopathologic Features of Tubular Carcinoma

Infiltrative "tubule-like," "tear drop," glands, with angular profiles
Glandular lumen patent
Single layer of neoplastic epithelium
Uniform columnar or cuboidal cells
Low-grade, round to oval, nuclei
Basally located nuclei
Even nuclear chromatin
Smooth nuclear membrane
Nucleoli inconspicuous
Mitoses rare, necrosis absent
Cytoplasmic snouts
Stroma rich in myofibroblasts, with elastosis
Calcifications in ~50%
Lymphovascular involvement rare
Perineural invasion rare
Negligible lymphocytic reaction

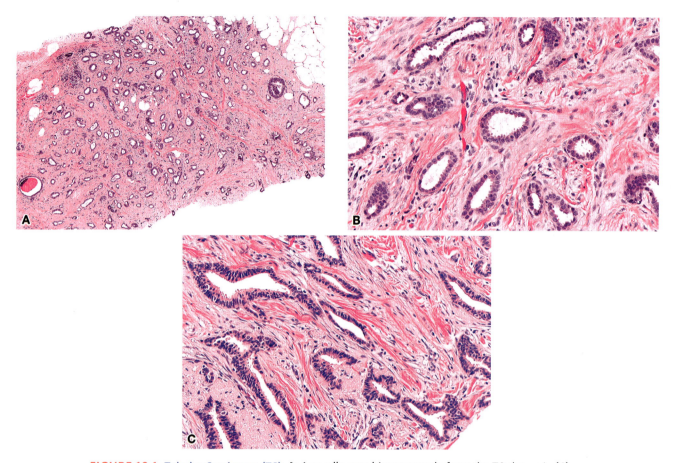

FIGURE 10.1 **Tubular Carcinoma (TC). A:** A needle core biopsy sample from the TC shown in **(C)**. **B:** The neoplastic glands are monostratified and embedded in the desmoplastic stroma. **C:** Note the angular profile of "tear drop"–shaped glands.

nuclear-to-cytoplasmic ratio. The cytoplasm tends to be abundant and has an amphophilic quality. The cells of atypical CCH have low-grade cytologic atypia, with round-to-oval nuclei, smooth nuclear membrane, and finely dispersed and homogeneous chromatin. The acini affected by CCC/CCH often contain dense secretions that can undergo calcification and are detected mammographically as fine punctate clustered calcifications. Blunt micropapillae, abortive cribriform spaces, and/or trabecular bars that alter the "flat" outline of the terminal duct lobular units (TDLUs) involved by atypical CCC constitute focal ADH.

ADH and DCIS with low nuclear grade and cribriform or micropapillary architecture often arise in the background of CCH with atypia (36,40). TC and columnar cell lesions are also often associated with classic lobular carcinoma in situ (LCIS) and atypical lobular hyperplasia (ALH)

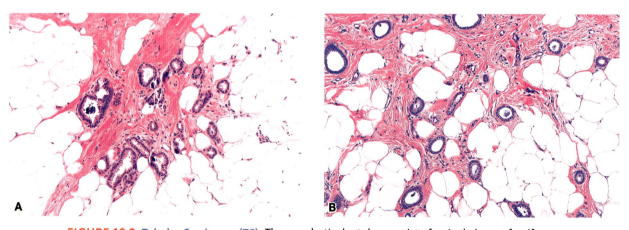

FIGURE 10.2 **Tubular Carcinoma (TC).** The neoplastic ductules consist of a single layer of uniform cuboidal cells. **A:** A normal terminal duct is shown on the left for contrast with the angular carcinomatous structures. **B:** This carcinoma is composed partly of glands with rounded shapes.

TUBULAR CARCINOMA 211

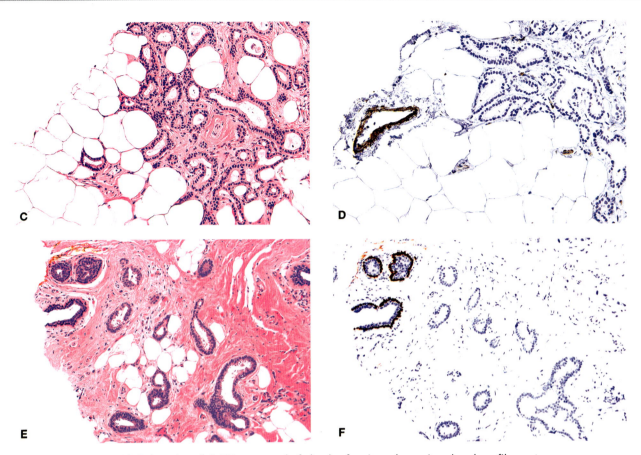

FIGURE 10.2 (*continued*) **C:** TC composed of glands of various shapes invades along fibrous trabeculae. **D:** Absence of myoepithelium is demonstrated by myosin immunostain. A blood vessel on the left is myosin-positive. **E:** TC invades fibroadipose tissue. **F:** Absence of myoepithelium is demonstrated by p63 immunostain.

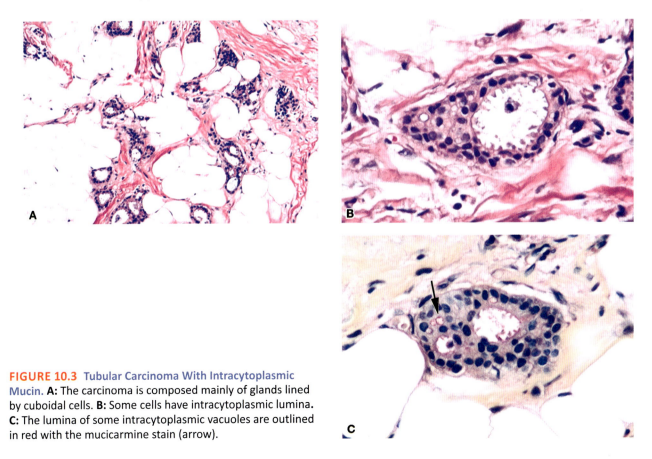

FIGURE 10.3 Tubular Carcinoma With Intracytoplasmic Mucin. A: The carcinoma is composed mainly of glands lined by cuboidal cells. **B:** Some cells have intracytoplasmic lumina. **C:** The lumina of some intracytoplasmic vacuoles are outlined in red with the mucicarmine stain (arrow).

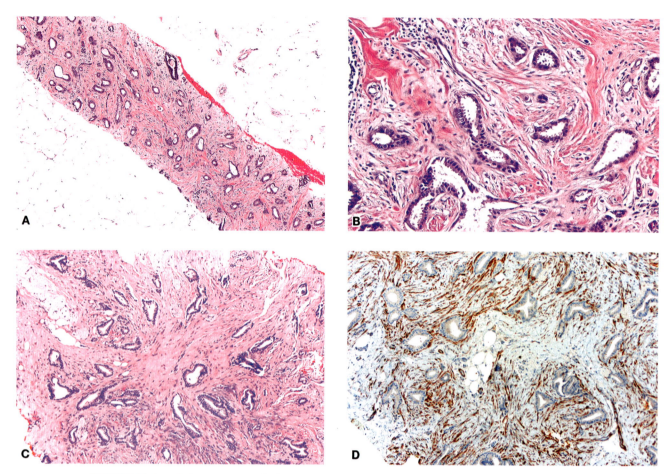

FIGURE 10.4 Tubular Carcinoma (TC) and Stromal Desmoplasia. A: The neoplastic glands of TC are admixed with abundant desmoplastic stroma in this needle core biopsy sample. **B:** At high-power examination, abundant desmoplastic stroma separates the neoplastic glands. Note the tear drop–shaped gland on the right and apical "snouts" around many neoplastic gland lumina. **C:** TC, with desmoplasia. **D:** Smooth muscle actin (SMA) highlights stromal myofibroblasts.

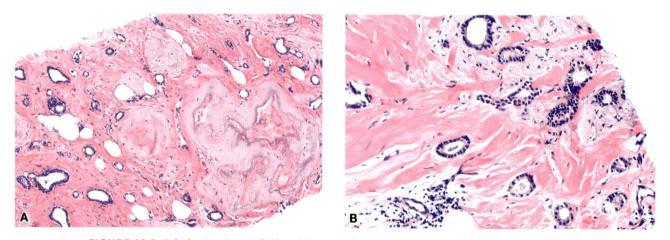

FIGURE 10.5 Tubular Carcinoma (TC) and Stromal Elastosis. A: The abundant elastotic stroma associated with this tubular carcinoma in a needle core biopsy sample simulates the elastotic core of a radial scar. The widely open lumina of the neoplastic glands are incompatible with a benign sclerosing lesion and support the diagnosis of TC. No myoepithelium was detected with immunostains for calponin and p63 (not shown). **B:** This NCB specimen from a nonpalpable tumor shows fibroelastotic tissue in the stroma of tubular carcinoma.

TUBULAR CARCINOMA **213**

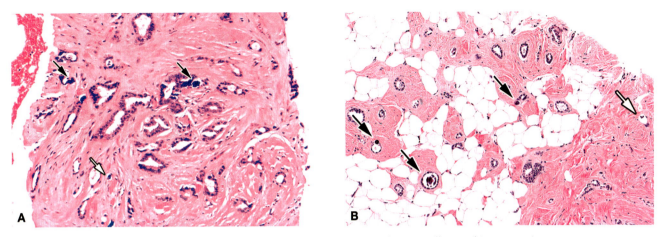

FIGURE 10.6 **Tubular Carcinoma and Calcifications. A, B:** These needle core biopsy specimens show small, evenly distributed glands with calcifications (black arrows). A minute stromal calcification is also present (white arrow).

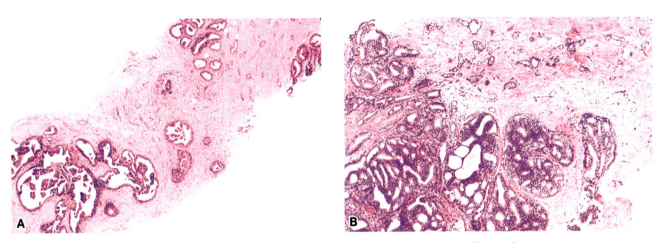

FIGURE 10.7 **Tubular Carcinoma (TC) With Intraductal Carcinoma.** Two-needle core biopsy specimens of TC (upper right) are shown. **A:** Papillary intraductal carcinoma. **B:** Cribriform intraductal carcinoma.

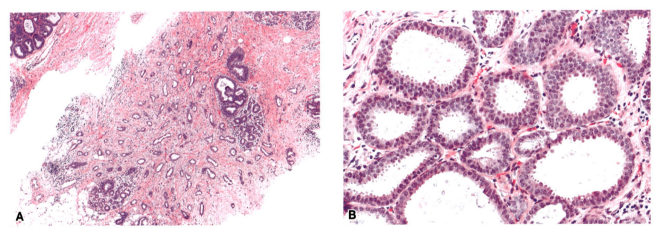

FIGURE 10.8 **Tubular Carcinoma (TC) and Columnar Cell Change. A:** In this needle core biopsy specimen, TC is accompanied by columnar cell change (CCC) with atypia. The carcinoma invades fat at the lower border. **B:** The acini involved by CCC with atypia are lined by a flat proliferation composed of two to three layers of the ductal epithelium with low-grade nuclear atypia. Many cells have apical cytoplasmic snouts protruding into the acinar lumina.

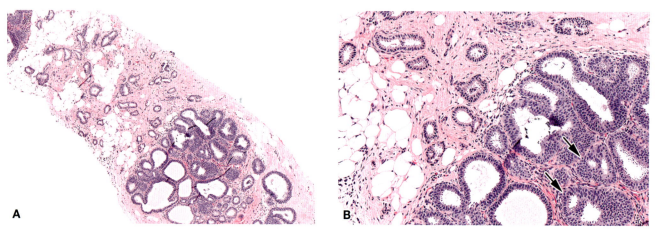

FIGURE 10.9 Tubular Carcinoma (TC) and Columnar Cell Change With Atypia. A: In this needle core biopsy specimen, TC is adjacent to lobules involved by columnar cell change with atypia. **B:** The haphazard and scattered distribution of the monostratified glands of the TC contrasts with the compact and lobulocentric arrangement of the cystic acini lined by multistratified columnar epithelium with low-grade nuclear atypia. Two glands with focal trabecular bars are diagnostic of atypical ductal hyperplasia (arrows).

(Figs. 10.10 and 10.11). This complex has been referred to as the "Rosen triad" (28) **(Fig. 10.11; Table 10.2)**. In a study of 14 TCs (35), 57% were associated with CCC with atypia (FEA), 50% with micropapillary ADH, 21% with low-grade DCIS, and 29% with ALH and/or classic LCIS. In a study of 102 TCs (11), TC was associated more frequently with columnar cell lesions (93%) than with usual ductal hyperplasia (UDH) (18%) or high-grade DCIS (1%). Columnar cell alterations coexisted with 89% of 27 TC in another series (36) and showed atypia in 22 cases; low-grade DCIS was present in 37% of cases. ALH and/or classic LCIS are/is found in 10% to 50% of cases of TC (11,28,35,36). These lesions are usually located near TC **(Figs. 10.10 and 10.11)** but can also occur separately in the ipsilateral or contralateral breast (also see section on Molecular Pathology).

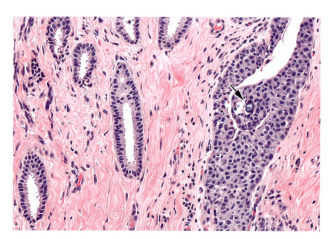

FIGURE 10.10 Tubular Carcinoma (TC) and Lobular Carcinoma In Situ (LCIS), Classic Type. TC glands (left) are adjacent to a focus of LCIS of the classic type in a duct (right). There is a calcification in the duct (arrow).

The identification of any of the aforementioned noninvasive lesions in an NCB specimen mandates careful evaluation to rule out the presence of TC and other low-grade invasive carcinomas. In particular, the proliferative nature of ADH and CCH, often coupled with ALH and/or classic LCIS, may distract from an inconspicuous focus on stromal invasion. In this setting, examination of the tissue cores at low-power magnification is helpful to identify foci of stromal desmoplasia containing the haphazardly distributed, widely patent, and irregular glands characteristic of TC. In contrast, acini involved by CCH with atypia retain a lobulocentric arrangement and are closely juxtaposed to one another with minimal intervening stroma. The acini of CCH with atypia have a cystic and open lumen, but the acinar profile has no angulated contour **(Fig. 10.9)**. At high magnification, CCC with atypia and TC show remarkable cytologic similarity, but the glands of TC have an irregular outline and are lined by the epithelium of variable height, devoid of myoepithelium and basement membrane. Clefts may be present around the glands of TC, at least focally **(Fig. 10.12)**. This morphologic feature, likely an artifact, is commonly associated with invasive carcinoma, whereas cleft-like spaces are usually not found around normal mammary epithelial structures and columnar cell lesions. Infiltration of the neoplastic glands into fat, with direct juxtaposition to adipocytes without intervening myoepithelium and basement membrane, is a feature associated with invasive carcinoma, including TC **(Fig. 10.12)**.

TC is characterized by a loss of **16q** (41). This chromosomal abnormality is also present in other low-grade mammary epithelial neoplastic lesions, namely CCH with atypia/FEA, ADH, low-grade DCIS, ALH and classic LCIS, well-differentiated IDC, and tubulolobular carcinoma (42). TC may also be associated with other benign proliferative lesions such as RSL (43,44).

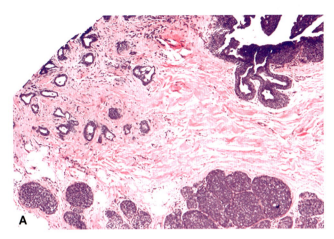
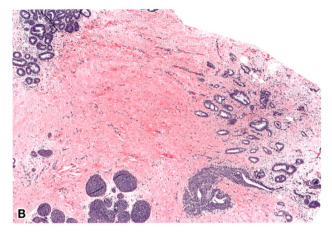
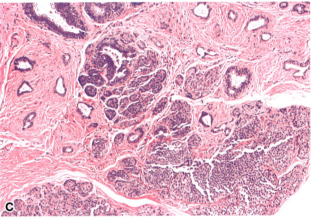

FIGURE 10.11 Tubular Carcinoma (TC), Lobular Carcinoma In Situ (LCIS), and Columnar Cell Change (Rosen Triad) in Needle Core Biopsy (NCB) Samples. **A:** The triad of TC (upper left), LCIS (center), and atypical columnar cell duct hyperplasia (lower left and lower right). **B:** Another example of the Rosen triad in which TC (right), LCIS (lower center), and columnar cell hyperplasia (CCH) (upper center) coexist in a NCB specimen. **C:** Yet another case of Rosen triad. LCIS (left), TC (center), and CCH (right).

Immunohistochemistry

The glands of TC lack a myoepithelial cell layer **(Figs. 10.12-10.14)**. Myosin and p63 are the most reliable myoepithelial markers for the diagnosis of stromal invasion. Staining for smooth muscle actin (SMA), albeit sensitive, is difficult to interpret because of substantial reactivity in the myofibroblasts comprising the desmoplastic stroma **(Fig. 10.13D)**. A commercially available cocktail of antibodies, that is, ADH5, targeting myoepithelial and epithelial antigens and optimized for dual chromogenic detection (brown chromogen: nuclear p63 and basal cytokeratins CK5 and CK14; red chromogen: luminal cytokeratins CK7 and CK18) **(Fig. 10.15)** might be particularly useful when the invasive carcinoma present in the NCB material is limited, but its sensitivity for the detection of TC has not been specifically investigated. The basement membrane is usually absent around the glands of TC. Immunostaining of basement membrane components is usually not recommended owing to difficulties in interpretation.

TABLE 10.2
The Rosen Triad

Tubular carcinoma
Lobular carcinoma in situ, almost always of the classic type
Columnar cell change/hyperplasia (almost always without atypia)

Biomarkers

More than 90% of TC are strongly and diffusely positive for estrogen receptor (ER) (6,9-13,15,17,29,45) **(Fig. 10.16)**. Progesterone receptor (PR) is detected in 69% to 75% of TC (10,11,15,45,46). All TCs studied by Rakha et al (11) were negative for HER2 and p53. Oakley et al (47) reported that none of the 55 TCs studied by fluorescence *in situ* hybridization exhibited *ERBB2* (HER2) gene amplification. Considering the bland histomorphology and indolent behavior of TC, it is recommended to carefully reassess the diagnosis for any carcinoma classified as TC that is found to be HER2 (+). TC is negative for S-100, CK5/6, and EGFR. Epithelial membrane antigen (EMA) decorates the luminal aspect of the cell membrane of the neoplastic epithelium.

Differential Diagnosis of Tubular Carcinoma

Well-differentiated Invasive Ductal Carcinoma

IDC (grade I) has complex architecture in more than 10% of the tumor and/or consists of glands with two or more cell layers **(Figs. 10.17 and 10.18)**. The outline of the glands of grade I IDC tends to be irregular and not as sharply defined as for a TC. The glands tend to be more clustered in some parts of the tumor and sparser in others, whereas the glands of TC are somewhat more evenly dispersed amid the desmoplastic stroma, despite having a haphazard distribution. The stroma of grade I IDC is often less cellular and abundant

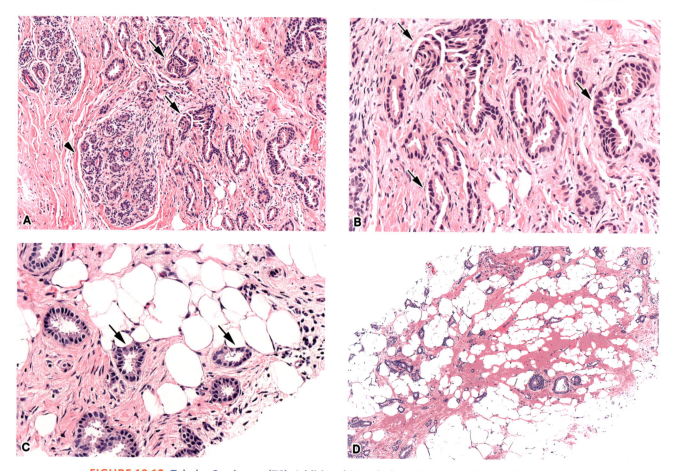

FIGURE 10.12 Tubular Carcinoma (TC), Additional Morphologic Features of Stromal Invasion.
A, B: Few cleft-like spaces adjacent to neoplastic glands, with no intervening basement membrane (arrows). Cleft-like spaces are not seen near normal glands and ducts, or a layer of the basement membrane is interposed between the cleft and the normal gland epithelium (arrowhead) **(A)**.
C: Small neoplastic glands that abut adipocytes (arrows) without an intervening basement membrane are diagnostic of stromal invasion. **D:** TC amid adipose tissue.

than in TC. Pure tubular morphology in an NCB sample does not guarantee that the rest of the lesion has the same morphology, and definitive diagnosis requires evaluation of the entire tumor **(see Tables 10.3-10.5)**.

Tubulolobular Carcinoma

A tubulolobular carcinoma is an invasive carcinoma with foci of tubular-like and invasive lobular-like growth patterns **(Fig. 10.19)**. The identification of neoplastic cells in linear

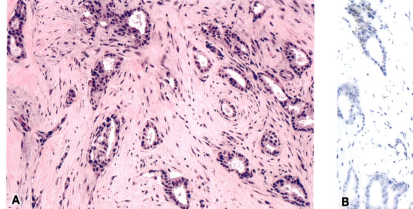
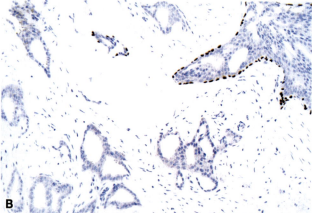

FIGURE 10.13 Tubular Carcinoma (TC), Immunohistochemistry. **A:** The tumor is composed of angular glands in the scleroelastotic stroma. **B:** Myoepithelial nuclei immunoreactive for p63 surround a duct with low-grade cribriform intraductal carcinoma in the upper right corner. p63 reactivity is not present around the glands of the TC.

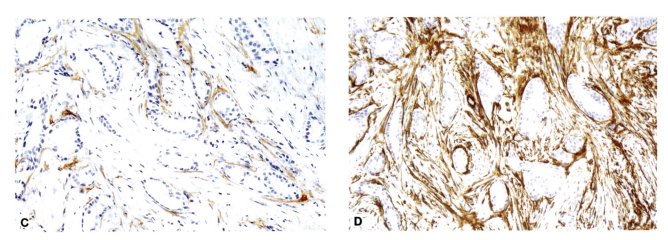

FIGURE 10.13 (*continued*) **C:** The CD10 immunostain shown here is difficult to interpret because of cross-reactivity with the stroma. The lack of discrete staining around the tumor glands suggests the absence of myoepithelium. **D:** The smooth muscle actin (SMA) immunostain shows strong stromal reactivity. The presence or absence of myoepithelium cannot be determined with the SMA stain in this situation.

arrays separates tubulolobular carcinoma from TC. Because the percentage of tubular and lobular components necessary for this diagnosis is not defined, the term is used inconsistently. Carcinomas with tubular and invasive lobular areas are part of the spectrum of low-grade epithelial mammary neoplasia (37,42) and are often associated with low-grade precursor lesions (48-50). Invasive carcinomas reported in the literature as tubulolobular range from 0.3 to 2.5 cm in greatest dimension (mean size about 1.3 cm) (48-50). Multifocality was noted in 19% (49) and 29% (48) of tubulolobular carcinoma versus 10% (49) and 20% (48) of TC in two studies. Tubulolobular carcinoma is strongly immunoreactive for ER and PR (48,50). It is only rarely HER2-positive (50). Most tubulolobular carcinomas show membranous reactivity for E-cadherin (49,50), a finding supportive of ductal differentiation thereof.

Microglandular Adenosis

Microglandular adenosis (MGA) (also see Chapter 6) is a rare benign epithelial lesion. MGA is an infiltrative proliferation of small glands lined by cytologically benign monostratified epithelium, devoid of myoepithelium, but surrounded by a basement membrane **(Fig. 10.20)**. The glands are small, round to oval, and have a smooth contour. The epithelium is cuboidal, has a uniform height within each individual gland, and has pale-to-clear cytoplasm. The lumen of the glands is open and often contains dense and homogenous eosinophilic secretions (which can rarely harbor calcifications). The stroma surrounding MGA shows neither desmoplasia nor any lymphocytic infiltrate. MGA may or may not be confined amid fibrous tissue and may extend into adipose tissue **(Fig. 10.20)**. MGA has been reported only in women. Surgical excision of a radiologic target that yields MGA at NCB is standard practice. TC can closely mimic MGA, but its glands tend to be open and angulated, and they are embedded in desmoplastic and/or elastotic stroma **(Fig. 10.21)**.

Sclerosing and/or Tubular Adenosis

Sclerosing adenosis (SA) is a lobulocentric proliferation of benign small glands and ductules in the sclerotic stroma.

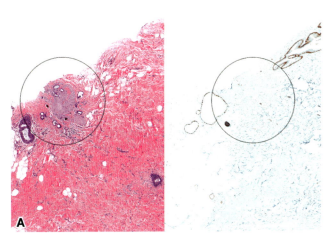
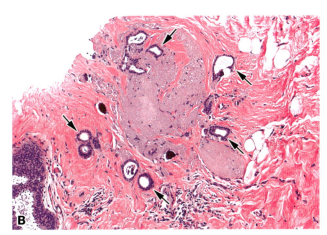

FIGURE 10.14 Tubular Carcinoma (TC), Immunohistochemistry. **A:** At low magnification view, this TC is barely noticeable as a few round small glands in a small focus of stromal elastosis (circle). The calponin stain highlights the myoepithelium in the normal ducts (right), but the TC shows no reactivity (circle). **B:** On closer examination, the neoplastic glands are cytologically bland (arrows). Stromal and glandular calcifications are present.

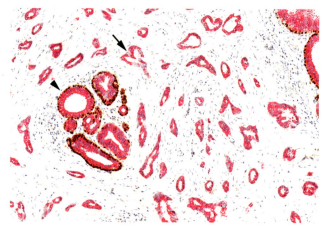

FIGURE 10.15 Tubular Carcinoma (TC), Immunohistochemistry. This image shows the pattern of staining of TC with a commercially available cocktail of antibodies for the detection of myoepithelial and epithelial markers in the same tissue section using two different chromogens. The brown chromogen highlights the nuclei (p63) and the cytoplasm (basal cytokeratin 5 and 14) of myoepithelial cells in normal glands (arrowhead). The red-pink chromogen for luminal cytokeratins 7 and 18 decorates the cytoplasm of the epithelial cells comprising normal ducts and lobules as well as the invasive carcinoma. Focally, heterogeneous staining intensity in the neoplastic glandular epithelium is evident in some of the glands (arrow).

Although a few scattered glands retain a round open lumen, most glands have a compressed or only minimally patent lumen. Tubular adenosis (TA) consists of elongated benign tubules that tend to be more infiltrative and open than those of SA **(Fig. 10.22)**. The glands and tubules of SA and/or TA are surrounded by spindly myoepithelium that can be highlighted with myoepithelial stains, whereas myoepithelial cells are absent around the glands of TC. A conspicuous layer of eosinophilic basement membrane usually encircles all glands and tubules of SA and TA. The stroma admixed with SA and/or TA is not desmoplastic **(Table 10.1)** (also see Chapter 6).

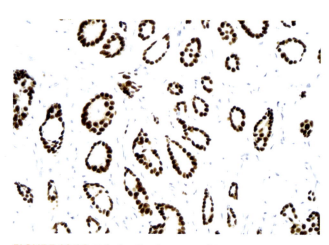

FIGURE 10.16 Tubular Carcinoma and Estrogen Receptor. Nuclei in the carcinomatous glands are strongly and diffusely immunoreactive for the estrogen receptor.

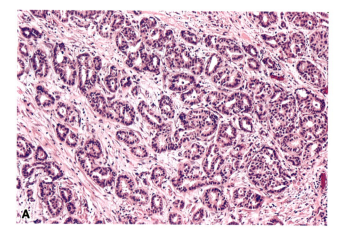
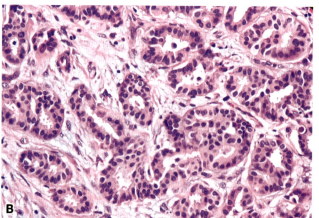

FIGURE 10.17 Well-differentiated Invasive Ductal Carcinoma. A, B: The glandular pattern is more complex than in tubular carcinoma. Intraglandular epithelial proliferation is evident.

Radial Scar/Radial Sclerosing Lesion

A RSL is a benign sclerosing lesion composed of adenosis and duct hyperplasia or papilloma, often accompanied by cysts. Stromal elastosis is a feature of many RSLs **(Fig. 10.22)**. Compared with a RSL, TC tends to have more open glands, stromal desmoplasia, and infiltrative growth at the periphery of the lesion. The use of a panel of myoepithelial markers inclusive of calponin and p63 is recommended for the evaluation of any diagnostically problematic sclerosing lesion. ADH5, a commercially available antibody cocktail (p63, basal cytokeratins CK5 and CK14, luminal cytokeratins CK7 and CK18), is suitable for visualization of epithelial and myoepithelial cells in the same tissue section **(Fig. 10.15)** and can distinguish benign sclerosing lesions and TC. Whenever immunohistochemical stains for myoepithelial markers are performed, a contemporaneous hematoxylin and eosin (H&E)-stained recut slide should always be prepared (51).

Treatment and Prognosis

Patients with TC usually undergo surgical excision of the lesion to obtain clear margins. Mastectomy is rarely performed. In a study based on SEER data, 82.4% of 4,477 patients with TC diagnosed between 1992 and 2007 underwent breast-conserving surgery, and only 17% had a mastectomy (4).

TUBULAR CARCINOMA

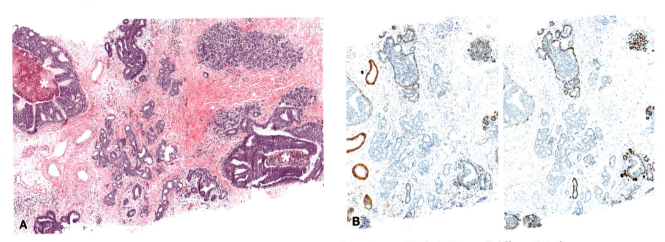

FIGURE 10.18 **Well-differentiated Invasive Ductal Carcinoma (IDC). A:** This well-differentiated IDC with cribriform architecture mimics lobular involvement by intraductal carcinoma. The neoplastic glands are adjacent and connected without much intervening stroma. Minimal stromal desmoplasia is present. Two ducts are involved by cribriform ductal carcinoma in situ with central necrosis (white asterisks). **B:** Immunostaining for calponin (left) and p63 (right) demonstrates the absence of myoepithelium around the glands of this well-differentiated IDC.

TABLE 10.3
Glandular Features in the Differential Diagnosis of Tubular Carcinoma, Microglandular Adenosis, and Grade I Invasive Ductal Carcinoma

Feature	Tubular Carcinoma	Microglandular Adenosis	Invasive Ductal Carcinoma, Low Grade
Shape	"Tear drop"	Round	Ovoid, rounded
Distribution	Rather uniform	Usually uniform	Rather haphazard
Myoepithelial layer	Absent	Absent	Rare
Basement membrane	Absent	Present	Absent
Glandular secretions	Uncommon	Rounded, dense, PAS (+)	Rare
Desmoplasia[a]	Prominent	Absent+	Present
Calcifications	~50%	Uncommon	Usually present

PAS, periodic acid–Schiff.
[a]Fibroelastosis.

TABLE 10.4
Epithelial Features in the Differential Diagnosis of Tubular Carcinoma, Microglandular Adenosis, and Grade I Invasive Ductal Carcinoma

Feature	Tubular Carcinoma	Microglandular Adenosis	Invasive Ductal Carcinoma, Low Grade
Cell layers	Single	Single	Single, focally more than one
Cell shape	Columnar/cuboidal	Cuboidal	Columnar
Cytoplasm	Amphophilic	Clear	Amphophilic
Apical snouts	Common	Absent	Variable
Nuclear grade	Grade I-II	Grade I	Grade I-II
Mitoses	Uncommon	Absent	Rare

TABLE 10.5
Immunohistochemistry in the Differential Diagnosis of Tubular Carcinoma, Microglandular Adenosis, and Grade I Invasive Ductal Carcinoma

Immunostain	Tubular Carcinoma	Microglandular Adenosis	Invasive Ductal Carcinoma, Low Grade
ER	(+), diffuse, strong	(−)	(+)
PR	(+), diffuse, strong	(−)	(+)
HER2	(−)	(−)	(−)
S-100	(−)	(+)	(−)
Myoepithelial markers[a]	(−)	(−)	(−)
Basement membrane[b]	(−)	(+)	(−)

[a]Smooth muscle actin, CD10, calponin, DOG1, smooth muscle myosin heavy chain, p40, p63.
[b]Collagen IV, laminin. Also reticulin stain.

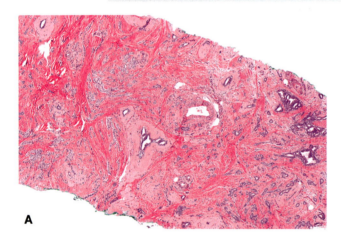
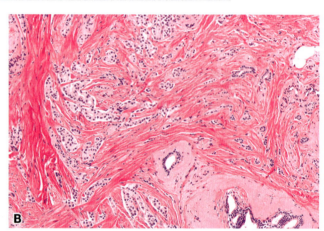

FIGURE 10.19 Tubulolobular Carcinoma (TC). A: The invasive carcinoma in this needle core biopsy specimen consists of small individual neoplastic glands (right) transitioning into small cords and trabeculae with lobular features (left). **B:** A higher-magnification view of the lobular-appearing component with typical TC glands (right).

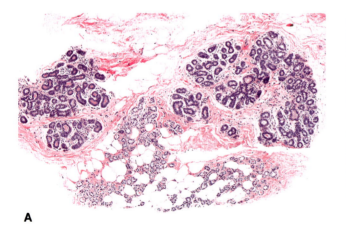
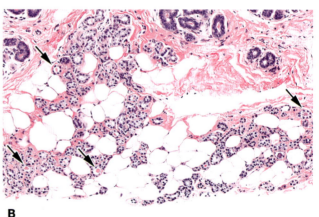

FIGURE 10.20 Microglandular Adenosis (MGA). A: A small glandular proliferation invasive into adipose tissue is present in this needle core biopsy. **B:** The glands are round to oval. They are lined by cuboidal monostratified epithelium with pale cytoplasm and inconspicuous nuclei. A few glands contain eosinophilic secretion (arrows). This lesion was strongly S-100 positive and negative for estrogen receptors (not shown). This pattern of immunoreactivity distinguishes MGA from tubular carcinoma.

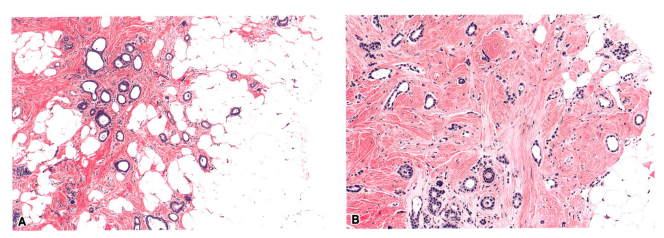

FIGURE 10.21 **Microglandular Adenosis-Like Tubular Carcinoma (TC).** **A:** The TC in this needle core biopsy sample is partly composed of small round-to-oval glands. It has elastotic stroma with only minimal desmoplasia. A few of the glands have angulated profiles. This lesion was strongly positive for estrogen receptors (not shown). **B:** Round and angular glands are shown in the TC surrounding an atrophic lobule (lower center).

Most patients with TC treated with breast-conserving surgery receive adjuvant radiotherapy. In an analysis of SEER data (14), 56.1% of 6,465 patients with TC diagnosed between 1992 and 2007 were treated with breast-conserving surgery and radiation therapy, whereas 23.6% had breast-conserving surgery but did not receive radiation. The investigators reported a 5-year overall survival (OS) benefit associated with radiotherapy following breast-conserving surgery (95% vs 90%, respectively), with a hazard ratio of 1.368 for patients who did not receive it. Other studies have confirmed the benefit of adjuvant radiotherapy following breast-conserving surgery in patients with TC (6-10,12-14,17,52). Notably, in one study, three patients with stage I TC and no evidence of extensive DCIS or LVI who were

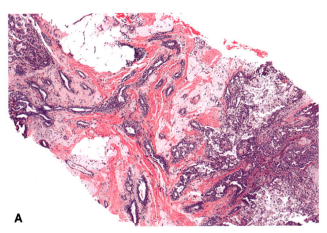

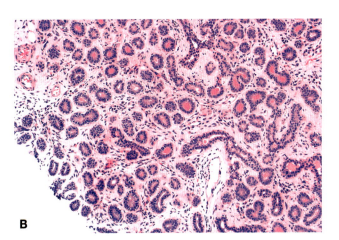

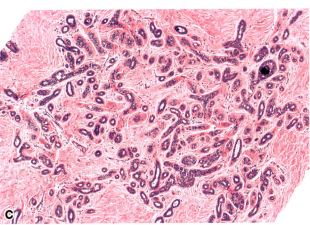

FIGURE 10.22 **Mimics of Tubular Carcinoma: Radial Scar, Tubular Adenoma, and Tubular Adenosis (TA).** **A:** The lumens of the ducts and glands in the elastotic nidus of this radial scar are compressed, consistent with a sclerosing process. **B:** Tubular adenoma shows a compact aggregate of uniform rounded glands amid minimal stroma. **C:** TA shows elongated benign tubules that tend to be more infiltrative and open than those of sclerosing adenosis.

prospectively treated by surgical excision with at least 1 cm wide clear margin and no adjuvant radiation or systemic therapy developed a local recurrence within 5 years (53).

The frequency of axillary lymph node (ALN) metastases ranges from 5% (12,13) to 25% (5). Metastatic TC usually involves only one to two lymph nodes (LNs) (11). In a retrospective analysis of sentinel lymph node (SLN) biopsy in 234 patients with TC (54), 2.5% of patients had macrometastases, and 6.4% had micrometastases. The median size of TC with SLN metastases was 12.17 versus 9.39 mm for TC not involving SLN(s). All patients with macrometastases had a TC greater than 1 cm in size, and the latter parameter was the only feature significantly associated with LN involvement in multivariate analysis. SLN biopsy is usually performed in patients with TC and may be performed if the tumor is larger than 1 cm (54), or if there is multifocal TC. Be that as it may, the case for omitting sentinel node biopsy at the time of tumor excision in invasive carcinomas that exhibit a predominant tubular growth pattern on preoperative biopsy is being increasingly made (55).

According to SEER data, 90.5% of women diagnosed with TC presented at stage I, 8.9% at stage II, 0.4% at stage III, and 0.2% at stage IV (4). A compilation of Netherlands registry data found that 70% of 3,456 patients with TC presented at stage I, 26% at stage II, 2% at stage III, and 1% at stage IV (3).

Adjuvant chemotherapy is rarely administered to patients with TC, and at present there is no evidence indicating that it is beneficial. The percentage of patients with TC who receive adjuvant hormonal therapy ranges from 10% to 90% (6-13,15,17). Even though TC theoretically constitutes an ideal target for hormonal therapy owing to the high expression of ER, available data do not suggest a substantial benefit associated with hormonal therapy.

A review of studies with follow-up data (6-13,15,17) shows a local recurrence rate ranging from 1% (17) to 13% (9), with most large series reporting a local recurrence rate of 4% to 7% (7,8,10,11). Rakha et al (11) compared the outcomes and local recurrence rates in 102 patients with TCs and 212 patients with grade I IDCs. The median follow-up time was 127 months. Local recurrence developed in 7% of patients with TC compared with 25% of patients with grade I IDC. None of the patients with TC died of disease, compared with 9% of patients with grade I IDC. Even when the analysis was limited to sub-centimeter tumors, patients with TC had a longer disease-free survival (DFS) and breast carcinoma-specific survival than patients with grade I IDC (11). Liu et al (10) also reported that patients with TC treated with breast conservation therapy had a lower rate of distant metastases (1% vs 13%) and breast cancer–specific death (1% vs 10%) than patients with IDC. A study (6) of 248 patients with unilateral and unicentric TC reported a survival rate of 96.3% at 5 years, 79.1% at 10 years, and 73.1% at 15 years. Several contemporary series with long-term follow-up report no deaths attributable to TC (7,8,10,11,45,48,56). In a retrospective study of 8,091 patients with TC, in the SEER database from 2000 to 2013, the 10-year breast cancer–specific survival and overall survival were 98.1 and 82.0%, respectively (57). The hazard ratio of breast cancer–specific mortality in patients of 50 years or older with ER+/PR+ tumors was 0.58 for TC compared with IFDC of no special type (4).

Overall, TC has an exceedingly good prognosis, which justifies separating it from other forms of low-grade IFDCs.

Molecular Pathology

The available morphologic, immunohistochemical, and molecular studies support the model of progression from lower-grade "preneoplastic" lesions to well-differentiated invasive carcinoma. Whole-arm loss of 16q likely represents one of the earliest steps in pathogenesis of the latter. 16q alterations have been identified in the lesions that comprise the "Rosen triad," that is, TC, LCIS, and columnar cell lesions (28,58). Simpson et al identified frequent recurrent loss of 16q in CCC, atypical CCH, ALH, low-grade DCIS, and well-differentiated invasive breast carcinoma (59). de Boer et al demonstrated lesions ranging from CCC to ADH and low-grade invasive carcinoma increasingly showed whole-arm losses of 16q along this spectrum of "low-grade breast neoplasia family" (60). These studies support the hypothesis of columnar cell lesions representing a nonobligate precursor toward the evolution of well-differentiated invasive carcinomas, including TC. Be that as it may, the "precursor" aspect of this "family" of lesions ought not to be overemphasized, as the risk of advancement of disease among such lesions is quite low (61). Factors that influence which of these lesions will progress, if at all, remain unidentified at this time.

As stated above, TC shares many of the same chromosomal alterations (including loss of 16q and gain of 1q) as reported in other well-differentiated invasive breast carcinomas. Notably, at a transcriptome level, TC shows upregulation of genes involved in estrogen signaling and downregulation of proliferation and cell cycle genes—molecular alterations not observed in other low-grade invasive carcinomas (62).

The clinical utility of Oncotype (21-gene recurrence score assay) testing, which predicts the likelihood of distant recurrence and chemotherapy benefit in early-stage, ER (+), HER2 (−) breast carcinomas, has been questioned (63,64).

REFERENCES

1. Foote FW Jr. Surgical pathology of cancer of the breast. In *Cancer of the Breast*. Edited by Parsons WH. Springfield, IL, Charles C. Thomas, 1959.
2. Northridge ME, Rhoads GG, Wartenberg D, Koffman D. The importance of histologic type on breast cancer survival. *J Clin Epidemiol*. 1997;50:283-290.
3. Louwman MW, Vriezen M, van Beek MW, et al. Uncommon breast tumors in perspective: incidence, treatment and survival in the Netherlands. *Int J Cancer*. 2007;121:127-135.
4. Li CI. Risk of mortality by histologic type of breast cancer in the United States. *Horm Cancer*. 2010;1:156-165.
5. Gunhan-Bilgen I, Oktay A. Tubular carcinoma of the breast: mammographic, sonographic, clinical and pathologic findings. *Eur J Radiol*. 2007;61:158-162.
6. Fritz P, Bendrat K, Sonnenberg M, et al. Tubular breast cancer. A retrospective study. *Anticancer Res*. 2014;34:3647-3656.
7. Livi L, Paiar F, Meldolesi E, et al. Tubular carcinoma of the breast: outcome and loco-regional recurrence in 307 patients. *Eur J Surg Oncol*. 2005;31:9-12.
8. Sullivan T, Raad RA, Goldberg S, et al. Tubular carcinoma of the breast: a retrospective analysis and review of the literature. *Breast Cancer Res Treat*. 2005;93:199-205.

9. Vo T, Xing Y, Meric-Bernstam F, et al. Long-term outcomes in patients with mucinous, medullary, tubular, and invasive ductal carcinomas after lumpectomy. *Am J Surg.* 2007;194:527-531.

10. Liu GF, Yang Q, Haffty BG, Moran MS. Clinical-pathologic features and long-term outcomes of tubular carcinoma of the breast compared with invasive ductal carcinoma treated with breast conservation therapy. *Int J Radiat Oncol Biol Phys.* 2009;75:1304-1308.

11. Rakha EA, Lee AH, Evans AJ, et al. Tubular carcinoma of the breast: further evidence to support its excellent prognosis. *J Clin Oncol.* 2010;28:99-104.

12. Fedko MG, Scow JS, Shah SS, et al. Pure tubular carcinoma and axillary nodal metastases. *Ann Surg Oncol.* 2010;17(suppl 3):338-342.

13. Hansen CJ, Kenny L, Lakhani SR, et al. Tubular breast carcinoma: an argument against treatment de-escalation. *J Med Imaging Radiat Oncol.* 2012;56:116-122.

14. Li B, Chen M, Nori D, et al. Adjuvant radiation therapy and survival for pure tubular breast carcinoma—experience from the SEER database. *Int J Radiat Oncol Biol Phys.* 2012;84:23-29.

15. Colleoni M, Rotmensz N, Maisonneuve P, et al. Outcome of special types of luminal breast cancer. *Ann Oncol.* 2012;23:1428-1436.

16. Nagtegaal ID, Allgood PC, Duffy SW, et al. Prognosis and pathology of screen-detected carcinomas: how different are they? *Cancer.* 2011;117:1360-1368.

17. Javid SH, Smith BL, Mayer E, et al. Tubular carcinoma of the breast: results of a large contemporary series. *Am J Surg.* 2009;197:674-677.

18. Leibman AJ, Lewis M, Kruse B. Tubular carcinoma of the breast: mammographic appearance. *AJR Am J Roentgenol.* 1993;160:263-265.

19. Vega A, Garijo F. Radial scar and tubular carcinoma. Mammographic and sonographic findings. *Acta Radiol.* 1993;34:43-47.

20. Frouge C, Tristant H, Guinebretiere JM, et al. Mammographic lesions suggestive of radial scars: microscopic findings in 40 cases. *Radiology.* 1995;195:623-625.

21. Yilmaz R, Bayramoglu Z, Emirikci S, et al. MR imaging features of tubular carcinoma: preliminary experience in twelve masses. *Eur J Breast Health.* 2018;14:39-45.

22. Li CI, Daling JR, Malone KE, et al. Relationship between established breast cancer risk factors and risk of seven different histologic types of invasive breast cancer. *Cancer Epidemiol Biomarkers Prev.* 2006;15:946-954.

23. Burga AM, Fadare O, Lininger RA, Tavassoli FA. Invasive carcinomas of the male breast: a morphologic study of the distribution of histologic subtypes and metastatic patterns in 778 cases. *Virchows Arch.* 2006;449:507-512.

24. Couto E, Banks E, Reeves G, et al. Family history and breast cancer tumour characteristics in screened women. *Int J Cancer.* 2008;123:2950-2954.

25. Flesch-Janys D, Slanger T, Mutschelknauss E, et al. Risk of different histological types of postmenopausal breast cancer by type and regimen of menopausal hormone therapy. *Int J Cancer.* 2008;123:933-941.

26. McDivitt RW, Boyce W, Gersell D. Tubular carcinoma of the breast. Clinical and pathological observations concerning 135 cases. *Am J Surg Pathol.* 1982;6:401-411.

27. Mitnick JS, Gianutsos R, Pollack AH, et al. Tubular carcinoma of the breast: sensitivity of diagnostic techniques and correlation with histopathology. *AJR Am J Roentgenol.* 1999;172:319-323.

28. Brandt SM, Young GQ, Hoda SA. The "Rosen Triad": tubular carcinoma, lobular carcinoma in situ, and columnar cell lesions. *Adv Anat Pathol.* 2008;15:140-146.

29. Winchester DJ, Sahin AA, Tucker SL, Singletary SE. Tubular carcinoma of the breast. Predicting axillary nodal metastases and recurrence. *Ann Surg.* 1996;223:342-347.

30. Thurman SA, Schnitt SJ, Connolly JL, et al. Outcome after breast-conserving therapy for patients with stage I or II mucinous, medullary, or tubular breast carcinoma. *Int J Radiat Oncol Biol Phys.* 2004;59:152-159.

31. Carstens PH, Huvos AG, Foote FW Jr, Ashikari R. Tubular carcinoma of the breast: a clinicopathologic study of 35 cases. *Am J Clin Pathol.* 1972;58:231-238.

32. Deos PH, Norris HJ. Well-differentiated (tubular) carcinoma of the breast. A clinicopathologic study of 145 pure and mixed cases. *Am J Clin Pathol.* 1982;78:1-7.

33. Peters GN, Wolff M, Haagensen CD. Tubular carcinoma of the breast. Clinical pathologic correlations based on 100 cases. *Ann Surg.* 1981;193:138-149.

34. Cserni G. Histological type and typing of breast carcinomas and the WHO classification changes over time. *Pathologica.* 2020;112:25-41.

35. Kunju LP, Ding Y, Kleer CG. Tubular carcinoma and grade 1 (well-differentiated) invasive ductal carcinoma: comparison of flat epithelial atypia and other intra-epithelial lesions. *Pathol Int.* 2008;58:620-625.

36. Aulmann S, Elsawaf Z, Penzel R, et al. Invasive tubular carcinoma of the breast frequently is clonally related to flat epithelial atypia and low-grade ductal carcinoma in situ. *Am J Surg Pathol.* 2009;33:1646-1653.

37. Abdel-Fatah TM, Powe DG, Hodi Z, et al. High frequency of coexistence of columnar cell lesions, lobular neoplasia, and low grade ductal carcinoma in situ with invasive tubular carcinoma and invasive lobular carcinoma. *Am J Surg Pathol.* 2007;31:417-426.

38. Rosen PP. Columnar cell hyperplasia is associated with lobular carcinoma in situ and tubular carcinoma. *Am J Surg Pathol.* 1999;23:1561.

39. van Deurzen CHM, Denkert C, Purdie CA. Tubular carcinoma. In: Brogi E, ed. *Breast Tumours WHO Classification of Tumours.* Vol 2. 5th ed. International Agency for Research on Cancer; 2019:119-122.

40. Collins LC, Achacoso NA, Nekhlyudov L, et al. Clinical and pathologic features of ductal carcinoma in situ associated with the presence of flat epithelial atypia: an analysis of 543 patients. *Mod Pathol.* 2007;20:1149-1155.

41. Waldman FM, Hwang ES, Etzell J, et al. Genomic alterations in tubular breast carcinomas. *Hum Pathol.* 2001;32:222-226.

42. Abdel-Fatah TM, Powe DG, et al. Morphologic and molecular evolutionary pathways of low nuclear grade invasive breast cancers and their putative precursor lesions: further evidence to support the concept of low nuclear grade breast neoplasia family. *Am J Surg Pathol.* 2008;32:513-523.

43. Linell F, Ljungberg O. Breast carcinoma. Progression of tubular carcinoma and a new classification. *Acta Pathol Microbiol Scand A.* 1980;88:59-60.

44. Linell F, Ljungberg O, Andersson I. Breast carcinoma. Aspects of early stages, progression and related problems. *Acta Pathol Microbiol Scand Suppl.* 1980:1-233.

45. Diab SG, Clark GM, Osborne CK, et al. Tumor characteristics and clinical outcome of tubular and mucinous breast carcinomas. *J Clin Oncol.* 1999;17:1442-1448.

46. Fasano M, Vamvakas E, Delgado Y, et al. Tubular carcinoma of the breast: immunohistochemical and DNA flow cytometric profile. *Breast J.* 1999;5:252-255.

47. Oakley GJ 3rd, Tubbs RR, Crowe J, et al. HER-2 amplification in tubular carcinoma of the breast. *Am J Clin Pathol.* 2006;126:55-58.

48. Green I, McCormick B, Cranor M, Rosen PP. A comparative study of pure tubular and tubulolobular carcinoma of the breast. *Am J Surg Pathol.* 1997;21:653-657.

49. Wheeler DT, Tai LH, Bratthauer GL, et al. Tubulolobular carcinoma of the breast: an analysis of 27 cases of a tumor with a hybrid morphology and immunoprofile. *Am J Surg Pathol.* 2004;28:1587-1593.

50. Esposito NN, Chivukula M, Dabbs DJ. The ductal phenotypic expression of the E-cadherin/catenin complex in tubulolobular carcinoma of the breast: an immunohistochemical and clinicopathologic study. *Mod Pathol.* 2007;20:130-138.

51. Hoda SA, Rosen PP. Contemporaneous H&E sections should be standard practice in diagnostic immunopathology. *Am J Surg Pathol.* 2007;31:1627.

52. Haffty BG, Perrotta PL, Ward B, et al. Conservatively treated breast cancer: outcome by histologic subtype. *Breast J.* 1997;3:7-14.

53. Lim M, Bellon JR, Gelman R, et al. A prospective study of conservative surgery without radiation therapy in select patients with stage I breast cancer. *Int J Radiat Oncol Biol Phys.* 2006;65:1149-1154.

54. Dejode M, Sagan C, Campion L, et al. Pure tubular carcinoma of the breast and sentinel lymph node biopsy: a retrospective multi-institutional study of 234 cases. *Eur J Surg Oncol.* 2013;39:248-254.

55. Rosen PR, Groshen S, Saigo PE, et al. A long-term follow-up study of survival in stage I (T1N0M0) and stage II (T1N1M0) breast carcinoma. *J Clin Oncol.* 1989;7:355-366.

56. Ramzi S, Hyett EL, Wheal AS, Cant PJ. The case for the omission of axillary staging in invasive breast carcinoma that exhibits a predominant tubular growth pattern on preoperative biopsy. *Breast J.* 2018;24:493-500.

57. Sun JY, Zhou J, Zhang WW, et al. Tubular carcinomas of the breast: an epidemiologic study. *Future Oncol.* 2018;14:3037-3047.

58. Tirkkonen M, Tanner M, Karhu R, et al. Molecular cytogenetics of primary breast cancer by CGH. *Genes Chromosomes Cancer.* 1998;21:177-184.

59. Simpson PT, Gale T, Reis-Filho JS, et al. Columnar cell lesions of the breast: the missing link in breast cancer progression? A morphological and molecular analysis. *Am J Surg Pathol.* 2005;29:734-746.

60. de Boer M, Verschuur-Maes AHJ, Buerger H, et al. Role of columnar cell lesions in breast carcinogenesis: analysis of chromosome 16 copy number changes by multiplex ligation-dependent probe amplification. *Mod Pathol.* 2018;31:1816-1833.

61. Collins LC. Precursor lesions of the low-grade breast neoplasia pathway. *Surg Pathol Clin.* 2018;11:177-197.

62. Lopez-Garcia MA, Geyer FC, Natrajan R, et al. Transcriptomic analysis of tubular carcinomas of the breast reveals similarities and differences with molecular subtype-matched ductal and lobular carcinomas. *J Pathol.* 2010;222:64-75.

63. Turashvili G, Brogi E, Morrow M, et al. The 21-gene recurrence score in special histologic subtypes of breast cancer with favorable prognosis. *Breast Cancer Res Treat.* 2017;165:65-76.

64. Wilson PC, Chagpar AB, Cicek AF, et al. Breast cancer histopathology is predictive of low-risk Oncotype Dx recurrence score. *Breast J.* 2018;24:976-980.

11

Papillary Carcinoma

ELAINE W. ZHONG AND SYED A. HODA

INTRODUCTION

Papillary carcinoma represents a form of breast carcinoma in which the neoplastic cells proliferate on an arborizing skeleton of fibrovascular fronds. Some papillary carcinomas have cystic areas. In cases showing minimal cyst formation, the underlying fronds may not be obvious; consequently, one can appreciate the papillary architecture based on the underlying fibrovascular stromal network.

Owing to their complex and variable morphology and shifting diagnostic criteria, papillary carcinomas are diagnostically challenging for many pathologists (1,2). Correct categorization on core biopsy can be especially difficult. Papillary carcinomas account for less than 1% of breast carcinomas in women (3-5) and 2% to 8% in men (6,7). Like other types of breast carcinoma, papillary carcinoma occurs in both noninvasive and invasive forms. Noninvasive papillary carcinomas include papillary ductal carcinoma in situ (DCIS), encapsulated papillary carcinoma (EPC), and solid papillary carcinoma (SPC).

CLINICAL FEATURES

Papillary carcinomas usually occur in adults older than 50 years. On average, women with papillary carcinomas are older than women with other types of breast carcinoma; mean ages range from 63 to 71 years. Small series and case reports document the occurrence of papillary carcinomas in women as young as 20 years and as old as 103 years (8). Men can develop papillary carcinomas of all subtypes and span the same age range (9).

Nearly 50% of papillary carcinomas arise in the central part of the breast. The most common presentation is a mass, with an average size of 2 to 3 cm. At least one-third of patients report discharge from the nipple. Patients with centrally located papillary carcinomas experience bleeding from the nipple more often than do women with papillomas. Paget disease rarely occurs in association with papillary carcinoma, but it may do so if the carcinoma involves a lactiferous duct.

Imaging studies of papillary carcinomas frequently display round, oval, or lobulated masses (10-12). Irregularity of the contour suggests the presence of an invasive component. Studies may also display multinodular densities in a segmental distribution, sometimes confined to a single quadrant (12). Most papillary carcinomas do not contain abundant calcifications; however, punctate calcifications can mark the associated intraductal component (13), and coarse, irregular calcifications may develop in areas of sclerosis or resolved hemorrhage. Sonography typically demonstrates masses that appear well defined, solid or mixed solid, and cystic, heterogeneous, and hypoechoic with posterior enhancement (11,12,14). MRI of SPC most often demonstrates nonmass, clumped, or mass with rim enhancement patterns (15), whereas EPC can appear as a cystic mass with mural nodules and a fluid level indicating hemorrhage (16).

HISTOPATHOLOGIC EVALUATION

Growth of the neoplastic cells on fibrovascular fronds represents the *sine qua non* of papillary carcinoma. Further subclassification is facilitated by the evaluation of the myoepithelial cell component. The following morphologic features characterize the histopathology of papillary carcinomas and provide the basis for distinguishing the latter from papillomas (see also **Table 11.1**).

Types of Cells

Malignant ductal cells constitute the entire epithelial population of papillary carcinomas, whereas benign luminal and myoepithelial cells compose the epithelium of papillomas. The epithelial cells in papillary carcinomas typically grow in a disorderly fashion, including loss of nuclear polarity with respect to the basement membrane and uneven stratification of the cells **(Fig. 11.1)**. The nuclei exhibit varying degrees of atypia, and the tumor cells sometimes have cytoplasmic "snouts" at the luminal surface **(Fig. 11.2)**. The cells can form papillary, micropapillary, cribriform, or solid arrangements identical to those of conventional DCIS **(Fig. 11.3)**. Rare low-grade papillary carcinomas have an orderly frond-forming structure and minimal epithelial stratification **(Fig. 11.4)**. One may have difficulty distinguishing such cases from papillomas based on hematoxylin and eosin (H&E)-stained sections of needle core biopsy (NCB) samples, but the morphologic features of the lesional cells identify them as malignant and thereby establish the diagnosis of papillary carcinoma.

Myoepithelial cells, which are distributed relatively uniformly and proportionately within the epithelium of papillomas, are characteristically absent from invasive papillary carcinoma as well as most noninvasive papillary carcinomas.

PAPILLARY CARCINOMA

TABLE 11.1
Differential Diagnosis of Papilloma and Noninvasive Papillary Carcinoma

	Papilloma	Papillary DCIS	Solid Papillary Carcinoma	Encapsulated Papillary Carcinoma
Epithelium	Bland, heterogeneous, often with apocrine metaplasia	Uniform, monotonous	Uniform, monotonous, often neuroendocrine or mucinous	Uniform, monotonous
Myoepithelium*	Peripheral and along FVC	Peripheral	Peripheral/absent	Absent
Architecture	Broad, blunt FVC	Slender FVC, may coexist with other patterns	Multinodular round solid nests embedded with inconspicuous FVC	Usually single nodule, with "capsule," slender FVC, cribriform

*peripheral: at the circumference/perimeter. FVC, fibrovascular cores.

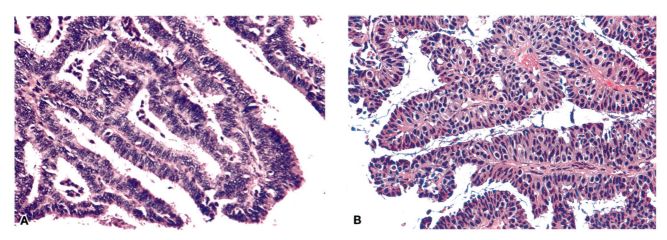

FIGURE 11.1 Papillary Carcinoma. A: The columnar cells in this papillary carcinoma demonstrate high nuclear-to-cytoplasmic ratios and inconsistent positioning of the nuclei with respect to the basement membrane. **B:** This needle core biopsy specimen from a 55-year-old woman shows irregular stratification of the neoplastic cells and mucin between the fronds.

The presence of myoepithelial cells in parts of a papillary lesion does not exclude the diagnosis of papillary carcinoma (17,18). Papillary DCIS and sometimes SPC maintain a layer of myoepithelial cells surrounding the involved duct.

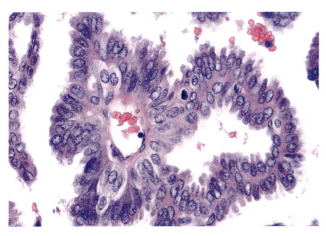

FIGURE 11.2 Papillary Carcinoma. The cytoplasm of the carcinoma cells forms apical blebs. A mitotic figure is present (upper center).

Noninvasive papillary carcinomas containing numerous myoepithelial cells may represent papillomas partly overtaken by carcinoma (*vide infra*) (19). Myoepithelium may persist in segments of residual epithelium or as a layer beneath the carcinomatous population.

Lefkowitz et al (20) drew attention to the presence of cuboidal cells with abundant clear or faintly eosinophilic cytoplasm (globoid cells) in some papillary carcinomas. Situated near the basement membrane, these cells occur singly, in small clusters, or in solid and cribriform aggregates **(Fig. 11.5)**. The proximity of the cuboidal cells to the basement recalls the appearance of myoepithelial cells or pagetoid spread of carcinoma. Both the basal cuboidal and superficial columnar cells are immunoreactive for cytokeratin, and the basal cells do not display reactivity for smooth muscle actin (SMA) or p63. This pattern is referred to as *dimorphic papillary carcinoma*.

Nuclei

The lesional cells of papillary carcinomas demonstrate the cytologic features of conventional DCIS. These features vary according to the grade of the carcinoma; however,

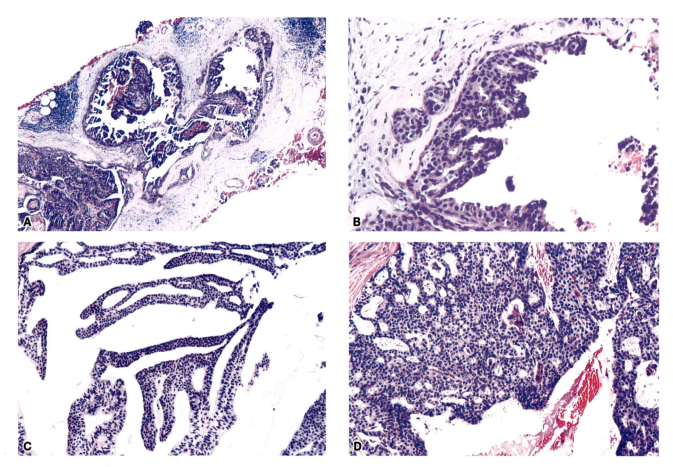

FIGURE 11.3 Papillary Ductal Carcinoma In Situ (DCIS). Various growth patterns are represented in these needle core biopsy specimens. **A, B:** Papillary and micropapillary DCIS are seen. Myoepithelial cells represented by oval nuclei arranged parallel to the basement membrane lie beneath the micropapillary carcinoma in **(B)**. **C:** Arborizing micropapillary DCIS with low nuclear grade is shown. **D:** A cribriform pattern is evident.

alterations common to all grades include an increase in the size of the cells and their nuclei, hyperchromasia of the nuclei, and an increase in the nuclear-to-cytoplasmic ratio. In low-grade papillary carcinomas, the cells appear uniform. Rare high-grade papillary carcinomas demonstrate conspicuous cellular pleomorphism and mitotic activity. The presence of more than an occasional mitotic figure in a papillary tumor suggests the diagnosis of papillary carcinoma.

Apocrine Metaplasia

Although the cells of papillary carcinoma sometimes have eosinophilic cytoplasm or secretory "snouts," papillary carcinomas do not contain the usual, cytologically bland apocrine cells commonly seen in papillomas. The presence of benign apocrine metaplasia provides strong evidence to support the diagnosis of papilloma, but its absence does not favor a diagnosis of papillary carcinoma.

Glandular Pattern

The cribriform pattern characteristic of low-grade DCIS occurs in many papillary carcinomas. One must distinguish it from the *complex glandular pattern*, a back-to-back arrangement of glands within the stalk of a papilloma. To make this distinction, one should look for stromal elements between the glands. Cribriform spaces form within aggregates of carcinoma cells unsupported by a surrounding stroma, whereas thin strands of collagen and slender capillaries encompass each of the glands that compose the complex glandular pattern.

Stroma

Although all noninvasive papillary carcinomas possess fibrovascular stroma, it usually appears less conspicuous than the stroma seen in papillomas. Many cases deviate from this generalization (21), and occasionally papillary carcinomas contain prominent stalks of sclerotic fibrous stroma **(Fig. 11.6)**. The character of the stroma within the lesion is not by itself a reliable differentiating diagnostic feature.

Scarring frequently occurs at the periphery of papillary tumors. This process can entrap both benign glands and those harboring in situ carcinoma. The resulting appearance simulates invasive carcinoma and makes the recognition of minimal invasion difficult. Caution should be taken not to overinterpret glands within the scar, especially in an NCB.

PAPILLARY CARCINOMA 227

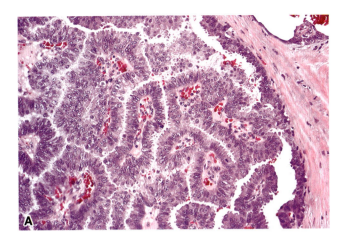
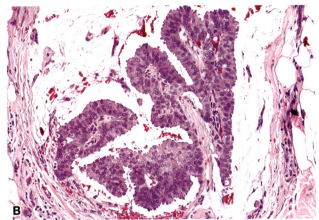
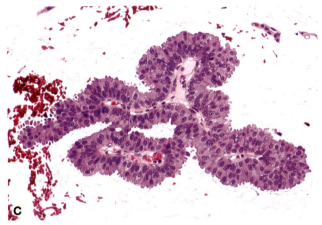

FIGURE 11.4 Papillary Carcinoma, In Situ and Invasive. These needle core biopsy samples show an orderly papillary carcinoma. **A:** Intraductal papillary carcinoma with mucin formation. **B, C:** Frond-forming invasive papillary carcinoma with mucin. Note the stroma in the invasive papillary fronds.

Epithelial Proliferations in Adjacent Ducts

When one finds it difficult to diagnose an orderly papillary tumor, the study of epithelial proliferations in nearby structures often helps to establish the diagnosis. The presence of papillary, cribriform, or solid DCIS in adjacent ducts or lobules usually indicates that the papillary lesion also contains carcinoma. Study of an epithelial proliferation situated on the wall of the duct harboring a papillary tumor can also shed light on the nature of the epithelial cells within the papillary portion.

Other Findings

Some papillary carcinomas, in particular SPCs, contain signet ring cells, intracellular mucin **(Fig. 11.7)**, or extracellular mucin **(Figs. 11.4 and 11.8)**. Alcian blue, mucicarmine, and periodic acid–Schiff stains will highlight mucin not easily seen on H&E stains. Papillomas rarely produce detectable mucin; thus, the presence of intraepithelial mucin in a papillary tumor should raise suspicion for papillary carcinoma.

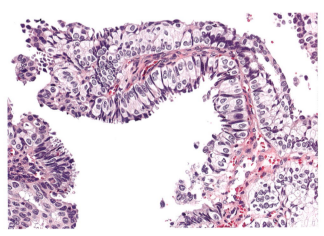

FIGURE 11.5 Dimorphic Papillary Carcinoma. Basal cells with abundant pale cytoplasm mingle with compressed columnar cells with scant eosinophilic cytoplasm. The juxtaposition is most apparent near the left border.

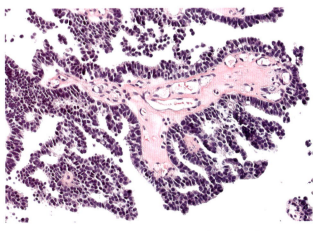

FIGURE 11.6 Papillary Carcinoma With Sclerotic Stroma. Dense collagen forms the stroma in this papillary carcinoma.

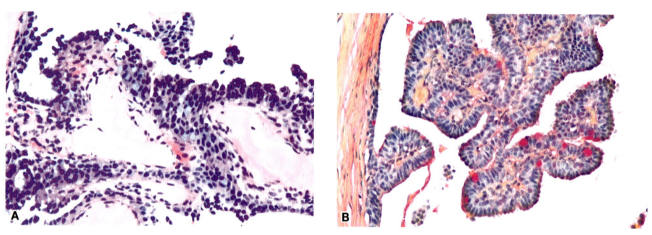

FIGURE 11.7 Papillary Carcinoma With Intracytoplasmic Mucin. A: Intracytoplasmic mucin is represented by discrete pale blue vacuoles. **B:** The mucicarmine stain colors the mucin magenta.

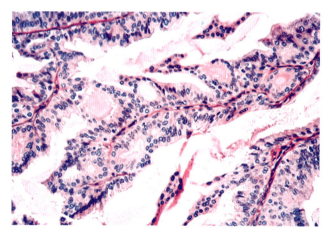

FIGURE 11.8 Papillary Carcinoma With Extracellular Mucin. This papillary carcinoma has a micropapillary structure and abundant mucin between the papillary fronds.

When present, the calcifications in papillary carcinomas often occupy the spaces enclosed by the malignant cells **(Fig. 11.9)**. Calcifications can form in the stromal cores of both papillary carcinomas and papillomas.

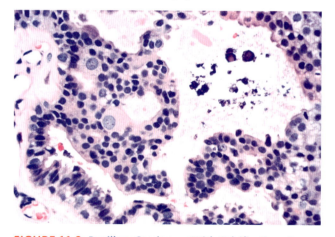

FIGURE 11.9 Papillary Carcinoma With Calcification. Granular calcifications are present in a duct lumen in this needle core biopsy specimen containing papillary carcinoma with a micropapillary pattern.

IMMUNOHISTOCHEMISTRY

More than 90% of papillary carcinomas express the estrogen and progesterone receptors (ER and PR), but those composed of apocrine or high-grade cells do not stain for these receptors (and usually do not express HER2).

Although it is usually possible to identify myoepithelial cells on H&E-stained sections, immunohistochemical staining provides a more reliable method for detecting them **(Fig. 11.10)**. Cytoplasmic markers of myoepithelial cells include CD10, DOG1, SMA, calponin, smooth muscle myosin heavy chain (SMMHC), and cytokeratin 5/6 (CK5/6). These markers cross-react with stromal myofibroblasts and vascular structures to varying degrees. The transcription factor p63 (and p40) stains nuclei of myoepithelial cells but does not react with those of stromal cells; however, the marker can also stain the nuclei of occasional high-grade carcinomas (22), and it regularly stains the nuclei of squamous cells. The position of spuriously staining epithelial cells (apart from the basement membrane) and the round or oval shapes of their nuclei identify these cells as epithelial rather than myoepithelial. Whenever possible, it is prudent to employ a panel composed of p63 and two or more cytoplasmic markers when investigating the presence of myoepithelial cells in a papillary tumor (23-25). Double immunostaining for epithelial and myoepithelial cells can be useful in this regard.

As with atypical ductal hyperplasia (ADH) and conventional DCIS, high-molecular-weight cytokeratin molecules (CK5/6, CK14, 34βE12) are absent or diminished in the neoplastic cells of papillary carcinomas (18,26,27). These are useful for distinguishing hyperplastic ductal cells involving a papilloma from neoplastic ductal proliferations with a papillary growth pattern. Rabban et al (26) reported the absence of reactivity for CK5/6 in the epithelium of 14 SPCs. CK5/6 antibodies did stain residual nonneoplastic epithelial cells and myoepithelial cells, and they also stained hyperplastic ductal cells strongly. Tan et al (27) reported that CK5/6 had higher sensitivity and specificity for distinguishing papillomas from papillary carcinomas than did CK14 and 34βE12.

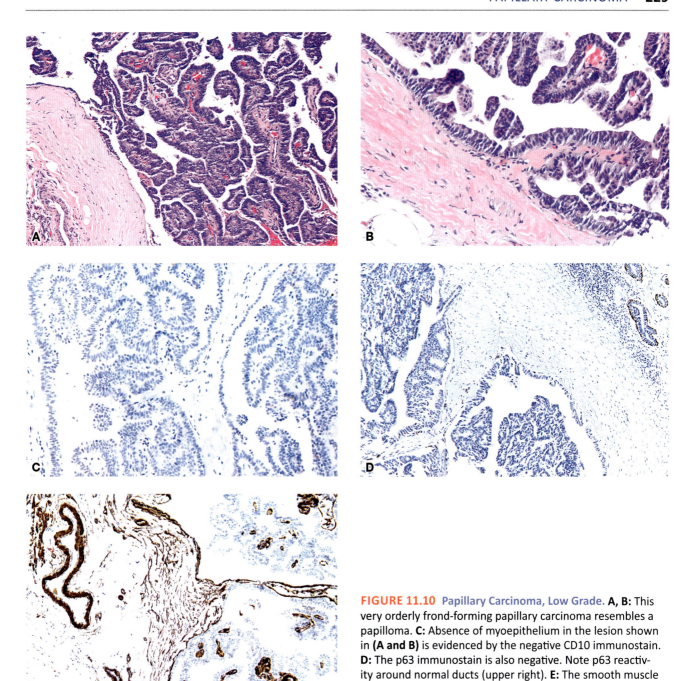

FIGURE 11.10 Papillary Carcinoma, Low Grade. A, B: This very orderly frond-forming papillary carcinoma resembles a papilloma. C: Absence of myoepithelium in the lesion shown in (A and B) is evidenced by the negative CD10 immunostain. D: The p63 immunostain is also negative. Note p63 reactivity around normal ducts (upper right). E: The smooth muscle actin immunostain highlights stromal cells and vascular structures. No myoepithelial reactivity is evident.

Tse et al (18) observed that moderate to strong staining for CK14 in 50% or more of the epithelial cells resulted in 100% specificity for identifying benign epithelial proliferations involving papillomas. Strong epithelial expression of CK5/6, CK14, or 34βE12 should cast doubt on a diagnosis of papillary carcinoma (except those that are high grade). Multiple studies have shown that the use of myoepithelial stains and ER on NCB samples of papillary tumors greatly increases diagnostic accuracy and concordance (17,28,29).

Wang et al (30) found that many cells of papillary carcinomas express cyclin D1, but only a few cells of papillomas do so. In this investigation, papillomas demonstrated high expression of CK5/6 and low expression of cyclin D1, whereas papillary carcinomas yielded the opposite results. In one study (31), 32 of 33 (97%) papillomas showed strong staining for CD133, whereas only 3 of 33 (9%) stained strongly.

Although these special studies can help to clarify the diagnosis of papillary tumors in certain settings, the distinction between a papilloma with unusual features and a papillary carcinoma remains difficult when examining specimens obtained by NCB. Fragments of florid ductal hyperplasia can suggest the diagnosis of DCIS in an NCB sample, and epithelial clusters entrapped in the stromal fragments of a benign sclerosing papillary lesion can mimic invasive carcinoma. Moreover, because carcinoma may only focally involve a papillary tumor, the absence of carcinoma in an NCB specimen showing a seemingly benign papilloma might simply represent incomplete sampling of a papilloma harboring carcinoma.

PATTERNS OF PAPILLARY CARCINOMA

Papillary Ductal Carcinoma In Situ

Papillary DCIS is one pattern of DCIS, typically seen alongside other patterns **(Fig. 11.3)**. It consists of delicate fibrovascular cores lined by malignant cells within a duct. Myoepithelial cells are present at the perimeter of the involved duct and not within the papillary fronds.

Encapsulated Papillary Carcinoma

EPC is a circumscribed papillary neoplasm, generally a single expansive tumor nodule, sometimes within a cystic space (intracystic), and/or surrounded by a variably thick fibrous "capsule" **(Fig. 11.11)**. The architecture ranges from overtly papillary with arborizing fronds to predominantly cribriform. A significant solid component should raise the differential of SPC.

The designation *EPC* arose from immunohistochemical studies of myoepithelial markers by Hill and Yeh (24). These investigators found five papillary carcinomas with "no staining or only focal staining of a basal [myoepithelial cell] layer" for calponin, SMMHC, and p63. Other investigations (23,32,33) yielded similar results, and the contributors to the fifth edition of the WHO classification of tumors of the breast (34) have taken up this usage. According to this edition, EPCs by definition display low- or intermediate-grade cytologic features.

The infiltrative nature of EPC remains controversial. For example, Rakha et al (32) wrote "...most [EPCs] are indolent invasive carcinoma, with a small proportion that may be *in situ*," whereas Esposito et al (35) stated "...[EPCs] are confined within an intact basement membrane and are thus *in situ* carcinomas." A study of invasion-associated matrix metalloproteinase expression found that EPCs have an expression pattern intermediate between that of DCIS and invasive carcinoma (36). This type of papillary carcinoma can elicit histopathologic uncertainty regarding the presence of invasion. Rare instances of axillary nodal metastases have been detected in cases in which frank invasion was not detected (35,37,38). One patient suffered pleural and brain metastases (39). However, the possibility that occult infiltrative foci in these cases were missed cannot be ruled out.

Approximately 3% (32) to 9.5% (40) of carcinomas resembling EPC demonstrate high-grade attributes. The findings of high-grade nuclear features and/or increased mitotic activity in these tumors are associated with larger size, triple-negative or HER2-positive phenotype, and stromal invasion (41,42). Pending larger studies with more extensive follow-up, it has been recommended that such "high-grade EPCs" be regarded as invasive carcinomas (34).

Solid Papillary Carcinoma

SPCs are well circumscribed and often multinodular tumors consisting of ducts nearly or completely filled by solid proliferation of neoplastic ductal cells supported by cores of fibrovascular stroma **(Figs. 11.12 and 11.13)**. The stromal network in the cellular areas is often inconspicuous. Collagenization of the periductal stroma, present to a variable degree, can distort the entrapped ducts to form ribbons or trabeculae of neoplastic cells, which one can mistake for invasive carcinoma or a radial sclerosing lesion. If the neoplastic cells extend into adjacent ducts, they usually display the cytologic and architectural features seen in the dominant portion of the carcinoma.

SPCs frequently exhibit neuroendocrine differentiation, a feature not seen in EPCs. The cells are monotonous, with

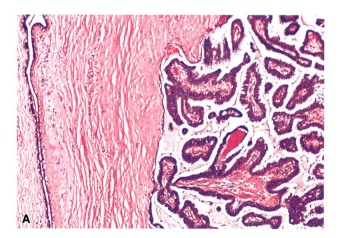
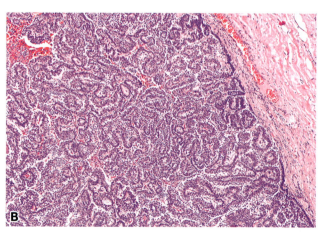

FIGURE 11.11 Encapsulated Papillary Carcinoma. A: This papillary tumor massively distends a duct space and is surrounded by collagenized fibrous tissue, with "intracystic" pattern. The epithelium consists of atypical columnar cells. **B:** Another example of encapsulated papillary carcinoma.

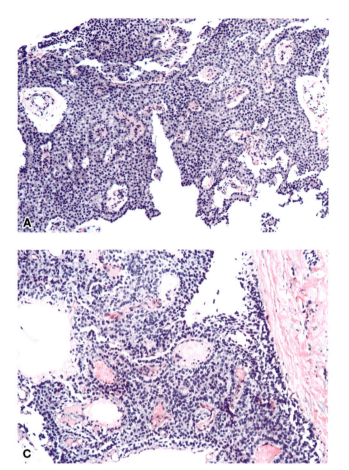
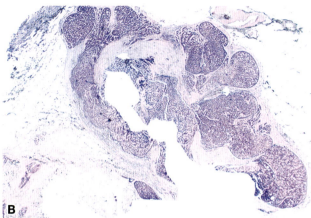

FIGURE 11.12 **Solid Papillary Carcinoma. A:** A needle core biopsy (NCB) specimen shows solid areas of in situ carcinoma arranged around fibrovascular stromal cores. The tumor cells have vacuolated amphophilic cytoplasm and well-differentiated round nuclei. One could mistake this specimen for invasive carcinoma if one failed to appreciate the basic papillary structure. **B:** A low magnification view illustrates the tumor in the excision specimen. **C:** An area at the periphery of the excised tumor duplicates the appearance of the carcinoma in the NCB specimen.

"salt and pepper" chromatin and oval-to-spindle shapes, and the cytoplasmic borders sometimes clearly stand out. In uncommon cases, a spindle morphology predominates (43). The neoplastic cells usually demonstrate low-grade atypia **(Fig. 11.14)**, but intermediate- and high-grade cytologic features occur in a minority of cases (35). Eccentric positioning of the nuclei results in a plasmacytoid appearance **(Fig. 11.14D)**. The cytoplasm usually appears eosinophilic or amphophilic and granular. In many cases, the cytoplasm contains mucin, either in the form of minuscule droplets or large vacuoles that create signet ring cells. Mitotic figures may be seen; but calcifications, cribriform spaces, and necrosis are not characteristic. Cells abutting the stroma sometimes line up to form a palisade pattern. Evidence of

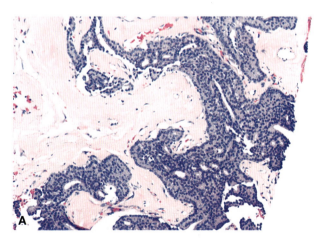
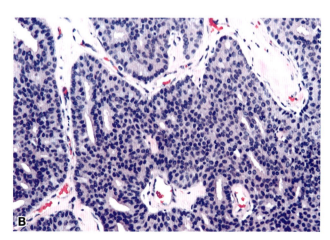

FIGURE 11.13 **Solid Papillary Carcinoma (SPC). A:** Collagenized stroma in this needle core biopsy specimen has distorted the structure of an in situ SPC. This pattern might be mistaken for an invasive carcinoma with a trabecular arrangement if one failed to appreciate the papillary character of the lesion. Spaces formed by separation of the epithelium from the stroma are common in SPC. **B:** This part of the lesion has a cribriform structure.

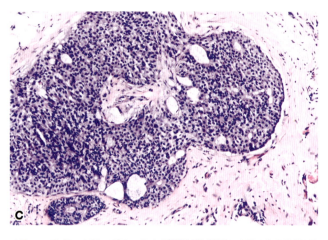
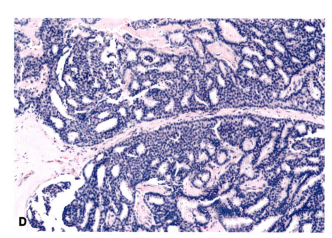
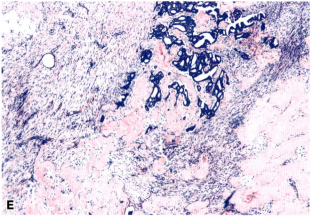

FIGURE 11.13 (*continued*) **C:** Cribriform ductal carcinoma in situ is also present in the excision. **D:** SPC is present in a duct at the periphery of the excision specimen. **E:** One can see an area in the center of the excised tumor showing a reactive stromal proliferation resulting from the needle core biopsy. Disrupted glands in the granulation tissue may be mistaken for invasive carcinoma.

neuroendocrine differentiation takes the form of immunoreactivity for synaptophysin, chromogranin, or INSM1 (44,45) **(Fig. 11.14F and G)**, or the detection of dense core granules. SPCs may also demonstrate neuroendocrine differentiation at the gene expression level (46,47).

The presence of myoepithelium around the periphery of a solid papillary tumor supports the diagnosis of noninvasive SPC, but focal or even complete absence of peripheral myoepithelium does not establish the presence of invasion (see **Table 11.1**). An irregular cribriform, tubular, or mucinous pattern that extends beyond the perimeter of the tumor represents a persuasive diagnostic feature of invasion **(Fig. 11.15)**. The diagnosis of SPC should be further qualified as in situ or invasive.

One sometimes observes extracellular mucin in the spaces formed by the carcinoma cells or between the neoplastic

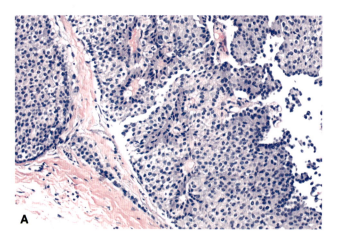
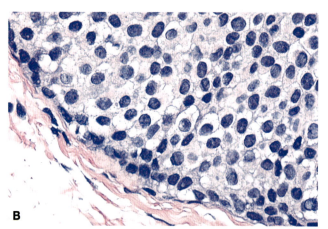

FIGURE 11.14 Solid Papillary Carcinoma (SPC) With Neuroendocrine Differentiation. **A:** In this needle core biopsy specimen, the in situ carcinoma contains small cords of fibrovascular stroma, which make it possible to recognize the papillary character of the tumor. The circumscribed border typifies solid papillary ductal carcinoma in situ with endocrine differentiation. **B:** This magnified view demonstrates uniform cells with mosaic-like distinct borders.

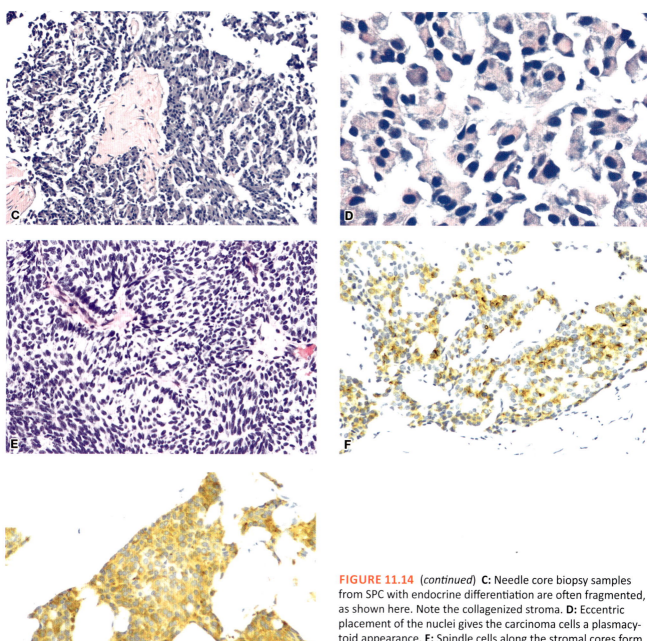

FIGURE 11.14 (*continued*) C: Needle core biopsy samples from SPC with endocrine differentiation are often fragmented, as shown here. Note the collagenized stroma. D: Eccentric placement of the nuclei gives the carcinoma cells a plasmacytoid appearance. E: Spindle cells along the stromal cores form palisades. F, G: Cytoplasmic reactivity for chromogranin (F) and synaptophysin (G) in another case of SPC with neuroendocrine differentiation.

cells and the adjacent stroma (Fig. 11.16). This phenomenon can occur within the tumor, adjacent to fibrovascular stalks, and at the border of tumor cell clusters. Larger accumulations may surround or disrupt portions of the epithelium. These pools of mucin should not be interpreted as invasive mucinous carcinoma unless they contain detached malignant cells and extend into the adjacent stroma.

Characteristics that may be useful for distinguishing between EPC and SPC are summarized in **Table 11.2**. Occasionally, a papillary carcinoma exhibits overlapping features of SPC and EPC (9,48,49), which precludes classification even on excision (Fig. 11.17). Limited sampling of a hybrid tumor may not capture all patterns. On NCB, "noninvasive papillary carcinoma with features suggestive of EPC/SPC" may be documented.

Invasive Papillary Carcinoma

Most invasive carcinomas arising in association with papillary DCIS, EPC, or SPC are conventional *invasive ductal carcinomas of no special type* (IDC NST), consisting of irregular jigsaw puzzle-like growths infiltrating fibrous or fibrofatty stroma and lacking papillary fronds. Only rare invasive carcinomas that show invasive glands containing papillary formations (in >90% of the tumor) are designated *invasive papillary carcinomas* (Fig. 11.18).

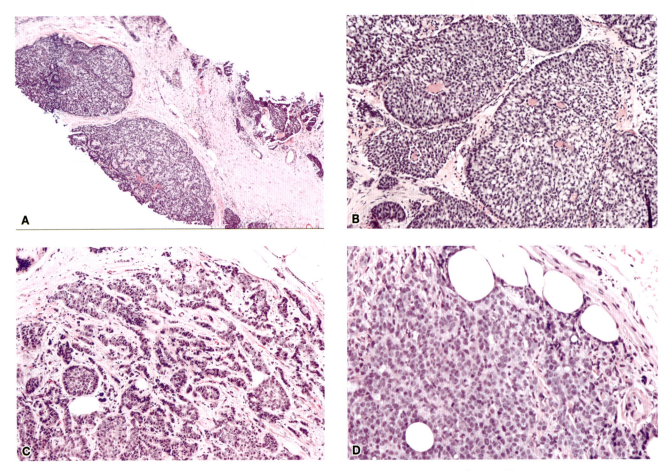

FIGURE 11.15 **Solid Papillary Carcinoma (SPC) With Invasion. A, B:** A needle core biopsy specimen showing SPC with signet ring cells, which were positive with the mucicarmine stain. Some glandular areas in the lower left of **(B)** have uneven borders, but invasion is not definite. **C:** The excision specimen contained this area of invasive carcinoma. Note the distinctly different growth patterns of the noninvasive and invasive components. **D:** Invasion of fat with a solid growth pattern in another example of SPC.

Carcinoma cells growing on a branching framework form a more or less compact mass, sometimes with cystic regions, that dissects into the surrounding tissue. Cribriform, tubular, and mucinous foci may also be present in the invasive component. The nuclear grade is low or intermediate in over 80% of cases (5).

Although the invasive nature of papillary carcinomas is usually obvious, the recognition of minimal invasion can

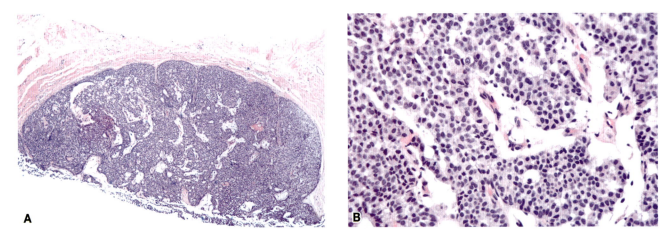

FIGURE 11.16 **Solid Papillary Carcinoma (SPC) With Mucinous Differentiation and Invasion. A:** This needle core biopsy specimen shows a well-circumscribed nodule of SPC. **B:** Mucin accumulation is evident between the neoplastic epithelium and fibrovascular stroma.

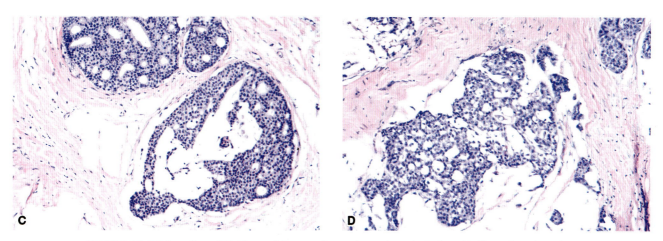

FIGURE 11.16 (*continued*) **C:** The excision specimen shown here includes cribriform ductal carcinoma in situ (upper border) as well as mucin in and partially around a duct (center). The presence of mucin in the stroma is not diagnostic of invasive carcinoma. **D:** Invasive mucinous carcinoma consists of extracellular mucin surrounding irregular groups of carcinoma cells in the stroma.

TABLE 11.2
Differential Diagnosis of Encapsulated Papillary Carcinoma and Solid Papillary Carcinoma

Histopathologic Features	EPC	SPC
Tumor nodule(s)	Single	Multiple
Architecture	Cystic, cribriform, papillary	Solid
"Capsule"	Prominent, thick	Ill-defined, thin
Internal fibrovascular cores	Prominent	Inconspicuous
Neoplastic cells	Columnar	Polygonal
Neuroendocrine features	Absent	Present
Extracellular mucin	Uncommon	Common
Unequivocal invasion	Uncommon	More common

EPC, encapsulated papillary carcinoma; SPC, solid papillary carcinoma.

Adapted from Patel A, Hoda RS, Hoda SA. Papillary breast tumors: continuing controversies and commentary on WHO's 2019 criteria and classification. *Int J Surg Pathol* 2022;30(2):124-137. doi:10.1177/10668969211035843

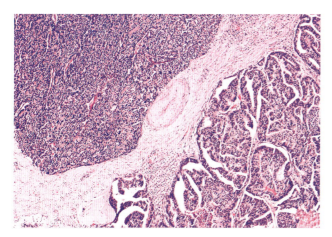

FIGURE 11.17 **Hybrid Papillary Carcinoma.** This tumor demonstrates morphologic features of both solid papillary carcinoma (upper left) and papillary ductal carcinoma in situ (lower right).

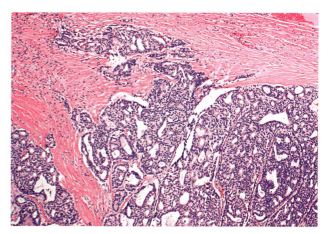

FIGURE 11.18 **Invasive Papillary Carcinoma.** The periphery of this papillary carcinoma shows irregular extension into the stroma, perpendicular to the contour of the tumor, diagnostic of invasion. The invasive component retains a papillary architecture.

be difficult. Fibrosis, hemorrhage, and chronic inflammatory cell infiltrate surround many papillary carcinomas. The finding of epithelial clusters within these areas presents a challenge. Groups of neoplastic cells distributed parallel to layers of reactive stroma at the border of a papillary carcinoma usually represent cells entrapped in distorted preexisting glands rather than invasive carcinoma. Perpendicular extension of the suspicious cells beyond the zone of reactive changes into the mammary parenchyma offers the most reliable histologic evidence of invasion. Immunohistochemical staining for myoepithelial cells can clarify uncertain cases, especially when coupled with a stain for keratin. A change in the pattern of growth also strongly suggests the presence of invasion. When scant sampling precludes a more precise diagnosis, "fragments of papillary carcinoma (without definitive invasion)" are sufficient to prompt excision.

TALL CELL CARCINOMA WITH REVERSED POLARITY

A variant of papillary carcinoma termed *tall cell carcinoma with reversed polarity* (erstwhile "SPC resembling the tall cell variant of papillary thyroid neoplasm") has been described (50,51) **(Fig. 11.19)**. The carcinoma cells grow in solid, papillary, and cribriform aggregates. The glands typically contain densely eosinophilic, homogeneous material with scalloped borders that resembles thyroid colloid. The neoplastic cells have columnar-to-cuboidal shapes, slightly pleomorphic oval nuclei, and eosinophilic granular cytoplasm. The nuclei may sit next to the luminal membranes, an orientation referred to as "reversed polarity." The nuclei have angular contours, grooves, and eosinophilic pseudoinclusions, and some nuclei appear clear. Psammoma bodies may be noted. Most examples express CK7 and calretinin (52), but staining for EMA, GATA3, mammaglobin, and GCDFP-15 has yielded variable results. Most do not express ER or PR (50,51). Hotspot point mutations in *IDH2* are characteristic (53,54). Despite morphologic similarities to the tall cell variant of papillary thyroid carcinoma (55), this entity does not express TTF-1 or thyroglobulin, nor does it display mutations of *RET* or *BRAF*.

OTHER PATTERNS

Carcinoma Involving a Papilloma

Papillomas harboring DCIS display remnants of preexisting benign as well as malignant ductal cells. The intermingling of benign and malignant cells can make the diagnosis of this type of papillary lesion difficult, especially based on the small and fragmented samples provided by NCBs. Signs of an underlying papilloma include blunt bulky fronds composed of dense acellular collagen, collections of histiocytes within stromal cores, and segments of epithelium containing well-arranged bland luminal and myoepithelial cells. To make a diagnosis of carcinoma in the presence of an underlying papilloma, one must find a sizable region (3 mm) in which the growth pattern and cytologic features constitute one of the established patterns of DCIS **(Fig. 11.20)**. A more limited focus can be classified as papilloma with ADH. Foci of atypia or carcinoma can typically be highlighted by stains for estrogen receptor (strongly positive) and CK5/6 (negative).

The presence of a papilloma should not distract from the diagnosis of malignancy or atypia. In multiple studies, the relative risk for the development of subsequent carcinoma in women with papilloma with ADH was 4 to 7.5 times the risk of women with papilloma without ADH/DCIS (56,57). The risk further increased when the atypia involved multiple papillomas. Underdiagnosis of such lesions is likely to result in inadequate treatment, as reflected in the outcomes in these reports.

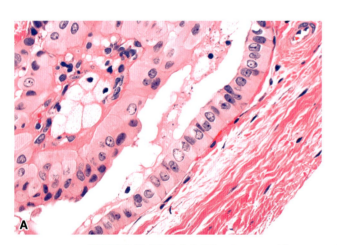 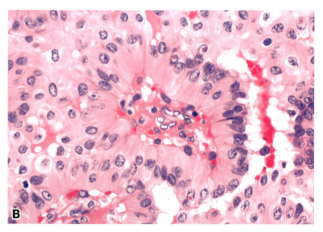

FIGURE 11.19 Tall Cell Carcinoma With Reversed Polarity. A: Cells at least twice as tall as wide with eosinophilic cytoplasm line fibrovascular cores. An aggregate of foamy macrophages is present. **B:** The nuclei are oval with small nucleoli and chromatin clearing and are characteristically polarized away from the fibrovascular cores.

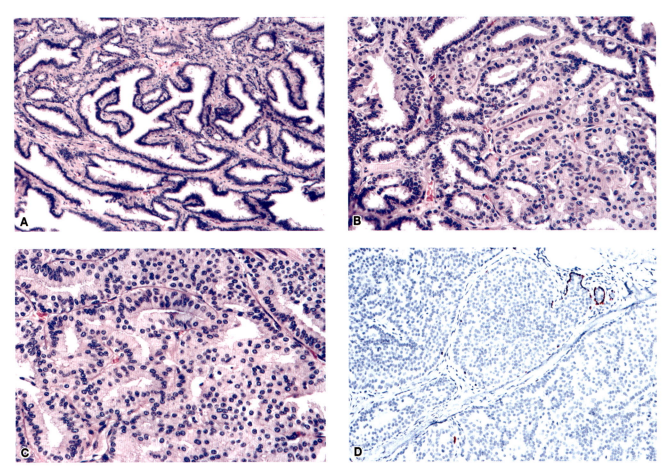

FIGURE 11.20 **Papillary Carcinoma Arising in a Papilloma.** Several areas in a single tumor are shown. **A:** This papilloma has a thin uniform layer of cuboidal and low-columnar cells overlying a prominent layer of myoepithelial cells and broad strands of stroma. **B:** An enlarged view from another region shows mingling of atypical ductal cells and normal luminal cells. In the region dominated by the atypical ductal cells (right), one has difficulty recognizing myoepithelial cells, and the stromal strands appear slenderer. **C:** The carcinoma cells form cribriform structures. Note the persisting arborizing stroma and the virtual absence of myoepithelial cells. **D:** The p63 immunostain reveals that this focus of solid ductal carcinoma in situ lacks myoepithelial cells. A few residual myoepithelial cells remain (upper right).

Infarction in Papillary Tumors

Both papillary carcinomas and papillomas can undergo infarction (ie, ischemic necrosis) either spontaneously or after a needling procedure **(Fig. 11.21A and B)**. In many examples of this phenomenon, the structure of the lesion becomes so altered that one cannot differentiate a papillary carcinoma from a papilloma using H&E-stained sections. Immunostains can help to resolve uncertainties if the reactivity of the pertinent antigens remains. For example, preserved reactivity for keratin may highlight the structure of the tumor **(Fig. 11.21C)**, and reactivity for p63 may reveal the presence of myoepithelial cells.

Epithelial Displacement

Papillary tumors subjected to needle aspiration or core biopsy before excision can exhibit alterations that complicate the recognition of invasion. The best microscopic clues to such manipulation are the presence of fresh hemorrhage and granulation tissue associated with the fragmentation of the lesion. One can find single tumor cells or compact cell clusters in regions of hemorrhage or granulation tissue formation along the track of the needle. These foci abut normal fat cells or, less commonly, fibrous stroma. In this clinical setting, one should regard these detached cells as a procedural artifact rather than evidence of invasion. These displaced cells can make their way into capillaries and lymphatic vessels. One should report this uncommon finding because it may be misinterpreted as evidence of invasive carcinoma in some instances (58). Clusters of invasive papillary carcinoma cells are particularly prone to shrinkage artifacts, and they often seem to lie in spaces simulating lymphatic tumor emboli. Strict criteria for the diagnosis of lymphatic invasion should be applied in such cases.

Epithelial displacement associated with needling procedures is further discussed in Chapter 25.

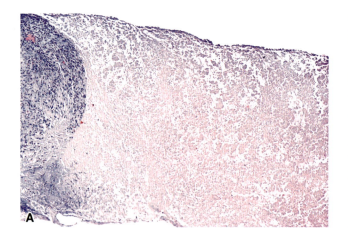
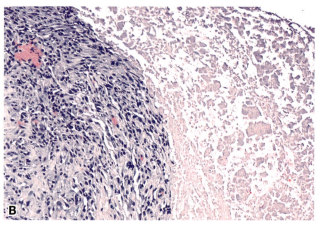
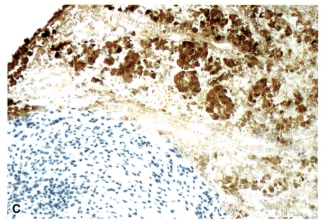

FIGURE 11.21 Infarcted Papillary Tumor, Probably Carcinoma. A, B: The needle core biopsy sample consists of infarcted tumor. Stroma with inflammatory cells is shown on the left. **C:** Papillary clusters of epithelial cells in the infarcted tissue are highlighted by the CK7 immunostain.

Metastatic Papillary Carcinoma in Breast

Purely papillary morphology is relatively rare in invasive breast carcinomas and relatively common in malignancies originating in other organs, such as the lung, pancreas, thyroid (59), kidney (60), and müllerian organs. The rare papillary pattern of prostatic carcinoma can present as a metastasis in the male breast (61). In the absence of DCIS, one may consider immunohistochemical staining for GATA3, SOX10, and/or TRPS1 to support breast origin (also see Chapter 22).

MOLECULAR STUDIES

Papillary carcinoma subtypes are overall similar at the genomic level. They have fewer genomic aberrations than grade- and ER-matched IDC NST (46) and similar patterns of changes, including 16q loss and *PIK3CA* mutations (40). However, there are a few distinctions. EPC and SPC differ in expression levels in less than 0.2% of genes, namely those involved in cell organization, migration, angiogenesis, and homeostasis (46). Unsupervised hierarchical clustering of microarray gene expression data using two different algorithms showed that EPCs clustered separately from SPCs, wherein the former were predominantly luminal A and the latter luminal B. Compared with SPC, EPC had decreased expression of genes related to neuroendocrine differentiation, including *RET*, *ASCL1*, and *DOK7*, as well as cell migration genes *PLAT* and *CTSF* (46). SPC also shares transcriptomic features with cellular mucinous carcinoma (62).

PROGNOSIS AND TREATMENT

Changing terminology, disagreement about the invasive nature of the lesions, variation in the evaluation and treatment of patients, and short follow-up intervals make it difficult to make detailed recommendations regarding the management of papillary carcinoma. Patients with papillary carcinomas generally experience good prognosis (3,5,63). A study by Zheng et al using data from the SEER database showed that after controlling for patient age, tumor size, histologic grade, hormone receptor profile, and lymph node metastases, patients with invasive papillary carcinoma had comparable survival to those with IDC NST (5). In a study of 284 patients with invasive papillary carcinoma, only four (1.4%) of the patients died of their papillary carcinoma (3).

The prognosis for patients with SPC is relatively favorable. In most cases of noninvasive SPC described in the literature, the patients remained free of metastatic carcinoma. Axillary lymph node and systemic metastases develop at a noticeable rate in patients with invasive SPC (64). In about one-half of the reported cases, the axillary metastases resembled the primary SPC; in the others, coexisting invasive carcinomas gave rise to the metastatic foci. At least seven deaths have been attributed to SPCs (65,66). Assessment of nine EPCs and five SPCs by a validated 21-gene assay yielded mostly low recurrence scores (≤17) (67).

The definitive treatment of patients with papillary carcinomas has ranged from excision to modified radical mastectomy, and a minority of patients have received radiation and systemic therapy. This variation in treatment coupled with uncertainties regarding the interpretation of certain histologic findings makes it difficult to formulate generic, well-founded treatment recommendations. Papillary carcinomas without frank invasion are considered to behave similarly to conventional DCIS and are presently managed accordingly. Complete excision of the carcinoma would seem prudent in all cases. Features such as the patient's age and the size and grade of the invasive component could help to determine the need for sampling of axillary lymph nodes and for the use of radiation and systemic therapy (68,69).

REFERENCES

1. Patel A, Hoda RS, Hoda SA. Papillary breast tumors: continuing controversies and commentary on WHO's 2019 criteria and classification. *Int J Surg Pathol.* 2022;30:124-137.
2. Rakha EA, Ellis IO. Diagnostic challenges in papillary lesions of the breast. *Pathology.* 2018;50:100-110.
3. Liu ZY, Liu N, Wang YH, et al. Clinicopathologic characteristics and molecular subtypes of invasive papillary carcinoma of the breast: a large case study. *J Cancer Res Clin Oncol.* 2013;139:77-84.
4. Zhang J, Zhang T, Wu N, et al. Intracystic papillary carcinoma of the breast: experience of a major Chinese cancer center. *Pathol Res Pract.* 2018;214:579-585.
5. Zheng YZ, Hu X, Shao ZM. Clinicopathological characteristics and survival outcomes in invasive papillary carcinoma of the breast: a seer population-based study. *Sci Rep.* 2016;6:24037.
6. Burga AM, Fadare O, Lininger RA, et al. Invasive carcinomas of the male breast: a morphologic study of the distribution of histologic subtypes and metastatic patterns in 778 cases. *Virchows Arch.* 2006;449:507-512.
7. Giordano SH, Cohen DS, Buzdar AU, et al. Breast carcinoma in men: a population-based study. *Cancer.* 2004;101:51-57.
8. Mogal H, Brown DR, Isom S, et al. Intracystic papillary carcinoma of the breast: a SEER database analysis of implications for therapy. *Breast.* 2016;27:87-92.
9. Zhong E, Cheng E, Goldfischer M, et al. Papillary lesions of the male breast: a study of 117 cases and brief review of the literature demonstrate a broad clinicopathologic spectrum. *Am J Surg Pathol.* 2020;44:68-76.
10. Estabrook A, Asch T, Gump F, et al. Mammographic features of intracystic papillary lesions. *Surg Gynecol Obstet.* 1990;170:113-116.
11. McCulloch GL, Evans AJ, Yeoman L, et al. Radiological features of papillary carcinoma of the breast. *Clin Radiol.* 1997;52:865-868.
12. Schneider JA. Invasive papillary breast carcinoma: mammographic and sonographic appearance. *Radiology.* 1989;171:377-379.
13. Soo MS, Williford ME, Walsh R, et al. Papillary carcinoma of the breast: imaging findings. *AJR Am J Roentgenol.* 1995;164:321-326.
14. Silva R, Ferrozzi F, Paties C. Invasive papillary carcinoma in elderly women: sonographic and mammographic features. *AJR Am J Roentgenol.* 1992;159:898-899.
15. You C, Peng W, Shen X, et al. Solid papillary carcinoma of the breast: magnetic resonance mammography, digital mammography, and ultrasound findings. *J Comput Assist Tomogr.* 2018;42:771-775.
16. Jiang T, Tang W, Gu Y, et al. Magnetic resonance imaging features of breast encapsulated papillary carcinoma. *J Comput Assist Tomogr.* 2018;42:536-541.
17. Reisenbichler ES, Balmer NN, Adams AL, et al. Luminal cytokeratin expression profiles of breast papillomas and papillary carcinomas and the utility of a cytokeratin 5/p63/cytokeratin 8/18 antibody cocktail in their distinction. *Mod Pathol.* 2011;24:185-193.
18. Tse GM, Tan PH, Lui PC, et al. The role of immunohistochemistry for smooth-muscle actin, p63, CD10 and cytokeratin 14 in the differential diagnosis of papillary lesions of the breast. *J Clin Pathol.* 2007;60:315-320.
19. Moritani S, Ichihara S, Hasegawa M, et al. Uniqueness of ductal carcinoma in situ of the breast concurrent with papilloma: implications from a detailed topographical and histopathological study of 50 cases treated by mastectomy and wide local excision. *Histopathology.* 2013;63:407-417.
20. Lefkowitz M, Lefkowitz W, Wargotz ES. Intraductal (intracystic) papillary carcinoma of the breast and its variants: a clinicopathological study of 77 cases. *Hum Pathol.* 1994;25:802-809.
21. Yamaguchi R, Tanaka M, Tse GM, et al. Broad fibrovascular cores may not be an exclusively benign feature in papillary lesions of the breast: a cautionary note. *J Clin Pathol.* 2014;67:258-262.
22. Stefanou D, Batistatou A, Nonni A, et al. P63 expression in benign and malignant breast lesions. *Histol Histopathol.* 2004;19:465-471.
23. Collins LC, Carlo VP, Hwang H, et al. Intracystic papillary carcinomas of the breast: a reevaluation using a panel of myoepithelial cell markers. *Am J Surg Pathol.* 2006;30:1002-1007.
24. Hill CB, Yeh IT. Myoepithelial cell staining patterns of papillary breast lesions: from intraductal papillomas to invasive papillary carcinomas. *Am J Clin Pathol.* 2005;123:36-44.
25. Nicolas MM, Wu Y, Middleton LP, et al. Loss of myoepithelium is variable in solid papillary carcinoma of the breast. *Histopathology.* 2007;51:657-665.
26. Rabban JT, Koerner FC, Lerwill MF. Solid papillary ductal carcinoma in situ versus usual ductal hyperplasia in the breast: a potentially difficult distinction resolved by cytokeratin 5/6. *Hum Pathol.* 2006;37:787-793.
27. Tan PH, Aw MY, Yip G, et al. Cytokeratins in papillary lesions of the breast: is there a role in distinguishing intraductal papilloma from papillary ductal carcinoma in situ? *Am J Surg Pathol.* 2005;29:625-632.
28. Douglas-Jones A, Shah V, Morgan J, et al. Observer variability in the histopathological reporting of core biopsies of papillary breast lesions is reduced by the use of immunohistochemistry for CK5/6, calponin and p63. *Histopathology.* 2005;47:202-208.
29. Grin A, O'Malley FP, Mulligan AM. Cytokeratin 5 and estrogen receptor immunohistochemistry as a useful adjunct in identifying atypical papillary lesions on breast needle core biopsy. *Am J Surg Pathol.* 2009;33:1615-1623.
30. Wang Y, Zhu JF, Liu YY, et al. An analysis of cyclin d1, cytokeratin 5/6 and cytokeratin 8/18 expression in breast papillomas and papillary carcinomas. *Diagn Pathol.* 2013;8:8.
31. Lin CH, Liu CH, Wen CH, et al. Differential CD133 expression distinguishes malignant from benign papillary lesions of the breast. *Virchows Arch.* 2015;466:177-184.
32. Rakha EA, Gandhi N, Climent F, et al. Encapsulated papillary carcinoma of the breast: an invasive tumor with excellent prognosis. *Am J Surg Pathol.* 2011;35:1093-1103.
33. Wynveen CA, Nehhozina T, Akram M, et al. Intracystic papillary carcinoma of the breast: an in situ or invasive tumor? results of immunohistochemical analysis and clinical follow-up. *Am J Surg Pathol.* 2011;35:1-14.
34. Allison KH, Brogi E, Ellis IO, et al. *Breast Tumours: WHO Classification of Tumours.* 5th ed. IARC Press; 2019.
35. Esposito NN, Dabbs DJ, Bhargava R. Are encapsulated papillary carcinomas of the breast in situ or invasive? A basement membrane study of 27 cases. *Am J Clin Pathol.* 2009;131:228-242.
36. Rakha EA, Tun M, Junainah E, et al. Encapsulated papillary carcinoma of the breast: a study of invasion associated markers. *J Clin Pathol.* 2012;65:710-714.
37. Mulligan AM, O'Malley FP. Metastatic potential of encapsulated (intracystic) papillary carcinoma of the breast: a report of 2 cases with axillary lymph node micrometastases. *Int J Surg Pathol.* 2007;15:143-147.
38. Solorzano CC, Middleton LP, Hunt KK, et al. Treatment and outcome of patients with intracystic papillary carcinoma of the breast. *Am J Surg.* 2002;184:364-368.
39. Kitahara M, Hozumi Y, Takeuchi N, et al. Distant metastasis after surgery for encapsulated papillary carcinoma of the breast: a case report. *Case Rep Oncol.* 2020;13:1196-1201.
40. Duprez R, Wilkerson PM, Lacroix-Triki M, et al. Immunophenotypic and genomic characterization of papillary carcinomas of the breast. *J Pathol.* 2012;226:427-441.
41. Liu X, Wu H, Teng L, et al. High-grade encapsulated papillary carcinoma of the breast is clinicopathologically distinct from low/intermediate-grade neoplasms in Chinese patients. *Histol Histopathol.* 2019;34:137-147.
42. Rakha EA, Varga Z, Elsheik S, et al. High-grade encapsulated papillary carcinoma of the breast: an under-recognized entity. *Histopathology.* 2015;66:740-746.
43. Tang F, Wei B, Tian Z, et al. Invasive mammary carcinoma with neuroendocrine differentiation: histological features and diagnostic challenges. *Histopathology.* 2011;59:106-115.
44. Kudo N, Takano J, Kudoh S, et al. INSM1 immunostaining in solid papillary carcinoma of the breast. *Pathol Int.* 2021;71:51-59.
45. Zhong E, Pareja F, Hanna MG, et al. Expression of novel neuroendocrine markers in breast carcinomas: a study of INSM1, ASCL1, and POU2F3. *Hum Pathol.* 2022;127:102-111.
46. Piscuoglio S, Ng CK, Martelotto LG, et al. Integrative genomic and transcriptomic characterization of papillary carcinomas of the breast. *Mol Oncol.* 2014;8:1588-1602.
47. Rosen LE, Gattuso P. Neuroendocrine tumors of the breast. *Arch Pathol Lab Med.* 2017;141:1577-1581.
48. Cui X, Wei S. Composite encapsulated papillary carcinoma and solid papillary carcinoma. *Pathol Int.* 2015;65:133-137.
49. Solanki MH, Derylo AF, Visotcky AM, et al. Encapsulated and solid papillary carcinomas of the breast: tumors in transition from in situ to invasive? *Breast J.* 2019;25:539-541.
50. Eusebi V, Damiani S, Ellis IO, et al. Breast tumor resembling the tall cell variant of papillary thyroid carcinoma: report of 5 cases. *Am J Surg Pathol.* 2003;27:1114-1118.
51. Foschini MP, Asioli S, Foreid S, et al. Solid papillary breast carcinomas resembling the tall cell variant of papillary thyroid neoplasms: a unique invasive tumor with indolent behavior. *Am J Surg Pathol.* 2017;41:887-895.
52. Alsadoun N, MacGrogan G, Truntzer C, et al. Solid papillary carcinoma with reverse polarity of the breast harbors specific morphologic, immunohistochemical and molecular profile in comparison with other benign or malignant papillary lesions of the breast: a comparative study of 9 additional cases. *Mod Pathol.* 2018;31:1367-1380.

240 CHAPTER 11

53. Chiang S, Weigelt B, Wen HC, et al. IDH2 mutations define a unique subtype of breast cancer with altered nuclear polarity. *Cancer Res.* 2016;76:7118-7129.

54. Pareja F, da Silva EM, Frosina D, et al. Immunohistochemical analysis of IDH2 R172 hotspot mutations in breast papillary neoplasms: applications in the diagnosis of tall cell carcinoma with reverse polarity. *Mod Pathol.* 2020;33:1056-1064.

55. Zhong E, Scognamiglio T, D'Alfonso T, et al. Breast tumor resembling the tall cell variant of papillary thyroid carcinoma: molecular characterization by next-generation sequencing and histopathological comparison with tall cell papillary carcinoma of thyroid. *Int J Surg Pathol.* 2019;27:134-141.

56. Lewis JT, Hartmann LC, Vierkant RA, et al. An analysis of breast cancer risk in women with single, multiple, and atypical papilloma. *Am J Surg Pathol.* 2006;30:665-672.

57. Page DL, Salhany KE, Jensen RA, et al. Subsequent breast carcinoma risk after biopsy with atypia in a breast papilloma. *Cancer.* 1996;78:258-266.

58. Youngson BJ, Cranor M, Rosen PP. Epithelial displacement in surgical breast specimens following needling procedures. *Am J Surg Pathol.* 1994;18:896-903.

59. Worapongpaiboon R, Vongsaisuwon M. Breast metastasis of papillary thyroid carcinoma. *BMJ Case Rep.* 2022;15:e251081.

60. Gupta D, Merino MI, Farhood A, et al. Metastases to breast simulating ductal carcinoma in situ: report of two cases and review of the literature. *Ann Diagn Pathol.* 2001;5:15-20.

61. Washburn ER, Weyant GW, Yang XJ, et al. A rare case of prostatic ductal adenocarcinoma presenting as papillary metastatic carcinoma of unknown primary: a case report and review of the literature. *Hum Pathol.* 2016;6:26-31.

62. Weigelt B, Geyer FC, Horlings HM, et al. Mucinous and neuroendocrine breast carcinomas are transcriptionally distinct from invasive ductal carcinomas of no special type. *Mod Pathol.* 2009;22:1401-1414.

63. Huang K, Appiah L, Mishra A, et al. Clinicopathologic characteristics and prognosis of invasive papillary carcinoma of the breast. *J Surg Res.* 2021;261:105-112.

64. Guo S, Wang Y, Rohr J, et al. Solid papillary carcinoma of the breast: a special entity needs to be distinguished from conventional invasive carcinoma avoiding over-treatment. *Breast.* 2016;26:67-72.

65. Nassar H, Qureshi H, Adsay NV, et al. Clinicopathologic analysis of solid papillary carcinoma of the breast and associated invasive carcinomas. *Am J Surg Pathol.* 2006;30:501-507.

66. Tariq MU, Idress R, Qureshi MB, et al. Solid papillary carcinoma of breast; a detailed clinicopathological study of 65 cases of an uncommon breast neoplasm with literature review. *Breast J.* 2020;26:211-215.

67. Turashvili G, Brogi E, Morrow M, et al. The 21-gene recurrence score in special histologic subtypes of breast cancer with favorable prognosis. *Breast Cancer Res Treat.* 2017;165:65-76.

68. Fayanju OM, Ritter J, Gillanders WE, et al. Therapeutic management of intracystic papillary carcinoma of the breast: the roles of radiation and endocrine therapy. *Am J Surg.* 2007;194:497-500.

69. Louwman MW, Vriezen M, van Beek MW, et al. Uncommon breast tumors in perspective: incidence, treatment and survival in the Netherlands. *Int J Cancer.* 2007;121:127-135.

12

Medullary Carcinoma and Related Carcinomas

RAZA S. HODA AND SYED A. HODA

The term *medullary* (from Latin: pith, marrow, ie, bone marrow-like) alludes to the soft nature of the tumor—as opposed to the scirrhous (ie, firm) feel of most invasive breast carcinomas. Other terms which have been used in the past for medullary carcinoma are "bulky," "lymphoepithelioma-like," "neo-mammary," and "solid circumscribed" carcinomas.

Medullary carcinoma refers to a well-circumscribed carcinoma composed of higher-grade mitotically active cells arranged in syncytia, with scant stroma and a prominent lymphoplasmacytic infiltrate. The term *atypical medullary carcinoma* was introduced to describe carcinomas that have some, but not all, defining characteristic features of medullary

carcinoma. Atypical medullary carcinoma has also been classified as *invasive ductal carcinomas with medullary features*. The (rather mystifying) evolution of medullary carcinoma as successively outlined by the World Health Organization (WHO) in all five of its iterations is summarized in **Table 12.1**.

The 5th edition of *WHO Classification of Tumors of the Breast* recommends that medullary carcinoma be included in the spectrum of invasive carcinoma of no special type (specifically as "invasive breast carcinoma of no special type with medullary pattern") characterized by predominance of stromal tumor–infiltrating lymphocytes and high-grade nuclei (1). This movement away from the diagnostic category

---

TABLE 12.1

Evolution of Medullary Carcinoma Over 50+ Years (1968-2019) in Successive Editions of World Health Organization (WHO) Classification of Breast Tumors

1st, 1968
Medullary carcinoma (ca): "…with minimal amount of fibrous tissue stroma, which may or may not show lymphoid infiltration…cells are arranged in syncytial masses and do not show a great deal of hyperchromatism or variation in nuclear size. The tumors may be rich in mitoses."

2nd, 1981
Medullary ca: "… poorly differentiated cells with scant stroma and prominent lymphoid infiltration…. Tumor cells are large with vesicular nuclei, prominent nucleoli, and indistinct cytoplasmic outlines…Tumor borders should be histologically blunt."

3rd, 2003
Medullary ca: "…five morphological traits: 1. syncytial architecture should be observed in over 75% of the tumour mass. 2. Glandular or tubular structures are not present. 3. Diffuse lymphoplasmacytic stromal infiltrate is a conspicuous features. 4. Carcinoma cells are usually round with abundant cytoplasm. 5. Complete histological circumscription of the tumor is best seen under low magnification." **Atypical medullary ca:** "predominantly syncytial architecture with only two or three of the other criteria…"

4th, 2012
Ca with medullary features: "…include medullary carcinomas, atypical medullary ca, and a subset of invasive carcinomas of no special type… demonstrate all or some of the following features: a circumscribed or pushing border, a syncytial growth pattern, cells with high-grade nuclei, and prominent lymphoid infiltrate"[a]

5th, 2019
Medullary ca eliminated as an entity: "diagnosing classic medullary ca…a *challenge*" (however, proposal to use "invasive breast carcinoma of no special type with medullary pattern.") Medullary ca is included in the spectrum of invasive ca of no special type characterized by predominance of stromal tumor–infiltrating lymphocytes and high-grade nuclei, ie, regarded as part of spectrum of tumor-infiltrating lymphocytes-rich breast ca.

1st edition: Scarff RW, Torloni H, eds. *International Histological Classification of Tumors. No 2—Histological Typing of Breast Tumors*. World Health Organization; 1968. **2nd edition:** *International Histological Classification of Tumors. No 2—Histological Typing of Breast Tumors*. 2nd ed. World Health Organization; 1981. **3rd edition:** Tavassoli FA, Devilee P, eds. *World Health Organization Classification of Tumors. Pathology and Genetics of Tumours of the Breast*. IARC Press; 2003. **4th edition:** Lakhani SR, Ellis IO, Schnitt SJ, et al, eds. *WHO Classification of Tumors of the Breast. Carcinomas With Medullary Features*. 4th ed. IARC Press; 2012. **5th edition:** Editorial Board, ed. *WHO Classification of Tumor WHO Classification of Tumors*. 5th ed. IARC; 2019.

[a]Entities combined since "diagnostic criteria are difficult to apply," *notwithstanding persistence of three different International Classification of Disease codes for the respective entities.*

of medullary seems regrettable because well-conducted clinical follow-up studies continue to demonstrate the favorable prognosis afforded by this type of breast carcinoma. It would be a shame to abandon the diagnosis of medullary carcinoma at a time when contemporary genomic studies offer the opportunity for a greater understanding of this type of tumor and improved specificity of its diagnosis. Until investigators have fully explored this group of tumors at the genetic level, it seems preferable to continue to classify certain carefully characterized carcinomas as medullary.

CLINICAL PRESENTATION

Medullary carcinoma constitutes fewer than 5% of breast carcinomas in most series (2-5). Patients as young as 21 years (6) and as old as 95 years (7) with medullary carcinomas have been reported. This broad range of ages notwithstanding, patients with medullary carcinoma tend to be relatively young. The mean age in several series ranges from 45 to 54 years (6,8-10). Medullary carcinoma is rare in the male breast (11).

The site and size distribution of medullary carcinoma do not differ from those of other common types of breast carcinomas. Medullary carcinoma is uncommon among patients with bilateral mammary carcinoma. On the other hand, bilateral carcinomas have been found in 3% to 12% of patients with medullary carcinoma (2,7,12). Synchronous or metachronous medullary carcinoma involving both breasts is uncommon (7,12).

Ipsilateral axillary lymph nodes tend to be enlarged in patients with medullary carcinoma because of marked reactive hyperplasia, even in the absence of nodal metastases. This phenomenon may lead to *clinical* upstaging (13). The relative ease of detecting the enlarged hyperplastic lymph nodes accounts for the larger number of lymph nodes retrieved from axillary dissections in patients with medullary carcinoma compared with specimens from patients with other types of carcinoma (14).

IMAGING STUDIES

Imaging studies of medullary carcinomas typically demonstrate a dense, round or oval mass with lobulated borders without calcifications (15). The circumscribed edges of medullary carcinoma can lead to it being misinterpreted as fibroadenoma. Imaging studies cannot differentiate medullary carcinoma from circumscribed non-medullary carcinoma (16). A mass with an irregular or jagged margin is highly unlikely to be a medullary carcinoma.

GROSS PATHOLOGY

On gross examination, medullary carcinoma is a relatively soft discrete tumor that could be mistaken for a fibroadenoma. A distinct edge usually outlines the mass and demarcates it from adjacent tissues; however, a marked peritumoral lymphoplasmacytic infiltrate at the perimeter of a carcinoma may blur the edge of the tumor. Medullary carcinoma has a lobulated or nodular structure on the cut section. Necrosis can lead to the formation of cysts in larger tumors.

HISTOPATHOLOGY

Despite the long-standing and relatively well-known diagnostic criteria of medullary carcinoma **(Table 12.2)**, the entity has suffered from varying degrees of interobserver diagnostic variability (17,18). Be that as it may, it is necessary to strictly adhere to established histopathologic criteria if the diagnosis of medullary carcinoma is to be predictive of a relatively favorable prognosis (7,8). Although alternative criteria (including some with imprecise boundaries) have been proposed, those set forth by Ridolfi et al (8) remain the most reliable for detecting survival differences between true medullary, atypical medullary, and non-medullary carcinomas (19).

Medullary carcinoma is defined by the following constellation of histopathologic features: prominent lymphoplasmacytic infiltrate, circumscription (with "pushing" margins), growth in sheets (with a syncytial pattern), high (poorly differentiated)-nuclear grade, and a high mitotic rate. A tumor must display all of these features to qualify for the diagnosis of medullary carcinoma. The tumor may be termed as *infiltrating ductal carcinoma with medullary features/atypical medullary carcinoma* when most, but not all, of these findings are present. Tumors in the latter category have some histopathologic features of medullary carcinoma but also show one or more of the following variations: invasive growth at the perimeter of the tumor, sparse or diminished lymphoplasmacytic reaction, low-grade nuclei, low-mitotic rate, or conspicuous glandular, trabecular, or papillary growth. Invasive ductal carcinomas with medullary features can display immunohistochemical findings seen in typical medullary carcinomas, but they do so less frequently.

The *lymphoplasmacytic reaction* must involve the periphery and be present diffusely within the tumor. Tumors with negligible *lymphoplasmacytic* infiltrate are best excluded from the diagnosis of medullary carcinoma. The internal lymphoplasmacytic infiltrate tends to be limited to fibrovascular stroma between syncytial zones of tumor cells.

TABLE 12.2
Medullary Carcinoma

Key Histopathologic Features

1. Syncytial pattern of growth in >75% of tumors
2. Lack of glandular structures
3. Diffusely prominent lymphoplasmacytic infiltrate
4. Nuclear pleomorphism, moderate to marked
5. High mitotic rate
6. Broad "pushing" borders with microscopic circumscription

From Ridolfi RL, Rosen PP, Port A, et al. Medullary carcinoma of the breast: a clinicopathologic study with 10 yr follow-up. *Cancer.* 1977;40:1365-1385.

Medullary carcinomas may occasionally be largely devoid of stroma, and the lymphoplasmacytic infiltrate may be intermingled with carcinoma (**Figs. 12.1-12.4**).

The amount of the lymphoplasmacytic infiltrate may vary, but it should appear at least moderately intense at the interface of the carcinoma with the mammary parenchyma and in the adjacent tissue. In the typical case, the lymphoplasmacytic reaction encompasses adjacent benign ducts and lobules, as well as those occupied by in situ carcinoma, in the vicinity of the dominant tumor. These secondary peripheral alterations are so common in medullary carcinoma that the diagnosis thereof may be questioned in their absence.

The lymphoplasmacytic infiltrate may be composed almost entirely of either lymphocytes (mostly of the peripheral T cell type) or plasma cells (generally of the IgA-producing type), but one most often finds a mixture of these cells. Bässler et al (20) reported that lymphocytes predominated at the periphery of medullary carcinomas, whereas plasma cells represented the preponderant inflammatory cell in the center of the carcinoma. This phenomenon does not occur in every case. Since marked lymphocytic infiltrates can occur in non-medullary invasive ductal carcinomas, this finding does not have diagnostic significance. A predominance of plasma cells, on the other hand, favors the diagnosis of medullary carcinoma. Neutrophils and eosinophils can be found in a medullary carcinoma, especially in the presence of necrosis or cystic degeneration, but these types of inflammatory cells are never dominant. Rarely, the lymphocytic infiltrate gives rise to germinal centers within the tumor or in the surrounding tissue. Hence, one cannot rely on the presence of germinal centers as evidence that one is dealing with metastatic carcinoma in a lymph node.

Tumoral circumscription refers to the convex "pushing" border of the invasive carcinoma (rather than the periphery of the surrounding lymphoplasmacytic reaction). In medullary carcinoma, the edge of the tumor habitually shows a smooth, rounded contour that appears to push aside the breast parenchyma rather than infiltrate it (**Fig. 12.2**). Consequently, nonneoplastic glandular or fatty breast tissue should not be found within the body of the invasive carcinoma. In assessing the margin of the carcinoma, one must not confuse the extension of inflammatory cells into the surrounding parenchyma with invasion of glandular (or adipose) tissue by the carcinoma. Tumor growth in trabecular, dendritic, or dispersed patterns is not consistent with the diagnosis of medullary carcinoma.

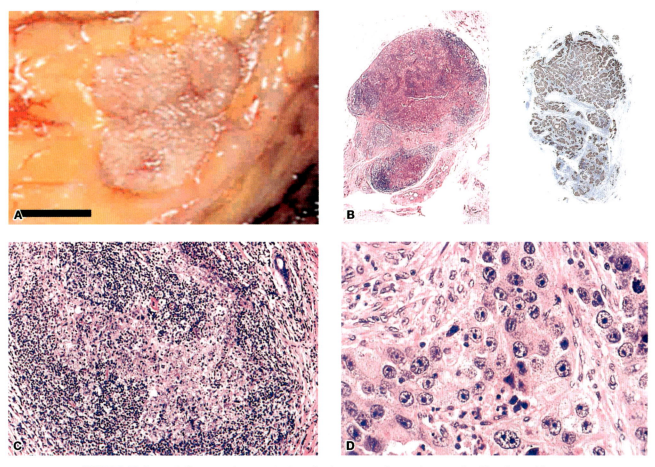

FIGURE 12.1 Medullary Carcinoma. A: Grossly, the tumor shows circumscribed borders with a lobulated cut surface (bar: 1 cm). **B:** Tumor borders are rounded. Adipocytes are present between circumscribed tumor nodules. **C:** Syncytial pattern of growth with indistinct cell borders of high-grade carcinoma cells. **D:** Prominent nucleoli are obvious in the high-grade carcinoma cells.

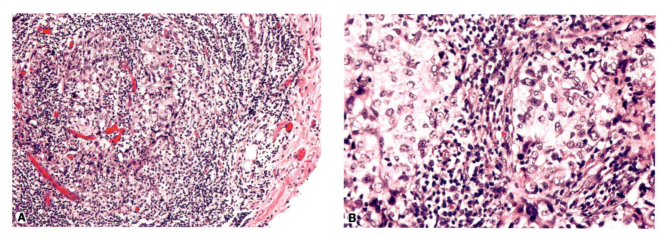

FIGURE 12.2 Medullary Carcinoma. A, B: This needle core biopsy shows a diffuse lymphoplasmacytic infiltrate between syncytial masses of high-grade carcinoma.

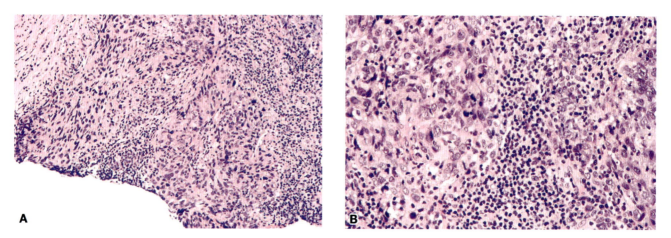

FIGURE 12.3 Medullary Carcinoma. A, B: This needle core biopsy shows well-defined "pushing" (convex) border.

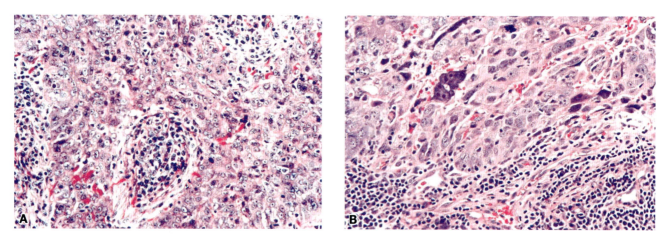

FIGURE 12.4 Medullary Carcinoma. A: The carcinoma cells form bands surrounded by an inflammatory cell reaction. The latter is mainly composed of plasma cells. Borders of individual carcinoma cells are indistinct (form "syncytia") and possess high-grade nuclei. **B:** A multinucleated tumor giant cell is present.

A *syncytial growth pattern* refers to the formation of broad, irregular, and interanastamosing sheets or islands of carcinoma cells in which the borders of individual cells are indistinct (**Fig. 12.3**). The appearance sometimes resembles that of a poorly differentiated squamous carcinoma. Giant cells, including some simulating syncytiotrophoblast, may be present—particularly at the periphery of the tumor. A tumor that is otherwise characteristic may be accepted as a medullary carcinoma if it has minor components of trabecular, glandular, alveolar, or papillary growth. Such foci may have a diminished lymphoplasmacytic infiltrate and fibrosis, and appear distinct from the medullary growth pattern. It has been reported that overall survival and relapse-free survival are directly related to the extent of the syncytial component (21). Although there was not a significant difference in outcome between patients with 75% and 90% syncytial growth, survival was diminished when less than 75% of a tumor was syncytial, and the difference was most marked at and below the 50% level. These data justify the requirement for at least a 75% syncytial component for a diagnosis of medullary carcinoma.

High nuclear grade and *high mitotic rate* are related characteristics of medullary carcinoma. Typically, the tumor cells have pleomorphic nuclei with coarse chromatin and prominent nucleoli (the cytologic "delicacy" has been likened to that of embryonal carcinoma). Pyknotic nuclei of degenerating cells are easily found. The tumor is rich in mitoses. Abnormal mitotic figures are common.

Multiple other microscopic features may be found in medullary carcinomas. The presence of one or more of these secondary histopathologic characteristics can be helpful to support the diagnosis of medullary carcinoma. These ancillary microscopic features include in situ carcinoma, squamous metaplasia, pseudosarcomatous metaplasia, and tumoral necrosis. The intratumoral fibrous component is usually scant.

The presence of ductal carcinoma in situ (DCIS) does not exclude the diagnosis of medullary carcinoma. DCIS is typically found at its periphery, often has a solid growth pattern, and only rarely contains calcifications. It is also not unusual for the carcinoma to extend into lobules (ie, "lobular cancerization"). Foci of intraductal and intralobular carcinoma are more frequent in larger tumors. DCIS is accompanied by prominent lymphoplasmacytic infiltrate. This inflammatory infiltrate can obscure lobular cancerization. DCIS cells are cytologically similar to those of the medullary carcinoma.

Expansile growth of in situ carcinoma in ducts and lobules leads to the formation of secondary tumor nodules around the main mass. These peripheral nodules have the appearance of smaller "satellite" medullary carcinomas (22). Fibrofatty mammary stroma may persist between nodules at the margin of the tumor. One should not interpret the presence of these satellite foci as evidence of invasion. Coalescence of these nodules and their incorporation into the expanding main mass account for the macroscopic nodular appearance of medullary carcinomas.

Rarely, one may encounter a lesion consisting only of DCIS showing the histologic features of DCIS usually found at the periphery of a medullary carcinoma. Such foci typically have the high-grade cytologic features that characterize medullary carcinoma and a solid growth pattern with central necrosis. The intense lymphoplasmacytic reaction can make it difficult to identify invasive carcinoma. There is no definite proof that these lesions constitute in situ form of medullary carcinoma, but this possibility can be inferred from uncommon examples of medullary carcinoma composed largely of DCIS with only a minor invasive component.

Metaplastic changes occur in a minority of medullary carcinomas and usually involve only a part of the lesion. Squamous metaplasia has been found in 16% of medullary carcinomas (8). Osseous, cartilaginous, and spindle cell metaplasia are much less common. Bizarre epithelial giant cells can be found (**Fig. 12.4**). It remains unclear whether the cytologically bizarre appearance of these cells reflects a metaplastic or a degenerative phenomenon.

Necrosis can develop in medullary carcinomas within zones of syncytial epithelial growth and squamous metaplasia. Expansion of these foci leads to the formation of clefts and cysts. The pattern of cystic degeneration resembles the process encountered in squamous carcinomas.

DIAGNOSING MEDULLARY CARCINOMA ON NEEDLE CORE BIOPSY SAMPLING

Some, but not all, criteria for diagnosing medullary carcinoma can be evident on samplings via needle core biopsy. These include the presence of syncytial pattern of growth, lack of glandular structures, prominent lymphoplasmacytic infiltrate, higher-grade nuclei, and high mitotic rate. Obviously, the broad "pushing" borders of the tumor cannot be ascertained on such limited sampling. Thus, the diagnosis of medullary carcinoma can be suggested, but not established, on core biopsy. Accurate testing of biomarkers should be ensured in all such tumors to devise appropriate management strategies.

DIFFERENTIATING MEDULLARY CARCINOMA WITH METASTASIS TO INTRAMAMMARY LYMPH NODE

The differential diagnosis of medullary carcinoma includes the entities of atypical medullary carcinoma and high-grade invasive carcinomas with prominent lymphoid infiltrate (vide supra). Differentiating between medullary carcinoma and metastasis to an intramammary lymph node can be problematic—especially in needle core biopsy sampling. Findings that can be helpful in this context are listed in **Table 12.3**.

IMMUNOHISTOCHEMISTRY

Most medullary carcinomas express cytokeratin (CK), and stain with CK~AE1/AE3 cocktail. Investigators have tested medullary carcinomas for the presence of specific CKs such as CK4, CK5/6, CK7, CK14, CK8/18, CK19, and CK20; however, these studies have not yielded consistent findings. Thus, one cannot rely on the expression of any of the types of CK to distinguish medullary carcinomas from

TABLE 12.3

Differential Diagnosis of Medullary Carcinoma and Metastatic Carcinoma in Intramammary Lymph Node

Feature	Medullary Carcinoma	Metastatic Carcinoma in Intramammary Lymph Node[a]
Lymph node capsule	(−)	(±)
Subcapsular sinus	(−)	(±)
Lymphoid follicles	(±)	(+)
Associated in situ carcinoma	(±)	(−)
Antecedent evidence of lymph node[b]	(−)	(+)
Benign breast glands amid lymphoid cells	(±)	(−)

[a]Tumor cells could be obscured by lymphoid cells.
[b]On prior imaging.

non-medullary carcinomas. Immunoreactivity for HLA-DR, GATA3, EMA, and E-cadherin is typically demonstrable in medullary carcinomas. Staining for mammaglobin or GCDFP-15 can be encountered in occasional cases (23-26).

Rodríguez-Pinilla et al (25) observed that carcinomas classified as invasive ductal carcinoma with medullary features display immunohistochemical features characteristic of basal-like carcinomas (BLCs) more often than do high-grade conventional invasive ductal carcinomas (62.9% vs 18.9% of cases). Jacquemier et al (26) observed that 71% of medullary carcinomas expressed EGFR, whereas only 37% of invasive ductal carcinoma did so, and Vincent-Salomon et al (27) reported similar results. Jacquemier et al (26) also found that 44% of medullary carcinomas expressed S-100, but only 24% of non-medullary high-grade ductal carcinomas did so.

Fewer than 10% of medullary carcinomas are ER (+) or PR (+) (24), and only a small percentage of medullary carcinoma express HER2 (26,28-30).

Medullary carcinoma with an exceptionally abundant lymphoplasmacytic reaction may resemble lymphoepithelial carcinomas that arise at other sites (31). These and other characteristics have suggested that the Epstein-Barr virus (EBV) might play a role in the pathogenesis of medullary carcinoma; however, a study of 10 medullary carcinomas using IHC, in situ hybridization, and PCR failed to detect evidence of EBV (32). A lymphoepithelioma-like tumor studied by Naidoo and Chetty (31) was also negative for EBV.

BRCA MUTATIONS AND MEDULLARY CARCINOMA

Medullary carcinomas constitute between 11% (33) and 19% (34) of *BRCA1*-associated breast carcinomas. Moreover, one can find *BRCA1* mutations in patients with medullary carcinomas more frequently than in patients with other varieties of breast carcinomas. Without knowledge of family histories, Eisinger et al (34) tested 18 medullary carcinomas selected from a hospital registry and discovered *BRCA1* nonsense mutations in two tumors (11%), 7 times the frequency of such mutations in the general population. In neither case did the patient report a family history of heritable breast carcinoma. The 11% detection rate is higher than that encountered when using early onset as a criterion for genetic testing. This observation suggests that the diagnosis of medullary carcinoma could represent an indication of *BRCA* testing (35). Those with germline *BRCA2* mutations only infrequently show medullary features. The main pathologic differences in carcinomas associated with *BRCA1* and *BRCA2* are outlined in **Table 12.4**.

PROGNOSIS AND TREATMENT

Patients with medullary carcinoma tend to have a lower frequency of axillary lymph node metastases than patients with either invasive ductal carcinoma with medullary features or usual invasive ductal carcinoma (2,3,6,8,36,37). When there is nodal involvement it is usually limited to a few nodes in the low axillary group. The prognosis of patients with "small" node-negative medullary carcinoma is particularly favorable, with disease-free survival of 90% or better (6,8). When nodal metastases are present, the involvement of three or fewer lymph nodes is typical (2,6,36,38,39). The survival results for stage II, $T_1N_1M_0$ medullary carcinoma have also been exceptionally good at 10 years (5) and 20 years of follow-up. Most deaths occur within 5 years of diagnosis. Although patients with stage II medullary carcinoma have a more favorable prognosis than equivalent patients with non-medullary carcinoma, tumor size and nodal status are still significant determinants of disease-free survival (36).

TABLE 12.4

Clinicopathologic Features of Invasive Breast Carcinomas Characteristically Encountered in *BRCA1* and *BRCA2* Mutation Carriers

Feature	*BRCA1*	*BRCA2*
Type of carcinoma	Medullary type, others	Non-medullary types
Grade	3	2 or 3
Lymphoplasmacytic infiltrate	(+)	(−)
ER and PR	(−)	(+)
HER2	(−)	(−)
CK5/6 and CK14	(+)	(−)
DCIS	(±)	(+)
LCIS	(±)	(+)
Metastatic sites	Visceral organs and brain	Soft tissue and bone

LCIS, lobular carcinoma in situ.

Patients whose medullary carcinomas are more than 3 cm, or who have four or more involved lymph nodes have higher recurrence rates—not appreciably different from the recurrence rates of patients with conventional invasive ductal carcinoma (8).

Recurrences tend to occur early in the clinical course of patients with medullary carcinoma, with few women having recurrences or dying 5 years or more after the time of diagnosis (6,8,36,40). This phenomenon is observed equally in stage I and stage II patients. Most initial recurrences are systemic, but local recurrence has been observed even in patients treated by radical or modified radical mastectomy. Survival after systemic recurrence tends to be brief, regardless of the site of the initial metastasis (36), although an occasional patient may benefit from resection of a solitary metastasis (6).

In most reported cases of medullary carcinoma, surgical treatment consisted of mastectomy. There is little reported experience with the use of breast-conserving surgery and radiotherapy in this setting. Combined data from 2 institutions included 27 women with medullary carcinoma treated by breast-conserving surgery and radiotherapy (41). In this series, the local recurrence rate was 4%, the 5-year overall survival was 90%, and relapse-free survival was 92% at 5 years. A series of 1,008 patients treated by breast conservation with radiotherapy at Yale University included 17 women with medullary carcinoma (42). None of the patients developed a systemic recurrence, but there were five local breast recurrences (29%) after a median follow-up of nearly 17 years. The longest interval to recurrence was 18 years.

Breast conservation with excision and radiation seems to represent a reasonable form of therapy for medullary carcinoma—especially for tumors that span less than 3 cm. A sentinel lymph node biopsy is appropriate. Indications for systemic adjuvant therapy are controversial. Although it has been suggested that adjuvant systemic therapy can be omitted for patients with stage $T_1N_0M_0$ true medullary carcinoma, those who question the specificity of the diagnosis (1) are likely to recommend therapy similar to that offered to patients with conventional invasive ductal carcinoma. This dichotomous approach is reflected in the NCCN 2011 Guidelines which recommended that medullary carcinomas be treated as other invasive carcinomas (43), whereas the St. Gallen Consensus Guidelines for the same year recommended that node-negative medullary carcinomas need not require adjuvant chemotherapy (44). Notably, the NCCN 2022 (45) and the St. Gallen/Vienna 2021 (46) Guidelines do not specifically address the management of medullary carcinoma.

MOLECULAR ASPECTS

Genomic instability is common in medullary carcinoma. Gains in 1q and 8q and losses in X are common, as are gains and losses on array CGH analyses, and recurrent gains in 10p, 9p; and 16q 4p losses; and 1q, 8p, 10p, and 12p amplicons (27). Among other genetic alterations, Romero and colleagues found statistically significant overexpression of *BCLG*, a proapoptotic gene, in cases of medullary carcinoma compared with cases of BLC and triple-negative breast carcinoma (TNBC). At a transcription level, studies demonstrate that medullary carcinoma belongs to the basal-like, immunomodulatory, and luminal androgen receptor triple-negative breast carcinoma molecular subgroups (47-49).

Mutations of the *TP53* tumor suppressor gene are common (observed in approximately 75% of cases). Microsatellite instability (a feature of carcinomas with "medullary" morphology in the colon) is not present in medullary carcinoma of the breast (50). Gene profiling studies show that medullary carcinomas typically cluster in the basal-like group and the tumors are triple-negative (ER-negative, PR-negative, and HER2-negative).

Parenthetically, it should be stated that immune signatures as evident in gene expression profiling studies correlate with better outcomes in invasive triple-negative carcinomas with a marked lymphocytic response (51). This finding recapitulates those of the original papers which defined the entity—decades back.

RELATIONSHIP BETWEEN MEDULLARY, TRIPLE-NEGATIVE, AND BASAL-LIKE CARCINOMAS

Medullary carcinoma is a TNBC *and* a BLC **(Fig. 12.5)**. TNBC and BLC encompass largely similar, but nonidentical, breast carcinoma (52,53), and both are characterized by high degree of genomic instability. Triple-negativity refers to a tumor being ER (−), PR (−), and HER2 (−). The term BLC refers to the similarity of some pathologic characteristics between BLC and "basally located" myoepithelial cells. Tumors that are both TNBC and BLC include metaplastic carcinomas (including spindle, squamous, and matrix-producing ones), as well as adenoid cystic and secretory carcinomas. The latter two carcinomas include adenoid cystic and secretory carcinomas (both of which also occur in the salivary glands and are regarded as "translocation-associated carcinomas"—involving MYB-NFIB and *ETV6-NTRK3*, respectively). Carcinomas which are TNBC but not BLC include some of those that are androgen receptor (+); whereas those which are BLC but not TNBC are uncommon and include those rare BLC that are ER (+) and HER2 (+).

TNBC is defined by protein expression, and BLC by mRNA expression. TNBC categorization is possible via immunohistochemistry routinely performed for biomarkers on invasive carcinomas; however, definitive classification of BLC requires mRNA-based gene expression profiling. The latter technique is not readily available in most centers and is costly. "Surrogate" immunohistochemical testing to identify BLC has been proposed (an alternative that is imperfect at best). Such testing utilizes "basal" CKs and EGFR, as well as P-cadherin and vimentin. "Basal" CKs are those that stain myoepithelial cells and include CK5, CK14, and CK17, as well as CK5/6. In any event, the definitive classification of a tumor as TNBC or BLC is *not* useful for routine clinical decision-making.

Clinically, tumors in these categories comprise 10% to 15% of all invasive breast carcinomas and are relatively more common in younger women, and in African-American and Hispanic-American women. *BRCA1*-associated carcinomas are commonly TNBC and BLC. Tumors in both groups of neoplasms usually present as palpable masses. Microscopically, these tumors show well-defined "pushing" borders, high-grade nuclei, and a prominent lymphoid infiltrate. Both TNBC and BLC show higher expression of programmed death ligand (PD-L1) than other breast carcinomas.

At each stage, TNBC and BLC have less favorable prognosis; but these tumors also show complete pathologic response to aggressive chemotherapy in one-third to one-half of cases. Metastases preferentially occur to internal organs and the brain. Nodal involvement is relatively less frequent.

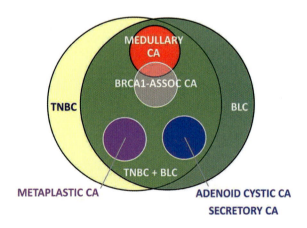

FIGURE 12.5 **Medullary Carcinoma: Relationship to Triple-Negative Breast Carcinoma (TNBC) and Basal-Like Carcinoma (BLC).** Medullary carcinoma is commonly associated (assoc) with *BRCA1*. Not all TNBC are BLC, and not all BLC are TNBC. Metaplastic carcinoma is typically both TNBC and BLC. "Translocation-associated" carcinomas (ie, adenoid cystic and secretory carcinomas) are also usually both TNBC and BLC. CA, carcinoma. (Reference: Hicks DG, Lester SC. *Diagnostic Pathology: Breast*. 3rd ed. Elsevier; 2021.)

REFERENCES

1. Editorial Board, ed. *WHO Classification of Tumor*. 5th ed. IARC; 2019.
2. Rapin V, Contesso G, Mouriesse H, et al. Medullary breast carcinoma: a reevaluation of 95 cases of breast cancer with inflammatory stroma. *Cancer*. 1988;61:2503-2510.
3. Li CI, Uribe DJ, Daling JR. Clinical characteristics of different histologic types of breast cancer. *Br J Cancer*. 2005;93:1046-1052.
4. Rosen PP, Saigo PE, Braun DW Jr, Weathers E, DePalo A. Predictors of recurrence in stage I ($T_1N_0M_0$) breast carcinoma. *Ann Surg*. 1981;193:15-25.
5. Rosen PP, Saigo PE, Braun DW, Weathers E, Kinne DW. Prognosis in stage II ($T_1N_1M_0$) breast cancer. *Ann Surg*. 1981;194:576-584.
6. Wargotz ES, Silverberg SG. Medullary carcinoma of the breast: a clinicopathologic study with appraisal of current diagnostic criteria. *Hum Pathol*. 1988;19:1340-1346.
7. Maier WP, Rosemond GP, Goldman LI, Kaplan GF, Tyson RR. A ten year study of medullary carcinoma of the breast. *Surg Gynecol Obstet*. 1977;144:695-698.
8. Ridolfi RL, Rosen PP, Port A, Kinne D, Miké V. Medullary carcinoma of the breast: a clinicopathologic study with 10 year follow-up. *Cancer*. 1977;40:1365-1385.
9. Rosen PP, Lesser ML, Senie RT, Duthie K. Epidemiology of breast carcinoma IV: age and histologic tumor type. *J Surg Oncol*. 1982;19:44-51.
10. Rosen PP, Lesser ML, Kinne DW. Breast carcinoma at the extremes of age: a comparison of patients younger than 35 years and older than 75 years. *J Surg Oncol*. 1985;28:90-96.
11. Martinez SR, Beal SH, Canter RJ, Chen SL, Khatri VP, Bold RJ. Medullary carcinoma of the breast: a population-based perspective. *Med Oncol*. 2011;28:738-744.
12. Lesser ML, Rosen PP, Kinne DW. Multicentricity and bilaterality in invasive breast carcinoma. *Surgery*. 1982;91:234-240.
13. Neuman ML, Homer MJ. Association of medullary carcinoma with reactive axillary adenopathy. *AJR Am J Roentgenol*. 1996;167:185-186.
14. Rosen PP, Lesser ML, Kinne DW, Beattie EJ. Discontinuous or "skip" metastases in breast carcinoma: analysis of 1228 axillary dissections. *Ann Surg*. 1983;197:276-283.

15. Jeong SJ, Lim HS, Lee JS, et al. Medullary carcinoma of the breast: MRI findings. *AJR Am J Roentgenol.* 2012;198:W482-W487.
16. Tominaga J, Hama H, Kimura N, Takahashi S. MR imaging of medullary carcinoma of the breast. *Eur J Radiol.* 2009;70:525-529.
17. Gaffey MJ, Mills SE, Frierson HF Jr, et al. Medullary carcinoma of the breast: interobserver variability in histopathologic diagnosis. *Mod Pathol.* 1995;8:31-38.
18. Rubens JR, Lewandrowski KB, Kopans DB, Koerner FC, Hall DA, McCarthy KA. Medullary carcinoma of the breast: overdiagnosis of a prognostically favorable neoplasm. *Arch Surg.* 1990;125:601-604.
19. Jensen ML, Kiaer H, Andersen J, Jensen V, Melsen F. Prognostic comparison of three classifications for medullary carcinomas of the breast. *Histopathology.* 1997;30:523-532.
20. Bässler R, Dittmann AM, Dittrich M. Mononuclear stromal reactions in mammary carcinoma, with special reference to medullary carcinomas with a lymphoid infiltrate: analysis of 108 cases. *Virchows Arch A Pathol Anat Histol.* 1981;393:75-91.
21. Pedersen L, Schiodt T, Holck S, Zedeler K. The prognostic importance of syncytial growth pattern in medullary carcinoma of the breast. *APMIS.* 1990;98:921-926.
22. Reyes C, Nadji M. The immunophenotype of nodular variant of medullary carcinoma of the breast. *Appl Immunohistochem Mol Morphol.* 2015;23:624-627.
23. Reyes C, Gomez-Fernandez C, Nadji M. Metaplastic and medullary mammary carcinomas do not express mammaglobin. *Am J Clin Pathol.* 2012;137:747-752.
24. Wendroth SM, Mentrikoski MJ, Wick MR. GATA3 expression in morphologic subtypes of breast carcinoma: a comparison with gross cystic disease fluid protein 15 and mammaglobin. *Ann Diagn Pathol.* 2015;19:6-9.
25. Rodríguez-Pinilla SM, Rodriguez-Gil Y, Moreno-Bueno G, et al. Sporadic invasive breast carcinomas with medullary features display a basal-like phenotype: an immunohistochemical and gene amplification study. *Am J Surg Pathol.* 2007;31:501-508.
26. Jacquemier J, Padovani L, Rabayrol L, et al. Typical medullary breast carcinomas have a basal/myoepithelial phenotype. *J Pathol.* 2005;207:260-268.
27. Vincent-Salomon A, Gruel N, Lucchesi C, et al. Identification of typical medullary breast carcinoma as a genomic subgroup of basal-like carcinomas, a heterogeneous new molecular entity. *Breast Cancer Res.* 2007;9:R24.
28. Rosen PP, Lesser ML, Arroyo CD, Cranor M, Borgen P, Norton L. Immunohistochemical detection of HER2/neu in patients with axillary lymph node negative breast carcinoma: a study of epidemiologic risk factors, histologic features, and prognosis. *Cancer.* 1995;75:1320-1326.
29. Bertucci F, Finetti P, Cervera N, et al. Gene expression profiling shows medullary breast cancer is a subgroup of basal breast cancers. *Cancer Res.* 2006;66:4636-4644.
30. Flucke U, Flucke MT, Hoy L, et al. Distinguishing medullary carcinoma of the breast from high-grade hormone receptor-negative invasive ductal carcinoma: an immunohistochemical approach. *Histopathology.* 2010;56:852-859.
31. Naidoo P, Chetty R. Lymphoepithelioma-like carcinoma of the breast with associated sclerosing lymphocytic lobulitis. *Arch Pathol Lab Med.* 2001;125:669-672.
32. Lespagnard L, Cochaux P, Larsimont D, Degeyter M, Velu T, Heimann R. Absence of Epstein-Barr virus in medullary carcinoma of the breast as demonstrated by immunophenotyping, in situ hybridization and polymerase chain reaction. *Am J Clin Pathol.* 1995;103:449-452.
33. Lakhani SR, Gusterson BA, Jacquemier J, et al. The pathology of familial breast cancer: histological features of cancers in families not attributable to mutations in BRCA1 or BRCA2. *Clin Cancer Res.* 2000;6:782-789.
34. Eisinger F, Jacquemier J, Charpin C, et al. Mutations at BRCA1: the medullary breast carcinoma revisited. *Cancer Res.* 1998;58:1588-1592.
35. Eisinger F, Nogues C, Birnbaum D, Jacquemier J, Sobol H. BRCA1 and medullary breast cancer. *JAMA.* 1998;280:1227-1228.
36. Reinfuss M, Stelmach A, Mitus J, Rys J, Duda K. Typical medullary carcinoma of the breast: a clinical and pathological analysis of 52 cases. *J Surg Oncol.* 1995;60:89-94.
37. Mitze M, Goepel E. [Prognostic factors in medullary breast cancer]. *Geburtshilfe Frauenheilkd.* 1989;49:635-641.
38. Dendale R, Vincent-Salomon A, Mouret-Fourme E, et al. Medullary breast carcinoma: prognostic implications of p53 expression. *Int J Biol Markers.* 2003;18:99-105.
39. Fisher ER, Kenny JP, Sass R, Dimitrov NV, Siderits RH, Fisher B. Medullary cancer of the breast revisited. *Breast Cancer Res Treat.* 1990;16:215-229.
40. Bloom HJ, Richardson WW, Field JR. Host resistance and survival in carcinoma of breast: a study of 104 cases of medullary carcinoma in a series of 1,411 cases of breast cancer followed for 20 years. *Br Med J.* 1970;3:181-188.
41. Kurtz JM, Jacquemier J, Torhorst J, et al. Conservation therapy for breast cancers other than infiltrating ductal carcinoma. *Cancer.* 1989;63:1630-1635.
42. Haffty BG, Perrotta PL, Ward B, et al. Conservatively treated breast cancer: outcome by histologic subtype. *Breast J.* 1997;3:7-14.
43. NCCN Guidelines Version 2.2011. *Breast cancer.* Accessed December 22, 2011. www.nccn.org/professionals/physician.pdf
44. Goldhirsch A, Wood WC, Coates AS, et al. Strategies for subtypes—dealing with the diversity of breast cancer: highlights of the St. Gallen International Expert Consensus on the primary therapy of early breast cancer 2011. *Ann Oncol.* 2011;22:1736-1747.
45. Gradishar WJ, Moran MS, Abraham J, et al. Breast cancer, version 3.2022, NCCN clinical practice guidelines in oncology. *J Natl Compr Canc Netw.* 2022;20:691-722.
46. Thomssen C, Balic M, Harbeck N, Gnant M. St. Gallen/Vienna 2021: a brief summary of the consensus discussion on customizing therapies for women with early breast cancer. *Breast Care (Basel).* 2021;16:135-143.
47. Romero P, Benhamo V, Deniziaut G, et al. Medullary breast carcinoma, a triple-negative breast cancer associated with BCLG overexpression. *Am J Pathol.* 2018;188:2378-2391.
48. Wang DY, Jiang Z, Ben-David Y, Woodgett JR, Zacksenhaus E. Molecular stratification within triple-negative cancer subtypes. *Sci Rep.* 2019;9:19107.
49. Lehmann BD, Jovanović B, Chen X, et al. Refinement of triple-negative breast cancer molecular subtypes: implications for neoadjuvant chemotherapy selection. *PLoS One.* 2016;11:e0157368. doi:10.1371/journal.pone.0157368
50. Osin P, Lu YJ, Stone J, et al. Distinct genetic and epigenetic changes in medullary breast cancer. *Int J Surg Pathol.* 2003;11:153-158.
51. Sabatier R, Finetti P, Cervera N, et al. A gene expression signature identifies two prognostic subgroups of basal breast cancer. *Breast Cancer Res Treat.* 2011;126:407-420.
52. Derakhshan F, Reis-Filho JS. Pathogenesis of triple-negative breast cancer. *Annu Rev Pathol.* 2022;17:181-204.
53. Borri F, Granaglia A. Pathology of triple negative breast cancer. *Semin Cancer Biol.* 2021;72:136-145.

Metaplastic Carcinomas, Including Low-Grade Adenosquamous Carcinoma

13

RAZA S. HODA AND SYED A. HODA

METAPLASTIC CARCINOMA

Metaplastic carcinomas are malignant neoplasms of epithelial origin that exhibit nonglandular morphology, such as squamous, spindle cell, chondroid, or osseous. These phenotypic alterations represent genomic dedifferentiation, ie, "epithelial to mesenchymal transition" (1). "Metaplastic carcinoma" is a generic term and is imprecise—because it encompasses a broad range of morphology. Thus, the term should not be used as a diagnosis *without* mention of the type of metaplasia(s) present in a particular case. There are no criteria regarding the extent of metaplasia required to diagnose such carcinomas. Metaplastic carcinomas of the breast are typically "triple-negative" (ie, estrogen receptor [ER]: negative, progesterone [PR]: negative, and human epidermal growth factor receptor 2 [HER2]: negative) and, with a few notable exceptions (discussed later), have an unfavorable prognosis.

Metaplastic carcinomas are rare. In a study based on the National Cancer Database, metaplastic carcinomas constituted 0.24% of 365,464 breast malignant tumors diagnosed between 2001 and 2003 (2). Metaplastic carcinomas can occur in women of any age, but peri- or postmenopausal women are affected more commonly (2-21). In one study (2), the mean age at diagnosis was 61 years, with 13.5% of cases occurring in women greater than 80 years of age, and 8% in women less than 40 years of age. Other series report younger median age (22), or no age differences (12) compared with women with invasive ductal carcinomas (IDC). Most (>70%) metaplastic carcinomas occur in White women (2,8). This tumor does not affect men. Rare cases have been reported in *BRCA1* germline mutation carriers (13,23-25).

Most patients present with a unilateral, rapidly growing palpable tumor. The mean and median size (3-4 cm) tend to be greater than that of IDC. Larger lesions can become fixed to the chest wall or ulcerate the overlying skin.

On imaging, metaplastic carcinomas tend to be more nodular and less infiltrative than IDC (19,22). They show relatively fewer calcifications and lesser acoustic shadowing (22). Calcifications are present in about 20% (19), and these are often present in the associated ductal carcinoma in situ (DCIS). Rarely, carcinomas with chondroid and osseous metaplasia with calcifications are detected mammographically (26-29). On ultrasound examination, metaplastic carcinomas have parallel orientation to the overlying skin in 97% of the cases, complex echogenicity in 81%, irregular shape in 60%, posterior acoustic enhancement in 50%, and lobulated margin in 41% (19). Common MRI findings include irregular heterogeneous enhancing mass, with an irregular shape (52.4%) and edges (57%). High T2-weighted signal intensity is detected in ~60% of the cases (19), correlating with necrosis (27) and chondroid areas (28). The tumors are highly metabolic on PET scan. Cystic areas may be present, especially in tumors with squamous metaplasia. Hemorrhagic foci can occur, especially in tumors with choriocarcinoma.

The diagnosis of metaplastic carcinoma requires evidence of epithelial origin and/or differentiation such as identification of DCIS and/or IDC and/or positive reactivity for keratin and/or (myo)epithelial markers. Metaplastic changes are commonly associated with high-grade invasive carcinomas but can also occur in other types of carcinoma. The extent of metaplasia varies from focal to complete. The transition from carcinomatous to metaplastic elements ("phenotypic switch") may be gradual or abrupt. DCIS is identified in 10% (30) to 65% (31) of cases and tends to have higher-grade nuclei. Rarely, lobular carcinoma in situ (LCIS) or atypical lobular hyperplasia (ADH) is found. A papillary or sclerosing lesion may be present in the vicinity of a metaplastic carcinoma, especially metaplastic spindle cell carcinoma (MSCC) or low-grade adenosquamous carcinoma (LGASC). Tumor-infiltrating lymphocytes (TILs) (ie, chronic inflammatory cell infiltrate at the periphery and within the tumor) can be prominent.

Metaplastic carcinomas encompass a wide morphologic spectrum, more evident in excisions than in needle core biopsies (NCB). In excisions, extensive sampling is required to assess all possible types of metaplasia. Nonetheless, a definitive diagnosis of metaplastic carcinoma can be rendered in most cases on NCB material.

Notably, metaplastic carcinoma is the most important consideration in the differential diagnosis of spindle cell tumors in the breast (32). Traditionally, metaplastic carcinomas are divided into carcinomas with squamous and/or spindle cell metaplasia, and those with heterologous component(s), such as chondromyxoid and/or osseous. Metaplastic LGASC exhibits characteristic histology and indolent clinical behavior. Of note, IDC with osteoclast-like giant cells is *not* a metaplastic carcinoma (because the giant cells are of nonneoplastic histiocytic nature).

SQUAMOUS CELL CARCINOMA

Mammary squamous cell carcinoma (SCC) resembles SCC at other sites **(Figs. 13.1 and 13.2)**. This diagnosis applies to carcinomas in which the squamous component represents ≥90% of the tumor. Consequently, this diagnosis cannot be definitively rendered on NCB. A spindle cell component may be present, but it may be difficult to distinguish from the associated reactive stroma, especially in NCB. Some tumor cells can display marked cytoplasmic clearing. The neoplastic spindle cells are usually immunoreactive for high-molecular-weight and basal cytokeratins (CKs), such as 34βE12 (K903), CK14, CK5/6, and for p63. A prominent mixed inflammatory cell infiltrate is often present, especially in keratinized and necrotic areas **(Figs. 13.1 and 13.2)**. This finding accounts for the occasional misinterpretation of SCC as an abscess. Rarely, the associated DCIS also shows squamous morphology **(Fig. 13.3)**. Squamous metaplasia can be associated with a variety of benign mammary lesions **(Fig. 13.4)**, including radial scar and papilloma. SCC arising in malignant phyllodes tumors (PTs) have been reported (33,34).

Differential Diagnosis at Needle Core Biopsy

A definitive diagnosis of primary SCC of the breast is possible only after a *metastasis from an extramammary primary site*, such as lung and cervix, and *secondary extension from the overlying skin* has been ruled out (35-37). SCCs primary in all organs are GATA3-positive; hence, this immunostain cannot be used to confirm mammary primary.

METAPLASTIC SPINDLE CELL CARCINOMA

Metaplastic spindle cell carcinomas (MSCC) are usually classified into two groups: higher-grade ("fibrosarcoma-like") and lower-grade ("fibromatosis-like"). These two types of MSCC show dissimilar differential diagnoses and clinical behaviors.

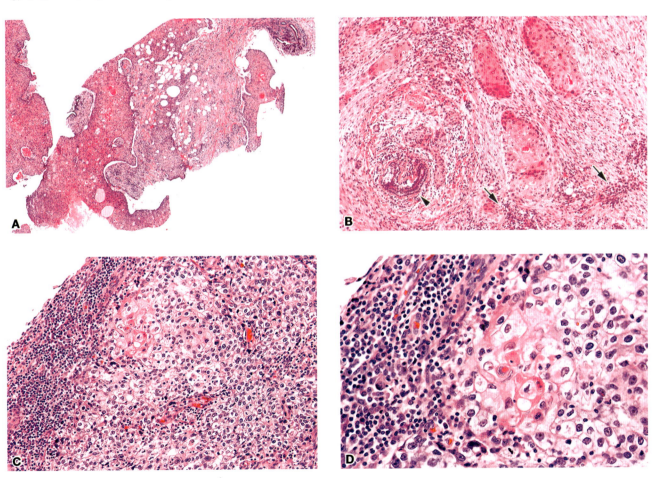

FIGURE 13.1 Invasive Carcinoma With Squamous-Type Morphology. A: A needle core biopsy (NCB) from a 3-cm mass in the breast of a 66-year-old woman shows a carcinoma with squamous morphology, well to moderately differentiated. **B:** The carcinoma consists of squamous nests with low-grade nuclear atypia amid desmoplastic stroma. Lymphocytes are also noted (arrows). A benign duct is present (arrowhead). **C, D:** Another NCB showing squamous differentiation in a poorly differentiated invasive duct carcinoma.

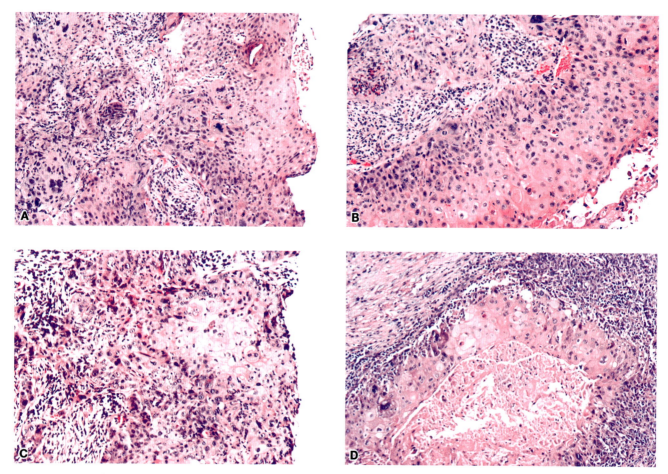

FIGURE 13.2 Invasive Squamous Carcinoma. A, B: A needle core biopsy showing well to moderately differentiated invasive squamous carcinoma. **C:** A part of the same tumor with poorly differentiated squamous carcinoma. **D:** An area in the excised tumor duplicates the appearance of the squamous carcinoma. Note cystic degeneration and prominent lymphoplasmacytic infiltrate.

Higher-Grade Metaplastic Spindle Cell Carcinoma

Most or all higher-grade MSCC consists of spindle cells with intermediate- to high-grade nuclei. Tumor cellularity is moderate to marked **(Fig. 13.5)**. Mitoses are identified and are usually numerous. Necrosis is common. The appearance can be "fibrosarcoma-like." Focal areas of squamous differentiation, DCIS, and IDC may be identified (**Fig. 13.5**); however, most cases have no obvious epithelial component, especially on NCB. In one study (38), DCIS was present

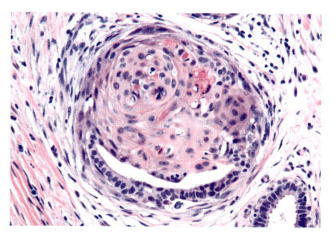

FIGURE 13.3 Squamous Cell Carcinoma In Situ. This needle core biopsy sample shows two contiguous ducts occupied by well-differentiated keratinizing squamous carcinoma.

FIGURE 13.4 Squamous Metaplasia in a Hyperplastic Duct. Benign squamous metaplasia tends to be reactive to inflammatory changes in the vicinity and is more common in ducts closer to the nipple.

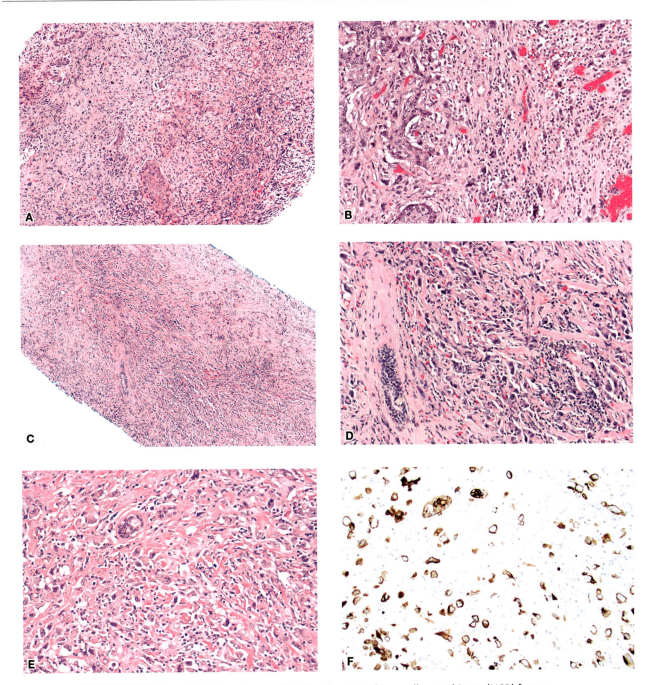

FIGURE 13.5 **Metaplastic Carcinoma, High Grade. A, B:** This needle core biopsy (NCB) from a rapidly growing breast mass of a 34-year-old woman shows high-grade spindle cell and epithelial components. **B:** The carcinomatous component consists of irregular clusters, whereas the sarcomatoid component is composed of bizarre spindle cells. **C-F:** NCB and excision of a breast mass of an 85-year-old woman. The NCB shows a high-grade malignant spindle and epithelioid neoplasm **(C, D)**. The tumor in the excision has high-grade morphology **(E)**. The neoplastic spindle cells are positive for cytokeratin 34βE12 **(F)**.

in excisions in 14% of cases. Usual ductal hyperplasia can be present at the periphery of the dominant tumor. Immunostains for epithelial markers, such as CK 34βE12, CK14, CK 5/6, CK18, and p63, can be positive, but the expression of epithelial markers in MSCC with intermediate- and high-grade morphology may be focal and weak, even at excision, and may be negative for epithelial markers on NCB. Positivity for GATA3 has been reported (39) (**Fig. 13.5**).

Differential Diagnosis at Needle Core Biopsy

The focal identification of an elongated epithelial-lined duct amid a portion of hypercellular stroma may be the only evidence differentiating *high-grade malignant phyllodes tumor* from MSCC with intermediate- or high-grade morphology (see Chapter 7). NCB sampling of areas of stromal expansion or overgrowth in a borderline or malignant PT may yield no ductal component. Furthermore, neoplastic cells of PTs may be focally positive for CKs (40). PTs are usually positive for CD34, whereas MSCCs are usually CD34-negative (41). S-100 can be positive in some MSCCs and PTs (41). A malignant tumor composed entirely of spindle cells having no epithelial component or frond-like architecture cannot be reliably classified on NCB, and both MSCC and malignant PT should be included in the differential diagnosis. Focal staining for CK favors MSCC, but caution is recommended when CK-positivity is focal, or is limited to epithelium near necrotic foci, and evident only with one of the CKs less sensitive for MSCC (eg, CAM5.2). It is worth noting that the definitive diagnosis of MSCC, a triple-negative breast cancer (TNBC), on NCB may lead to treatment with neoadjuvant chemotherapy.

Primary sarcomas of the breast are rare (see Chapter 20). A clinical history of prior ipsilateral breast carcinoma treated with breast-conserving surgery and radiotherapy is often obtained in cases of radiation-induced sarcoma. Sporadic primary mammary angiosarcomas tend to occur in young women, can show solid growth, and are positive for CD31 and ERG and negative for CKs. Focal positivity for CKs has been reported (42), particularly in epithelioid angiosarcoma. p63-positivity has also been reported in angiosarcoma (43,44). Clinical history is important to rule out sarcoma metastatic from an extramammary site.

The differential diagnosis of any epithelioid and spindle cell malignant tumor includes *melanoma* and requires appropriate immunohistochemical workup. S-100 can be positive in some MSCC with intermediate- and high-grade morphology (41). SOX10, a Schwann cell and melanocytic marker, has been detected in some metaplastic carcinomas (45) (**Fig. 13.5**).

Low-Grade ("Fibromatosis-Like") Metaplastic Spindle Cell Carcinoma

MSCC with dense, keloid-like areas of fibrosis, storiform pattern, and minimal cytologic atypia is referred to as "fibromatosis-like" (46) or "low grade" (47) or "lower grade" (**Figs. 13.6-13.8**). Such tumors often show deceptively bland nuclear features, heterogeneous cellularity, with abrupt juxtaposition of hypercellular and hypocellular areas.

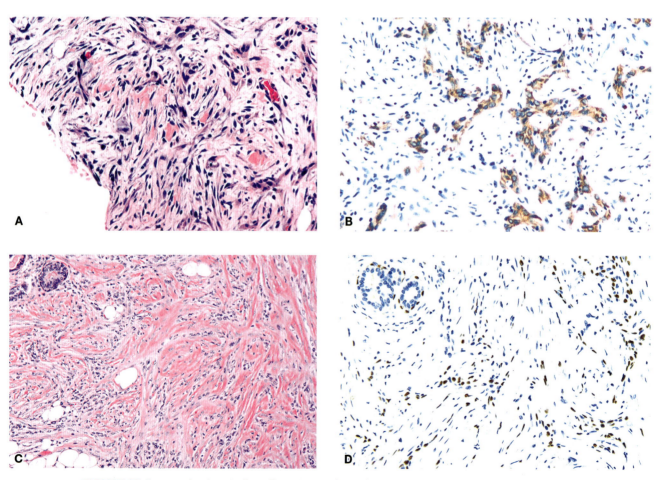

FIGURE 13.6 Metaplastic Spindle Cell Carcinoma (MSCC), Low-Grade Fibromatosis-Like. **A:** The bland spindle cells comprising this low-grade MSCC are arranged in short haphazard fascicles. The storiform pattern is suggestive of metaplastic carcinoma. Some spindle cells have epithelioid morphology and are arranged in structures that resemble capillaries. Cytokeratin AE1/AE3 reactivity highlights the epithelioid cells **(B)**. **C, D:** A spindle cell metaplastic carcinoma with bands of keloid-like collagen. The neoplastic spindle cells shown in **(C)** display nuclear reactivity for p63 **(D)**.

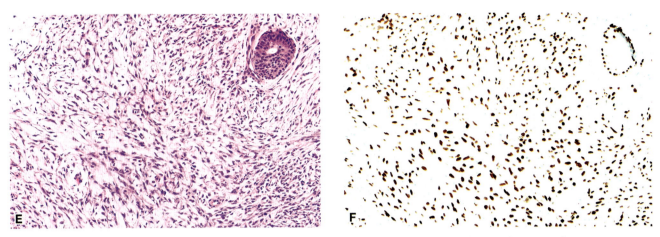

FIGURE 13.6 (*continued*) **E, F:** Another spindle cell metaplastic carcinoma. The neoplastic spindle cells shown in (**E**) display p63-positivity (**F**).

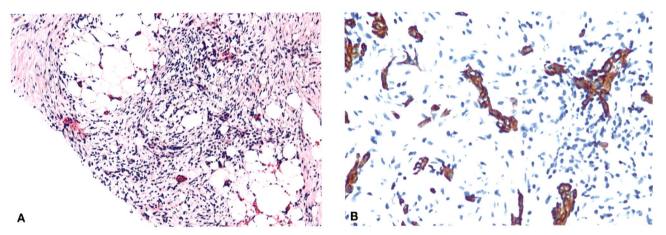

FIGURE 13.7 **Metaplastic Spindle Cell Carcinoma, Low-Grade Fibromatosis-Like.** A tumor that resembles an inflammatory lesion. **A:** The pattern of infiltration into fat and lymphocytic reaction were mistaken for fat necrosis. **B:** Cytokeratin 34βE12 expression is demonstrated in some spindle cells.

Collagenized fibrosis can be extensive. The tumor can be hypocellular and may be particularly paucicellular in its center. The neoplastic cells are arranged in short interlacing fascicles and tend to be inconspicuous, with ill-defined cell borders, minimal cytoplasm, and elongated nuclei. In the more cellular areas, the spindle cells may have more abundant and denser cytoplasm (appear "epithelioid") and are arranged in short cords. These epithelioid foci are usually positive for CKs with a characteristic linear and branching arrangement (**Figs. 13.6 and 13.7**). Rare atypical spindle cells with

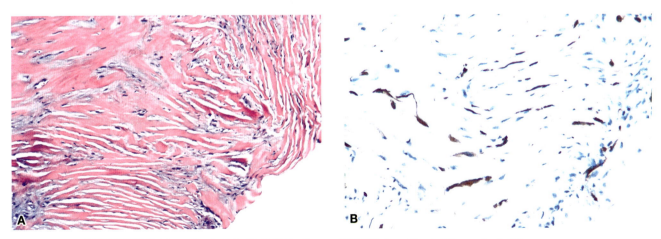

FIGURE 13.8 **Metaplastic Spindle Cell Carcinoma (MSCC), Low-Grade Fibromatosis-Like.** **A, B:** Low-grade MSCC that is fibromatosis-like. Some spindle cells are immunoreactive for cytokeratin 34βE12 (**B**).

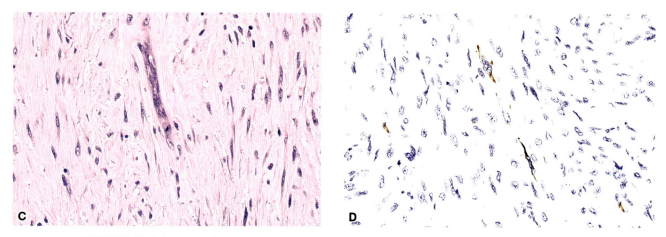

FIGURE 13.8 (continued). **C, D:** Another low-grade metaplastic spindle cell carcinoma that is fibromatosis-like. Rare spindle cells are positive for cytokeratin AE1/AE3 **(D)**.

enlarged and hyperchromatic nuclei may be identified; however, the overall nuclear grade tends to be lower. Mitoses are sparse, ranging from less than 2 mitoses/10 high-power field (HPFs) to less than 5 mitoses/10 HPFs (46,47). Mitoses are more common in cellular areas. Chronic inflammatory cell infiltrate is scattered throughout the tumor and at its periphery (Figs. 13.6 and 13.7). Lower-grade DCIS (46,47), classic LCIS (47), and ADH (3,46) have been described in association with such carcinomas; however, ductal hyperplasia of the "gynecomastia type" is a common intraductal epithelial alteration. Lower-grade MSCC can be associated with papillomata (47,48), complex sclerosing lesions (CSLs), and florid papillomatosis of nipple (so-called "nipple adenoma") (49,50).

Differential Diagnosis at Needle Core Biopsy

Fibromatosis may arise in the breast (primary mammary fibromatosis) or extend into the breast from the chest wall. Fibromatosis tends to occur in women of reproductive age, whereas metaplastic carcinoma is most common in peri- and postmenopausal women, but there are exceptions. The lesional spindle cells are arranged in broad, sweeping fascicles and display minimal cytologic atypia. Fibromatosis may closely resemble lower-grade spindle cell metaplastic carcinoma—hence the alternate term for the latter: "fibromatosis-like" **(Table 13.1)**. Mitoses are infrequent, and most cases show diffuse nuclear staining for β-catenin **(Fig. 13.9)**. Focal nuclear staining for β-catenin has been documented in ~25% of metaplastic carcinomas, as well as in most PTs

TABLE 13.1
Low-Grade ("Fibromatosis-Like") Spindle Cell Carcinoma Versus Mammary Fibromatosis

Features	LGSCC[a] (Fibromatosis-Like)	Mammary Fibromatosis[b]
Incidence	Rare (~0.2%)	Rare (~0.2%)
Structure	Infiltrative	Infiltrative
Cellularity	Low to moderate	Typically low
Lesional spindle cells	Elongated, bland	Elongated, bland, in "bands"
Ductal elements	Round, comma, squamoid	Absent
Lesional squamous cells[c]	"Pearl" & "onion skin"-like	Absent
"Epithelioid cells"	Between spindle cells	Absent
Stromal cell mitoses	−/+	±
Nuclear hyperchromasia	Mild, focal	Minimal
Nuclear atypia	+	±
Nucleoli	Minuscule	Inconspicuous
Tumor stroma	Sclerotic, elastotic	Edematous
Collagen in background	+	+
DCIS	±	−

(continued)

TABLE 13.1
Low-Grade ("Fibromatosis-Like") Spindle Cell Carcinoma Versus Mammary Fibromatosis *(continued)*

Features	LGSCC[a] (Fibromatosis-Like)	Mammary Fibromatosis[b]
DCIS and sclerosing lesion in vicinity	±	−
Inflammatory cells	At edge, "cannonball"-like	At edge
Vasculature	Inconspicuous	Prominent

DCIS, ductal carcinoma in situ; LGSCC, low-grade spindle cell carcinoma.

[a]Please see **Table 13.2** also.

[b]Proliferation of fibroblasts and myofibroblasts amid collagen. The relatively uniform lesional spindle cells are elongated and bland and form broad sweeping fascicles. The latter infiltrate native, usually inactive, breast parenchyma.

[c]Usually constitute minor (<5%) component of the tumor mass.

(51). Thus, focal and weak nuclear staining for β-catenin in a cytologically bland spindle cell breast lesion on NCB should be interpreted cautiously. *Nodular fasciitis*, a transient lesion related to *USP6* gene rearrangement (52), and *inflammatory pseudotumor*, a benign neoplasm associated with *ALK1* gene overexpression (53), are infrequent in the breast (see Chapter 20). Prominent inflammatory cell infiltrate is present in both. Also, both lesions are negative for CKs. *Myofibroblastoma* (see Chapter 20) are usually circumscribed, exhibit no cytologic atypia, do not express CKs, and may be positive for ER. Scattered mast cells are common; however, chronic inflammatory cell infiltrate is uncommon.

METAPLASTIC CARCINOMA WITH HETEROLOGOUS ELEMENTS

Metaplastic carcinoma with heterologous elements shows cartilaginous and/or osseous and/or other types of "mesenchymal" matrix (54). Some carcinomas show only matrix production **(Fig. 13.10)**, whereas others have foci that resemble

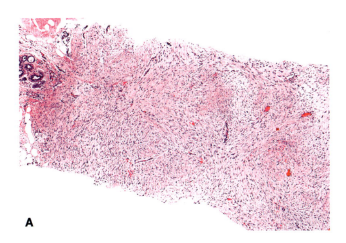

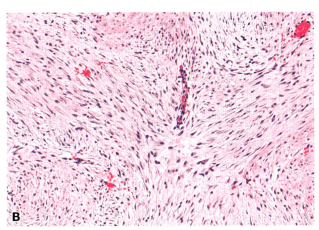

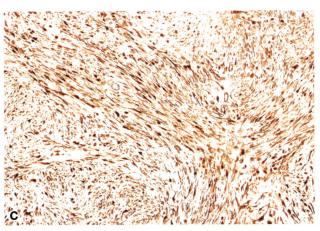

FIGURE 13.9 Primary Mammary Fibromatosis. A, B: This needle core biopsy sampled a breast mass in a 32-year-old woman. The spindle cell proliferation is cytologically bland and arranged in broad sweeping fascicles. Blood vessels are conspicuous. **C:** A β-catenin stain decorates the cytoplasm and the nuclei of the lesional cells; p63 and cytokeratins were negative (not shown). These findings support the diagnosis of fibromatosis.

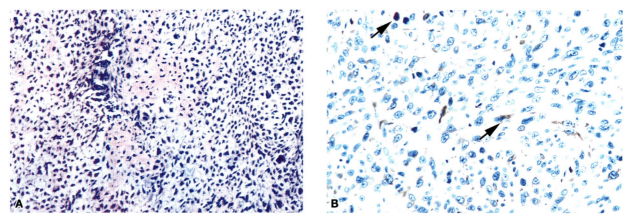

FIGURE 13.10 **Metaplastic Carcinoma, Osteocartilaginous Metaplasia. A:** The tumor has poorly formed osteoid and chondroid matrix. **B:** Cytokeratin CAM5.2 expression is demonstrated in spindle and round cells (arrows).

cartilage **(Fig. 13.11)**. Osteosarcomatous, rhabdomyosarcomatous, liposarcomatous, and angiosarcomatous metaplasia are uncommon **(Fig. 13.12)**. Epithelial foci with glandular and/or squamous morphology may be present. Myxoid areas are also common **(Fig. 13.13)**. Metaplastic matrix-producing carcinoma is one of the most common types of heterologous differentiation and shows *direct transition from glandular elements to "matrix"—without an intervening spindle cell zone.*

In a series evaluating resections of matrix-producing carcinomas (21), chondromyxoid or chondroid matrix constituted greater than 40% of the tumor mass in nearly one-third of the cases. The neoplastic cells within the matrix had low-grade nuclei in 72%, but 94% of the cells of the associated invasive carcinomas had high-grade nuclei. Approximately 60% showed necrosis, and 25% had foci of lymphovascular involvement (21). Squamous differentiation was present in ~40% in another series (26). Some high-grade carcinomas with a dominant central acellular (necrotic/fibrotic) zone qualify for the designation of metaplastic carcinoma (55,56) **(Fig. 13.14)**.

Nearly, all matrix-producing metaplastic carcinomas are "triple-negative" (26,57) and are positive for S-100, p63, and calponin (26,57). Lymph node (LN) metastases occur in 20% to 45% of cases (21,26,58) and can be matrix-producing (26). Distant metastases can also show matrix production. DCIS associated with matrix-producing metaplastic carcinomas has solid, cribriform, or micropapillary architecture, intermediate or high nuclear grade, and necrosis (26). Matrix-producing DCIS is exceedingly rare. Some matrix-producing metaplastic carcinomas arise in association with microglandular adenosis (57,59,60).

Differential Diagnosis at Needle Core Biopsy

The matrix present in some metaplastic carcinoma may focally resemble mucin and raise the differential diagnosis of *mucinous carcinoma*, especially on NCB **(Fig. 13.13)**. Although sometimes mucin-positivity can be demonstrated in the stroma, the matrix-producing tumor cells do not contain intracellular mucin. Metaplastic matrix-producing carcinomas are strongly and diffusely positive for S-100 and are negative for ER, whereas most mucinous carcinomas are strongly and diffusely positive for ER and are negative for S-100. *Pleomorphic adenoma* of the breast is a rare benign biphasic (epithelial and myoepithelial) neoplasm similar to its counterpart in the salivary glands **(Fig. 13.15)**. The

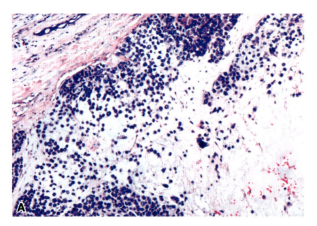
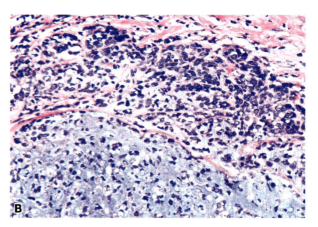

FIGURE 13.11 **Metaplastic Carcinoma, Matrix-Producing Type. A, B:** This tumor is characterized by carcinoma cells with direct transition to cartilaginous-like matrix—without an intervening spindle cell component. The matrix could be mistaken for mucin.

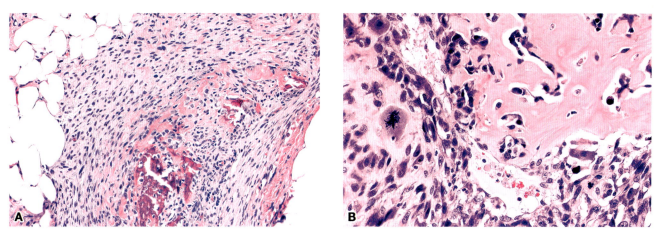

FIGURE 13.12 Metaplastic Carcinoma With Osteoid Matrix. A, B: Two cases with metaplastic osteoid production in a carcinoma. Note high-grade nuclei in the carcinoma cells with an atypical mitosis (left center).

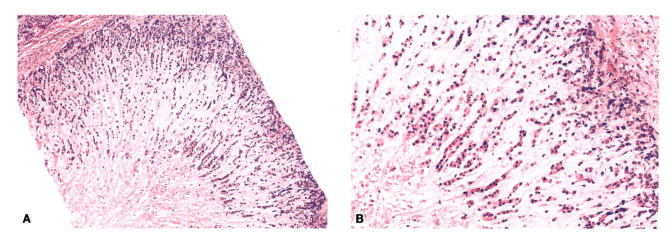

FIGURE 13.13 Metaplastic Carcinoma, Matrix-Producing Type. A, B: Tumor cells with relatively higher-grade nuclei are present at the periphery of the tumor, and tumor cells with lower-grade nuclei in the matrix-producing area.

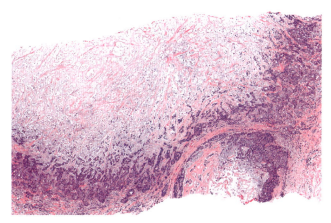

FIGURE 13.14 Metaplastic Matrix-Producing Carcinoma With Central Zone of Necrosis: This needle core biopsy shows a high-grade carcinoma with central necrosis. Viable carcinoma has a ring-like distribution at the periphery of the tumor.

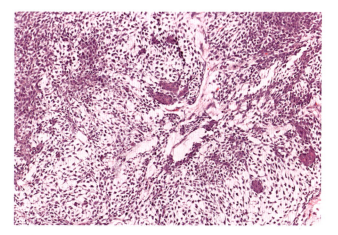

FIGURE 13.15 Mixed Tumor (Pleomorphic Adenoma). This primary neoplasm of the breast resembles a mixed tumor (pleomorphic adenoma) of the salivary glands. It consists of benign epithelial and myoepithelial cells amid stromal matrix.

lesional cells are cytologically bland. Given its similarity to metaplastic matrix-producing carcinoma, pleomorphic adenoma of breast is sometimes mistaken for the latter on NCB (61). Cases of matrix-producing metaplastic carcinoma arising from pleomorphic adenoma have been reported (62). Thus, the definitive diagnosis of pleomorphic adenoma should only be rendered on examination of the entire tumor.

Metastatic chondrosarcoma and osteosarcoma may rarely involve the breast. Obviously, the clinical history is crucial. Some *metaplastic carcinomas with acantholytic pattern* may simulate *pseudoangiomatous stromal hyperplasia* (PASH) or *angiosarcoma* **(Fig. 13.16)**. In some cases, the acantholytic appearance of some MSCC may be caused by poor tissue fixation.

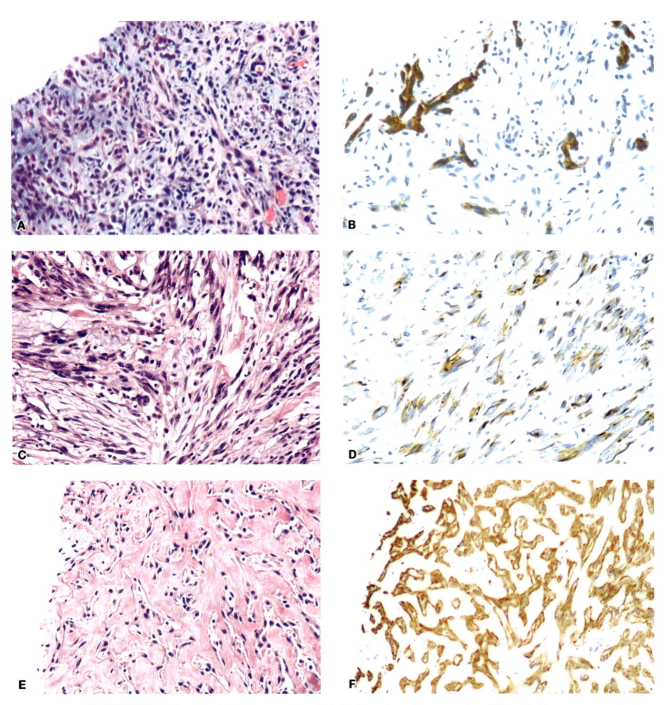

FIGURE 13.16 Metaplastic Carcinoma, Acantholytic (Pseudoangiosarcomatous) Type. **A, B:** Epithelial elements form slender, serpiginous strands. **B:** Cytokeratin AE1/AE3 immunoreactivity is present. **C, D:** Spaces have formed between spindle cells in this tumor. **D:** There is immunoreactivity for cytokeratin CK7 in the tumor shown in **C**. **E, F:** The fully developed acantholytic pattern is evident. This lesion could be mistaken for pseudoangiomatous stromal hyperplasia. **F:** Pronounced cytokeratin 34βE12 reactivity in the tumor shown in **E**.

METAPLASTIC CARCINOMA WITH CHORIOCARCINOMATOUS MORPHOLOGY

Metaplastic carcinomas with choriocarcinomatous areas are most uncommon. They can occur at any age and have no specific presenting features (63-67). These tumors tend to be hemorrhagic. Syncytiotrophoblasts (large, multinucleated, pleomorphic cells that express β-HCG) are present. A cytotrophoblastic component is usually less conspicuous. The identification of an associated IDC or of DCIS supports mammary origin of the tumor.

Differential Diagnosis at Needle Core Biopsy

The differential diagnosis of this rare form of metaplastic carcinoma at NCB includes metastatic choriocarcinoma. Clinical information regarding recent pregnancy or a hydatidiform mole or a choriocarcinoma should be sought. Choriocarcinoma, although aggressive in histologic appearance, usually has an excellent response to chemotherapy.

METASTATIC METAPLASTIC BREAST CARCINOMA

Metaplastic mammary carcinomas tend to follow an aggressive clinical course and develop distant metastases, especially to the lung and the brain. Distant metastases may occur in the absence of axillary nodal involvement. Metastatic MSCC can demonstrate epithelial or metaplastic or both phenotypes. Separate metastases of the same metaplastic carcinoma may show different morphologies (30) or even display heterologous elements not identified in the index tumor (68). Metastases of metaplastic carcinoma with chondroid or osseous metaplasia to bone can be diagnostically challenging. History of metaplastic breast carcinoma is fundamental to avoid misdiagnosis at this, and at any other, site. Comparative histologic review of the primary tumor is always desirable in this setting. GATA3, SOX10, and TRPS1 immunostains can be useful in this regard (39).

IMMUNOHISTOCHEMISTRY OF METAPLASTIC CARCINOMA

Metaplastic carcinomas typically acquire various degrees of immunoreactivity with "mesenchymal" markers while retaining some epithelial immunostaining. The former is illustrated by vimentin staining in these carcinomas and the latter by the ubiquitous use of multiple cytokeratins in the workup of metaplastic carcinoma.

Cytokeratins

The expression of CKs in metaplastic carcinomas varies among different tumors and can be heterogeneous within a lesion. Thus, the diagnostic workup needs to include a broad panel of CKs (38,69). Cytokeratin MNF116, 34βE12 (K903),

CK5/6, CK14, and CK17 are among the CKs that are useful to document epithelial differentiation. Some MSCC are only positive for high-molecular-weight cytokeratins (CK14 and CK17). MSCCs with intermediate- and high-grade morphology are least positive for CKs. In such cases, the reactivity for CKs may be focal or even absent, especially on NCB. Conversely, lower-grade MSCC is usually positive for CKs, especially CK5/6, CK14, and 34βE12, with a characteristic linear and reticular pattern. One study detected MNF116 in 93% of all MSCC (38). CK14 is positive in 30% (41) to 90% of MSCCs (38,70). Other CKs that are expressed in sarcomatous areas of MSCC include 34βE12 (41,71), CK5 (41), and CK5/6 (70,71). Cytokeratin AE1:AE3 stained only 28% (41) to 41% (38) of MSCCs. Similarly, CAM5.2 decorated only 30% (41) to 40% (38) of cases. Epithelial membrane antigen (EMA) was positive in 43% of MSCCs (38). CK7 and CK19 are positive less frequently (41). CK AE1:AE3 stained 38% of 21 matrix-producing metaplastic carcinomas (26).

Myoepithelial Antigens

Most metaplastic carcinomas are positive for p63 (38,71,72). In particular, p63 is expressed in 60% to 90% of MSCCs (38,71-73). In one study (72), the sensitivity and specificity of p63 for the diagnosis of metaplastic carcinoma was 86.7% and 99.4%, respectively. Most fibroepithelial tumors and primary mammary sarcomas are negative for p63 (72), but reactivity for p63 has been documented in some malignant PTs (74). The expression of p63 in nonmammary soft tissue tumors is rare (44) and has been detected in osseous (75) and vascular tumors (43). Focal CK and/or EMA expression sometimes occurs in vascular tumors, particularly in epithelioid angiosarcomas (42). Therefore, the use of vascular markers, such as ERG, FLI1, and CD31, should be included in the diagnostic workup of a p63-positive well-vascularized spindle cell breast lesion suspected to be angiosarcoma. Tumors with ambiguous morphology and sparse staining for p63 and CKs require thorough evaluation. Typically, metaplastic carcinomas show stronger and more diffuse positivity for p63 and CKs than sarcomas. CD10, myosin, and smooth muscle actin (SMA) are often expressed in the sarcomatoid areas of some metaplastic carcinomas, although less consistently than p63 (41,73,76). CD10 is detected in 50% of malignant PTs (77). A CD10-positive variant of mammary sarcoma has also been described (78). Focal CD10 positivity has also been detected in vascular tumors (79).

ER, PR, and HER2

Metaplastic carcinomas usually are "triple-negative." Focal positivity for ER and/or HER2 is usually confined to the neoplastic epithelial component (18,70,71,80).

Epidermal Growth Factor Receptor is detected in some metaplastic carcinomas, especially in carcinomas with squamous morphology. This finding may have therapeutic implications. One study (81) identified no EGFR-activating mutations in 303 TNBC.

GATA3 was detected in 54% of metaplastic carcinomas in a study (39); thus, GATA3 can be useful to support mammary origin of metastases of a metaplastic carcinoma (39). GATA3 is also expressed in 86% of urothelial carcinomas, in 2% of endometrial carcinomas, and also in other tumors (82,83).

Snail (SNAI1) and other EMT-related proteins are expressed in metaplastic carcinomas. The sensitivity of Snail for the diagnosis of metaplastic carcinoma has been reported to be 100%, but specificity to be 3.8% (10).

Matrix Components

Laminin 5 b3 and χ2 chains decorated 80% to 95% cases of metaplastic carcinoma in two series, but also a few PTs (71,84). These markers were less useful than p63 in the diagnosis of metaplastic carcinoma (84). *ab-crystallin* was detected in 86% of 29 metaplastic carcinomas (85), predominantly in the carcinomatous component. Another study (86) found positive *ab*-crystallin only in 20% of metaplastic carcinomas.

SOX10 is a transcription factor regarded as highly specific for Schwann cell and melanocytic origin. In one study, SOX10 was detected in 46% of 13 metaplastic carcinomas, including 5 of 6 matrix-producing metaplastic carcinomas, and 1 of 3 spindle and squamous metaplastic carcinomas (45).

TRPS1

Trichorhinophalangeal syndrome type 1 is emerging as a highly sensitive and specific marker for breast carcinoma, especially TNBC. Ai et al reported on immunohistochemical expression of TRPS1 in 479 breast carcinomas and found that TRPS1 and GATA3 had comparable positive expression in ER-positive (98% vs 95%) and HER2-positive (87% vs 88%) breast carcinomas (87). TRPS1 was highly expressed in TNBC and was expressed more than GATA3 in metaplastic (86% vs 21%) and nonmetaplastic (86% vs 51%) TNBC. In addition, TRPS1 expression was evaluated in 1,234 cases of solid tumor from various organs. In contrast to the high expression of GATA3 in urothelial carcinoma, TRPS1 showed absent or minimal expression in urothelial and other carcinomas.

Of note, Han et al have recently reported that an immunohistochemical panel comprised of OSCAR (a broad-spectrum CK), CK14, and p63 is an efficient one for diagnosing MSCC with a sensitivity 97.9% (88). Conversely, Rakha et al found that 8 of 140 (~6%) metaplastic breast carcinomas lacked expression of all CKs tested (89).

TREATMENT AND PROGNOSIS OF METAPLASTIC CARCINOMA

Most reported series of metaplastic carcinoma are retrospective or include relatively limited numbers of cases or provide only minimal histologic information. In 2022, Yang et al reported a meta-analysis of nine cohort or case-control studies of metaplastic breast carcinomas. These studies had been published between 2010 and 2020 (90). Treatment was not assessed. Compared with TNBC patients, the hazard ratios for 5-year disease-free survival and 5-year overall survival

of those with metaplastic carcinomas were 1.64 (95% confidence interval [CI] 1.36-1.98; $P < .001$) and 1.52 (95% CI 1.27-1.81; $P < .001$), respectively. Patients with metaplastic carcinoma had worse prognosis than those with TNBC-negative carcinomas. Most patients with the latter presented at ≥50 years of age, with larger (>5) cm masses, and negative LNs. There were no statistically significant differences in the occurrence of distant metastasis.

Approximately 20% of patients in two epidemiologic series (2,8) had nodal metastases. About 60% of patients presented with stage II disease, and 10% to 14% (8) with stage III. Surgical treatment involved mastectomy in 55% of the cases (2). Radiotherapy was administered to 43% (2), greater than 50% received chemotherapy, and 6% underwent hormone-modulating therapy (2). Based on Surveillance, Epidemiology, and End Results (SEER) data (8), overall survival (OS) at 5 years was 81% for stage I, 59% for stage II, 67% for stage III, and 18% for stage IV. Disease-specific survival (DSS) at 5 years was 93% for patients with stage I disease, 67% for stage II, 71% for stage III, and 20% for stage IV. In another SEER data–based study (14), 38.6% of 1,501 patients with metaplastic carcinoma received radiotherapy. Ten-year OS and DSS for all patients were 53.2% and 68.3%, respectively. Radiotherapy improved OS (64%) and overall DSS (74%).

Most patients with metaplastic carcinoma receive chemotherapy regimens used for usual breast carcinomas, but some patients receive sarcoma-specific chemotherapy. It is unclear which chemotherapy regimen is more effective. The use of neoadjuvant chemotherapy has been reported in some series (6,8,9,11,18), but the pathologic complete response (pCR) rate was only 10% in one study (8).

MSCC of high grade have the worst prognosis among all metaplastic carcinomas. About 50% of patients in published series underwent mastectomy (4,17). In one series, (17) 22% had nodal involvement. Nearly all patients received chemotherapy (4,17). In a series with a median follow-up time of 36 months (4), 47% of the patients developed local recurrence, including 57% of patients who did not receive radiotherapy at initial diagnosis, and only 10% of patients who did. Approximately one-third of patients died of disease between 4 and 91 months after treatment, two patients were alive with disease at 9 and 87 months, and another patient developed a distant recurrence. In another series (17), 80% of the patients received chemotherapy, 68% received radiotherapy, and 10% hormonal therapy. At a median follow-up of 30 months, 28% of the patients developed a locoregional recurrence, 40% developed distant metastases, and 21% had both; 40% of the patients died of disease. Patients with MSCC had decreased DFS when compared with patients with TNBC matched by age, stage, tumor grade, chemotherapy, and radiation therapy. The 5-year DFS for patients with stage I to III MSCC was 44% (vs 74% in the control group) and 53% for patients with stage I to II MSCC (vs 87% in the control group).

The first series of patients with *lower-grade (fibromatosis-like) MSCC* (46) reported a 44% rate of local recurrence at

METAPLASTIC CARCINOMAS, INCLUDING LOW-GRADE ADENOSQUAMOUS CARCINOMA 263

a median time of 15.5 months after initial surgery, but no distant metastases or deaths from disease were reported. Subsequent studies (3,38,47) have documented lung metastases and death caused by disease in a few patients. Two patients were alive with disease at 35 and 42 months of follow-up (38). Overall, lower-grade MSCCs appear to have a relatively more indolent behavior than the rapidly aggressive MSCCs with intermediate- or high-grade morphology.

In published series, about 40% to 60% of patients with *metaplastic carcinoma with chondroid and/or osteoid matrix* have undergone mastectomy (21,26,58). LN metastases have been detected in 23% to 45% of patients (21,26,58) and were purely chondroid in 60% of cases (26). In one series (21), 43% of patients received postmastectomy radiation, and most patients received chemotherapy. Approximately twenty percent of patients in another study (58) developed local recurrence or distant metastases within 2 years of initial treatment, and four died of disease. The overall 5-year survival rate was 60%. In this study, patients with matrix-producing metaplastic carcinoma had a more favorable prognosis than control patients with IDC. In yet another series (26), the median patient survival was 38.6 months. In a relatively recent series of 32 patients with matrix-producing metaplastic carcinomas (21), 22% developed locoregional recurrence, and 31% developed distant metastases at a median time of 28 months. At a median follow-up time of 29 months, 25% of patients died because of disease.

A notable caveat regarding prognosis of metaplastic carcinoma is that although the prognosis of metaplastic carcinoma is influenced partly by *stage* at diagnosis, these carcinomas have a lower frequency of nodal metastases (ie, lower stage).

LOW-GRADE ADENOSQUAMOUS CARCINOMA

Low-grade adenosquamous carcinoma (LGASC) is an unusual, and uncommon, diagnostically challenging variant of metaplastic mammary carcinoma. Several case series and case reports of LGASC have been published (91); however, this number likely underestimates the true incidence of LGASC (because it is possible that some, if not most, LGASCs are underdiagnosed). Mucoepidermoid carcinoma of the breast is distinct from LGASC—and is histologically similar to the eponymous tumor in the salivary gland (with mucinous, squamous, and "intermediate" cells set in a solid and cystic pattern).

LGASC occurs in peri- or postmenopausal women, although there are reports thereof in much younger women (92,93). Two patients were pregnant at the time of diagnosis (93). One patient with LGASC was a *BRCA1* germline mutation carrier (94); two others had a family history of breast carcinoma (93), and another two had personal histories of ipsilateral breast carcinoma (93). A patient had bilateral florid papillomatosis of nipple, and another subsequently developed a CSL in the contralateral breast (93).

Most LGASCs present as a palpable breast mass, and some are detected on mammography. LGASCs may originate in the retroareolar region. Rarely, nipple discharge is the presenting symptom (93). Mammography can detect LGASC, but the findings are nonspecific. Ultrasound examination of a 5-cm tumor was reported as inconclusive (92). The average size of LGASC is about 2.0 cm (range 0.5-5.0 cm).

LGASC is a variant of metaplastic carcinoma with biphasic (epithelial and myoepithelial/squamous) differentiation (91,95). Four types of cells are present: ductal epithelial, squamous metaplastic, myoepithelial, and spindle cells. Please see **Table 13.2**. These tumors lie amid desmoplastic stroma

---

TABLE 13.2

Histopathologic Constituents of Low-Grade Adenosquamous Carcinoma

a. Epithelial (ductal) cells
Present in ducts, some of which are compressed with minimal and collapsed lumina
Some ducts may be rounded or ovoid or "tadpole-like" or "solid"
Nuclear grade is low/intermediate, and mitoses are rare
Epithelial cells may be multilayered or appear in isolated minute "epithelioid" clusters
Some ducts show squamous cell metaplasia
Low-molecular-weight cytokeratins (Cam 5.2, CK8, CK18) are variably positive
Some inner ("luminal") cells are strongly CK-positive ("core staining")
"Core staining" observed in at least some ducts, to variable degree, in ~50% of cases

b. Squamous cells
Present within ducts or seemingly per se
Form "pearl-like" or "onion skin–like" structures
Nuclear grade is low/intermediate, and mitoses are rare
Keratinization may occur, and keratinous cysts can form
p63-positive, p40-positive (some spindle cells are also variably positive for p63 and p40)

TABLE 13.2
Histopathologic Constituents of Low-Grade Adenosquamous Carcinoma *(continued)*

c. **Myoepithelial cells**
   Variably identified at perimeter of some epithelial cell–lined ducts
   Nuclear grade is low-intermediate
   p63-positive, CK5/14-positive, other myoepithelial markers are variably positive
   Myoepithelial cells may resemble spindle cells, and vice versa, at perimeter of ducts

d. **Spindle cells**
   Comprise the dominant component of the tumor in most cases
   Lie amid variably dense collagen and (myo)fibroelastic stroma
   Spindle cells appear to merge with periductal myoepithelial cells
   Nuclear grade is low, and mitoses are rare
   Spindle cells are variably hypercellular
   Some spindle cells may be neoplastic, and others may be reactive
   High-molecular-weight cytokeratins (CK5/6 and CK14) are variably positive
   Muscle markers (actin, calponin, myosin, etc.) show "lamellar" periductal staining (in 50% of cases)

e. **Collagenous Background**
   Background stroma is variably myofibroblastic and fibrocollagenous
   May also show elastosis

(Figs. 13.17-13.19). The tumor infiltrates normal ducts and lobules The squamous metaplasia ranges from focal and inconspicuous to substantial. Syringoma-like foci and microcysts containing keratotic debris can be present. The neoplastic squamous cells bear low- to intermediate-grade nuclei, with scattered apoptosis and rare mitoses. Tumoral necrosis is uncommon. The spindle cells around the squamous foci often show a distinctively lamellar arrangement and in some areas

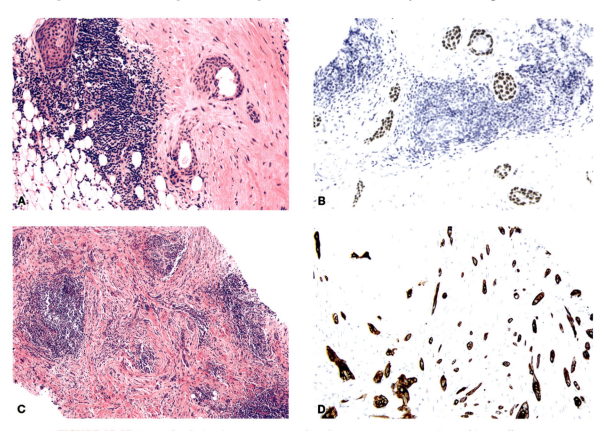

FIGURE 13.17 Metaplastic Carcinoma, Low-Grade Adenosquamous Type. **A, B:** This needle core biopsy sample is from a nonpalpable, mammographically detected stellate tumor. The nests of carcinoma cells with squamous differentiation are accompanied by a lymphocytic infiltrate **(A)**. Nuclear reactivity for p63 in areas of squamous differentiation **(B)**. **C, D:** There are cords and clusters of cells with squamoid and glandular differentiation **(C)**. A prominent lymphocytic infiltrate is present. Tumor cells are immunoreactive for the cytokeratin 34βE12 **(D)**.

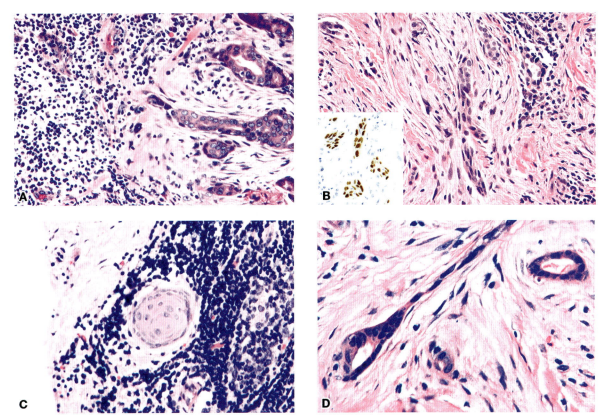

FIGURE 13.18 Metaplastic Carcinoma, Low-Grade Adenosquamous Type. Images from various tumors are shown. **A:** Neoplastic glands and cords are shown in association with tumor-infiltrating lymphocytes. **B:** Cords of epithelial elements are present amid relatively cellular stroma. Inset shows p63-positivity in tumor cells. **C:** In another area of the specimen, a squamous pearl is enveloped by lymphocytes. **D:** Tadpole-like and well-formed tubular-like neoplastic glands are present.

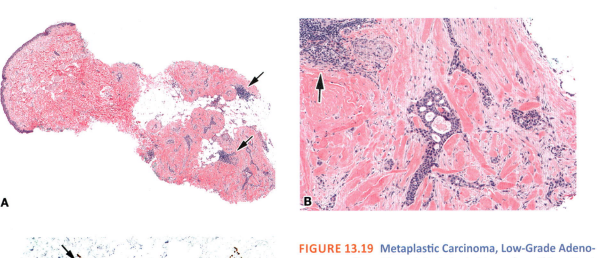

FIGURE 13.19 Metaplastic Carcinoma, Low-Grade Adenosquamous Type. The original nipple biopsy from this patient was misdiagnosed as a syringoma. The tumor recurred 2 years later deep in the nipple. The images in **A-C** illustrate the tumor recurrence. **A:** The lesion shows no involvement of the superficial dermis. Aggregates of lymphocytes are associated with the tumor (arrows). **B:** A few neoplastic glands and squamous clusters are present in desmoplastic stroma. An aggregate of lymphocytes is present (arrow). **C:** p63 stain highlights the myoepithelial cells around the neoplastic glands and in the stroma. A few clusters are composed entirely of p63-positive cells (arrows). A neoplastic cluster shows incomplete circumferential staining for p63 (arrowhead).

appear to merge with the lesional myoepithelium/epithelium. Transition of LGASC to higher-grade MSCC is rare (93,96-97). LGASC is typically TNBC (albeit with favorable prognosis). Rarely, the tumor is low-positive for ER (1% to <10%).

DCIS can be associated with LGASC and sometimes displays apocrine features. The infiltrating glands of LGASC may show a peripheral myoepithelial cell layer (or myoepithelial differentiation), and in some cases it is difficult to distinguish DCIS from infiltrating carcinoma. LGASC tends to arise in association with sclerosing lesions, such as florid papillomatosis of nipple, adenomyoepithelioma, papilloma, radial sclerosing lesion (RSL), or sclerosing adenosis (95,98,99). The strikingly prominent desmoplasia associated with LGASC is a feature useful in the differential diagnosis with nonneoplastic sclerosing lesions. The latter show a much lesser degree of desmoplasia.

Differential Diagnosis of LGASC

The diagnosis of LGASC is especially challenging in NCB samples, because the characteristic findings can be focal and subtle (98). Disorganized squamous cords and duct-like structures surrounded by spindle cells in a lamellar arrangement should raise the differential diagnosis of LGASC. In some cases, the neoplastic epithelial clusters consist of a few cells with eosinophilic and squamoid cytoplasm, admixed with fibrotic or elastotic stroma.

Syringoma closely resembles LGASC, both morphologically and immunohistochemically, but it does not show cytologic atypia, apoptosis, and dyskeratosis. Syringoma arises primarily in the skin, usually involves the superficial dermis, and rarely extends into the breast parenchyma. In contrast, LGASC arises primarily within the breast and may rarely involve the skin secondarily. The differential diagnosis between syringoma and LGASC is particularly challenging when the latter arises in the nipple (**Fig. 13.19**).

Sclerosing lesions such as an RSL and a CSL closely mimic LGASC. Furthermore, LGASC tends to arise in association with a sclerosing lesion. Therefore, it is good practice to consider LGASC in evaluating sclerosing lesions—particularly in NCBs. Compared with RSL, LGASC usually shows an overtly infiltrative pattern. The neoplastic glands and squamous nests of LGASC display nuclear atypia (at least mild), apoptosis, and rare mitoses. These findings are uncommon in RSL. Furthermore, the periductal lamellar fibrosis typically associated with LGASC is not present in RSL. An inflammatory cell infiltrate is often present at the periphery of LGASC.

Immunoreactivity Pattern of LGASC

LGASCs do not exhibit predictable immunoreactivity for epithelial and myoepithelial markers (93,97). This staining "pattern" has been described as being "consistently inconsistent." (93) AE1:3, CK5/6, CK7, CK14, and CK17 staining has been reported in the epithelial clusters in ~50% of cases, but less-frequent staining for cytokeratin 34βE12 (35%) and CAM5.2 (10%). Some epithelial clusters are CK-negative. The epithelial clusters of LGASC are seemingly surrounded by myoepithelium. Complete circumferential staining for p63, SMMHC, SMA, CD10, and calponin was found only in 11% of the cases in one series (93). The stroma associated with LGASC usually exhibits no reactivity for CKs, although the presence of rare CK7-positive epithelioid stromal cells and 34βE12- and SMA-positive spindle cells has been reported (93). p63-Positive stromal cells are not present. Stromal staining for SMMHC was identified in 53% of cases and for calponin in 57% (93). LGASC is positive for EGFR (in ~50%) of cases. Familiarity with the different patterns of immunoreactivity of LGASC is necessary to avoid misinterpretation.

Prognosis and Treatment of LGASC

LGASC has excellent prognosis. The primary clinical concern is local recurrence, rather than nodal involvement or distant metastases. The only documented report of systemic disease caused by LGASC pertains to a 33-year-old woman with an 8-cm primary breast carcinoma and lung metastases at presentation (91). A patient with locally recurrent disease developed hemithorax and died of the disease 8.4 years after diagnosis. About 50% of women who were treated initially by excision developed ipsilateral recurrence 1 to 3.5 years after the initial treatment and required mastectomy (91). A case of LGASC misdiagnosed initially on NCB as syringomatous adenoma of nipple recurred after 5 years as a large mass requiring mastectomy (93). The surgical management of LGASC is similar to that of other types of invasive carcinomas. Radiotherapy can be used after breast-conserving surgery. At this time, the role of chemotherapy in LGASC remains undetermined.

MOLECULAR PATHOLOGY OF METAPLASTIC CARCINOMA

The molecular pathology profile of MSCC, including that of LGASC, is evolving (100-106). Multiple molecular studies support the view that the epithelial and non-epithelial components of MSCC, despite each being genetically complex, are clonally related and originate from the same stem cell (70,80). MSCC are typically "triple-negative." Intrinsic gene profiling classifies the tumors as basal-like or claudin-low. High frequency of mutations, amplification, and activation have been reported. Transcriptional profile of these tumors is similar to, but distinct from, other "basal-like" carcinomas. MSCC harbor somatic mutations, most frequently in *TP53, PIK3CA,* and *PTEN*. Accordingly, the potential role of novel targeted therapies is emerging.

In LGASC, similar gene amplifications have been found in the epithelial and spindle/stromal components, suggesting that at least a proportion of the latter are malignant. *PIK3CA* mutations are found in about one-half of LGASC cases. EGFR amplification has also been reported therein. The overexpression of PD-L1 and TILs in these tumors suggests an endogenous immune response and offers a possible rationale for therapeutic immunomodulation.

REFERENCES

1. Kalluri R, Weinberg RA. The basics of epithelial-mesenchymal transition. *J Clin Invest.* 2009;119:1420-1428.
2. Pezzi CM, Patel-Parekh L, Cole K, et al. Characteristics and treatment of metaplastic breast cancer: analysis of 892 cases from the National Cancer Database. *Ann Surg Oncol.* 2007;14:166-173.
3. Kurian KM, Al-Nafussi A. Sarcomatoid/metaplastic carcinoma of the breast: a clinicopathological study of 12 cases. *Histopathology.* 2002;40:58-64.
4. Davis WG, Hennessy B, Babiera G, et al. Metaplastic sarcomatoid carcinoma of the breast with absent or minimal overt invasive carcinomatous component: a misnomer. *Am J Surg Pathol.* 2005;29:1456-1463.
5. Barnes PJ, Boutilier R, Chiasson D, et al. Metaplastic breast carcinoma: clinical-pathologic characteristics and HER2/neu expression. *Breast Cancer Res Treat.* 2005;91:173-178.
6. Beatty JD, Atwood M, Tickman R, et al. Metaplastic breast cancer: clinical significance. *Am J Surg.* 2006;191:657-664.
7. Dave G, Cosmatos H, Do T, et al. Metaplastic carcinoma of the breast: a retrospective review. *Int J Radiat Oncol Biol Phys.* 2006;64:771-775.
8. Hennessy BT, Giordano S, Broglio K, et al. Biphasic metaplastic sarcomatoid carcinoma of the breast. *Ann Oncol.* 2006;17:605-613.
9. Luini A, Aguilar M, Gatti G, et al. Metaplastic carcinoma of the breast, an unusual disease with worse prognosis: the experience of the European Institute of Oncology and review of the literature. *Breast Cancer Res Treat.* 2007;101:349-353.
10. Nassar A, Sookhan N, Santisteban M, et al. Diagnostic utility of snail in metaplastic breast carcinoma. *Diagn Pathol.* 2010;5:76.
11. Okada N, Hasebe T, Iwasaki M, et al. Metaplastic carcinoma of the breast. *Hum Pathol.* 2010;41:960-970.
12. Park HS, Park S, Kim JH, et al. Clinicopathologic features and outcomes of metaplastic breast carcinoma: comparison with invasive ductal carcinoma of the breast. *Yonsei Med J.* 2010;51:864-869.
13. Gwin K, Buell-Gutbrod R, Tretiakova M, et al. Epithelial-to-mesenchymal transition in metaplastic breast carcinomas with chondroid differentiation: expression of the E-cadherin repressor Snail. *Appl Immunohistochem Mol Morphol.* 2010;18:526-531.
14. Tseng WH, Martinez SR. Metaplastic breast cancer: to radiate or not to radiate? *Ann Surg Oncol.* 2011;18:94-103.
15. Bae SY, Lee SK, Koo MY, et al. The prognoses of metaplastic breast cancer patients compared to those of triple-negative breast cancer patients. *Breast Cancer Res Treat.* 2011;126:471-478.
16. Chen IC, Lin CH, Huang CS, et al. Lack of efficacy to systemic chemotherapy for treatment of metaplastic carcinoma of the breast in the modern era. *Breast Cancer Res Treat.* 2011;130:345-351.
17. Lester TR, Hunt KK, Nayeemuddin KM, et al. Metaplastic sarcomatoid carcinoma of the breast appears more aggressive than other triple receptor-negative breast cancers. *Breast Cancer Res Treat.* 2012;131:41-48.
18. Lee H, Jung SY, Ro JY, et al. Metaplastic breast cancer: clinicopathological features and its prognosis. *J Clin Pathol.* 2012;65:441-446.
19. Choi BB, Shu KS. Metaplastic carcinoma of the breast: multimodality imaging and histopathologic assessment. *Acta Radiol.* 2012;53:5-11.
20. Alvarenga CA, Paravidino PI, Alvarenga M, et al. Reappraisal of immunohistochemical profiling of special histological types of breast carcinomas: a study of 121 cases of eight different subtypes. *J Clin Pathol.* 2012;65:1066-1071.
21. Downs-Kelly E, Nayeemuddin KM, Albarracin C, et al. Matrix-producing carcinoma of the breast: an aggressive subtype of metaplastic carcinoma. *Am J Surg Pathol.* 2009;33:534-541.
22. Yang WT, Hennessy B, Broglio K, et al. Imaging differences in metaplastic and invasive ductal carcinomas of the breast. *AJR Am J Roentgenol.* 2007;189:1288-1293.
23. Rashid MU, Shah MA, Azhar R, et al. A deleterious BRCA1 mutation in a young Pakistani woman with metaplastic breast carcinoma. *Pathol Res Pract.* 2011;207:583-586.
24. Suspitsin EN, Sokolenko AP, Voskresenskiy DA, et al. Mixed epithelial mesenchymal metaplastic carcinoma (carcinosarcoma) of the breast in BRCA1 carrier. *Breast Cancer.* 2011;18:137-140.
25. Ashida A, Fukutomi T, Tsuda H, et al. Atypical medullary carcinoma of the breast with cartilaginous metaplasia in a patient with a BRCA1 germline mutation. *Jpn J Clin Oncol.* 2000;30:30-32.
26. Gwin K, Wheeler DT, Bossuyt V, et al. Breast carcinoma with chondroid differentiation: a clinicopathologic study of 21 triple negative (ER−, PR−, Her2/neu−) cases. *Int J Surg Pathol.* 2010;18:27-35.
27. Velasco M, Santamaria G, Ganau S, et al. MRI of metaplastic carcinoma of the breast. *AJR Am J Roentgenol.* 2005;184:1274-1278.
28. Shin HJ, Kim HH, Kim SM, et al. Imaging features of metaplastic carcinoma with chondroid differentiation of the breast. *AJR Am J Roentgenol.* 2007;188:691-696.
29. Park JM, Han BK, Moon WK, et al. Metaplastic carcinoma of the breast: mammographic and sonographic findings. *J Clin Ultrasound.* 2000;28:179-186.
30. Kaufman MW, Marti JR, Gallager S, et al. Carcinoma of the breast with pseudosarcomatous metaplasia. *Cancer.* 1984;53:1908-1917.
31. Wargotz ES, Norris HJ. Metaplastic carcinomas of the breast: V. Metaplastic carcinoma with osteoclastic giant cells. *Hum Pathol.* 1990;21:1142-1150.
32. Anderson WJ, Fletcher CDM. Mesenchymal lesions of the breast. *Histopathology.* 2023;82:83-94.
33. Sugie T, Takeuchi E, Kunishima F, et al. A case of ductal carcinoma with squamous differentiation in malignant phyllodes tumor. *Breast Cancer.* 2007;14:327-332.
34. Ramdass MJ, Dindyal S. Phyllodes breast tumour showing invasive squamous-cell carcinoma with invasive ductal, clear-cell, secretory, and squamous components. *Lancet Oncol.* 2006;7:880.
35. Bauer TW, Rostock RA, Eggleston JC, Baral E. Spindle cell carcinoma of the breast: four cases and review of the literature. *Hum Pathol.* 1984;15:147-152.
36. Leiman G. Squamous carcinoma of the breast: diagnosis by aspiration cytology. *Acta Cytol.* 1982;26:201-209.
37. DeLair DF, Corben AD, Catalano JP, et al. Non-mammary metastases to the breast and axilla: a study of 85 cases. *Mod Pathol.* 2013;26:343-349.
38. Carter MR, Hornick JL, Lester S, et al. Spindle cell (sarcomatoid) carcinoma of the breast: a clinicopathologic and immunohistochemical analysis of 29 cases. *Am J Surg Pathol.* 2006;30:300-309.
39. Cimino-Mathews A, Subhawong AP, Illei PB, et al. GATA3 expression in breast carcinoma: utility in triple-negative, sarcomatoid, and metastatic carcinomas. *Hum Pathol.* 2013;44:1341-1349.
40. Chia Y, Thike AA, Cheok PY, et al. Stromal keratin expression in phyllodes tumors of the breast: a comparison with other spindle cell breast lesions. *J Clin Pathol.* 2012;65:339-347.
41. Dunne B, Lee AH, Pinder SE, et al. An immunohistochemical study of metaplastic spindle cell carcinoma, phyllodes tumor and fibromatosis of the breast. *Hum Pathol.* 2003;34:1009-1015.
42. Miettinen M, Fetsch JF. Distribution of keratins in normal endothelial cells and a spectrum of vascular tumors: implications in tumor diagnosis. *Hum Pathol.* 2000;31:1062-1067.
43. Kallen ME, Nunes Rosado FG, Gonzalez AL, et al. Occasional staining for p63 in malignant vascular tumors: a potential diagnostic pitfall. *Pathol Oncol Res.* 2012;18:97-100.
44. Jo VY, Fletcher CD. p63 immunohistochemical staining is limited in soft tissue tumors. *Am J Clin Pathol.* 2011;136:762-766.
45. Cimino-Mathews A, Subhawong AP, Elwood H, et al. Neural crest transcription factor Sox10 is preferentially expressed in triple-negative and metaplastic breast carcinomas. *Hum Pathol.* 2013;44:959-965.
46. Gobbi H, Simpson JF, Borowsky A, et al. Metaplastic breast tumors with a dominant fibromatosis-like phenotype have a high risk of local recurrence. *Cancer.* 1999;85:2170-2182.
47. Sneige N, Yaziji H, Mandavilli SR, et al. Low-grade (fibromatosis-like) spindle cell carcinoma of the breast. *Am J Surg Pathol.* 2001;25:1009-1016.
48. Rekhi B, Shet TM, Badwe RA, et al. Fibromatosis-like carcinoma-an unusual phenotype of a metaplastic breast tumor associated with a micropapilloma. *World J Surg Oncol.* 2007;5:24.
49. Gobbi H, Simpson JF, Jensen RA, et al. Metaplastic spindle cell breast tumors arising within papillomas, complex sclerosing lesions, and nipple adenomas. *Mod Pathol.* 2003;16:893-901.
50. Denley H, Pinder SE, Tan PH, et al. Metaplastic carcinoma of the breast arising within complex sclerosing lesion: a report of five cases. *Histopathology.* 2000;36:203-209.
51. Lacroix-Triki M, Geyer FC, Lambros MB, et al. Beta-catenin/Wnt signaling pathway in fibromatosis, metaplastic carcinomas and phyllodes tumors of the breast. *Mod Pathol.* 2010;23:1438-1448.
52. Erickson-Johnson MR, Chou MM, Evers BR, et al. Nodular fasciitis: a novel model of transient neoplasia induced by MYH9-USP6 gene fusion. *Lab Invest.* 2011;91:1427-1433.
53. Lawrence B, Perez-Atayde A, Hibbard MK, et al. TPM3-ALK and TPM4-ALK oncogenes in inflammatory myofibroblastic tumors. *Am J Pathol.* 2000;157:377-384.
54. Wargotz ES, Norris HJ. Metaplastic carcinomas of the breast. I. Matrix-producing carcinoma. *Hum Pathol.* 1989;20:628-635.
55. Tsuda H, Takarabe T, Hasegawa F, et al. Large, central acellular zones indicating myoepithelial tumor differentiation in high-grade invasive ductal carcinomas as markers of predisposition to lung and brain metastases. *Am J Surg Pathol.* 2000;24:197-202.
56. Tsuda H, Takarabe T, Hasegawa T, et al. Myoepithelial differentiation in high-grade invasive ductal carcinomas with large central acellular zones. *Hum Pathol.* 1999;30:1134-1139.
57. Shui R, Bi R, Cheng Y, et al. Matrix-producing carcinoma of the breast in the Chinese population: a clinicopathological study of 13 cases. *Pathol Int.* 2011;61:415-422.
58. Chhieng C, Cranor M, Lesser ME, et al. Metaplastic carcinoma of the breast with osteocartilaginous heterologous elements. *Am J Surg Pathol.* 1998;22:188-194.
59. Rosenblum MK, Purrazzella R, Rosen PP. Is microglandular adenosis a precancerous disease? A study of carcinoma arising therein. *Am J Surg Pathol.* 1986;10:237-245.
60. Geyer FC, Lacroix-Triki M, Colombo PE, et al. Molecular evidence in support of the neoplastic and precursor nature of microglandular adenosis. *Histopathology.* 2012;60:E115-E130.
61. Rakha EA, Aleskandarany MA, Samaka RM, et al. Pleomorphic adenoma-like tumor of the breast. *Histopathology.* 2016;68:405-410.
62. Hayes MM, Lesack D, Girardet C, et al. Carcinoma ex-pleomorphic adenoma of the breast. Report of three cases suggesting a relationship to metaplastic carcinoma of matrix-producing type. *Virchows Arch.* 2005;446:142-149.

63. Saigo PE, Rosen PP. Mammary carcinoma with "choriocarcinomatous" features. *Am J Surg Pathol.* 1981;5:773-778.
64. Resetkova E, Sahin A, Ayala AG, et al. Breast carcinoma with choriocarcinomatous features. *Ann Diagn Pathol.* 2004;8:74-79.
65. Canbay E, Bozkurt B, Ergul G, et al. Breast carcinoma with choriocarcinomatous features. *Breast J.* 2010;16:202-203.
66. Siddiqui NH, Cabay RJ, Salem F. Fine-needle aspiration biopsy of a case of breast carcinoma with choriocarcinomatous features. *Diagn Cytopathol.* 2006;34:694-697.
67. Akbulut M, Zekioglu O, Ozdemir N, et al. Fine needle aspiration cytology of mammary carcinoma with choriocarcinomatous features: a report of 2 cases. *Acta Cytol.* 2008;52:99-104.
68. Chell SE, Nayar R, De Frias DV, et al. Metaplastic breast carcinoma metastatic to the lung mimicking a primary chondroid lesion: report of a case with cytohistologic correlation. *Ann Diagn Pathol.* 1998;2:173-180.
69. Adem C, Reynolds C, Adlakha H, et al. Wide spectrum screening keratin as a marker of metaplastic spindle cell carcinoma of the breast: an immunohistochemical study of 24 patients. *Histopathology.* 2002;40:556-562.
70. Reis-Filho JS, Milanezi F, Steele D, et al. Metaplastic breast carcinomas are basal-like tumors. *Histopathology.* 2006;49:10-21.
71. Carpenter PM, Wang-Rodriguez J, Chan OT, et al. Laminin 5 expression in metaplastic breast carcinomas. *Am J Surg Pathol.* 2008;32:345-353.
72. Koker MM, Kleer CG. p63 expression in breast cancer: a highly sensitive and specific marker of metaplastic carcinoma. *Am J Surg Pathol.* 2004;28:1506-1512.
73. Leibl S, Gogg-Kammerer M, Sommersacher A, et al. Metaplastic breast carcinomas: are they of myoepithelial differentiation? Immunohistochemical profile of the sarcomatoid subtype using novel myoepithelial markers. *Am J Surg Pathol.* 2005;29:347-353.
74. Cimino-Mathews A, Sharma R, Illei PB, et al. A subset of malignant phyllodes tumors express p63 and p40: a diagnostic pitfall in breast core needle biopsies. *Am J Surg Pathol.* 2014;38:1689-1696.
75. Kallen ME, Sanders ME, Gonzalez AL, et al. Nuclear p63 expression in osteoblastic tumors. *Tumour Biol.* 2012;33:1639-1644.
76. Popnikolov NK, Ayala AG, Graves K, et al. Benign myoepithelial tumors of the breast have immunophenotypic characteristics similar to metaplastic matrix-producing and spindle cell carcinomas. *Am J Clin Pathol.* 2003;120:161-167.
77. Tse GM, Tsang AK, Putti TC, et al. Stromal CD10 expression in mammary fibroadenomas and phyllodes tumors. *J Clin Pathol.* 2005;58:185-189.
78. Leibl S, Moinfar F. Mammary NOS-type sarcoma with CD10 expression: a rare entity with features of myoepithelial differentiation. *Am J Surg Pathol.* 2006;30:450-456.
79. Weinreb I, Cunningham KS, Perez-Ordonez B, et al. CD10 is expressed in most epithelioid hemangioendotheliomas: a potential diagnostic pitfall. *Arch Pathol Lab Med.* 2009;133:1965-1968.
80. Reis-Filho JS, Milanezi F, Carvalho S, et al. Metaplastic breast carcinomas exhibit EGFR, but not HER2, gene amplification and overexpression: immunohistochemical and chromogenic in situ hybridization analysis. *Breast Cancer Res.* 2005;7:R1028-R1035.
81. Bossuyt V, Fadare O, Martel M, et al. Remarkably high frequency of EGFR expression in breast carcinomas with squamous differentiation. *Int J Surg Pathol.* 2005;13:319-327.
82. Liu H, Shi J, Wilkerson ML, et al. Immunohistochemical evaluation of GATA3 expression in tumors and normal tissues: a useful immunomarker for breast and urothelial carcinomas. *Am J Clin Pathol.* 2012;138:57-64.
83. Miettinen M, McCue PA, Sarlomo-Rikala M, et al. GATA3: a multispecific but potentially useful marker in surgical pathology: a systematic analysis of 2500 epithelial and nonepithelial tumors. *Am J Surg Pathol.* 2014;38:13-22.
84. D'Alfonso TM, Ross DS, Liu YF, et al. Expression of p40 and laminin 332 in metaplastic spindle cell carcinoma of the breast compared with other malignant spindle cell tumors. *J Clin Pathol.* 2015;68:516-521.

85. Sitterding SM, Wiseman WR, Schiller CL, et al. AlphaB-crystallin: a novel marker of invasive basal-like and metaplastic breast carcinomas. *Ann Diagn Pathol.* 2008;12:33-40.
86. Tsang JY, Lai MW, Wong KH, et al. AlphaB-crystallin is a useful marker for triple negative and basal breast cancers. *Histopathology.* 2012;61:378-386.
87. Ai D, Yao J, Yang F, et al. TRPS1: a highly sensitive and specific marker for breast carcinoma, especially for triple-negative breast cancer. *Mod Pathol.* 2021;34:710-719.
88. Han M, Zhang H, Dabbs DJ. Best practice (efficient) immunohistologic panel for diagnosing metaplastic breast carcinoma. *Appl Immunohistochem Mol Morphol.* 2021;29:265-269.
89. Rakha EA, Quinn CM, Foschini MP, et al. Metaplastic carcinomas of the breast without evidence of epithelial differentiation: a diagnostic approach for management. *Histopathology.* 2021;78:759-771.
90. Yang X, Tang T, Zhou T. Prognosis and clinicopathological characteristics of metaplastic breast cancer: a meta-analysis. *Medicine (Baltimore).* 2022;101(49):e32226. doi:10.1097/MD.0000000000032226
91. Rosen PP, Ernsberger D. Low-grade adenosquamous carcinoma: a variant of metaplastic mammary carcinoma. *Am J Surg Pathol.* 1987;11:351-358.
92. Agrawal A, Saha S, Ellis IO, et al. Adenosquamous carcinoma of breast in a 19 years old woman: a case report. *World J Surg Oncol.* 2010;8:44.
93. Kawaguchi K, Shin SJ. Immunohistochemical staining characteristics of low-grade adenosquamous carcinoma of the breast. *Am J Surg Pathol.* 2012;36(7):1009-1020.
94. Noel JC, Buxant F, Engohan-Aloghe C. Low-grade adenosquamous carcinoma of the breast—a case report with a BRCA1 germline mutation. *Pathol Res Pract.* 2010;206:511-513.
95. Van Hoeven KH, Drudis T, Cranor ML, et al. Low-grade adenosquamous carcinoma of the breast: a clinocopathologic study of 32 cases with ultrastructural analysis. *Am J Surg Pathol.* 1993;17:248-258.
96. Suster S, Moran CA, Hurt MA. Syringomatous squamous tumors of the breast. *Cancer.* 1991;67:2350-2355.
97. Geyer FC, Lambros MB, Natrajan R, et al. Genomic and immunohistochemical analysis of adenosquamous carcinoma of the breast. *Mod Pathol.* 2010;23:951-960.
98. Wilsher JW. Significance of adenosquamous proliferation in breast lesions. *J Clin Pathol.* 2021;74:559-567.
99. Foschini MP, Pizzicannella G, Peterse JL, et al. Adenomyoepithelioma of the breast associated with low-grade adenosquamous and sarcomatoid carcinomas. *Virchows Arch.* 1995;427:243-250.
100. Khoury T. Metaplastic breast carcinoma revisited; subtypes determine outcomes: comprehensive pathologic, clinical, and molecular review. *Surg Pathol Clin.* 2022;15:159-174.
101. McCart Reed AE, Kalaw EM, Lakhani SR. An update on the molecular pathology of metaplastic breast cancer. *Breast Cancer (Dove Med Press).* 2021;13:161-170.
102. Zhai J, Giannini G, Ewalt MD, et al. Molecular characterization of metaplastic breast carcinoma via next-generation sequencing. *Hum Pathol.* 2019;86:85-92.
103. Tray N, Taff J, Adams S. Therapeutic landscape of metaplastic breast cancer. *Cancer Treat Rev.* 2019;79:101888. doi:10.1016/j.ctrv.2019.08.004
104. McMullen ER, Zoumberos NA, Kleer CG. Metaplastic breast carcinoma: update on histopathology and molecular alterations. *Arch Pathol Lab Med.* 2019;143:1492-1496.
105. Krings G, Chen YY. Genomic profiling of metaplastic breast carcinomas reveals genetic heterogeneity and relationship to ductal carcinoma. *Mod Pathol.* 2018;31:1661-1674.
106. Bataillon G, Fuhrmann L, Girard E, et al. High rate of *PIK3CA* mutations but no *TP53* mutations in low-grade adenosquamous carcinoma of the breast. *Histopathology.* 2018;73:273-283.

Mucinous Carcinoma

RAZA S. HODA AND SYED A. HODA

Mucinous carcinoma (MC), occasionally still referred to as "colloid" carcinoma, is composed of neoplastic epithelial clusters admixed with extracellular mucin. The latter should comprise at least 90% of the tumor to qualify for the designation of MC. The terms *mixed* ("impure") *mucinous carcinoma* or *invasive carcinoma with mucinous features* are used for tumors with a mucinous component comprising less than 90% of the lesion. Mention of mucinous differentiation should be included in the diagnostic report of an invasive carcinoma with lesser mucinous component. MC has a relatively good prognosis. The prognosis of mixed MC and invasive carcinoma with mucinous differentiation is not as favorable as that for MC.

CLINICAL PRESENTATION

In most series, MC constitutes less than 2% of all breast carcinomas (1-8). A mucinous component of variable extent may be present in up to 2% of other breast carcinomas.

Women with MC are usually older than those with non-MC (1,5,6,8-14). Although MC can occur at any age (range 25-85) (11), the median and the mean age at diagnosis of 11,422 patients with MC in a study based on 1973 to 2002 Surveillance, Epidemiology, and End Results (SEER) data (11) were 71 and 68.3 years, respectively, significantly higher than that for patients with invasive ductal carcinoma (IDC; $P < .01$). More than 80% of patients with MC are postmenopausal (8,11). Most studies (15-17) have found no significant difference in the age distribution and median age of women with MC and mixed MC, although in one series (13) the mean age of patients with MC was 75 years (range 59-90) versus 65 years (range 35-89) for patients with mixed MC ($P = .02$).

MC does not appear to be associated with familial breast carcinoma (18) or with *BRCA1* germline mutation carrier status (19). Lacroix-Triki et al (20) found no evidence of microsatellite instability (MSI) associated with Lynch syndrome in MC. This type of carcinoma is most frequent among Caucasian women (2,11,19,21). In a study based on 1992 to 2007 SEER data (2), 78.5% of women with MC were non-Hispanic Whites. MC can also occur in men. The incidence of MC in males was 0.5% between 1973 and 2002 (11) and 2% between 1985 and 2000 (22). In a series of 759 primary invasive mammary carcinomas in men (23), 21 (2.8%) were MCs and 26 (3.4%) were mixed MCs.

MC usually presents as a unifocal soft palpable mass, or either as a mammographic mass or architectural distortion (12,24,25). In one study (26), 44.6% of 56 MCs were self-detected, 37.5% were detected at mammographic screening, and 17.9% were first identified at clinical examination. A palpable mass was the presenting symptom in 87% of cases in another series (27). Primary MC can also arise in ectopic breast tissue, including the axilla and vulva.

Imaging

Tumors with a high mucin content tend to be mammographically and sonographically lobulated and circumscribed (25,28-30). In one series, the sensitivity of mammograms was 76.5% for the detection of MC versus 100% for mixed MCs (31). Only 37.5% of MCs in another series were first detected at mammographic screening (26). Mammographically detected calcifications in MC are found in up to 40% of MCs (12,27,30,32,33). Calcifications can also occur in adjacent ductal carcinoma in situ (DCIS) (14,34) or in a concurrent mucocele-like lesion (MLL) (35). On ultrasound examination, MC can be isoechogenic to mammary adipose tissue (36). In one study, the sensitivity of ultrasound was 94.7% for MC versus 100% for mixed MCs (31). Dhillon et al (30) reported that 39% of mammographically evident MCs ranging in size from 5 to 20 mm (mean: 11 mm) were not evident on ultrasound. In the same series (30), 38% of MCs were not recognized as abnormal when first encountered in a mammogram or at ultrasound. Nonetheless, patients with delayed diagnosis had no lymph node (LN) metastases at excision.

The differential diagnosis of MC on ultrasound examination includes fibroadenoma, benign cysts, and circumscribed carcinomas including those that are matrix-producing or have a large central acellular zone (37). MC has a gradually enhancing contrast pattern and high signal intensity on T2-weighted images at magnetic resonance imaging (MRI) (38,39). MC and fibroadenomas may not appear dissimilar on MRI (40). In general, mucinous lesions that are well circumscribed are more likely to be pure MC than mixed MC.

Size

In a study based on 1973 to 2002 SEER data (11), MC had a mean size of 2.2 cm, a median size of 1.6 cm, and 83.2% of tumors measured ≤ 3.0 cm or less. More than 50% of MCs in

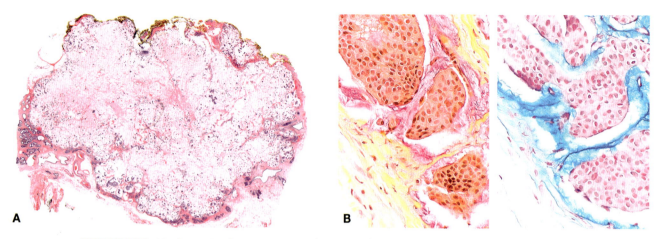

FIGURE 14.1 Mucinous Carcinoma. A: More than 90% of this neoplasm shows mucinous features. There are clusters of carcinoma cells floating amid mucin. **B:** Extracellular mucin is less evident at the edge of this neoplasm and is highlighted via histochemical stains: mucicarmine (left panel) and Alcian blue (right panel).

a contemporary series measured 2 cm or less (12,16,17,21). MCs that span greater than 5 cm were observed in only 2.8% (17) and 4.9% (12) of cases in two studies. The mean size of MC without LN metastases was 1.5 cm versus 2.6 cm for MC with LN involvement (21). MCs are typically smaller than IDC (11,12) and mixed MCs (15-17).

Histopathology

MC is composed of at least 90% of abundant extracellular mucin admixed with invasive neoplastic epithelial cells **(Fig. 14.1)**. The latter seem to "float in a sea of mucin." The mucinous component of a mixed MC constitutes less than 90% of the tumor **(Fig. 14.2)**. Extensive sampling of paucicellular MCs, composed almost entirely of extracellular mucin, may be required to detect the neoplastic epithelium **(Figs. 14.1-14.6)**. The carcinoma cells of MC are arranged in a variety of patterns, including trabecular, festoon-like, cribriform, alveolar, micropapillary, and papillary **(Fig. 14.4)**. The extent of MC should be based on the greatest dimension of the stromal mucin with free-floating malignant cells.

Most MCs are well circumscribed, display "pushing" margins, and are well to moderately differentiated. In a study based on SEER data (11), 53% of the tumors were well differentiated, 38% were moderately differentiated, and 9% were poorly differentiated. MCs with high nuclear grade are rare (16) and have worse prognosis (11). In view of the latter, *poorly differentiated MCs should be classified as invasive ductal carcinoma with mucinous differentiation*. Calcifications associated with MC tend to be coarse and irregular. The pools of mucin may or may not show capillary channels (so-called "neovascularization").

Onken et al (41) evaluated mucin neovascularization on hematoxylin and eosin (H&E) sections of 140 needle core biopsy (NCB) containing mucin-producing lesions

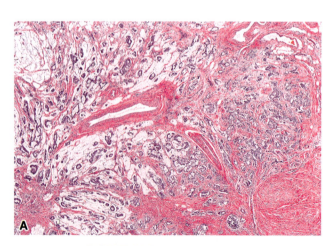
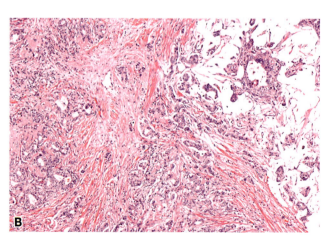

FIGURE 14.2 Mixed Mucinous Carcinoma (MC). A, B: In these mixed MCs, the mucinous component (represented by clusters of carcinoma cells floating amid mucin) represents less than 90% of the tumor.

MUCINOUS CARCINOMA 271

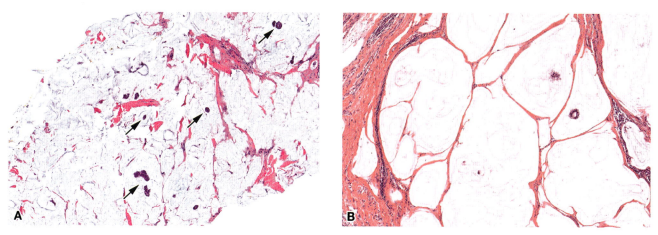

FIGURE 14.3 Mucinous Carcinoma (MC), Hypocellular. A, B: Only minute and sparse clusters of carcinoma cells (arrows in **A**) are present in these MCs.

including 52 MC, 17 mucinous DCIS, and 71 MLLs. In 116 cases with adequate residual material (42 MC, 16 mucinous DCIS, and 58 MLL), mucin neovascularization was studied via CD31 immunostains. Neovascularization of mucin, defined as delicate, thin-walled microvessels in mucin, unassociated with fibrous septae, was present more frequently in MC than in MLL (69.2% vs 14.1%; $P = .0001$). The difference in frequency of mucin neovascularization between MC and MLL was even greater on CD31 immunostains (97.6% vs 13.8%, $P < .00001$). The sensitivity, specificity, positive predictive value, and negative predictive value of mucin neovascularization for categorizing a lesion as MC were 69.2%, 85.8%, 78.3%, and 79.2%, respectively, for H&E sections and 97.6%, 86.2%, 83.7%, and 98.0%, respectively, for CD31 immunostains. Based on this study, evaluation of mucin neovascularization may be helpful in distinguishing between MC and MLL.

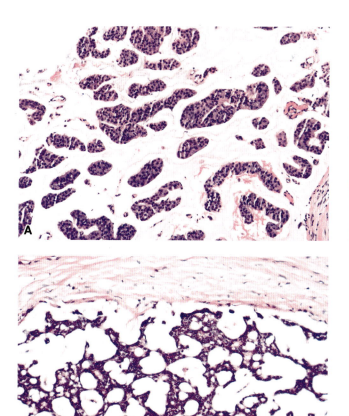

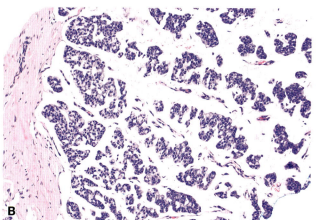

FIGURE 14.4 Mucinous Carcinoma, Variable Architectural Pattern. Needle core biopsies showing different architectural patterns. **A:** Trabecular pattern. **B:** Festoon ("garland") pattern. **C:** Cribriform pattern.

MC can be morphologically subclassified into three morphologic **types A, B, and AB** by Capella et al (42). The hypocellular type A MCs are those having abundant extracellular mucin, with epithelium distributed in loose "trabeculae and ribbons or festoons." The hypercellular type B MCs have less abundant extracellular mucin and consist of tighter "solid sheets" of cells with intracytoplasmic mucin, with often granular cytoplasm. Type AB MCs have "indeterminate" features and constitute approximately 20% of cases. Patients with type A MC tend to be younger than those with type B MC. This classification has *not* been proven to be prognostically significant (5). In one contrarian series (16), type A MCs were found to be smaller than those of type B (1.4 vs 1.9 cm, respectively), had lower rates of lymphovascular involvement (LVI) (3% vs 25%) and LN metastases (8% vs 25%), and were less often human epidermal growth factor receptor 2 (HER2) positive (5.4% vs 25%). The subtyping of MC into A, B, or AB morphology is occasionally difficult (43), but this matter does not seem to be of great importance, as this subclassification appears to be of *no* clinical relevance. Based on cumulative evidence, it appears that hypercellular (type B) MC and some forms of solid papillary and neuroendocrine carcinomas may comprise a spectrum of related lesions, and that hypocellular (type A) MC likely comprises a distinctive entity.

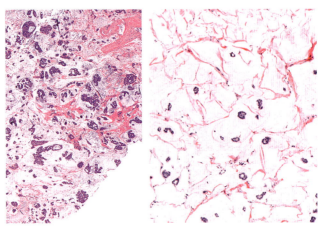

FIGURE 14.5 Mucinous Carcinoma (MC), Variable Cellularity. On needle core biopsy, this MC shows numerous cohesive clusters of carcinoma cells admixed with extracellular mucin (left panel). On excisional biopsy, the MC appears relatively hypocellular with more abundant mucin (right panel).

In **micropapillary variant of MC**, the micropapillae are arranged either in relatively small and tightly cohesive clusters or in ring-like structures in a space filled

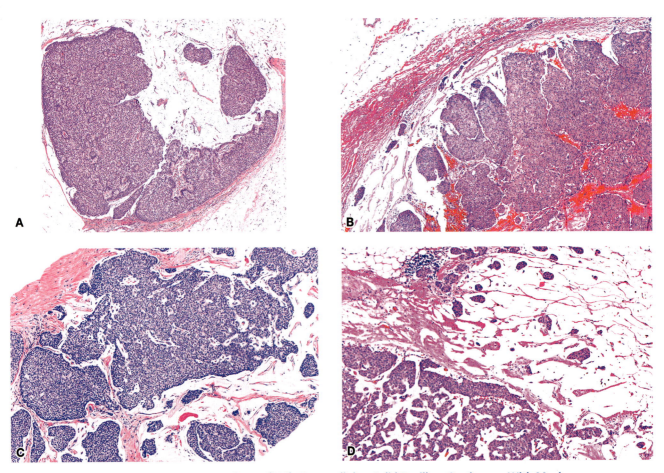

FIGURE 14.6 Mucinous Carcinoma (MC), Hypercellular: Solid Papillary Carcinoma, With Mucinous Differentiation. **A-D:** The MC in these examples of solid papillary carcinoma shows variable proportions of solid papillary growth and extracellular mucin.

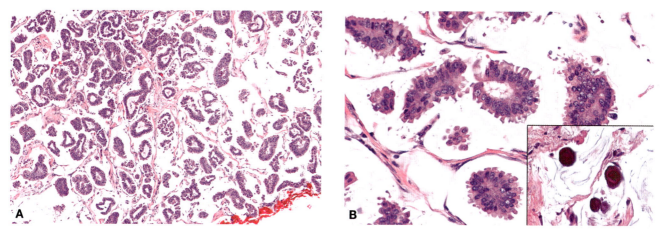

FIGURE 14.7 **Mucinous Carcinoma (MC) With Micropapillary Pattern. A, B:** The MC in this needle core biopsy has micropapillary features, best appreciated at high magnification (**B**). Note associated psammomatous calcifications (inset).

with mucin (16,43,44) **(Fig. 14.7)**. Psammomatous calcifications are common. Invasive micropapillary carcinoma is characterized by extracellular mucin and an "inside-out" appearance leading to "reversed polarity" of its constituent cells. A micropapillary component was recognized in 66.6% (45), 35% (44), and 20% (16) of MC in three separate series, but the proportion of MC with micropapillary morphology required for diagnosis was not defined. In one series (16), MC with and without a micropapillary component had similar average size (1.7 and 1.65 cm, respectively), but patients with a micropapillary component were younger (47 vs 60 years, respectively). Three of the five (60%) MCs with LN metastases had a micropapillary component, versus only 14% of MCs without LN involvement (16). In another series (46), LVI was present in 9/15 (60%) micropapillary MCs, and LN metastases occurred in 33% of cases. One of 13 patients with follow-up information developed a chest wall recurrence 9 months after mastectomy. Liu et al (47) found that 134 patients with MC composed of micropapillary clusters in at least 50% of the tumor were significantly younger (median age 46 years), had more frequent LN involvement (35%), and significantly reduced 10-year overall survival (OS) and relapse-free survival compared to 397 patients with pure MC with absent or less than 50% micropapillary component. Micropapillary MCs are usually ER-positive and HER2-negative. MCs that show LVI and are HER2-positive are more likely to be of the micropapillary type.

Signet ring cell MC is characterized by the presence of extracellular mucin with prominent signet ring cells arranged in large solid clusters or as single cells. The presence of intracellular (ie, intracytoplasmic) mucin can be highlighted via mucicarmine stains. This type of tumor is more common in MC with neuroendocrine features **(Fig. 14.8)**. **Solid papillary carcinoma** is commonly associated with MC **(Fig. 14.6)**. These tumors typically are hypercellular, display neuroendocrine morphology, and usually express neuroendocrine markers. **Invasive lobular carcinoma** can be rarely associated with mucinous features (48).

Ductal Carcinoma In Situ in Mucinous Carcinoma

DCIS is identified in two-thirds to 92.5% of MC (14,15,34), and such DCIS is only uncommonly high grade **(Fig. 14.9)**. In one series, the nuclear grade of DCIS associated with MC was low in 29.3% of cases, intermediate in 61%, and high in 9.8% (34). DCIS with necrosis was present in 17% (14) to 30% (34) of the cases. DCIS with high nuclear grade was more common in association with type B MC and mixed MC (14). In one study (34), 86% of DCIS near MC contained intraluminal mucin, and the latter showed neovascularization in 70% of the cases.

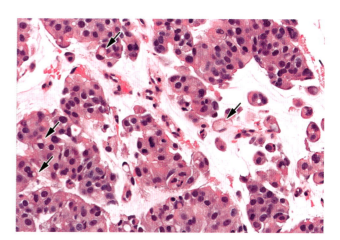

FIGURE 14.8 **Mucinous Carcinoma (MC), Hypercellular With Signet Ring Cells.** This needle core biopsy from a 40-year-old woman shows a hypercellular MC. The carcinoma cells are somewhat noncohesive. Capillaries are evident in the mucin. Some neoplastic cells show signet ring morphology (arrows).

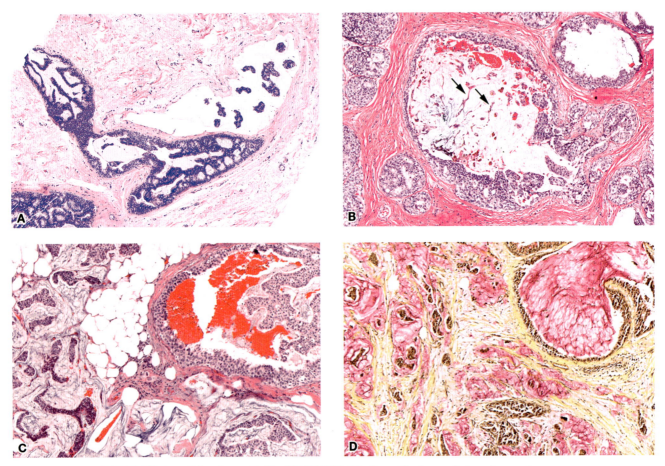

FIGURE 14.9 **Ductal Carcinoma In Situ (DCIS) With Mucinous Features. A:** Invasive carcinoma is associated with micropapillary DCIS. Both components of the carcinoma, in situ and invasive, show mucinous features. **B:** DCIS with mucinous features. The mucin present within the lumen of a duct involved by DCIS has numerous capillaries (arrows). This finding was present near a focus of mucinous carcinoma (MC, not shown). Neovascularization of the mucin in DCIS does *not* constitute unequivocal evidence of invasive carcinoma. **C, D:** In this case, the mucin associated with both components of this MC, DCIS and invasive, is highlighted by mucicarmine stains (**D**).

Neovascularization of the mucin in the lumen of ducts involved by DCIS does not imply stromal invasion (41).

Mucocele-Like Lesions

MLL, a rare entity first described by Rosen in 1986 (35), consists of mucin-containing cysts that rupture and discharge the mucin into the adjacent stroma **(Figs. 14.10-14.14)**. NCBs yielding an MLL are uncommon, with only 35 cases (0.38%) identified among 9,286 image-guided NCB specimens obtained between 2006 and 2013 at one institution (54). Most subsequent series of MLL report an incidence of less than 1%. Rarely, MLLs present as palpable tumors and appear as well-circumscribed and lobulated lesions on mammography. An increasing number of nonpalpable, smaller MLLs are detected only by mammography as clustered calcifications without a mass, or as mass-lesions with calcifications (49-54). Ultrasonography shows a hypoechoic, round or lobulated, solid or cystic tumor, sometimes with an ill-defined margin (55-57). A sonographic mass was detected in 7/17 (41%) MLLs and complex cysts in 6/17 (36%). In one series (51), calcifications constituted the dominant radiologic abnormality in 84.6% MLLs, and ultrasound examination was negative in 8 of 13 cases. The type of calcifications in MLL (dispersed or clustered, fine or coarse, homogeneous or pleomorphic) is not always predictable of association with atypia or with in situ carcinoma (53).

MLL is characterized by abundant pools of extracellular mucin in the mammary stroma. The process is almost always associated with two processes: (a) exuberant production of mucin by ducts in its immediate vicinity and (b) extravasation of mucin into stroma. The epithelium that lines the cystically dilated, mucin-filled ducts can either be inactive, or hyperplastic, or atypical, or malignant **(Figs. 14.10-14.14)** and is the key determinant of the clinical behavior of MLL.

Per se, the presence of the extravasated mucin is seemingly inconsequential, although it is certainly eye-catching. This could explain the low upgrade rate of radiology-pathology concordant non-atypical MLL. In some cases, the lining

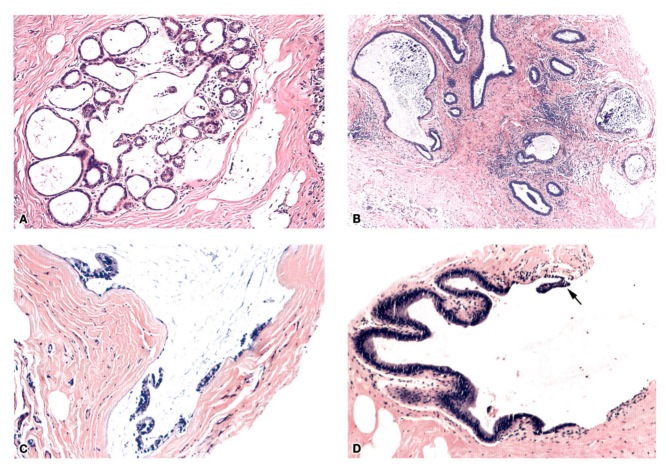

FIGURE 14.10 Mucocele-Like Lesions Involving Lobules, Ducts, and Associated Mucin-Filled Cysts. A: In this mucocele-like lesion, mucin is present within the acinar lumina of this *lobule*. Note the associated extravasation of mucin into the stroma (with calcifications). There is neither cytologic nor architectural atypia. **B:** In another mucocele-like lesion, the mucin is present within the lumen of *ducts*. There is also associated extravasation of mucin. The lesion shows calcifications. **C, D:** In this mucocele-like lesion, part of the epithelium lining the mucin-filled duct has become detached from the wall of the duct and has "curled up" (arrow, in **D**).

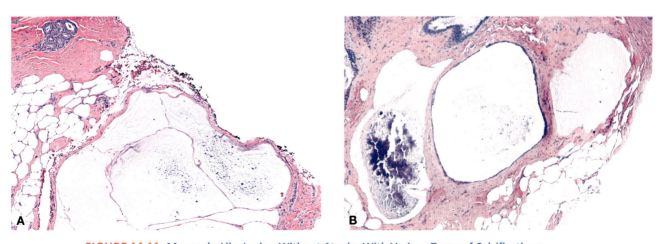

FIGURE 14.11 Mucocele-Like Lesion Without Atypia, With Various Types of Calcifications.
A: Mucocele-like lesion with simple cyst and extravasated mucin-containing fine calcifications.
B: Another mucocele-like lesion with simple mucin-filled cysts and extravasated mucin-containing fine as well as coarse calcifications.

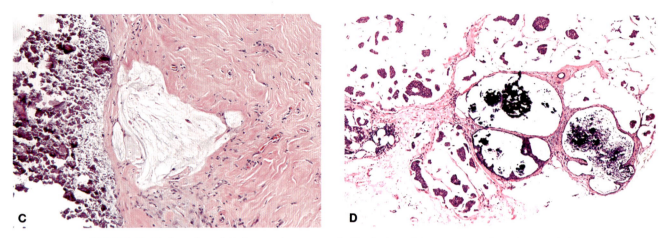

FIGURE 14.11 (*continued*) **C:** Yet another mucocele-like lesion with extravasated mucin-containing coarse calcifications. **D:** Invasive mucinous carcinoma and DCIS with mucinous features show different types of calcification.

epithelia may become detached from the ductal wall and either "curl up" or lose connection with the ductal wall and lie free within the mucin-filled cystic cavity. Fibrous septa may traverse some MLL, and in rare cases capillary channels do the same. The epithelium lining the ducts in an MLL without atypia is, for the most part, flat or cuboidal (**Fig. 14.10**). Epithelial atypia in MLL ranges from columnar cell change (CCC) with atypia/flat epithelial atypia (FEA) to DCIS (35,58,59) (**Figs. 14.11-14.13**). Verschuur-Maes and Van Diest (60) found acellular stromal mucin in 19/20 (90%) NCB samples targeting mammographic calcifications associated with mucinous CCC. Atypical ductal hyperplasia

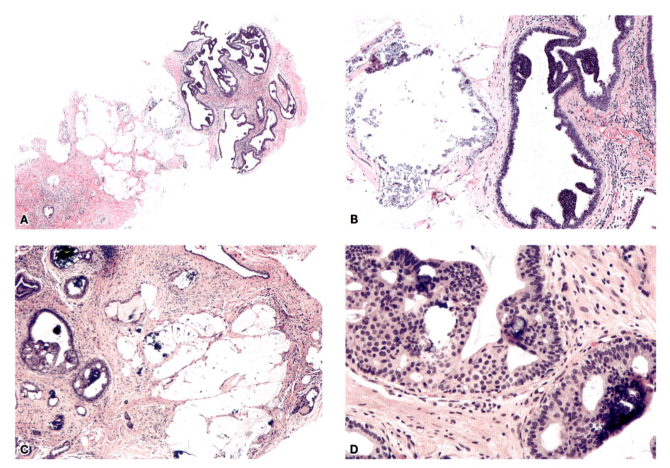

FIGURE 14.12 Mucocele-Like Lesion With Atypical Ductal Hyperplasia (ADH). **A, B:** ADH with extravasated mucin and calcifications, at lower and higher magnification. **C, D:** Another case of ADH with extravasated mucin and coarse calcifications, at lower and higher magnification.

MUCINOUS CARCINOMA 277

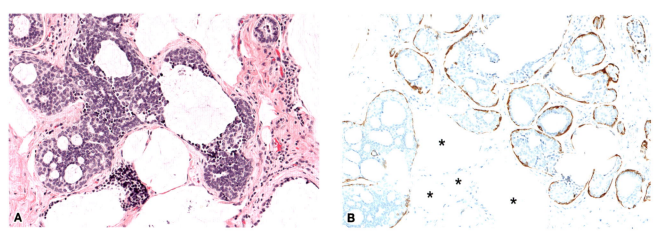

FIGURE 14.13 **Mucocele-Like Lesion With Ductal Carcinoma In Situ (DCIS).** **A:** Mucin is present in the lumen of cribriform DCIS involving a few ducts. The acellular mucin pools present in the stroma show relatively regular outlines. **B:** Calponin immunostain highlights myoepithelium around the DCIS. The stromal mucin pools (asterisks) are difficult to appreciate in the immunostained preparation.

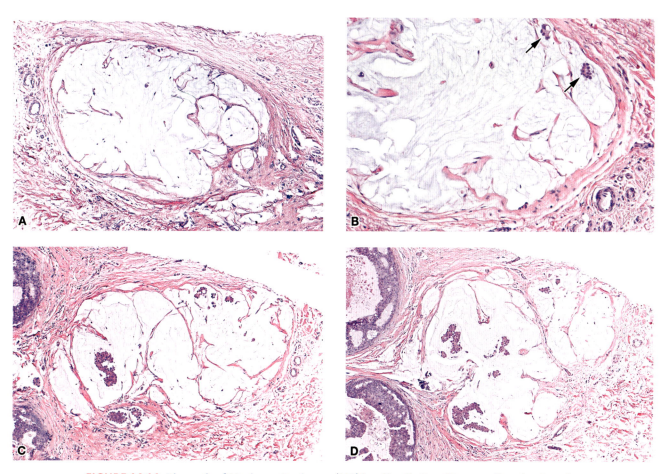

FIGURE 14.14 **Diagnosis of Mucinous Carcinoma (MC) in a Needle Core Biopsy on Examination of "Deeper" Levels of a Mucocele-Like Lesion.** **A:** Mucocele-like lesion is identified. The acellular mucin pools present in the stroma have relatively smooth outlines. Note ingrowth of capillary channels ("neovascularization") in the mucin. **B:** The first "deeper" level shows rare minuscule clusters of uniform epithelial cells (arrows). **C:** The second "deeper" level shows relatively larger clusters of free-floating uniform epithelial cells. The findings are suspicious for MC. **D:** The third "deeper" level shows relatively larger clusters of free-floating uniform epithelial cells. DCIS with mucinous features is evident (in **C** and **D**). Invasive MC can be unequivocally diagnosed (in **C** and **D**).

TABLE 14.1

Factors to Consider Following the Diagnosis of Mucocele-Like Lesion on Needle Core Biopsy

Factor	Consider Clinical/Radiologic Observation	Consider Surgery
Associated atypia or worse[a]	No	Yes
Radiology-Pathology	Concordant	Discordant
Imaging studies	Nonsuspicious	Suspicious
Clinically	Asymptomatic	Symptomatic
Extent[b]	Smaller; ie, <5 mm	Larger; ie, >5 mm
Mass-forming	No	Yes

[a]The clinical behavior of an MLL is almost certainly related to the epithelium composing the lesion or lying in its vicinity.
[b]On imaging or on needle core biopsy. References: 48,53,54,73-77.

(ADH) was present in three cases. Variable types and amounts of calcifications are often present in the mucin of an MLL **(Figs. 14.10-14.13)**. See text later and **Table 14.1** for additional discussion of MLL—particularly with regard to management.

HISTOCHEMISTRY AND IMMUNOHISTOCHEMISTRY

Mucin is the defining feature of MC. *MUC2* is expressed in more than 80% of MC (61,62) but has also been identified in benign mucinous lesions (60). Immunohistochemical detection of *MUC2* has no application in the diagnostic evaluation of MC. Intracellular mucin may not be histochemically demonstrable in MC cells. Likewise, intracytoplasmic mucin is only rarely identified in the cells of benign MLL.

Most MCs are strongly and diffusely positive for **estrogen receptor (ER) and progesterone receptor (PR)** (10,12,16,63,64). In a review of 1992 to 2007 SEER data (2), 84% of MCs were ER^+/PR^+, 12.7% ER^+/PR^-, 0.5% ER^-/PR^+, and 2.8% ER^-/PR^-. One study (12) detected ER in 73.4% MCs and PR in 65.4% MCs; the rate of hormone receptor positivity was significantly higher in MC than in control tumors ($P < .001$). In another study (16), 95% of MCs were ER-positive, 84% PR-positive, and 9% **HER2**-positive; 91% of mixed MCs were ER-positive, 87% PR-positive, and 33% HER2-positive. Although most MCs are HER2-negative, a small proportion (<5%) overexpress HER2 (10,64). **Androgen receptor (AR)** was detected in 80.5% of MCs in one study (65). In another series, AR expression was significantly lower in MC than in IDC of no special type (NST) (21.7% vs 51.4%, respectively; $P = .01$) (66).

Ki-67 staining was reported as low in 77% (67) and 91.4% (64) of MC cases; moderate/intermediate in 5.7% (64) and 23% (67), and high (>30%) in only one case (2.9%) (64). The mean and median percentage of Ki-67-immunoreactive tumor cells was 16.8 and 15, respectively (68).

Nuclear staining for **WT1**, an antigen expressed in leukemias and in solid tumors of the urogenital tract, has been detected in 63.7% (64) and 65% (69) of MCs in two series. Staining intensity was weak in 33% of the cases, moderate in 62% of the cases, and strong in only one (5%) case (69). WT1 staining was significantly associated with low tumor grade ($P = .01$) and low cellularity ($P = .01$). WT1 was also detected in 11/33 (33%) mixed MCs, with similar expression in mucinous and non-mucinous components (69).

MCs, especially those that are hypercellular, often have growth patterns reminiscent of a neuroendocrine tumor. Scopsi et al (5) detected neuroendocrine markers (neuron-specific enolase [NSE], synaptophysin, and chromogranins A and B) in most MCs. Neuroendocrine features and/or differentiation in MC does not appear to have prognostic significance, although at least one study has documented an association with favorable histologic parameters (70).

DIFFERENTIAL DIAGNOSIS OF MUCINOUS LESIONS

A definitive diagnosis of MC requires evaluation of the entire lesion and cannot be rendered based on limited sample obtained via NCB. Several entities are worthy considerations in the differential diagnosis of MC **(Figs. 14.15 and 14.16)**.

The **large solid nests of hypercellular MC** can sometimes raise the differential diagnosis of DCIS. The finding of mucin-filled clefts around the free-floating tumor clusters constitutes evidence of stromal invasion (14). In this setting, the use of myoepithelial stains is not always helpful (14).

A diagnostic problem can arise when **DCIS with mucin** coexists with stromal mucin devoid of carcinoma. Evaluation

MUCINOUS CARCINOMA 279

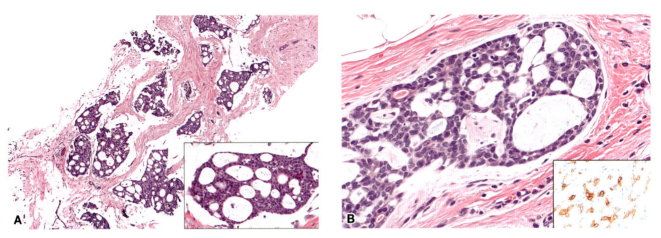

FIGURE 14.15 Mucinous Carcinoma (MC) and Adenoid Cystic Carcinoma (ACC). A: This MC with cribriform architecture in this needle core biopsy resembles an ACC. **B:** An ACC with its characteristic cribriform architecture is shown here for comparison. The basophilic matter in the duct is basement membrane material. Inset shows the epithelial cells of ACC to be positive for CK7.

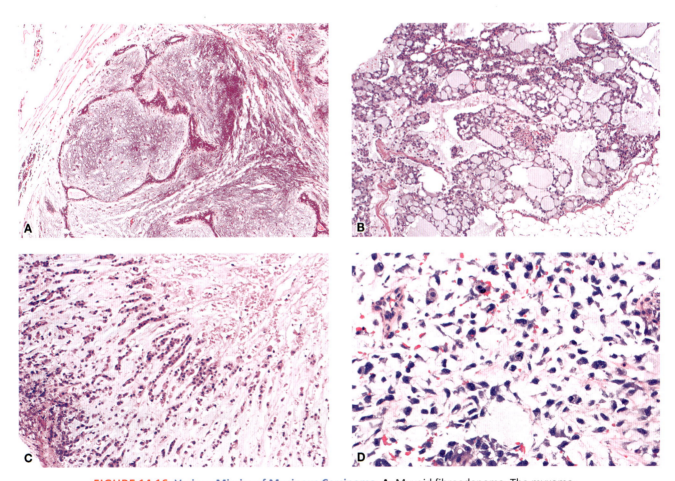

FIGURE 14.16 Various Mimics of Mucinous Carcinoma. A: Myxoid fibroadenoma. The myxomatous stroma can simulate mucin in this benign tumor. **B:** Secretory carcinoma. Note absence of free-floating neoplastic epithelial cells amid the intraluminal mucin. **C:** Matrix-producing metaplastic carcinoma. The matrix of this tumor can simulate mucin. The linear and trabecular array of the neoplastic epithelial cells amid the matrix is typical of this entity. **D:** Myxoid stromal change in a mammary sarcoma. The tumor cells bear high-grade nuclei and are rarely epithelioid in appearance.

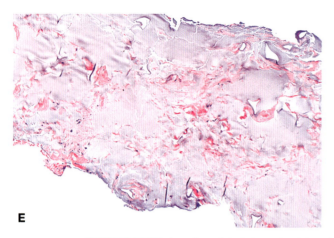 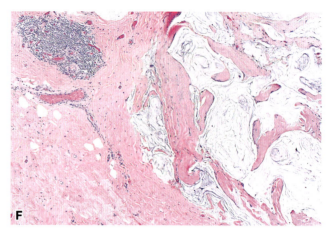

FIGURE 14.16 (*continued*) **E:** Polyacrylamide gel injected into the breast for cosmetic augmentation is evident in this core biopsy of a palpable mass. This type of gel resembles acellular mucin. **F:** Stromal mucin devoid of epithelium in this core biopsy of the "tumor bed" from a patient with invasive ductal (non-mucinous) carcinoma status post neoadjuvant chemotherapy. No residual carcinoma was identified on examination of multiple "levels" of the core biopsy and in the subsequent mastectomy.

of H&E-stained deeper "levels" in equivocal cases may be helpful in "finding" carcinoma cells. Mucin extruded into the stroma from benign cysts following tissue trauma is in the differential diagnosis of such lesions. The presence of carcinoma cells amid stromal mucin—unassociated with healing biopsy site or linear needle track–related changes—is required for definitive diagnosis of MC in such cases.

Mucocele-like lesion is the most important consideration in the differential diagnosis of MC. In practical terms, particularly with regard to MLL encountered in NCBs, the ducts in the immediate vicinity of the MLL should be carefully evaluated. Examination of additional "serials," "levels," or "deepers" taken from the corresponding tissue block is prudent whenever these ducts appear to be inactive or hyperplastic (yet non-atypical). Of course, excisional biopsy of the lesional area is indicated whenever an MLL associated with ADH or DCIS is present in an NCB.

Free-floating malignant cells amid mucin should be diagnosed as MC. Stromal mucin devoid of epithelium is an exceedingly rare finding in NCB; however, this finding can be encountered status post neoadjuvant chemotherapy (NACT; even in cases wherein the primary tumor was nonmucinous). The mucin in benign MLL is typically "clean" (ie, devoid of debris). Histiocytes and inflammatory cells may be rarely present.

Excisional biopsies following NCB occasionally show extracellular deposits of mucin admixed with benign epithelial strips. In such cases, the findings that favor the diagnosis of artifactual detachment over MC include lack of epithelial atypia, epithelium arranged in clusters or strips. The immunohistochemical identification of myoepithelial cells within the benign epithelia supports artifactual detachment. In this setting, lack of myoepithelium, however, does not constitute evidence of stromal invasion. If malignant cells are identified in the mucin, additional evidence of invasion is usually present, including bulbous outlines of mucin pools, papillary arrangement of the epithelial clusters (14), presence of a few myofibroblasts and/or capillaries in the mucin pools, and focal inflammatory infiltrate (71,72). In some instances, it may not be possible to definitively distinguish between artifactual detachment and (micro)invasive MC, particularly if the epithelium shows some atypical features. Cytokeratin immunostain can be useful to identify epithelial cells in stromal mucin pools apparently devoid of epithelium. Notably, MC cells may occasionally have abundant pale cytoplasm that can mimic histiocytes.

The upgrade rate (from NCB to excision) of benign MLL has been the subject of several studies. Until about a decade or so back, excision was recommended for all MLL diagnosed on NCB; however, recent studies increasingly indicate that those MLL that show radiology-pathology concordance and are without atypia can be followed up without undergoing surgery. Based on cumulative data, approximately one-third to one-half of MLL diagnosed on NCB material exhibit no atypia. As stated earlier, the behavior of an MLL is almost certainly related to the epithelium in the lesion or lying in its vicinity.

Some of the studies dealing with upgrade rates did not separately report the rate of NCB with or without atypia and/or did not comment on the radiologic-pathologic concordance between the histologic findings in the NCB and the radiologic characteristics of the target lesion (48,53,54,73–77). The relatively recent well-conducted study by Moseley et al evaluated 50 MLL identified on core biopsies from two institutions, including 36 with no atypia and 14 with limited atypia (77). The radiologic targets were calcifications in 74% of the cases, calcifications with associated mass or density in 16%, and mass in 10%. One of the 16 excised lesions without atypia on NCB, which was a mass lesion, was upgraded to MC on excision. Of the 12 excised lesions with limited atypia, none were upgraded on excision. Among the non-excised lesions, 20 without atypia had a median follow-up of 61 months, and 2 with limited atypia had follow-up of 97 and 109 months. None of these 22 patients developed any lesion on follow-up. The upgrade rate was 2% in this cohort, 3% for lesions without atypia, and 0% for lesions with limited atypia. The authors concluded that clinicoradiologic follow-up can be appropriate when an MLL without atypia is identified on NCB for a nonmass lesion with pathologic-radiologic concordance.

The key factors that should be considered in managing an MLL diagnosed on NCB are listed in **Table 14.1**. Notably, smaller (<5 mm), incidentally diagnosed, and nonmass-forming MLLs are much less likely to be upgraded (48,53,54,73-77). Based on published data, excision is recommended following NCB diagnosis of MLL with atypia (ADH or atypical columnar cell hyperplasia) and/or if the radiologic and pathologic findings of the NCB are discordant. Excision of a non-atypical MLL in an NCB can be omitted whenever there is radiologic-pathologic concordance. In this regard, it should be kept in mind that *the upgrade rate in a radiology-pathology concordant non-atypical MLL is less than 3%.*

Mucinous cystadenocarcinoma of the breast is a rare variant of breast carcinoma with favorable prognosis despite showing a basal-like phenotype **(Fig. 14.17)**. The tumor is typically multicystic. The cysts are lined by relatively uniform tall columnar cells with abundant intracytoplasmic mucin. The tumor is histopathologically similar to that observed in its ovarian counterpart.

Nodular mucinosis is an extremely rare entity, usually presenting in young women. Pathologically, it consists of a myxoid (mucoid-type) mass of loosely placed benign spindle cells (78). The lesion is of uncertain histogenesis and presents as an asymptomatic, usually superficially located, tumor in the subareolar region. A possible myofibroblastic origin has been suggested.

Cystic hypersecretory lesions of the breast (see Chapter 17) may bear superficial similarity to MLLs because of the presence of cystically dilated lumina filled with secretion. The latter consists of homogeneous material that resembles thyroid colloid. The dense hypersecretory material tends to fracture along parallel lines, resulting in the characteristic "shutter" pattern reminiscent of "Venetian blinds." In contrast, on H&E staining, mucin has pale, gray to blue color and is seemingly "translucent."

Secretory carcinoma (see Chapter 17) is a rare variant of breast carcinoma and harbors a characteristic chromosomal fusion gene (*ETV6-NTRK3*). The carcinoma has amphophilic or pale eosinophilic intraluminal secretion, which often looks "bubbly." Intracellular secretion can also occur, but secretions are not present in the stroma. Most secretory carcinomas are positive for pan-TRK and S-100 and are negative for ER and PR. MCs are usually positive for ER and PR and negative for pan-TRK and S-100.

A brief discussion of other uncommon tumors that may be considered in the differential diagnosis of MC, especially

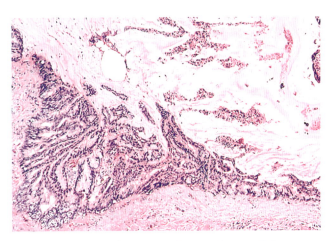

FIGURE 14.17 Mucinous Cystadenocarcinoma of the Breast. This cystic tumor is characterized by intracytoplasmic and extracellular mucin and is lined by columnar cells. The findings in this breast tumor are similar to those observed in ovarian mucinous cystadenocarcinoma.

in the limited sampling of NCBs, follows. **Adenoid cystic carcinoma** (ACC) (see Chapter 16) with delicate myxoid matrix can simulate MC with cribriform growth, but the matrix is devoid of cells. ACC is a biphasic (epithelial and myoepithelial) carcinoma composed of p63-positive myoepithelial cells and CK7-positive epithelial cells **(Fig. 14.15)**; it is typically positive for MYB and is negative for ER and PR. **Mucoepidermoid carcinoma** of the breast features both mucinous cells and extracellular mucin, resembling its commoner counterpart in the salivary glands. The tumor is commonly triple-negative. **Pleomorphic adenoma** of the breast (see Chapter 5) is a rare benign tumor that most likely represents a variant of adenomyoepithelioma. It often has areas of myxoid stroma that contain spindly myoepithelial cells. **Metaplastic matrix-producing carcinoma** contains focal or diffuse areas of myxoid change. The cells of this type of metaplastic carcinoma tend to have higher nuclear grade, are irregularly distributed, and do not form cohesive clusters (see Chapter 13). **Squamous cell carcinoma with prominent myxoid stroma** can also, at least focally, mimic MC (79). **Metastases from an extramammary MC** (see Chapter 22) have been reported in the breast. Immunostains can be helpful in the differential diagnosis whenever a non-mammary primary MC is in the differential diagnosis. Mammary primary MCs are GATA3+ and ER+; ovarian primary MCs are CK20+ and WT1, pulmonary primary MCs are CK7+ and TTF1+; and colonic primary MCs are CDX2+. Comparative histopathologic review with the primary may obviate the need for immunostains. A variety of **benign or malignant spindle cell lesions with myxoid stroma** (including myxoid fibroadenoma, myxoma, neurofibroma with prominent myxoid change, and a variety of sarcomas) can focally resemble MC, especially when sampled via NCB. In such lesions, the myxoid stroma is admixed with benign-appearing spindle cells of either myofibroblastic or other stromal origin.

Lastly, **foreign material** (including hydrophilic polyacrylamide gel) can resemble extracellular mucin. Clues to the correct diagnosis include a slightly different tinctorial quality and a foreign body–type giant cell reaction (72). The latter feature tends to be evident at the perimeter of the foreign substance and may be underrepresented in an NCB sample. Injection of hydrophilic polyacrylamide gel for breast augmentation has been used in some regions, including Eastern Europe and Asia. Polyacrylamide hydrogel resembles mucin in tinctorial quality and translucency (80). Over time, the material can cause breast nodularity and deformity **(Fig. 14.16)**. Clinical history is of foremost importance in these cases. The gel used during sonographic examination can be present in NCB-acquired *histologic* samples; however, it is relatively more common in fine needle aspiration (FNA)-derived *cytologic* material. Parenthetically, it may be stated that excision of breast lesions that yield **acellular mucin on FNA sampling**, even in the absence of epithelial atypia, is prudent.

TREATMENT AND PROGNOSIS

The relatively favorable prognosis of MC is supported by the results of numerous studies (1,2,5,11,12,17,21,31,81-83); however, few studies have used a uniform definition for MC. Pure MCs tend to be smaller than tumors with a mixed MC pattern. Patients with pure MC have a lower frequency of axillary lymph node (ALN) metastases (5,13). Nodal metastases are uncommon in MC, which span less than 1 cm. In one study (21), node-positive patients had a mean tumor size of 2.7 cm compared to 1.5 cm for node-negative patients ($P = .0003$), and none of the 31 patients with tumor size less than 1 cm had LN metastasis. Larger tumor size correlates significantly with LN involvement (11,21).

In contemporary series (12,16,17,21,31,82,83), patients with node-negative MC range from 74% to 83% of the cases. Positive nodal status was the most significant predictor of worse prognosis in a large SEER data–based study of 11,422 patients with MC (11). In two studies (10,81), patients with node-positive MC were significantly more likely to develop recurrent MC. In another study (8), the number of involved nodes was the only significant predictor of patient death ($P = .02$). Ranade et al (16) reported that 18.5% of MCs had sentinel lymph node (SLN) metastases versus 16% of mixed MCs. Non-SLNs were positive in 14% of MCs versus 39% of mixed MCs. MCs can exhibit uncommon metastatic patterns, including pseudomyxoma peritonei.

The primary treatment of MC has typically been breast-conserving surgery in 15.4% to 81.1% of the cases (12,17,21,31,82). Most, appropriately selected, patients treated with breast-conserving surgery also received adjuvant radiotherapy (17,21,31,81,82). In a study based on SEER data (11), adjuvant radiotherapy was associated with a minor survival advantage observed only on univariate analysis. Adjuvant hormonal therapy was administered to patients with MC in 41% to 81.6% of the cases (12,17,31,81,82).

Barkly et al (21) specified that hormonal therapy constituted the only adjuvant treatment in 54% of MC patients.

Per 2022 National Comprehensive Cancer Network (NCCN) guidelines, the management of pure MC (with favorable prognostic features) depends mainly on its size and the presence as well as extent of axillary nodal metastasis (84). To be associated with favorable prognosis, the MC should be "pure" (>90% on excision, not on NCB), should not be high grade, and should be negative for HER2. Adjuvant endocrine therapy should be *considered* for risk reduction in ER-positive MC less than 3.0 cm, and adjuvant endocrine therapy should be used for those that span 3.0 cm or more. Micrometastasis or lesser degree of axillary nodal involvement should not influence management. Adjuvant endocrine therapy and chemotherapy should be used for those MC of any size with nodal metastasis that spans greater than 2 mm. Cases of MC in which the prognostic features are not favorable should be managed as IDC.

Follow-up analysis of MC in one series found that adjuvant chemotherapy is not necessarily indicated for node-negative MC measuring 3 cm or less (85). Adjuvant chemotherapy for treatment of MC was used in only 3% to 13% of patients in three series from Western countries (21,81,82), but seems more commonly adopted in Eastern countries, where three series reported its use in 40.8% to 63.7% of patients (12,17,31). MCs that overexpress HER2, however, are suitable for HER2-targeted treatment in the adjuvant or neoadjuvant settings. In one older series published more than 30 years ago, the clinical response of 12 MCs treated with NACT was significantly poorer than that for IDC, with minimal reduction in the mean tumor size (86).

When compared with patients who have IDC or IDC with mucinous features, women with pure MC have had a better recurrence-free survival (RFS) 5 and 10 years after mastectomy (5,9,87). In a series of patients treated by lumpectomy (81) combined with radiotherapy in 90% of cases, hormonal therapy in 41% of cases, and chemotherapy in 13% of cases, local recurrence and locoregional recurrence rates were both 5%, lower than that for IDC (8% and 10%, respectively). The disease-free survival (DFS) was 91.6% at 5 years and 75.3% at 10 years. The OS rate was 91.8% at 5 years and 74.5% at 10 years. In a study based on 1973 to 2002 SEER data (11), the 10-, 15-, and 20-year survival for 11,422 patients with MC was 89%, 85%, and 81%, respectively, compared to 72% (10-year survival), 66% (15-year survival), and 62% (20-year survival) for 338,479 patients with IDC. Scopsi et al (5) reported no deaths because of disease among 25 patients with node-negative MC. In a series of patients treated between 1997 and 2005 (82), 143 patients with MC had 93% 5-year DFS and 96.3% OS.

MC can develop late metastases (9,85,88,89), even up to 25 and 30 years (90,91) after diagnosis. In a series with a mean follow-up of 16 years (9), 42% of the deaths because of disease in MC patients occurred 12 years or more after diagnosis. Relatively small MCs neither show propensity for late recurrence (92,93) nor fatal outcome (6).

The prognostic factors that are relevant for most types of breast carcinoma also apply to MC (11). Recurrence is least likely for patients with smaller tumors and no LN metastases (21). The prognostic significance of neuroendocrine differentiation in MC has not been established at this time.

The use of NACT in MCs is uncommon in the current era of de-escalated treatment. Pathologic assessment after NACT can demonstrate marked reduction in tumor cellularity, but persistent space-occupying mucin pools rarely show acellular mucin. One series of MC treated by NACT showed less than 1% tumor cellularity in three of seven cases, and 5% to 10% cellularity in three cases in both the treated breast LN and ALNs (94).

MOLECULAR PATHOLOGY OF MUCINOUS CARCINOMA

Based on published studies (20,64,95,96), the key molecular pathology features of MC can be summarized as follows. MCs display a relatively low level of genomic instability and show relatively few chromosomal losses or gains. Based on array-based comparative genomic hybridization (CGH) profile, pure MC are homogeneous and cluster together, separately from IDC—and less frequently harbor gains of 1q and 16p, and losses of 10q and 22q than grade- and ER-matched IDCs. MC typically classifies as luminal type A by transcriptional profiling studies. MCs show lower *PIK3CA* and *TP53* mutation rates. Most MCs generate a low Oncotype 21-gene recurrence score (<25). Hypercellular MCs show a molecular profile rather similar to those of IDC with neuroendocrine features. MSI, a common feature of colonic MC, is uncommon in mammary MC. Absence of *KRAS*, *NRAS*, and *BRAF* mutations has been demonstrated in mammary mucinous cystadenocarcinoma.

REFERENCES

1. Louwman MW, Vriezen M, van Beek MW, et al. Uncommon breast tumors in perspective: incidence, treatment and survival in the Netherlands. *Int J Cancer*. 2007;121:127-135.
2. Li CI. Risk of mortality by histologic type of breast cancer in the United States. *Horm Cancer*. 2010;1:156-165.
3. Albrektsen G, Heuch I, Thoresen SO. Histological type and grade of breast cancer tumors by parity, age at birth, and time since birth: a register-based study in Norway. *BMC Cancer*. 2010;10:226.
4. Rasmussen BB, Rose C, Christensen IB. Prognostic factors in primary mucinous breast carcinoma. *Am J Clin Pathol*. 1987;87:155-160.
5. Scopsi L, Andreola S, Pilotti S, et al. Mucinous carcinoma of the breast: a clinicopathologic, histochemical, and immunocytochemical study with special reference to neuroendocrine differentiation. *Am J Surg Pathol*. 1994;18:702-711.
6. Toikkanen S, Kujari H. Pure and mixed mucinous carcinomas of the breast: a clinicopathologic analysis of 61 cases with long-term follow-up. *Hum Pathol*. 1989;20:758-764.
7. Avisar E, Khan MA, Axelrod D, et al. Pure mucinous carcinoma of the breast: a clinicopathological correlation study. *Ann Surg Oncol*. 1998;5:447-451.
8. Komenaka IK, El-Tamer MB, Troxel A, et al. Pure mucinous carcinoma of the breast. *Am J Surg*. 2004;187:528-532.
9. Rosen PP, Wang T-Y. Colloid carcinoma of the breast: analysis of 64 patients with long-term follow-up. *Am J Clin Pathol*. 1980;73:30.
10. Diab SG, Clark GM, Osborne CK, et al. Tumor characteristics and clinical outcome of tubular and mucinous breast carcinomas. *J Clin Oncol*. 1999;17:1442-1448.
11. Di Saverio S, Gutierrez J, Avisar E. A retrospective review with long term follow up of 11,400 cases of pure mucinous breast carcinoma. *Breast Cancer Res Treat*. 2008;111:541-547.
12. Cao AY, He M, Liu ZB, et al. Outcome of pure mucinous breast carcinoma compared to infiltrating ductal carcinoma: a population-based study from China. *Ann Surg Oncol*. 2012;19:3019-3027.
13. Paramo JC, Wilson C, Velarde D, et al. Pure mucinous carcinoma of the breast: is axillary staging necessary? *Ann Surg Oncol*. 2002;9:161-164.
14. Kryvenko ON, Chitale DA, Yoon J, et al. Precursor lesions of mucinous carcinoma of the breast: analysis of 130 cases. *Am J Surg Pathol*. 2013;37:1076-1084.
15. Fentiman IS, Millis RR, Smith P, et al. Mucoid breast carcinomas: histology and prognosis. *Br J Cancer*. 1997;75:1061-1065.
16. Ranade A, Batra R, Sandhu G, et al. Clinicopathological evaluation of 100 cases of mucinous carcinoma of breast with emphasis on axillary staging and special reference to a micropapillary pattern. *J Clin Pathol*. 2010;63:1043-1047.
17. Bae SY, Choi MY, Cho DH, et al. Mucinous carcinoma of the breast in comparison with invasive ductal carcinoma: clinicopathologic characteristics and prognosis. *J Breast Cancer*. 2011;14:308-313.
18. Li CI, Daling JR, Malone KE, et al. Relationship between established breast cancer risk factors and risk of seven different histologic types of invasive breast cancer. *Cancer Epidemiol Biomarkers Prev*. 2006;15:946-954.
19. Work ME, Andrulis IL, John EM, et al. Risk factors for uncommon histologic subtypes of breast cancer using centralized pathology review in the Breast Cancer Family Registry. *Breast Cancer Res Treat*. 2012;134:1209-1220.
20. Lacroix-Triki M, Lambros MB, Geyer FC, et al. Absence of microsatellite instability in mucinous carcinomas of the breast. *Int J Clin Exp Pathol*. 2010;4:22-31.
21. Barkley CR, Ligibel JA, Wong JS, et al. Mucinous breast carcinoma: a large contemporary series. *Am J Surg*. 2008;196:549-551.
22. Hodgson NC, Button JH, Franceschi D, et al. Male breast cancer: is the incidence increasing? *Ann Surg Oncol*. 2004;11:751-755.
23. Burga AM, Fadare O, Lininger RA, et al. Invasive carcinomas of the male breast: a morphologic study of the distribution of histologic subtypes and metastatic patterns in 778 cases. *Virchows Arch*. 2006;449:507-512.
24. Cardenosa G, Doudna C, Eklund GW. Mucinous (colloid) breast cancer: clinical and mammographic findings in 10 patients. *AJR Am J Roentgenol*. 1994;162:1077-1079.
25. Lam WW, Chu WC, Tse GM, et al. Sonographic appearance of mucinous carcinoma of the breast. *AJR Am J Roentgenol*. 2004;182:1069-1074.
26. Newcomer LM, Newcomb PA, Trentham-Dietz A, et al. Detection method and breast carcinoma histology. *Cancer*. 2002;95:470-477.
27. Liu H, Tan H, Cheng Y, et al. Imaging findings in mucinous breast carcinoma and correlating factors. *Eur J Radiol*. 2011;80:706-712.
28. Conant EF, Dillon RL, Palazzo J, et al. Imaging findings in mucin-containing carcinomas of the breast: correlation with pathologic features. *AJR Am J Roentgenol*. 1994;163:821-824.
29. Goodman DN, Boutross-Tadross O, Jong RA. Mammographic features of pure mucinous carcinoma of the breast with pathological correlation. *Can Assoc Radiol J*. 1995;46:296-301.
30. Dhillon R, Depree P, Metcalf C, et al. Screen-detected mucinous breast carcinoma: potential for delayed diagnosis. *Clin Radiol*. 2006;61:423-430.
31. Park S, Koo J, Kim JH, et al. Clinicopathological characteristics of mucinous carcinoma of the breast in Korea: comparison with invasive ductal carcinoma-not otherwise specified. *J Korean Med Sci*. 2010;25:361-368.
32. Wilson TE, Helvie MA, Oberman HA, et al. Pure and mixed mucinous carcinoma of the breast: pathologic basis for differences in mammographic appearance. *AJR Am J Roentgenol*. 1995;165:285-289.
33. Ruggieri A, Scola F, Schepps B. Mucinous carcinoma of the breast: mammographic findings. *Breast Dis*. 1995;8:353-361.
34. Gadre SA, Perkins GH, Sahin AA, et al. Neovascularization in mucinous ductal carcinoma in situ suggests an alternative pathway for invasion. *Histopathology*. 2008;53:545-553.
35. Rosen PP. Mucocele-like tumors of the breast. *Am J Surg Pathol*. 1986;10:464-469.
36. Memis A, Ozdemir N, Parildar M, et al. Mucinous (colloid) breast cancer: mammographic and US features with histologic correlation. *Eur J Radiol*. 2000;35:39-43.
37. Yamaguchi R, Tanaka M, Mizushima Y, et al. "High-grade" central acellular carcinoma and matrix-producing carcinoma of the breast: correlation between ultrasonographic findings and pathological features. *Med Mol Morphol*. 2011;44:151-157.
38. Kawashima M, Tamaki Y, Nonaka T, et al. MR imaging of mucinous carcinoma of the breast. *AJR Am J Roentgenol*. 2002;179:179-183.
39. Okafuji T, Yabuuchi H, Sakai S, et al. MR imaging features of pure mucinous carcinoma of the breast. *Eur J Radiol*. 2006;60:405-413.
40. Miller RW, Harms S, Alvarez A. Mucinous carcinoma of the breast: potential false-negative MR imaging interpretation. *AJR Am J Roentgenol*. 1996;167:539-540.
41. Onken AM, Collins LC, Schnitt SJ. Mucin neovascularization as a diagnostic aid to distinguish mucinous carcinomas from mucocele-like lesions in breast core needle biopsies. *Am J Surg Pathol*. 2022;46:637-642.
42. Capella C, Eusebi V, Mann B, et al. Endocrine differentiation in mucoid carcinoma of the breast. *Histopathology*. 1980;4:613-630.
43. Cserni G. Histological type and typing of breast carcinomas and the WHO classification changes over time. *Pathologica*. 2020;112:25-41.
44. Bal A, Joshi K, Sharma SC, et al. Prognostic significance of micropapillary pattern in pure mucinous carcinoma of the breast. *Int J Surg Pathol*. 2008;16:251-256.

45. Shet T, Chinoy R. Presence of a micropapillary pattern in mucinous carcinomas of the breast and its impact on the clinical behavior. *Breast J*. 2008;14:412-420.
46. Barbashina V, Corben AD, Akram M, et al. Mucinous micropapillary carcinoma of the breast: an aggressive counterpart to conventional pure mucinous tumors. *Hum Pathol*. 2013;44(8):1577-1585.
47. Liu F, Yang M, Li Z, et al. Invasive micropapillary mucinous carcinoma of the breast is associated with poor prognosis. *Breast Cancer Res Treat*. 2015;151:443-451.
48. Cserni G, Floris G, Koufopoulos N, et al. Invasive lobular carcinoma with extracellular mucin production-a novel pattern of lobular carcinomas of the breast. Clinico-pathological description of eight cases. *Virchows Arch*. 2017;471:3-12.
49. Ramsaroop R, Greenberg D, Tracey N, et al. Mucocele-like lesions of the breast: an audit of 2 years at Breast Screen Auckland (New Zealand). *Breast J*. 2005;11:321-325.
50. Kim JY, Han BK, Choe YH, et al. Benign and malignant mucocele-like tumors of the breast: mammographic and sonographic appearances. *AJR Am J Roentgenol*. 2005;185:1310-1316.
51. Farshid G, Pieterse S, King JM, et al. Mucocele-like lesions of the breast: a benign cause for indeterminate or suspicious mammographic microcalcifications. *Breast J*. 2005;11:15-22.
52. Leibman AJ, Staeger CN, Charney DA. Mucocelelike lesions of the breast: mammographic findings with pathologic correlation. *AJR Am J Roentgenol*. 2006;186:1356-1360.
53. Carkaci S, Lane DL, Gilcrease MZ, et al. Do all mucocele-like lesions of the breast require surgery? *Clin Imaging*. 2011;35:94-101.
54. Ha D, Dialani V, Mehta TS, et al. Mucocele-like lesions in the breast diagnosed with percutaneous biopsy: is surgical excision necessary? *AJR Am J Roentgenol*. 2015;204:204-210.
55. Kim Y, Takatsuka Y, Morino H. Mucocele-like tumor of the breast: a case report and assessment of aspirated cytological specimens. *Breast Cancer*. 1998;5:317-320.
56. Yeoh GP, Cheung PS, Chan KW. Fine-needle aspiration cytology of mucocele-like tumors of the breast. *Am J Surg Pathol*. 1999;23:552-559.
57. Park YJ, Kim EK. A pure mucocele-like lesion of the breast diagnosed on ultrasonography-guided core-needle biopsy: is imaging follow-up sufficient? *Ultrasonography*. 2015;34:133-138.
58. Ro JY, Sneige N, Sahin AA, et al. Mucocelelike tumor of the breast associated with atypical ductal hyperplasia or mucinous carcinoma: a clinicopathologic study of seven cases. *Arch Pathol Lab Med*. 1991;115:137-140.
59. Hamele-Bena D, Cranor ML, Rosen PP. Mammary mucocele-like lesions: benign and malignant. *Am J Surg Pathol*. 1996;20:1081-1085.
60. Verschuur-Maes AH, Van Diest PJ. The mucinous variant of columnar cell lesions. *Histopathology*. 2011;58:847-853.
61. Rakha EA, Boyce RW, Abd El-Rehim D, et al. Expression of mucins (MUC1, MUC2, MUC3, MUC4, MUC5AC and MUC6) and their prognostic significance in human breast cancer. *Mod Pathol*. 2005;18:1295-1304.
62. O'Connell JT, Shao ZM, Drori E, et al. Altered mucin expression is a field change that accompanies mucinous (colloid) breast carcinoma histogenesis. *Hum Pathol*. 1998;29:1517-1523.
63. Shousha S, Coady AT, Stamp T, et al. Oestrogen receptors in mucinous carcinoma of the breast: an immunohistological study using paraffin wax sections. *J Clin Pathol*. 1989;42:902-905.
64. Lacroix-Triki M, Suarez PH, MacKay A, et al. Mucinous carcinoma of the breast is genomically distinct from invasive ductal carcinomas of no special type. *J Pathol*. 2010;222:282-298.
65. Collins LC, Cole KS, Marotti JD, et al. Androgen receptor expression in breast cancer in relation to molecular phenotype: results from the Nurses' Health Study. *Mod Pathol*. 2011;24:924-931.
66. Cho LC, Hsu YH. Expression of androgen, estrogen and progesterone receptors in mucinous carcinoma of the breast. *Kaohsiung J Med Sci*. 2008;24:227-232.
67. Kato N, Endo Y, Tamura G, et al. Mucinous carcinoma of the breast: a multifaceted study with special reference to histogenesis and neuroendocrine differentiation. *Pathol Int*. 1999;49:947-955.
68. Alvarenga CA, Paravidino PI, Alvarenga M, et al. Reappraisal of immunohistochemical profiling of special histological types of breast carcinomas: a study of 121 cases of eight different subtypes. *J Clin Pathol*. 2012;65:1066-1071.
69. Domfeh AB, Carley AL, Striebel JM, et al. WT1 immunoreactivity in breast carcinoma: selective expression in pure and mixed mucinous subtypes. *Mod Pathol*. 2008;21:1217-1223.
70. Tse GM, Ma TK, Chu WC, et al. Neuroendocrine differentiation in pure type mammary mucinous carcinoma is associated with favorable histologic and immunohistochemical parameters. *Mod Pathol*. 2004;17:568-572.
71. Molavi D, Argani P. Distinguishing benign dissecting mucin (stromal mucin pools) from invasive mucinous carcinoma. *Adv Anat Pathol*. 2008;15:1-17.
72. Tan PH, Tse GM, Bay BH. Mucinous breast lesions: diagnostic challenges. *J Clin Pathol*. 2008;61:11-19.
73. Rakha EA, Shaaban AM, Haider SA, et al. Outcome of pure mucocele-like lesions diagnosed on breast core biopsy. *Histopathology*. 2013;62:894-898.
74. Wang J, Simsir A, Mercado C, et al. Can core biopsy reliably diagnose mucinous lesions of the breast? *Am J Clin Pathol*. 2007;127:124-127.
75. Begum SM, Jara-Lazaro AR, Thike AA, et al. Mucin extravasation in breast core biopsies—clinical significance and outcome correlation. *Histopathology*. 2009;55:609-617.
76. Sutton B, Davion S, Feldman M, et al. Mucocele-like lesions diagnosed on breast core biopsy: assessment of upgrade rate and need for surgical excision. *Am J Clin Pathol*. 2012;138:783-788.
77. Moseley TW, Shah SS, Nguyen CV, et al. Clinical management of mucocele-like lesions of the breast with limited or no epithelial atypia on core biopsy: experience from two institutions. *Ann Surg Oncol*. 2019;26:3478-3488.
78. Sanati S, Leonard M, Khamapirad T, et al. Nodular mucinosis of the breast: a case report with pathologic, ultrasonographic, and clinical findings and review of the literature. *Arch Pathol Lab Med*. 2005:129:e58-e61.
79. Foschini MP, Fulcheri E, Baracchini P, et al. Squamous cell carcinoma with prominent myxoid stroma. *Hum Pathol*. 1990;21:859-865.
80. Lau PP, Chan AC, Tsui MH. Diagnostic cytological features of polyacrylamide gel injection augmentation mammoplasty. *Pathology*. 2009;41:443-447.
81. Vo T, Xing Y, Meric-Bernstam F, et al. Long-term outcomes in patients with mucinous, medullary, tubular, and invasive ductal carcinomas after lumpectomy. *Am J Surg*. 2007;194:527-531.
82. Colleoni M, Rotmensz N, Maisonneuve P, et al. Outcome of special types of luminal breast cancer. *Ann Oncol*. 2012;23:1428-1436.
83. Komaki K, Sakamoto G, Sugano H, et al. The morphologic feature of mucus leakage appearing in low papillary carcinoma of the breast. *Hum Pathol*. 1991;22:231-236.
84. Accessed July 25, 2023. http://www.nccn.org/professionals/physician_gls/pdf/breast.pdf
85. Maibenco DC, Weiss LK, Pawlish KS, et al. Axillary lymph node metastases associated with small invasive breast carcinomas. *Cancer*. 1999;85:1530-1536.
86. Rosen PP, Groshen S, Kinne DW. Survival and prognostic factors in node-negative breast cancer: results of long-term follow-up studies. *J Natl Cancer Inst Monogr*. 1992;(11):159-162.
87. Nagao T, Kinoshita T, Hojo T, et al. The differences in the histological types of breast cancer and the response to neoadjuvant chemotherapy: the relationship between the outcome and the clinicopathological characteristics. *Breast*. 2012;21:289-295.
88. Andre S, Cunha F, Bernardo M, et al. Mucinous carcinoma of the breast: a pathologic study of 82 cases. *J Surg Oncol*. 1995;58:162-167.
89. Wulsin JH, Schreiber JT. Improved prognosis in certain patterns of carcinoma of the breast: colloid, medullary with lymphoid stroma, and intraductal. *Arch Surg*. 1962;85:791-800.
90. Clayton F. Pure mucinous carcinomas of breast: morphologic features and prognostic correlates. *Hum Pathol*. 1986;17:34-38.
91. Lee YT, Terry R. Surgical treatment of carcinoma of the breast: i: pathological finding and pattern of relapse. *J Surg Oncol*. 1983;23:11-15.
92. Komaki K, Sakamoto G, Sugano H, et al. Mucinous carcinoma of the breast in Japan: a prognostic analysis based on morphologic features. *Cancer*. 1988;61:989-996.
93. Scharnhorst D, Huntrakoon M. Mucinous carcinoma of the breast: recurrence 30 years after mastectomy. *South Med J*. 1988;81:656-657.
94. Didonato R, Shapiro N, Koenigsberg T, et al. Invasive mucinous carcinoma of the breast and response patterns after neoadjuvant chemotherapy. *Histopathology*. 2018;72:965-973.
95. Jain E, Kumar A, Jain R, Sharma S. Primary mucinous cystadenocarcinoma of the breast: a rare case report with review of literature. *Int J Surg Pathol*. 2021;29:740-746.
96. Pareja F, Lee JY, Brown DN, et al. The genomic landscape of mucinous breast cancer. *J Natl Cancer Inst*. 2019;111:737-741.

Apocrine Carcinoma

ELAINE W. ZHONG AND SYED A. HODA

INTRODUCTION

Apocrine cells are a common metaplastic phenomenon in the breast. They have abundant, dense, eosinophilic cytoplasm and large round nuclei with prominent nucleoli. Apocrine lesions of the breast include apocrine metaplasia—a type of fibrocystic change (FCC)—and atypical and neoplastic apocrine epithelial proliferations (1,2). The relationship between the aforementioned lesions remains unclear. Except for apocrine metaplasia, the identification of "apocrine" lesions has limited reproducibility, and some regard "apocrine" morphology as a nonspecific alteration.

Aside from morphologic features, an "apocrine" immunohistochemical (IHC) profile has been described as negative for both estrogen receptor (ER) and progesterone receptor (PR), and positive for androgen receptor (AR) (3). Based on gene profiling studies, the "molecular apocrine" subtype of breast carcinoma is a constituent of the luminal androgen receptor subset of triple-negative breast carcinomas (4) characterized by a high rate of AR signaling, high rate of *HER2* amplification, and enrichment of genes involved in amino acid and fatty acid metabolism (5,6). Notably, morphologic, IHC, and molecular "apocrine" tumors are identified by different criteria and only partially overlap (7).

In this chapter, the designation of "apocrine carcinoma" is used for carcinomas with predominantly (>90%) apocrine morphology. The 2019 edition of the *WHO Classification of Breast Tumours* refers to these as "carcinomas with apocrine differentiation." Cells with apocrine morphology can also be found in some other subtypes of carcinomas.

CLINICAL FEATURES

Carcinomas with apocrine features represent 1% (8) of all breast carcinomas. The incidence of carcinomas having apocrine cytomorphology in at least 90% of the tumor is unknown. These carcinomas can occur at any age, but most arise in postmenopausal women (8-13). The mean age of patients with invasive apocrine carcinoma in two series was 58.5 years (12) and 67.4 years (14), 5 to 10 years older than women with nonapocrine invasive ductal carcinoma. Apocrine carcinomas are rare in men. Breast lesions in patients with Cowden syndrome (germline *PTEN* mutation) often have apocrine features (15,16) but not exclusively. Apocrine carcinoma is not specifically linked to Cowden syndrome.

Clinical and imaging findings are similar to those in patients with nonapocrine carcinomas. Bilateral apocrine carcinomas are uncommon. Apocrine ductal carcinoma in situ (DCIS) can be mass-forming, often involves sclerosing lesions such as radial sclerosing lesion (RSL) and sclerosing adenosis (SA) (17), and can mimic invasive carcinoma clinically, radiologically, and microscopically. Calcifications are common in invasive apocrine carcinomas, apocrine DCIS, and atypical apocrine adenosis (AAA). In one PET/CT imaging study, invasive apocrine carcinomas (21 cases) had the highest mean maximum standardized uptake value out of 498 primary breast carcinomas (18).

HISTOPATHOLOGIC EVALUATION

Apocrine Metaplasia

Apocrine metaplasia is a benign epithelial alteration that is part of FCCs. It often involves benign cysts and has a papillary or micropapillary configuration (**Fig. 15.1**). In the absence of a true papilloma/papillary lesion, the qualification of "papillary" should not be used for apocrine metaplasia in the report of a needle core biopsy (NCB) specimen, as it might trigger an unnecessary excision. Calcium oxalate crystals with characteristic "broken glass" appearance are typically associated with benign apocrine metaplasia and are common in apocrine cysts (**Fig. 15.1D**). Mammographically, they are usually detected as "milk of calcium," and might be the target of NCB. Rarely, psammomatous calcifications can also occur in apocrine cysts (**Fig. 15.1E**).

Atypical Apocrine Proliferations

Atypical apocrine proliferations that are not frankly neoplastic often occur in the context of sclerosing lesions, such as papilloma, RSL, and SA (apocrine adenosis) (**Figs. 15.2 and 15.3**), and can raise the differential diagnosis of apocrine DCIS. The atypical cells are cytologically similar to those of low-grade or even intermediate-grade apocrine DCIS, including at least a 3-fold variation in nuclear size with hyperchromasia and prominent nucleoli (19). However, the proliferation lacks the expansive growth, complex architecture, necrosis, mitoses, and/or sheer extent required for the diagnosis of apocrine DCIS (19,20). The term *atypical apocrine adenosis* (AAA) has been suggested for these lesions (21).

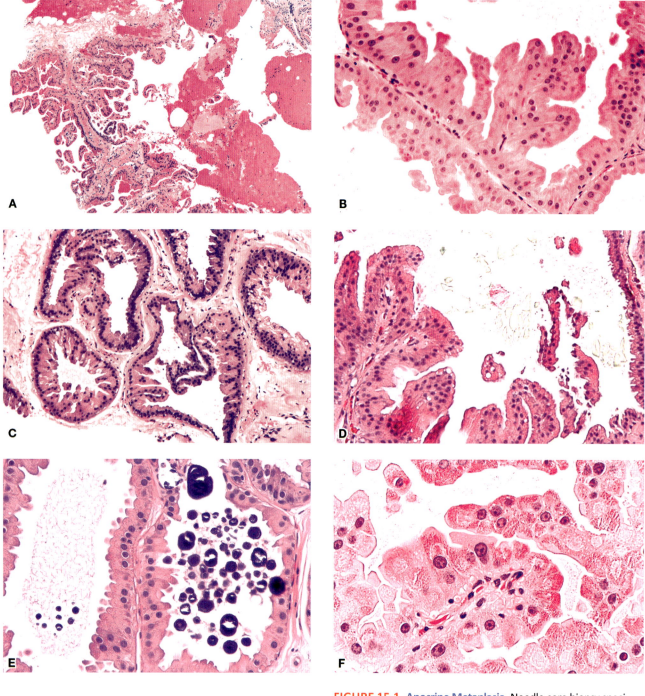

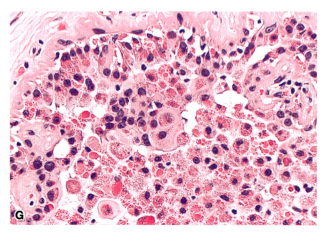

FIGURE 15.1 Apocrine Metaplasia. Needle core biopsy specimens showing different apocrine lesions. **A, B:** Cystic papillary apocrine metaplasia is composed of cells with abundant eosinophilic cytoplasm, small round nuclei, and punctate nucleoli. The nuclei are regularly and evenly distributed with respect to the basement membrane. **C:** These glands are lined by a single layer of columnar cells with evenly spaced, basally oriented nuclei. The eosinophilia seen in **(A)** and **(B)** and the basophilia in **(C)** reflect different staining properties in apocrine lesions. **D:** Apocrine metaplasia with oxalate calcifications showing the characteristic "broken glass" appearance. **E:** Cystic apocrine metaplasia with psammomatous calcifications. **F:** Benign apocrine metaplastic cells. Note the concentration of apocrine granules toward the apical portion of the cells. **G:** Benign apocrine metaplastic cells, with degenerative changes. Note apocrine cells with prominent pink granules lining the duct and also loosely clustered in the ductal lumen.

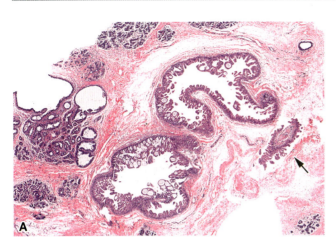 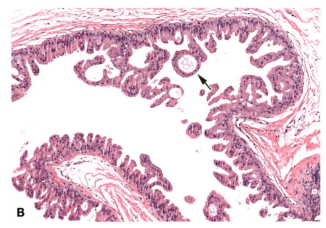

FIGURE 15.2 Apocrine Metaplasia With Atypia. A: Two ducts are involved by an atypical apocrine proliferation. A detached papillary fragment lined by micropapillary apocrine epithelium is also present (arrow). **B:** The apocrine epithelium is arranged in micropapillae and focally shows incipient bridge formation. Focal "button-hole" arrangement is seen (arrow).

Given the intrinsic difficulties in the interpretation of atypical apocrine proliferations, a cautious diagnostic approach is recommended, particularly in the evaluation of NCB material. AAA is also discussed in Chapter 6.

Apocrine Ductal Carcinoma In Situ

Apocrine DCIS has the same architectural patterns as nonapocrine DCIS **(Figs. 15.4-15.7)**. Involvement of lobules is common. Intermediate- to high-grade neoplastic apocrine cells have enlarged, hyperchromatic, and often pleomorphic nuclei, with prominent, and sometimes multiple and irregular, nucleoli. Binucleation and intranuclear inclusions are common. The nuclear chromatin is coarse and clumped, or deeply basophilic and smudged. Three-fold or greater variation of the nuclear diameter in adjacent neoplastic cells is common (19).

High-grade apocrine DCIS can have densely eosinophilic cytoplasm, often shows necrosis, and can resemble squamous DCIS, but it lacks keratin formation. Light blue mucoid cytoplasm can be seen on hematoxylin and eosin (H&E)-stained preparations. Low-grade apocrine DCIS is less common and more difficult to recognize. The nuclei are slightly larger than those of benign apocrine metaplastic cells, and the chromatin is denser; nucleoli are present but inconspicuous **(Fig. 15.7)**. The cytoplasm of neoplastic apocrine cells is usually abundant and shows dense eosinophilia; it can also be granular. Cytoplasmic vacuolization or clearing may be present in atypical apocrine lesions, but it is prominent in apocrine carcinomas. The diagnosis of low-grade apocrine DCIS rests on the identification of expansive growth and/or complex and rigid architectural patterns characteristic of DCIS. This diagnosis can be challenging, especially based on the review of NCB material. The differential diagnosis includes apocrine atypia and apocrine metaplasia.

Apocrine DCIS often harbors calcifications, which are coarse, heterogeneous, and associated with necrosis in high-grade DCIS; and are punctate and small in low-grade

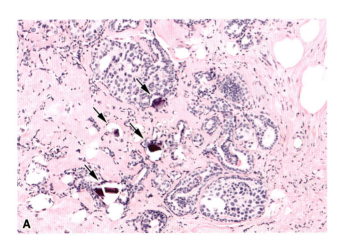 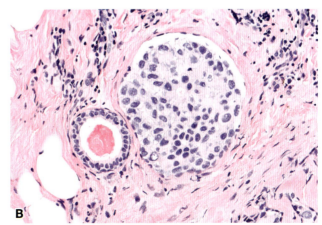

FIGURE 15.3 Apocrine Metaplasia With Atypia in a Radial Scar. A, B: A few sclerosed acini are minimally expanded by atypical apocrine cells. Calcifications are also present in **(A)** (arrows). The apocrine cytologic atypia is evident in **(B)**, compared to the normal epithelium in an adjacent acinus.

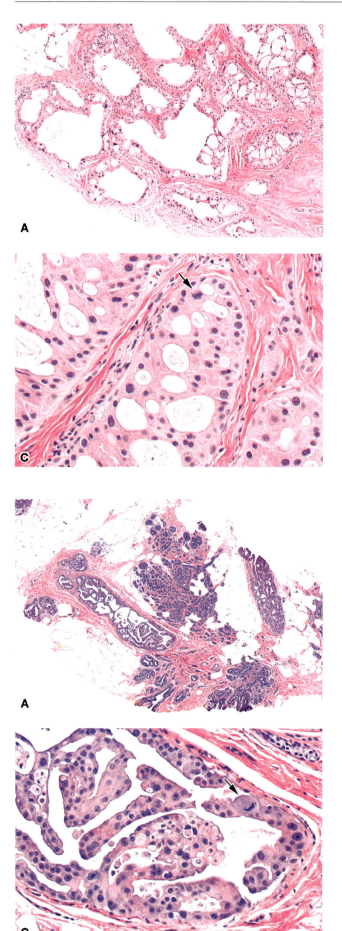

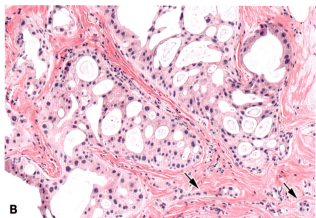

FIGURE 15.4 **Apocrine Ductal Carcinoma In Situ (DCIS), Intermediate-Grade, in a Radial Scar. A:** This needle core biopsy material shows the periphery of a radial scar with focal DCIS. The elastotic center of the radial scar is on the right. **B:** The glands involved by apocrine DCIS are expanded and show cribriform architecture. Few nests of carcinoma near the elastotic center of the radial scar simulate stromal invasion (arrows). **C:** The DCIS has intermediate nuclear grade. A mitotic figure is present (arrow). No evidence of invasive carcinoma was present in this case.

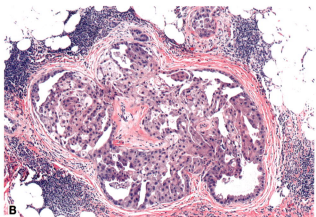

FIGURE 15.5 **Apocrine Ductal Carcinoma In Situ (DCIS), Intermediate-Grade, in a Sclerosing Lesion. A:** This needle core biopsy material shows a sclerosing lesion with apocrine DCIS. **B:** An expanded duct is involved by apocrine DCIS with intermediate nuclear grade. Periductal fibrosis and inflammation are present. **C:** A few cells have large nuclei with prominent nucleoli. A mitotic figure is present (arrow).

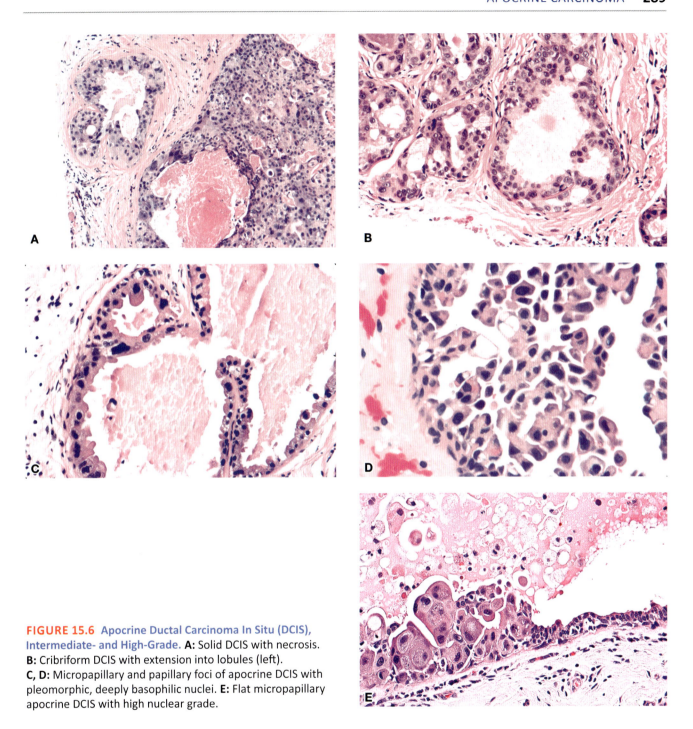

FIGURE 15.6 Apocrine Ductal Carcinoma In Situ (DCIS), Intermediate- and High-Grade. A: Solid DCIS with necrosis. **B:** Cribriform DCIS with extension into lobules (left). **C, D:** Micropapillary and papillary foci of apocrine DCIS with pleomorphic, deeply basophilic nuclei. **E:** Flat micropapillary apocrine DCIS with high nuclear grade.

DCIS. Periductal fibrosis and inflammation are common near ducts and lobules involved by apocrine DCIS or atypical apocrine epithelium. Foam cells (histiocytes with foamy cytoplasm) can be present in ducts involved by apocrine DCIS **(Fig. 15.8)** and may mimic invasive carcinoma with histiocytoid features when present in the stroma adjacent to apocrine DCIS.

Apocrine DCIS and AAA often arise in or around sclerosing lesions, such as RSL and SA (17). Papillary lesions often harbor apocrine metaplasia, and apocrine DCIS can be papillary and/or arise in a papillary lesion.

When evaluating a papillary apocrine lesion, it is critical to determine whether the apocrine epithelial proliferation has cytologic and architectural atypia. Without these, the absence of myoepithelium alone does not justify a diagnosis of invasive carcinoma **(Fig. 15.9)**. Cytologically benign cystic and papillary apocrine lesions with little to no detectable myoepithelium have been described (22-24). Conversely, IHC stains for cytokeratin and myoepithelial markers are usually useful for detecting minute invasive foci near apocrine DCIS and in cases of apocrine DCIS involving a sclerosing lesion.

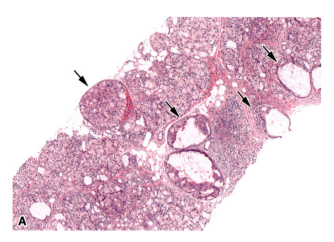 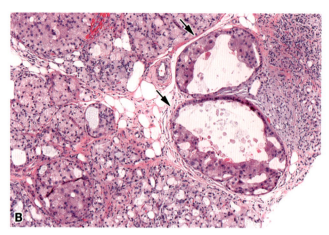

FIGURE 15.7 Invasive and In Situ Apocrine Carcinoma, Low Nuclear Grade. A, B: This needle core biopsy sample from a breast mass in an 80-year-old woman shows invasive apocrine carcinoma with low nuclear grade. Solid and cribriform apocrine ductal carcinoma in situ of low nuclear grade is present in a few scattered ducts (arrows). Minimal stromal inflammation is noted.

Apocrine Lobular Carcinoma In Situ

Apocrine cytoplasmic features can also be seen in lobular carcinoma in situ (LCIS) (25). In particular, the apocrine variant of pleomorphic LCIS (AP-LCIS) is characterized by relatively large "pleomorphic" cells with abundant eosinophilic and occasionally granular cytoplasm, intercellular dyscohesion, necrosis, and calcifications **(Fig. 15.10)** (26). AP-LCIS displays greater genomic instability and complexity than nonapocrine pleomorphic LCIS (27,28).

Invasive Apocrine Carcinoma

Most invasive apocrine carcinomas are poorly differentiated with high-grade cytomorphology **(Fig. 15.11)** (8,9). They typically consist of medium or small tumor nests. Tumor-infiltrating lymphocytes are common **(Fig. 15.12)**. Papillary **(Fig. 15.13)** or micropapillary **(Fig. 15.14)** morphology is encountered. The uncommon histiocytoid variant consists of large polygonal cells with abundant foamy or eosinophilic cytoplasm (29); closely resembles invasive pleomorphic lobular carcinoma but shows membranous reactivity for E-cadherin. Lymphovascular invasion (LVI) is present in 30% to 50% of cases of apocrine carcinoma (8,30,31). Notably, "occult carcinomas" (those that present with axillary metastases) are commonly of the apocrine type. In some cases, invasive apocrine carcinoma and invasive lobular carcinoma are closely associated. Some apocrine carcinomas can have foci of clear-cell morphology. Focal mucicarmine staining may be identified **(Fig. 15.15)**. Cells with apocrine morphology can also occur in some mucinous, micropapillary, encapsulated papillary (32), and invasive

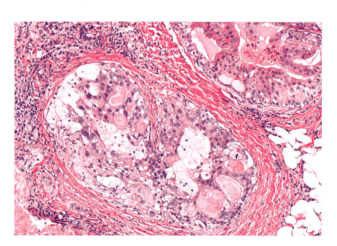 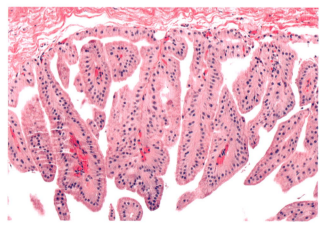

FIGURE 15.8 Foam Cells Admixed With Apocrine Carcinoma. This needle core biopsy sample from a breast mass in a 56-year-old woman shows solid and cribriform ductal carcinoma in situ (DCIS) with low nuclear grade. Stromal inflammation is also present. Foam cells are present in ducts involved by apocrine DCIS.

FIGURE 15.9 Atypical Cystic and Papillary Apocrine Lesion. This 3-cm cystic and papillary lesion in the breast of a 47-year-old woman consisted entirely of apocrine cells with no cytologic atypia, arranged in long and filiform papillae. No mitoses or necrosis were present. The entire lesion was devoid of myoepithelium when studied with immunohistochemical stains (not shown).

APOCRINE CARCINOMA 291

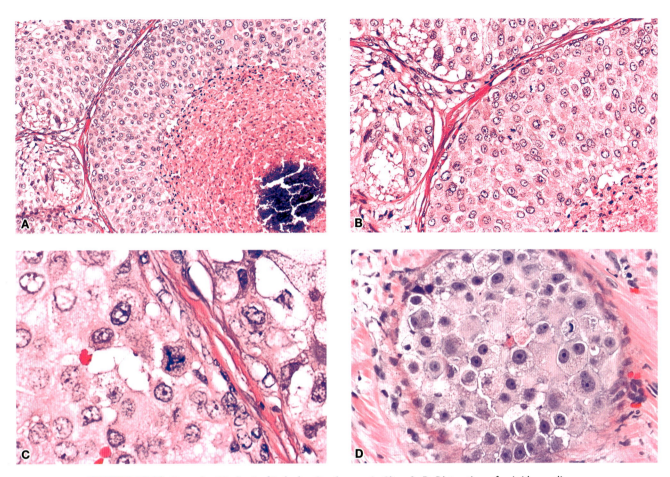

FIGURE 15.10 **Apocrine Variant of Lobular Carcinoma In Situ. A, B:** Distention of acini by malignant cells and central necrosis with calcifications. **C:** Atypical (tripolar) mitosis and nuclear pleomorphism. **D:** Eosinophilic cytoplasm with fine granules in rare cells (center). Note prominent nucleoli.

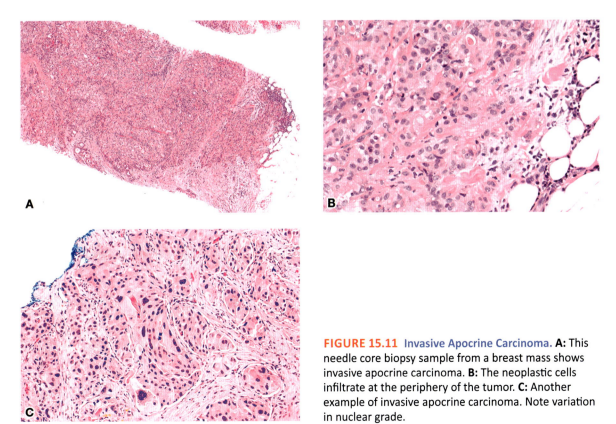

FIGURE 15.11 **Invasive Apocrine Carcinoma. A:** This needle core biopsy sample from a breast mass shows invasive apocrine carcinoma. **B:** The neoplastic cells infiltrate at the periphery of the tumor. **C:** Another example of invasive apocrine carcinoma. Note variation in nuclear grade.

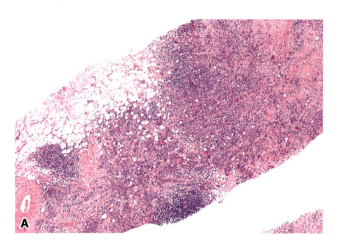
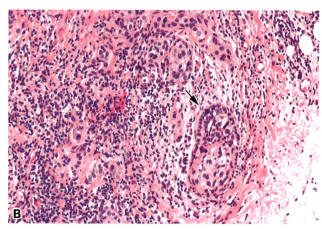

FIGURE 15.12 Invasive Apocrine Carcinoma With Tumor-Infiltrating Lymphocytes. A: This needle core biopsy sample from a breast mass shows invasive apocrine carcinoma with an abundant inflammatory infiltrate. **B:** The inflammatory cells almost mask the invasive carcinoma. A focus of solid apocrine ductal carcinoma in situ is also present (arrow).

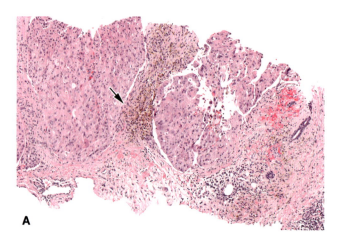
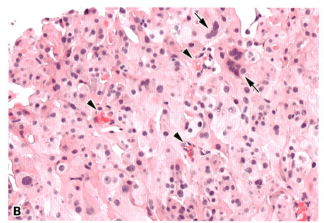

FIGURE 15.13 Invasive Apocrine Carcinoma With Solid Papillary Architecture. A: This needle core biopsy sample from a breast mass in a 56-year-old woman shows invasive papillary apocrine carcinoma. Hemosiderin is present in the stroma (arrow), consistent with prior hemorrhage. **B:** The neoplastic cells have solid growth and low cytologic atypia. A few multinucleated cells are present (arrows). Fibrovascular cores are evident (arrowheads).

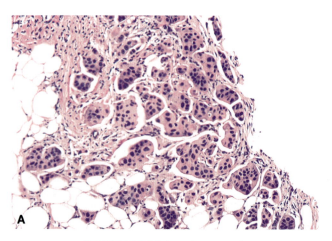
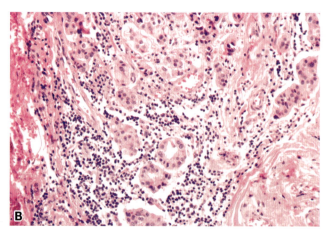

FIGURE 15.14 Invasive Apocrine Carcinoma With Micropapillary Architecture. A: The invasive apocrine carcinoma in this needle core biopsy specimen forms micropapillary clusters. **B:** Another invasive apocrine duct carcinoma forming glands and micropapillae. A stromal lymphocytic reaction is evident.

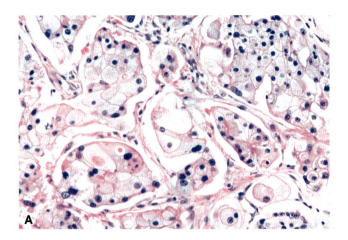
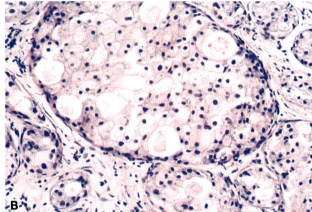
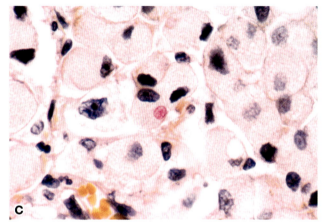

FIGURE 15.15 Apocrine Carcinoma, Clear-Cell Type. A: An invasive apocrine carcinoma with marked cytoplasmic clearing. **B:** Cribriform intraductal carcinoma. **C:** Intracytoplasmic mucin is a magenta spot in one cell (mucicarmine stain).

lobular carcinomas, especially invasive lobular carcinoma of the pleomorphic type (5,26,33). A definitive diagnosis of apocrine carcinoma is not possible based on the review of the small tissue sample obtained at NCB.

IMMUNOHISTOCHEMISTRY

Estrogen Receptor, Progesterone Receptor, Androgen Receptor, and Human Epidermal Growth Factor Receptor 2

Apocrine metaplastic cells are AR-positive but ER- and PR-negative. Most invasive apocrine carcinomas are negative or minimally positive for ER and PR (13,34–37), but some are ER-positive and/or PR-positive (9,13). AR is detected in most apocrine carcinomas, but it is expressed in other subtypes of breast carcinoma, including 95% of ER-positive carcinomas and about 50% of ER-negative carcinomas (38). Some authors consider as "pure apocrine" carcinomas only those with ER- and PR-negative, AR-positive immunoprofile, similar to apocrine metaplasia (8,37), and regard those carcinomas with apocrine morphology that are ER-positive and/or AR-positive as "apocrine-like." Nearly 50% of "pure apocrine" carcinomas are HER2-positive (8,9,13,37).

All apocrine DCIS in one study (39) were AR-positive. Low-grade DCIS were ER- and PR-negative, and about 10% of intermediate- and high-grade apocrine DCIS were ER-positive and/or PR-positive.

Gross Cystic Disease Fluid Protein 15, GATA3, Cytokeratins, and Other Antigens

Gross cystic disease fluid protein 15 (GCDFP-15) is expressed not only in most intraductal and invasive apocrine carcinomas (30,40) but also in other subtypes of breast carcinoma (40), including some carcinomas with neuroendocrine differentiation (41), as well as in the fluid of benign breast cysts. Other antigens associated with apocrine differentiation like uroplakin (42), HMG-CoA reductase (43), and GGT-1 (44) are even less specific and do not have diagnostic applications at present.

α-Methylacyl-CoA racemase (AMACR), a prostate carcinoma biomarker, was recently reported to be overexpressed in both in situ and invasive apocrine carcinoma of the breast (45). AMACR is superior in specificity and comparable in sensitivity to GCDFP-15 for apocrine carcinoma.

In one study (34), most apocrine DCIS and invasive carcinomas were negative for ER, PR, BCL2, and GATA3, akin to apocrine metaplasia, but another group detected

GATA3 in most apocrine carcinomas (40). Apocrine carcinomas tend to be immunoreactive for carcinoembryonic antigen (CEA) and are usually negative to focally positive for S-100 protein. Apocrine carcinomas are almost always positive for cytokeratins, including CK7, CK8, CK18, and CK19 (46,47). In one study, 50% of the carcinomas with apocrine features were CK20-positive, whereas all nonapocrine carcinomas were CK20-negative. None of the carcinomas with apocrine features in this study was positive for CK5/6 or CK14. Reactivity for p53 is detected in 46% (48) to 75% of invasive apocrine carcinomas and in 40% (39) to 100% (48) of apocrine DCIS, but it is not found in benign apocrine cysts (48). EGFR (epidermal growth factor receptor) was detected in 62% of apocrine carcinomas, with expression in 76% of "pure apocrine" and 29% of "apocrine-like" carcinomas (37). EGFR expression in "pure apocrine" carcinoma was inversely correlated with HER2 positivity (37). Apocrine carcinomas are negative for TTF1 and napsin A, but nonspecific granular cytoplasmic immunostaining can be seen (49). Some apocrine carcinoma may contain mucicarmine-positive secretions **(Fig. 15.15C)**. Rarely, intracytoplasmic mucin accumulation results in signet ring-type cells.

DIFFERENTIAL DIAGNOSIS IN NEEDLE CORE BIOPSY MATERIAL

Metastasis From an Extramammary Site

The differential diagnosis in an NCB sample with no DCIS includes metastasis of a carcinoma primary at an extramammary site, such as pulmonary adenocarcinoma **(Fig. 15.16)**, cutaneous apocrine carcinoma, epithelioid melanoma, or renal cell carcinoma. See also Chapter 22.

Apocrine Ductal Carcinoma In Situ in Sclerosing Lesion Mimics Invasive Carcinoma

Stromal invasion is always best assessed at the periphery of a tumor, and the examination should focus on the interface between the carcinoma and the adjacent breast parenchyma. In the absence of stromal invasion, the stroma around the sclerosing lesion typically lacks reactive desmoplasia and inflammation, and a continuous layer of basement membrane is often evident. The identification of focal stromal elastosis in the center of the lesion suggests the possibility of

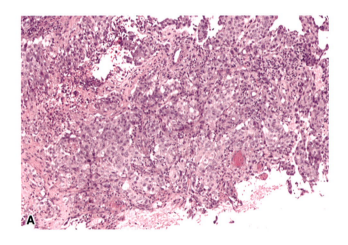

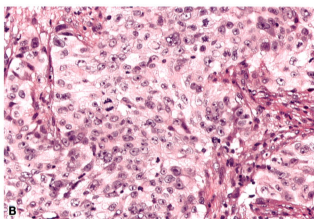

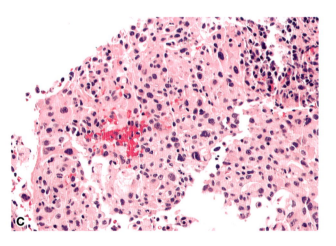

FIGURE 15.16 Metastatic Carcinoma Mimics Triple-negative Apocrine Breast Carcinoma. **A:** A needle core biopsy (NCB) specimen from a 2.5-cm superficial mass in the breast of an 80-year-old woman. No breast parenchyma or ductal carcinoma in situ is present. **B:** The carcinoma is poorly differentiated. The neoplastic cells have large and pleomorphic nuclei, with prominent nucleoli. The carcinoma was not reactive for estrogen receptor, progesterone receptor, and human epidermal growth factor receptor 2. **C:** The NCB specimen of a stellate lung lesion found at imaging workup a few weeks later. The carcinoma in the lung morphologically resembles the carcinoma in **(A)** and **(B)**. Immunohistochemical stains conducted in parallel on the material from the breast and lung lesions showed that both were positive for TTF1 and napsin, whereas negative for gross cystic disease fluid protein 15 and GATA3 (not shown), demonstrating pulmonary origin for the breast lesion.

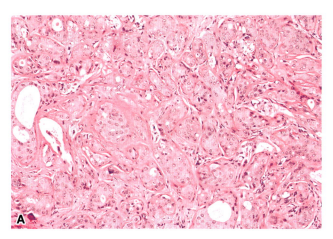
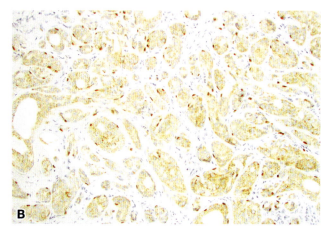

FIGURE 15.17 Ductal Carcinoma In Situ (DCIS) Involving a Sclerosing Lesion Mimics Invasive Carcinoma. A: The carcinoma in this needle core biopsy specimen mimics stromal invasion. The swirling arrangement of the neoplastic epithelium, the presence of basement membranes around the tumor nests, and the absence of stromal desmoplasia suggest the possibility of DCIS involving a sclerosing lesion. **B:** A p63 immunostain highlights the myoepithelial nuclei around the carcinoma, confirming the diagnosis of DCIS.

an underlying radial scar. In questionable cases, IHC stains for myoepithelial markers (e.g. calponin and p63) may be helpful to document the noninvasive nature of the carcinoma **(Fig. 15.17)**.

Radiation Changes

Irradiated glandular epithelium is characterized by nuclear enlargement, binucleation, intranuclear inclusions, and cytoplasmic vacuolization. These changes are relatively more pronounced in apocrine metaplastic cells. Focal necrosis sometimes is present in the lumen of acini in NCB specimens obtained shortly after the completion of breast irradiation. All of these changes closely mimic apocrine atypia and apocrine DCIS. Cell proliferation is not part of the alterations secondary to radiation treatment, and irradiated epithelium usually consists of a single layer of cells, with no epithelial expansion, and shows no mitotic activity **(Fig. 15.18)**. Whenever possible, it is recommended to compare the morphology of the pretreatment carcinoma with that of the posttreatment specimen. In questionable cases, a conservative approach is recommended, which may include surgical

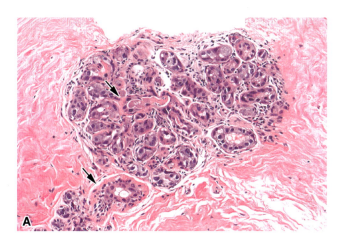
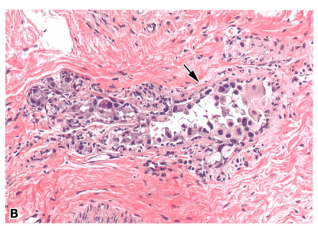

FIGURE 15.18 Radiation Changes. A, B: This needle core biopsy specimen sampled calcification in the breast of a patient who completed radiation therapy 6 months earlier for the treatment of low-grade ductal carcinoma in situ (DCIS). Coarse stromal calcifications were identified (not shown). Two lobules are shown. The epithelium shows nuclear enlargement and hyperchromasia. The differential diagnosis includes lobular involvement of apocrine DCIS. Although the epithelial alterations involve adjacent cells, no proliferation is present. Thickened basement membranes are noted around the acini, consistent with radiation therapy (arrows). Morphologic comparison with the prior low-grade DCIS supported the interpretation of radiation changes in metaplastic apocrine epithelium.

Oncocytic Neoplasms

Invasive breast carcinomas with oncocytic pattern (characterized ultrastructurally by abundant mitochondria, strong immunoreactivity with an antimitochondrial antibody, and typically negativity for GCDFP-15 and AR) are extremely rare in the breast (50). Definitive diagnosis of an oncocytic neoplasm requires evaluation of the entire tumor.

Tall Cell Carcinoma With Reversed Polarity

The abundant eosinophilic cytoplasm and variably solid, papillary, or cystic architecture of this rare breast tumor may raise the differential diagnosis of lower-grade apocrine carcinoma. Both tumors are usually triple-negative or weakly hormone receptor-positive. Cells at least twice as tall as wide, colloid-like cyst material, and apical nuclei with intranuclear grooves support the diagnosis of tall cell carcinoma with reversed polarity.

Granular Cell Tumor

Granular cell tumor (GCT) closely mimics invasive apocrine carcinoma clinically, radiologically, and microscopically. The lesional cells are admixed with sclerotic, but not desmoplastic, stroma. The cytoplasm is abundant and has a characteristic and diffuse granularity because of the presence of abundant lysosomes. The nuclei tend to be small, with no visible nucleoli, and usually lack any atypia **(Fig. 15.19)**. Lymphocytes tend to be rare in GCT but are common in apocrine carcinoma. GCT is strongly CD68-positive but negative for CK-AE1/AE3, whereas apocrine carcinoma is CK-AE1/AE3-positive and CD68-negative. Both tumors are negative for ER and PR. S-100 is strongly and diffusely positive in GCT, but it can also show some reactivity in apocrine carcinoma, although the staining tends to be focal and less intense.

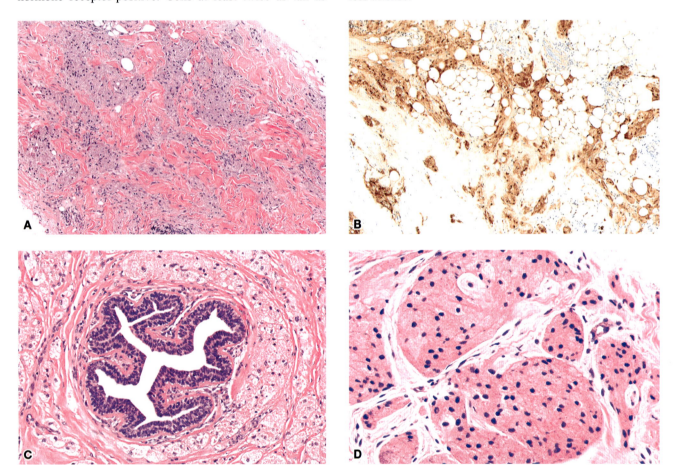

FIGURE 15.19 **Granular Cell Tumor. A, B:** This needle core biopsy specimen sampled a mammographic area of architectural distortion. The lesion consists of irregularly distributed aggregates of cells with abundant granular cytoplasm admixed with sclerotic stroma. The tumor cells are positive for S-100 **(B)** and negative for cytokeratins (not shown), consistent with the diagnosis. **C:** Another example of granular cell tumor surrounding a benign mammary duct, in a pattern that mimics invasive carcinoma. **D:** The cells of granular cell tumor have abundant amphophilic granular cytoplasm and small nuclei.

TREATMENT AND PROGNOSIS

Atypical Apocrine Adenosis

It is unclear whether AAA is a risk factor for the subsequent development of carcinoma. Carter and Rosen (19) reported no carcinomas in 51 patients with index atypical sclerosing apocrine lesions and a mean follow-up of 35 months. In another series, of 37 patients with a mean follow-up of 8.7 years (21) 11% of women with apocrine adenosis developed carcinoma (3 ipsilateral, 1 contralateral). In a recent study of 37 patients with AAA treated at the Mayo Clinic (51) with a median follow-up of 14 years, 8% of the patients developed carcinoma, including 2 ipsilateral invasive carcinomas and 1 contralateral DCIS. None of the carcinomas had apocrine morphology.

Based on current data, patients with atypical apocrine lesions should be managed clinically with the same follow-up regimen as those with nonapocrine atypical proliferative lesions. The effectiveness of selective ER modulators on atypical apocrine lesions (which are typically ER-negative) has not been determined.

A lesion yielding AAA at NCB should be surgically excised for its complete and definitive evaluation. A recent study evaluating the upgrade at surgical excision of AAA reported no upgrades to carcinoma (52) (please see also Chapter 6).

Apocrine Ductal Carcinoma In Situ

Apocrine DCIS appears to have the same clinical course as nonapocrine DCIS. Management includes surgical excision and radiation therapy or mastectomy. Hormonal modulation therapy is indicated if at least 1% of apocrine DCIS cells express ER.

Invasive Apocrine Carcinoma

Studies have found that the prognosis of invasive apocrine mammary carcinoma is similar to that of nonapocrine invasive ductal carcinoma (12). One group (10) studied 29 triple-negative apocrine carcinomas and found LVI in 24% of patients, and lymph node (LN) metastases in 45%. The 5-year overall survival (OS) was 92%, and the disease-free survival (DFS) was 83.7% at 5 years and 67% at 10 years. One group (8) reported that pure apocrine carcinomas had worse DFS than nonapocrine carcinomas (HR 1.7), whereas apocrine-like carcinomas and nonapocrine carcinomas had similar DFS and OS. Among triple-negative carcinomas, the outcome of apocrine carcinomas is similar to or better than that of triple-negative invasive ductal carcinomas of no special type (10,14,53-56).

The prognosis of invasive apocrine carcinoma is determined by conventional prognostic factors such as grade, tumor size, and nodal status. Carcinomas with apocrine differentiation are usually strongly and diffusely AR-positive. Rakha et al (57) reported that AR-positive triple-negative

breast carcinomas had higher nuclear grade, and higher rate of recurrent disease and distant metastases. In a cohort of postmenopausal patients with ER-positive breast carcinoma, AR expression was associated with significantly reduced breast cancer–specific mortality (HR 0.68) and overall mortality (HR 0.70) by multivariate analysis (58). In the same study, however, postmenopausal women with ER-*negative* and AR-positive breast carcinoma, such as apocrine carcinomas, had significantly *increased* breast cancer-specific mortality (HR 1.59).

At present, patients with triple-negative, AR-positive metastatic breast carcinomas can be treated with AR-antagonist drugs not only in the context of a clinical trial, but also occasionally outside of a trial. Enzalutamide and bicalutamide, potent AR inhibitors approved for the treatment of patients with metastatic prostate carcinoma, have demonstrated efficacy and safety in patients with advanced triple-negative breast carcinoma in multiple clinical trials (59-61). Specific correlation with apocrine morphology has not been studied.

REFERENCES

1. Quinn CM, D'Arcy C, Wells C. Apocrine lesions of the breast. *Virchows Arch.* 2022;480:177-189.
2. Vranic S, Schmitt F, Sapino A, et al. Apocrine carcinoma of the breast: a comprehensive review. *Histol Histopathol.* 2013;28:1393-1409.
3. Selim AG, Wells CA. Immunohistochemical localisation of androgen receptor in apocrine metaplasia and apocrine adenosis of the breast: relation to oestrogen and progesterone receptors. *J Clin Pathol.* 1999;52:838-841.
4. Lehmann BD, Bauer JA, Chen X, et al. Identification of human triple-negative breast cancer subtypes and preclinical models for selection of targeted therapies. *J Clin Invest.* 2011;121:2750-2767.
5. D'Arcy C, Quinn CM. Apocrine lesions of the breast: part 2 of a two-part review. Invasive apocrine carcinoma, the molecular apocrine signature and utility of immunohistochemistry in the diagnosis of apocrine lesions of the breast. *J Clin Pathol.* 2019;72:7-11.
6. Farmer P, Bonnefoi H, Becette V, et al. Identification of molecular apocrine breast tumours by microarray analysis. *Oncogene.* 2005;24:4660-4671.
7. Gromov P, Espinoza JA, Gromova I. Molecular and diagnostic features of apocrine breast lesions. *Expert Rev Mol Diagn.* 2015;15:1011-1022.
8. Dellapasqua S, Maisonneuve P, Viale G, et al. Immunohistochemically defined subtypes and outcome of apocrine breast cancer. *Clin Breast Cancer.* 2013;13:95-102.
9. Alvarenga CA, Paravidino PI, Alvarenga M, et al. Reappraisal of immunohistochemical profiling of special histological types of breast carcinomas: a study of 121 cases of eight different subtypes. *J Clin Pathol.* 2012;65:1066-1071.
10. Montagna E, Maisonneuve P, Rotmensz N, et al. Heterogeneity of triple-negative breast cancer: histologic subtyping to inform the outcome. *Clin Breast Cancer.* 2013;13:31-39.
11. Ogiya A, Horii R, Osako T, et al. Apocrine metaplasia of breast cancer: clinicopathological features and predicting response. *Breast Cancer.* 2010;17:290-297.
12. Tanaka K, Imoto S, Wada N, et al. Invasive apocrine carcinoma of the breast: clinicopathologic features of 57 patients. *Breast J.* 2008;14:164-168.
13. Tsutsumi Y. Apocrine carcinoma as triple-negative breast cancer: novel definition of apocrine-type carcinoma as estrogen/progesterone receptor-negative and androgen receptor-positive invasive ductal carcinoma. *Jpn J Clin Oncol.* 2012;42:375-386.
14. Mills MN, Yang GQ, Oliver DE, et al. Histologic heterogeneity of triple negative breast cancer: a national cancer centre database analysis. *Eur J Cancer.* 2018;98:48-58.
15. Banneau G, Guedj M, MacGrogan G, et al. Molecular apocrine differentiation is a common feature of breast cancer in patients with germline PTEN mutations. *Breast Cancer Res.* 2010;12:R63.
16. Schrager CA, Schneider D, Gruener AC, et al. Clinical and pathological features of breast disease in Cowden's syndrome: an underrecognized syndrome with an increased risk of breast cancer. *Hum Pathol.* 1998;29:47-53.
17. Moritani S, Ichihara S, Hasegawa M, et al. Topographical, morphological and immunohistochemical characteristics of carcinoma in situ of the breast involving sclerosing adenosis. two distinct topographical patterns and histological types of carcinoma in situ. *Histopathology.* 2011;58:835-846.
18. Arslan E, Cermik TF, Trabulus FDC, et al. Role of 18F-FDG PET/CT in evaluating molecular subtypes and clinicopathological features of primary breast cancer. *Nucl Med Commun.* 2018;39:680-690.

19. Carter DJ, Rosen PP. Atypical apocrine metaplasia in sclerosing lesions of the breast: a study of 51 patients. *Mod Pathol.* 1991;4:1-5.
20. Asirvatham JR, Falcone MM, Kleer CG. Atypical apocrine adenosis: diagnostic challenges and pitfalls. *Arch Pathol Lab Med.* 2016;140:1045-1051.
21. Seidman JD, Ashton M, Lefkowitz M. Atypical apocrine adenosis of the breast: a clinicopathologic study of 37 patients with 8.7-year follow-up. *Cancer.* 1996;77:2529-2537.
22. Cserni G. Lack of myoepithelium in apocrine glands of the breast does not necessarily imply malignancy. *Histopathology.* 2008;52:253-255.
23. Cserni G. Benign apocrine papillary lesions of the breast lacking or virtually lacking myoepithelial cells-potential pitfalls in diagnosing malignancy. *APMIS.* 2012;120:249-252.
24. Tramm T, Kim JY, Tavassoli FA. Diminished number or complete loss of myoepithelial cells associated with metaplastic and neoplastic apocrine lesions of the breast. *Am J Surg Pathol.* 2011;35:202-211.
25. D'Arcy C, Quinn C. Apocrine lesions of the breast: part 1 of a two-part review: benign, atypical and in situ apocrine proliferations of the breast. *J Clin Pathol.* 2019;72:1-6.
26. Zhong E, Solomon JP, Cheng E, et al. Apocrine variant of pleomorphic lobular carcinoma in situ: further clinical, histopathologic, immunohistochemical, and molecular characterization of an emerging entity. *Am J Surg Pathol.* 2020;44:1092-1103.
27. Chen YY, Hwang ES, Roy R, et al. Genetic and phenotypic characteristics of pleomorphic lobular carcinoma in situ of the breast. *Am J Surg Pathol.* 2009;33:1683-1694.
28. Shin SJ, Lal A, De Vries S, et al. Florid lobular carcinoma in situ: molecular profiling and comparison to classic lobular carcinoma in situ and pleomorphic lobular carcinoma in situ. *Hum Pathol.* 2013;44:1998-2009.
29. Eusebi V, Foschini MP, Bussolati G, et al. Myoblastomatoid (histiocytoid) carcinoma of the breast. A type of apocrine carcinoma. *Am J Surg Pathol.* 1995;19:553-562.
30. Kasashima S, Kawashima A, Ozaki S, et al. Expression of 5alpha-reductase in apocrine carcinoma of the breast and its correlation with clinicopathological aggressiveness. *Histopathology.* 2012;60:E51-E57.
31. Matsuo K, Fukutomi T, Tsuda H, et al. Apocrine carcinoma of the breast: clinicopathological analysis and histologic subclassification of 12 cases. *Breast Cancer.* 1998;5:279-284.
32. Seal M, Wilson C, Naus GJ, et al. Encapsulated apocrine papillary carcinoma of the breast—a tumour of uncertain malignant potential: report of five cases. *Virchows Arch.* 2009;455:477-483.
33. Eusebi V, Magalhaes F, Azzopardi JG. Pleomorphic lobular carcinoma of the breast: an aggressive tumor showing apocrine differentiation. *Hum Pathol.* 1992;23:655-662.
34. Celis JE, Cabezon T, Moreira JM, et al. Molecular characterization of apocrine carcinoma of the breast: validation of an apocrine protein signature in a well-defined cohort. *Mol Oncol.* 2009;3:220-337.
35. Honma N, Takubo K, Akiyama F, et al. Expression of oestrogen receptor-beta in apocrine carcinomas of the breast. *Histopathology.* 2007;50:425-433.
36. Niemeier LA, Dabbs DJ, Beriwal S, et al. Androgen receptor in breast cancer: expression in estrogen receptor-positive tumors and in estrogen receptor-negative tumors with apocrine differentiation. *Mod Pathol.* 2010;23:205-212.
37. Vranic S, Tawfik O, Palazzo J, et al. EGFR and HER-2/neu expression in invasive apocrine carcinoma of the breast. *Mod Pathol.* 2010;23:644-653.
38. Collins LC, Cole KS, Marotti JD, et al. Androgen receptor expression in breast cancer in relation to molecular phenotype: results from the nurses' health study. *Mod Pathol.* 2011;24:924-931.
39. Leal C, Henrique R, Monteiro P, et al. Apocrine ductal carcinoma in situ of the breast: histologic classification and expression of biologic markers. *Hum Pathol.* 2001;32:487-493.

40. Wendroth SM, Mentrikoski MJ, Wick MR. GATA3 expression in morphologic subtypes of breast carcinoma: a comparison with gross cystic disease fluid protein 15 and mammaglobin. *Ann Diagn Pathol.* 2015;19:6-9.
41. Sapino A, Righi L, Cassoni P, et al. Expression of apocrine differentiation markers in neuroendocrine breast carcinomas of aged women. *Mod Pathol.* 2001;14:768-776.
42. Tajima S, Koda K. Uroplakin II expression in breast carcinomas showing apocrine differentiation: putting some emphasis on invasive pleomorphic lobular carcinoma as a potential mimic of urothelial carcinoma at metastatic sites. *Dis Markers.* 2016;2016:2940496.
43. Celis JE, Gromov P, Moreira JM, et al. Apocrine cysts of the breast: biomarkers, origin, enlargement, and relation with cancer phenotype. *Mol Cell Proteomics.* 2006;5:462-483.
44. Choi J, Jung WH, Koo JS. Clinicopathologic features of molecular subtypes of triple negative breast cancer based on immunohistochemical markers. *Histol Histopathol.* 2012;27:1481-1493.
45. Nakamura H, Kukita Y, Kunimasa K, et al. Alpha-methylacyl-CoA racemase: a useful immunohistochemical marker of breast carcinoma with apocrine differentiation. *Hum Pathol.* 2021;116:39-48.
46. Alvarenga CA, Paravidino PI, Alvarenga M, et al. Expression of CK19 in invasive breast carcinomas of special histologic types: implications for the use of one-step nucleic acid amplification. *J Clin Pathol.* 2011;64:493-497.
47. Shao MM, Chan SK, Yu AM, et al. Keratin expression in breast cancers. *Virchows Arch.* 2012;461:313-322.
48. Moriya T, Sakamoto K, Sasano H, et al. Immunohistochemical analysis of Ki-67, p53, p21, and p27 in benign and malignant apocrine lesions of the breast: its correlation to histologic findings in 43 cases. *Mod Pathol.* 2000;13:13-18.
49. Vitkovski T, Chaudhary S, Sison C, et al. Aberrant expression of napsin A in breast carcinoma with apocrine features. *Int J Surg Pathol.* 2016;24:377-381.
50. Ragazzi M, de Biase D, Betts CM, et al. Oncocytic carcinoma of the breast: frequency, morphology and follow-up. *Hum Pathol.* 2011;42:166-175.
51. Fuehrer N, Hartmann L, Degnim A, et al. Atypical apocrine adenosis of the breast: long-term follow-up in 37 patients. *Arch Pathol Lab Med.* 2012;136:179-182.
52. Calhoun BC, Booth CN. Atypical apocrine adenosis diagnosed on breast core biopsy: implications for management. *Hum Pathol.* 2014;45:2130-2135.
53. Arciero CA, Diehl AH 3rd, Liu Y, et al. Triple-negative apocrine carcinoma: a rare pathologic subtype with a better prognosis than other triple-negative breast cancers. *J Surg Oncol.* 2020;122:1232-1239.
54. Dreyer G, Vandorpe T, Smeets A, et al. Triple negative breast cancer: clinical characteristics in the different histological subtypes. *Breast.* 2013;22:761-766.
55. Meattini I, Pezzulla D, Saieva C, et al. Triple negative apocrine carcinomas as a distinct subtype of triple negative breast cancer: a case-control study. *Clin Breast Cancer.* 2018;18:e773-e780.
56. Zhao S, Ma D, Xiao Y, et al. Clinicopathologic features and prognoses of different histologic types of triple-negative breast cancer: a large population-based analysis. *Eur J Surg Oncol.* 2018;44:420-428.
57. Rakha EA, El-Sayed ME, Green AR, et al. Prognostic markers in triple-negative breast cancer. *Cancer.* 2007;109:25-32.
58. Hu R, Dawood S, Holmes MD, et al. Androgen receptor expression and breast cancer survival in postmenopausal women. *Clin Cancer Res.* 2011;17:1867-1874.
59. Gucalp A, Tolaney S, Isakoff SJ, et al. Phase II trial of bicalutamide in patients with androgen receptor-positive, estrogen receptor-negative metastatic breast cancer. *Clin Cancer Res.* 2013;19:5505-5512.
60. Schwartzberg LS, Yardley DA, Elias AD, et al. A phase I/Ib study of enzalutamide alone and in combination with endocrine therapies in women with advanced breast cancer. *Clin Cancer Res.* 2017;23:4046-4054.
61. Traina TA, Miller K, Yardley DA, et al. Enzalutamide for the treatment of androgen receptor-expressing triple-negative breast cancer. *J Clin Oncol.* 2018;36:884-890.

16

Adenoid Cystic Carcinoma

ELAINE W. ZHONG AND SYED A. HODA

Mammary adenoid cystic carcinoma (ACC) is morphologically similar to its counterpart in the salivary glands but has a more indolent behavior. Most ACCs of the breast and salivary glands carry a characteristic *MYB-NFIB* fusion gene, which results from a *t*(6;9)(q22-23;p23-24) translocation (1-3).

CLINICAL FEATURES

ACC is one of the least common forms of primary mammary carcinoma (4,5), accounting for less than 0.1% of breast carcinomas (5,6) and 11.5% of all ACCs in the body (5). The incidence rate of ACC was relatively constant between 1977 and 2006 (5,7).

ACC occurs in women of any age, but the mean and median ages of patients with ACC range from 50 to 63 years in various studies (5,7-10). Between 70% and 96% of women with ACC in three separate series (7,11,12) were postmenopausal. Most (78%-87%) women with ACC are non-Hispanic White (5,9,12). ACC can occur in males, including adolescent males, and constituted 1% of 759 primary breast carcinomas in men in one series (13). No association with familial syndromes has been described.

ACC presents as a palpable, discrete, and firm mass in about 80% of cases (12). Pain (12,14,15) and tenderness (15) are rare presenting symptoms and have not been specifically correlated with the histologic finding of perineural invasion. Even though ACC frequently arises in the subareolar region or centrally in the breast (7), nipple discharge and Paget disease are rare presenting symptoms. The most frequent sites of ACC are the upper outer quadrant and the retroareolar region (7). ACC is usually unifocal, and only rarely consists of two or more distinct foci (12,16). Bilateral ACC is uncommon.

IMAGING FEATURES

ACC presents mammographically as a well-defined lobulated mass or an ill-defined lesion (17); a mammographic spiculated mass can also be observed (15). Only 18% of ACCs in one series (12) were detected by mammography; in another study (17), 87.5% of ACCs were mammographically detected. Calcifications are rarely associated with ACC.

The sonographic appearance of ACC is that of a heterogeneous or hypoechoic mass (15,17). Eight of nine ACCs studied sonographically (17) appeared as irregularly shaped hypoechoic or heterogeneous masses, oriented parallel to the skin, with no echogenic halo or posterior shadowing. Doppler sonography detected only minimal flow signal around and within the tumor. One tumor presented as an 8-mm hypoechoic nodule suggestive of an intramammary lymph node (LN) (18).

MRI is helpful for defining the extent of the ACC, especially in a dense breast (17). ACC tends to be irregular or lobulated, with rapid and heterogeneous enhancement (17).

Most ACCs measure between 1 and 3 cm. In a recent series of 31 ACCs (19), the mean tumor size was 2.7 cm (range: 0.6-15 cm); the mean size of ACC with classic histology was 2.9 cm (range: 0.7-12 cm), and that of ACC with solid basaloid morphology was 2.6 cm (range: 0.6-15 cm). In another series of six cases of solid basaloid ACC (20), the mean tumor size was 2 cm.

HISTOPATHOLOGIC EVALUATION

ACC is composed of glandular epithelium (adenoid component) and basaloid/myoepithelial cells, which produce a variable amount of myxoid or eosinophilic basement membrane material (**Figs. 16.1 and 16.2**) that collect in the glandular lumens (cystic component). These components are heterogeneously distributed within any given tumor and produce different morphologic appearances, including cribriform, tubular, reticular, solid, insular, and other patterns. ACC often shows intratumoral heterogeneity and sometimes can be difficult to recognize in the limited material obtained by needle core biopsy (NCB).

Cribriform Morphology

Classic ACCs have a predominantly cribriform glandular arrangement that closely mimics invasive or in situ cribriform carcinoma (**Fig. 16.1**), especially when the basaloid element and basement membrane material are sparse.

Tubular Morphology

This pattern consists of infiltrative glands lined by a luminal epithelial cell layer and one or more abluminal myoepithelial cell layers. The glands may be round or elongated and irregular.

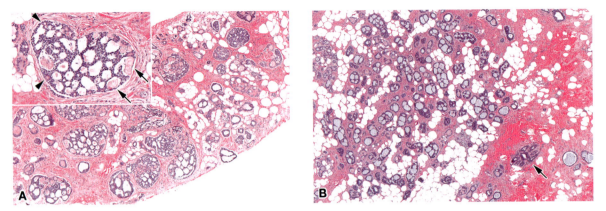

FIGURE 16.1 Adenoid Cystic Carcinoma (ACC), Cribriform Growth Pattern. A: A needle core biopsy specimen showing nests of predominantly cribriform ACC. Cribriform growth with basement membrane spherules (arrows) and small glandular lumina (arrowheads) are shown in the inset. **B:** The surgically excised tumor has similar morphology. Note the diffuse infiltrative growth pattern and lack of stromal desmoplasia. A small duct is also present (arrow).

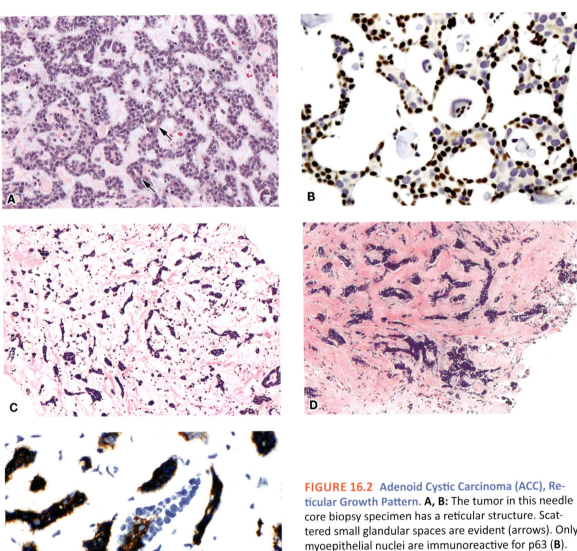

FIGURE 16.2 Adenoid Cystic Carcinoma (ACC), Reticular Growth Pattern. A, B: The tumor in this needle core biopsy specimen has a reticular structure. Scattered small glandular spaces are evident (arrows). Only myoepithelial nuclei are immunoreactive for p63 (**B**). **C:** Small cords and clusters of carcinoma cells float within basement membrane material in another reticular ACC. **D, E:** Crush artifact in another core biopsy obscures the cytology of this high-grade carcinoma; CD117 (**E**) supports the diagnosis of ACC.

Reticular Morphology

The carcinoma consists of trabeculae with a nearly linear arrangement, surrounded by expanded extracellular basement membrane matrix, often with myxoid to mucoid tinctorial quality. Scattered minute glands are visible (**Fig. 16.2**). Occasionally, different patterns coexist in the same case (**Fig. 16.3**).

Solid Basaloid Morphology

Solid growth of the basaloid cells yields a pattern referred to as the "solid variant of ACC with basaloid features" (21) or solid basaloid ACC (**Fig. 16.4**). The neoplastic cells have scant cytoplasm, relatively large hyperchromatic nuclei, and frequent mitoses. Scattered small glands are usually appreciable, as well as focal minute eosinophilic deposits of basement membrane material.

Ro et al (22) suggested that ACC be stratified into three grades based on the proportion of solid growth within the lesion: grade I, no solid elements; grade II, less than 30% solid growth; and grade III, solid areas composing more than 30% of the tumor. The authors (22) found that grade II and III tumors tended to be larger and were more likely to have recurrences than grade I tumors. The grading scheme proposed by Ro et al (22) was not prognostically significant in a subsequent study (23).

Metaplastic Alterations

Some ACCs have focal sebaceous metaplasia or squamous differentiation. Adenomyoepitheliomatous (24,25) and syringomatous areas can be present. Adipocytic differentiation and myofibroblastic hyperplasia can also occur in the stroma of ACC. A high-grade solid basaloid ACC showed morphologic transition into a metaplastic spindle cell and glandular adenocarcinoma with melanomatous differentiation (26). Another solid basaloid ACC merged with a "small cell carcinoma" (27).

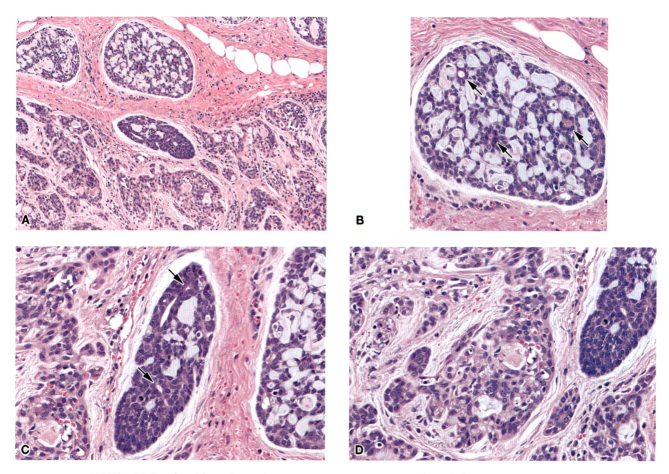

FIGURE 16.3 Adenoid Cystic Carcinoma, Coexisting Patterns. **A:** Three different growth patterns are present in this tumor. **B:** The cribriform pattern in this nest mimics cribriform ductal carcinoma in situ. Few small glandular lumina are evident (arrows), and there are numerous spherules of basophilic basement membrane material. **C:** A small nest has solid growth with scattered glandular lumina (arrows). Cribriform (right) and reticular (left) patterns are also represented. **D:** The prevalent growth pattern in this field is reticular. The solid basaloid nest in **(C)** is partially represented in the right upper corner.

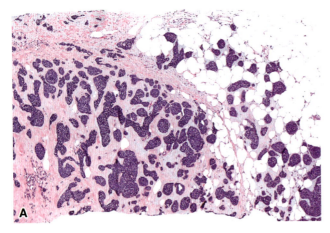
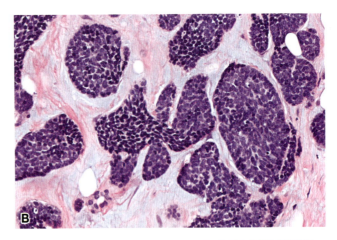
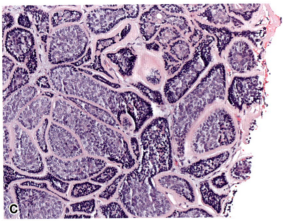
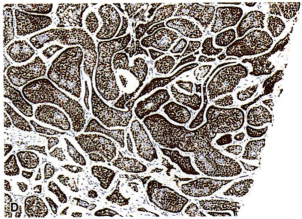
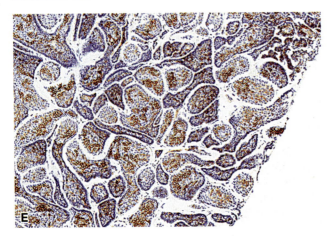

FIGURE 16.4 Adenoid Cystic Carcinoma (ACC), Solid Basaloid Pattern. A: The carcinoma consists of solid nests composed of hyperchromatic cells. The stroma around the neoplastic nests is hypocellular, with a focally pale blue tinctorial quality. **B:** At higher magnification, the neoplastic cells show basaloid morphology. The pale blue staining of the stroma around the invasive nests is a feature commonly associated with high-grade ACC and should not be mistaken for stromal mucin. **C-E:** Needle core biopsy of a solid basaloid ACC with closely packed nests surrounded by thick basement membrane reminiscent of cylindroma. p63 **(D)** and CD117 **(E)** highlight the biphasic cell population.

Perineural and Lymphovascular Invasion

In contrast to salivary gland ACC, perineural and lymphovascular invasion (LVI) are uncommon in mammary ACC with classic morphology, and it is rarely detected in NCB material. Shrinkage artifact is common, especially in fibrotic portions of ACC, and can mimic LVI (**Fig. 16.5**). Three of six solid basaloid ACCs in one series (20) had LVI, including two tumors that also showed perineural invasion.

Adenoid Cystic Carcinoma In Situ

In situ or intraductal ACC is occasionally encountered in the breast (5,10,28). ACC in situ lacks the periductal cuff of cellular myxoid stroma that typically surrounds the nests of invasive ACC, but this finding can be subtle. Calponin decorates the native myoepithelium of the ducts and acini harboring in situ ACC, but it is absent within and around the nests of invasive ACC. Lobules and ducts adjacent to invasive ACC can display adenoid cystic traits, with small cylindromatous areas, which represent in situ carcinoma (**Fig. 16.6**).

Other Associated Lesions

Associations with various benign lesions have been reported, including microglandular adenosis (MGA) (29,30), tubular adenosis (31), fibroadenoma (32), and adenomyoepithelioma

ADENOID CYSTIC CARCINOMA 303

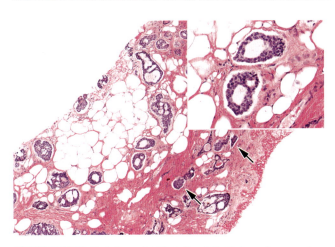

FIGURE 16.5 Shrinkage Artifact Can Mimic Lymphovascular Invasion. Shrinkage artifact around nests of adenoid cystic carcinoma (ACC) is common and can simulate lymphovascular invasion (arrows). On high-power examination (inset), the space around the nests of ACC is devoid of endothelium.

(AME) (33). The relationship between these entities and ACCs is unclear at this time.

Patients with ACC can also develop other types of breast carcinoma in the same or opposite breast coincidentally or asynchronously. Merging of ACC with well-differentiated estrogen receptor (ER)-positive invasive ductal carcinoma has been observed (**Fig. 16.7**).

IMMUNOHISTOCHEMISTRY

Glandular Cells

The glandular (luminal) cells of ACC are positive for CK7, CEA, EMA, CK5/6, CK8/18, and CD117/CKIT (**Fig. 16.8**) (34). These cells are focal in solid basaloid ACC. In most solid basaloid ACCs, CK7 highlights scattered and glandular lumina (19), but some cases show diffuse staining for CK7 (20).

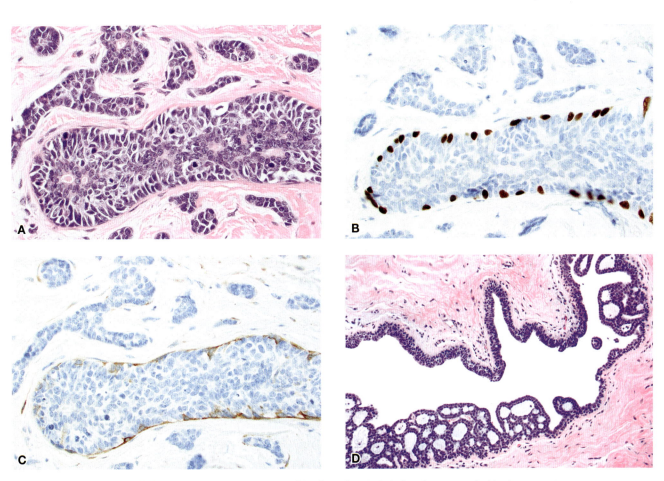

FIGURE 16.6 Adenoid Cystic Carcinoma (ACC) In Situ. A-C: A duct is surrounded by basement membrane and contains a biphasic population of neoplastic cells with intermediate- to high-grade nuclei, similar to those of the adjacent small invasive nests. Immunohistochemical staining for p63 (**B**) and calponin (**C**) highlights the native myoepithelial cells around the duct involved by carcinoma in situ, whereas the adjacent invasive nests are negative for both antigens. **D:** Cribriform intraductal ACC partially involving a duct. Invasive ACC was present elsewhere in the specimen.

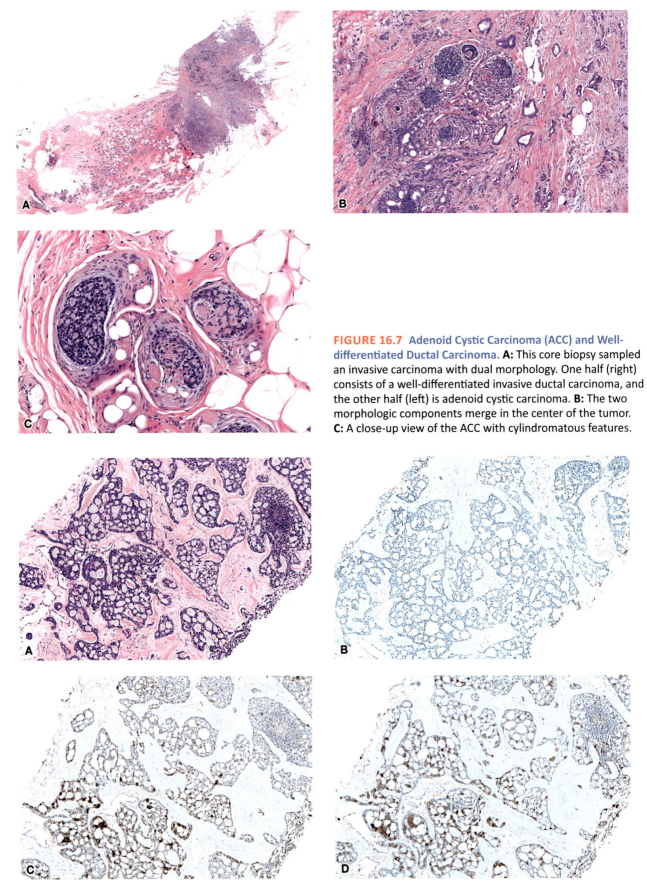

FIGURE 16.7 Adenoid Cystic Carcinoma (ACC) and Well-differentiated Ductal Carcinoma. A: This core biopsy sampled an invasive carcinoma with dual morphology. One half (right) consists of a well-differentiated invasive ductal carcinoma, and the other half (left) is adenoid cystic carcinoma. B: The two morphologic components merge in the center of the tumor. C: A close-up view of the ACC with cylindromatous features.

FIGURE 16.8 Adenoid Cystic Carcinoma (ACC), Immunohistochemistry. The ACC (A) is negative for ER (B) and shows positive reactivity for CK7 (C) and CD117 (D) in the epithelial component, and for smooth muscle myosin (SMM) (partial) (E) and p63 (F) in the myoepithelial/basaloid cells.

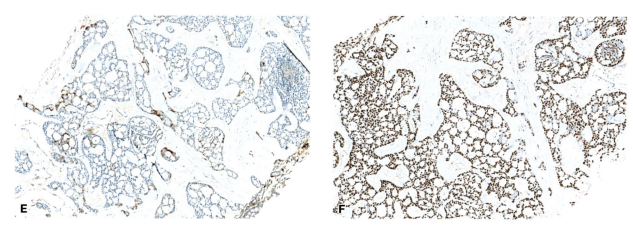

FIGURE 16.8 (continued)

Basaloid Cells

The basaloid (myoepithelial) cells of ACC express the myoepithelial markers p63 (**Figs. 16.2 and 16.8**) (34,35), smooth muscle actin (SMA) (35), and maspin (36) but show little or no reactivity for calponin (35), smooth muscle myosin heavy chain (21,35) (**Fig. 16.8**), or CD10 (37). The basaloid cells are also positive for basal keratins CK14 and CK17 (3). CK5/6 is notably negative in the myoepithelial cells of classic ACC (34,38). Glandular and myoepithelial cells stain with keratin 34βE12, albeit not uniformly. Most solid basaloid ACCs are diffusely positive for p63, but some cases are p63-negative or only focally positive (20), including cases with documented *MYB* rearrangement by fluorescence in situ hybridization (FISH) (19). The basement membrane material stains for type IV collagen and laminin.

Estrogen Receptor, Progesterone Receptor, Androgen Receptor, and Human Epidermal Growth Factor Receptor 2

Most ACCs are negative for ER (3,6,34), progesterone receptor (PR), androgen receptor (AR) (39), and human epidermal growth factor receptor 2 (HER2) (34). Limited positivity for ER has been detected in some ACCs (12,17,21,40). Based on its triple-negative profile and reactivity for basal cytokeratins, ACC qualifies as a "basal-like" triple-negative breast carcinoma, but it differs from other "basal-like" mammary carcinomas in that it harbors a characteristic genetic alteration and has a relatively good prognosis.

SOX10

Like most other basal-like breast carcinomas (41), ACC expresses SOX10, in the nuclei of both the epithelial and myoepithelial cells (42,43).

Ki67

Ki67 staining in ACC ranges from 4% to 70%, depending on the tumor grade, with a trend to a higher positivity in higher-grade tumors (40). In one study (44), three ACCs with a low Ki67 index and no expression of p53 protein had no LN involvement, whereas a fourth tumor with a high Ki67 index and p53 expression presented with LN metastases. Other investigators found that the Ki67 index is not significantly related to prognosis (23).

CD117/KIT

CK117 (KIT), a transmembrane tyrosine kinase receptor encoded by the protooncogene *c-KIT* located on chromosome 4(q11-12), is involved in the regulation of cell growth and is expressed in normal mammary glandular epithelium. Mammary ACC is typically CD117-positive (3,34,35,40,45) (**Fig. 16.8**). CD117 staining in cribriform ACC is reported to be limited to the epithelial component (34,45); however, diffuse positivity in all (epithelial and myoepithelial/basaloid) cells was detected in some laboratories and may be antibody- and/or protocol-dependent. CD117 decorates nearly all cells in solid basaloid ACC (34,45). CD117 is negative in ductal carcinoma in situ (DCIS), invasive cribriform carcinoma, and the benign epithelium associated with collagenous spherulosis (CS) (35). However, it is occasionally expressed in AME (46) and basal-like invasive ductal carcinoma of no special type.

MYB

In the breast, MYB IHC (immunohistochemistry) is sensitive and specific for ACC (47,48). Immunohistochemical evidence of nuclear MYB expression (**Fig. 16.9**), predominantly in the basaloid/myoepithelial cells, is detected in both *MYB-NFIB* fusion-positive and fusion-negative ACC. In the absence of

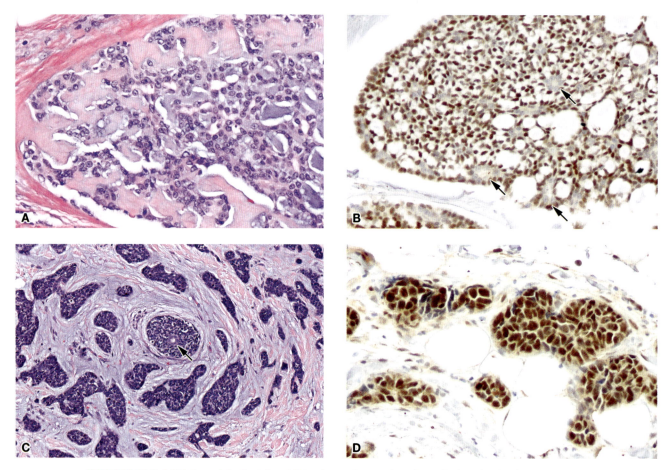

FIGURE 16.9 MYB Reactivity in Adenoid Cystic Carcinoma (ACC). **A:** The basaloid cells of this ACC with cribriform pattern express MYB protein **(B)**. The glandular cells appear negative (arrows). **C:** The basaloid cells in this solid basaloid ACC express strong nuclear reactivity for the MYB protein **(D)**. A small glandular lumen is identified in **(C)** (arrow).

the appropriate tumor morphology, weak or focal MYB immunoreactivity is not diagnostic of ACC, as this can be seen in some triple-negative breast carcinomas and CS (48).

DIFFERENTIAL DIAGNOSIS IN NEEDLE CORE BIOPSY MATERIAL

Invasive Cribriform Carcinoma and Cribriform Ductal Carcinoma In Situ

Invasive cribriform carcinoma is a monophasic ER-positive adenocarcinoma and has no myoepithelial component or intrinsic matrix deposition. Cribriform DCIS shows no internal reactivity for myoepithelial markers, but it is usually surrounded by myoepithelium and basement membrane that are normal components of the duct wall.

Carcinoma With Neuroendocrine Features

Solid basaloid ACC can mimic invasive or in situ solid-papillary carcinoma. The presence of scattered cytokeratin (CK)-positive small glands and focal basement membrane deposits admixed with the solid basaloid proliferation supports the diagnosis of ACC. The differential diagnosis of solid basaloid ACC should be considered whenever an invasive carcinoma with apparent neuroendocrine morphology is negative for ER and PR. The stroma associated with solid basaloid ACC can have a pale blue tinctorial quality that mimics stromal mucin (**Fig. 16.10**). Neuroendocrine markers, such as chromogranin and synaptophysin, are negative in ACC.

Small Cell Carcinoma

Solid basaloid ACC with necrosis can closely resemble a high-grade neuroendocrine carcinoma (small cell carcinoma) primary in the breast or metastatic from another site. In contrast to small cell carcinoma, solid basaloid ACC is TTF1-negative. In addition, ACC has no detectable neuroendocrine differentiation with immunohistochemical stains. In a study of basaloid, small cell, and ACCs of the oropharynx (49), staining for high-molecular-weight keratin 34βE12 was present in basaloid carcinomas and ACCs but absent in small cell carcinomas. The diagnostic utility of 34βE12 staining in the differential diagnosis of ACC and small cell carcinoma in breast NCB material has not been evaluated. A case of ACC merging with small cell carcinoma has been reported (27).

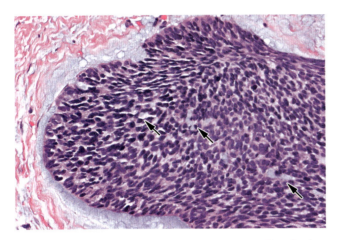

FIGURE 16.10 Solid Adenoid Cystic Carcinoma (ACC). The basaloid cells of this ACC are surrounded by a pale blue rim of basement membrane–like material that superficially resembles stromal mucin. Note that the same pale blue material is also present within the carcinoma (arrows).

High-Grade Carcinoma Arising in Microglandular Adenosis

High-grade carcinoma arising in MGA can resemble the solid basaloid variant of ACC. MGA and MGA-associated carcinomas are characteristically negative for all myoepithelial markers, whereas solid basaloid ACC is typically positive for p63 and SMA.

Adenomyoepithelioma

ACC can arise in association with AME. Both lesions are biphasic (epithelial and myoepithelial), and sometimes they can be difficult to differentiate. The myoepithelial cells of AME are calponin-positive, whereas the basaloid/myoepithelial cells of ACC are typically calponin-negative (see Chapter 5).

Collagenous Spherulosis

CS (see Chapter 4) is a lobular alteration in which benign acini are admixed with globoid deposits of eosinophilic and/or myxoid basement membrane material produced by the myoepithelium. Atypical lobular hyperplasia (ALH) and classic lobular carcinoma in situ (LCIS) frequently involve CS. The combination of glands and spherules of basement membrane material surrounded by myoepithelium found in CS may simulate a cribriform ACC, especially in limited NCB material. The myoepithelium surrounding the spherules of CS reacts with p63, SMA, calponin, and smooth muscle myosin heavy chain, but the latter two antigens are not typically expressed in the basaloid/myoepithelial cells of ACC (35). CS is negative for CD117/KIT (34,35,40,44,45) **(Table 16.1)**.

Small Tubular Proliferations

A limited sample of ACC consisting predominantly of the tubular pattern may raise the differential diagnosis of other proliferations of small infiltrative tubules. Tubular carcinoma is positive for ER and PR and has no myoepithelial component. Typical MGA consists of cytologically bland cells with clear or amphophilic cytoplasm, rather than basaloid cells, and is also negative for myoepithelial markers (other than S-100). Low-grade adenosquamous carcinoma variably expresses myoepithelial markers; the presence of spindle cells highlighted via myosin and calponin surrounding the glands in a lamellar arrangement suggests this diagnosis.

Others

ACC arising in the nipple can resemble a syringomatous adenoma, a benign lesion that does not produce Paget disease. A cylindroma of the skin overlying the breast can also simulate a mammary ACC if one overlooks its superficial location and cutaneous origin. In contrast to ACC, syringomatous adenoma and cylindroma show no cytologic atypia. ACC with conspicuous basement membrane material compressing the glandular elements can simulate invasive lobular carcinoma.

TABLE 16.1
Differential Immunostaining in Adenoid Cystic Carcinoma and Collagenous Spherulosis

	ACC		CS	
	Epithelium	Myoepithelium	Epithelium	Myoepithelium
p63	Negative	Positive	Negative	Positive
SMA	Negative	Positive	Negative	Positive
Calponin	Negative	Negative (typically)	Negative	Positive
SMM-HC	Negative	Negative (typically)	Negative	Positive
CD10	Negative	Negative (typically)	Negative	Positive
ER and PR	Negative	Negative	Positive (scattered)	Negative
CD117/KIT	Positive	Negative/positive	Negative/positive (rare)	Negative
MYB	Positive	Positive	Negative/positive (rare)	Negative

ACC, adenoid cystic carcinoma; CS, collagenous spherulosis.

Metastasis

In patients with a clinical history of extramammary ACC, it is important from both a treatment and prognostic perspective to distinguish primary ACC of the breast from a metastasis. Cases of metastatic ACC to the breast from the salivary gland (50,51) and the cervix (52) have been reported. Morphology and IHC (including GATA3) (53) are often indistinguishable. Salivary ACC is more likely to demonstrate perineural invasion. Ultimately, clinical history is the key.

MOLECULAR TESTING

Molecular testing is seldom required to render the diagnosis of ACC but it can help resolve morphologically ambiguous cases. The canonical *MYB-NFIB* fusion can be demonstrated by FISH or sequencing. ACCs lacking this fusion occasionally harbor *MYB* amplification or *MYBL1* (*MYB*-like-1) rearrangement and overexpression (54). Rare cases with *BRAF* mutation, including *BRAF* V600E, have been reported (55). In a subset of ACCs, the genetic driver has yet to be identified.

Among the solid basaloid subtype, *MYB* rearrangements are seen in less than 20% of cases, despite a high rate of MYB IHC positivity (56). Mutations in *NOTCH* genes and chromatin remodelers such as *CREBBP*, *ARID1A*, and *KMT2C* are present in a subset of cases (56,57). High-grade transformation in classic ACC is also associated with NOTCH pathway, tyrosine kinase receptor, and chromatin remodeler alterations, but unlike in common forms of triple-negative breast cancer *TP53* mutation is generally absent (58).

PROGNOSIS AND MANAGEMENT

Breast-conserving surgery is the preferred primary therapy for mammary ACC (11,12,34,59,60), with the exception of large tumors that require a mastectomy to achieve a negative margin (12). ACC tends to show peripheral infiltration beyond the obvious tumor mass, and wide excision margins are usually recommended (14,23).

Adjuvant radiotherapy is recommended in patients treated with breast-conserving surgery. In a study (59) of 376 women with mammary ACC recorded in the SEER database for the years 1988 to 2005, 53% of 227 patients treated surgically with lumpectomy received adjuvant radiotherapy and showed a survival benefit of 12.4% at 5 years and 19.7% at 10 years compared with patients who were not treated with radiotherapy. Radiotherapy was administered to 66% of 61 patients in one series (12), including 35 patients who received whole-breast irradiation after breast-conserving surgery. After a median follow-up of 79 months, local recurrence developed in 5.7% of the patients who received radiotherapy and in 33% of the patients who did not receive radiotherapy.

ACC rarely metastasizes to LNs. In one study (12), none of the 51 patients with ACC who underwent axillary LN dissection or sentinel LN biopsy had LN involvement. Only 4.9% of 244 women with mammary ACC were treated between 1988 and 2006 and recorded in the California Cancer Registry (5) and 5.1% of 703 women with ACC in the National Cancer Database between 1998 and 2008 (7) had axillary LN metastases. The mean tumor size of ACC with LN metastases was 3.7 cm (range: 1.4-7.7 cm) versus 2.2 cm (range: 0.1-8 cm) for ACC without LN metastases, but the difference was not statistically significant (5). Axillary LN involvement usually carries an adverse prognosis, even though distant metastases can occur independent of LN involvement.

Adjuvant chemotherapy is rarely administered to patients with ACC. Only 11.3% of 933 patients with ACC in the 1998 to 2008 National Cancer Database received chemotherapy versus 45.4% of all patients with breast carcinoma treated in the same period ($P < .0001$) (9). In one series (12), only 24.5% of 61 women with ACC received adjuvant chemotherapy, and none of the 18 patients in another series did (34). Hormonal therapy is usually not prescribed for ACC, as most are hormone receptor-negative. In a study of 23 patients (11), 70% had no adjuvant therapy, 26% had hormonal therapy, and only one patient received chemotherapy.

The overall survival of 61 patients with ACC in the Rare Cancer Network (12) was 94% and 86% at 5 and 10 years, respectively, and the corresponding disease-free survival was 82% and 74%. In one study (5), women with ACC had a relative cumulative survival advantage of approximately 20% after 10 years of follow-up when compared with women with breast carcinoma in general. In another study (9), a patient with ACC treated only by radiotherapy died of disease 2 years after diagnosis. Two patients initially treated with breast-conserving surgery developed local recurrence after 11 and 13 years and were treated surgically; both patients were alive 16 and 19 years after treatment.

All patients with distant metastases have had pulmonary involvement, which usually occurred 6 to 12 years after initial diagnosis (9,61), although some patients developed metastases earlier (19). Other sites of distant metastases include bone (22), liver (22,62), brain (61,63), and kidneys (64).

Overall, patients with mammary ACC have a very good prognosis with a low risk of systemic metastases and death because of ACC.

Although data on the prognosis of ACC with solid basaloid morphology are limited, there is evidence that this variant is clinically more aggressive. Compared with classic ACC, solid basaloid ACC demonstrates higher rates of LN involvement (19-21,57), higher rates of local recurrence and distant metastasis (19,56), and significantly shorter disease-free survival (57,65). In one series of 104 women with mammary ACC, 14% of those with solid basaloid ACC had LN metastasis (vs 0% of classic ACC) and their median invasive disease-free survival was 46.5 months (vs 151.8 months) (57). It should be emphasized that this is a biologically distinct variant, for which axillary staging should be considered.

REFERENCES

1. Brill LB II, Kanner WA, Fehr A, et al. Analysis of MYB expression and MYB-NFIB gene fusions in adenoid cystic carcinoma and other salivary neoplasms. *Mod Pathol*. 2011;24:1169-1176.
2. Persson M, Andren Y, Mark J, et al. Recurrent fusion of MYB and NFIB transcription factor genes in carcinomas of the breast and head and neck. *Proc Natl Acad Sci U S A*. 2009;106:18740-18744.

3. Wetterskog D, Lopez-Garcia MA, Lambros MB, et al. Adenoid cystic carcinomas constitute a genomically distinct subgroup of triple-negative and basal-like breast cancers. *J Pathol*. 2012;226:84-96.

4. McClenathan JH, de la Roza G. Adenoid cystic breast cancer. *Am J Surg*. 2002;183:646-649.

5. Thompson K, Grabowski J, Saltzstein SL, et al. Adenoid cystic breast carcinoma: is axillary staging necessary in all cases? Results from the California Cancer Registry. *Breast J*. 2011;17:485-489.

6. Marchio C, Weigelt B, Reis-Filho JS. Adenoid cystic carcinomas of the breast and salivary glands (or "The strange case of Dr Jekyll and Mr Hyde" of exocrine gland carcinomas). *J Clin Pathol*. 2010;63:220-228.

7. Ghabach B, Anderson WF, Curtis RE, et al. Adenoid cystic carcinoma of the breast in the United States (1977 to 2006): a population-based cohort study. *Breast Cancer Res*. 2010;12:R54.

8. Delanote S, Van den Broecke R, Schelfhout VR, et al. Adenoid cystic carcinoma of the breast in a 19-year-old girl. *Breast*. 2003;12:75-77.

9. Kulkarni N, Pezzi CM, Greif JM, et al. Rare breast cancer: 933 adenoid cystic carcinomas from the National Cancer Data Base. *Ann Surg Oncol*. 2013;20:2236-2241.

10. Rosen PP. Adenoid cystic carcinoma of the breast. A morphologically heterogeneous neoplasm. *Pathol Annu*. 1989;24(Pt 2):237-254.

11. Arpino G, Clark GM, Mohsin S, et al. Adenoid cystic carcinoma of the breast: molecular markers, treatment, and clinical outcome. *Cancer*. 2002;94:2119-2127.

12. Khanfir K, Kallel A, Villette S, et al. Management of adenoid cystic carcinoma of the breast: a Rare Cancer Network study. *Int J Radiat Oncol Biol Phys*. 2012;82:2118-2124.

13. Burga AM, Fadare O, Lininger RA, et al. Invasive carcinomas of the male breast: a morphologic study of the distribution of histologic subtypes and metastatic patterns in 778 cases. *Virchows Arch*. 2006;449:507-512.

14. Hodgson NC, Lytwyn A, Bacopulos S, et al. Adenoid cystic breast carcinoma: high rates of margin positivity after breast conserving surgery. *Am J Clin Oncol*. 2010;33:28-31.

15. Sarnaik AA, Meade T, King J, et al. Adenoid cystic carcinoma of the breast: a review of a single institution's experience. *Breast J*. 2010;16:208-210.

16. Montagna E, Maisonneuve P, Rotmensz N, et al. Heterogeneity of triple-negative breast cancer: histologic subtyping to inform the outcome. *Clin Breast Cancer*. 2013;13:31-39.

17. Glazebrook KN, Reynolds C, Smith RL, et al. Adenoid cystic carcinoma of the breast. *AJR Am J Roentgenol*. 2010;194:1391-1396.

18. Saqi A, Mercado CL, Hamele-Bena D. Adenoid cystic carcinoma of the breast diagnosed by fine-needle aspiration. *Diagn Cytopathol*. 2004;30:271-274.

19. D'Alfonso TM, Mosquera JM, MacDonald TY, et al. MYB-NFIB gene fusion in adenoid cystic carcinoma of the breast with special focus paid to the solid variant with basaloid features. *Hum Pathol*. 2014;45:2270-2280.

20. Foschini MP, Rizzo A, De Leo A, et al. Solid variant of adenoid cystic carcinoma of the breast: a case series with proposal of a new grading system. *Int J Surg Pathol*. 2016;24:97-102.

21. Shin SJ, Rosen PP. Solid variant of mammary adenoid cystic carcinoma with basaloid features: a study of nine cases. *Am J Surg Pathol*. 2002;26:413-420.

22. Ro JY, Silva EG, Gallager HS. Adenoid cystic carcinoma of the breast. *Hum Pathol*. 1987;18:1276-1281.

23. Kleer CG, Oberman HA. Adenoid cystic carcinoma of the breast: value of histologic grading and proliferative activity. *Am J Surg Pathol*. 1998;22:569-575.

24. Spyrou A, Katsourakis A, Chytas D, et al. Combination of adenomyoepithelioma and adenoid cystic carcinoma of the breast: a case report of an uncommon histopathological entity. *Am J Case Rep*. 2022;23:e934391.

25. Yang Y, Wang Y, He J, et al. Malignant adenomyoepithelioma combined with adenoid cystic carcinoma of the breast: a case report and literature review. *Diagn Pathol*. 2014;9:148.

26. Noske A, Schwabe M, Pahl S, et al. Report of a metaplastic carcinoma of the breast with multi-directional differentiation: an adenoid cystic carcinoma, a spindle cell carcinoma and melanoma. *Virchows Arch*. 2008;452:575-579.

27. Cabibi D, Cipolla C, Maria Florena A, et al. Solid variant of mammary "adenoid cystic carcinoma with basaloid features" merging with "small cell carcinoma." *Pathol Res Pract*. 2005;201:705-711.

28. Wells J, Ozerdem U, Scognamiglio T, et al. Invasive mammary adenoid cystic carcinoma with an intraductal component. *Breast J*. 2016;22:233-234.

29. Acs G, Simpson JF, Bleiweiss IJ, et al. Microglandular adenosis with transition into adenoid cystic carcinoma of the breast. *Am J Surg Pathol*. 2003;27:1052-1060.

30. Shin SJ, Simpson PT, Da Silva L, et al. Molecular evidence for progression of microglandular adenosis (MGA) to invasive carcinoma. *Am J Surg Pathol*. 2009;33:496-504.

31. Da Silva L, Buck L, Simpson PT, et al. Molecular and morphological analysis of adenoid cystic carcinoma of the breast with synchronous tubular adenosis. *Virchows Arch*. 2009;454:107-114.

32. Blanco M, Egozi L, Lubin D, et al. Adenoid cystic carcinoma arising in a fibroadenoma. *Ann Diagn Pathol*. 2005;9:157-159.

33. Van Dorpe J, De Pauw A, Moerman P. Adenoid cystic carcinoma arising in an adenomyoepithelioma of the breast. *Virchows Arch*. 1998;432:119-122.

34. Azoulay S, Lae M, Freneaux P, et al. KIT is highly expressed in adenoid cystic carcinoma of the breast, a basal-like carcinoma associated with a favorable outcome. *Mod Pathol*. 2005;18:1623-1631.

35. Rabban JT, Swain RS, Zaloudek CJ, et al. Immunophenotypic overlap between adenoid cystic carcinoma and collagenous spherulosis of the breast:

potential diagnostic pitfalls using myoepithelial markers. *Mod Pathol*. 2006;19:1351-1357.

36. Reis-Filho JS, Milanezi F, Silva P, et al. Maspin expression in myoepithelial tumors of the breast. *Pathol Res Pract*. 2001;197:817-821.

37. Cabibi D, Giannone AG, Belmonte B, et al. CD10 and HHF35 actin in the differential diagnosis between collagenous spherulosis and adenoid-cystic carcinoma of the breast. *Pathol Res Pract*. 2012;208:405-409.

38. Nakai T, Ichihara S, Kada A, et al. The unique luminal staining pattern of cytokeratin 5/6 in adenoid cystic carcinoma of the breast may aid in differentiating it from its mimickers. *Virchows Arch*. 2016;469:213-222.

39. Vranic S, Gatalica Z, Deng H, et al. ER-alpha36, a novel isoform of ER-alpha66, is commonly over-expressed in apocrine and adenoid cystic carcinomas of the breast. *J Clin Pathol*. 2011;64:54-57.

40. Mastropasqua MG, Maiorano E, Pruneri G, et al. Immunoreactivity for c-kit and p63 as an adjunct in the diagnosis of adenoid cystic carcinoma of the breast. *Mod Pathol*. 2005;18:1277-1282.

41. Yoon EC, Wang G, Parkinson B, et al. TRPS1, GATA3, and SOX10 expression in triple-negative breast carcinoma. *Hum Pathol*. 2022;125:97-107.

42. Ivanov SV, Panaccione A, Nonaka D, et al. Diagnostic SOX10 gene signatures in salivary adenoid cystic and breast basal-like carcinomas. *Br J Cancer*. 2013;109:444-451.

43. Yang C, Zhang L, Sanati S. SOX10 is a sensitive marker for breast and salivary gland adenoid cystic carcinoma: immunohistochemical characterization of adenoid cystic carcinomas. *Breast Cancer (Auckl)*. 2019;13:1178223419842185.

44. Pastolero G, Hanna W, Zbieranowski I, et al. Proliferative activity and p53 expression in adenoid cystic carcinoma of the breast. *Mod Pathol*. 1996;9:215-219.

45. Crisi GM, Marconi SA, Makari-Judson G, et al. Expression of c-kit in adenoid cystic carcinoma of the breast. *Am J Clin Pathol*. 2005;124:733-739.

46. Hungermann D, Buerger H, Oehlschlegel C, et al. Adenomyoepithelial tumours and myoepithelial carcinomas of the breast—a spectrum of monophasic and biphasic tumours dominated by immature myoepithelial cells. *BMC Cancer*. 2005;5:92.

47. Cimino-Mathews A. Novel uses of immunohistochemistry in breast pathology: interpretation and pitfalls. *Mod Pathol*. 2021;34:62-77.

48. Poling JS, Yonescu R, Subhawong AP, et al. MYB labeling by immunohistochemistry is more sensitive and specific for breast adenoid cystic carcinoma than MYB labeling by FISH. *Am J Surg Pathol*. 2017;41:973-979.

49. Morice WG, Ferreiro JA. Distinction of basaloid squamous cell carcinoma from adenoid cystic and small cell undifferentiated carcinoma by immunohistochemistry. *Hum Pathol*. 1998;29:609-612.

50. Khazai L, Falcon S, Rosa M. Metastatic salivary duct carcinoma to the breast. *Breast J*. 2016;22:461-463.

51. Krucoff KB, Shammas RL, Stoecker M, et al. Rare breast metastasis from adenoid cystic carcinoma of the submandibular gland. *BMJ Case Rep*. 2018;2018:bcr2017223345.

52. Surer Budak E, Yildirim S, Yildiz S, et al. Two uncommon sites of metastasis: breast and hypophysis metastases of head and neck adenoid cystic carcinoma detected by FDG PET/CT. *Mol Imaging Radionucl Ther*. 2017;26:120-123.

53. Schwartz LE, Begum S, Westra WH, et al. GATA3 immunohistochemical expression in salivary gland neoplasms. *Head Neck Pathol*. 2013;7:311-315.

54. Kim J, Geyer FC, Martelotto LG, et al. MYBL1 rearrangements and MYB amplification in breast adenoid cystic carcinomas lacking the MYB-NFIB fusion gene. *J Pathol*. 2018;244:143-150.

55. Wetterskog D, Wilkerson PM, Rodrigues DN, et al. Mutation profiling of adenoid cystic carcinomas from multiple anatomical sites identifies mutations in the RAS pathway, but no KIT mutations. *Histopathology*. 2013;62:543-550.

56. Masse J, Truntzer C, Boidot R, et al. Solid-type adenoid cystic carcinoma of the breast, a distinct molecular entity enriched in NOTCH and CREBBP mutations. *Mod Pathol*. 2020;33:1041-1055.

57. Schwartz CJ, Brogi E, Marra A, et al. The clinical behavior and genomic features of the so-called adenoid cystic carcinomas of the solid variant with basaloid features. *Mod Pathol*. 2022;35:193-201.

58. Fusco N, Geyer FC, De Filippo MR, et al. Genetic events in the progression of adenoid cystic carcinoma of the breast to high-grade triple-negative breast cancer. *Mod Pathol*. 2016;29:1292-1305.

59. Coates JM, Martinez SR, Bold RJ, et al. Adjuvant radiation therapy is associated with improved survival for adenoid cystic carcinoma of the breast. *J Surg Oncol*. 2010;102:342-347.

60. Millar BA, Kerba M, Youngson B, et al. The potential role of breast conservation surgery and adjuvant breast radiation for adenoid cystic carcinoma of the breast. *Breast Cancer Res Treat*. 2004;87:225-232.

61. Koller M, Ram Z, Findler G, et al. Brain metastasis: a rare manifestation of adenoid cystic carcinoma of the breast. *Surg Neurol*. 1986;26:470-472.

62. Gillie B, Kmeid M, Asarian A, et al. Adenoid cystic carcinoma of the breast with distant metastasis to the liver and spleen: a case report. *J Surg Case Rep*. 2020;2020:rjaa483.

63. Silva I, Tome V, Oliveira J. Adenoid cystic carcinoma of the breast with cerebral metastisation: a clinical novelty. *BMJ Case Rep*. 2011;2011:bcr0820114692.

64. Mhamdi HA, Kourie HR, Jungels C, et al. Adenoid cystic carcinoma of the breast—an aggressive presentation with pulmonary, kidney, and brain metastases: a case report. *J Med Case Rep*. 2017;11:303.

65. Slodkowska E, Xu B, Kos Z, et al. Predictors of outcome in mammary adenoid cystic carcinoma: a multi-institutional study. *Am J Surg Pathol*. 2020;44:214-223.

Other Special Types of Invasive Breast Carcinoma

17

ELAINE W. ZHONG AND SYED A. HODA

INTRODUCTION

Breast carcinomas can exhibit a variety of distinctive histologic patterns. Per the *World Health Organization (WHO) Classification of Tumours* (1), the category of pure invasive carcinoma of special type should be reserved for those tumors in which at least 90% of the entire excised carcinoma demonstrates the characteristic growth pattern. This criterion cannot be applied in needle core biopsy (NCB) specimens; therefore, one can reasonably diagnose "invasive ductal carcinoma with X features" based on examination of limited sampling in an NCB.

Some of the special variants—namely cystic hypersecretory, glycogen-rich, and lipid-rich carcinoma and mammary carcinoma with osteoclast-like giant cells—may or may not truly represent distinctive entities. More studies will be needed to determine whether these should be considered clinically distinct types of carcinomas.

INVASIVE MICROPAPILLARY CARCINOMA

Invasive micropapillary carcinoma is a distinctive form of ductal carcinoma in which the tumor cells grow in morule-like clusters creating an "exfoliative appearance" (2). This growth pattern may be found throughout the lesion (*pure invasive micropapillary carcinoma*) or as part of an otherwise conventional invasive ductal carcinoma (*mixed invasive micropapillary carcinoma*). Pure invasive micropapillary carcinomas account for 0.9% to 2% of the cases in two study groups, each consisting of approximately 1,000 breast carcinomas (3,4). Mixed invasive micropapillary carcinoma occurs more commonly. For example, Pettinato et al (5) observed a micropapillary pattern in 3.8% of 1,635 breast carcinomas, and Luna-Moré et al (6) detected micropapillary differentiation in 27 of 986 (2.7%) consecutive breast carcinomas.

Clinical Features

The reported age at diagnosis ranges from 25 to 92 years, and the mean ages in several series fall in the sixth decade. Patients with lesions composed of more than 50% invasive micropapillary carcinoma tend to be older than patients with less extensive micropapillary growth (6). The literature contains only a few well-documented reports of pure invasive micropapillary carcinoma in men (7-9).

The majority of patients present with a palpable mass. Less frequently, routine imaging reveals a suspicious density, an irregular mass, a region of calcifications, or another suspicious finding (10,11).

The reported carcinomas span from 0.1 to 11 cm. Tumors with more than 50% micropapillary growth tend to be larger (mean size 6 cm) than those with a lesser amount of this pattern (mean size 3.5 cm) (6). The presence of multiple nodules has been noted (5).

Histopathologic Evaluation

The invasive carcinoma cells are cuboidal to columnar and contain finely granular or dense, eosinophilic cytoplasm, with intermediate- to high-grade nuclei. The tumor cells grow in minute clusters, which have serrated peripheral borders and sometimes surround central lumina (**Fig. 17.1**). The clusters lack fibrovascular cores and exhibit an "inside-out" arrangement, with the nucleus facing the outer surface of the cluster. The appearance has been described as "hollow balls of cells." No true papillary structure is evident. Uncommon variants feature microcystic dilatation of lumina within cell clusters and apocrine change. Mucin may be present. Necrosis and lymphocytic infiltration are not typical features; however, large tumors may undergo necrosis, and a lymphoid infiltrate may permeate the stroma. Microcalcifications, sometimes with psammomatous features, are variably present.

A clear space outlined by stroma surrounds each tumor cell cluster. An endothelial lining is not present. These spaces are usually attributed to shrinkage of the clusters during tissue fixation. The presence of these retraction spaces in NCB of breast carcinoma has been found to be highly predictive of lymph node metastasis (12). The spaces generally appear empty, but in some instances mucinous material has been demonstrated using special stains (6). The stroma consists of dense collagenous tissue or a network of delicate collagen bundles. Myxoid stroma has been noted in a minority of cases. The sponge-like pattern of spaces filled by tumor cell clusters is duplicated in metastatic foci.

The proclivity of the carcinoma to grow in a sponge-like pattern makes it difficult to identify lymphatic tumor emboli. By using antibodies to factor VIII and CD31 to mark

OTHER SPECIAL TYPES OF INVASIVE BREAST CARCINOMA 311

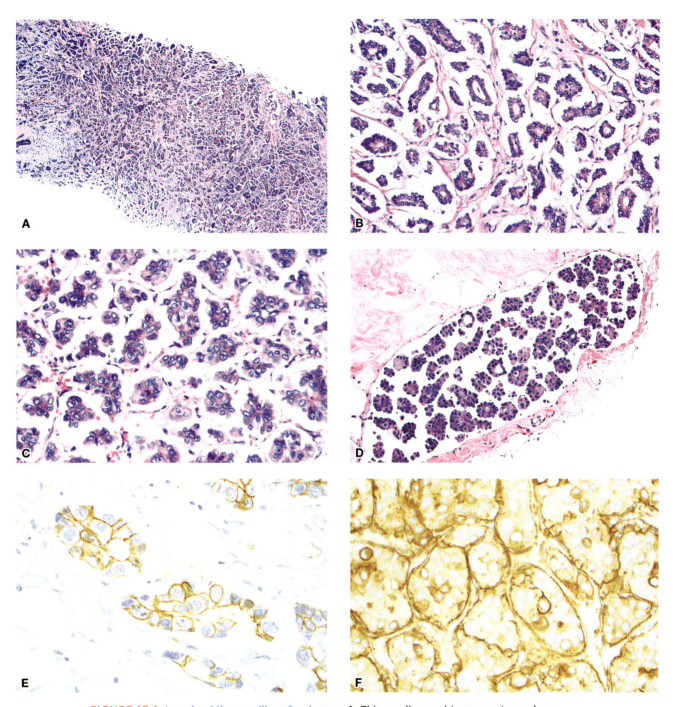

FIGURE 17.1 Invasive Micropapillary Carcinoma. A: This needle core biopsy specimen shows small nests of carcinoma cells outlined by clear spaces. **B, C:** The "inside-out" pattern consists of morule-like solid clusters of tumor cells with serrated outer borders. The spaces between the carcinoma cells and the stroma are devoid of secretion. **D:** Clusters of invasive micropapillary carcinoma occupy the lumen of a lymphatic vessel. **E:** The neoplastic cells show a characteristic "basolateral" or "U-shaped" staining pattern for HER2. According to the American Society of Clinical Oncology/College of American Pathologists (ASCO/CAP) guidelines, this pattern of staining is equivocal (2+) and HER2 FISH is required to rule out *ERBB2* amplification. **F:** EMA decorates the stroma-facing surface of micropapillary tumor clusters, documenting reverse polarity.

vascular endothelium, Pettinato et al (5) demonstrated lymphovascular invasion in 63% of tumors. Intravascular carcinoma cells form micropapillary clusters similar to invasive primary carcinoma.

Mixed invasive micropapillary carcinomas usually show a sharp demarcation between the micropapillary and conventional components. The latter typically has the conventional ductal pattern, but invasive mucinous, lobular, cribriform, metaplastic, and tubular types have been reported (11,13-16).

Ductal carcinoma in situ (DCIS) coexists with invasive carcinoma in most cases. In pure invasive micropapillary carcinoma, the DCIS usually has a micropapillary or cribriform architecture, but solid DCIS sometimes occurs. The noninvasive cells usually possess intermediate-grade nuclei. Prominent necrosis tends to occur in tumors with only a focal invasive micropapillary pattern, and the carcinoma cells in these cases usually have high-grade nuclei. Calcifications are sometimes found in the noninvasive component.

Ultrastructure and Immunohistochemistry

Ultrastructural study has revealed microvilli on the cell surfaces that border the clear spaces. This finding suggests that the cells are oriented as though the spaces around the tumor cell clusters were glandular lumina (6). The distribution of mucin-1 (MUC-1) glycoprotein (aka epithelial membrane antigen, EMA) supports this interpretation. MUC-1 localizes to the apical cell membrane in conventional, gland-forming breast carcinomas, where the glycoprotein contributes to the formation of lumina. In invasive micropapillary carcinoma, MUC-1 localizes on the stroma-facing external surfaces of papillary tumor clusters (adjacent to the surrounding stroma) (6,17). This reversal of cell polarity has also been observed in intralymphatic clusters of micropapillary carcinoma (18,19).

Most cases of invasive micropapillary carcinoma stain for E-cadherin, although Pettinato et al (5) noted that reactivity was limited to cell membranes between carcinoma cells ("basolateral") and that the cell membranes abutting the stroma (apical portion) did not stain. This pattern is a "mirror image" of that seen with MUC-1. In one series (20), all 12 examples of invasive micropapillary carcinoma stained for GATA3. The tumors typically do not stain for cytokeratin (CK)5/6, CK14, CK20, EGFR, or c-kit. The majority of invasive micropapillary carcinomas are immunoreactive for estrogen receptor (ER) and progesterone receptor (PR), and human epidermal growth factor receptor 2 (HER2) overexpression or gene amplification occurs in 10% to 50% of the cases (8,11,21). HER2 immunohistochemical staining in some micropapillary carcinomas yields U-shaped basolateral staining that spares the luminal cell membrane. This pattern should be regarded as equivocal; and the tumor should be "reflexed" to in situ hybridization (22,23). A minority of cases (5%-10%) are triple-negative.

Differential Diagnosis

The differential diagnosis of invasive micropapillary carcinoma includes conventional invasive ductal carcinoma with prominent retraction of the malignant cells from the stroma and metastatic (nonmammary) micropapillary carcinoma. The carcinoma cells in commonplace invasive carcinoma with prominent retraction artifact do not display the complete reversal of cell polarity characteristic of invasive micropapillary carcinoma, nor do they exhibit strong peripheral linear membrane staining for EMA. One can detect focal (<5%) peripheral linear membrane EMA staining in as many as 50% of conventional invasive carcinomas (24) and robust linear membrane staining in clusters of conventional carcinoma cells within lymphatic vessels (18,19). Staining for EMA must be evaluated carefully whenever the diagnosis of invasive micropapillary carcinoma is suspected.

The ovary represents the most common origin of metastatic micropapillary carcinoma in the breast. Other possible sites include the lung, urinary bladder, and colon. The presence of an intraductal component serves as strong evidence to support primary breast carcinoma. In the absence of an in situ component, immunohistochemical staining for CA-125 and WT1 may help to distinguish an ovarian carcinoma from a mammary carcinoma. Lee et al (25) observed membranous staining for CA-125 in 18% of invasive micropapillary breast carcinomas and cytoplasmic staining for the protein in 3% of the same group. This marker was identified in more than 90% of serous papillary ovarian carcinomas, usually in 80% to 100% of the cells. WT1 nuclear staining was found in 26% of invasive micropapillary breast carcinomas, typically in fewer than 10% of cells, and weak cytoplasmic staining, at high magnification, was seen in 59% of the tumors. Only 1 of 34 invasive micropapillary breast carcinomas displayed both nuclear reactivity for WT1 and cytoplasmic reactivity for CA-125. The presence of diffuse nuclear expression of WT1 and strong staining for CA-125 of a micropapillary carcinoma in the breast strongly favors the diagnosis of metastatic ovarian carcinoma. Detection of proteins suggestive of Müllerian origin such as PAX8 and PAX2 or those typical of mammary origin such as mammaglobin and GATA3 (26,27) may also help in this regard. The results of immunohistochemical staining for other markers and clinical investigations will usually exclude the diagnosis of metastatic carcinoma originating from the lung, urinary bladder, and other sites (27).

Uncommon examples of invasive micropapillary carcinoma feature the presence of abundant extracellular mucin. Whole-exome sequencing has suggested that such carcinomas represent a convergent phenotype between invasive micropapillary and mucinous carcinoma (28). It may be difficult to distinguish such tumors (which have been termed *invasive micropapillary mucinous carcinoma*) from conventional mucinous carcinomas. The tumor cell clusters in conventional mucinous carcinoma usually exhibit a smooth outer contour rather than the serrated shape seen in invasive micropapillary carcinoma. Furthermore, the cell clusters in the former do not display the "inside-out" micropapillary arrangement characteristic of the latter. In contrast to conventional mucinous carcinomas, 20% of micropapillary mucinous carcinomas are HER2-positive (14).

Prognosis and Treatment

Compared to conventional invasive ductal carcinoma of similar size and receptor status, invasive micropapillary carcinomas tend to present at higher stage, more often have an intermediate or high histologic grade, and have a higher likelihood of lymphovascular invasion and metastasis to local lymph nodes (29). Despite these unfavorable features, the 5-year disease-specific survival and overall survival of patients with invasive micropapillary carcinoma did not differ from those of patients with conventional breast carcinoma in a large study using the Surveillance, Epidemiology, and End Results (SEER) database (29). In one study (16), patients with stage I invasive micropapillary mucinous carcinoma experienced the same overall survival and recurrence-free survival as patients with pure conventional mucinous carcinoma. Patients with higher-stage (II and III) invasive micropapillary mucinous carcinoma had survival rates between those of patients with pure mucinous carcinoma and conventional invasive micropapillary carcinoma.

The propensity of micropapillary carcinoma to spread to axillary lymph nodes necessitates careful staging of the axilla. Recommendation for treatment usually follows that of conventional invasive ductal carcinomas.

INVASIVE CRIBRIFORM CARCINOMA

Invasive cribriform carcinoma consists of lower-grade carcinoma cells growing in cribriform, and also tubular, patterns. Whether or not invasive cribriform carcinoma represents a low-grade variant of invasive ductal carcinoma or a specific subtype of carcinoma remains to be established. Fewer than 4% of invasive mammary carcinomas are invasive cribriform carcinomas (30-33).

Clinical Features

The ages of the female patients ranged from 7 to 91 years. Three reported patients were men (32,34,35). Choi et al (36) described a 6-cm invasive cribriform carcinoma occupying a 10-cm malignant phyllodes tumor in a 62-year-old woman.

In a study of eight cases, mammograms revealed spiculated masses spanning 20 to 35 mm in four patients (37). Two of these carcinomas contained calcifications, as did the carcinoma described by Nishimura et al (35). Invasive cribriform carcinomas do not have consistent sonographic findings (35,38). Some cases exhibit findings typically seen in benign breast lesions such as parallel orientation and lack of acoustic shadowing (34). Magnetic resonance imaging (MRI) performed on one tumor displayed findings compatible with a carcinoma (38). Data from several studies suggest that a minority of invasive cribriform carcinomas are multifocal (31,33).

Histopathologic Evaluation

Invasive cribriform carcinoma exhibits essentially the same sieve-like growth pattern that characterizes conventional cribriform DCIS, albeit with an infiltrative pattern. The rounded and angular masses of uniform, well-differentiated tumor cells are embedded in variable amounts of collagenous stroma. Sharply outlined, round, or oval glandular spaces are haphazardly distributed throughout these tumor aggregates, creating a fenestrated appearance (**Fig. 17.2**). The invasive cribriform pattern should be accorded a score of 1 for tubule formation (even though cribriform architecture does not display typical tubule formation), and as such invasive cribriform carcinomas are generally Nottingham grade 1 tumors. Variable amounts of mucin occupy the lumina (39), which may also contain calcifications (40). The in situ carcinoma also has a cribriform pattern in most, but not all, invasive cribriform carcinomas.

Besides displaying a cribriform pattern, invasive cribriform carcinomas can show areas of tubular growth (**Fig. 17.3**), and such foci can comprise a substantial

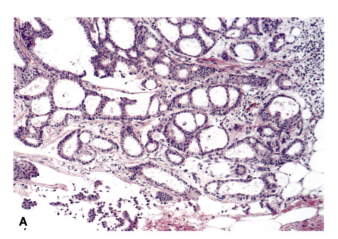 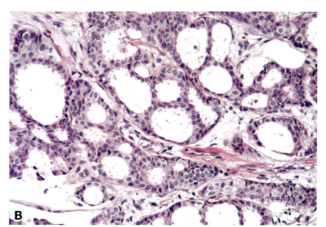

FIGURE 17.2 **Invasive Cribriform Carcinoma. A, B:** The invasive carcinoma in this needle core biopsy specimen has a cribriform structure composed of round or oval glandular spaces formed by thin, rigid bands of tumor cells with low-grade nuclei.

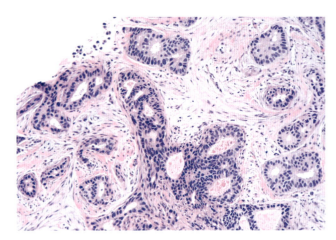

FIGURE 17.3 Invasive Cribriform Carcinoma. In the region shown, the cribriform carcinoma in this needle core biopsy specimen has tubular features.

proportion of the lesion (31-33). The presence of regions showing a tubular pattern does not itself justify the use of the diagnosis of tubular carcinoma. Tumors composed of both cribriform and tubular areas in which each pattern accounts for more than 10% of the mass should be classified as mixed cribriform and tubular carcinomas. When the tubular pattern represents more than 90% of the mass, one should render the diagnosis of tubular carcinoma if the cytologic and architectural features of the tubules are appropriate. Most NCB specimens do not provide sufficient material to allow one to evaluate the proportions of these two patterns. Notably, pure invasive cribriform carcinoma is far less common than tubular carcinoma.

Immunohistochemistry

Demir et al (34) reported that 16 of 16 invasive cribriform carcinomas were both ER-positive and PR-positive. Others have reported positive staining for ER, variable staining for PR, and lack of staining for HER2 (35,41,42), although rare HER2-positive examples have been reported (33,34).

Differential Diagnosis

Invasive cribriform carcinoma should be distinguished from adenoid cystic carcinoma. Cribriform growth of an invasive cribriform carcinoma produces a fenestrated structural pattern that lacks the cylindromatous components composed of basement membrane material characteristic of adenoid cystic carcinoma. Although adenoid cystic carcinomas can contain regions showing prominent cribriform pattern (43), one should not interpret the presence of such regions in an adenoid cystic carcinoma as evidence of a component of invasive cribriform carcinoma. Occasionally, invasive cribriform carcinoma simulates in situ cribriform carcinoma; irregular contours of the cribriform structures, infiltration into fat, and absence of peripheral myoepithelial cells aid the diagnosis.

Prognosis and Treatment

The majority of patients described in published reports were treated by mastectomy and axillary dissection. The authors of three studies concluded that patients with invasive cribriform carcinoma were less likely to develop axillary lymph node metastases than women with invasive ductal carcinoma (32,33). One case report (41) documents spread to an internal mammary lymph node without involvement of the axillary sentinel lymph node.

Deaths attributable to classic invasive cribriform carcinoma did not occur among 34 patients studied by Page et al (31) with follow-up intervals of 10 to 21 years. One patient was alive with recurrent invasive cribriform carcinoma, and another died of metastases from a contralateral carcinoma. Venable et al (32) reported a disease-free survival of 100% among 45 patients with invasive cribriform carcinoma followed up for 1 to 5 years. In the study of Cong et al (44), one of eight patients with invasive cribriform carcinoma developed a local recurrence, but the other seven remained free of carcinoma with a median follow-up of 38 months.

Using the SEER database, Liu et al (45) compared clinical and pathologic findings of more than 600 invasive cribriform carcinomas with those of invasive ductal carcinoma. The investigators found that invasive cribriform carcinomas were relatively smaller, less likely to involve lymph nodes, more often positive for ER and PR, and less often positive for HER2 than were conventional invasive carcinomas. Approximately 60% of patients in this study were treated with breast conservation therapy. Patients with invasive cribriform carcinoma experienced greater disease-specific survival and overall survival than those with conventional carcinomas. The improvement in survival appears to depend on the more favorable staging and receptor profile of invasive cribriform carcinoma. When corrected for these confounding features, patients with invasive cribriform carcinoma did not show more favorable survival than those with conventional carcinomas.

The foregoing data suggest that breast conservation therapy is feasible if an adequate excision can be achieved, but the possibility of encountering multifocal lesions should be borne in mind. Axillary staging by sentinel lymph node mapping is appropriate.

SECRETORY CARCINOMA

Secretory carcinoma features abundant pink or amphophilic intracellular and extracellular (ie, within the cytoplasm of the carcinoma cells and the lumina of the spaces formed by the carcinoma cells) secretory material—similar to its counterpart in the salivary gland. Although secretory carcinoma is an uncommon (<0.2%) type of breast carcinoma, and the majority of cases occur in adults, it is the most common breast carcinoma in children. The cytologic and histopathologic characteristics of the lesion are alike in patients of all ages.

Secretory carcinoma is the only breast carcinoma with the balanced translocation t(12;15)(p13;q25), resulting in the *ETV6-NTRK3* gene fusion tyrosine kinase product.

Clinical Features

Secretory carcinoma affects individuals throughout life. The reported ages of females with secretory carcinoma range from 2 to 96 years (46,47). Male patients exhibit a similar age range (3-79 years) (48,49). There is a dearth of cases of secretory carcinoma in girls 10 to 15 years of age, and cases in males cluster in the pediatric and adolescent age groups.

Most patients describe a painless, circumscribed mass that may have been present for one or more years. A subareolar tumor is most common in prepubertal girls and males of all ages because their breast tissue is localized in this region. Among women, the upper outer quadrant is the most common location. Secretory carcinoma usually grows as a single mass, but rare cases present with two or more nodules (50,51). Secretory carcinomas have arisen in axillary breast tissue (52,53) and from adnexal glands of the axillary skin (54). Nipple discharge is uncommon.

Pregnancy has not been implicated in the development of secretory carcinoma, nor has there been any clinical evidence of a hormonal abnormality that would explain the secretory properties of this carcinoma. Be that as it may, secretory carcinoma developed in the breast of a male-to-female transsexual individual, who had undergone "long-term cross-sex hormone treatment" of an unspecified nature (55).

Associated breast conditions have been described in a few cases. Gynecomastia accompanied a minority of the secretory carcinomas in male patients. The coexistence of juvenile papillomatosis (JP) and secretory carcinoma has been reported (56), but the evidence presented to substantiate the diagnosis of JP is not convincing in several other reports.

Mammography typically reveals a discrete tumor with smooth or irregular borders (50,57,58), which one could mistake for fibroadenoma or papilloma. Sonography discloses a solid, hypoechoic to isoechoic mass, which may have a microlobulated border (50,59).

Secretory carcinoma usually forms a circumscribed, firm mass, which may be lobulated; rarely, the tumor has infiltrative margin. The tumors tend to be 3 cm or smaller in greatest dimension (60), although carcinomas spanning 10 cm were reported in two women (61,62) and another spanning 12.5 cm was reported in a man (63).

Histopathologic Evaluation

Like other forms of ductal carcinoma, secretory carcinoma may exhibit an intraductal component. Kameyama et al (58) described a purely noninvasive form of secretory carcinoma. Most commonly, the DCIS has a papillary or cribriform pattern of growth, but solid foci and, rarely, central necrosis may also be found. The invasive component tends to form a compact mass subdivided by fibrous septa. The borders of the carcinoma usually appear circumscribed, but overtly infiltrative growth is sometimes present. The neoplastic cells grow in papillary, microcystic, and glandular formations.

The tumor cells vary from secretory to apocrine in their appearance. Cells of a secretory nature possess pale to clear, pink or amphophilic cytoplasm that contains abundant secretion. The low-grade nuclei vary from small to modest in size, and their chromatin from dark and finely dispersed to pale and granular (**Fig. 17.4**). Nuclei with pale chromatin usually contain minute, uniform nucleoli. Cells with apocrine features contain granular, eosinophilic cytoplasm and nuclei with features similar to those of conventional apocrine cells (**Fig. 17.5**). Both types of cells can be found in a carcinoma, although one type or the other can predominate. On occasion, cells with apocrine features growing in a solid pattern comprise most of the tumor and thereby obscure the secretory nature of the carcinoma. The cells do not display noticeable mitotic activity or necrosis. Calcifications in the neoplastic glands or the stroma are uncommon.

Secretion accumulates in the tumor cells, in the glands formed by the tumor cells, and in the microcystic spaces associated with the tumor cells. The secretory material appears pale pink or amphophilic with hematoxylin and eosin (H&E) staining, and it often contains lacunae, which

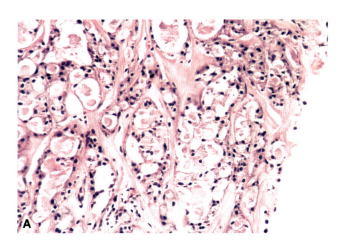 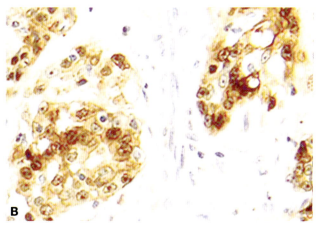

FIGURE 17.4 **Secretory Carcinoma.** This needle core biopsy specimen comes from a circumscribed 2-cm tumor in a 68-year-old woman. **A:** The carcinoma has the characteristic microcystic architecture. The tumor cells in this example have small, low-grade nuclei. **B:** S-100 is positive in secretory carcinoma.

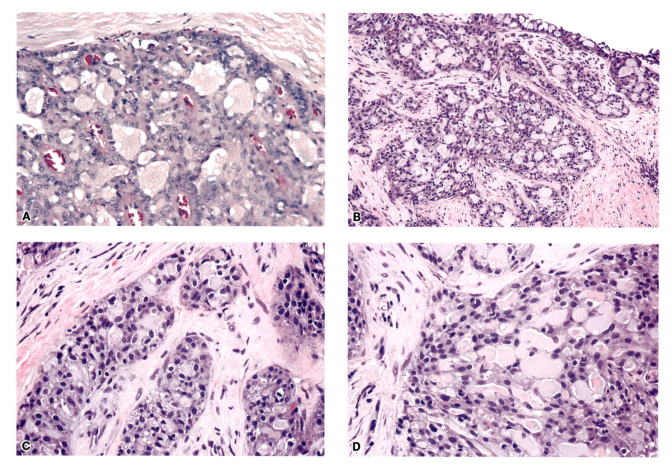

FIGURE 17.5 Secretory Carcinoma With Apocrine Cytology. A: The lesion has a well-circumscribed border and a microcystic growth pattern. The nuclei have prominent nucleoli typically associated with apocrine differentiation. **B-D:** Secretory carcinoma in needle core biopsy samples from a 41-year-old woman. Note the apocrine cytologic features, the irregular shapes of the microcystic spaces, and the dense secretions.

create a "bubbly" appearance. The secretion stains with the periodic acid–Schiff (PAS) and Alcian blue methods, and PAS staining persists after diastase digestion. The secretory material reacts variably for mucicarmine. The secretion in microcystic areas resembles thyroid colloid and that which accumulates in cystic hypersecretory lesions of the breast (**Fig. 17.6**).

Differential Diagnosis

Pathologists should not have difficulty recognizing secretory carcinoma when they have sufficient material to study. It may require excision of the mass to provide an adequate sample, but the diagnosis can be suspected in a needle aspiration or NCB specimen (50). Other lesions to consider include cystic hypersecretory carcinoma (CHC), apocrine carcinoma, microglandular adenosis (MGA), and "acinic cell carcinoma."

In most CHCs, DCIS constitutes either the exclusive or the dominant component. It gives rise to dilated ducts and acini lined by cells that possess intermediate- to high-grade nuclei and lack prominent cytoplasmic vacuolization. Apocrine carcinomas do not demonstrate the evidence of secretory activity seen in secretory carcinomas. MGA consists of an orderly proliferation of uniform small, round glands displaying open lumina, lined by small uniform cells with bland nuclei and encircled by basement membrane. "Acinic cell carcinoma" (64) is composed of cells with abundant granular cytoplasm in solid, microglandular, and microcystic formations; and is usually associated with MGA. The cells stain for salivary-type amylase, a protein not characteristic of secretory carcinomas, but "acinic cell carcinomas" fail to stain for acidophilin seen in secretory carcinomas (65).

Immunohistochemistry and Molecular Studies

The results of staining for cellular markers do not differ among secretory carcinomas from females and males nor among tumors from children and adults. Strong staining for α-lactalbumin has been reported (66). The carcinoma cells stain for CK, EMA, E-cadherin, mammaglobin, and, with rare exceptions (67), S-100 protein and SOX10. One report (68) documents nuclear staining for p63 in three of seven cases and staining of the cytoplasm and secretory material

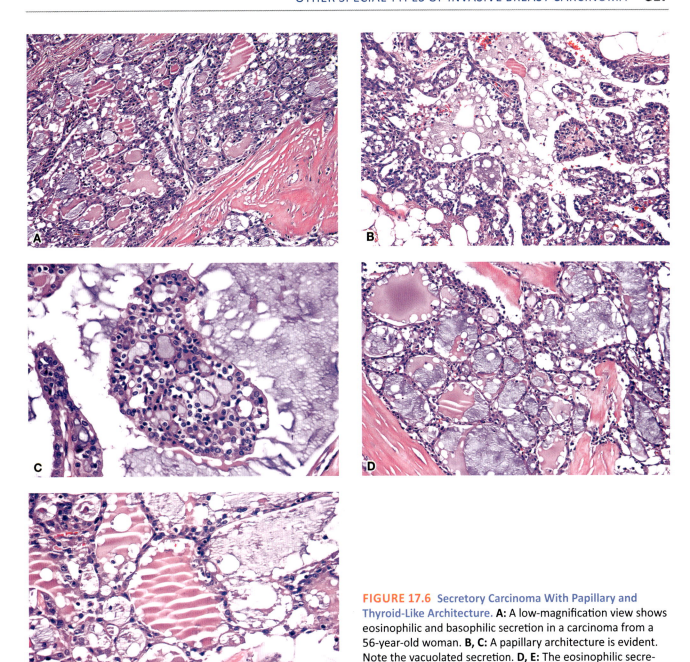

FIGURE 17.6 **Secretory Carcinoma With Papillary and Thyroid-Like Architecture. A:** A low-magnification view shows eosinophilic and basophilic secretion in a carcinoma from a 56-year-old woman. **B, C:** A papillary architecture is evident. Note the vacuolated secretion. **D, E:** The eosinophilic secretion with peripheral scalloping and parallel linear cracking resembles thyroid colloid and the secretion in cystic hypersecretory lesions of the breast.

for p63 in the remaining four cases. The latter observation may reflect the secretory nature of the carcinoma cells. Variable reactivity for carcinoembryonic antigen (CEA) and gross cystic disease fluid protein 15 (GCDFP-15) has been observed.

Most secretory carcinomas lack ER and PR, but weak expression is not uncommon. Three reported carcinomas did not express androgen receptor (48,55,69). Strong expression of HER2 protein has been detected in at least two secretory carcinomas (51,70).

Tognon et al (71) and Euhus et al (72) described the presence of the *ETV6-NTRK3* fusion gene (previously detected in congenital fibrosarcoma and cellular congenital mesoblastic nephroma) in secretory carcinomas. Using fluorescence in situ hybridization (FISH), sequencing of reverse transcriptase-polymerase chain reaction (RT-PCR) products, and immunoprecipitation, evidence of this oncoprotein was found in 12 of 13 (92%) secretory carcinomas and in only 1 of 50 (2%) invasive ductal carcinomas (71). The single conventional invasive carcinoma that demonstrated fusion transcripts contained regions with features suggestive of secretory carcinoma. Testing of other cases of secretory carcinoma and of commonplace breast carcinomas has confirmed the presence of this fusion gene in most secretory carcinomas and the absence of the gene in conventional breast carcinomas (73) and several other lesions with features similar to those of secretory carcinoma (65). Pan-TRK is a novel immunohistochemical antibody for *NTRK* family gene rearrangements and is sensitive and specific in the breast for secretory carcinoma (74).

Prognosis and Treatment

Axillary lymph node metastases have been observed in approximately one-third of all patients (60), but the risk in males is approximately 50% (49). The risk of nodal involvement in children is at least as great as it is in adults (75). The metastatic deposits rarely involve more than three lymph nodes. Metastatic foci display the characteristic features of secretory carcinoma. Sentinel lymph node biopsy is indicated for studying the axilla. Distant metastases following primary treatment are unusual but have been reported in both male and female patients, most commonly to the liver, lung, and bones (76-78).

In most patients, secretory carcinoma shows an indolent clinical course (60,70). A study using the SEER database revealed a 10-year cause-specific survival of 91.4% (60). The treatment of secretory carcinoma is surgical, but the optimal extent of surgery and use of adjuvant therapies remain undetermined. Until about two decades ago, most adult patients were treated with mastectomy, whereas excision was the preferred treatment in children (75). Local recurrence in residual breast tissue after mastectomy has been reported (79). Currently, in postmenarchal girls and women, local excision suffices for smaller lesions, but quadrantectomy may be necessary to obtain negative margins around larger tumors. Because of the small size of the male breast, surgical excision usually constitutes a mastectomy. The value of postoperative irradiation and adjuvant systemic therapy, radiotherapy, and chemotherapy in the treatment of recurrent or metastatic secretory carcinoma has not been determined.

The role of adjuvant therapy with TRK inhibitors (eg, larotrectinib or entrectinib), which have shown antitumor activity in other TRK fusion-positive malignancies, is being explored in secretory carcinoma (80).

CYSTIC HYPERSECRETORY CARCINOMA

First described by Rosen and Scott (81), CHC displays cysts containing eosinophilic secretory material. The latter bears a striking resemblance to thyroid colloid. CHC exists on a spectrum of cystic hypersecretory lesions from hyperplasia, hyperplasia with atypia, in situ carcinoma, to invasive carcinoma. The majority of cases have been DCIS.

Clinical Features

The age distribution of CHC ranges from 34 to 79 years. The mean age falls in the sixth or seventh decade (82,83). All patients have been women. The presenting symptom is usually a mass or other palpable abnormality. Nipple discharge occurs rarely and can appear bloody (84). Paget disease of the nipple was present in one case (85).

Radiologic imaging has not revealed distinctive findings. Mammograms of cases with invasive components have shown a region of increased density with trabecular thickening (86), an irregular asymmetric density (84), and spiculated masses with calcifications (87). Sonography may reveal a heterogeneous lesion with internal septations and lobulations, suggestive of an abscess (88).

Histopathologic Evaluation

The microscopic hallmark of all types of cystic hypersecretory lesions is the presence of cysts that contain eosinophilic secretion similar in appearance to thyroid colloid (**Fig. 17.7**). The homogeneous and virtually acellular secretion often retracts from the surrounding epithelium, resulting in a smooth or scalloped edge. Folds, linear cracks, or punched out holes occur in the secretion. The linear cracks in the secretions have been likened to "Venetian blinds." Positive reactions of the cyst contents for CEA, α-lactalbumin, and mucin have been observed. The secretion stains with the PAS method but does not stain for thyroglobulin. Disruption of cysts results in discharge of their contents into the stroma, eliciting an intense inflammatory reaction consisting of lymphocytes, histiocytes, and sometimes giant cells. Scant fine needle aspiration or NCB samples may capture only inflammatory cells and acellular proteinaceous material (88).

In CHC, the epithelium of involved cystic ducts grows as micropapillary DCIS (**Fig. 17.7E-F**). One often observes a spectrum of architectural patterns of the noninvasive component within a single case. The formations range from short, knobby epithelial tufts to complex branching fronds, which may traverse the duct lumen. The so-called Roman arch, or bridging pattern, commonly seen in micropapillary DCIS is uncommon in hypersecretory lesions, but the solid pattern can occur. Fibrovascular stroma within the micropapillary fronds is only rarely present. Ducts with DCIS may not contain the characteristic colloid-like secretion.

The cells in the fronds of micropapillary DCIS have crowded, hyperchromatic nuclei with sparse cytoplasm. The nuclei display an intermediate or high grade, with irregular contours and prominent nucleoli, and intranuclear inclusions. One does not see secretory material within the cytoplasm of the tumor cells, but the presence of frayed, apical cell borders and cytoplasmic blebs suggests secretory activity. Calcifications form within ducts in many cases.

Most invasive carcinomas encountered in this setting have been poorly differentiated ductal carcinomas with a solid growth pattern. The nuclei in the invasive carcinoma cells usually have a clear vacuolated appearance similar to that of the cells in papillary thyroid carcinoma. Scattered lymphocytes often mingle with the invasive carcinoma (84). The carcinoma cells do not display noticeable evidence of secretory activity. The metastases in the axillary lymph nodes of two patients displayed cystic elements that contained eosinophilic secretions (83).

OTHER SPECIAL TYPES OF INVASIVE BREAST CARCINOMA 319

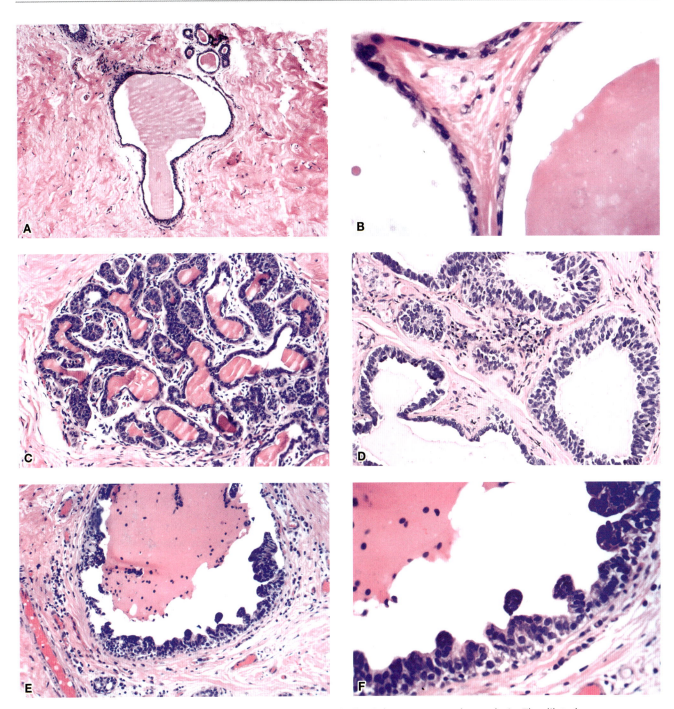

FIGURE 17.7 Cystic Hypersecretory Lesions. A, B: Cystic hypersecretory hyperplasia. The dilated ducts in two needle core biopsy specimens contain dense, eosinophilic secretion, which retracts from the inconspicuous epithelium. The secretion has developed cracks and small punctate holes. The cystic spaces are lined by a single layer of flat cells. **C:** Cystic hypersecretory hyperplasia in lobules. **D:** Cystic hypersecretory hyperplasia with atypia. Note marked epithelial crowding with loss of basal polarity. **E, F:** Cystic hypersecretory ductal carcinoma in situ. Low micropapillary fronds with hyperchromatic nuclei line the wall of this dilated duct. The retracted eosinophilic secretion has a scalloped border.

CHC usually coexists with other cystic hypersecretory lesions, most commonly *cystic hypersecretory hyperplasia* (CHH) (82,83). In CHH, orderly columnar epithelial cells with round to oval vesicular nuclei and eosinophilic cytoplasm, often with apical blebs, line the cysts (**Fig. 17.7A-C**). When the lining cells display cytologic atypia, the lesion is termed *cystic hypersecretory hyperplasia with atypia*. Atypical features in this setting are epithelial crowding sometimes resulting in micropapillary structures, hyperchromasia, and enlargement of nuclei, which may contain nucleoli (**Fig. 17.7D**). One occasionally observes cysts lined by a single layer of inconspicuous, flat, cuboidal, or low columnar cells with bland nuclei and scant cytoplasm. This form of cystic hypersecretory lesion, referred to as *cystic hypersecretory change*, does not commonly coexist with CHC.

The finding of areas with the typical features of CHH, sometimes with atypia, associated with CHC suggests that these processes are related, but convincing evidence of progression through these stages has not yet been observed. Review of prior biopsies from women with CHC has disclosed various lesions, including seemingly unrelated common proliferative changes as well as CHH and CHC. Follow-up of eight patients with CHH revealed subsequent breast carcinoma in two cases. One woman developed a fatal contralateral invasive ductal carcinoma that lacked cystic hypersecretory features. The other patient had DCIS separate from CHH in a biopsy specimen and residual CHH in the mastectomy specimen. Bogomoletz (89) described a 55-year-old woman who was well without recurrence 6 years after excision of a 7-cm focus of CHH.

The mammary lobules adjacent to cystic hypersecretory lesions often exhibit hypersecretory changes that include the accumulation of secretion in glandular lumina. This lobular abnormality may occur as an isolated finding in the absence of a fully developed cystic hypersecretory lesion, an observation that suggests that hypersecretory lesions may originate in such foci.

A few examples of intraductal CHC have been encountered in which there is pronounced vacuolization of the cytoplasm of the carcinoma cells and secretion, a pattern reminiscent of pregnancy-like hyperplasia (PLH). Secretion of the type found in a cystic hypersecretory lesion may be found in glands lined by epithelium showing the appearance of PLH. Moreover, one occasionally encounters cases wherein CHH or CHC and PLH coexist, and aspects of the two conditions seem to overlap when this occurs (90,91). This convergence is usually marked by cytologic and architectural atypia, which may be severe. Rarely, the proliferative and cytologic abnormalities warrant a diagnosis of CHC that has features of PLH (91). The relationship between cystic hypersecretory lesions and PLH has not been elucidated.

Immunohistochemistry

In the small number of cases of CHC studied, the carcinoma cells have not stained for CK5 or CK14 (82). Many of the tumors stained for ER, and a lesser number stained for PR (82,84). Three of ten cases in one report (84) stained for androgen receptor. At least five reported CHCs showed overexpression of HER2 (84,88,92). Staining for p63, smooth muscle myosin heavy chain, and CK5 failed to detect myoepithelial cells around the cysts in one case of CHC and another of CHH (82).

Differential Diagnosis

The differential diagnosis of CHC includes fibrocystic changes (FCCs), conventional micropapillary DCIS, JP, secretory carcinoma, and tall cell carcinoma with reversed polarity. The eosinophilic secretions that fill cysts of FCC do not stain as densely as the contents of the cysts in cystic hypersecretory lesions; furthermore, the former lack the scalloping and linear cracking characteristic of the latter. Lipid-laden histiocytes usually sit in the cysts of FCC, but they do not do so in hypersecretory cysts. Cells lining the cysts of FCC do not display the atypia demonstrated by the cells of CHC. The usual examples of micropapillary DCIS do not contain secretions like those seen in CHC, and the carcinoma cells display lower nuclear grade, in contrast to the higher grade of nuclei seen in CHC. The intraductal component of CHC grows in a predominantly micropapillary architecture and does not blend with areas showing a cribriform pattern as conventional micropapillary DCIS does. The large cysts seen in JP contain secretory material like that seen in FCC. The benign apocrine cells and bland ductal cells lining the cysts of JP do not resemble the atypical cells seen in CHC. Secretory carcinoma is a low-grade carcinoma in which eosinophilic secretions accumulate within cells and in microcystic spaces created by the carcinoma cells. The tumor cells contain the characteristic *ETV6-NTRK3* fusion gene. Tall cell carcinoma with reversed polarity, another breast tumor with thyroid colloid-like secretions, demonstrates solid papillary or follicular growth and columnar cells with apically polarized nuclei.

Prognosis and Treatment

Complete histologic examination of the lesional area is prudent if CHH is present in an NCB to exclude concurrent carcinoma (93). Some lesions have been misclassified as fibrocystic change, and the true nature of the process became apparent only after the lesion recurred (81).

The clinical course of intraductal CHC does not differ from that of other forms of DCIS. All patients had negative lymph nodes. Therapeutic options for women with noninvasive CHC are similar to those available for women with other forms of DCIS. There have only been rare recurrences in women treated by mastectomy alone after a mean follow-up of 8 years and extending in one case to 23 years (83,84). Breast recurrence has also been reported after excision alone. Too few patients have been treated by excision and radiotherapy to assess this form of treatment.

Because several women with invasive CHC had metastases in axillary lymph nodes (83,84,92), sentinel node biopsy is indicated when invasive carcinoma is present. A patient who presented with locally advanced carcinoma and died of her carcinoma 9 months later stands as the single reported death from CHC (83) to date. Adjuvant chemotherapy is prudent when poorly differentiated invasive carcinoma is present.

MAMMARY CARCINOMA WITH OSTEOCLAST-LIKE GIANT CELLS

Benign osteoclast-like giant cells can be seen as a component of several otherwise conventional types of mammary carcinoma. The presence of these cells defines such a carcinoma as *mammary carcinoma with osteoclast-like giant cells*. Since the first series was published in 1979 (94), numerous cases of this type of mammary carcinoma have been reported.

Clinical Features

The clinical features of this uncommon (<0.1%) form of breast carcinoma are similar to those of breast carcinoma generally. Patients' ages range from 28 to 88 years, and the mean age at diagnosis in the largest series is 43.8 years (95). One reported case affected a man (95). Multifocal lesions were clinically described in three cases (96,97). Bilateral primary carcinomas with osteoclast-like giant cells are exceedingly rare (95,98).

On mammography and ultrasonography, the well-circumscribed margin of most tumors simulates a benign lesion such as cyst or fibroadenoma (97,99). MRI of one carcinoma exhibited "rich vascularity, especially in the periphery" (100). Reported maximum dimensions range from 0.5 to 10 cm. The mean size in one series was 1.7 cm (95).

Histopathologic Evaluation

Most of these lesions are invasive ductal carcinomas of conventional type (**Fig. 17.8**). The publication of Zhou et al (95) tabulates the types of carcinomas showing osteoclast-like giant cells in 112 published cases. A cribriform growth pattern occurs relatively more often than among ductal carcinomas (101), and metaplastic carcinomas constitute

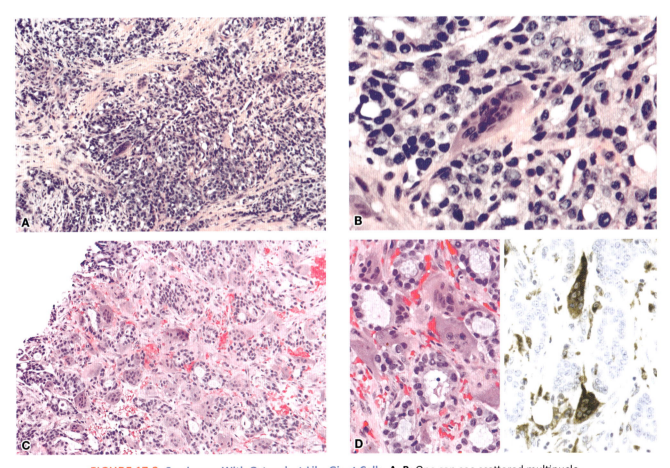

FIGURE 17.8 Carcinoma With Osteoclast-Like Giant Cells. A, B: One can see scattered multinucleate osteoclast-like giant cells in this invasive, poorly differentiated ductal carcinoma. The tumor shown in this needle core biopsy (NCB) specimen is unusual because it lacks the typical stromal elements, which include erythrocytes, hemosiderin, and lymphocytes. **C:** The invasive ductal carcinoma in another NCB specimen contains many osteoclast-like giant cells nestled among the neoplastic glands. Extravasated erythrocytes populate the stroma. **D:** The nuclei of the osteoclast-like giant cells differ from those of the neoplastic cells **(left panel)**. The osteoclast-like giant cells stain for KP1 **(right panel)**.

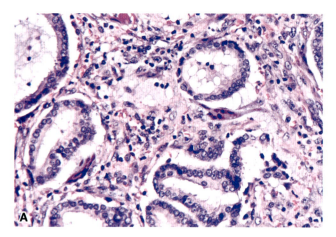 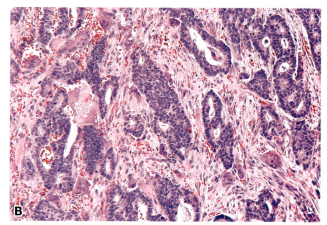

FIGURE 17.9 Carcinomas With Osteoclast-Like Giant Cells. A: This infiltrating ductal carcinoma with osteoclast-like giant cells has a well-differentiated glandular pattern and the characteristic stroma. The giant cells are attenuated and apposed to the outer surfaces of the glands. **B:** The stroma of this low-grade invasive ductal carcinoma with a cribriform structure contains osteoclast-like giant cells and many red blood cells.

another frequently seen type (95,102-104). Uncommon patterns include well-differentiated (**Fig. 17.9**) or tubular (101,103,105), lobular (94,98,106), squamous, papillary (94), apocrine, mucinous (107), neuroendocrine (108,109), and invasive micropapillary (110) carcinomas. Rarely, the carcinoma has a glandular pattern reminiscent of infiltrating colonic carcinoma. One case with prominent clear cells has been described (111). When present, the DCIS has the appearance of one of the conventional variants, usually cribriform, solid, or papillary. Osteoclast-like giant cells are not always present in the associated DCIS. It is uncommon to find osteoclast-like giant cells in DCIS in the absence of an invasive lesion (112).

The osteoclast-like giant cells range from 20 to 180 μm in diameter, and they number from fewer than 1 to more than 10 per high-power field. The giant cells contain abundant cytoplasm and many evenly distributed and usually centrally located oval nuclei, some of which contain small nucleoli. The giant cells tend to cluster close to the edges of carcinomatous glands or in the intervening stroma and may be found in the glandular lumina. The stroma typically contains histiocytes whose cytologic features resemble those of the giant cells. The extravasated erythrocytes and hemosiderin, found in the vascular stroma in most cases, reflect episodes of hemorrhage. Erythrophagocytosis by the giant cells is uncommon, and they contain little hemosiderin. Fibroblastic reaction, collagenization, and lymphocytic infiltration are variably present. It has been hypothesized that the giant cells form in response to tumor neoangiogenesis. The latter may be prominent in these tumors. Notably, bone formation (ie, presence of osteoid) is not a feature.

Osteoclast-like giant cells are found in some but not all metastases. The presence of osteoclast-like giant cells within intralymphatic carcinomatous emboli (99) suggests that these stromal cells can be transported to regional lymph nodes and to distant metastases.

Immunohistochemistry

The immunohistochemical profile of the carcinoma cells depends on the type of the carcinoma. The malignant cells typically stain for CK and often stain for EMA. Staining for CEA, ER, PR, GCDFP-15, and HER2 has yielded variable results. In one group of tumors in which the carcinoma was of ductal type (95), all of the 36 cases demonstrated a luminal phenotype (ER-positive and/or PR-positive).

The giant cells stain for markers of macrophages such as α_1-antitrypsin and CD68 (KP1) and for proteins found in osteoclasts such as acid phosphatase and tartrate-resistant acid phosphatase. These results suggest that the giant cells represent a specific type of histiocyte with osteoclastic features.

Differential Diagnosis

The differential diagnosis includes several non-carcinomatous lesions. Megakaryocytes in myeloid metaplasia in the breast might be mistaken for osteoclast-like giant cells. The lesion of extramedullary hematopoiesis has abundant myeloid elements in various stages of maturation, a feature not found in carcinomas with osteoclast-like giant cells. Granulomatous foci in inflammatory conditions such as sarcoidosis or coexistent with carcinoma also contain giant cells. The giant cells in these situations do not resemble osteoclasts and the lesions have a granulomatous pattern. The multinucleated stromal giant cells, which occasionally occur in fibroepithelial tumors, lack the relatively abundant cytoplasm seen in the osteoclast-like giant cells associated with mammary carcinomas.

Prognosis and Treatment

Primary treatment in many reports was mastectomy with axillary dissection, but breast conservation with radiotherapy has been used more recently (95). One patient was offered adjuvant chemotherapy based on an Oncotype DX recurrence score (RS) of 23—however, it should be cautioned that non-carcinoma inflammatory cells such as osteoclast-like giant cells may falsely increase the RS (113). Axillary lymph node metastases have been reported in a small proportion of cases, and metastases to the lungs and other sites have also been reported (94,95). Nearly two-thirds of reported patients have remained alive and well, but most follow-up does not extend beyond 5 years (95,97,103,105).

SMALL CELL CARCINOMA

Carcinoma resembling small cell neuroendocrine carcinoma of the lung is an especially uncommon variant of breast carcinoma. Breast large cell neuroendocrine carcinomas are seldom reported and poorly studied. The diagnosis of primary small cell mammary carcinoma can be rendered only if a nonmammary site is excluded as a source of metastasis to the breast or an in situ component is histologically demonstrated. Several reports fail to meet these criteria, and others do not provide sufficient details to substantiate the diagnosis of mammary small cell carcinoma. Moreover, one should reserve the diagnosis of small cell carcinoma for tumors displaying both the characteristic morphologic features and diffuse immunohistochemical evidence of neuroendocrine differentiation. Mammary carcinomas that stain for neuroendocrine markers while showing conventional morphologic features, and carcinomas composed of small cells that do not display evidence of neuroendocrine differentiation should *not* be classified as small cell carcinomas.

Clinical Features

The ages of patients with mammary small cell carcinoma range from 25 (108) to 99 years (114). The mean is 64 years. With the exception of two cases (115,116), all patients have been women. Small cell carcinoma typically forms a single mass, but multiple nodules have been described (117,118). Patients with small cell carcinoma frequently present with advanced disease: according to a SEER registry analysis, 42% presented with localized disease, 39% with locoregional disease, and 19% with distant metastasis (119).

Mammograms of patients with small cell carcinomas reveal well-defined or irregular masses with borders often described as microlobulated. Using sonography, the masses appear solid, and MRI displays early enhancement (120-124). The pattern of enhancement on computed tomography and MRI scans may be indicative of extensive DCIS (125). Gallium-68 PET/CT, a technique for somatostatin-expressing neuroendocrine tumors, can aid in detection and exclusion of extramammary primary sites (126).

Histopathologic Evaluation

The histologic characteristics of mammary small cell carcinomas are similar to those of small cell carcinomas arising in other organs. The noninvasive component usually consists of small cells with scant cytoplasm and hyperchromatic nuclei. These cells may constitute the entire noninvasive neoplastic population, as they did in five of the nine cases reported by Shin et al (120), or the small cells may represent one component of an in situ carcinoma with mixed features. The two types of neoplastic cells sometimes mingle in such a way that the non-small cell component surrounds the small cell carcinoma cells. Invasive small cell carcinoma also frequently presents as a component of a mixed carcinoma with areas of poorly differentiated invasive ductal carcinoma (127) or other histologic types (127-131). Squamous metaplasia may occur.

The invasive component typically consists of patternless sheets and clusters of cells that often contain zones of coagulative necrosis and foci of hemorrhage (**Fig. 17.10**). Regions sometimes display architectural patterns of a neuroendocrine nature: organoid groups, trabeculae, or rosette-like structures surrounded by delicate blood vessels and stroma. The neoplastic cells appear small and round, polygonal, or spindly and are prone to crush artifact, especially on NCB. They contain round to oval nuclei, homogeneous dark chromatin, inconspicuous nucleoli, and scant cytoplasm. The nuclear-to-cytoplasmic ratio is high. Nuclear molding can be seen, but it usually does not appear as prominent in histologic sections as it does in cytologic specimens (127). Mitotic figures abound in most examples, and mitotic counts as high as 10 per high-power field have been recorded (121). Disruption of nuclei occasionally leads to deposition of the nuclear material in the walls of blood vessels (the "Azzopardi effect"). Lymphovascular involvement often appears prominent.

The cells of small cell carcinoma can involve the epidermis in a pagetoid pattern (127,132), but Paget disease of the nipple has not been reported.

Immunohistochemistry

No consistent pattern of immunoreactivity in mammary small cell carcinomas has been reported. With rare exceptions (121,133,134), almost all cases have stained for CK AE1/AE3, CK7, and CAM 5.2. Most failed to stain for CK20, and the results of staining for CK5/6 and 34βE12 have been variable or negative. Staining for EMA usually yields a positive reaction, whereas testing for GCDFP-15 usually does not. Except for two examples (135,136), small cell carcinomas have expressed E-cadherin. The latter observation suggests that the majority of mammary small cell carcinomas are ductal in their nature.

Among proteins suggestive of neuroendocrine differentiation, synaptophysin, chromogranin A, and INSM1 are preferred (137,138). Staining for neuron-specific enolase, gastrin-releasing peptide (bombesin), serotonin, PGP9.5, CD56, and leu 7 has produced variable results (127,128,134,136,139).

A few investigators reported the staining results of both noninvasive and invasive components of small cell carcinomas. The two components displayed similar staining properties in two tumors (132,139), but in two other instances, the noninvasive and invasive cells exhibited different staining reactions (130,140).

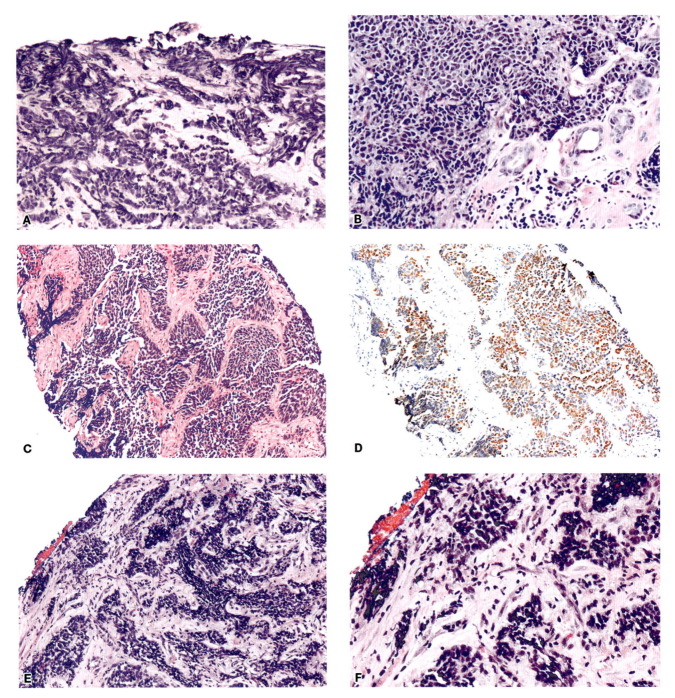

FIGURE 17.10 **Small Cell Neuroendocrine Carcinoma. A:** This needle core biopsy (NCB) specimen shows small carcinoma cells growing in ill-defined bands. Characteristic crush artifact is evident at the edge of the tumor. **B:** The excision specimen from the tumor shown in **A** shows small cell carcinoma infiltrating the mammary parenchyma and in situ carcinoma in a terminal duct lobular unit (**C**). **C:** NCB of a small cell carcinoma in the breast of a 55-year-old woman. The carcinoma was triple-negative with a Ki67-based proliferation rate of >95%. INSM1 (**D**) was diffusely and strongly positive. **E, F:** Invasive small cell carcinoma with a trabecular growth pattern is present in this NCB sample.

Small cell carcinomas demonstrate variable immunoreactivity for ER and PR. About 30% to 60% of cases have expressed ER, and slightly more have stained for PR. These are significantly higher rates than in pulmonary small cell carcinoma (141). Except for four tumors (115,136,142,143), the carcinomas have not overexpressed HER2.

Because a small cell carcinoma in the breast sometimes represents a metastasis rather than a primary carcinoma, investigators have studied the expression of TTF-1 and CD117 in bona fide mammary small cell carcinomas. Eight of 19 reported mammary small cell carcinomas stained for TTF-1 (121-123,125,130,132,136,140,143,144), and researchers detected CD117 in three out of four tumors (120,124,135,145). Mammary tumors can also show the same alterations of *RB1* as pulmonary tumors (146). These findings make clear that one cannot rely on the presence of these markers to distinguish a mammary small cell carcinoma from a metastasis from a pulmonary small cell carcinoma or one from another site. Notably, *PIK3CA* mutations are common in mammary small cell carcinoma and virtually absent in pulmonary small cell carcinoma. This finding may be diagnostically useful and may have therapeutic implications (141).

Differential Diagnosis

Neuroendocrine neoplasms (NENs) of the breast have been defined in the WHO 2019 classification (1) as carcinomas with greater than 90% neuroendocrine histologic features and "extensive expression" of chromogranin and/or synaptophysin. Those with less than diffuse findings are designated "invasive carcinoma with neuroendocrine features." To harmonize with schemas in other organ systems, breast NENs have been classified into two types: neuroendocrine "tumors" (grade 1 and 2) and neuroendocrine carcinomas (grade 3). All three grades of NENs are invasive carcinomas. Notably, solid papillary carcinoma, among others, may express neuroendocrine markers. Positivity for the latter does not, per se, have any prognostic or therapeutic implications. As such, routine staining of breast carcinomas for neuroendocrine markers is not recommended, and prognostic and predictive factors are those of non-neuroendocrine breast carcinomas and not of NENs of other organ systems. See **Table 17.1** for a summary of WHO classification of NENs.

The differential diagnosis of mammary small cell carcinoma includes lymphomas, certain sarcomas, and metastatic carcinomas. Evaluation of the growth pattern and cytologic features of the malignant cells, the presence of noninvasive carcinoma, and the results of immunohistochemical stains for epithelial and lymphoid proteins should allow one to exclude the diagnosis of a lymphoproliferative malignancy. Sarcomas such as Ewing sarcoma, osteosarcoma, mesenchymal chondrosarcoma, and synovial sarcoma would belong in the differential diagnosis in certain cases. Evaluation of problematic tumors via immunohistochemical staining and genetic studies allows one to exclude these possibilities. Pathologists must keep in mind that mammary small cell carcinomas can stain for CD99 (133,135), a protein usually present in the aforementioned mesenchymal tumors.

Pure primary small cell carcinoma is rare in the breast but comparatively common in other organs. To exclude the possibility of a metastatic lesion, pathologists should sample the specimen extensively to detect an in situ component. When the primary site is in doubt, clinicians should undertake a careful search for evidence of a primary carcinoma in another organ. The lung stands out as the most likely primary source for metastatic small cell carcinoma in the breast, and the mammary metastasis may be the first manifestation of an occult pulmonary small cell carcinoma. Spread from a Merkel cell carcinoma of the skin represents another possibility, the diagnosis of which can be facilitated by staining for CK20 and neurofilaments (139,147). In most reported examples of metastatic nonmammary small cell carcinoma in the breast (130), the existence of an extramammary primary was known.

Prognosis and Treatment

The small number of cases, the variation in inclusion criteria and treatment, and the short duration of follow-up prevent one from drawing secure conclusions regarding

---

TABLE 17.1

WHO's Classification of Neuroendocrine Neoplasms of the Breast (1)

		Neuroendocrine Tumor	Neuroendocrine Carcinoma
Synonym		**Carcinoid**	**Small cell carcinoma**
Nuclear grade		1 or 2	3
Architecture		Typical carcinoid-like	Solid, dense
Cytology	Cell shape	Plasmacytoid, spindle, polygonal	Small, molded together
	Cytoplasm	Finely granular, amphophilic	Minimal
	Nuclear chromatin	"Salt and pepper"	Hyperchromatic
	Proliferation rate	Low	High, >90%
IHC	ER	++	+/−
	HER2	−	−
	GATA3	+++	++
	Chromogranin	++	++
	Synaptophysin	+	++

ER, estrogen receptor; HER2, human epidermal growth factor receptor 2; IHC, immunohistochemistry; WHO, World Health Organization.

either the prognosis or the optimum treatment of patients with mammary small cell carcinoma. Most, including large SEER database studies, support a poor prognosis of small cell carcinoma compared with stage-matched invasive ductal carcinoma (114,148,149). Compared to its lung counterpart, breast small cell carcinoma presents at an earlier stage and has a relatively favorable prognosis (119,150). Among the patients in published reports, approximately 20% succumbed to the carcinoma during intervals from 3 months (132) to approximately 2 years (120), and approximately 20% developed recurrences during the same interval yet remained alive with disease. Finally, about one-half of the patients followed up for 3 months (127) to 49 months (128) remained free of carcinoma. Prognosis is substantially dependent on tumor size and stage at clinical diagnosis (127).

Surgery followed by chemotherapy may cure patients with early-stage disease (127), but it is unclear whether radiation therapy improves survival (119,151). Neoadjuvant chemotherapy may benefit patients with locally advanced carcinomas (152). In some settings, protocols akin to those for pulmonary small cell carcinoma are being implemented (153,154).

GLYCOGEN-RICH CARCINOMA

Malignant cells containing abundant glycogen compose this variety of mammary carcinoma. Extraction of glycogen during tissue processing leaves the cytoplasm of these carcinomas vacuolated or completely clear in routine sections. In a SEER database analysis, about 0.01% of 1,251,584 breast carcinomas were classified as clear cell, glycogen-rich carcinomas (155,156).

Clinical Features

The age of reported patients with glycogen-rich carcinoma ranges from 31 to 81 years (157,158). The patients presented with a mass accompanied by skin dimpling, nipple retraction, or pain.

Both in situ and invasive lesions may be detected by mammography (159) and sonography (160). The images often reveal an oval solid and cystic mass (158), which may contain calcifications (158,161). MRI has shown an irregular mass with internal high signal intensity and peritumoral edema on T2-weighted imaging (160).

Most tumors measure between 2 and 5 cm; the largest spanned "about 15 cm" (161). The mean sizes in two series were 3 cm (157) and 3.2 cm (158). The carcinoma can form multifocal or multicentric masses (162).

Histopathologic Evaluation

Glycogen-rich carcinomas grow in both noninvasive and invasive forms. The noninvasive component can create papillary, solid, cribriform, micropapillary, and intracystic patterns. Cytoplasmic clearing appears most evident in solid areas, in which the cells exhibit intermediate-grade nuclei. Those in cribriform and micropapillary regions usually have low-grade nuclei and less often appear water-clear. The neoplastic cells can undergo focal necrosis, but abundant central necrosis associated with high-grade nuclei does not commonly occur. In most cases, one can detect small regions in which the cells contain eosinophilic, granular, or apocrine features.

The invasive component usually exhibits the growth pattern of a conventional invasive ductal carcinoma. The tumor cells form sheets, cords, solid nests, or papillary structures, but the formation of ductular structure occurs only rarely. A linear pattern consisting of strands of cells resembling invasive lobular carcinoma may be seen, and glycogen-rich variants of tubular, medullary, micropapillary, and neuroendocrine carcinomas have been described (155,157,163,164). The cells exhibit sharply defined borders and polygonal rather than rounded contours. The cytoplasm is clear or, less often, finely granular or foamy. Like the noninvasive component, the invasive carcinoma sometimes contains foci in which the cells have eosinophilic and granular cytoplasm that suggests an apocrine nature, and these cells often form a continuum with the clear cells. Observers have noted PAS-positive, diastase-resistant, intracytoplasmic hyaline droplets in rare cases (159). The nuclei appear hyperchromatic and sometimes contain clumped chromatin and nucleoli (**Fig. 17.11**). Mitotic figures are easily identified in most cases. One report (165) recorded the presence of 65 mitotic figures in 10 high-power fields. Large tumors often show necrosis. The carcinoma cells can invade lymphovascular channels. The histologic appearance of the primary tumor is duplicated in the metastases, which also contain abundant glycogen (166).

Immunohistochemistry

The cytoplasm of glycogen-rich carcinomas yields a positive, diastase-labile reaction with the PAS stain. The tumor cells are reactive for CK7, CK AE1/AE3, CK8/18, CAM 5.2, and E-cadherin and variably or weakly reactive for

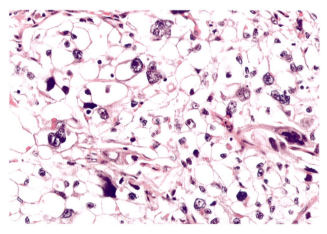

FIGURE 17.11 Glycogen-Rich Carcinoma. The neoplastic cells have pale eosinophilic or clear cytoplasm.

CK19, CK34βE12, and EMA. Glycogen-rich carcinomas do not display a consistent pattern of staining for hormone receptors. The reported frequency of ER and PR expression varies from 35% to 62%, and 12% to 43% of cases have stained for HER2 (157,158,167).

Differential Diagnosis

The differential diagnosis of glycogen-rich carcinoma includes both benign and malignant mammary and extramammary neoplasms. The clear cell type of hidradenoma (eccrine acrospiroma) shares the presence of many glycogen-laden clear cells with glycogen-rich carcinoma; however, hidradenomas are centered in the dermis; have well-defined, smooth contours; and consist of uniform bland cells. Atypical and malignant hidradenomas pose greater challenges in differential diagnosis. Myoepithelial cells with clear cytoplasm can dominate in uncommon examples of mammary adenomyoepithelioma. Detection of a second population consisting of glandular cells and immunohistochemical markers for myoepithelial cells may help to distinguish such a tumor from glycogen-rich carcinoma.

Among the types of primary mammary carcinomas, lipid-rich, secretory, histiocytoid lobular, and apocrine carcinomas exhibit certain features that simulate the appearance of glycogen-rich carcinoma. Lipid-rich carcinomas contain lipid rather than glycogen. Secretory carcinomas feature microcystic spaces containing mucin and eosinophilic secretions. Invasive lobular carcinomas of the histiocytoid type possess intracytoplasmic mucin rather than glycogen. Apocrine carcinomas can contain clear cells, and focal apocrine features are identified in the majority of glycogen-rich carcinomas. This association suggests that glycogen-rich carcinoma might constitute a variant of apocrine carcinoma (159). Notwithstanding these overlapping findings and the possibility of an etiologic relationship, the usual apocrine carcinoma contains intracytoplasmic, diastase-resistant eosinophilic granules, a finding that does not characterize glycogen-rich carcinomas.

Metastatic clear cell carcinomas can mimic the appearance of glycogen-rich carcinoma. Carcinoma of the kidney is the most notable culprit in this regard. Rare cases of angiomyolipoma, a lesion of the clear cell "sugar" tumor family, of the breast have been reported (168,169).

Finally, the mere presence of glycogen in a mammary carcinoma does not establish the diagnosis of glycogen-rich carcinoma, because Fisher et al (155) found that 58% of breast carcinomas lacking clear cells contained intracytoplasmic glycogen. To substantiate the diagnosis of glycogen-rich carcinoma, one must both observe the characteristic morphologic findings and establish the presence of abundant glycogen by histochemical means.

Prognosis and Treatment

In one series (158), 46% of patients had metastatic carcinoma in axillary lymph nodes. The limited follow-up data suggest that the prognosis of patients with glycogen-rich mammary carcinoma is similar to that of invasive ductal carcinoma when analyzed on a stage- and grade-matched basis (155,156,158,159). Treatment recommendations should probably follow those proposed for conventional breast carcinomas. Radiation in the setting of breast-conserving surgery has improved survival (156).

LIPID-RICH CARCINOMA

This rare variant of infiltrating ductal carcinoma features large cells with abundant cytoplasmic lipid, which imparts a vacuolated or foamy appearance to the cytoplasm. The tumor was first described in a case report by Aboumrad et al (170) as *lipid-secreting carcinoma*; later, Ramos and Taylor (171) proposed the less committal term, *lipid-rich carcinoma*.

Clinical Features

With rare exceptions (172), all adult patients have been women between the ages of 22 and 81 years. One patient was a 10-year-old girl (173). Most patients presented with a palpable mass. Attachment to the skin with dimpling, retraction, ulceration, and *peau d'orange* has been reported.

Mammography revealed masses in most patients and calcifications in about 40% (174). Although the tumors contain a large proportion of lipid, they are of higher density than the adjacent tissues. Ultrasonography and MRI in one patient demonstrated findings suspicious for malignancy (175).

Histopathologic Evaluation

In most cases, there is a predominantly invasive carcinoma composed of sheets, nests, and cords of large, polygonal cells, which may have poorly defined borders. Two examples seemed to represent an entirely noninvasive form (175,176). van Bogaert and Maldague (177) described three histopathologic patterns created by the malignant cells. The *histiocytoid pattern*, which represents the most common variety, consists of large cells with pale foamy cytoplasm and small dark nuclei that lack pleomorphism (**Fig. 17.12**). Cells with large, irregular, and bubbly microvacuoles, pleomorphic nuclei, and prominent nucleoli characterize the *sebaceous pattern* of lipid-rich carcinoma. The third pattern consists of cells with *apocrine* qualities. The latter possess abundant, finely granular, eosinophilic cytoplasm and nuclei with coarse chromatin and prominent nucleoli. Cells with these different appearances sometimes mingle in a single carcinoma. These overlapping cytologic features raise the possibility of common biology with apocrine carcinoma (178) and glycogen-rich carcinoma (176).

One can usually detect mitotic figures without difficulty, and the carcinomas usually belong to the category of histologic grade 2 or 3. Scalloping of the nuclei by the cytoplasmic vacuoles can simulate the appearance of sebaceous cells or brown fat. Unusual histologic findings include focal

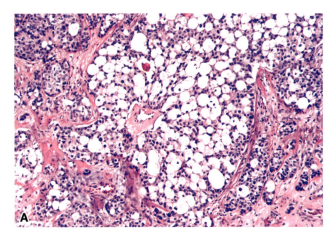
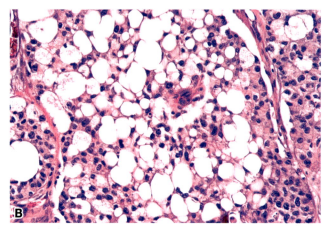

FIGURE 17.12 Lipid-Rich Carcinoma. **A, B:** The carcinoma cells contain prominent cytoplasmic vacuoles resulting from extraction of lipid during tissue processing. (Courtesy of Dr. Frank Brazza.)

chondroid metaplasia (179) and cytologic findings similar to those in pregnancy-like change (180).

Histochemistry and Immunohistochemistry

The cytoplasmic vacuolization arises because histologic processing extracts the cytoplasmic lipid. To document the presence of lipid, one can employ Oil Red O or Sudan III stains using frozen sections of fresh tissue or tissue processed in a fashion that preserves cytoplasmic lipids. Lipid-rich carcinomas do not stain with PAS, Alcian blue, or mucicarmine stains.

These carcinomas do not stain for CK5/6, CK14, S-100 protein, SMA, or p63. Staining for E-cadherin, CK7, mammaglobin, and CEA was observed in one case (181). The results of studies of ER and PR expression vary. Staining for α-lactalbumin, lactoferrin, EMA, and adipophilin has been reported. Most investigators report little or no detection of ER but modest expression of PR. Many cases showed strong membrane staining for HER2 and amplification of the *ERBB2* gene (174,180-182).

Differential Diagnosis

The diagnosis of lipid-rich carcinoma requires the presence of two types of evidence: the characteristic cellular features, which include clear, pale, or vacuolated cytoplasm, and intracytoplasmic lipid demonstrated by special studies. Neither type of evidence alone can establish the diagnosis of lipid-rich carcinoma. The most commonly encountered carcinomas that resemble lipid-rich carcinoma include glycogen-rich carcinoma, apocrine carcinoma, and secretory carcinoma. Myoepithelial carcinoma and liposarcoma might also enter into consideration. The cytoplasm of glycogen-rich carcinomas appears clear rather than foamy and it contains diastase-sensitive, PAS-positive glycogen rather than lipid. Apocrine carcinomas typically stain strongly for androgen receptors and GCDFP-15, whereas lipid-rich carcinomas may not. In secretory carcinomas, PAS-positive, Alcian blue–positive acid mucopolysaccharides form cytoplasmic vacuoles, and genetic studies demonstrate the characteristic fusion gene. Myoepithelial carcinomas express characteristic proteins not seen in lipid-rich carcinomas, and the cells of liposarcoma do not commonly express CK.

The accumulated information notwithstanding, the nature of lipid-rich carcinoma remains undefined.

Treatment and Prognosis

The prognosis of lipid-rich carcinoma seems to be poor, with 2- and 5-year overall survival of 64.6% and 33.2%, respectively, in the largest series to date (174). Axillary nodal metastases have been found in 70% of cases at presentation (183), mostly associated with tumors measuring greater than 3 cm, and 80% of patients developed distant metastasis within 2 years of follow-up (183). Patients with nodal metastases at the time of diagnosis have a poor prognosis, but those with negative lymph nodes have survived as long as 20 years (180). Treatment of patients with lipid-rich carcinoma has been by mastectomy and axillary dissection in most cases, but breast-conserving surgery could be an alternative in appropriate situations. Systemic chemotherapy and HER2-targeted therapy can also be instrumental (174,184).

OTHER RARE TYPES OF CARCINOMA

Other rare types of mammary carcinoma include so-called acinic cell carcinoma (185), mucoepidermoid carcinoma (186), oncocytic carcinoma (187), polymorphous adenocarcinoma (188), and sebaceous carcinoma (189). For tall cell carcinoma with reversed polarity, see Chapter 11. Please see *Rosen's Breast Pathology* (5th ed.) for a full discussion of these tumors.

Although one might suspect one of these diagnoses when examining an NCB specimen, it would require a thorough evaluation of the excised specimen to make a secure diagnosis of such rare types of mammary carcinoma.

REFERENCES

1. Allison KH, Brogi E, Ellis IO, et al. *WHO Classification of Breast Tumours.* 5th ed. IARC; 2019.
2. Fisher ER, Palekar AS, Redmond C, et al. Pathologic findings from the National Surgical Adjuvant Breast Project (protocol no. 4). VI. Invasive papillary cancer. *Am J Clin Pathol.* 1980;73:313-322.
3. Gunhan-Bilgen I, Zekioglu O, Ustun EE, et al. Invasive micropapillary carcinoma of the breast: clinical, mammographic, and sonographic findings with histopathologic correlation. *AJR Am J Roentgenol.* 2002;179:927-931.
4. Guo X, Chen L, Lang R, et al. Invasive micropapillary carcinoma of the breast: association of pathologic features with lymph node metastasis. *Am J Clin Pathol.* 2006;126:740-746.
5. Pettinato G, Manivel CJ, Panico L, et al. Invasive micropapillary carcinoma of the breast: clinicopathologic study of 62 cases of a poorly recognized variant with highly aggressive behavior. *Am J Clin Pathol.* 2004;121:857-866.
6. Luna-More S, Gonzalez B, Acedo C, et al. Invasive micropapillary carcinoma of the breast. A new special type of invasive mammary carcinoma. *Pathol Res Pract.* 1994;190:668-674.
7. Erhan Y, Erhan Y, Zekioglu O. Pure invasive micropapillary carcinoma of the male breast: report of a rare case. *Can J Surg.* 2005;48:156-157.
8. Marchio C, Iravani M, Natrajan R, et al. Genomic and immunophenotypical characterization of pure micropapillary carcinomas of the breast. *J Pathol.* 2008;215:398-410.
9. Trepant AL, Hoorens A, Noel JC. Pure invasive micropapillary carcinoma of the male breast: report of a rare case with C-MYC amplification. *Pathol Res Pract.* 2014;210:1164-1166.
10. Alsharif S, Daghistani R, Kamberoglu EA, et al. Mammographic, sonographic and MR imaging features of invasive micropapillary breast cancer. *Eur J Radiol.* 2014;83:1375-1380.
11. Yun SU, Choi BB, Shu KS, et al. Imaging findings of invasive micropapillary carcinoma of the breast. *J Breast Cancer.* 2012;15:57-64.
12. Acs G, Paragh G, Chuang ST, et al. The presence of micropapillary features and retraction artifact in core needle biopsy material predicts lymph node metastasis in breast carcinoma. *Am J Surg Pathol.* 2009;33:202-210.
13. Aggarwal G, Reid MD, Sharma S. Metaplastic variant of invasive micropapillary breast carcinoma: a unique triple negative phenotype. *Int J Surg Pathol.* 2012;20:488-493.
14. Barbashina V, Corben AD, Akram M, et al. Mucinous micropapillary carcinoma of the breast: an aggressive counterpart to conventional pure mucinous tumors. *Hum Pathol.* 2013;44:1577-1585.
15. Chen L, Fan Y, Lang RG, et al. Breast carcinoma with micropapillary features: clinicopathologic study and long-term follow-up of 100 cases. *Int J Surg Pathol.* 2008;16:155-163.
16. Liu F, Yang M, Li Z, et al. Invasive micropapillary mucinous carcinoma of the breast is associated with poor prognosis. *Breast Cancer Res Treat.* 2015;151:443-451.
17. Nassar H, Pansare V, Zhang H, et al. Pathogenesis of invasive micropapillary carcinoma: role of MUC1 glycoprotein. *Mod Pathol.* 2004;17:1045-1050.
18. Acs G, Esposito NN, Rakosy Z, et al. Invasive ductal carcinomas of the breast showing partial reversed cell polarity are associated with lymphatic tumor spread and may represent part of a spectrum of invasive micropapillary carcinoma. *Am J Surg Pathol.* 2010;34:1637-1646.
19. Adams SA, Smith ME, Cowley GP, et al. Reversal of glandular polarity in the lymphovascular compartment of breast cancer. *J Clin Pathol.* 2004;57:1114-1117.
20. Wendroth SM, Mentrikoski MJ, Wick MR. GATA3 expression in morphologic subtypes of breast carcinoma: a comparison with gross cystic disease fluid protein 15 and mammaglobin. *Ann Diagn Pathol.* 2015;19:6-9.
21. Yamaguchi R, Tanaka M, Kondo K, et al. Characteristic morphology of invasive micropapillary carcinoma of the breast: an immunohistochemical analysis. *Jpn J Clin Oncol.* 2010;40:781-787.
22. Stewart RL, Caron JE, Gulbahce EH, et al. HER2 immunohistochemical and fluorescence in situ hybridization discordances in invasive breast carcinoma with micropapillary features. *Mod Pathol.* 2017;30:1561-1566.
23. Wolff AC, Hammond ME, Hicks DG, et al. Recommendations for human epidermal growth factor receptor 2 testing in breast cancer: American Society of Clinical Oncology/College of American Pathologists clinical practice guideline update. *J Clin Oncol.* 2013;31:3997-4013.
24. Kuba S, Ohtani H, Yamaguchi J, et al. Incomplete inside-out growth pattern in invasive breast carcinoma: association with lymph vessel invasion and recurrence-free survival. *Virchows Arch.* 2011;458:159-169.
25. Lee AH, Paish EC, Marchio C, et al. The expression of Wilms' tumour-1 and CA125 in invasive micropapillary carcinoma of the breast. *Histopathology.* 2007;51:824-828.
26. Chivukula M, Dabbs DJ, O'Connor S, et al. PAX 2: a novel Mullerian marker for serous papillary carcinomas to differentiate from micropapillary breast carcinoma. *Int J Gynecol Pathol.* 2009;28:570-578.
27. Lotan TL, Ye H, Melamed J, et al. Immunohistochemical panel to identify the primary site of invasive micropapillary carcinoma. *Am J Surg Pathol.* 2009;33:1037-1041.
28. Pareja F, Selenica P, Brown DN, et al. Micropapillary variant of mucinous carcinoma of the breast shows genetic alterations intermediate between those of mucinous carcinoma and micropapillary carcinoma. *Histopathology.* 2019;75:139-145.
29. Chen AC, Paulino AC, Schwartz MR, et al. Population-based comparison of prognostic factors in invasive micropapillary and invasive ductal carcinoma of the breast. *Br J Cancer.* 2014;111:619-22.
30. Branca G, Ieni A, Barresi V, et al. An updated review of cribriform carcinomas with emphasis on histopathological diagnosis and prognostic significance. *Oncol Rev.* 2017;11:317.
31. Page DL, Dixon JM, Anderson TJ, et al. Invasive cribriform carcinoma of the breast. *Histopathology.* 1983;7:525-536.
32. Venable JG, Schwartz AM, Silverberg SG. Infiltrating cribriform carcinoma of the breast: a distinctive clinicopathologic entity. *Hum Pathol.* 1990;21:333-338.
33. Zhang W, Zhang T, Lin Z, et al. Invasive cribriform carcinoma in a Chinese population: comparison with low-grade invasive ductal carcinoma-not otherwise specified. *Int J Clin Exp Pathol.* 2013;6:445-457.
34. Demir S, Sezgin G, Sari AA, et al. Clinicopathological analysis of invasive cribriform carcinoma of the breast, with review of the literature. *Ann Diagn Pathol.* 2021;54:151794.
35. Nishimura R, Ohsumi S, Teramoto N, et al. Invasive cribriform carcinoma with extensive microcalcifications in the male breast. *Breast Cancer.* 2005;12:145-148.
36. Choi Y, Lee KY, Jang MH, et al. Invasive cribriform carcinoma arising in malignant phyllodes tumor of breast: a case report. *Korean J Pathol.* 2012;46:205-209.
37. Stutz JA, Evans AJ, Pinder S, et al. The radiological appearances of invasive cribriform carcinoma of the breast. Nottingham breast team. *Clin Radiol.* 1994;49:693-695.
38. Lim HS, Jeong SJ, Lee JS, et al. Sonographic findings of invasive cribriform carcinoma of the breast. *J Ultrasound Med.* 2011;30:701-705.
39. Wells CA, Ferguson DJ. Ultrastructural and immunocytochemical study of a case of invasive cribriform breast carcinoma. *J Clin Pathol.* 1988;41:17-20.
40. Shousha S, Schoenfeld A, Moss J, et al. Light and electron microscopic study of an invasive cribriform carcinoma with extensive microcalcification developing in a breast with silicone augmentation. *Ultrastruct Pathol.* 1994;18:519-523.
41. Gatti G, Pruneri G, Gilardi D, et al. Report on a case of pure cribriform carcinoma of the breast with internal mammary node metastasis: description of the case and review of the literature. *Tumori.* 2006;92:241-243.
42. Gjerdrum LM, Lauridsen MC, Sorensen FB. Breast carcinoma with osteoclast-like giant cells: morphological and ultrastructural studies of a case with review of the literature. *Breast.* 2001;10:231-236.
43. Rosen PP. Adenoid cystic carcinoma of the breast. A morphologically heterogeneous neoplasm. *Pathol Annu.* 1989;24 Pt 2:237-254.
44. Cong Y, Qiao G, Zou H, et al. Invasive cribriform carcinoma of the breast: a report of nine cases and a review of the literature. *Oncol Lett.* 2015;9:1753-1758.
45. Liu XY, Jiang YZ, Liu YR, et al. Clinicopathological characteristics and survival outcomes of invasive cribriform carcinoma of breast: a SEER population-based study. *Medicine (Baltimore).* 2015;94:e1309.
46. Gong P, Xia C, Yang Y, et al. Clinicopathologic profiling and oncologic outcomes of secretory carcinoma of the breast. *Sci Rep.* 2021;11:14738.
47. Noh WC, Paik NS, Cho KJ, et al. Breast mass in a 3-year-old girl: differentiation of secretory carcinoma versus abnormal thelarche by fine needle aspiration biopsy. *Surgery.* 2005;137:109-110.
48. Alenda C, Aranda FI, Segui FJ, et al. Secretory carcinoma of the male breast: correlation of aspiration cytology and pathology. *Diagn Cytopathol.* 2005;32:47-50.
49. Ding J, Jiang L, Gan Y, et al. A rare case of secretory breast carcinoma in a male adult with axillary lymph node metastasis. *Int J Clin Exp Pathol.* 2015;8:3322-3327.
50. Beatty SM, Orel SG, Kim P, et al. Multicentric secretory carcinoma of the breast in a 35-year-old woman: mammographic appearance and the use of core biopsy in preoperative management. *Breast J.* 1998;4:200-203.
51. Diallo R, Schaefer KL, Bankfalvi A, et al. Secretory carcinoma of the breast: a distinct variant of invasive ductal carcinoma assessed by comparative genomic hybridization and immunohistochemistry. *Hum Pathol.* 2003;34:1299-1305.
52. Li D, Xiao X, Yang W, et al. Secretory breast carcinoma: a clinicopathological and immunophenotypic study of 15 cases with a review of the literature. *Mod Pathol.* 2012;25:567-575.
53. Shin SJ, Sheikh FS, Allenby PA, et al. Invasive secretory (juvenile) carcinoma arising in ectopic breast tissue of the axilla. *Arch Pathol Lab Med.* 2001;125:1372-1374.
54. Brandt SM, Swistel AJ, Rosen PP. Secretory carcinoma in the axilla: probable origin from axillary skin appendage glands in a young girl. *Am J Surg Pathol.* 2009;33:950-953.
55. Grabellus F, Worm K, Willruth A, et al. ETV6-NTRK3 gene fusion in a secretory carcinoma of the breast of a male-to-female transsexual. *Breast.* 2005;14:71-74.
56. Rosen PP, Holmes G, Lesser ML, et al. Juvenile papillomatosis and breast carcinoma. *Cancer.* 1985;55:1345-1352.
57. de Bree E, Askoxylakis J, Giannikaki E, et al. Secretory carcinoma of the male breast. *Ann Surg Oncol.* 2002;9:663-667.
58. Kameyama K, Mukai M, Iri H, et al. Secretory carcinoma of the breast in a 51-year-old male. *Pathol Int.* 1998;48:994-997.
59. Paeng MH, Choi HY, Sung SH, et al. Secretory carcinoma of the breast. *J Clin Ultrasound.* 2003;31:425-429.
60. Horowitz DP, Sharma CS, Connolly E, et al. Secretory carcinoma of the breast: results from the survival, epidemiology and end results database. *Breast.* 2012;21:350-353.

61. Din NU, Idrees R, Fatima S, et al. Secretory carcinoma of breast: clinicopathologic study of 8 cases. *Ann Diagn Pathol*. 2013;17:54-57.
62. Yildirim E, Turhan N, Pak I, et al. Secretory breast carcinoma in a boy. *Eur J Surg Oncol*. 1999;25:98-99.
63. Woto-Gaye G, Kasse AA, Dieye Y, et al. [Secretory breast carcinoma in a man. A case report with rapid evolution unfavorable]. *Ann Pathol*. 2004;24:432-435; quiz 393.
64. Damiani S, Pasquinelli G, Lamovec J, et al. Acinic cell carcinoma of the breast: an immunohistochemical and ultrastructural study. *Virchows Arch*. 2000;437:74-81.
65. Osako T, Takeuchi K, Horii R, et al. Secretory carcinoma of the breast and its histopathological mimics: value of markers for differential diagnosis. *Histopathology*. 2013;63:509-519.
66. Lamovec J, Bracko M. Secretory carcinoma of the breast: light microscopical, immunohistochemical and flow cytometric study. *Mod Pathol*. 1994;7:475-479.
67. Lae M, Freneaux P, Sastre-Garau X, et al. Secretory breast carcinomas with ETV6-NTRK3 fusion gene belong to the basal-like carcinoma spectrum. *Mod Pathol*. 2009;22:291-298.
68. Choi J, Kim D, Koo JS. Secretory carcinoma of breast demonstrates nuclear or cytoplasmic expression in p63 immunohistochemistry. *Int J Surg Pathol*. 2012;20:367-372.
69. Lambros MB, Tan DS, Jones RL, et al. Genomic profile of a secretory breast cancer with an ETV6-NTRK3 duplication. *J Clin Pathol*. 2009;62:604-612.
70. Jacob JD, Hodge C, Franko J, et al. Rare breast cancer: 246 invasive secretory carcinomas from the National Cancer Data Base. *J Surg Oncol*. 2016;113:721-725.
71. Tognon C, Knezevich SR, Huntsman D, et al. Expression of the ETV6-NTRK3 gene fusion as a primary event in human secretory breast carcinoma. *Cancer Cell*. 2002;2:367-376.
72. Euhus DM, Timmons CF, Tomlinson GE. ETV6-NTRK3—Trk-ing the primary event in human secretory breast cancer. *Cancer Cell*. 2002;2:347-348.
73. Makretsov N, He M, Hayes M, et al. A fluorescence in situ hybridization study of ETV6-NTRK3 fusion gene in secretory breast carcinoma. *Genes Chromosomes Cancer*. 2004;40:152-157.
74. Harrison BT, Fowler E, Krings G, et al. Pan-TRK immunohistochemistry: a useful diagnostic adjunct for secretory carcinoma of the breast. *Am J Surg Pathol*. 2019;43:1693-1700.
75. Rosen PP, Cranor ML. Secretory carcinoma of the breast. *Arch Pathol Lab Med*. 1991;115:141-144.
76. Hoda RS, Brogi E, Pareja F, et al. Secretory carcinoma of the breast: clinicopathologic profile of 14 cases emphasising distant metastatic potential. *Histopathology*. 2019;75:213-224.
77. Lian J, Wang LX, Guo JH, et al. Secretory breast carcinoma in a female adult with liver metastasis: a case report and literature review. *Diagn Pathol*. 2021;16:89.
78. Tang H, Zhong L, Jiang H, et al. Secretory carcinoma of the breast with multiple distant metastases in the brain and unfavorable prognosis: a case report and literature review. *Diagn Pathol*. 2021;16:56.
79. Mies C. Recurrent secretory carcinoma in residual mammary tissue after mastectomy. *Am J Surg Pathol*. 1993;17:715-721.
80. Cocco E, Scaltriti M, Drilon A. NTRK fusion-positive cancers and TRK inhibitor therapy. *Nat Rev Clin Oncol*. 2018;15:731-747.
81. Rosen PP, Scott M. Cystic hypersecretory duct carcinoma of the breast. *Am J Surg Pathol*. 1984;8:31-41.
82. D'Alfonso TM, Ginter PS, Liu YF, et al. Cystic hypersecretory (in situ) carcinoma of the breast: a clinicopathologic and immunohistochemical characterization of 10 cases with clinical follow-up. *Am J Surg Pathol*. 2014;38:45-53.
83. Guerry P, Erlandson RA, Rosen PP. Cystic hypersecretory hyperplasia and cystic hypersecretory duct carcinoma of the breast. Pathology, therapy, and follow-up of 39 patients. *Cancer*. 1988;61:1611-1620.
84. Skalova A, Ryska A, Kajo K, et al. Cystic hypersecretory carcinoma: rare and poorly recognized variant of intraductal carcinoma of the breast. Report of five cases. *Histopathology*. 2005;46:43-49.
85. Sahoo S, Gopal P, Roland L, et al. Cystic hypersecretory carcinoma of the breast with Paget disease of the nipple: a diagnostic challenge. *Int J Surg Pathol*. 2008;16:208-212.
86. Resetkova E, Padula A, Albarracin CT, et al. Pathologic quiz case: a large, ill-defined cystic breast mass. Invasive cystic hypersecretory duct carcinoma. *Arch Pathol Lab Med*. 2005;129:e79-e80.
87. Park JM, Seo MR. Cystic hypersecretory duct carcinoma of the breast: report of two cases. *Clin Radiol*. 2002;57:312-315.
88. Chitti S, Misra S, Ahuja A, et al. Invasive cystic hypersecretory carcinoma of the breast. *Autops Case Rep*. 2022;12:e2021375.
89. Bogomoletz WV. [Cystic hypersecretory hyperplasia of the breast. A rare diagnosis in breast pathology]. *Ann Pathol*. 1994;14:131-132.
90. Shin SJ, Rosen PP. Pregnancy-like (pseudolactational) hyperplasia: a primary diagnosis in mammographically detected lesions of the breast and its relationship to cystic hypersecretory hyperplasia. *Am J Surg Pathol*. 2000;24:1670-1674.
91. Shin SJ, Rosen PP. Carcinoma arising from preexisting pregnancy-like and cystic hypersecretory hyperplasia lesions of the breast: a clinicopathologic study of 9 patients. *Am J Surg Pathol*. 2004;28:789-793.
92. Sun J, Wang X, Wang C. Invasive cystic hypersecretory carcinoma of the breast: a rare variant of breast cancer: a case report and review of the literature. *BMC Cancer*. 2019;19:31.
93. Singh K, Falkenberry S, Eklund B, et al. Cystic hypersecretory hyperplasia of breast. *Int J Surg Pathol*. 2018;26:432-433.
94. Agnantis NT, Rosen PP. Mammary carcinoma with osteoclast-like giant cells. A study of eight cases with follow-up data. *Am J Clin Pathol*. 1979;72:383-389.
95. Zhou S, Yu L, Zhou R, et al. Invasive breast carcinomas of no special type with osteoclast-like giant cells frequently have a luminal phenotype. *Virchows Arch*. 2014;464:681-688.
96. Richter G, Uleer C, Noesselt T. Multifocal invasive ductal breast cancer with osteoclast-like giant cells: a case report. *J Med Case Rep*. 2011;5:85.
97. Saimura M, Fukutomi T, Tsuda H, et al. Breast carcinoma with osteoclast-like giant cells: a case report and review of the Japanese literature. *Breast Cancer*. 1999;6:121-126.
98. Iacocca MV, Maia DM. Bilateral infiltrating lobular carcinoma of the breast with osteoclast-like giant cells. *Breast J*. 2001;7:60-65.
99. Holland R, van Haelst UJ. Mammary carcinoma with osteoclast-like giant cells. Additional observations on six cases. *Cancer*. 1984;53:1963-1973.
100. Shishido-Hara Y, Kurata A, Fujiwara M, et al. Two cases of breast carcinoma with osteoclastic giant cells: are the osteoclastic giant cells pro-tumoural differentiation of macrophages? *Diagn Pathol*. 2010;5:55.
101. Ohashi R, Hayama A, Matsubara M, et al. Breast carcinoma with osteoclast-like giant cells: a cytological-pathological correlation with a literature review. *Ann Diagn Pathol*. 2018;33:1-5.
102. Lee JS, Kim YB, Min KW. Metaplastic mammary carcinoma with osteoclast-like giant cells: identical point mutation of p53 gene only identified in both the intraductal and sarcomatous components. *Virchows Arch*. 2004;444:194-197.
103. Tavassoli FA, Norris HJ. Breast carcinoma with osteoclastlike giant cells. *Arch Pathol Lab Med*. 1986;110:636-639.
104. Wargotz ES and Norris HJ. Metaplastic carcinomas of the breast: V. Metaplastic carcinoma with osteoclastic giant cells. *Hum Pathol*. 1990;21:1142-1150.
105. Ichijima K, Kobashi Y, Ueda Y, et al. Breast cancer with reactive multinucleated giant cells: report of three cases. *Acta Pathol Jpn*. 1986;36:449-457.
106. Pena-Jaimes L, Gonzalez-Garcia I, Reguero-Callejas ME, et al. Pleomorphic lobular carcinoma of the breast with osteoclast-like giant cells: a case report and review of the literature. *Diagn Pathol*. 2018;13:62.
107. Nielsen BB, Kiaer HW. Carcinoma of the breast with stromal multinucleated giant cells. *Histopathology*. 1985;9:183-193.
108. Cozzolino I, Ciancia G, Limite G, et al. Neuroendocrine differentiation in breast carcinoma with osteoclast-like giant cells. Report of a case and review of the literature. *Int J Surg*. 2014;12(Suppl 2):S8-S11.
109. Fadare O, Gill SA. Solid neuroendocrine carcinoma of the breast with osteoclast-like giant cells. *Breast J*. 2009;15:205-206.
110. Marchio C, Pietribiasi F, Castiglione R, et al. "Giants in a Microcosm": multinucleated giant cells populating an invasive micropapillary carcinoma of the breast. *Int J Surg Pathol*. 2015;23:654-655.
111. Zagelbaum NK, Ward MF 2nd, Okby N, et al. Invasive ductal carcinoma of the breast with osteoclast-like giant cells and clear cell features: a case report of a novel finding and review of the literature. *World J Surg Oncol*. 2016;14:227.
112. Krishnan C, Longacre TA. Ductal carcinoma in situ of the breast with osteoclast-like giant cells. *Hum Pathol*. 2006;37:369-372.
113. Irelli A, Sirufo MM, Quaglione GR, et al. Invasive ductal breast cancer with osteoclast-like giant cells: a case report based on the gene expression profile for changes in management. *J Pers Med*. 2021;11:156.
114. Wang J, Wei B, Albarracin CT, et al. Invasive neuroendocrine carcinoma of the breast: a population-based study from the surveillance, epidemiology and end results (SEER) database. *BMC Cancer*. 2014;14:147.
115. Jiang J, Wang G, Lv L, et al. Primary small-cell neuroendocrine carcinoma of the male breast: a rare case report with review of the literature. *Onco Targets Ther*. 2014;7:663-666.
116. Jundt G, Schulz A, Heitz PU, et al. Small cell neuroendocrine (oat cell) carcinoma of the male breast. Immunocytochemical and ultrastructural investigations. *Virchows Arch A Pathol Anat Histopathol*. 1984;404:213-221.
117. Jochems L, Tjalma WA. Primary small cell neuroendocrine tumour of the breast. *Eur J Obstet Gynecol Reprod Biol*. 2004;115:231-223.
118. Rineer J, Choi K, Sanmugarajah J. Small cell carcinoma of the breast. *J Natl Med Assoc*. 2009;101:1061-1064.
119. Hare F, Giri S, Patel JK, et al. A population-based analysis of outcomes for small cell carcinoma of the breast by tumor stage and the use of radiation therapy. *Springerplus*. 2015;4:138.
120. Hojo T, Kinoshita T, Shien T, et al. Primary small cell carcinoma of the breast. *Breast Cancer*. 2009;16:68-71.
121. Kitakata H, Yasumoto K, Sudo Y, et al. A case of primary small cell carcinoma of the breast. *Breast Cancer*. 2007;14:414-419.
122. Latif N, Rosa M, Samian L, et al. An unusual case of primary small cell neuroendocrine carcinoma of the breast. *Breast J*. 2010;16:647-651.
123. Mariscal A, Balliu E, Diaz R, et al. Primary oat cell carcinoma of the breast: imaging features. *AJR Am J Roentgenol*. 2004;183:1169-1171.
124. Yamaguchi R, Tanaka M, Otsuka H, et al. Neuroendocrine small cell carcinoma of the breast: report of a case. *Med Mol Morphol*. 2009;42:58-61.
125. Amano M, Ogura K, Ozaki Y, et al. Two cases of primary small cell carcinoma of the breast showing non-mass-like pattern on diagnostic imaging and histopathology. *Breast Cancer*. 2015;22:437-441.
126. Sampaio Vieira T, Borges Faria D, Souto Moura C, et al. Incidental finding of a breast carcinoma on Ga-68-DOTA-1-Nal3-octreotide positron emission tomography/computed tomography performed for the evaluation of a pancreatic neuroendocrine tumor: a case report. *Medicine (Baltimore)*. 2018;97:e11878.

127. Shin SJ, DeLellis RA, Ying L, et al. Small cell carcinoma of the breast: a clinicopathologic and immunohistochemical study of nine patients. *Am J Surg Pathol*. 2000;24:1231-1238.
128. Kawasaki T, Bussolati G, Castellano I, et al. Small-cell carcinoma of the breast with squamous differentiation. *Histopathology*. 2013;63:739-741.
129. Kinoshita S, Hirano A, Komine K, et al. Primary small-cell neuroendocrine carcinoma of the breast: report of a case. *Surg Today*. 2008;38:734-738.
130. Salman WD, Harrison JA, Howat AJ. Small-cell neuroendocrine carcinoma of the breast. *J Clin Pathol*. 2006;59:888.
131. Sridhar P, Matey P, Aluwihare N. Primary carcinoma of breast with small-cell differentiation. *Breast*. 2004;13:149-151.
132. Christie M, Chin-Lenn L, Watts MM, et al. Primary small cell carcinoma of the breast with TTF-1 and neuroendocrine marker expressing carcinoma in situ. *Int J Clin Exp Pathol*. 2010;3:629-633.
133. Hoang MP, Maitra A, Gazdar AF, et al. Primary mammary small-cell carcinoma: a molecular analysis of 2 cases. *Hum Pathol*. 2001;32:753-757.
134. Salmo EN, Connolly CE. Primary small cell carcinoma of the breast: report of a case and review of the literature. *Histopathology*. 2001;38:277-278.
135. Bergman S, Hoda SA, Geisinger KR, et al. E-cadherin-negative primary small cell carcinoma of the breast. Report of a case and review of the literature. *Am J Clin Pathol*. 2004;121:117-121.
136. Yamamoto J, Ohshima K, Nabeshima K, et al. Comparative study of primary mammary small cell carcinoma, carcinoma with endocrine features and invasive ductal carcinoma. *Oncol Rep*. 2004;11:825-831.
137. Lavigne M, Menet E, Tille JC, et al. Comprehensive clinical and molecular analyses of neuroendocrine carcinomas of the breast. *Mod Pathol*. 2018;31:68-82.
138. Zhong E, Pareja F, Hanna MG, et al. Expression of novel neuroendocrine markers in breast carcinomas: a study of INSM1, ASCL1, and POU2F3. *Hum Pathol*. 2022;127:102-111.
139. Adegbola T, Connolly CE, Mortimer G. Small cell neuroendocrine carcinoma of the breast: a report of three cases and review of the literature. *J Clin Pathol*. 2005;58:775-778.
140. Ersahin C, Bandyopadhyay S, Bhargava R. Thyroid transcription factor-1 and "basal marker"—expressing small cell carcinoma of the breast. *Int J Surg Pathol*. 2009;17:368-372.
141. McCullar B, Pandey M, Yaghmour G, et al. Genomic landscape of small cell carcinoma of the breast contrasted to small cell carcinoma of the lung. *Breast Cancer Res Treat*. 2016;158:195-202.
142. An JK, Woo JJ, Kang JH, et al. Small-cell neuroendocrine carcinoma of the breast. *J Korean Surg Soc*. 2012;82:116-119.
143. Ge QD, Lv N, Cao Y, et al. A case report of primary small cell carcinoma of the breast and review of the literature. *Chin J Cancer*. 2012;31:354-358.
144. Shin SJ, DeLellis RA and Rosen PP. Small cell carcinoma of the breast—additional immunohistochemical studies. *Am J Surg Pathol*. 2001;25:831-832.
145. Yamasaki T, Shimazaki H, Aida S, et al. Primary small cell (oat cell) carcinoma of the breast: report of a case and review of the literature. *Pathol Int*. 2000;50:914-918.
146. Bean GR, Najjar S, Shin SJ, et al. Genetic and immunohistochemical profiling of small cell and large cell neuroendocrine carcinomas of the breast. *Mod Pathol*. 2022;35:1349-1361.
147. Bobos M, Hytiroglou P, Kostopoulos I, et al. Immunohistochemical distinction between Merkel cell carcinoma and small cell carcinoma of the lung. *Am J Dermatopathol*. 2006;28:99-104.
148. Cloyd JM, Yang RL, Allison KH, et al. Impact of histological subtype on long-term outcomes of neuroendocrine carcinoma of the breast. *Breast Cancer Res Treat*. 2014;148:637-644.
149. Wei B, Ding T, Xing Y, et al. Invasive neuroendocrine carcinoma of the breast: a distinctive subtype of aggressive mammary carcinoma. *Cancer*. 2010;116:4463-4473.
150. Subramanian J, Vamsidhar V, Goodgame BW, et al. Distinctive characteristics of extrapulmonary small cell carcinoma: a Surveillance Epidemiology and End Results (SEER) analysis. *J Clin Oncol*. 2008;26:22106.
151. Grossman RA, Pedroso FE, Byrne MM, et al. Does surgery or radiation therapy impact survival for patients with extrapulmonary small cell cancers? *J Surg Oncol*. 2011;104:604-612.
152. Ochoa R, Sudhindra A, Garcia-Buitrago M, et al. Small-cell cancer of the breast: what is the optimal treatment? A report and review of outcomes. *Clin Breast Cancer*. 2012;12:287-292.
153. Angarita FA, Rodriguez JL, Meek E, et al. Locally-advanced primary neuroendocrine carcinoma of the breast: case report and review of the literature. *World J Surg Oncol*. 2013;11:128.
154. Inno A, Bogina G, Turazza M, et al. Neuroendocrine carcinoma of the breast: current evidence and future perspectives. *Oncologist*. 2016;21:28-32.
155. Fisher ER, Tavares J, Bulatao IS, et al. Glycogen-rich, clear cell breast cancer: with comments concerning other clear cell variants. *Hum Pathol*. 1985;16:1085-1090.
156. Zhou Z, Kinslow CJ, Hibshoosh H, et al. Clinical features, survival and prognostic factors of glycogen-rich clear cell carcinoma (GRCC) of the breast in the U.S. population. *J Clin Med*. 2019;8:246.
157. Akbulut M, Zekioglu O, Kapkac M, et al. Fine needle aspiration cytology of glycogen-rich clear cell carcinoma of the breast: review of 37 cases with histologic correlation. *Acta Cytol*. 2008;52:65-71.

158. Ma X, Han Y, Fan Y, et al. Clinicopathologic characteristics and prognosis of glycogen-rich clear cell carcinoma of the breast. *Breast J*. 2014;20:166-173.
159. Hayes MM, Seidman JD, Ashton MA. Glycogen-rich clear cell carcinoma of the breast. A clinicopathologic study of 21 cases. *Am J Surg Pathol*. 1995;19:904-911.
160. Eun NL, Cha YJ, Son EJ, et al. Clinical imaging of glycogen-rich clear cell carcinoma of the breast: a case series with literature review. *Magn Reson Med Sci*. 2019;18:238-242.
161. Martin-Martin B, Berna-Serna JD, Sanchez-Henarejos P, et al. An unusual case of locally advanced glycogen-rich clear cell carcinoma of the breast. *Case Rep Oncol*. 2011;4:452-457.
162. Salemis NS. Intraductal glycogen-rich clear cell carcinoma of the breast: a rare presentation and review of the literature. *Breast Care (Basel)*. 2012;7:319-321.
163. Di Tommaso L, Pasquinelli G, Portincasa G, et al. [Glycogen-rich clear-cell breast carcinoma with neuroendocrine differentiation features]. *Pathologica*. 2001;93:676-680.
164. Gurbuz Y, Ozkara SK. Clear cell carcinoma of the breast with solid papillary pattern: a case report with immunohistochemical profile. *J Clin Pathol*. 2003;56:552-554.
165. Sato A, Kawasaki T, Kashiwaba M, et al. Glycogen-rich clear cell carcinoma of the breast showing carcinomatous lymphangiosis and extremely aggressive clinical behavior. *Pathol Int*. 2015;65:674-676.
166. Hull MT, Warfel KA. Glycogen-rich clear cell carcinomas of the breast. A clinicopathologic and ultrastructural study. *Am J Surg Pathol*. 1986;10:553-559.
167. Kuroda H, Sakamoto G, Ohnisi K, et al. Clinical and pathological features of glycogen-rich clear cell carcinoma of the breast. *Breast Cancer*. 2005;12:189-195.
168. Damiani S, Chiodera P, Guaragni M, et al. Mammary angiomyolipoma. *Virchows Arch*. 2002;440:551-552.
169. Govender D, Sabaratnam RM, Essa AS. Clear cell "sugar" tumor of the breast: another extrapulmonary site and review of the literature. *Am J Surg Pathol*. 2002;26:670-675.
170. Aboumrad MH, Horn RC Jr, Fine G. Lipid-secreting mammary carcinoma. Report of a case associated with Paget's disease of the nipple. *Cancer*. 1963;16:521-525.
171. Ramos CV, Taylor HB. Lipid-rich carcinoma of the breast. A clinicopathologic analysis of 13 examples. *Cancer*. 1974;33:812-819.
172. Mazzella FM, Sieber SC, Braza F. Ductal carcinoma of male breast with prominent lipid-rich component. *Pathology*. 1995;27:280-283.
173. Balik E, Taneli C, Cetinkursun S, et al. Lipid secreting breast carcinoma in childhood: a case report. *Eur J Pediatr Surg*. 1993;3:48-49.
174. Shi P, Wang M, Zhang Q, et al. Lipid-rich carcinoma of the breast. A clinico-pathological study of 49 cases. *Tumori*. 2008;94:342-346.
175. Nagata Y, Hanagiri T, Ono K, et al. A non-invasive form of lipid-secreting carcinoma of the breast. *Breast Cancer*. 2012;19:83-87.
176. Kurisu Y, Tsuji M, Shibayama Y, et al. Intraductal lipid-rich carcinoma of the breast with a component of glycogen-rich carcinoma. *J Breast Cancer*. 2012;15:135-138.
177. van Bogaert LJ, Maldague P. Histologic variants of lipid-secreting carcinoma of the breast. *Virchows Arch A Pathol Anat Histol*. 1977;375:345-353.
178. Moritani S, Ichihara S, Hasegawa M, et al. Intracytoplasmic lipid accumulation in apocrine carcinoma of the breast evaluated with adipophilin immunoreactivity: a possible link between apocrine carcinoma and lipid-rich carcinoma. *Am J Surg Pathol*. 2011;35:861-867.
179. Varga Z, Robl C, Spycher M, et al. Metaplastic lipid-rich carcinoma of the breast. *Pathol Int*. 1998;48:912-916.
180. Kimura A, Miki H, Yuri T, et al. A case report of lipid-rich carcinoma of the breast including histological characteristics and intrinsic subtype profile. *Case Rep Oncol*. 2011;4:275-280.
181. Machalekova K, Kajo K, Bencat M. Unusual occurrence of rare lipid-rich carcinoma and conventional invasive ductal carcinoma in the one breast: case report. *Case Rep Pathol*. 2012;2012:387045.
182. Guan B, Wang H, Cao S, et al. Lipid-rich carcinoma of the breast clinicopathologic analysis of 17 cases. *Ann Diagn Pathol*. 2011;15:225-232.
183. Reis-Filho JS, Fulford LG, Lakhani SR, et al. Pathologic quiz case: a 62-year-old woman with a 4.5-cm nodule in the right breast. Lipid-rich breast carcinoma. *Arch Pathol Lab Med*. 2003;127:e396-e398.
184. Umekita Y, Yoshida A, Sagara Y, et al. Lipid-secreting carcinoma of the breast: a case report and review of the literature. *Breast Cancer*. 1998;5:171-173.
185. Limite G, Di Micco R, Esposito E, et al. Acinic cell carcinoma of the breast: review of the literature. *Int J Surg*. 2014;12(Suppl 1):S35-S39.
186. Ye RP, Liao YH, Xia T, et al. Breast mucoepidermoid carcinoma: a case report and review of literature. *Int J Clin Exp Pathol*. 2020;13:3192-3199.
187. Ragazzi M, de Biase D, Betts CM, et al. Oncocytic carcinoma of the breast: frequency, morphology and follow-up. *Hum Pathol*. 2011;42:166-175.
188. Asioli S, Marucci G, Ficarra G, et al. Polymorphous adenocarcinoma of the breast. Report of three cases. *Virchows Arch*. 2006;448:29-34.
189. Huang X, Lin Y, Wu H, et al. Sebaceous carcinoma of the breast nipple: a case report and literature review. *Int J Clin Exp Pathol*. 2017;10:10571-10575.

18
Lobular Carcinoma In Situ and Atypical Lobular Hyperplasia

ELAINE W. ZHONG AND SYED A. HODA

TERMINOLOGY OF "LOBULAR" LESIONS

Foote and Stewart (1) coined the term "lobular carcinoma in situ" (LCIS) for a group of neoplastic lesions of the breast that occurred in the terminal ducts and lobules and were characterized by loss of cellular cohesion, presence of cytoplasmic vacuoles, pagetoid extension, and multifocality.

Classic LCIS (C-LCIS) refers to a pattern of LCIS in which the affected acini are minimally distended, and the affected lobules are generally scattered amid breast tissue (**Figs. 18.1-18.3**). In objective terms, distention is defined as "the presence of 8 or more cells in the cross-sectional diameter of an acinus" (2). C-LCIS may be populated by cells of type "A" or type "B."

Type "A" cells are smaller (<1.5 times size of lymphocyte) with minimal cytoplasm, low-grade nuclei, inconspicuous nucleoli, and extremely rare mitoses. Type "B" cells are larger (2 times the size of lymphocyte) with more cytoplasm, intermediate-grade nuclei, micronucleoli, and rare mitoses (**Fig. 18.4**).

The classification of C-LCIS into types "A" and "B" is of no known clinical significance; however, such categorization serves as a reminder that "some cytologic variation can be observed in *bona fide* cases of C-LCIS, and these features should not be over-interpreted as representing the

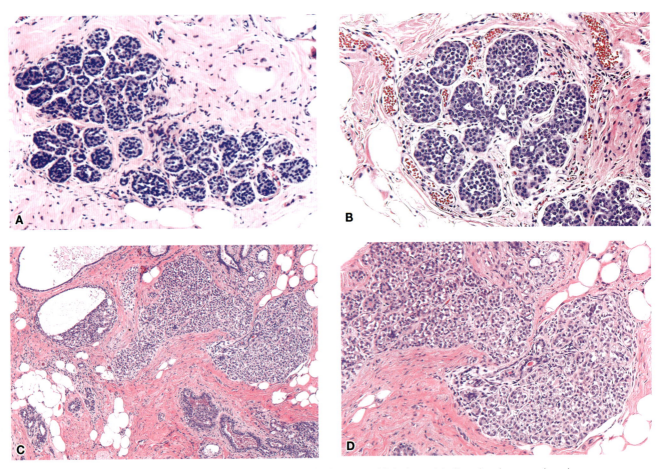

FIGURE 18.1 Lobular Carcinoma In Situ (LCIS). The normal lobular epithelium has been replaced by neoplastic cells that fill the acinar lumina in these needle core biopsy specimens. **A:** Two contiguous lobules are affected. The biopsy was performed for mammographically detected calcifications that were present in lobular glands not involved by in situ carcinoma. **B:** Magnified view of classic LCIS in a lobule is shown. **C, D:** Classic form of LCIS.

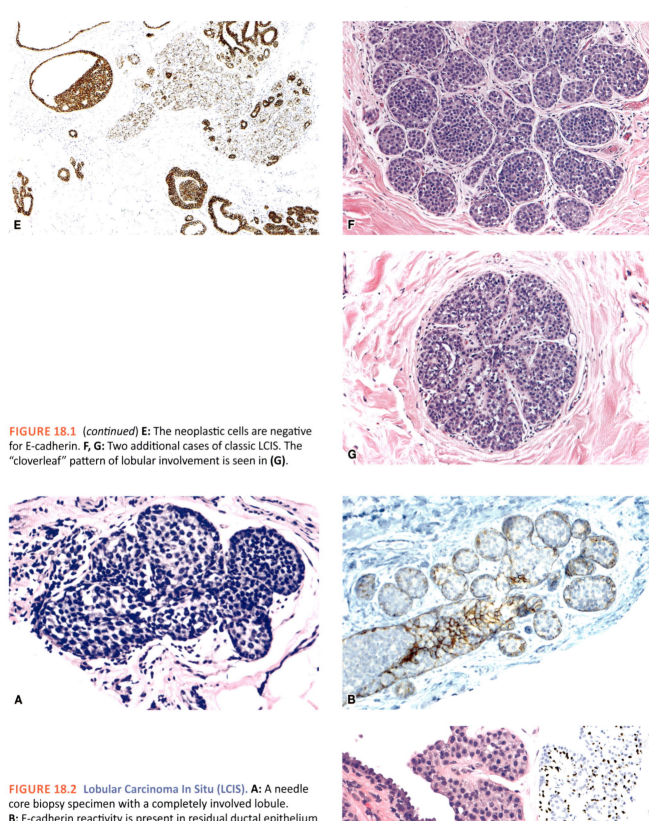

FIGURE 18.1 (*continued*) **E:** The neoplastic cells are negative for E-cadherin. **F, G:** Two additional cases of classic LCIS. The "cloverleaf" pattern of lobular involvement is seen in **(G)**.

FIGURE 18.2 Lobular Carcinoma In Situ (LCIS). **A:** A needle core biopsy specimen with a completely involved lobule. **B:** E-cadherin reactivity is present in residual ductal epithelium and in lobular myoepithelial cells in this example of LCIS in a terminal duct lobular unit. The neoplastic cells are not reactive. **C:** Another example of LCIS involving a terminal duct lobular unit. Top inset shows abundant presence of myoepithelial cells (p63-positive) around the LCIS. Bottom inset shows E-cadherin reactivity in myoepithelial cells and the absence of E-cadherin in the neoplastic cells. Such a lesion can be mistaken for myoepithelial hyperplasia.

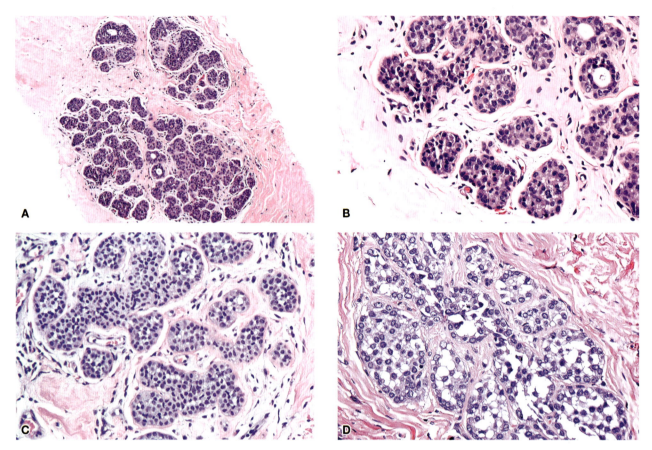

FIGURE 18.3 Lobular Carcinoma In Situ (LCIS). A, B: A needle core biopsy specimen with minimal diagnostic evidence. Approximately 85% of the lobular glands are involved. **C, D:** Loss of cohesion and focal cellular degeneration have resulted in the formation of spaces in some lobular glands. These are not true acinar lumina.

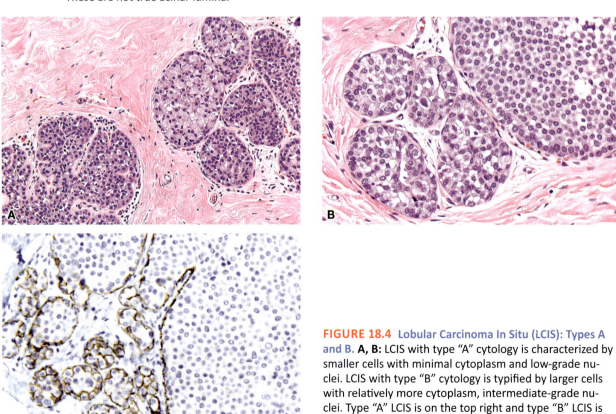

FIGURE 18.4 Lobular Carcinoma In Situ (LCIS): Types A and B. A, B: LCIS with type "A" cytology is characterized by smaller cells with minimal cytoplasm and low-grade nuclei. LCIS with type "B" cytology is typified by larger cells with relatively more cytoplasm, intermediate-grade nuclei. Type "A" LCIS is on the top right and type "B" LCIS is on the lower left in **(B)**. **C:** The E-cadherin immunostain is negative in both types of LCIS (same case as shown in **B**).

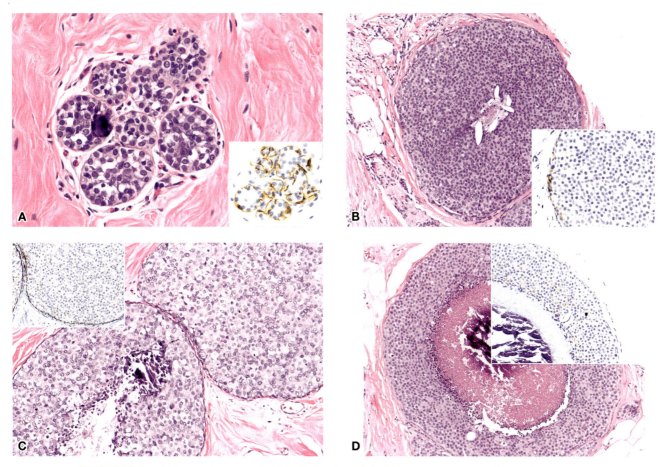

FIGURE 18.5 **Lobular Carcinoma In Situ (LCIS), Classic and Florid Patterns. A:** Low-grade neoplastic cells fill acini in this example of classic LCIS. This particular lesion has a calcification. **B:** A markedly enlarged duct is filled with a solid growth of florid LCIS with punctate central necrosis (insets show negativity for E-cadherin in each case). **C, D:** Two examples of florid LCIS with "macroacini," intermediate-grade nuclei, necrosis, and calcifications are shown. Insets show negativity for E-cadherin in each case.

pleomorphic variant of LCIS" (2). Nevertheless, in recent years, the cytologic classification of LCIS as "type A" and "type B" has been largely abandoned in favor of grouping into classic, florid, and pleomorphic variants.

LCIS can be architecturally as well as cytologically heterogeneous. Minimal distention of acini is the hallmark of C-LCIS, whereas confluent lobular involvement with marked distention of acini is observed in *florid LCIS* (F-LCIS). One proposed definition of F-LCIS requires at least 40 to 50 cells across the diameter of an acinus (3). The *pleomorphic variant of LCIS* (P-LCIS) is typically characterized by high-grade nuclei populating LCIS with florid-type features.

F-LCIS may be populated by cells of types "A" or "B" and can show central necrosis (**Figs. 18.5 and 18.6**). F-LCIS

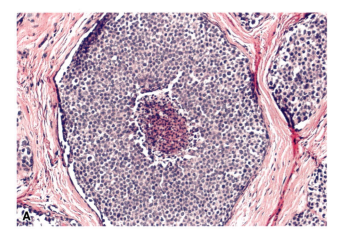
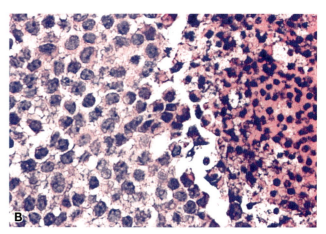

FIGURE 18.6 **Florid Lobular Carcinoma In Situ (LCIS). A:** A markedly enlarged duct is filled with a solid growth of florid LCIS. Central "comedo-type" necrosis is evident. **B:** This magnified view of the carcinoma shows necrosis and loss of cohesion between tumor cells.

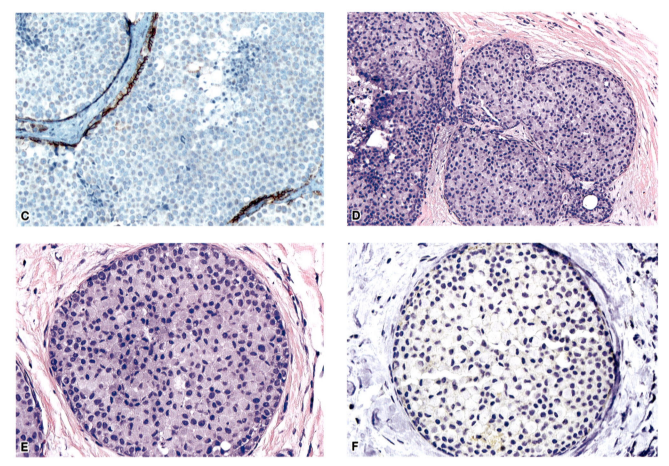

FIGURE 18.6 (*continued*) **C:** The LCIS is E-cadherin-negative. Reactivity is demonstrated in persisting myoepithelium. **D to F:** Another example of florid LCIS composed of cells with cytoplasmic mucin. The LCIS is E-cadherin-negative **(F)**.

with signet ring cells has also been described (4). F-LCIS shares several features with C-LCIS including some cytologic characteristics, loss of E-cadherin, gain of chromosome 1q, and loss of 16q; however, F-LCIS has been shown to demonstrate more genomic alterations than C-LCIS (5).

P-LCIS refers to a variant of LCIS in which there is diffuse involvement of contiguous lobules, and the individual acini are considerably distended. P-LCIS is populated by cells with variable size and shape (hence the designation: pleomorphic). P-LCIS cells are much larger (4 times the size of lymphocyte) and bear high-grade nuclei, irregular nuclear membranes, prominent nucleoli, and frequent mitoses. Central necrosis of the so-called "comedo" type usually accompanies P-LCIS. LCIS which is *cytologically* pleomorphic can be rarely found with classic *architectural* morphology in the vicinity of P-LCIS. Some cases of P-LCIS possess abundant eosinophilic (apocrine-type) cytoplasm and are referred to as apocrine P-LCIS (AP-LCIS) (6).

The issue of how much lobular involvement is necessary for the diagnosis of LCIS is of questionable relevance in the diagnosis of needle core biopsies (NCBs) that provide limited samples. Because the number of affected lobules in a biopsy has not proven to be related to the risk for subsequent carcinoma among patients not treated by mastectomy (7,8), there is presently no reason for drawing a distinction between one and two or more involved lobules (8). In some instances, the only evidence of a neoplastic lobular proliferation is one lobule in which some, but not all, acini are involved. It has been suggested, rather arbitrarily, that at least 50% (9) or 75% (10) of one lobule should be involved to establish a diagnosis of LCIS. Specimens with lesser lesions should be denoted *atypical lobular hyperplasia* (ALH).

The umbrella diagnostic term *lobular neoplasia* (LN), encompassing ALH and LCIS, was introduced by Haagensen et al (11) mainly for the purpose of avoiding overtreatment of the disease by removing the word "carcinoma" in an era when breast conservation therapy was uncommon (**Fig. 18.7**). This rationale is no longer valid. Furthermore, the spectrum of lesions encompassed by LN, from ALH to P-LCIS, is so broad as to render it a useless and misleading term.

Studies (12,13) have reported good interobserver agreement between general pathologists and specialized breast pathologists in the diagnosis of ALH ($\kappa = 0.62$), C-LCIS ($\kappa = 0.66$), and F-LCIS ($\kappa = 0.69$); however, poor to moderate agreement was observed for P-LCIS ($\kappa = 0.22\text{-}0.56$). It is probable that the presence of overt central necrosis in P-LCIS is the most likely reason for it to be mistaken for high-grade ductal carcinoma in situ (DCIS).

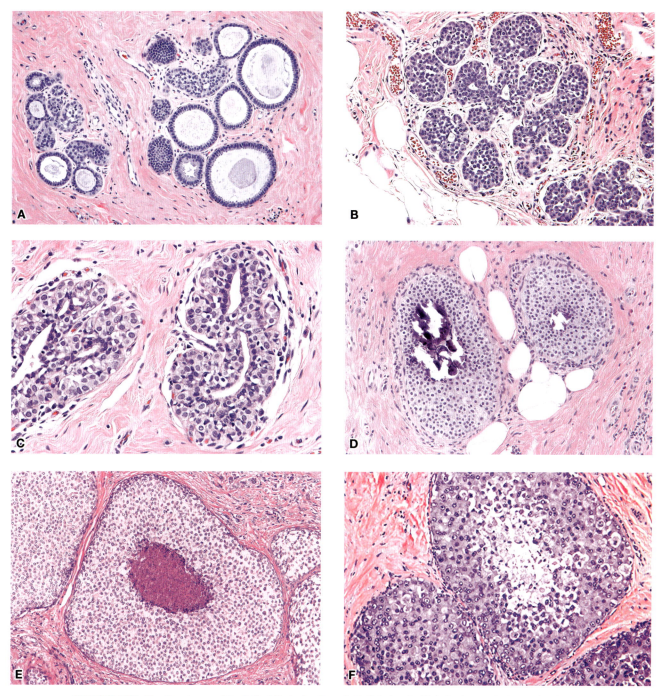

FIGURE 18.7 The Spectrum of So-Called "Lobular Neoplasia." **A:** Atypical lobular hyperplasia. **B:** Classic lobular carcinoma in situ (LCIS), type "A." **C:** Classic LCIS, type "B." **D:** Florid LCIS with calcifications. **E:** Florid LCIS with markedly distended acini, intermediate-grade nuclei, and central necrosis. **F:** Pleomorphic LCIS with markedly distended acini, high-grade nuclei, slightly apocrine cytoplasmic traits, and central necrosis.

CLINICAL FEATURES

C-LCIS is usually evident only on microscopic examination; it almost never forms a palpable tumor (14) and is rarely detectable by imaging. Typically, C-LCIS is discovered incidentally in breast tissue biopsied for lesions that produce masses or cause abnormalities on imaging studies. Calcifications are infrequently formed in C-LCIS, and when present are usually associated with another lesion. In particular, columnar cell alterations, which are predisposed to develop calcifications, often coexist with LCIS (15,16). Magnetic resonance imaging (MRI) sometimes shows non–mass enhancement (17) and may detect foci of ALH or LCIS, which are mammographically and sonographically occult (18,19). In one case report, dual-energy contrast-enhanced CT performed for evaluation of thoracic trauma in a 44-year-old patient incidentally detected a right breast mass, which was diagnosed on biopsy as LCIS (20). Histopathologic images and the LCIS subtype were not provided. Despite increasing sensitivity, no radiologic technique has proven to be a reliable method for detecting C-LCIS (8).

Exceptional situations exist in instances of F-LCIS and P-LCIS, the two variant forms of LCIS. These forms of LCIS show marked expansion of acini within lobules. F-LCIS and P-LCIS may involve the breast extensively (21) and can sometimes involve foci of sclerosing adenosis. Necrosis and calcification can be associated with F-LCIS and with nearly every case of P-LCIS. Additional imaging findings described in P-LCIS include mammographic distortion and regional clumped non-mass enhancement (22). F-LCIS and P-LCIS display a pattern and distribution more commonly encountered with DCIS rather than LCIS (23). Thus, the resultant appearance on mammography is likely to suggest DCIS.

LCIS is identified in 0.5% to 3% of benign breast biopsies (24,25). In a retrospective cohort analysis of a Surveillance, Epidemiology, and End Results (SEER) database, including 14,048 patients diagnosed with LCIS, a 38% increase in the incidence of LCIS was reported between 2000 and 2009, from 2.0 to 2.75 per 100,000 person-years (26), continuing the increase in incidence observed between 1978 and 1998 in U.S. population-based studies (27). The increase was highest among women 50 to 59 years of age. The increasing use and sensitivity of breast imaging leading to more frequent biopsies is probably the most important factor responsible for this trend (28).

Up to 25% of LCIS patients are postmenopausal at the time of first diagnosis (29). LCIS occurs infrequently in women younger than 35 years. In a consecutive series of more than 1,000 patients treated for breast carcinoma, the mean age of women with LCIS (53 years) was not significantly different from the mean age of patients who had invasive ductal carcinoma (57 years) (30).

Some conclusions based on the earliest studies of LCIS are still valid and provide invaluable insight into its behavior. These conclusions include the relatively high frequency of ipsilateral multicentric carcinoma, in 60% to 80% of patients (31), including occult invasive carcinoma in 5% to 6% of women who undergo mastectomy (32). LCIS is bilateral in 20% to 60% of biopsied cases (24). Urban (33) had reported finding LCIS in the contralateral breast in 40% of the cases when a random biopsy was performed even in the absence of any clinical abnormality. This procedure is rarely performed in current practice.

HISTOPATHOLOGIC EVALUATION

The anatomic distribution of LCIS in lobules and terminal ducts (and occasionally in ducts) as well as morphologic alterations in these structures influence the histopathologic appearance of LCIS in any given case. In the typical form, a population of neoplastic cells replaces the normal epithelium of acini within lobules. Intralobular ductules are also characteristically involved (**Fig. 18.8**). The LCIS cells must be

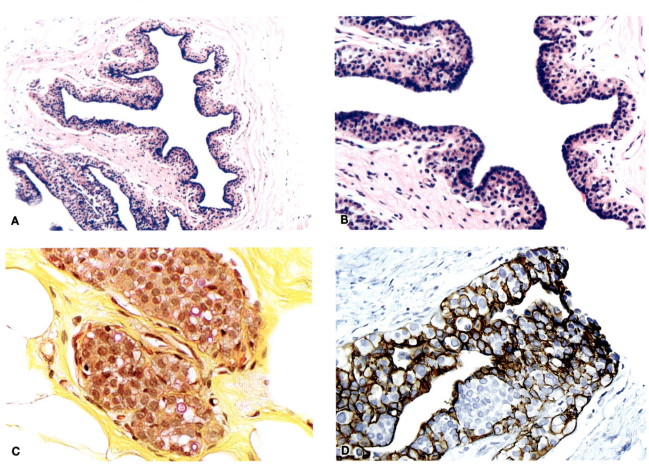

FIGURE 18.8 **Lobular Carcinoma In Situ (LCIS), Pagetoid Ductal and Partial Lobular Involvement.**
A, B: These dilated ducts involved by pagetoid spread of LCIS were found in a needle core biopsy specimen. **C:** Intracytoplasmic mucin is demonstrated with the mucicarmine stain in carcinoma cells. **D:** Pagetoid LCIS in this duct is highlighted by the absence of E-cadherin reactivity. The hyperplastic ductal epithelium is E-cadherin-positive.

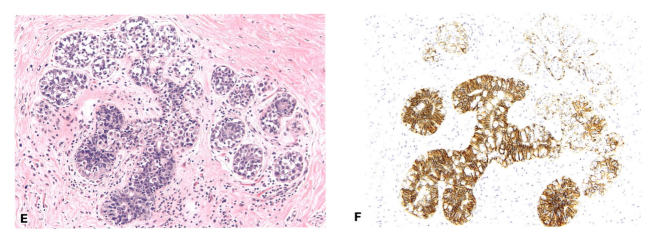

FIGURE 18.8 (*continued*) **E, F:** LCIS with partial (>50%) involvement of a lobule. E-cadherin immunostain (in **F**) shows reactivity limited to residual ductal cells.

sufficiently numerous to cause expansion of these structures. There may be enlargement of the entire lobule in comparison with uninvolved lobules in the adjacent breast tissues; however, lobular enlargement is not an absolute diagnostic criterion (**Fig. 18.9**). Lobular atrophy in postmenopausal women makes expansion of lobules an unreliable diagnostic feature in that patient group. If the diagnosis of LCIS is to be meaningful (ie, identifies a lesion associated with a substantial risk of invasive carcinoma), then the *architectural or quantitative finding of lobular enlargement* cannot

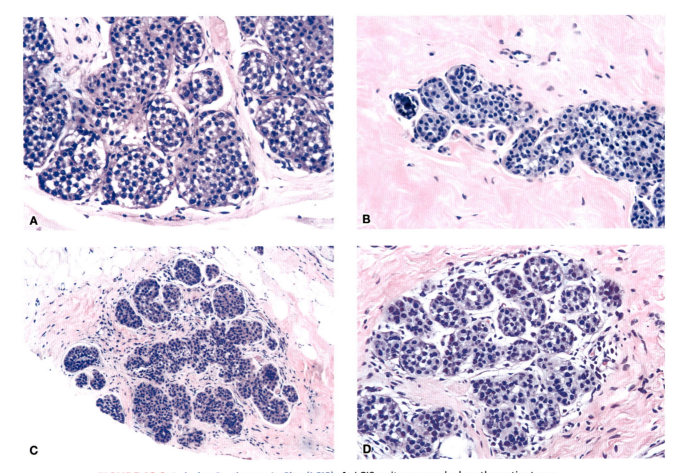

FIGURE 18.9 **Lobular Carcinoma In Situ (LCIS).** **A:** LCIS as it appeared when the patient was premenopausal. The lobular glands are fully expanded. **B:** LCIS as it appeared in a biopsy specimen taken from the same breast after the menopause. The lobules are markedly shrunken. One lobular gland contains a calcification. **C:** The only histopathologic lesion in this needle core biopsy specimen was this lobule with LCIS. **D:** This is one of several foci of LCIS found in the subsequent excisional biopsy specimen.

be regarded as the paramount diagnostic criterion in lesions that have reached an acceptable *qualitative level of cytologic abnormality*.

Loss of intercellular cohesion is a characteristic of LCIS, although this is not always readily apparent in acini filled and expanded by the process. When loss of cohesion is prominent, the resultant intercellular spaces may be mistaken for glandular lumina. Degenerative changes may also disrupt the cellular composition of LCIS. In these situations, the neoplastic cells are not arranged in a polarized fashion. The latter is a trait of non-neoplastic cells persisting around true glandular lumina. Loss of cohesion in LCIS is attributable to genetic alterations in the *CDH1* gene that are evidenced by greatly reduced, fragmented, or absent membrane E-cadherin immunoreactivity (34,35).

Intracytoplasmic vacuoles that contain mucin are present in some LCIS cells (**Fig. 18.10**). The presence of mucin can be highlighted with mucicarmine, Alcian blue, or periodic acid–Schiff (PAS) stains. A distinctive manifestation of this phenomenon is the formation of signet ring cells having a distended cytoplasmic vacuole that causes the nucleus to appear eccentric, crescentic, or indented. Signet ring cells can have low-, intermediate-, or high-grade nuclei. Intracytoplasmic mucin vacuoles are uncommon in ductal carcinoma cells and are also uncommon in hyperplastic lesions of ductal or lobular epithelium. Thus, the presence of intracellular mucin is an important but not a necessary criterion for the diagnosis of LCIS. Intracytoplasmic mucin is also present in LCIS with clear cell change.

Several uncommon cytologic features can be found in LCIS. Cytoplasmic pallor or cytoplasmic clearing occurs rarely. These cells may have intracytoplasmic mucin that is not restricted to vacuoles, an occurrence manifested by diffuse cytoplasmic staining with mucicarmine or Alcian blue stains. Apocrine change has been described in LCIS (36). Mucin in the cytoplasm of cells in apocrine LCIS is usually evident in hematoxylin and eosin (H&E)-stained sections as cytoplasmic amphophilia or basophilia. Apocrine LCIS often has pleomorphic cytology and tends to grow in a pagetoid manner into ducts where it can be difficult to distinguish from apocrine DCIS (**Fig. 18.11**) (6). However, apocrine LCIS is E-cadherin-negative, and it is often estrogen receptor (ER)-positive, whereas apocrine DCIS is E-cadherin-positive and almost always ER-negative. LCIS in atrophic lobules and

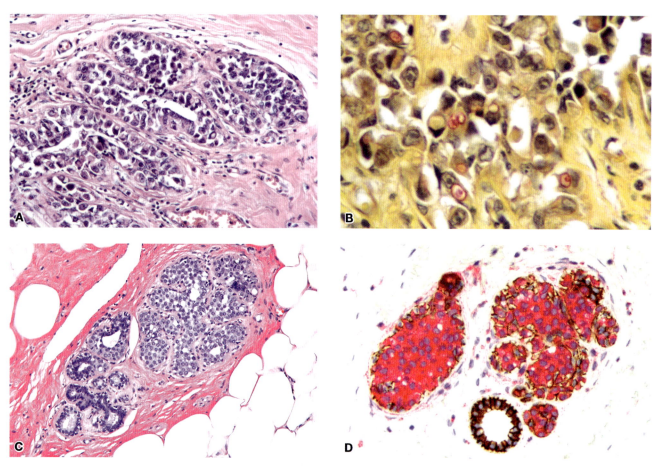

FIGURE 18.10 Lobular Carcinoma In Situ (LCIS), Postmenopausal. A, B: The lesion is characterized by loss of cohesion and shrinkage of the tumor cells in lobular glands. Intracytoplasmic mucin is demonstrated with the mucicarmine stain **(B)**. **C, D:** In this example of LCIS in the elderly, the entire lobule is small. The lesional cells are p120-positive (depicted by red cytoplasmic staining). Benign epithelial cells are strongly positive for E-cadherin (depicted by brown staining), and myoepithelial cells show weaker staining with E-cadherin (double immunostain with p120 and E-cadherin). The LCIS cells are not reactive for E-cadherin.

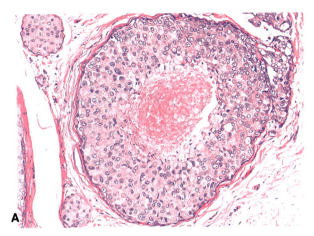 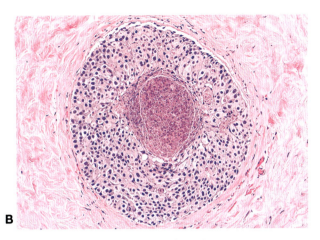

FIGURE 18.11 **Apocrine Pleomorphic Lobular Carcinoma In Situ (AP-LCIS) Versus Ductal Carcinoma In Situ (DCIS). A:** AP-LCIS. **B:** Solid apocrine (high-grade) DCIS. Note the cytologic and architectural similarity of the two lesions. Both show solid growth with central necrosis, pleomorphic high-grade nuclei, and cytoplasmic eosinophilia. E-cadherin immunostain (not shown) was positive in the tumor in (**A**) and negative in the tumor in (**B**).

terminal ducts of postmenopausal women sometimes features cells with dark, eosinophilic-to-basophilic cytoplasm and deeply basophilic, eccentric nuclei. This appearance is probably the result of cytoplasmic condensation associated with loss of cohesion and shrinkage of cells. These cells frequently contain intracytoplasmic mucin; they may resemble smooth muscle cells, and in that event have been referred to as *myoid* LCIS. In another variant, the cells of LCIS have a *mosaic* appearance that seemingly results from the presence of distinct cell borders between cells and prominent, round, centrally placed nuclei surrounded by pale cytoplasm (**Fig. 18.12**). Intracytoplasmic mucin vacuoles can usually be found in this type of LCIS.

LCIS typically involves terminal ductules as well as acinar units within the lobule (**Fig. 18.13**). In postmenopausal patients with atrophic lobules, ductal involvement may be the only manifestation of LCIS. The irregular configuration of ductules affected by LCIS has been described as "saw-toothed" or as resembling a cloverleaf. Pagetoid LCIS cells growing beneath the non-neoplastic ductal epithelium may be distributed continuously or discontinuously along the ductal system, undermining and ultimately displacing the native ductal epithelium. The cloverleaf pattern of LCIS sometimes involves the terminal ducts, seemingly without lobular involvement. The myoepithelial layer is preserved to a variable extent, and it may require p63 and other appropriate immunostains to confirm its presence. LCIS can be found in lesions with intra-acinar myoepithelial cell hyperplasia (37).

Pagetoid spread of LCIS may also be encountered in papillomas or radial sclerosing lesions. F-LCIS may proliferate to form a solid mass of tumor cells that fill and expand the ductal lumen and develop central necrosis and calcifications that are detectable in mammograms. A negative, weak, or fragmented E-cadherin immunostain distinguishes this pattern of F-LCIS from E-cadherin-positive solid high-grade DCIS (38).

Parenthetically, the *Rosen Triad* comprises LCIS, columnar cell changes, and tubular carcinoma, which frequently

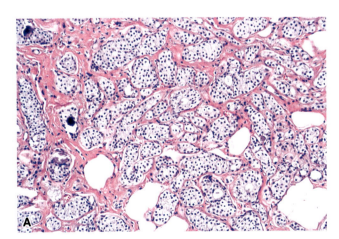 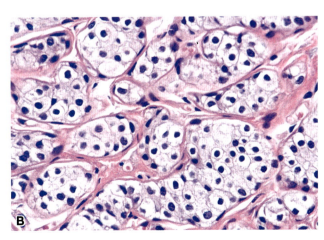

FIGURE 18.12 **Lobular Carcinoma In Situ (LCIS), Mosaic Pattern. A, B:** The lesion involves sclerosing adenosis. Calcifications are shown in (**A**). The cells have distinct cytoplasmic borders, abundant pale cytoplasm, and punctate centrally placed nuclei.

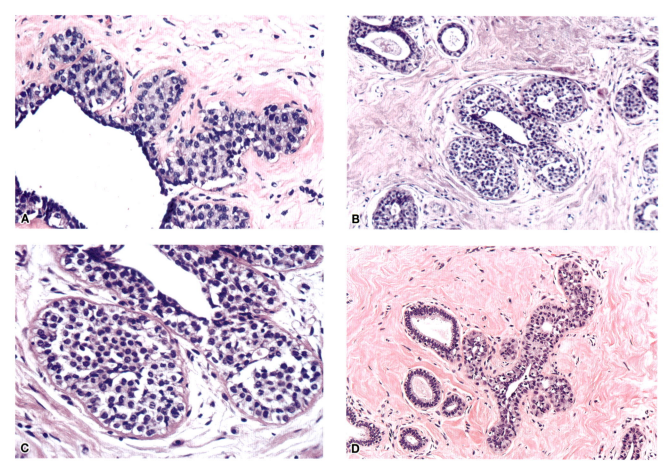

FIGURE 18.13 Lobular Carcinoma In Situ (LCIS), Ductal Involvement. A: The cloverleaf pattern of ductal involvement is shown. The presence of lobule-like structures around the perimeter of the duct suggests that the neoplasm arose de novo at this site. **B, C:** This small duct exhibits florid LCIS and pagetoid spread in adjacent ductules. **D:** Another example of LCIS with pagetoid spread into a terminal duct.

coexist (**Fig. 18.14**) (39). The latter two lesions are often responsible for mammographically detected calcifications in the absence of a palpable lesion. ALH and LCIS are commonly associated with various types of columnar change (**Fig. 18.15**). An instance of the Rosen Triad with LCIS of the signet ring cell type has been reported (40).

Lobular Carcinoma In Situ With Collagenous Spherulosis

An unusual pattern of ductal involvement occurs when LCIS develops in glands altered by collagenous spherulosis (41). This configuration mimics cribriform DCIS (**Fig. 18.16**).

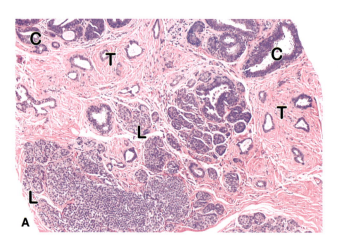
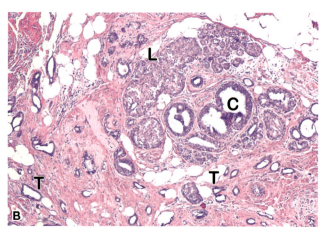

FIGURE 18.14 The Rosen Triad. A, B: Two examples of the "Rosen Triad" comprising lobular carcinoma in situ (labeled *L*), columnar cell changes (labeled *C*), and tubular carcinoma (labeled *T*) are shown. The entire triad is seen in a needle core biopsy sampling in **(A)**.

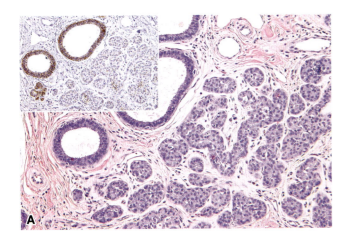
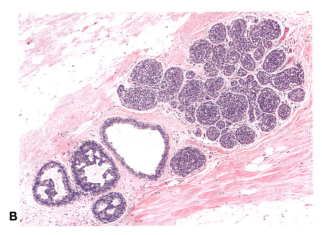
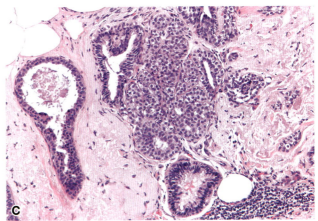

FIGURE 18.15 Lobular Carcinoma In Situ (LCIS)/Atypical Lobular Hyperplasia (ALH) and Columnar Cell Changes. A: LCIS associated with columnar cell change (inset shows E-cadherin negativity in LCIS and E-cadherin positivity in columnar cell change). **B:** LCIS associated with atypical columnar cell hyperplasia. **C:** ALH associated with columnar cell change.

However, myoepithelial cells outline the spherule material. The latter should be distinguished from true microlumina of cribriform DCIS. The neoplastic cells in such foci display loss of cohesion and intracytoplasmic vacuoles characteristic of lobular carcinoma. When LCIS involves collagenous spherulosis, myoepithelium can be highlighted with immunostains such as p63 and myosin. LCIS cells will be E-cadherin-negative. LCIS in collagenous spherulosis only rarely occurs as an isolated finding even in NCB samplings. In the series reported by Eisenberg and Hoda (41), LCIS was identified beyond the index lesion in 4 of 38 cases (14%). In this series, 22 of the 38 specimens were NCB samplings.

IMMUNOHISTOCHEMISTRY

The distinction between LCIS and DCIS on NCB sampling is of clinical significance because a subsequent excisional biopsy may not be performed for LCIS. Furthermore, there may be long-term implications for nonsurgical risk-reducing management. Immunohistochemical and histologic features of LCIS are listed in **Table 18.1**.

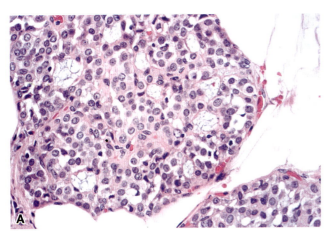
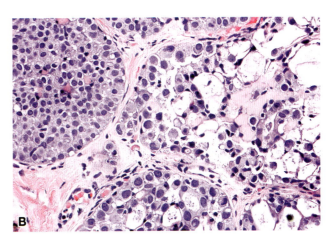

FIGURE 18.16 Lobular Carcinoma In Situ (LCIS) in Collagenous Spherulosis. A: LCIS is shown involving collagenous spherulosis above. Indistinct fibrillary material in the spherules contributes to the cribriform-like appearance. **B:** Pleomorphic LCIS in collagenous spherulosis.

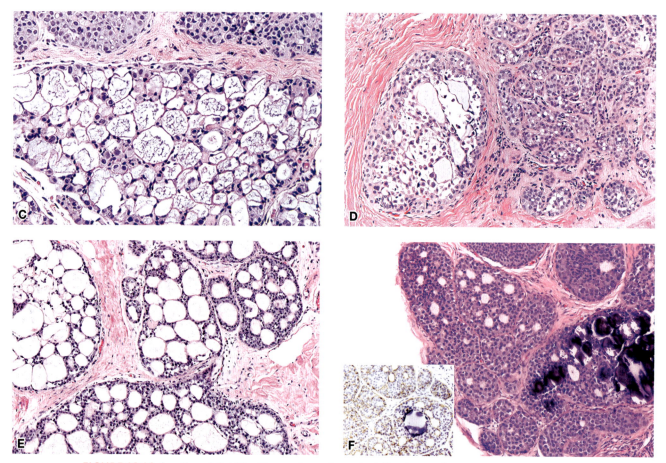

FIGURE 18.16 (*continued*) **C:** LCIS with apocrine traits and calcifications in degenerative collagenous spherulosis. **D:** LCIS in collagenous spherulosis with "mucoid" features. **E:** LCIS with collagenous spherulosis mimicking cribriform type of ductal carcinoma in situ (DCIS). **F:** LCIS in collagenous spherulosis that resembles cribriform/solid DCIS with calcifications. Inset shows absence of E-cadherin immunoreactivity.

TABLE 18.1
Histopathologic Features of Classic and Variant LCIS

	C-LCIS	F-LCIS	P-LCIS	AP-LCIS
Cytology	Type A (<1.5× size of lymphocyte) and Type B (2× size of lymphocyte)	Cytologic features of C-LCIS	Pleomorphic, >4× size of lymphocyte	Cytologic features of P-LCIS, eosinophilic granular cytoplasm, nucleoli
Architecture	>50% acini in TDLU filled and expanded	Marked distention of TDLU, 40-50 cells across	Variable	Variable
Calcifications	Uncommon	Variable	Variable	Variable
Necrosis	Uncommon	Variable	Present	Present
IHC ER	(+)	(+)	(+/−)	(−/+)
PR	(+)	(+)	(+/−)	(−/+)
HER2	(−)	(−)	(−/+)	(−/+)
E-cadherin	(−)	(−)	(−)	(−)
p120	Cytoplasmic	Cytoplasmic	Cytoplasmic	Cytoplasmic
Ki67	Low	Intermediate	High	High

AP-LCIS, apocrine pleomorphic lobular carcinoma in situ; C-LCIS, classic lobular carcinoma in situ; ER, estrogen receptor; F-LCIS, florid lobular carcinoma in situ; HER2, human epidermal growth factor receptor 2; IHC, immunohistochemistry; P-LCIS, pleomorphic lobular carcinoma in situ; PR, progesterone receptor; TDLU, terminal duct lobular unit.

C-LCIS is strongly and diffusely positive for ER and for progesterone receptor (PR) and only rarely expresses human epidermal growth factor receptor 2 (HER2) or p53 protein. F-LCIS shows a similar pattern of immunoreactivity. Khoury et al (42) reported the results of ancillary studies on P-LCIS. Seven of the 25 (28%) cases were negative for ER, nine (36%) were negative for PR, and five (20%) were negative for both ER and PR. Seven of the 17 cases (41%) were HER2-positive, and eight (47%) were equivocal for HER2 (fluorescence in situ hybridization was not reported). There were two triple-negative cases. AP-LCIS is even more likely to be negative for ER and PR and/or show HER2 expression (43,44).

The E-cadherin complex is composed of transmembrane E-cadherin protein and various catenins (including α-, β-, and p120 catenin). The catenins serve to anchor the E-cadherin protein to cytoplasmic actin filaments. When E-cadherin is defective or absent, its intracellular ligand p120 redistributes from its submembranous location to the cytoplasm. Notably, p120 immunoreactivity is evident in cytosol of ALH, LCIS, and invasive lobular carcinoma (ILC) cells. β-Catenin as well as α-catenin are absent in ALH and LCIS (12,45). LCIS is negative for E-cadherin in approximately 90% of all LCIS cases. It is important to ensure that there is cytoplasmic membrane positivity of E-cadherin in normal breast epithelium before interpreting the lack of lesional staining as negative.

Rarely, the cells of ALH or LCIS display weak, fragmented ("dot-like"), and discontinuous E-cadherin reactivity, which is substantially weaker than that observed in ductal epithelium, so-called "aberrant reactivity" (38,46-49) (**Fig. 18.17**). Approximately 10% of LCIS cases express E-cadherin in this fashion (50,51). Cases of LCIS that have aberrant E-cadherin reactivity may nonetheless be negative for β-catenin and show cytoplasmic p120—a finding that is consistent with loss of function of the E-cadherin and catenin complex (52) (**Fig. 18.18**). Aberrant reactivity for E-cadherin should not preclude the diagnosis of LCIS if the cytologic and histologic characteristics are indicative of lobular differentiation. It is notable that true E-cadherin negativity in carcinomas of ductal phenotype (except those of the metaplastic type) is rare (<1%) (53).

Some cases of LCIS show concomitant classic and pleomorphic cell types, both of which are E-cadherin-negative (35). Variable E-cadherin reactivity has been reported when different antibodies were used (46).

In some cases, apparent positivity of LCIS cells for E-cadherin may be due to admixture of non-neoplastic reactive

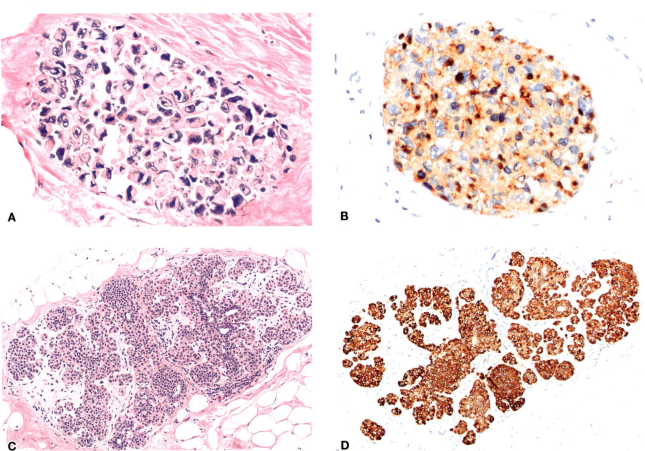

FIGURE 18.17 **E-cadherin Immunohistochemistry. A, B:** Pleomorphic lobular carcinoma in situ (LCIS) with aberrant ("dot-like") staining with E-cadherin. **C, D:** Classic LCIS with unusual diffuse membranous and cytoplasmic expression of E-cadherin. This finding should not preclude the diagnosis of LCIS in the setting of typical morphology.

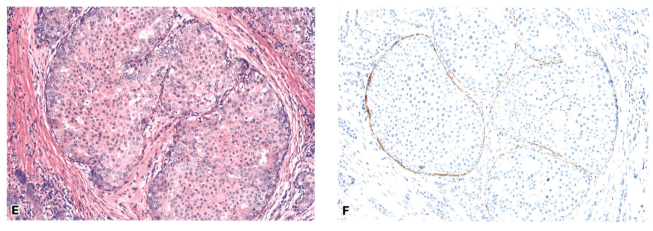

FIGURE 18.17 (*continued*) **E, F:** Solid in situ carcinoma with morphology indeterminate for ductal versus lobular differentiation. Negative E-cadherin supports the latter.

myoepithelial cells or residual ductal epithelial cells. Indeed, there may be marked intra-acinar myoepithelial proliferation in certain LCIS lesions (37). In such cases, E-cadherin shows negativity in LCIS and diffuse, albeit weak, positivity in myoepithelial cells. There is a potential for such biphasic staining to be misinterpreted and for the lesion to be misdiagnosed as mixed LCIS and DCIS.

MOLECULAR STUDIES

Approximately 60% of LCIS shows loss or inactivation of chromosome 16q22.1, the site of the *CDH1* gene (54,55). Inactivation via deletion, truncating mutation, or promoter methylation is most common. *CDH1* gene encodes E-cadherin, a transmembrane glycoprotein involved in intercellular

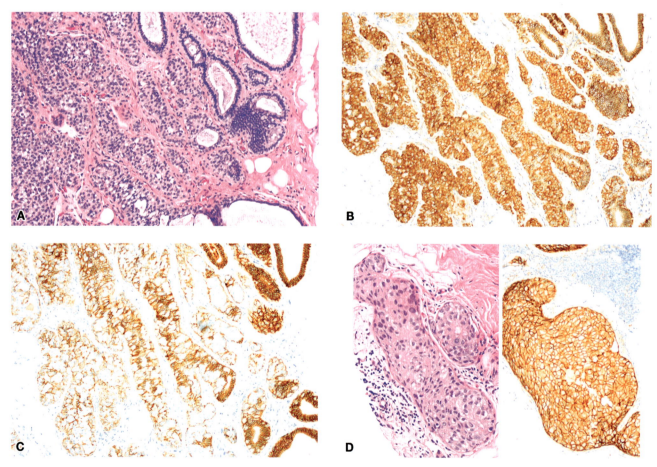

FIGURE 18.18 p120 immunohistochemistry. A to C: Classic lobular carcinoma in situ (LCIS) showing cytoplasmic expression of p120 (**B**), a result of dysfunctional cadherin-catenin complex. Note membranous staining in adjacent uninvolved ducts (upper right). E-cadherin (**C**) is negative in LCIS. **D:** In contrast, there is membranous expression of p120 in ductal carcinoma in situ.

adhesion. Notably, *CDH1* mutation status does not always correlate with E-cadherin expression (56), nor is it entirely specific to LCIS. Despite the high frequency of somatic *CDH1* mutations in LCIS, germline mutations are rarely detected in these patients (54,57). Germline *CHEK2* mutation was associated with pure LCIS in a targeted sequencing study of LCIS and ILC (58). Other chromosomal alterations common in the spectrum of low-grade mammary lesions such as −16p, −17p, −22q, and +6q are also observed in LCIS (59).

P-LCIS and AP-LCIS share alterations with C-LCIS but exhibit a more complex genetic profile (36). F-LCIS shows still more aberrations (60). Amplification of *CCND1* was more prevalent in P-LCIS than in C-LCIS in one study (36). AP-LCIS has not demonstrated any specific molecular alterations by massively parallel sequencing (6).

The data most closely linking LCIS to ILC come from molecular studies of the two lesions when they coexist. Multiple studies have demonstrated that concurrent LCIS and ILCs shared the same E-cadherin mutations and the same distribution of loss of heterozygosity, including loss of 16.q22.1 (35,55,61-63). These provide evidence that at least some LCIS are non-obligate precursors of ILC.

DIFFERENTIAL DIAGNOSIS

DCIS is the most frequent entity that is mistaken for LCIS, and vice versa. Low-grade solid DCIS can be mistaken for C-LCIS and F-LCIS (**Table 18.2**), and P-LCIS may be difficult to distinguish from high-grade DCIS. The E-cadherin immunostain is the most effective method to differentiate between LCIS and DCIS. C-LCIS, F-LCIS, and P-LCIS exhibit strong reactivity for the high-molecular-weight cytokeratin 34βE12 (K903). The latter is typically absent or weakly present in DCIS. The presence of cribriform,

papillary, or micropapillary architecture also suggests ductal differentiation.

Intraepithelial histiocytes can be confused with pagetoid LCIS. Histiocytes possess foamy cytoplasm, sometimes with lipofuscin or hemosiderin pigment, and relatively small dark nuclei. Intracytoplasmic mucin is typically absent from histiocytes, and the latter are not immunoreactive for cytokeratin. The overlying non-neoplastic epithelium is attenuated and flattened over intraepithelial histiocytes as well as over pagetoid spread of LCIS. Intraepithelial histiocytes may be relatively sparse, or they may form a continuous layer, which may be one or more cells thick. CD68 immunostain highlights histiocytes.

Epithelioid myoepithelial hyperplasia is more likely to be mistaken for pagetoid spread of LCIS than the presence of intraepithelial histiocytes. Epithelioid myoepithelial cells have abundant clear vesicular cytoplasm. Except in papillomas, hyperplastic myoepithelial cells tend to be distributed in a single layer, causing less attenuation of the overlying epithelium than pagetoid LCIS. Some "myoid" immunohistochemical properties are usually retained in epithelioid myoepithelial hyperplasia. p63 immunostain is reliable in this circumstance because nuclear reactivity is retained in epithelioid myoepithelial cells, whereas LCIS cells are p63-negative.

Coexistence of LCIS and DCIS in a single duct is a relatively unusual phenomenon (**Figs. 18.19 and 18.20**). When this occurs, LCIS often grows in a cloverleaf pattern around the perimeter of a ductal lumen that contains cytologically and histologically different DCIS. E-cadherin immunostaining is helpful in confirming the diagnosis of coexistent LCIS and DCIS in a single ductal lobular unit (38).

Lobules structurally altered by various other proliferative processes can harbor LCIS (41,64). Consequently, LCIS has been encountered in sclerosing adenosis, radial scars, collagenous spherulosis, fibroadenoma, phyllodes tumor, papilloma, and papillary carcinoma (**Fig. 18.21**). The demonstration of intracytoplasmic mucin droplets is helpful for distinguishing LCIS from florid adenosis. In all of the foregoing situations, the most reliable method for confirming the presence of LCIS is the demonstration of weak, fragmented, or absent E-cadherin immunoreactivity along with appropriate cytologic features.

LCIS in tubular adenosis and in sclerosing adenosis has a striking histologic appearance (**Fig. 18.22**). Most cases show a lobular configuration at low magnification, uninvolved sclerosing adenosis in neighboring tissue, and separate foci of unequivocal LCIS (65). Normal lobular architecture is markedly distorted in sclerosing lesions, and as a result it is difficult to exclude invasion when LCIS occurs in such foci (64). Careful inspection usually reveals the underlying adenosis pattern in which glandular units are surrounded by myoepithelial cells and basement membrane. The latter structure can be highlighted with reticulin stain and by laminin or type IV collagen immunostain. p63, CD10, calponin, and actin immunostains highlight the myoepithelial layer. The spindle-shaped myoepithelial cells persist in sclerosing adenosis, albeit in an extremely slender form, even when the

TABLE 18.2

Staining Patterns of Classic LCIS and Low-Grade Solid DCIS

	Classic LCIS	Low-Grade Solid DCIS
Mucin stains[a]	(+)	(−)
E-cadherin	(−)	(+)
β-Catenin	(−)	(+)
α-Catenin	(−)	(+)
p120 localization	(+) cytoplasmic	(+) membranous
Cytokeratin 34βE12	(+)	(−), or weakly (+)

DCIS, ductal carcinoma in situ; LCIS, lobular carcinoma in situ.
[a]Mucicarmine, Alcian blue, or periodic acid–Schiff (PAS) histochemical stains can be utilized.

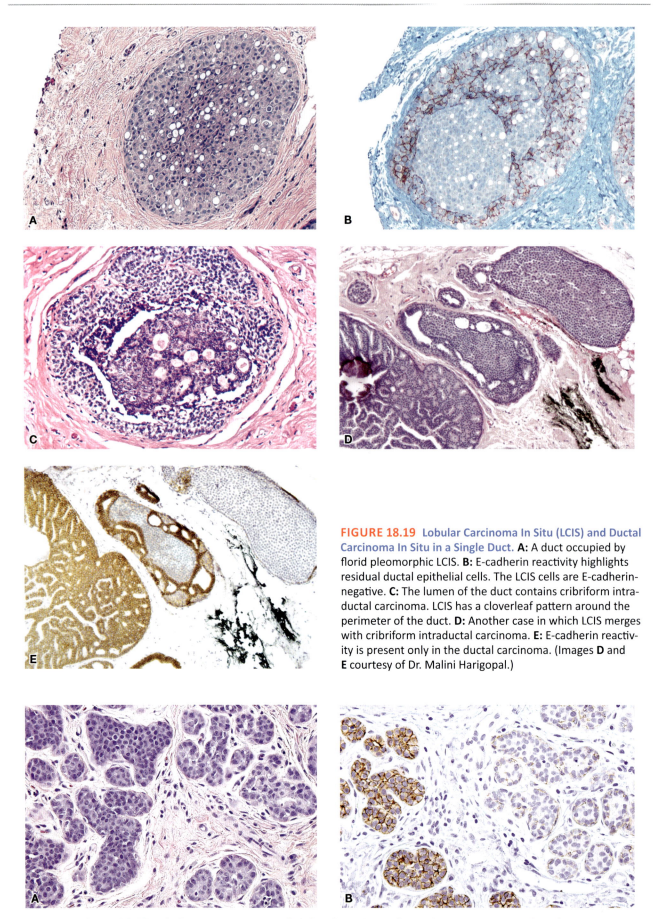

FIGURE 18.19 **Lobular Carcinoma In Situ (LCIS) and Ductal Carcinoma In Situ in a Single Duct. A:** A duct occupied by florid pleomorphic LCIS. **B:** E-cadherin reactivity highlights residual ductal epithelial cells. The LCIS cells are E-cadherin-negative. **C:** The lumen of the duct contains cribriform intraductal carcinoma. LCIS has a cloverleaf pattern around the perimeter of the duct. **D:** Another case in which LCIS merges with cribriform intraductal carcinoma. **E:** E-cadherin reactivity is present only in the ductal carcinoma. (Images **D** and **E** courtesy of Dr. Malini Harigopal.)

FIGURE 18.20 **Lobular Carcinoma In Situ (LCIS) in the Vicinity of Ductal Carcinoma In Situ (DCIS). A, B:** In this example, LCIS **(right)** and DCIS **(left)** of the solid type lie in juxtaposition. LCIS cells appear discohesive. E-cadherin differentiates LCIS (negative stain) from DCIS (positive staining).

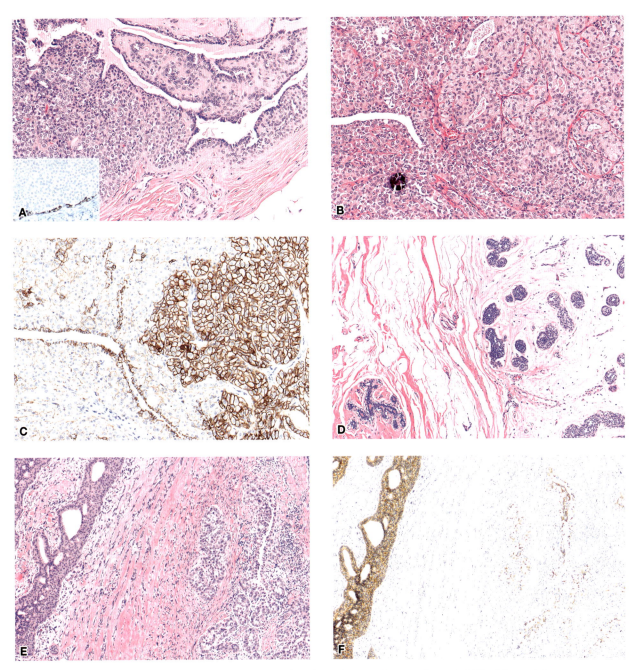

FIGURE 18.21 Lobular Carcinoma In Situ (LCIS) Involving Various Lesions. A: LCIS with partial involvement of an intraductal papilloma (inset shows negative E-cadherin staining in LCIS). **B, C:** LCIS with partial involvement of a solid papillary carcinoma. LCIS cells are negative for E-cadherin **(C)**. **D:** LCIS in a myxoid fibroadenoma. **E, F:** LCIS in a benign phyllodes tumor. There is moderate epithelial hyperplasia in the elongated ducts on the left. LCIS cells are negative for E-cadherin **(F)**.

lesion is colonized by LCIS (64). Invasive carcinoma cannot be diagnosed as long as the neoplastic cells remain confined to sclerosing adenosis.

MICROINVASIVE LOBULAR CARCINOMA

The diagnosis of ILC can be rendered by finding carcinoma cells in the stroma outside the confines of the periglandular myoepithelial cells and basement membrane (Figs. 18.23 and 18.24). Foci of microinvasive (<0.1 cm) carcinoma are more easily detected with double immunostaining, typically myoepithelial (myosin) and epithelial (cytokeratin).

Most lobules in premenopausal women are surrounded by fibrous stroma, but infrequently lobules are distributed amid adipose tissue. Lobules in fat are subject to the same histopathologic alterations that occur in parenchymal lobules, including the development of sclerosing adenosis and LCIS. These conditions may resemble invasive carcinoma.

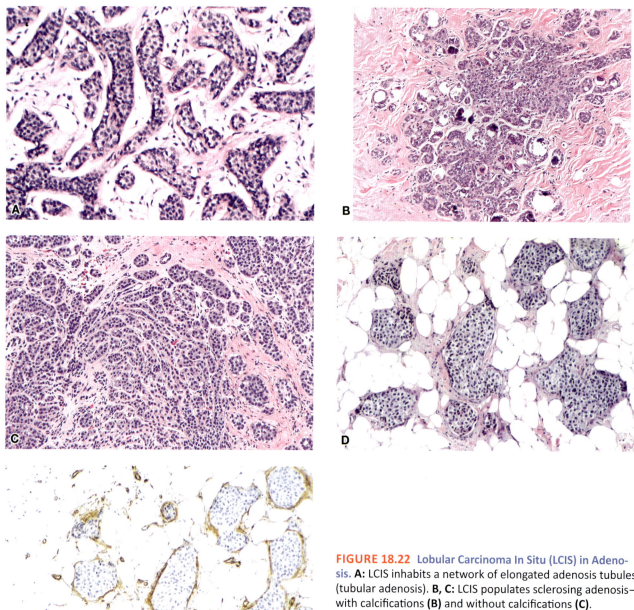

FIGURE 18.22 **Lobular Carcinoma In Situ (LCIS) in Adenosis. A:** LCIS inhabits a network of elongated adenosis tubules (tubular adenosis). **B, C:** LCIS populates sclerosing adenosis—with calcifications **(B)** and without calcifications **(C)**. **D, E:** Glandular structures occupied by LCIS are shown in fat. This pattern suggests invasive carcinoma. Each glandular structure is outlined by an actin-positive border indicative of a myoepithelial cell layer **(E)**. This supports the in situ nature of the lesion.

Important distinguishing features of LCIS in fat are the presence of well-circumscribed glands containing LCIS encircled by myoepithelial cells in contrast to the linear pattern of most ILC. However, the distinction between LCIS and the alveolar variant of ILC in fat can be difficult.

Ross and Hoda (66) published the clinicopathologic profile of 16 cases of microinvasive (<0.1 cm) lobular carcinoma. The mean age of patients with this rare disease was 52 (range: 41–65) years. Most (13/16) patients had presented with a radiographic abnormality. All cases of microinvasive lobular carcinoma were unilateral and were associated with LCIS. LCIS was of the classic type in 11 cases, florid type in 4, and pleomorphic type in 1. The mean number of microinvasive foci was 1.5 (range: 1–5). Axillary lymph node biopsies were negative in 13 of 13 cases. In a mean follow-up of 24 months, there was no evidence of recurrence or metastases. It is noteworthy that a "slight enhancement of stromal cellularity was the only histologic hint of microinvasive disease at low-power microscopy." This finding emphasizes the need for careful scrutiny of all cases of LCIS—especially in the limited samplings obtained on NCBs wherein such a subtle finding may not be readily evident.

PROGNOSIS

The diagnosis of LCIS confers a cumulative long-term risk of subsequent invasive carcinoma that averages about 1%

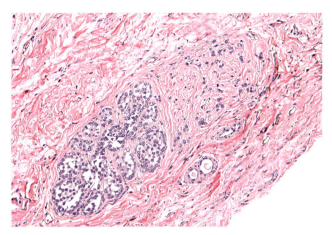

FIGURE 18.23 Microinvasive (<0.1 cm) Lobular Carcinoma Associated With Lobular Carcinoma In Situ of the Classic Type. Microinvasive lobular carcinoma cells have low-grade nuclei **(right)**.

per year and remains steady over time, resulting in a relative risk of up to 11-fold higher. The overall risk of invasive carcinoma can be summarized by the following easily remembered statistics: the risk increases by approximately 1% annually, with about 10% risk at 10 years and about 20% risk after 20 years.

Follow-up studies of LCIS have consisted of patients who were biopsied for palpable clinical abnormalities in which LCIS was an incidental, sometimes unrecognized, abnormality. The frequency of subsequent carcinoma (DCIS or invasive carcinoma) varied from 12% to 36.4%, 4 to 12 times the risk of control populations (1,8,27,67,68). Studies with longer follow-up tend to report a higher frequency of subsequent carcinoma. Variant LCIS (ie, P-LCIS and F-LCIS) is frequently not differentiated in these studies. In most studies, the risk of subsequent carcinoma was slightly higher in the ipsilateral than in the contralateral breast, although the difference has not been significant.

The choice of management for LCIS has ranged from bilateral mastectomy to surveillance with or without chemoprevention, complicating analysis of the disease biology. In a SEER analysis of 14,048 patients diagnosed with LCIS from 2000 to 2009, 16% of the patients had mastectomy, 74% underwent excision, and 10% underwent biopsy alone (26).

Several studies have prospectively assessed the follow-up of patients with LCIS following local excision. After approximately 5 years, in three studies, subsequent ipsilateral carcinoma developed in 7% to 17% of patients (69,70). In a recent long-term follow-up study, King et al (69) evaluated 1,060 women with a median prospective follow-up of 81 months (range 6-368). Subsequent carcinoma was detected in 150 (14%), consisting of invasive carcinoma in 65% and DCIS in 35%. Goldstein et al (48) reported actuarial rates for subsequent carcinoma of 7.8% after 10 years of follow-up and 15.4% after 20 years. Six of the subsequent 21 carcinomas (29%) developed 20 or more years after diagnosis.

Few studies have evaluated outcomes of NCB-proven C-LCIS cases that underwent surveillance alone; pooled data suggest that the rate of ipsilateral ILC is comparable (69,71,72), but longer follow-up is needed.

Predictors of Subsequent Invasion

Reliable pathologic predictors of increased risk for the subsequent development of carcinoma after biopsy-proven LCIS remain elusive. Multiple studies reported a greater risk in patients with LCIS which were of classic and pleomorphic types in comparison with patients who had LCIS of either type alone (8,11,73). Lesions with marked ductal distention, necrosis, and calcification are of special concern because the authors have found an unexpectedly high frequency of microinvasive carcinoma in such cases (74). Specimens with these features should be examined carefully with cytokeratin and E-cadherin immunostains accompanied by contemporaneous H&E-stained recuts. In a retrospective study by Goldstein et al (48), the presence of focal E-cadherin reactivity (present in 9 of 82 cases) was associated with a higher risk for developing subsequent carcinoma, earlier onset of carcinoma, and more frequent ductal carcinoma. This observation remains to be confirmed by other investigators. The risk of invasive recurrence for patients with C-LCIS is higher when LCIS has a proliferation rate greater than 10% as measured by Ki67 than if the proliferation rate is less than 10% (75).

Clinical and radiologic features may also be predictive. According to SEER data, African American women had significantly higher risk of developing invasive carcinoma after LCIS than White women (76). Metovic et al (73) found that among 122 patients with ALH or LCIS on biopsy, the features of Breast Imaging Reporting and Data System (BI-RADS) category 4 or 5 and age greater than 54 years were associated with upgrade at definitive surgery. Only lesions with BI-RADS category 5 and/or "high-grade LN"

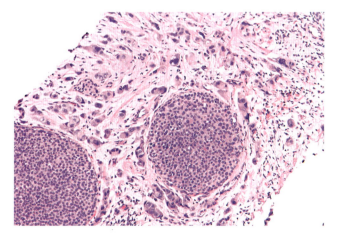

FIGURE 18.24 Pleomorphic Type of Invasive Lobular Carcinoma Associated With Lobular Carcinoma In Situ of the Classic Type. The invasive lobular carcinoma cells contain high-grade nuclei. Both invasive and in situ carcinoma cells were negative for E-cadherin (not shown).

were consistently treated with surgery. Other radiologic indications for excision in retrospective analyses have included mammographic calcifications, mass/distortion, or non-mass enhancement (77). On MRI, LCIS that presented as T2 hypointense or as linear or segmental non–mass enhancement was associated with a higher upgrade rate (78). In one study, the most important predictor of upgrade on excision was a synchronous mass lesion (79). The needle gauge, number of cores obtained, number of cores affected, and number of lobules involved have not been shown to correlate with upgrade (73,80).

ATYPICAL LOBULAR HYPERPLASIA

There are no specific clinical features associated with the diagnosis of ALH. The clinical indications for biopsy are the same as those that lead to the detection of LCIS: a palpable lesion or an imaging abnormality. ALH is usually an incidental finding not specifically associated with the abnormality that prompted the biopsy.

The epithelial proliferation in ALH has some features of LCIS, but is not sufficiently developed to qualify for the latter diagnosis (**Figs. 18.25-18.27**). There are no universally accepted criteria for the distinction between ALH and LCIS. Qualitative and quantitative factors must be considered. It has been suggested that the diagnosis of ALH be made if less than 50% (9) or 75% (10) of the affected lobule shows the features of LCIS.

ALH is characterized by the presence, within one or more lobules, of abnormal cells similar to those found in LCIS. In the least conspicuous configuration, these cells replace a portion of the normal lobular glandular epithelium, effacing some lumina. The acini are not enlarged at this level of proliferation. As the process evolves, the accumulation of a greater number of cells causes progressive acinar expansion, but the borders of individual acini and intralobular ductules remain indistinct in ALH. Clear delineation of intralobular acinar units filled by the abnormal cell population is an important feature that characterizes LCIS and reflects the accumulation of enough neoplastic cells to cause the individual glands to have a distinct configuration.

Similar criteria apply to the diagnosis of lobular proliferations in terminal ductal structures. These alterations tend to create a cloverleaf pattern similar to LCIS. The peripheral

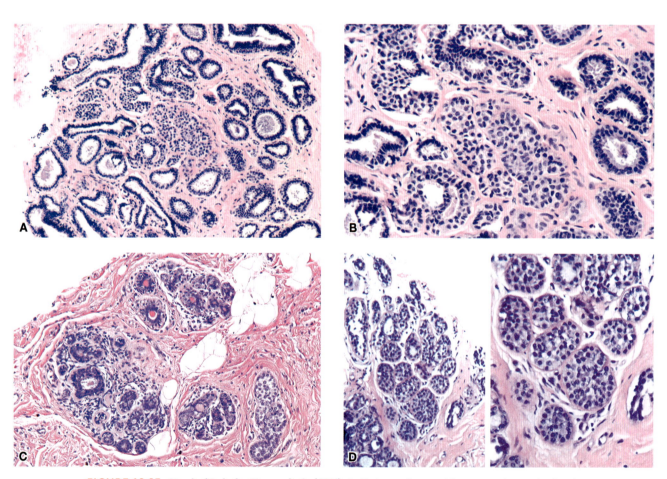

FIGURE 18.25 **Atypical Lobular Hyperplasia (ALH). A, B:** A needle core biopsy specimen obtained for calcifications revealed tubular carcinoma. One of the additional tissue samples had this focus of ALH in adenosis. **C:** ALH **(lower right)** next to normal lobules in a needle core biopsy sample. **D:** One partially involved lobule is present at the edge of this needle core biopsy specimen. The procedure was performed for calcifications that were present in sclerosing adenosis next to the ALH in a premenopausal patient.

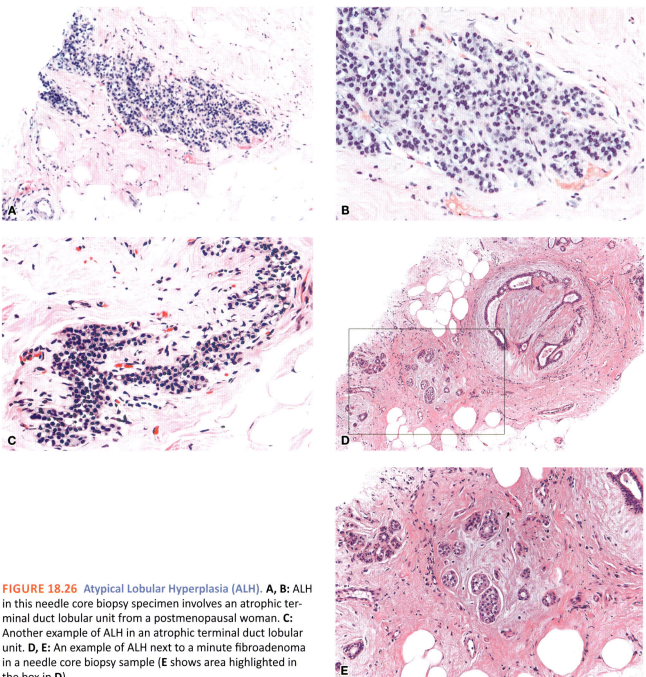

FIGURE 18.26 **Atypical Lobular Hyperplasia (ALH). A, B:** ALH in this needle core biopsy specimen involves an atrophic terminal duct lobular unit from a postmenopausal woman. **C:** Another example of ALH in an atrophic terminal duct lobular unit. **D, E:** An example of ALH next to a minute fibroadenoma in a needle core biopsy sample (**E** shows area highlighted in the box in **D**).

lobule-like bulges are sometimes inhabited by a mixture of normal and neoplastic cells. ALH of terminal ducts may also occur in a solid form that develops when the neoplastic growth is distributed in a continuous layer around the ductal lumen. ALH is E-cadherin-negative and genetically similar to LCIS (81).

Estimates of the risk for subsequent carcinoma in women with ALH are clouded by the absence of a clear definition for this lesion. Some investigators who did not distinguish between ALH and LCIS have reported relative risk estimates for both lesions under the heading of LN (11). The relative risk for developing carcinoma after the finding of ALH is 2.6 times the expected frequency when compared to age-matched controls (68), approximately half that of LCIS. The risk is higher in women with a family history of breast carcinoma, when there is ductal involvement by the ALH (82), and when there is coexistent atypical *ductal* hyperplasia (ADH) (68). The distinction between ALH and LCIS remains valuable for the purpose of patient counseling (3).

IS EXCISIONAL BIOPSY ALWAYS INDICATED AFTER THE NEEDLE CORE BIOPSY DIAGNOSIS OF LOBULAR CARCINOMA IN SITU?

The management of a patient with LCIS in a mammographically directed NCB specimen is a relatively recent concern. Some of the many reports evaluating the management of

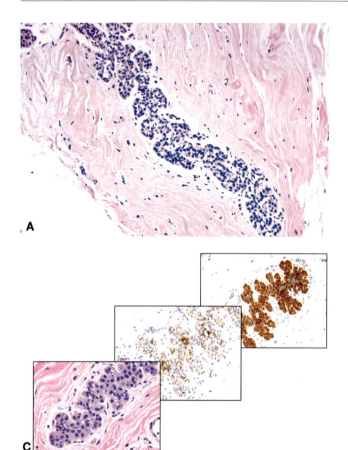
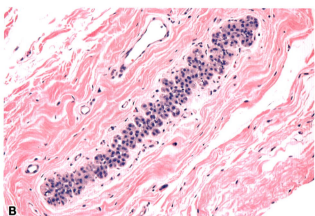

FIGURE 18.27 **Atypical Lobular Hyperplasia, Ductal Involvement. A:** Atypical lobular hyperplasia in a duct from a postmenopausal patient cut in a longitudinal plane. **B, C:** Another example of lobular carcinoma in situ with ductal involvement in an elderly woman. The lesional cells are negative for E-cadherin **(center figure)** and show cytoplasmic positivity for p120 **(upper right)** in C.

LCIS and ALH after diagnosis by an NCB were summarized by Rendi et al (83). This review of 18 studies found that the excision rate varied from 41% to 89%, with no data for this factor in three reports and excisions in less than 50% of cases in six other reports. Eight of the 18 studies included instances of P-LCIS or "mixed CIS." Some investigators lumped ALH and LCIS under the term "lobular neoplasia." The limitations inherent in these reports are representative of most studies that have been undertaken to determine how often and under which conditions excisional biopsy of LCIS is beneficial.

Earlier reports had observed an "upgrade rate" (either DCIS or invasive carcinoma on subsequent excision) of 20% to 50% after NCB diagnosis of LCIS or ALH (77,84-87). A summary of these and other studies (including a total of 140 patients with LCIS diagnosed in an NCB specimen who later underwent surgical biopsy) was compiled by Arpino et al (88). Carcinoma, either intraductal or invasive, was found in 40 cases (26%). These data support a recommendation to perform a surgical biopsy in most patients after LCIS is detected in an NCB specimen (89). The final decision for the management of individual patients may be influenced by clinical and imaging factors. Londero et al (90) and Brem et al (91) reported that the likelihood of finding intraductal or invasive carcinoma in a surgical biopsy was greater if the mammogram was classified as BI-RADS 4 or 5 than if it was BI-RADS 3. Based on their study of 1,315 consecutive NCB specimens at Memorial Hospital in New York City,

Liberman et al (74) proposed that surgical biopsy should be performed when a core biopsy specimen contains LCIS accompanied by a "high-risk" proliferative lesion, when F-LCIS resembling DCIS is present, or if there is discordance between histopathologic and imaging findings.

More recent series have generally reported a lower upgrade rate of less than 10% in consecutive cases of C-LCIS (19,92-95). The lower upgrade rate most likely reflects increasing adoption of a multidisciplinary approach to disease management with enhanced assessment of radiologic-pathologic concordance as well as careful exclusion of other high-risk lesions. It is evident that not all patients with an NCB diagnosis of C-LCIS or ALH require excisional biopsy and that a more nuanced approach is required.

Upgrade Rate of Variant Lobular Carcinoma In Situ

Reports of follow-up studies of LCIS diagnosed by NCB have not always identified the LCIS as classic, florid, or pleomorphic type, and in some instances they have not clearly distinguished between LCIS and ALH. In a recently published series, P-LCIS has been reported to have a higher upgrade rate, between 25% and 60% (21,96). Chivukula et al (97) studied a series of patients with P-LCIS diagnosed by NCB. Subsequent surgical excisions revealed residual P-LCIS in 10 (83%) and ILC in 3 of the 12 cases (25%). One invasive carcinoma was classified as classic, one as pleomorphic, and one as classic/pleomorphic. In a meta-analysis that included 42 patients with P-LCIS on NCB from five studies, Pieri et al showed an upgrade rate of 33% (98). The combined results of additional studies show that the incidence of invasive carcinoma on excision after P-LCIS diagnosed on NCB in 45 patients was 44% (20/45) (21,86,99-102). All three patients with P-LCIS on NCB in another series were found to have invasive carcinoma upon excision (ie, the upgrade rate was 100%) (67). These data support the performance of an excisional biopsy after the diagnosis of P-LCIS on NCB sampling. Until the clinicopathologic and biologic significance of F-LCIS are fully characterized, an excisional biopsy should follow the NCB diagnosis of this variant of LCIS (3).

Radiologic-Pathologic Concordance

Because most cases of LCIS that are currently diagnosed on NCBs are performed for an abnormality found on imaging studies, radiologic-pathologic correlation is an important element in the decision to perform an excisional biopsy thereafter. This entails determination of whether there is concordance between the intended target lesion and findings in the NCB.

A *concordant biopsy* is one wherein the histopathologic findings provide adequate explanation for the target on imaging, typically calcifications in LCIS (or in benign tissue) or fibroadenomas (with incidental LCIS within or beyond the benign tumor). Notably, calcifications can be associated with all variants of LCIS, and therefore the findings could be concordant on NCB (99).

A *discordant biopsy* is one wherein the histopathologic findings do not provide adequate explanation for the imaging abnormality (typically: insufficient explanation for a mass, inadequate sampling, no calcifications in NCB).

In a carefully conducted study at Memorial Sloan Kettering Cancer Center, Murray et al (19) found that excisional biopsy identified carcinoma in 3% (2 of 72) of concordant cases, and excisions in discordant cases yielded carcinoma in 38% (3/8) of the cases. The two carcinomas found in concordant cases included one low-grade DCIS and one grade 1 invasive carcinoma, each of which spanned 2 mm. Additional studies assessing for radiologic-pathologic concordance reported upgrade rates of 4.4% (3/68) (83) and 3.4% (3/87) (80).

IS EXCISIONAL BIOPSY INDICATED AFTER A NEEDLE CORE BIOPSY DIAGNOSIS OF ATYPICAL LOBULAR HYPERPLASIA?

Many of the foregoing limitations in the data about LCIS also hinder our understanding of the optimal management of ALH diagnosed in an NCB sample. This is illustrated in some of the following reports.

Lechner et al (87) reported the results of a multi-institutional study that included 154 (0.5%) instances of ALH in 32,424 NCB specimens. Excisional biopsies, performed in

only 84 of the 154 cases of ALH (55%), revealed ILC in 3 (4%) and DCIS in 4 (5%). A review of 6,081 consecutive breast NCB procedures performed at two institutions uncovered 20 (0.3%) cases of ALH (85). Excisional biopsies performed in 14 of the 20 cases revealed DCIS in 2 cases. The six patients who did not have an excisional biopsy had not developed clinical evidence of carcinoma after a mean follow-up of 36 months, an exceedingly short time in the context of ALH. Cangiarella et al (103) reviewed 24 publications that described 393 patients with ALH, among whom 51 (13%) were found to have DCIS or invasive carcinoma in a subsequent excisional biopsy. Lower upgrade rates of 2% to 3.4% were reported in smaller studies (94,104,105).

Close clinical and radiologic follow-up ought to be ensured in all cases of ALH or LCIS diagnosed on NCB that are not subjected to excisional biopsy. Larger tissue sampling (status post NCB with LCIS or ALH) via use of vacuum-assisted biopsy has been proposed as an alternative to excisional biopsy in select cases (106). The optimal management of ALH and LCIS diagnosed on NCB remains an area of active research (7,80,93,107,108).

TREATMENT SUMMARY

In view of these heterogeneous data, definitive conclusions are somewhat tenuous, but some indications seem to be reasonably well substantiated with respect to performing an excisional biopsy in certain circumstances after an NCB diagnosis of LCIS. These are as follows:

a. When the imaging and biopsy findings are discordant (eg, calcifications seen on mammogram are not present in the NCB specimen)
b. Patients at significantly increased risk for breast carcinoma such as those with concurrent or prior ADH, a family history of breast carcinoma, positive BRCA status, or contralateral breast carcinoma
c. The presence of P-LCIS or F-LCIS, even if the NCB findings are concordant with imaging

Hormone chemoprevention with tamoxifen, raloxifene, or aromatase inhibitors reduces the risk of subsequent carcinoma in women with C-LCIS by over 50% (109,110). In a prospective study of 1,004 women who chose surveillance instead of surgery after a diagnosis of LCIS, King et al (69) reported that the incidence of subsequent carcinoma was significantly reduced among those entered into a chemoprevention program. The assignment of patients was not randomized, with 173 choosing chemoprevention and 831 opting for surveillance alone. Overall, the annual incidence of carcinoma during surveillance follow-up with or without chemoprevention was 2%. The 10-year cumulative risk for subsequent carcinoma among those in the chemoprevention group was 7% compared to 21% in the surveillance-alone group. The investigators did not distinguish between subgroups of patients with C-LCIS, F-LCIS, and P-LCIS, but it is likely that the majority of patients had C-LCIS.

These data strongly support the use of chemoprevention in women with LCIS who choose follow-up surveillance.

Various aspects of the clinical management of P-LCIS were summarized by Murray et al (111) and Masannat et al (112). Surgical excision with clear margins, similar to DCIS, is the preferred approach (113). According to the National Comprehensive Cancer Network (NCCN) guidelines, the optimal width of margins for P-LCIS is "not known," and that for F-LCIS is not mentioned (114). In a review of 16,002 patients with LCIS (variant unspecified) from a SEER database, the addition of radiation did not confer survival advantage over excision alone (115). There are insufficient data to support the routine use of adjuvant radiation therapy for LCIS of any type (116).

LOBULAR CARCINOMA IN SITU: PRECURSOR LESION OR MARKER OF INVASIVE CARCINOMA?

The concept that LCIS is simply a "marker" lesion has been widely promoted. The impression created by this idea is that LCIS is a proliferative abnormality associated with an increased risk for the development of invasive breast carcinoma, but, in contrast to DCIS, LCIS does not itself progress to invasive carcinoma. This misperception is now falling into disfavor. There is ample cumulative evidence to support the conclusion that LCIS is a direct precursor to ILC and possibly also in a minority of instances to invasive ductal carcinoma (eg, mixed ductal and lobular and tubulolobular), although this progression is not observed in most patients with LCIS.

It appears that progression of LCIS to the invasive phenotype is less frequent and takes longer than in DCIS. Because LCIS and DCIS coexist in a number of patients, it is not surprising that some of them might develop invasive ductal carcinoma sooner and therefore more frequently than ILC. This phenomenon most likely reflects differences in the rates of progression of the two diseases so that the earlier appearance of invasive ductal carcinoma results in treatment before the LCIS has had an opportunity to evolve into ILC.

LCIS is a heterogeneous disease in both cytologic and architectural terms. The relationships of these differences to prognosis or to the risk of disease progression have not been well characterized. As discussed earlier, data linking C-LCIS to ILC come from molecular studies of the two lesions when they coexist (35,61,63,117). Additional evidence against LCIS as a "marker" lesion has come from the recognition of the florid and pleomorphic variants of LCIS characterized by marked glandular expansion with a tendency to necrosis and calcification.

Contrary to the widely held perception that LCIS is an incidental lesion, F-LCIS and P-LCIS are likely to present with calcifications and a mammographic pattern that resembles DCIS. The paradigm of LCIS as an incidental "marker" lesion does not fit well with this clinical presentation and the histopathologic findings. The advocacy for more aggressive management of P-LCIS is based largely on observations

that (a) P-LCIS is commonly concurrent with invasive carcinoma and (b) molecular studies show similarities between P-LCIS and invasive pleomorphic lobular carcinoma. Much of the foregoing is also true for F-LCIS. The authors are of the opinion that these variant forms of LCIS should be treated as DCIS, at least with respect to local surgical control in the conserved breast.

REFERENCES

1. Foote FW, Stewart FW. Lobular carcinoma in situ: a rare form of mammary cancer. *Am J Pathol.* 1941;17:491-496.3.
2. King TA, Reis-Filho JS. Lobular neoplasia. *Surg Oncol Clin N Am.* 2014;23: 487-503.
3. Wen HY, Brogi E. Lobular carcinoma in situ. *Surg Pathol Clin.* 2018;11:123-145.
4. Alvarado-Cabrero I, Picon Coronel G, Valencia Cedillo R, et al. Florid lobular intraepithelial neoplasia with signet ring cells, central necrosis and calcifications: a clinicopathological and immunohistochemical analysis of ten cases associated with invasive lobular carcinoma. *Arch Med Res.* 2010;41:436-441.
5. Shin SJ, Lal A, De Vries S, et al. Florid lobular carcinoma in situ: molecular profiling and comparison to classic lobular carcinoma in situ and pleomorphic lobular carcinoma in situ. *Hum Pathol.* 2013;44:1998-2009.
6. Zhong E, Solomon JP, Cheng E, et al. Apocrine variant of pleomorphic lobular carcinoma in situ: further clinical, histopathologic, immunohistochemical, and molecular characterization of an emerging entity. *Am J Surg Pathol.* 2020;44: 1092-1103.
7. Atkins KA, Cohen MA, Nicholson B, et al. Atypical lobular hyperplasia and lobular carcinoma in situ at core breast biopsy: use of careful radiologic-pathologic correlation to recommend excision or observation. *Radiology.* 2013;269:340-347.
8. Mackaren G, Yacoub LK, Lee AKC, et al. Effects of screening on detection of lobular carcinoma in situ of the breast: nonspecificity of mammography and physical examination. *Breast Dis.* 1994;7:339-345.
9. Page DL, Andersen TJ, ed. *Diagnostic Histopathology of the Breast.* Churchill Livingstone; 1987.
10. Rosen PP. Lobular carcinoma in situ and intraductal carcinoma of the breast. In: McDivitt RW, Oberman HA, Ozello L, et al., eds. *The Breast.* Williams & Wilkins; 1984:59-105.
11. Haagensen CD, Lane N, Lattes R, et al. Lobular neoplasia (so-called lobular carcinoma in situ) of the breast. *Cancer.* 1978;42:737-769.
12. Gomes DS, Porto SS, Rocha RM, et al. Usefulness and limitations of E-cadherin and beta-catenin in the classification of breast carcinomas in situ with mixed pattern. *Diagn Pathol.* 2013;8:114.
13. Singh K, Paquette C, Kalife ET, et al. Evaluating agreement, histological features, and relevance of separating pleomorphic and florid lobular carcinoma in situ subtypes. *Hum Pathol.* 2018;78:163-170.
14. Christiano JG, Duncan LD, Bell JL. Lobular carcinoma in situ of the breast presenting as a discrete mass. *Am Surg.* 2012;78:E38-E40.
15. Carley AM, Chivukula M, Carter GJ, et al. Frequency and clinical significance of simultaneous association of lobular neoplasia and columnar cell alterations in breast tissue specimens. *Am J Clin Pathol.* 2008;130:254-258.
16. Rosen PP. Columnar cell hyperplasia is associated with lobular carcinoma in situ and tubular carcinoma. *Am J Surg Pathol.* 1999;23:1561.
17. Amos B, Chetlen A, Williams N. Atypical lobular hyperplasia and lobular carcinoma in situ at core needle biopsy of the breast: an incidental finding or are there characteristic imaging findings? *Breast Dis.* 2016;36:5-14.
18. Chikarmane SA, Harrison BT, Giess CS, et al. Lobular neoplasia detected at MRI-guided biopsy: imaging findings and outcomes. *Clin Imaging.* 2021;78: 171-178.
19. Murray MP, Luedtke C, Liberman L, et al. Classic lobular carcinoma in situ and atypical lobular hyperplasia at percutaneous breast core biopsy: outcomes of prospective excision. *Cancer.* 2013;119:1073-1079.
20. Erdemir AG, Durhan G, Akpinar E. Lobular carcinoma in situ incidentally detected by dual-energy computed tomography. *Balkan Med J.* 2022;39: 218-219.
21. Flanagan MR, Rendi MH, Calhoun KE, et al. Pleomorphic lobular carcinoma in situ: radiologic-pathologic features and clinical management. *Ann Surg Oncol.* 2015;22:4263-4269.
22. Savage JL, Jeffries DO, Noroozian M, et al. Pleomorphic lobular carcinoma in situ: imaging features, upgrade rate, and clinical outcomes. *AJR Am J Roentgenol.* 2018;211:462-467.
23. Fadare O, Dadmanesh F, Alvarado-Cabrero I, et al. Lobular intraepithelial neoplasia [lobular carcinoma in situ] with comedo-type necrosis: a clinicopathologic study of 18 cases. *Am J Surg Pathol.* 2006;30:1445-1453.
24. Allison KH, Brogi E, Ellis IO, et al. *WHO Classification of Breast Tumours.* 5th ed. IARC; 2019.
25. Rosen PP, Kosloff C, Lieberman PH, et al. Lobular carcinoma in situ of the breast. Detailed analysis of 99 patients with average follow-up of 24 years. *Am J Surg Pathol.* 1978;2:225-251.
26. Portschy PR, Marmor S, Nzara R, et al. Trends in incidence and management of lobular carcinoma in situ: a population-based analysis. *Ann Surg Oncol.* 2013; 20:3240-3246.

27. Li CI, Anderson BO, Daling JR, et al. Changing incidence of lobular carcinoma in situ of the breast. *Breast Cancer Res Treat*. 2002;75:259-268.
28. Ginter PS, D'Alfonso TM. Current concepts in diagnosis, molecular features, and management of lobular carcinoma in situ of the breast with a discussion of morphologic variants. *Arch Pathol Lab Med*. 2017;141:1668-1678.
29. Rosen PP, Senie RT, Farr GH, et al. Epidemiology of breast carcinoma: age, menstrual status, and exogenous hormone usage in patients with lobular carcinoma in situ. *Surgery*. 1979;85:219-224.
30. Rosen PP, Lesser ML, Senie RT, et al. Epidemiology of breast carcinoma IV: age and histologic tumor type. *J Surg Oncol*. 1982;19:44-51.
31. Powers RW, O'Brien PH, Kreutner A, Jr. Lobular carcinoma in situ. *J Surg Oncol*. 1980;13:269-273.
32. Shah JP, Rosen PP, Robbins GF. Pitfalls of local excision in the treatment of carcinoma of the breast. *Surg Gynecol Obstet*. 1973;136:721-725.
33. Urban JA. Biopsy of the "normal" breast in treating breast cancer. *Surg Clin North Am*. 1969;49:291-301.
34. Moll R, Mitze M, Frixen UH, et al. Differential loss of E-cadherin expression in infiltrating ductal and lobular breast carcinomas. *Am J Pathol*. 1993;143:1731-1742.
35. Vos CB, Cleton-Jansen AM, Berx G, et al. E-cadherin inactivation in lobular carcinoma in situ of the breast: an early event in tumorigenesis. *Br J Cancer*. 1997;76:1131-1133.
36. Chen YY, Hwang ES, Roy R, et al. Genetic and phenotypic characteristics of pleomorphic lobular carcinoma in situ of the breast. *Am J Surg Pathol*. 2009;33:1683-1694.
37. Shousha S. In situ lobular neoplasia of the breast with marked myoepithelial proliferation. *Histopathology*. 2011;58:1081-1085.
38. Acs G, Lawton TJ, Rebbeck TR, et al. Differential expression of E-cadherin in lobular and ductal neoplasms of the breast and its biologic and diagnostic implications. *Am J Clin Pathol*. 2001;115:85-98.
39. Brandt SM, Young GQ, Hoda SA. The "Rosen Triad": tubular carcinoma, lobular carcinoma in situ, and columnar cell lesions. *Adv Anat Pathol*. 2008;15:140-146.
40. Bezic J, Gugic D. Signet ring lobular carcinoma in situ as a part of the "Rosen Triad" (tubular carcinoma, columnar cell hyperplasia, and lobular carcinoma in situ). *Turk Patoloji Derg*. 2013;29:134-137.
41. Eisenberg RE, Hoda SA. Lobular carcinoma in situ with collagenous spherulosis: clinicopathologic characteristics of 38 cases. *Breast J*. 2014;20:440-441.
42. Khoury T, Karabakhtsian RG, Mattson D, et al. Pleomorphic lobular carcinoma in situ of the breast: clinicopathological review of 47 cases. *Histopathology*. 2014;64:981-993.
43. Kuba MG, Murray MP, Coffey K, et al. Morphologic subtypes of lobular carcinoma in situ diagnosed on core needle biopsy: clinicopathologic features and findings at follow-up excision. *Mod Pathol*. 2021;34:1495-1506.
44. Lien HC, Chen YL, Juang YL, et al. Frequent alterations of HER2 through mutation, amplification, or overexpression in pleomorphic lobular carcinoma of the breast. *Breast Cancer Res Treat*. 2015;150:447-455.
45. Morrogh M, Andrade VP, Giri D, et al. Cadherin-catenin complex dissociation in lobular neoplasia of the breast. *Breast Cancer Res Treat*. 2012;132:641-652.
46. Choi YJ, Pinto MM, Hao L, et al. Interobserver variability and aberrant E-cadherin immunostaining of lobular neoplasia and infiltrating lobular carcinoma. *Mod Pathol*. 2008;21:1224-1237.
47. Goldstein NS, Bassi D, Watts JC, et al. E-cadherin reactivity of 95 noninvasive ductal and lobular lesions of the breast. Implications for the interpretation of problematic lesions. *Am J Clin Pathol*. 2001;115:534-542.
48. Goldstein NS, Kestin LL, Vicini FA. Clinicopathologic implications of E-cadherin reactivity in patients with lobular carcinoma in situ of the breast. *Cancer*. 2001;92:738-747.
49. Jacobs TW, Pliss N, Kouria G, et al. Carcinomas in situ of the breast with indeterminate features: role of E-cadherin staining in categorization. *Am J Surg Pathol*. 2001;25:229-236.
50. Harigopal M, Shin SJ, Murray MP, et al. Aberrant E-cadherin staining patterns in invasive mammary carcinoma. *World J Surg Oncol*. 2005;3:73.
51. Lee AH. Use of immunohistochemistry in the diagnosis of problematic breast lesions. *J Clin Pathol*. 2013;66:471-477.
52. Dabbs DJ, Schnitt SJ, Geyer FC, et al. Lobular neoplasia of the breast revisited with emphasis on the role of E-cadherin immunohistochemistry. *Am J Surg Pathol*. 2013;37:e1-e11.
53. de Deus Moura R, Wludarski SC, Carvalho FM, et al. Immunohistochemistry applied to the differential diagnosis between ductal and lobular carcinoma of the breast. *Appl Immunohistochem Mol Morphol*. 2013;21:1-12.
54. Etzell JE, Devries S, Chew K, et al. Loss of chromosome 16q in lobular carcinoma in situ. *Hum Pathol*. 2001;32:292-296.
55. Sakr RA, Schizas M, Carniello JV, et al. Targeted capture massively parallel sequencing analysis of LCIS and invasive lobular cancer: repertoire of somatic genetic alterations and clonal relationships. *Mol Oncol*. 2016;10:360-370.
56. Grabenstetter A, Mohanty AS, Rana S, et al. E-cadherin immunohistochemical expression in invasive lobular carcinoma of the breast: correlation with morphology and CDH1 somatic alterations. *Hum Pathol*. 2020;102:44-53.
57. Schrader KA, Masciari S, Boyd N, et al. Germline mutations in CDH1 are infrequent in women with early-onset or familial lobular breast cancers. *J Med Genet*. 2011;48:64-68.
58. Petridis C, Arora I, Shah V, et al. Frequency of pathogenic germline variants in CDH1, BRCA2, CHEK2, PALB2, BRCA1, and TP53 in sporadic lobular breast cancer. *Cancer Epidemiol Biomarkers Prev*. 2019;28:1162-1168.

59. Reis-Filho JS, Lakhani SR. The diagnosis and management of pre-invasive breast disease: genetic alterations in pre-invasive lesions. *Breast Cancer Res*. 2003;5:313-319.
60. Boldt V, Stacher E, Halbwedl I, et al. Positioning of necrotic lobular intraepithelial neoplasias (LIN, grade 3) within the sequence of breast carcinoma progression. *Genes Chromosomes Cancer*. 2010;49:463-470.
61. Hwang ES, Nyante SJ, Yi Chen Y, et al. Clonality of lobular carcinoma in situ and synchronous invasive lobular carcinoma. *Cancer*. 2004;100:2562-2572.
62. Rieger-Christ KM, Pezza JA, Dugan JM, et al. Disparate E-cadherin mutations in LCIS and associated invasive breast carcinomas. *Mol Pathol*. 2001;54:91-97.
63. Sarrio D, Moreno-Bueno G, Hardisson D, et al. Epigenetic and genetic alterations of APC and CDH1 genes in lobular breast cancer: relationships with abnormal E-cadherin and catenin expression and microsatellite instability. *Int J Cancer*. 2003;106:208-215.
64. Richards D, Ayala AA, Wu Y, et al. Carcinoma in situ involving sclerosing adenosis on core biopsy: diagnostic pearls to aid the practicing clinician and avoid overtreatment. *Oncol Ther*. 2020;8:81-89.
65. Cui X, Wei S. Carcinoma in situ involving sclerosing adenosis: seeking the salient histological characteristics to prevent overdiagnosis. *Ann Clin Lab Sci*. 2017;47:529-534.
66. Ross DS, Hoda SA. Microinvasive (T1mic) lobular carcinoma of the breast: clinicopathologic profile of 16 cases. *Am J Surg Pathol*. 2011;35:750-756.
67. Niell B, Specht M, Gerade B, et al. Is excisional biopsy required after a breast core biopsy yields lobular neoplasia? *AJR Am J Roentgenol*. 2012;199:929-935.
68. Page DL, Schuyler PA, Dupont WD, et al. Atypical lobular hyperplasia as a unilateral predictor of breast cancer risk: a retrospective cohort study. *Lancet*. 2003;361:125-129.
69. King TA, Pilewskie M, Muhsen S, et al. Lobular carcinoma in situ: a 29-year longitudinal experience evaluating clinicopathologic features and breast cancer risk. *J Clin Oncol*. 2015;33:3945-3952.
70. Ottesen GL, Graversen HP, Blichert-Toft M, et al. Lobular carcinoma in situ of the female breast. Short-term results of a prospective nationwide study. The danish breast cancer cooperative group. *Am J Surg Pathol*. 1993;17:14-21.
71. Laws A, Katlin F, Nakhlis F, et al. Atypical lobular hyperplasia and classic lobular carcinoma in situ can be safely managed without surgical excision. *Ann Surg Oncol*. 2022;29:1660-1667.
72. Matar R, Sevilimedu V, Park A, et al. Comparison of outcomes for classic-type lobular carcinoma in situ managed with surgical excision after core biopsy versus observation. *Ann Surg Oncol*. 2022;29:1670-1679.
73. Metovic J, Abate SO, Borella F, et al. The lobular neoplasia enigma: management and prognosis in a long follow-up case series. *World J Surg Oncol*. 2021;19:80.
74. Liberman L, Sama M, Susnik B, et al. Lobular carcinoma in situ at percutaneous breast biopsy: surgical biopsy findings. *AJR Am J Roentgenol*. 1999;173:291-299.
75. Pallis L, Wilking N, Cedermark B, et al. Receptors for estrogen and progesterone in breast carcinoma in situ. *Anticancer Res*. 1992;12:2113-2115.
76. Dania V, Liu Y, Ademuyiwa F, et al. Associations of race and ethnicity with risk of developing invasive breast cancer after lobular carcinoma in situ. *Breast Cancer Res*. 2019;21:120.
77. Pride RM, Jimenez RE, Hoskin TL, et al. Upgrade at excisional biopsy after a core needle biopsy diagnosis of classic lobular carcinoma in situ. *Surgery*. 2021;169:644-648.
78. Cha E, Ambinder EB, Oluyemi ET, et al. High-risk lesions in the breast diagnosed by MRI-guided core biopsy: upgrade rates and features associated with malignancy. *Breast Cancer Res Treat*. 2022;196:517-525.
79. Middleton LP, Grant S, Stephens T, et al. Lobular carcinoma in situ diagnosed by core needle biopsy: when should it be excised? *Mod Pathol*. 2003;16:120-129.
80. Chaudhary S, Lawrence L, McGinty G, et al. Classic lobular neoplasia on core biopsy: a clinical and radio-pathologic correlation study with follow-up excision biopsy. *Mod Pathol*. 2013;26:762-771.
81. Mastracci TL, Tjan S, Bane AL, et al. E-cadherin alterations in atypical lobular hyperplasia and lobular carcinoma in situ of the breast. *Mod Pathol*. 2005;18:741-751.
82. Page DL, Dupont WD, Rogers LW. Ductal involvement by cells of atypical lobular hyperplasia in the breast: a long-term follow-up study of cancer risk. *Hum Pathol*. 1988;19:201-207.
83. Rendi MH, Dintzis SM, Lehman CD, et al. Lobular in-situ neoplasia on breast core needle biopsy: imaging indication and pathologic extent can identify which patients require excisional biopsy. *Ann Surg Oncol*. 2012;19:914-921.
84. Crisi GM, Mandavilli S, Cronin E, et al. Invasive mammary carcinoma after immediate and short-term follow-up for lobular neoplasia on core biopsy. *Am J Surg Pathol*. 2003;27:325-333.
85. Foster MC, Helvie MA, Gregory NE, et al. Lobular carcinoma in situ or atypical lobular hyperplasia at core-needle biopsy: is excisional biopsy necessary? *Radiology*. 2004;231:813-819.
86. Hussain M, Cunnick GH. Management of lobular carcinoma in-situ and atypical lobular hyperplasia of the breast—a review. *Eur J Surg Oncol*. 2011;37:279-289.
87. Lechner MC, Jackman RJ, Brem RF, et al. Lobular carcinoma in situ and atypical lobular hyperplasia at percutaneous biopsy with surgical correlation: a multi-institutional study. *Radiology*. 1999;213:106-106.
88. Arpino G, Allred DC, Mohsin SK, et al. Lobular neoplasia on core-needle biopsy—clinical significance. *Cancer*. 2004;101:242-250.
89. Cohen MA. Cancer upgrades at excisional biopsy after diagnosis of atypical lobular hyperplasia or lobular carcinoma in situ at core-needle biopsy: some reasons why. *Radiology*. 2004;231:617-621.

90. Londero V, Zuiani C, Linda A, et al. Lobular neoplasia: core needle breast biopsy underestimation of malignancy in relation to radiologic and pathologic features. *Breast*. 2008;17:623-630.

91. Brem RF, Lechner MC, Jackman RJ, et al. Lobular neoplasia at percutaneous breast biopsy: variables associated with carcinoma at surgical excision. *AJR Am J Roentgenol*. 2008;190:637-641.

92. Crary IL, Parker EU, Lowry KP, et al. Risk of lobular neoplasia upgrade with synchronous carcinoma. *Ann Surg Oncol*. 2022;29:6350-6358.

93. D'Alfonso TM, Wang K, Chiu YL, et al. Pathologic upgrade rates on subsequent excision when lobular carcinoma in situ is the primary diagnosis in the needle core biopsy with special attention to the radiographic target. *Arch Pathol Lab Med*. 2013;137:927-935.

94. Sen LQ, Berg WA, Hooley RJ, et al. Core breast biopsies showing lobular carcinoma in situ should be excised and surveillance is reasonable for atypical lobular hyperplasia. *AJR Am J Roentgenol*. 2016;207:1132-1145.

95. Vora H, Kim S, Amersi F, et al. Lobular carcinoma in situ: a 15-year single institution review. *Am Surg*. 2017;83:1040-1044.

96. Fasola CE, Chen JJ, Jensen KC, et al. Characteristics and clinical outcomes of pleomorphic lobular carcinoma in situ of the breast. *Breast J*. 2018;24:66-69.

97. Chivukula M, Haynik DM, Brufsky A, et al. Pleomorphic lobular carcinoma in situ (PLCIS) on breast core needle biopsies: clinical significance and immunoprofile. *Am J Surg Pathol*. 2008;32:1721-1726.

98. Pieri A, Harvey J, Bundred N. Pleomorphic lobular carcinoma in situ of the breast: can the evidence guide practice? *World J Clin Oncol*. 2014;5:546-553.

99. Georgian-Smith D, Lawton TJ. Calcifications of lobular carcinoma in situ of the breast: radiologic-pathologic correlation. *AJR Am J Roentgenol*. 2001;176:1255-1259.

100. Lavoue V, Graesslin O, Classe JM, et al. Management of lobular neoplasia diagnosed by core needle biopsy: study of 52 biopsies with follow-up surgical excision. *Breast*. 2007;16:533-539.

101. Mahoney MC, Robinson-Smith TM, Shaughnessy EA. Lobular neoplasia at 11-gauge vacuum-assisted stereotactic biopsy: correlation with surgical excisional biopsy and mammographic follow-up. *AJR Am J Roentgenol*. 2006;187:949-954.

102. Pacelli A, Rhodes DJ, Amrami KK, et al. Outcome of atypical lobular hyperplasia and lobular carcinoma in situ diagnosed by core needle biopsy: clinical and surgical follow-up of 30 cases. *Am J Clin Pathol*. 2001;116:591-592.

103. Cangiarella J, Guth A, Axelrod D, et al. Is surgical excision necessary for the management of atypical lobular hyperplasia and lobular carcinoma in situ diagnosed on core needle biopsy? A report of 38 cases and review of the literature. *Arch Pathol Lab Med*. 2008;132:979-983.

104. Hwang H, Barke LD, Mendelson EB, et al. Atypical lobular hyperplasia and classic lobular carcinoma in situ in core biopsy specimens: routine excision is not necessary. *Mod Pathol*. 2008;21:1208-1216.

105. Muller KE, Roberts E, Zhao L, et al. Isolated atypical lobular hyperplasia diagnosed on breast biopsy: low upgrade rate on subsequent excision with long-term follow-up. *Arch Pathol Lab Med*. 2018;142:391-395.

106. Parkin CK, Garewal S, Waugh P, et al. Outcomes of patients with lobular in situ neoplasia of the breast: the role of vacuum-assisted biopsy. *Breast*. 2014;23:651-655.

107. Middleton LP, Sneige N, Coyne R, et al. Most lobular carcinoma in situ and atypical lobular hyperplasia diagnosed on core needle biopsy can be managed clinically with radiologic follow-up in a multidisciplinary setting. *Cancer Med*. 2014;3:492-499.

108. Shah-Khan MG, Geiger XJ, Reynolds C, et al. Long-term follow-up of lobular neoplasia (atypical lobular hyperplasia/lobular carcinoma in situ) diagnosed on core needle biopsy. *Ann Surg Oncol*. 2012;19:3131-3138.

109. Cuzick J, Sestak I, Forbes JF, et al. Use of anastrozole for breast cancer prevention (IBIS-II): long-term results of a randomised controlled trial. *Lancet*. 2020;395:117-122.

110. Goss PE, Ingle JN, Ales-Martinez JE, et al. Exemestane for breast-cancer prevention in postmenopausal women. *N Engl J Med*. 2011;364:2381-2391.

111. Murray L, Reintgen M, Akman K, et al. Pleomorphic lobular carcinoma in situ: treatment options for a new pathologic entity. *Clin Breast Cancer*. 2012;12:76-79.

112. Masannat YA, Bains SK, Pinder SE, et al. Challenges in the management of pleomorphic lobular carcinoma in situ of the breast. *Breast*. 2013;22:194-196.

113. Masannat YA, Husain E, Roylance R, et al. Pleomorphic LCIS what do we know? A UK multicenter audit of pleomorphic lobular carcinoma in situ. *Breast*. 2018;38:120-124.

114. National Comprehensive Cancer Network. Accessed August 8, 2023. http://www.nccn.org.

115. Cheng P, Huang Q, Shou J, et al. Treatment and survival outcomes of lobular carcinoma in situ of the breast: a SEER population based study. *Oncotarget*. 2017;8:103047-103054.

116. Morrow M, Schnitt SJ, Norton L. Current management of lesions associated with an increased risk of breast cancer. *Nat Rev Clin Oncol*. 2015;12:227-238.

117. Nayar R, Zhuang Z, Merino MJ, et al. Loss of heterozygosity on chromosome 11q13 in lobular lesions of the breast using tissue microdissection and polymerase chain reaction. *Hum Pathol*. 1997;28:277-282.

19

Invasive Lobular Carcinoma

ELAINE W. ZHONG AND SYED A. HODA

INTRODUCTION

Invasive lobular carcinoma (ILC) is the second most common histologic subtype of invasive breast carcinoma. The classic type of ILC (C-ILC) infiltrates mammary stroma either in linear cords or in a concentric pattern around native glands. The dyscohesive individual invasive carcinoma cells are relatively small with round-to-ovoid nuclei and minimal occasionally vacuolated cytoplasm. "Skip areas," that is, poorly delimited foci of invasive carcinoma separated by unremarkable mammary glandular and stromal tissue without desmoplastic reaction, impart the impression of multifocality. There is minimal disruption of the native mammary glandular architecture.

CLINICAL FEATURES

When the diagnosis is restricted to the histologic and cytologic features of an invasive carcinoma, as described in the preceding paragraph, less than 5% of carcinomas qualify for the diagnosis of C-ILC. If the classification is broadened to include variant forms, the frequency of ILC is as high as 10% to 14% of all invasive carcinomas (1-5). ILC occurs almost throughout the age range of breast carcinoma in adult women (28-86 years). Most studies have placed the median age at diagnosis between 51 and 65 years, slightly older than patients with invasive ductal carcinoma (IDC) (1,3,4,6). ILC is relatively more common among women older than 75 years than in women 35 years or younger (6-9).

A population-based study of women with invasive breast carcinoma diagnosed from 1987 to 1999 revealed that the incidence rate of lobular carcinoma increased during this period, particularly in women 50 years of age or older (5). Subsequent analysis of women in the United States between 1999 and 2004 revealed a decline in the age-adjusted incidence of ILC by 20.5% (10). These trends may be related to the use of hormone therapy (11). ILC of classic as well as pleomorphic types occurs, albeit rarely, in the male breast (12-16). Hereditary ILC can occur in patients or families with hereditary diffuse gastric carcinoma associated with deleterious germline *CDH1* mutations (17).

The presenting symptom of ILC in almost all cases is either a mass or a radiologically evident lesion. In a minority of cases, the only physical evidence of the neoplasm is vague thickening or diffuse nodularity of the breast.

Imaging

On *mammography*, ILC usually manifests as an ill-defined spiculated mass or architectural distortion (18-21); ILC is not prone to exhibit calcifications. Calcifications may be present coincidentally in benign proliferative lesions such as sclerosing adenosis associated with ILC (20). A lower frequency of calcifications detected by mammography has been reported in ILC than in ductal carcinomas (18,19,22). Exceptions are ILC associated with florid lobular carcinoma in situ (F-LCIS) or pleomorphic lobular carcinoma in situ (P-LCIS), both of which can show central necrosis and calcifications within glands (see Chapter 18). As such, pleomorphic ILC is less likely to be missed on imaging than C-ILC (23). In the screening setting, ILC is detected more often during intervals between examinations than by mammography (the so-called "*interval carcinomas*") (24). The mammographic size of ILC tends to be smaller when determined mammographically than grossly (25), although the latter methodology has its own disadvantages (26).

In 8% to 46% of cases, ILC is mammographically occult (22,27,28). The absence of well-defined margins and a tendency to form multiple subtle nodules of variable extent throughout the breast are features that hinder radiologic detection of ILC and lead to a false-negative interpretation of mammograms. Patients with a spiculated ILC are less likely to have residual carcinoma when re-excision is performed than are those with ill-defined or asymmetric lesions (29). A minority of ILCs present with mammographically round or ovoid tumors (27). The addition of tomosynthesis to digital mammography can improve detection of ILC by increasing conspicuity of the lesion margins and architectural distortion (30,31).

Ultrasonography has been useful for detecting multifocal and multicentric ILC (32), and it may be more accurate than mammography for predicting tumor size (33). The sensitivity of sonography for detecting ILC (89%-98%) is substantially higher than that of mammography (65%-71%) (34,35).

Multiple studies have demonstrated that *magnetic resonance imaging* (MRI) is more sensitive for ILC than either sonography or mammography. Mann et al (36) reported that MRI detected secondary foci of ipsilateral ILC that were not detected by sonography or mammography in 32% of cases, and occult contralateral carcinoma was detected in 7% of patients. Yeh et al (37) reported that tumor morphology as seen on MRI combined with quantitative measurement of gadolinium uptake was effective for detecting ILC in most cases. ILC enhances more slowly than IDC on MRI, but peak enhancement is similar (38). In the context of ILC, the effectiveness of MRI is somewhat diminished by the high rate of false-positives and overestimation of extent of disease.

Breast-specific gamma imaging (BSGI, also known as molecular breast imaging) has potential to be the most effective radiologic tool for the detection of ILC (39). There is particular interest in this technology for women with dense breasts, in whom ILC is frequently occult by conventional screening methods (40). Of the reported 41 breast malignancies detected only by supplemental BSGI, 24% were ILC (41-44). In a study by Brem et al (45) of 26 women with a total of 28 biopsy-proven ILC, BSGI was shown to have the highest sensitivity for the detection of ILC with a sensitivity of 93%, whereas mammography, sonography, and MRI showed sensitivities of 79%, 68%, and 83%, respectively. At present, BSGI has yet to gain widespread adoption in screening.

Bilaterality

Patients with ILC are reported to have a relatively high frequency of *bilateral* carcinoma when compared with women who have other types of carcinoma (46-49). The reported relative risk for contralateral carcinoma in women with ILC compared with those with IDC ranged from 1.6 to 2 (50,51). Synchronous and metachronous contralateral carcinomas have been described in 6% to 28% of ILC cases (3,49,52).

The reported incidence of subsequent contralateral carcinoma ranges from 1.0 (52,53) to 2.38 (54) per 100 women per year. There is some evidence that the frequency of bilaterality is higher in patients with classic ILC than in patients with the variant subtypes (54). A lobular component has been found in the majority of synchronous or metachronous contralateral carcinomas, and at least 50% of these have been invasive (52,53). Two series of random concurrent contralateral biopsies revealed intraductal carcinoma in 3% to 6% and invasive carcinoma in 2% to 10% of patients (55,56). Biopsies performed for clinical indications in an additional 22 cases in one of these series yielded intraductal carcinoma in 5% and invasive carcinoma in 32% (55). The probability of detecting contralateral invasive carcinoma was significantly greater in women who had multicentric ILC in the ipsilateral breast or who had ipsilateral lymph node metastases.

HISTOPATHOLOGIC EVALUATION

Several *growth patterns* may be encountered in lesions classified as C-ILC. The common denominator is the virtual absence of solid, alveolar, papillary, and gland-forming aggregates of cells. In the two-dimensional plane of a histologic section, the slender strands of cells are arranged in a linear fashion, with one or two cells across **(Fig. 19.1)**. If the tumor cells are arranged around ducts and lobules in a concentric fashion, the distribution is described as having a "targetoid" (or "bull's eye") appearance **(Fig. 19.2)**. In a

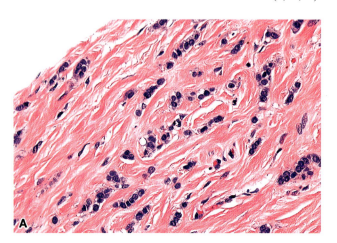

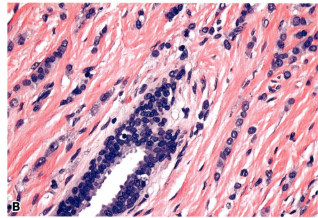

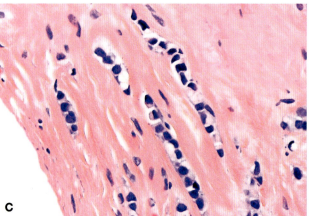

FIGURE 19.1 Histology and Cytology of Invasive Lobular Carcinoma, Classic Type. **A-C:** The "small" malignant cells with scant cytoplasm and dark, homogeneous nuclei are arranged in a linear pattern in these three different needle core biopsy specimens.

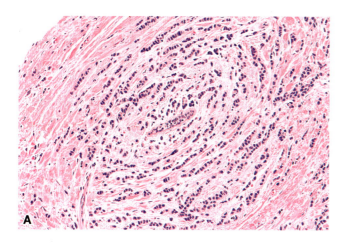
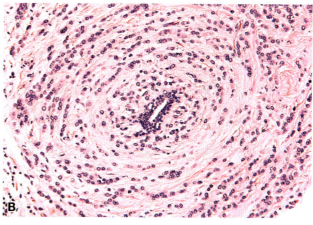
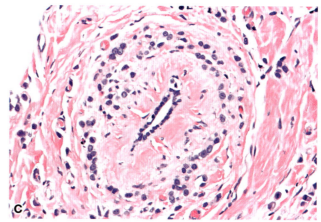

FIGURE 19.2 **Invasive Lobular Carcinoma, Classic Type With "Targetoid" Growth. A-C:** The linear infiltrates of carcinoma cells are distributed circumferentially around ducts. The "targetoid" ("bull's eye" or "satellitosis") appearance can occasionally be quite subtle, as seen in **(C)**.

minority of cases, the linear strand-forming pattern is not conspicuous, and the tumor cells tend to grow mainly in dispersed and disorderly foci **(Fig. 19.3)**. The tumor cells in such foci may be small enough to be mistaken for lymphocytes or plasma cells, especially in areas of fibrosis or amid adipose tissue when sections are examined at lower magnification in a frozen section or in a needle core biopsy (NCB) specimen **(Figs. 19.4 and 19.5)**. ILC is only

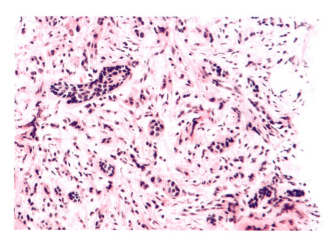

FIGURE 19.3 **Invasive Lobular Carcinoma, Classic Type.** The linear growth pattern is obscured by stromal reaction around a terminal duct and lobular glands in this needle core biopsy specimen.

rarely accompanied by a notable lymphocytic reaction **(Fig. 19.6)**, although the term "lymphoepithelioma-like carcinoma" has been applied to an ILC with prominent lymphocytic reaction (57).

Occasionally, the sample obtained in an NCB procedure contains minimal, inconspicuous evidence of ILC that can easily be overlooked or mistaken for a lymphocytic infiltrate (58) **(Figs. 19.7 and 19.8)**. When LCIS is identified in an NCB specimen, all sections should be vigilantly inspected for subtle foci of invasion. A cytokeratin immunostain can be helpful in detecting inconspicuous ILC **(Fig. 19.9)**.

All of the *cytologic appearances* found in LCIS may also be present in ILC. C-ILC consists of small, uniform cells with round nuclei and inconspicuous nucleoli. A variable proportion of cells have intracytoplasmic lumina **(Fig. 19.10)**. Mucin is demonstrable in these vacuoles with the mucicarmine and Alcian blue stains (59). When the secretion is prominent, the cells assume a signet ring configuration. The majority, but not all, of the so-called signet ring cell carcinomas are forms of ILC (3,60,61). Histiocytoid ILC is composed of cells with foamy vacuolated or finely granular cytoplasm consistent with apocrine differentiation (62,63). This variant may be difficult to distinguish from reactive histiocytic infiltrates or even histiocytic neoplasms, which can rarely show signet ring cell forms (64,65).

C-ILC exhibits negligible duct (gland) formation, cytologic blandness as well as monotony, and negligible mitotic

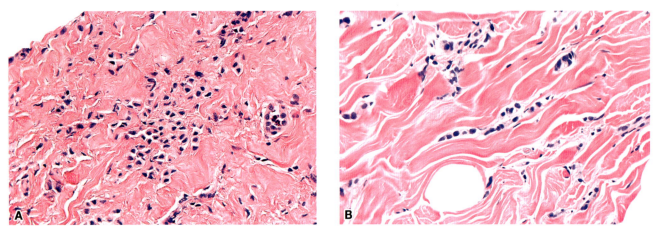

FIGURE 19.4 **Invasive Lobular Carcinoma, Classic Type, Obscured by Fibrosis. A, B:** The invasive carcinoma cells in these two needle core biopsy specimens are obscured by dense fibrosis and pseudoangiomatous stromal hyperplasia.

activity. As such, when C-ILCs are graded according to the Nottingham scheme, most are accorded grade 2 (usually 3+2+1).

Some *variants of ILC* (solid, alveolar, or trabecular) are based on architectural variance from the classic type. Other variants (signet ring cell, pleomorphic) differ in cytologic appearance **(Table 19.1)**. The typical pattern of linear and concentric infiltration of dyscohesive neoplastic cells is a common feature in some of these variants (3). One or more variants of ILC may coexist with C-ILC in cases that should be regarded as a *mixed group*. Areas of C-ILC with a linear pattern are found (at least focally) in most variant forms, but they may not be necessarily represented in an NCB sampling.

The *solid* type of ILC consists of compact nests or sheets of tumor cells **(Fig. 19.11)**. *Trabecular* ILC refers to

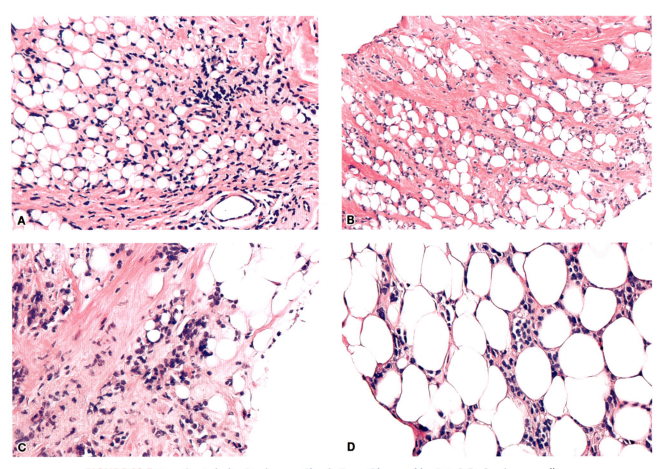

FIGURE 19.5 **Invasive Lobular Carcinoma, Classic Type, Obscured by Fat. A–D:** Carcinoma cells infiltrating fat in these four needle core biopsy specimens create an appearance that superficially resembles fat necrosis.

INVASIVE LOBULAR CARCINOMA   363

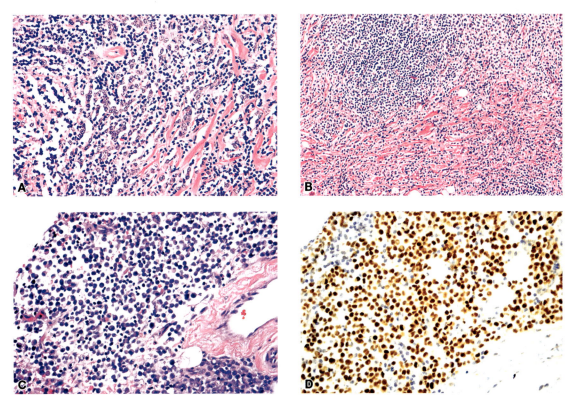

FIGURE 19.6 **Invasive Lobular Carcinoma (ILC) With Prominent Lymphocytic Reaction and "Plasmacytoid" Type of ILC. A, B:** The ILC cells have a linear growth pattern that is difficult to appreciate in the midst of the lymphocytic reaction. **C:** In this needle core biopsy specimen, the ILC cells display plasma cell-like cytology. **D:** The neoplastic cells of the case shown in **(C)** are strongly and diffusely immunoreactive for estrogen receptor.

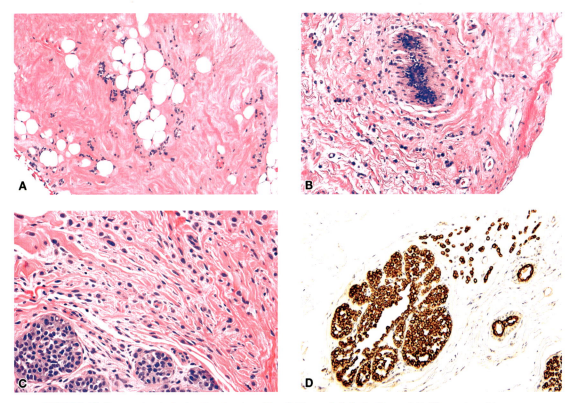

FIGURE 19.7 **Invasive Lobular Carcinoma, Classic Type, Subtle Lesions. A-D:** The only evidence of invasive carcinoma in these four needle core biopsies was subtle and inconspicuous foci, each of which spanned less than 1 mm. Microinvasive lobular carcinoma, next to lobular carcinoma in situ, is highlighted by the cytokeratin (CK7) immunostain in **(D)**.

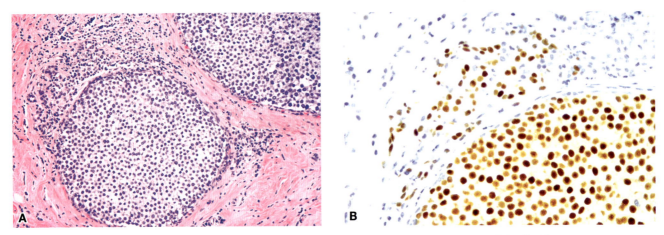

FIGURE 19.8 **Microinvasive Lobular Carcinoma. A, B:** Lobular carcinoma in situ of the florid type associated with a solitary focus of microinvasive lobular carcinoma. The latter is highlighted by the estrogen receptor immunostain (shown in **B**).

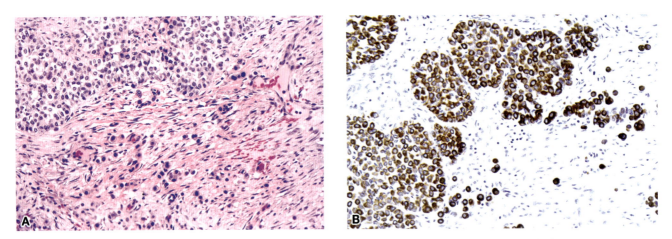

FIGURE 19.9 **In Situ and Invasive Lobular Carcinoma (ILC), Classic Type, in a Benign Phyllodes Tumor. A:** In situ lobular carcinoma is shown in enlarged lobules (top). The stroma contains "small" round cells suggestive of ILC. **B:** Scattered invasive carcinoma cells are highlighted with a cytokeratin (CK7) immunostain.

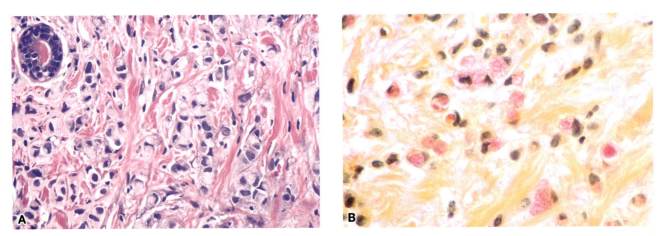

FIGURE 19.10 **Invasive Lobular Carcinoma (ILC) With Signet Ring Cells. A, B:** Signet ring cells are shown in this ILC found in a needle core biopsy specimen. The intracytoplasmic mucin in the signet ring cells is highlighted by a mucicarmine stain in **(B)**.

TABLE 19.1
Architectural and Cytologic Types of Invasive Lobular Carcinoma

Architectural Types
Classic
Solid
Alveolar
Trabecular
Mixed

Cytologic Types
Classic
Signet ring cell
Histiocytoid
Pleomorphic (including apocrine)
Mixed

Note: Tubulolobular carcinoma is classified as a ductal carcinoma, although LCIS is associated with around one-third of tubulolobular carcinomas.

tumors with prominent bands of more than two cells broad **(Fig. 19.12)**. Usually, the trabecular pattern is found in association with other variants, and the tumors are classified as mixed. The *alveolar* pattern of ILC is defined by rounded ("globular") aggregates of cells that may simulate LCIS, particularly in NCB sampling (66) **(Fig. 19.13)**. Recently, cases of ILC with growth patterns resembling solid-papillary and encapsulated papillary carcinoma have been described (67-70). LCIS coexists with about 85% of variant tumors. The observation that many examples of C-ILC have minor components of alveolar, tubular, trabecular, or solid growth is further evidence for classifying neoplasms that express these features prominently as variants of ILC. This conclusion is also supported by the fact that variant forms are not immunoreactive with E-cadherin. Tubulolobular carcinoma, however, is typically immunoreactive for E-cadherin and should be regarded as a variant of tubular carcinoma, rather than of lobular carcinoma (see Chapter 10).

Perineural invasion is uncommon in ILC but may occur when the lesion is either extensive or of the solid type. Lymphovascular involvement is rarely identified in ILC, and in some situations shrinkage artifacts may simulate carcinoma in lymphovascular spaces. When lymphovascular tumor

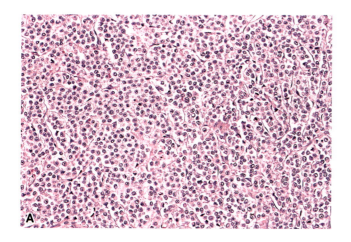

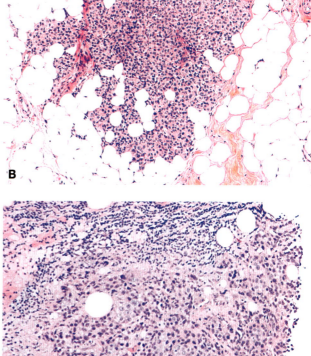

FIGURE 19.11 Invasive Lobular Carcinoma (ILC), Solid Variant. A: Solid growth pattern, albeit with loss of cohesion (a feature commonly present in ILC), is illustrated in this area. Slender strands of stroma are present. **B:** The tumor cells form a solid mass with uneven borders infiltrating fat (hematoxylin-phloxine-safranin). **C:** A needle core biopsy specimen in which the border of solid ILC is defined by a lymphocytic reaction.

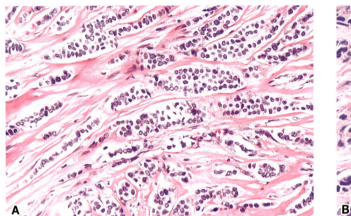
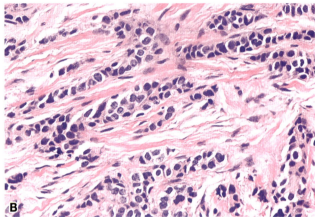

FIGURE 19.12 Invasive Lobular Carcinoma, Trabecular Variant. **A, B:** Both tumors shown here display a trabecular growth pattern formed by bands of cells. The latter are arrayed two to four cells across.

emboli are present, the tumor cells tend to form cohesive aggregates rather than being singly dispersed. This finding is significantly more prevalent in pleomorphic ILC (P-ILC) (19.2%) than in C-ILC (1%) (7).

About 15% of ILC consist entirely, or in part, of cells with relatively abundant cytoplasm and enlarged hyperchromatic nuclei **(Fig. 19.14)**. These distinctive cells have been referred to as *pleomorphic* (from Greek, *pleo*: more than one, *morphe*: form) lobular carcinoma (7,9,71). The cytoplasm of the cells in P-ILC may display apocrine or histiocytoid traits (63,71) **(Fig. 19.15)** and is usually associated with LCIS that is composed of cytologically similar pleomorphic cells (ie, P-LCIS). Most forms of ILC described previously as either histiocytoid or apocrine ought to qualify for the designation of P-ILC. Apocrine variant of P-LCIS, a recently characterized entity, may be associated with P-ILC with apocrine features (72). A low frequency of reactivity for estrogen receptor (ER) and progesterone receptor (PR) is

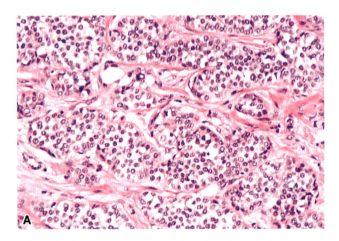
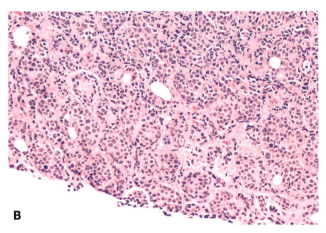
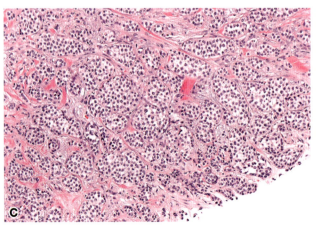

FIGURE 19.13 Invasive Lobular Carcinoma (ILC), Alveolar Type. **A:** The tumor cells form rounded masses that duplicate the appearance of lobular carcinoma in situ (LCIS). Immunostains for myoepithelial cells (not shown here) are useful to distinguish alveolar type of ILC and LCIS. **B-C:** Core biopsies performed for a mass **(B)** and distortion **(C)**. Despite the seemingly cohesive growth, the cytologic features are those of lobular carcinoma. Confirmatory E-cadherin was negative (not shown).

INVASIVE LOBULAR CARCINOMA 367

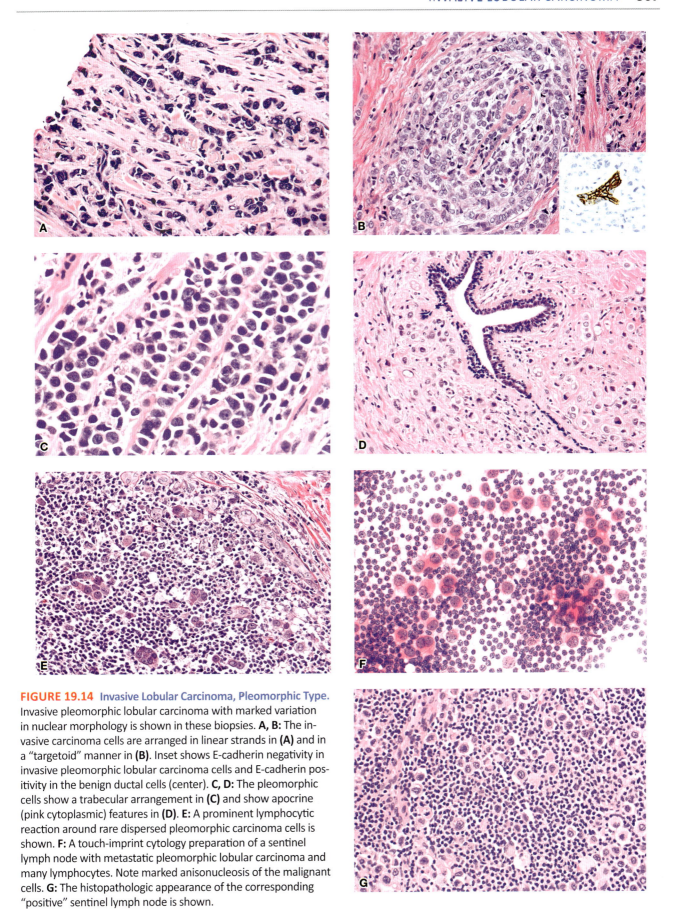

FIGURE 19.14 Invasive Lobular Carcinoma, Pleomorphic Type. Invasive pleomorphic lobular carcinoma with marked variation in nuclear morphology is shown in these biopsies. **A, B:** The invasive carcinoma cells are arranged in linear strands in **(A)** and in a "targetoid" manner in **(B)**. Inset shows E-cadherin negativity in invasive pleomorphic lobular carcinoma cells and E-cadherin positivity in the benign ductal cells (center). **C, D:** The pleomorphic cells show a trabecular arrangement in **(C)** and show apocrine (pink cytoplasmic) features in **(D)**. **E:** A prominent lymphocytic reaction around rare dispersed pleomorphic carcinoma cells is shown. **F:** A touch-imprint cytology preparation of a sentinel lymph node with metastatic pleomorphic lobular carcinoma and many lymphocytes. Note marked anisonucleosis of the malignant cells. **G:** The histopathologic appearance of the corresponding "positive" sentinel lymph node is shown.

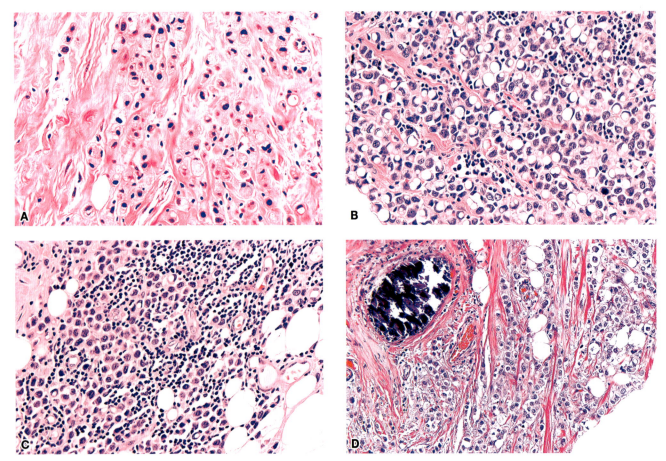

FIGURE 19.15 **Invasive Lobular Carcinoma (ILC), Pleomorphic Type With Variable Cytologic and Histologic Appearances. A:** These invasive pleomorphic lobular carcinoma cells show "histiocytoid" cytoplasm with a foamy appearance. **B:** This invasive pleomorphic lobular carcinoma has almost exclusively signet ring cell features. **C:** Another example of invasive pleomorphic lobular carcinoma showing neoplastic cells in minute aggregates amid lymphocytes. **D:** This invasive pleomorphic lobular carcinoma, associated with dense calcification, is infiltrative in linear arrays in a manner reminiscent of classic type of ILC.

found in P-ILC (9), and apocrine carcinomas are also typically not reactive for these receptors. Androgen receptors have been detected in pleomorphic lobular carcinomas (73) and are also typically present in apocrine carcinomas. P-ILC exhibits a relatively high nuclear grade and brisker mitotic rate; as such, per the Nottingham system, these carcinomas are accorded grade 3 (usually 3+3+2).

IMMUNOHISTOCHEMISTRY

About 95% of ILCs, both classic and variant types, exhibit nuclear immunoreactivity for ER and PR (**Fig. 19.16**). ILCs with apocrine differentiation are usually negative for hormone receptors (74). Human epidermal growth factor receptor 2 (HER2) is only rarely positive (ie, 3+, on a scale of 0 to 3+) in C-ILC (and LCIS) (51). Monhollen et al (9) detected *ERBB2* gene amplification in 37% of P-ILC. ILCs are typically positive for gross cystic disease fluid protein-15 (GCDFP-15, BRST2), particularly those with pleomorphic and signet ring cytology (71,75). ILC is typically negative for p53 (with the exception of some P-ILC) (8), p63, and vimentin (76). About 20% of ILCs are positive for CK5/6 (77); these cases tend to be negative for ER and may represent a "basal-like" subset of ILCs.

E-cadherin is an epithelium-associated molecule involved in cell-to-cell adhesion that acts as a tumor invasion suppressor gene. Unlike IDC, E-cadherin immunoreactivity is either markedly diminished or absent in approximately 90% of ILCs (78-80) (**Fig. 19.17**). The frequency is somewhat lower in variant ILCs. Loss of immunoreactivity for α-, β-, and λ-catenins also occurs in ILC (78). Loss of E-cadherin immunoreactivity is consistently observed in LCIS of classic, florid, and pleomorphic types in the presence or absence of concomitant ILC (81,82). The consequent defect in cell adhesion results in the characteristic dyscohesion of lobular carcinoma cells.

Since the E-cadherin staining pattern is so highly associated with histologic tumor type, lesions that depart from expected E-cadherin reactivity are described as having *aberrant E-cadherin staining* (83) (**Fig. 19.18**). This can consist of cytoplasmic, reduced intensity membranous, or partial,

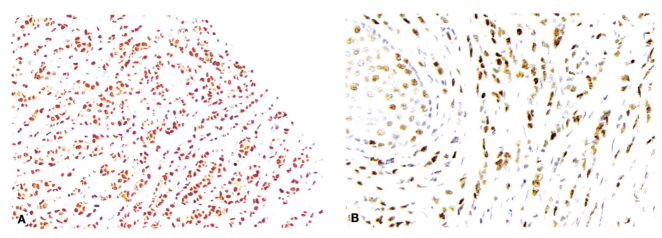

FIGURE 19.16 Invasive Lobular Carcinoma (ILC), Estrogen Receptors (ER). A: The characteristic strong and diffuse nuclear immunoreactivity for ER is evident in this classic type of ILC. This is the most common pattern of ER immunoreactivity in invasive classic lobular carcinoma. **B:** This immunostained section of another needle core biopsy specimen displays intermediate-to-strong nuclear immunoreactivity for ER in the majority of the ILC cells of the classic type. This is the second most common pattern of ER-positivity in ILC of the classic type.

fragmented, or granular membranous expression (84,85). Such aberrant expression has been observed in 16% to 23% of ILC (85,86). Da Silva et al (87) reported that the cadherin-catenin complex may not be functional in lobular carcinomas with aberrant E-cadherin expression. These authors concluded that when the hematoxylin and eosin (H&E) appearance is characteristic of lobular carcinoma, "positive staining for E-cadherin should not preclude a diagnosis of lobular in favor of ductal carcinoma." Conversely, up to 24% of ductal carcinomas may lose E-cadherin expression because of gene deletion or transcription defects (88,89).

Several additional immunohistochemical markers, including p120, β-catenin, and low-molecular-weight and high-molecular-weight cytokeratins, have been reported

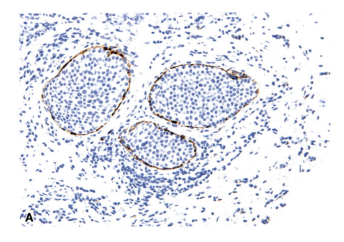

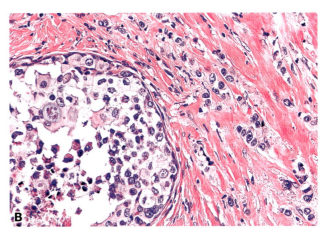

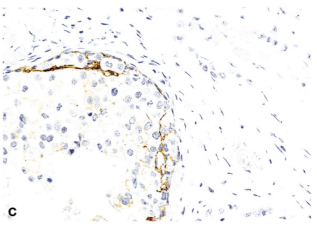

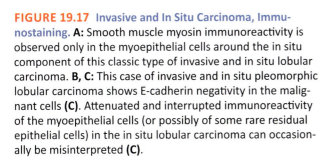

FIGURE 19.17 Invasive and In Situ Carcinoma, Immunostaining. A: Smooth muscle myosin immunoreactivity is observed only in the myoepithelial cells around the in situ component of this classic type of invasive and in situ lobular carcinoma. **B, C:** This case of invasive and in situ pleomorphic lobular carcinoma shows E-cadherin negativity in the malignant cells **(C)**. Attenuated and interrupted immunoreactivity of the myoepithelial cells (or possibly of some rare residual epithelial cells) in the in situ lobular carcinoma can occasionally be misinterpreted **(C)**.

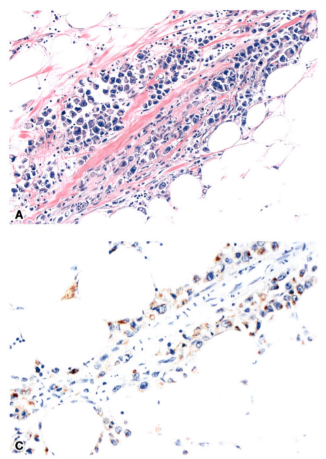

FIGURE 19.18 Invasive Lobular Carcinoma, Pleomorphic Type With Aberrant Staining. **A:** Invasive carcinoma with high-grade nuclear atypia. E-cadherin **(B)** and p120 **(C)** immunostains show aberrant "dot-like" and cytoplasmic (nonmembranous) staining. These findings are compatible with the diagnosis of lobular carcinoma.

to help distinguish between lobular and ductal carcinoma (Table 19.2) (90). Occasionally, a sampling of invasive carcinoma on NCB exhibits morphologic and immunohistochemical features that are neither definitively lobular nor ductal. It is generally acceptable to report such carcinomas as "invasive mammary carcinoma (with mixed ductal and lobular features)" and defer further characterization to excision. Data from 11 pathology laboratories in the United Kingdom and Ireland showed that of 1,112 carcinomas diagnosed as ILC or mixed ILC/IDC on NCB, on excision 76% were pure ILC, 14% were mixed ILC/IDC, and 10% were ultimately categorized as invasive ductal carcinomas of no special type (IDC NST) (91).

MOLECULAR STUDIES

Classic ILCs typically show loss of chromosomal arm 16q (including *CDH1*, the gene encoding E-cadherin), gain of material on 1q, and loss of 16p. In one study of paired LCIS and ILC samples from 24 patients, loss of the entire 16q arm was detected in all tumors, and it was concluded that "the striking similarity in genomic changes between the in situ and invasive components of these lesions clearly demonstrated the common clonality of the two lesions" (92). Pleomorphic ILCs exhibit similar alterations and also display amplification of 8q24 (*MYC*), 17q12 (*ERBB2*), and 20q13, which are archetypal changes of high-grade ductal carcinomas (93-95).

TABLE 19.2

Immunohistochemical Results for Invasive Ductal and Invasive Lobular Carcinoma

	Invasive Lobular Carcinoma	Invasive Ductal Carcinoma
E-cadherin	Negative	Positive
p120	Positive (cytoplasmic or punctate paranuclear)	Positive (membranous)
β-Catenin	Negative	Positive
HMW-CK (K903/34β12)	Positive (perinuclear)	Negative

HMW-CK, high-molecular-weight cytokeratin.

Inactivation of E-cadherin via *CDH1* gene alterations is the most commonly identified genetic alteration in ILC, in both classic (93) and pleomorphic (81) ILCs. *CDH1* loss at the DNA, mRNA, and protein level was identified in 95% of ILC in one study (96). Importantly, E-cadherin expression does not always correlate with *CDH1* mutational status. In a study of 202 cases of breast carcinoma with *CDH1* somatic alterations—predominantly truncations—identified by massively parallel sequencing, 155 were E-cadherin negative by immunohistochemistry (IHC) and 47 were at least partially E-cadherin positive (97). The presence of E-cadherin staining in carcinomas with *CDH1* truncation supported the notion of aberrant expression of a nonfunctional E-cadherin protein. Moreover, *CDH1* alterations have been reported in breast carcinomas that do not meet morphologic criteria for ILC, including 2% of IDC (84,96-98). Molecular findings, like IHC, must be interpreted in conjunction with morphology.

Other alterations enriched in ILC include mutations affecting *TBX3*, *FOXA1*, and *PTEN* leading to AKT activation (96,99). A molecular subtype-matched comparison of ILC and IDC by oligonucleotide arrays demonstrated in ILC downregulation of genes related to actin cytoskeleton remodeling, protein ubiquitin, DNA repair, cell adhesion, and transforming growth factor beta (TGF-β) signaling; and upregulation of transcription factors, lipid/prostaglandin biosynthesis genes, and cell migration genes (98). Classic and pleomorphic ILC were similar at the molecular level.

METASTATIC LOBULAR CARCINOMA

Metastatic deposits of ILC tend to duplicate the cytologic (and sometimes the architectural) features of the primary tumor **(Fig. 19.19)**. Axillary lymph node metastases derived from ILC of the classic type may be distributed largely in sinusoids, sparing lymphoid areas. If lymph node involvement is sparse, the distinction between tumor cells and histiocytes may be difficult to appreciate in H&E-stained NCB samples. Use of cytokeratin (CK) in this setting facilitates detection and precise determination of extent of involvement (100,101).

When compared with ductal carcinoma, there is a statistically significant greater frequency of metastases of lobular carcinoma to the peritoneum (102), meninges, gastrointestinal tract (103), and gynecologic organs, and a lower frequency of pulmonary metastases (104). Metastatic lobular

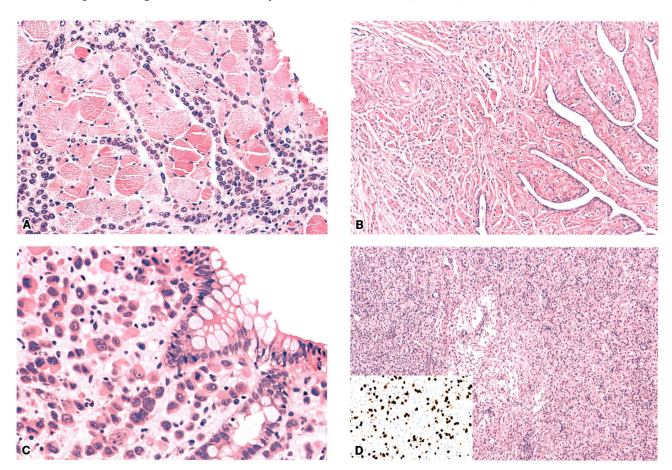

FIGURE 19.19 Metastatic Lobular Carcinoma. A: Lobular carcinoma with a linear growth pattern is shown infiltrating around fibers of skeletal muscle. **B:** Carcinoma cells are subtle in stroma of mucosal folds of the fallopian tube. **C:** Diffuse involvement of colonic mucosa. **D:** Metastatic lobular carcinoma in a meningioma, in a patient with history of breast carcinoma 5 years prior (inset: GATA3).

carcinoma cells can be rather difficult to identify in cytologic examination of pleural, ascitic, or cerebrospinal fluid. In the uterus, metastatic lobular carcinoma cells blend with normal endometrial stromal cells and may be overlooked in endometrial curettings (105). Metastatic lobular carcinoma has been described in endometrial polyps associated with tamoxifen therapy (106). Metastases involving the stomach can produce clinical and pathologic findings indistinguishable from those of a primary gastric carcinoma (107). ER immunoreactivity has been reported in primary gastric adenocarcinomas; however, in the appropriate clinical setting, diffusely strong immunoreactivity of carcinoma cells in gastric mucosa for ER and GATA3 favors metastatic lobular carcinoma (107). Isolated metastatic lobular carcinoma cells in the bone marrow may resemble normal hematopoietic elements (108). No significant differences have been found in the distribution of metastases between patients with the classic and variant patterns of ILC (3).

PROGNOSIS

At this time, size of ILC and nodal status remain the most important determinants of treatment and prognosis. Several studies have shown that the prognosis of nonpleomorphic ILC is similar to (90,109-113) or slightly better than (114,115) that of IDC when matched for grade and stage. However, others have indicated that the rate of local and distant metastasis is higher in ILC (116-118). Patients with classic ILC have a slightly better prognosis than those with variant forms as a group, but the differences have not been statistically significant.

Data from several studies suggest that the pleomorphic variant of ILC may have a less-favorable prognosis than classic variants (7,71,119). The prognosis of P-ILC has been related specifically to mitotic activity rather than nuclear pleomorphism (74). Monhollen et al (9) reported on 40 cases of P-ILC, which included 5 triple-negative cases and 14 HER2-positive cases. Older age and negative hormonal receptor status correlated significantly with worse clinical outcomes ($P < .03$). The 5-year recurrence-free and overall survival rates were 54.9% and 76.2%, respectively. Based on these data, the authors concluded that P-ILC has "hybrid clinicopathologic characteristics" between ILC and IDC.

The role of gene expression-based classifiers—for example, Oncotype DX and MammaPrint—is less well-established for ILC than for IDC (120,121). Analysis of 7,316 patients with ILC from the Surveillance, Epidemiology, and End Results (SEER) 2004 to 2013 database reported 8% of the group were high-risk, 71% intermediate-risk, and 21% low-risk. Adjuvant chemotherapy did not seem to confer a survival benefit in either the intermediate- or high-risk cohorts (122). Beumer et al (123) reported a significant association between high-risk MammaPrint result (seen in 24% of patients in their series) and poor clinical outcome. Studies characterizing the immune microenvironment and programmed death-ligand 1 (PD-L1) expression of ILC are limited (124,125). The utility and cost-effectiveness of these tests in ILC require more investigation.

TREATMENT

Successful treatment by breast conservation with radiotherapy is possible (21,112,126-130). Several studies indicate that survival and local recurrence rates for patients with ILC treated by breast conservation are similar to the result obtained for ductal carcinoma at 5 years of follow-up. However, there is an observed trend to later local recurrence of ILC compared with IDC, and more comprehensive data with longer follow-up is needed (131). Patients with multifocal ILC had a greater frequency of breast recurrence than those with unifocal tumors (129).

Limited information is available about the treatment of invasive pleomorphic lobular carcinoma by conservation therapy. If the latter option is exercised, P-LCIS ought to be viewed as being similar to high-grade ductal carcinoma in situ with respect to assessing margins.

ILC presents special challenges for management (132). ILC, when treated with conservative surgery, requires re-excision or mastectomy more frequently owing to margin-positivity (133). ILC can be successfully treated with conservative surgery, although accurate preoperative estimation of extent and multifocality of ILC, for example guided by MRI (134), may facilitate the goal.

ILC responds poorly to neoadjuvant chemotherapy when compared with IDC (135). Neoadjuvant letrozole has proven to be effective (136). Thus, determination of differentiation (ductal vs lobular) of invasive carcinoma in NCB samples can be of significance vis-à-vis initiation of appropriate treatment.

REFERENCES

1. Arpino G, Bardou VJ, Clark GM, Elledge RM. Infiltrating lobular carcinoma of the breast: tumor characteristics and clinical outcome. *Breast Cancer Res.* 2004;6:R149-R156.
2. Brogi E, Murray MP, Corben AD. Lobular carcinoma, not only a classic. *Breast J.* 2010;16(suppl 1):S10-S14.
3. DiCostanzo D, Rosen PP, Gareen I, Franklin S, Lesser M. Prognosis in infiltrating lobular carcinoma. An analysis of "classical" and variant tumors. *Am J Surg Pathol.* 1990;14:12-23.
4. Jacobs M, Fan F, Tawfik O. Clinicopathologic and biomarker analysis of invasive pleomorphic lobular carcinoma as compared with invasive classic lobular carcinoma: an experience in our institution and review of the literature. *Ann Diagn Pathol.* 2012;16:185-189.
5. Li CI, Anderson BO, Daling JR, Moe RE. Trends in incidence rates of invasive lobular and ductal breast carcinoma. *JAMA.* 2003;289:1421-1424.
6. Jung SP, Lee SK, Kim S, et al. Invasive pleomorphic lobular carcinoma of the breast: clinicopathologic characteristics and prognosis compared with invasive ductal carcinoma. *J Breast Cancer.* 2012;15:313-319.
7. Buchanan CL, Flynn LW, Murray MP, et al. Is pleomorphic lobular carcinoma really a distinct clinical entity? *J Surg Oncol.* 2008;98:314-317.
8. Middleton LP, Palacios DM, Bryant BR, Krebs P, Otis CN, Merino MJ. Pleomorphic lobular carcinoma: morphology, immunohistochemistry, and molecular analysis. *Am J Surg Pathol.* 2000;24:1650-1656.
9. Monhollen L, Morrison C, Ademuyiwa FO, Chandrasekhar R, Khoury T. Pleomorphic lobular carcinoma: a distinctive clinical and molecular breast cancer type. *Histopathology.* 2012;61:365-377.
10. Eheman CR, Shaw KM, Ryerson AB, Miller JW, Ajani UA, White MC. The changing incidence of in situ and invasive ductal and lobular breast carcinomas: United States, 1999-2004. *Cancer Epidemiol Biomarkers Prev.* 2009;18:1763-1769.
11. Chen CL, Weiss NS, Newcomb P, Barlow W, White E. Hormone replacement therapy in relation to breast cancer. *JAMA.* 2002;287:734-741.
12. Ishida M, Mori T, Umeda T, et al. Pleomorphic lobular carcinoma in a male breast: a case report with review of the literature. *Int J Clin Exp Pathol.* 2013;6:1441-1444.
13. Melo Abreu E, Pereira P, Marques JC, Esteves G. Invasive lobular carcinoma: a rare presentation in the male breast. *BMJ Case Rep.* 2016;2016:bcr2016215665.
14. Moten A, Obirieze A, Wilson LL. Characterizing lobular carcinoma of the male breast using the SEER database. *J Surg Res.* 2013;185:e71-e76.
15. Spencer JT, Shutter J. Synchronous bilateral invasive lobular breast cancer presenting as carcinomatosis in a male. *Am J Surg Pathol.* 2009;33:470-474.
16. Zahir MN, Minhas K, Shabbir-Moosajee M. Pleomorphic lobular carcinoma of the male breast with axillary lymph node involvement: a case report and review of literature. *BMC Clin Pathol.* 2014;14:16.

17. Corso G, Figueiredo J, La Vecchia C, et al. Hereditary lobular breast cancer with an emphasis on E-cadherin genetic defect. *J Med Genet*. 2018;55: 431-441.

18. Helvie MA, Paramagul C, Oberman HA, Adler DD. Invasive lobular carcinoma. Imaging features and clinical detection. *Invest Radiol*. 1993;28:202-207.

19. Le Gal M, Ollivier L, Asselain B, et al. Mammographic features of 455 invasive lobular carcinomas. *Radiology*. 1992;185:705-708.

20. Mendelson EB, Harris KM, Doshi N, Tobon H. Infiltrating lobular carcinoma: mammographic patterns with pathologic correlation. *AJR Am J Roentgenol*. 1989;153:265-271.

21. White JR, Gustafson GS, Wimbish K, et al. Conservative surgery and radiation therapy for infiltrating lobular carcinoma of the breast. The role of preoperative mammograms in guiding treatment. *Cancer*. 1994;74:640-647.

22. Krecke KN, Gisvold JJ. Invasive lobular carcinoma of the breast: mammographic findings and extent of disease at diagnosis in 184 patients. *AJR Am J Roentgenol*. 1993;161:957-960.

23. Jung HN, Shin JH, Han BK, Ko EY, Cho EY. Are the imaging features of the pleomorphic variant of invasive lobular carcinoma different from classic ILC of the breast? *Breast*. 2013;22:324-329.

24. Porter PL, El-Bastawissi AY, Mandelson MT, et al. Breast tumor characteristics as predictors of mammographic detection: comparison of interval- and screen-detected cancers. *J Natl Cancer Inst*. 1999;91:2020-2028.

25. Yeatman TJ, Cantor AB, Smith TJ, et al. Tumor biology of infiltrating lobular carcinoma. Implications for management. *Ann Surg*. 1995;222:549-559; discussion 559-61.

26. Varma S, Ozerdem U, Hoda SA. Complexities and challenges in the pathologic assessment of size (T) of invasive breast carcinoma. *Adv Anat Pathol*. 2014;21:420-432.

27. Evans WP, Warren Burhenne LJ, Laurie L, O'Shaughnessy KF, Castellino RA. Invasive lobular carcinoma of the breast: mammographic characteristics and computer-aided detection. *Radiology*. 2002;225:182-189.

28. Lopez JK, Bassett LW. Invasive lobular carcinoma of the breast: spectrum of mammographic, US, and MR imaging findings. *Radiographics*. 2009;29:165-176.

29. Porter AJ, Evans EB, Foxcroft LM, Simpson PT, Lakhani SR. Mammographic and ultrasound features of invasive lobular carcinoma of the breast. *J Med Imaging Radiat Oncol*. 2014;58:1-10.

30. Chamming's F, Kao E, Aldis A, et al. Imaging features and conspicuity of invasive lobular carcinomas on digital breast tomosynthesis. *Br J Radiol*. 2017;90:20170128.

31. Grubstein A, Rapson Y, Morgenstern S, et al. Invasive lobular carcinoma of the breast: appearance on digital breast tomosynthesis. *Breast Care (Basel)*. 2016;11:359-362.

32. Berg WA, Gilbreath PL. Multicentric and multifocal cancer: whole-breast US in preoperative evaluation. *Radiology*. 2000;214:59-66.

33. Skaane P, Skjørten F. Ultrasonographic evaluation of invasive lobular carcinoma. *Acta Radiol*. 1999;40:369-375.

34. Albayrak ZK, Onay HK, Karatağ GY, Karatağ O. Invasive lobular carcinoma of the breast: mammographic and sonographic evaluation. *Diagn Interv Radiol*. 2011;17:232-238.

35. Selinko VL, Middleton LP, Dempsey PJ. Role of sonography in diagnosing and staging invasive lobular carcinoma. *J Clin Ultrasound*. 2004;32:323-332.

36. Mann RM, Hoogeveen YL, Blickman JG, Boetes C. MRI compared to conventional diagnostic work-up in the detection and evaluation of invasive lobular carcinoma of the breast: a review of existing literature. *Breast Cancer Res Treat*. 2008;107:1-14.

37. Yeh ED, Slanetz PJ, Edmister WB, Talele A, Monticciolo D, Kopans DB. Invasive lobular carcinoma: spectrum of enhancement and morphology on magnetic resonance imaging. *Breast J*. 2003;9:13-18.

38. Mann RM, Veltman J, Huisman H, Boetes C. Comparison of enhancement characteristics between invasive lobular carcinoma and invasive ductal carcinoma. *J Magn Reson Imaging*. 2011;34:293-300.

39. Conners AL, Jones KN, Hruska CB, Geske JR, Boughey JC, Rhodes DJ. Direct-conversion molecular breast imaging of invasive breast cancer: imaging features, extent of invasive disease, and comparison between invasive ductal and lobular histology. *AJR Am J Roentgenol*. 2015;205:W374-W381.

40. Hruska CB. Molecular breast imaging for screening in dense breasts: state of the art and future directions. *AJR Am J Roentgenol*. 2017;208:275-283.

41. Hruska CB, Rhodes DJ, Collins DA, Tortorelli CL, Askew JW, O'Connor MK. Evaluation of molecular breast imaging in women undergoing myocardial perfusion imaging with Tc-99m sestamibi. *J Womens Health (Larchmt)*. 2012;21:730-738.

42. Rhodes DJ, Hruska CB, Conners AL, et al. Journal club: molecular breast imaging at reduced radiation dose for supplemental screening in mammographically dense breasts. *AJR Am J Roentgenol*. 2015;204:241-251.

43. Rhodes DJ, Hruska CB, Phillips SW, Whaley DH, O'Connor MK. Dedicated dual-head gamma imaging for breast cancer screening in women with mammographically dense breasts. *Radiology*. 2011;258:106-118.

44. Shermis RB, Wilson KD, Doyle MT, et al. Supplemental breast cancer screening with molecular breast imaging for women with dense breast tissue. *AJR Am J Roentgenol*. 2016;207:450-457.

45. Brem RF, Ioffe M, Rapelyea JA, et al. Invasive lobular carcinoma: detection with mammography, sonography, MRI, and breast-specific gamma imaging. *AJR Am J Roentgenol*. 2009;192:379-383.

46. Bernstein JL, Thompson WD, Risch N, Holford TR. Risk factors predicting the incidence of second primary breast cancer among women diagnosed with a first primary breast cancer. *Am J Epidemiol*. 1992;136:925-936.

47. Broët P, de la Rochefordière A, Scholl SM, et al. Contralateral breast cancer: annual incidence and risk parameters. *J Clin Oncol*. 1995;13:1578-1583.

48. Lesser ML, Rosen PP, Kinne DW. Multicentricity and bilaterality in invasive breast carcinoma. *Surgery*. 1982;91:234-240.

49. Mejdahl MK, Wohlfahrt J, Holm M, et al. Synchronous bilateral breast cancer: a nationwide study on histopathology and etiology. *Breast Cancer Res Treat*. 2020;182:229-238.

50. Horn PL, Thompson WD. Risk of contralateral breast cancer: associations with factors related to initial breast cancer. *Am J Epidemiol*. 1988;128:309-323.

51. Kollias J, Ellis IO, Elston CW, et al. Clinical and histological predictors of contralateral breast cancer. *Eur J Surg Oncol*. 1999;25:584-589.

52. Dixon JM, Anderson TJ, Page DL, et al. Infiltrating lobular carcinoma of the breast: an evaluation of the incidence and consequence of bilateral disease. *Br J Surg*. 1983;70:513-516.

53. Hislop TG, Elwood JM, Coldman AJ, et al. Second primary cancers of the breast: incidence and risk factors. *Br J Cancer*. 1984;49:79-85.

54. du Toit RS, Locker AP, Ellis IO, et al. Invasive lobular carcinomas of the breast—the prognosis of histopathological subtypes. *Br J Cancer*. 1989;60:605-609.

55. Simkovich AH, Sclafani LM, Masri M, et al. Role of contralateral breast biopsy in infiltrating lobular cancer. *Surgery*. 1993;114:555-557.

56. Smith BL, Bertagnolli M, Klein BB, et al. Evaluation of the contralateral breast. The role of biopsy at the time of treatment of primary breast cancer. *Ann Surg*. 1992;216:17-21.

57. Cristina S, Boldorini R, Brustia F, et al. Lymphoepithelioma-like carcinoma of the breast. An unusual pattern of infiltrating lobular carcinoma. *Virchows Arch*. 2000;437:198-202.

58. Ross DS and Hoda SA. Microinvasive (T1mic) lobular carcinoma of the breast: clinicopathologic profile of 16 cases. *Am J Surg Pathol*. 2011;35:750-756.

59. Cserni G, Floris G, Koufopoulos N, et al. Invasive lobular carcinoma with extracellular mucin production-a novel pattern of lobular carcinomas of the breast. Clinico-pathological description of eight cases. *Virchows Arch*. 2017;471:3-12.

60. Chatterjee D, Bal A, Das A, et al. Invasive duct carcinoma of the breast with dominant signet-ring cell differentiation: a microsatellite stable tumor with aggressive behavior. *Appl Immunohistochem Mol Morphol*. 2017;25:720-724.

61. Steinbrecher JS, Silverberg SG. Signet-ring cell carcinoma of the breast. The mucinous variant of infiltrating lobular carcinoma? *Cancer*. 1976;37:828-840.

62. Fujiwara M, Horiguchi M, Mori S, et al. Histiocytoid breast carcinoma: solid variant of invasive lobular carcinoma with decreased expression of both E-cadherin and CD44 epithelial variant. *Pathol Int*. 2005;55:353-359.

63. Tan PH, Harada O, Thike AA, et al. Histiocytoid breast carcinoma: an enigmatic lobular entity. *J Clin Pathol*. 2011;64:654-659.

64. Gould E, Perez J, Albores-Saavedra J, et al. Signet ring cell sinus histiocytosis. A previously unrecognized histologic condition mimicking metastatic adenocarcinoma in lymph nodes. *Am J Clin Pathol*. 1989;92:509-512.

65. Pathi R, Lawrence WD, Barroeta JE. Signet ring cell histiocytosis in axillary lymph nodes: a sheep in wolves' clothing? A potentially under-recognized pitfall in the diagnosis of metastatic breast cancer. *Breast J*. 2009;15:302-303.

66. Butler R, Pinsky R, Jorns JM. Alveolar variant of invasive lobular carcinoma in a fibroadenoma. *Breast J*. 2012;18:613-614.

67. Li X, Lin M, Xu J, et al. New variant of breast-invasive lobular carcinoma with solid and encapsulated papillary carcinoma growth pattern. *Breast Cancer*. 2021;28:1383-1388.

68. Motanagh SA, Muller KE. Invasive lobular carcinoma with papillary features: a newly described variant that poses a difficult histologic differential diagnosis. *Breast J*. 2020;26:1231-1233.

69. Rakha EA, Abbas A, Sheeran R. Invasive lobular carcinoma mimicking papillary carcinoma: a report of three cases. *Pathobiology*. 2016;83:221-227.

70. Zheng L, Saluja K, Guo T. Invasive lobular carcinoma mimicking encapsulated papillary carcinoma with a literature review: a rare variant detected serendipitously. *Int J Surg Pathol*. 2022;30(8):912-920.

71. Eusebi V, Magalhaes F, Azzopardi JG. Pleomorphic lobular carcinoma of the breast: an aggressive tumor showing apocrine differentiation. *Hum Pathol*. 1992;23:655-662.

72. Zhong E, Solomon JP, Cheng E, et al. Apocrine variant of pleomorphic lobular carcinoma in situ: further clinical, histopathologic, immunohistochemical, and molecular characterization of an emerging entity. *Am J Surg Pathol*. 2020;44:1092-1103.

73. Augros M, Buénerd A, Devouassoux-Shisheboran M, et al. [Infiltrating lobular carcinoma of the breast with histiocytoid features: three cases]. *Ann Pathol*. 2004;24:259-263; quiz 227.

74. Rakha EA, van Deurzen CH, Paish EC, et al. Pleomorphic lobular carcinoma of the breast: is it a prognostically significant pathological subtype independent of histological grade? *Mod Pathol*. 2013;26:496-501.

75. Dillon MF, Hill AD, Fleming FJ, et al. Identifying patients at risk of compromised margins following breast conservation for lobular carcinoma. *Am J Surg*. 2006;191:201-205.

76. Domagala W, Markiewski M, Kubiak R, et al. Immunohistochemical profile of invasive lobular carcinoma of the breast: predominantly vimentin and p53 protein negative, cathepsin D and oestrogen receptor positive. *Virchows Arch A Pathol Anat Histopathol*. 1993;423:497-502.

77. Fadare O, Wang SA, Hileeto D. The expression of cytokeratin 5/6 in invasive lobular carcinoma of the breast: evidence of a basal-like subset? *Hum Pathol*. 2008;39:331-336.

78. De Leeuw WJ, Berx G, Vos CB, et al. Simultaneous loss of E-cadherin and catenins in invasive lobular breast cancer and lobular carcinoma in situ. *J Pathol*. 1997;183:404-411.

79. Lehr HA, Folpe A, Yaziji H, et al. Cytokeratin 8 immunostaining pattern and E-cadherin expression distinguish lobular from ductal breast carcinoma. *Am J Clin Pathol*. 2000;114:190-196.

80. Morrogh M, Andrade VP, Giri D, et al. Cadherin-catenin complex dissociation in lobular neoplasia of the breast. *Breast Cancer Res Treat*. 2012;132:641-652.

81. Palacios J, Sarrio D, Garcia-Macias MC, et al. Frequent E-cadherin gene inactivation by loss of heterozygosity in pleomorphic lobular carcinoma of the breast. *Mod Pathol*. 2003;16:674-678.

82. Wahed A, Connelly J, Reese T. E-cadherin expression in pleomorphic lobular carcinoma: an aid to differentiation from ductal carcinoma. *Ann Diagn Pathol*. 2002;6:349-351.

83. Harigopal M, Shin SJ, Murray MP, et al. Aberrant E-cadherin staining patterns in invasive mammary carcinoma. *World J Surg Oncol*. 2005;3:73.

84. Dabbs DJ, Schnitt SJ, Geyer FC, et al. Lobular neoplasia of the breast revisited with emphasis on the role of E-cadherin immunohistochemistry. *Am J Surg Pathol*. 2013;37:e1-e11.

85. Rakha EA, Patel A, Powe DG, et al. Clinical and biological significance of E-cadherin protein expression in invasive lobular carcinoma of the breast. *Am J Surg Pathol*. 2010;34:1472-1479.

86. Sarrió D, Moreno-Bueno G, Hardisson D, et al. Epigenetic and genetic alterations of APC and CDH1 genes in lobular breast cancer: relationships with abnormal E-cadherin and catenin expression and microsatellite instability. *Int J Cancer*. 2003;106:208-215.

87. Da Silva L, Parry S, Reid L, et al. Aberrant expression of E-cadherin in lobular carcinomas of the breast. *Am J Surg Pathol*. 2008;32:773-783.

88. Canas-Marques R, Schnitt SJ. E-cadherin immunohistochemistry in breast pathology: uses and pitfalls. *Histopathology*. 2016;68:57-69.

89. Hajra KM, Chen DY, Fearon ER. The SLUG zinc-finger protein represses E-cadherin in breast cancer. *Cancer Res*. 2002;62:1613-1618.

90. de Deus Moura R, Wludarski SC, Carvalho FM, et al. Immunohistochemistry applied to the differential diagnosis between ductal and lobular carcinoma of the breast. *Appl Immunohistochem Mol Morphol*. 2013;21:1-12.

91. Naidoo K, Beardsley B, Carder PJ, et al. Accuracy of classification of invasive lobular carcinoma on needle core biopsy of the breast. *J Clin Pathol*. 2016;69:1122-1123.

92. Hwang ES, Nyante SJ, Yi Chen Y, et al. Clonality of lobular carcinoma in situ and synchronous invasive lobular carcinoma. *Cancer*. 2004;100:2562-2572.

93. McCart Reed AE, Kutasovic JR, Lakhani SR, et al. Invasive lobular carcinoma of the breast: morphology, biomarkers and 'omics. *Breast Cancer Res*. 2015;17:12.

94. Simpson PT, Reis-Filho JS, Lambros MB, et al. Molecular profiling pleomorphic lobular carcinomas of the breast: evidence for a common molecular genetic pathway with classic lobular carcinomas. *J Pathol*. 2008;215:231-244.

95. Vargas AC, Lakhani SR, Simpson PT. Pleomorphic lobular carcinoma of the breast: molecular pathology and clinical impact. *Future Oncol*. 2009;5:233-243.

96. Ciriello G, Gatza ML, Beck AH, et al. Comprehensive molecular portraits of invasive lobular breast cancer. *Cell*. 2015;163:506-519.

97. Grabenstetter A, Mohanty AS, Rana S, et al. E-cadherin immunohistochemical expression in invasive lobular carcinoma of the breast: correlation with morphology and CDH1 somatic alterations. *Hum Pathol*. 2020;102:44-53.

98. Weigelt B, Geyer FC, Natrajan R, et al. The molecular underpinning of lobular histological growth pattern: a genome-wide transcriptomic analysis of invasive lobular carcinomas and grade- and molecular subtype-matched invasive ductal carcinomas of no special type. *J Pathol*. 2010;220:45-57.

99. Trivedi H, Hamdani O, Thomas B, et al. Patient with lobular carcinoma of the breast and activating AKT1 E17K variant. *Acta Med Acad*. 2021;50:209-217.

100. Cserni G, Bianchi S, Vezzosi V, et al. The value of cytokeratin immunohistochemistry in the evaluation of axillary sentinel lymph nodes in patients with lobular breast carcinoma. *J Clin Pathol*. 2006;59:518-522.

101. Patel A, D'Alfonso T, Cheng E, et al. Sentinel lymph nodes in classic invasive lobular carcinoma of the breast: cytokeratin immunostain ensures detection, and precise determination of extent, of involvement. *Am J Surg Pathol*. 2017;41:1499-1505.

102. Inoue M, Nakagomi H, Nakada H, et al. Specific sites of metastases in invasive lobular carcinoma: a retrospective cohort study of metastatic breast cancer. *Breast Cancer*. 2017;24:667-672.

103. Zhao R, Li Y, Yu X, et al. Duodenal metastasis from recurrent invasive lobular carcinoma of breast: a case report and literature review. *Int J Clin Oncol*. 2012;17:160-164.

104. Borst MJ, Ingold JA. Metastatic patterns of invasive lobular versus invasive ductal carcinoma of the breast. *Surgery*. 1993;114:637-641; discussion 641-642.

105. Choi S, Joo JW, Do SI, et al. Endometrium-limited metastasis of extragenital malignancies: a challenge in the diagnosis of endometrial curettage specimens. *Diagnostics (Basel)*. 2020;10:150.

106. Houghton JP, Ioffe OB, Silverberg SG, et al. Metastatic breast lobular carcinoma involving tamoxifen-associated endometrial polyps: report of two cases and review of tamoxifen-associated polypoid uterine lesions. *Mod Pathol*. 2003;16:395-398.

107. Clinton LK, Plesec T, Goldblum JR, et al. Specific histopathologic features aid in distinguishing diffuse-type gastric adenocarcinoma from metastatic lobular breast carcinoma. *Am J Surg Pathol*. 2020;44:77-86.

108. Lyda MH, Tetef M, Carter NH, et al. Keratin immunohistochemistry detects clinically significant metastases in bone marrow biopsy specimens in women with lobular breast carcinoma. *Am J Surg Pathol*. 2000;24:1593-1599.

109. Fortunato L, Mascaro A, Poccia I, et al. Lobular breast cancer: same survival and local control compared with ductal cancer, but should both be treated the same way? Analysis of an institutional database over a 10-year period. *Ann Surg Oncol*. 2012;19:1107-1114.

110. Garcia-Fernandez A, Lain JM, Chabrera C, et al. Comparative long-term study of a large series of patients with invasive ductal carcinoma and invasive lobular carcinoma. Loco-regional recurrence, metastasis, and survival. *Breast J*. 2015;21:533-537.

111. Jayasinghe UW, Bilous AM, Boyages J. Is survival from infiltrating lobular carcinoma of the breast different from that of infiltrating ductal carcinoma? *Breast J*. 2007;13:479-485.

112. Moran MS, Yang Q, Haffty BG. The Yale University experience of early-stage invasive lobular carcinoma (ILC) and invasive ductal carcinoma (IDC) treated with breast conservation treatment (BCT): analysis of clinical-pathologic features, long-term outcomes, and molecular expression of COX-2, Bcl-2, and p53 as a function of histology. *Breast J*. 2009;15:571-578.

113. Viale G, Rotmensz N, Maisonneuve P, et al. Lack of prognostic significance of "classic" lobular breast carcinoma: a matched, single institution series. *Breast Cancer Res Treat*. 2009;117:211-214.

114. Bharat A, Gao F, Margenthaler JA. Tumor characteristics and patient outcomes are similar between invasive lobular and mixed invasive ductal/lobular breast cancers but differ from pure invasive ductal breast cancers. *Am J Surg*. 2009;198:516-519.

115. Wasif N, Maggard MA, Ko CY, et al. Invasive lobular vs. ductal breast cancer: a stage-matched comparison of outcomes. *Ann Surg Oncol*. 2010;17:1862-1869.

116. Adachi Y, Sawaki M, Hattori M, et al. Comparison of sentinel lymph node biopsy between invasive lobular carcinoma and invasive ductal carcinoma. *Breast Cancer*. 2018;25:560-565.

117. Chen Z, Yang J, Li S, et al. Invasive lobular carcinoma of the breast: a special histological type compared with invasive ductal carcinoma. *PLoS One*. 2017;12:e0182397.

118. Danzinger S, Hielscher N, Izsó M, et al. Invasive lobular carcinoma: clinicopathological features and subtypes. *J Int Med Res*. 2021;49:3000605211017039.

119. Zhang Y, Luo X, Chen M, et al. Biomarker profile of invasive lobular carcinoma: pleomorphic versus classic subtypes, clinicopathological characteristics and prognosis analyses. *Breast Cancer Res Treat*. 2022;194:279-295.

120. Allison KH, Kandalaft PL, Sitlani CM, et al. Routine pathologic parameters can predict Oncotype DX recurrence scores in subsets of ER positive patients: who does not always need testing? *Breast Cancer Res Treat*. 2012;131:413-424.

121. Kelly CM, Krishnamurthy S, Bianchini G, et al. Utility of oncotype DX risk estimates in clinically intermediate risk hormone receptor-positive, HER2-normal, grade II, lymph node-negative breast cancers. *Cancer*. 2010;116:5161-5167.

122. Kizy S, Huang JL, Marmor S, et al. Impact of the 21-gene recurrence score on outcome in patients with invasive lobular carcinoma of the breast. *Breast Cancer Res Treat*. 2017;165:757-763.

123. Beumer IJ, Persoon M, Witteveen A, et al. Prognostic value of MammaPrint® in invasive lobular breast cancer. *Biomark Insights*. 2016;11:139-146.

124. Desmedt C, Salgado R, Fornili M, et al. Immune infiltration in invasive lobular breast cancer. *J Natl Cancer Inst*. 2018;110:768-776.

125. Thompson ED, Taube JM, Asch-Kendrick RJ, et al. PD-L1 expression and the immune microenvironment in primary invasive lobular carcinomas of the breast. *Mod Pathol*. 2017;30:1551-1560.

126. Biglia N, Maggiorotto F, Liberale V, et al. Clinical-pathologic features, long term-outcome and surgical treatment in a large series of patients with invasive lobular carcinoma (ILC) and invasive ductal carcinoma (IDC). *Eur J Surg Oncol*. 2013;39:455-60.

127. Morrow M, Keeney K, Scholtens D, et al. Selecting patients for breast-conserving therapy: the importance of lobular histology. *Cancer*. 2006;106:2563-2568.

128. Santiago RJ, Harris EE, Qin L, et al. Similar long-term results of breast-conservation treatment for Stage I and II invasive lobular carcinoma compared with invasive ductal carcinoma of the breast: the University of Pennsylvania experience. *Cancer*. 2005;103:2447-2454.

129. Schnitt SJ, Connolly JL, Recht A, et al. Influence of infiltrating lobular histology on local tumor control in breast cancer patients treated with conservative surgery and radiotherapy. *Cancer*. 1989;64:448-454.

130. Yang C, Lei C, Zhang Y, et al. Comparison of overall survival between invasive lobular breast carcinoma and invasive ductal breast carcinoma: a propensity score matching study based on SEER DATABASE. *Front Oncol*. 2020;10:590643.

131. Anwar IF, Down SK, Rizvi S, et al. Invasive lobular carcinoma of the breast: should this be regarded as a chronic disease? *Int J Surg*. 2010;8:346-352.

132. Jacobs C, Ibrahim MF, Clemons M, et al. Treatment choices for patients with invasive lobular breast cancer: a doctor survey. *J Eval Clin Pract*. 2015;21:740-748.

133. Chung A, Gangi A, Amersi F, et al. Impact of consensus guidelines by the Society of Surgical Oncology and the American Society for Radiation Oncology on margins for breast-conserving surgery in stages 1 and 2 invasive breast cancer. *Ann Surg Oncol*. 2015;22(suppl 3):S422-S427.

134. Cocco D, ElSherif A, Wright MD, et al. Invasive lobular breast cancer: data to support surgical decision making. *Ann Surg Oncol*. 2021;28:5723-5729.

135. Marmor S, Hui JYC, Huang JL, et al. Relative effectiveness of adjuvant chemotherapy for invasive lobular compared with invasive ductal carcinoma of the breast. *Cancer*. 2017;123:3015-3021.

136. Dixon JM, Renshaw L, Dixon J, et al. Invasive lobular carcinoma: response to neoadjuvant letrozole therapy. *Breast Cancer Res Treat*. 2011;130:871-877.

20

Mesenchymal Lesions

ELAINE W. ZHONG AND SYED A. HODA

INTRODUCTION

The diagnosis of mesenchymal mammary lesions using needle core biopsy (NCB) specimens often challenges the pathologist. The limitations posed by the small size of the tissue samples and the overlapping features of many mesenchymal tumors impede the pathologist's ability to provide a specific diagnosis. This group of lesions spans a broad range of lineages, and from benign to locally aggressive to malignant. Difficulties include recognizing phyllodes tumor and metaplastic carcinoma, and distinguishing low-grade sarcoma from its benign counterparts. Making such distinctions usually requires evaluation of the excised mass to search for findings which are often focal, such as the presence of characteristic benign intralesional glandular tissue which would suggest the diagnosis of phyllodes tumor, and for immunohistochemical (IHC) evidence of epithelial differentiation which would point to the diagnosis of metaplastic carcinoma.

Despite these limitations, the study of specimens obtained by NCB can establish definitive diagnoses in certain cases and can narrow the range of possible diagnoses in most others. By integrating conventional morphologic findings with the results of IHC staining or molecular analysis **(Table 20.1)**, one can usually establish unequivocal diagnoses of granular cell tumor, fibromatosis, myofibroblastoma, schwannoma, solitary fibrous tumor (SFT), rhabdomyosarcoma, liposarcoma, synovial sarcoma, and others. Even if it is not possible to make a definitive diagnosis, the pathologist can often provide valuable information, including triaging for surgical excision.

Mammary sarcomas arise only rarely. According to data from the Surveillance, Epidemiology, and End Results (SEER) database, the annual incidence is 4.6 cases per million women (1). Women treated for breast carcinoma experience a slight increase in their risk for soft tissue sarcomas, and the use of irradiation further increases the risk for the development of angiosarcomas, undifferentiated pleomorphic sarcomas (UPSs), and other rare types of sarcoma within the irradiation field (2-4). It is difficult to determine the frequencies of the various types of mammary sarcomas because of the rather indiscriminate use in the literature of the generic term *stromal sarcoma*. As much as possible, one should employ the terminology used for extramammary sarcomas when referring to their mammary counterparts. The microscopic features of both are generally similar and depend on

TABLE 20.1

Recurrent Molecular Alterations in Mesenchymal Tumors of the Breast

Diagnosis	Molecular Findings
Angiolipoma	*PRKD2* mutation
Angiomyxoma/myxoma	*PRKAR1A* mutation
Atypical lipomatous tumor/ well-differentiated liposarcoma	*MDM2* and/or *CDK4* amplification
Dermatofibrosarcoma protuberans	t(17;22) *COL1A1-PDGFB*
Fibromatosis	*CTNNB1* mutation
Myofibroblastoma	13q (*RB1*) deletion
Myxoid liposarcoma	t(12;16) *FUS-DDIT3*
Nodular fasciitis	*USP6* rearrangement
Postirradiation angiosarcoma	*MYC* amplification
Solitary fibrous tumor	inv12 *NAB2-STAT6*
Spindle cell lipoma	13q (*RB1*) deletion

the nature of the neoplastic cells. Before making a diagnosis of mammary sarcoma, one must exclude more common entities such as phyllodes tumor with a dominant stromal component, metaplastic carcinoma, and certain benign stromal proliferations of mesenchymal cells.

(MYO)FIBROBLASTIC

Pseudoangiomatous Stromal Hyperplasia

Pseudoangiomatous stromal hyperplasia (PASH) is a benign stromal proliferation characterized by slit-like spaces within dense collagenous stroma. The term *pseudoangiomatous* was introduced by Vuitch et al (5) to acknowledge the vessel-like appearance of the proliferation, though it lacks endothelium or intraluminal blood cells. It has been suggested that the spaces in PASH are part of a "prelymphatic" pathway (6). Although typically an incidental finding, in some cases the lesion gives rise to a palpable or radiographically detected mass ("PASH tumor") simulating a neoplasm. Ibrahim et al (7)

375

found microscopic foci of PASH in 23% of 200 consecutive breast specimens, and Degnim et al (8) found evidence of PASH in 6% of 9,065 consecutive excision specimens showing only benign lesions.

Mammograms usually demonstrate a mass without calcification or, less frequently, a focal asymmetric density. The borders of the mass usually appear smooth, but the tumor can have spiculated or ill-defined margins. Ultrasound reveals a well-defined hypoechoic mass (9,10). Magnetic resonance imaging (MRI) most commonly demonstrates non-mass enhancement with persistent kinetics (11).

With rare exceptions, patients with PASH tumor have been females. The age at diagnosis ranges from 3 to 86 years, and the mean age in several series (5,10,12-14) ranges from 37 to 51 years. The pathogenesis is thought to be related to hormone imbalance. The majority of women are premenopausal, and postmenopausal women with PASH often have a history of hormone replacement therapy. Rare examples of PASH tumors have been described in children and adolescents. One of the youngest patients was a 3-year-old boy, who had a 5.5-cm tumor in the right breast (14)! Singh et al (15) described a menarchal 12-year-old girl with marked bilateral breast enlargement because of PASH. When it occurs in males, PASH usually represents an incidental component in 24% to 54% of gynecomastia (16,17), and 98% of samples showing PASH in men were associated with gynecomastia (18). Unusual examples include an 11-cm mass associated with gynecomastia in a 50-year-old man (19), and 10-cm masses in both axillae of a 44-year-old man (20).

Patients typically describe a palpable, painless, unilateral mass, which feels rubbery or firm. Although the lesion tends to arise in the upper outer quadrant, any part of the breast, including the subareolar region, can be affected (21). Rare examples are located in the axillary tail (13) or vulva (22). Occasional patients have had bilateral PASH. Diffuse breast enlargement is seen rarely, and rapid growth of the lesion may occur (23). *Peau d'orange* change and skin necrosis have been observed during pregnancy in patients who have massive breast enlargement caused by diffuse PASH (24).

The most striking histologic finding is a complex pattern of empty, often anastomosing spaces in dense collagenous stroma. These slits, visible at low magnification, typically involve the perilobular nonspecialized stroma. In florid cases, the pseudoangiomatous changes involve the intralobular specialized stroma as well **(Fig. 20.1)**.

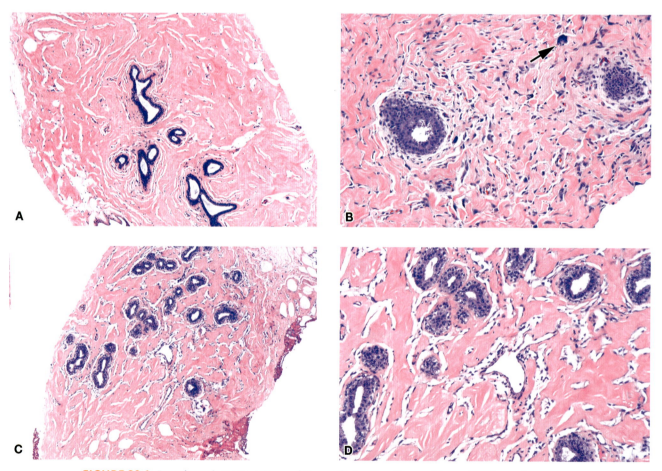

FIGURE 20.1 Pseudoangiomatous Stromal Hyperplasia. Needle core biopsy (NCB) specimens from three patients are shown. **A:** In this specimen, the myofibroblasts appear inconspicuous, and the slit-shaped spaces are largely unconnected. Collagen fibrils traverse some of the spaces. **B:** NCB demonstrates enlarged multinucleate cells (arrow). **C, D:** This pronounced pseudoangiomatous proliferation with connected spaces involves a lobule and the surrounding stroma.

Collagenization of intralobular stroma and attenuation of ducts can create an appearance that mimics fibroadenoma or artifactual "whirlies" (or "swirlies") **(Fig. 20.2)** (see Chapter 25). The spaces may contain a few red blood cells, and collagen fibrils may traverse the spaces. Basement membrane material is not demonstrable around the slit-like spaces. The stroma also contains genuine small blood vessels and capillaries.

Myofibroblasts distributed singly and discontinuously at the margins of the spaces resemble endothelial cells. The nuclei of the myofibroblasts usually appear attenuated and lack atypia and mitotic activity. Uncommonly, some lesional cells appear enlarged and have noticeably hyperchromatic or multiple nuclei. One can find these cells in patients with PASH and neurofibromatosis type I (NF1) (25), but the presence of multinucleated stromal giant cells is not limited to such patients (17). In an unusual variant of PASH, the myofibroblasts contain cytoplasmic inclusion bodies of the type found in digital fibromas (26).

When myofibroblasts accumulate in distinct relatively short bundles or fascicles, they give rise to the lesion known as *fascicular PASH* **(Fig. 20.3)**. The presence of these bundles attests to a more robust proliferation of the myofibroblasts. Examples of fascicular PASH showing extreme myofibroblastic proliferation resemble myofibroblastoma. This similarity becomes especially evident when the myofibroblasts have abundant cytoplasm and grow as localized tumors. Myoid differentiation can occur in isolated myofibroblasts. When this phenomenon occurs in many cells, the resulting nodule comes to resemble a leiomyoma.

Cytologic alterations of myofibroblasts are sometimes encountered in PASH and are denoted as *atypical PASH*. Pleomorphic nuclei can be found infrequently in PASH displaying conventional and fascicular patterns, and are sometimes accompanied by mitotic activity **(Fig. 20.4)** (27). Several instances of PASH tumors in which the myofibroblasts demonstrate marked cytologic atypia, multinucleation, and mitotic activity have been encountered in teenage girls. The significance of these findings is unknown at this time.

The myofibroblasts of PASH usually stain for CD34 and vimentin and show variable immunoreactivity for smooth muscle actin (SMA), muscle-specific actin, BCL2, desmin, and calponin. They are negative for cytokeratin and vascular markers such as factor VIII–related antigen, CD31, ERG, and D2-40. The results of studies of hormone receptor stains in PASH have varied. Bowman et al (12) found high rates of estrogen receptor (ER) and progesterone receptor (PR) immunoreactivity (79% and 63%, respectively), but most ER-positive cases showed only "occasional" positive cells. The propensity for PASH tumors to affect premenopausal women and postmenopausal women taking hormone replacement therapy and the frequent coexistence of PASH and gynecomastia also suggest hormonal pathogenesis.

Minute incidental foci of PASH do not warrant any treatment. Excision is commonly recommended for PASH that is clinically evident (or distressing), enlarging, or with discordant radiologic and pathologic findings. Among studies of patients who underwent surveillance only, an average of 10.4% of tumors continued to grow, whereas the rest remained unchanged or decreased (28,29). Most lesions that progressed were excised, and pathologic evaluation revealed PASH without atypical features (10,13). Rarely mastectomy may be necessary to control multiple recurrent tumors (15). Isolated case reports document the response of PASH to selective ER modulators (30,31).

Most patients have remained well after excision of PASH. Ipsilateral recurrences have been reported in 2% to 30% of the patients, and rare patients have experienced multiple ipsilateral recurrences (5). Recurrent lesions do not ordinarily exhibit increased cellularity or other atypical features; moreover, examples that have recurred do not differ in their histologic attributes from those that did not recur.

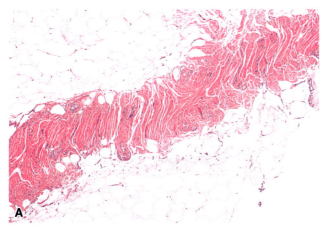 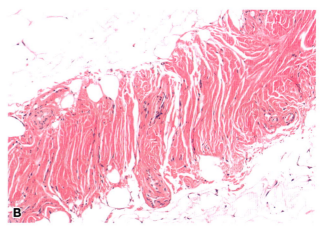

FIGURE 20.2 "Whirlies" or "Swirlies." **A, B:** An artifact of vacuum-assisted stereotactic core biopsy procurement commonly mistaken for pseudoangiomatous stromal hyperplasia. Note the absence of nuclei lining the slit-like spaces.

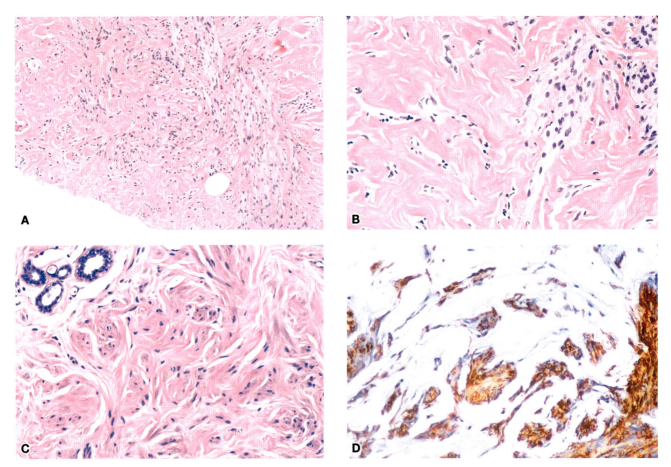

FIGURE 20.3 Pseudoangiomatous Stromal Hyperplasia, Fascicular. A: Myofibroblasts have formed distinct bundles with an interlacing pattern in this needle core biopsy (NCB). **B:** Another portion of the specimen shows pseudoangiomatous and fascicular elements. **C:** A fascicular pattern with myoid differentiation is shown. **D:** The myofibroblasts are immunoreactive for actin.

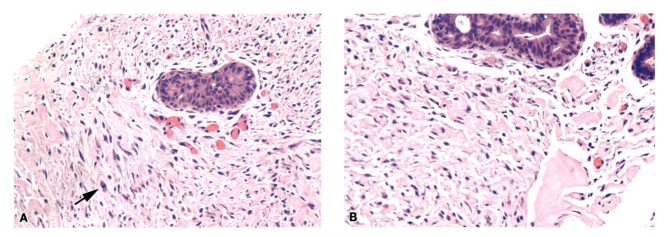

FIGURE 20.4 Atypical Pseudoangiomatous Stromal Hyperplasia, Fascicular. A, B: This needle core biopsy (NCB) was obtained from a 12-cm tumor in a 29-year-old woman. The stroma has occasional mitotic figures (arrow) and is focally cellular. The pseudoangiomatous pattern is maintained in the cellular foci. Ductal hyperplasia is also evident.

PASH is not associated with an increased risk of subsequent breast carcinoma (8), though they occasionally coincide (13).

Fibromatosis

Fibromatosis is an infiltrative, histologically low-grade, locally aggressive neoplasm composed of fibroblastic cells and variable amounts of collagen. Other terms applied to this lesion include extraabdominal desmoid and aggressive fibromatosis.

Patients with mammary fibromatosis range from 11 months to 83 years at diagnosis. The average age in most studies falls between 37 (32) and 50.3 (33) years. Females are more commonly affected than males. Patients typically present with a palpable, firm, painless tumor, which may suggest carcinoma on clinical examination. Dimpling or retraction of the skin may reinforce this clinical impression. Fibromatosis affects left and right breasts approximately equally. It rarely involves the subareolar region or axillary breast tissue (34). Several cases of bilateral mammary fibromatosis have been reported; in most of the cases, the bilateral tumors presented simultaneously (35).

Antecedent injury from trauma or surgery was noted in a few cases, and several examples developed following breast augmentation (32,36-39). The tumors came to attention after a mean interval of 3 years from the time of implant placement. Such tumors are typically unilateral and arise in or around the implant capsule. Current evidence does not suggest that the biomaterials by themselves cause fibromatosis. Rare examples of mammary fibromatosis have been associated with familial adenomatous polyposis (FAP), a condition of germline *APC* alteration in which somatic fibromatosis (desmoid tumor) frequently occurs. The family history of breast carcinoma mentioned in a few case reports is probably coincidental. Rarely, patients had invasive ductal carcinoma of the contralateral breast. A 22-year-old woman developed unilateral mammary fibromatosis 5 years after treatment of Hodgkin disease by chemotherapy alone (32). Despite the frequent association of abdominal desmoid tumors with pregnancy, only a few cases of mammary fibromatosis have been pregnancy-related and were likely coincidental.

Mammography reveals a stellate tumor that may be indistinguishable from carcinoma. Calcifications are rarely formed in mammary fibromatosis, but they may be present in a benign lesion such as sclerosing adenosis which has been engulfed by the tumor. The sizes of tumors vary from less than 1 to 17 cm and average 2.5 to 3.0 cm (32,33,40,41). Most examples of fibromatosis have a distinct stellate configuration; others are described as circumscribed or well-demarcated nodules.

The histologic features of mammary fibromatosis are similar to those of fibromatosis in extramammary sites. Although the mass often exhibits varied growth patterns, spindle cells and collagen constitute consistent components. The spindle cells are usually distributed in broad sheets, sometimes in a storiform configuration, or in interlacing bundles with a herringbone pattern. The cells usually have small, pale, oval or spindly, uniform nuclei **(Fig. 20.5A)**. Nuclear atypia and pleomorphism are uncommon. Mitotic figures are inconspicuous in most cases, although a rate of 3 mitotic figures per 10 high-power field (HPF) has been reported (32). Areas in which the collagenous element overshadows the spindle cells have a keloidal appearance **(Fig. 20.5B)**. In certain tumors, the center appears more fibrous than the periphery, whereas others exhibit more pronounced collagenization in the outer regions. Myxoid areas sometimes occur. Focal lymphocytic infiltrates, some with germinal centers, are found in nearly half of the tumors **(Fig. 20.5C,D)** and usually appear more prominent at the periphery. Smaller caliber blood vessels are evenly distributed throughout the tumor. Stromal calcification is rare.

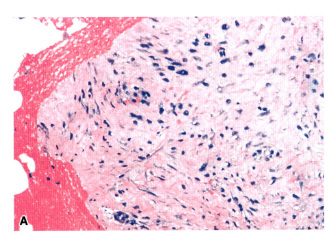
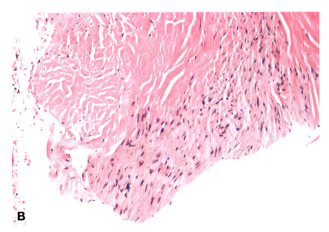

FIGURE 20.5 Fibromatosis. A: Needle core biopsy (NCB) shows average cellularity and mild stromal edema. The tumor cells have uniform round-to-oval nuclei. **B:** This NCB displays an area of dense collagenous tissue adjacent to a more cellular component of the mass. The slit-shaped spaces in the keloidal tissue resemble pseudoangiomatous stromal hyperplasia.

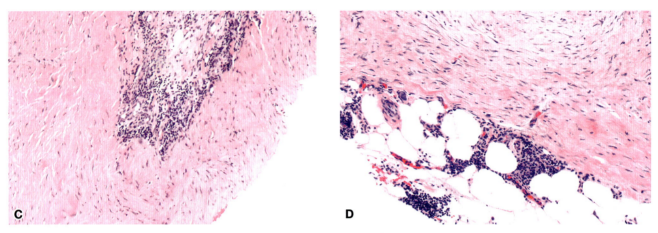

FIGURE 20.5 (*continued*) **C, D:** Perivascular and peripheral lymphoid aggregates are seen in these NCB specimens.

SMA-positive cytoplasmic inclusion bodies similar to those seen in infantile digital fibromatosis have been described in two mammary tumors that appear to be fibromatosis (42).

Regardless of *gross* circumscription, all fibromatoses have invasive stellate extensions into the surrounding parenchyma. It is generally possible to identify mammary ducts and lobules engulfed by these peripheral extensions **(Fig. 20.6)**. The appearance of these infiltrative areas may mimic a phyllodes tumor. Glandular parenchymal elements are less conspicuous or absent toward the center of the mass.

Rare cases of fibromatosis are limited to the mammary subcutaneous fat with little or no parenchymal involvement.

Nuclear localization of β-catenin, commonly seen in somatic fibromatosis, is also seen in mammary fibromatosis. Among 53 examples of mammary fibromatosis pooled from three series (33,40,43), 83% demonstrated nuclear β-catenin reactivity. The majority showed diffuse and intense nuclear staining, although occasional tumors demonstrated only focal reactivity. Concomitant cytoplasmic positivity is observed in 87% to 100% of mammary fibromatosis cases (43).

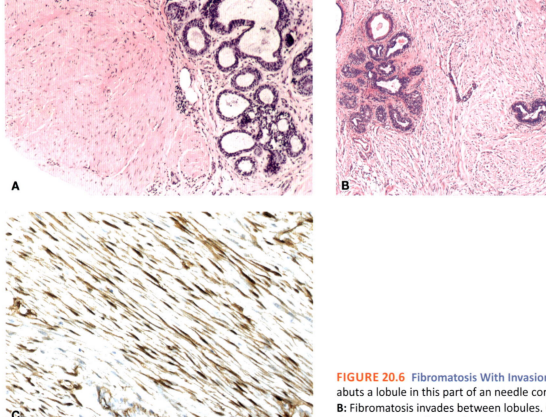

FIGURE 20.6 **Fibromatosis With Invasion. A:** The tumor abuts a lobule in this part of an needle core biopsy (NCB). **B:** Fibromatosis invades between lobules. **C:** β-catenin stain demonstrates nuclear and cytoplasmic reactivity.

Nuclear localization of β-catenin results from activation of Wnt signaling, most commonly because of sporadic *CTNNB1* exon 3 mutations (75%) (40) or *APC* inactivation (12%) (44). Nuclear staining for β-catenin is not specific to fibromatosis, as it can be seen in spindle cell metaplastic carcinomas (23%), phyllodes tumors (94% of benign, 57% of malignant), fibroadenomas, and even scars (43,45). The absence of β-catenin reactivity also does not exclude the diagnosis of fibromatosis.

The spindle cells of fibromatosis variably express SMA, actin, and desmin. Anecdotal observations suggest that actin and desmin reactivity may be more common in subcutaneous than in parenchymal fibromatosis. The tumor cells are negative for cytokeratin and seldom express CD34, ER, or PR.

It is important in cases of suspected fibromatosis to exclude low-grade fibromatosis-like metaplastic carcinoma. Both tumors are histologically low-grade without significant mitotic activity. Features favoring metaplastic carcinoma include mild to moderate nuclear atypia, epithelioid areas, ductal carcinoma in situ, and immunoreactivity for cytokeratins and p63. Because cytokeratin expression may be limited, a panel including multiple antibodies such as CK AE1/AE3, CK5/6, 34βE12, CK14, and CAM 5.2 are recommended. A predominantly lymphocytic inflammatory reaction occurs more diffusely in and around most metaplastic carcinomas than it does in fibromatosis. In a study of 26 excised fibromatoses, the use of β-catenin, CD34, high-molecular-weight keratins, and p63 IHC facilitated accurate NCB diagnosis in 22 (85%) of the cases (46).

Another important and challenging differential for mammary fibromatosis is reparative and reactive processes. Scars from healed fat necrosis, remote trauma, and surgery must be distinguished from fibromatosis. Calcifications are more likely to be associated with fat necrosis but can rarely occur in fibromatosis. Foreign body granulomas, sometimes with partly absorbed suture material, indicate prior surgery. If the patient has recurrent fibromatosis, reparative changes caused by an earlier operation may mingle with recurrent tumor, further complicating the diagnosis. In one study, 21 of 22 (95%) scars exhibited some degree of nuclear β-catenin expression, with diffuse expression in 16 cases (45). The presence of lymphoid infiltrates, which commonly occur at the periphery of fibromatosis, should not be mistaken for an inflammatory condition. In nodular fasciitis, inflammatory cells are dispersed more diffusely at the periphery as well as within the lesion. Myoid and multinucleated cells characteristically found in nodular fasciitis are not features of fibromatosis.

The recommended treatment is wide local excision. When a tumor is adherent to fascia, muscle, or skin, excision should be extended to include the involved tissue, and it may be necessary to perform a mastectomy to achieve adequate margins. Immediate reexcision of the biopsy site should be considered if the initial excision removed only a limited amount of tissue, or if the margins are positive. Reexcision seems especially important for lesions located deep in the breast or near the chest wall, because recurrences at these sites may be difficult to control. On the other hand, follow-up is preferable to reexcision for relatively superficial lesions or subareolar nodules, which might require excision of the nipple.

The frequency of local recurrence ranges from 23% to 29% (32,41). Although the risk of recurrence is higher in patients with positive margins, recurrences have been observed in cases with apparently negative margins. As such, radical resections and reexcisions for positive margins are discouraged by some (47). Most recurrences occur within 3 years of diagnosis; however, in a few instances, local recurrences were not detected for nearly a decade. Multiple recurrences have been documented (41). Histologic features such as cellularity, mitotic activity, and cellular pleomorphism do not seem to predict recurrence.

Irradiation, hormonal therapy, and chemotherapy have been used to treat fibromatosis arising outside the breast, but none of these approaches represents an established treatment for mammary fibromatosis.

Nodular Fasciitis

Nodular fasciitis is a benign reactive fibroblastic and myofibroblastic proliferation. Although it is a common tumor of the soft tissues, it only rarely affects the mammary gland. Most reports illustrate superficial, palpable nodules, but masses abutting the deep fascia have been described as well (48,49). Some descriptions (50) mention mammary glands at the edges of the masses.

Nodular fasciitis of the mammary region occurs in both females and males. The ages of the patients range from 15 to 84 years. Most patients present with a recently discovered, palpable firm mass, and they often describe rapid enlargement of the mass. Prior trauma is not usually mentioned.

The radiographic findings are often suspicious for carcinoma. Mammography demonstrates a high-density mass with spiculated or irregular margins, and ultrasonography reveals a hypoechoic mass with irregular borders (48,49,51). MRI may also suggest the presence of a malignancy (52). In a literature review by Squillaci et al (51), reported examples ranged from 1 to 7 cm with an average size of 2.4 cm.

The proliferative spindle cells form short bundles and fascicles randomly dispersed in a loose myxoid to collagenous stroma **(Fig. 20.7)**. The appearance is often described as having a feathery or tissue culture-like quality. Older lesions show greater collagenization. The spindle cells have bipolar to oval nuclei with delicate chromatin and micronucleoli. Cellularity is high in early lesions, and mitotic activity may be brisk but without atypical forms. Inflammatory cells, extravasated red blood cells, and prominent thin-walled vessels are present within the nodule. The borders of the mass are irregular. Benign ducts and lobules can become entrapped in the proliferation.

The spindle cells in nodular fasciitis are positive for SMA and muscle-specific actin. The proliferative cells do not stain for CD34, nuclear β-catenin, or keratin, but rare spindle cells may express CK AE1/AE3. Rearrangement of *USP6* is characteristic, most commonly *MYH9-USP6* fusion, which can be detected by fluorescence in situ hybridization (FISH) in challenging cases (53,54).

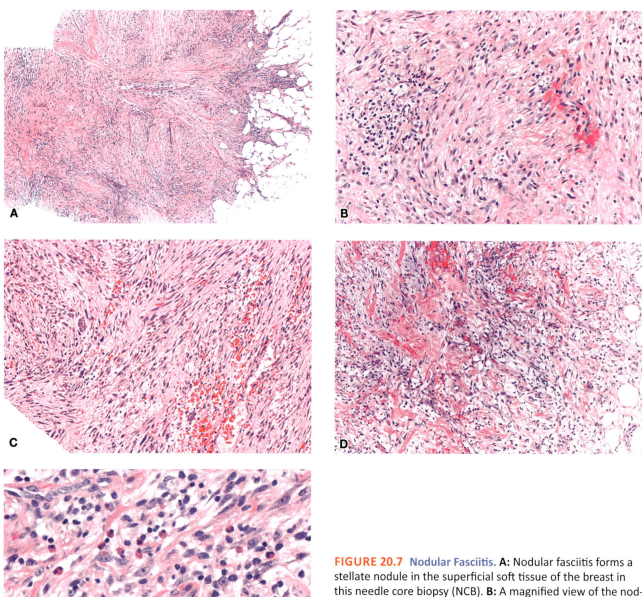

FIGURE 20.7 **Nodular Fasciitis. A:** Nodular fasciitis forms a stellate nodule in the superficial soft tissue of the breast in this needle core biopsy (NCB). **B:** A magnified view of the nodule shown in **(A)** demonstrates the uniform spindle cells and extravasated erythrocytes. **C:** An NCB of nodular fasciitis with prominent extravasated erythrocytes and nuclear hyperchromasia. **D, E:** NCB from another example of nodular fasciitis demonstrates the "feathery" growth pattern of the spindle cells **(D)** and the mixed inflammatory infiltrate **(E)**.

The differential diagnosis includes spindle cell carcinoma, fibromatosis, myofibroblastoma, and sarcoma. Notably, "pseudosarcomatous fasciitis" has been used as a synonym for nodular fasciitis. Spindle cell carcinoma can mimic the appearance of nodular fasciitis. The presence of nuclear atypia, clustered cell aggregates, or in situ carcinoma favors the former diagnosis. Some spindle cell carcinomas consist of bland cells that lack overt epithelial differentiation. IHC for cytokeratins and p63 can be helpful to clarify the diagnosis in such cases. Fibromatosis is characterized by longer, sweeping fascicles and greater infiltration of the surrounding parenchyma, and most cases display nuclear reactivity for β-catenin. Myofibroblastoma demonstrates more clearly defined fascicles intermixed with conspicuous bands of bright, eosinophilic collagen. The usual example appears sharply circumscribed and stains for CD34. The absence of nuclear atypia and pleomorphism helps to distinguish nodular fasciitis from sarcoma.

Nodular fasciitis is a benign, self-limited process. Several reports document spontaneous resolution of mammary lesions within 3 to 6 months from the time of diagnosis (48,49). A conservative approach that includes monitoring for several months may provide adequate management for some patients. Nevertheless, it may be difficult to exclude other diagnoses based on the findings in an NCB sample, and excision should be considered in most circumstances. Recurrence after surgical excision is rare.

Myofibroblastoma

Myofibroblastoma is a benign neoplasm composed of myofibroblasts. These spindle-shaped mesenchymal cells are minimally represented in virtually all tissues. Like myoepithelial cells, myofibroblasts can express actin and calponin, but only myoepithelial cells demonstrate immunoreactivity for high-molecular-weight cytokeratins and p63.

Myofibroblastomas typically afflict middle-aged to elderly patients (age range, 41-87; mean, seventh decade) (55,56). They are seen in younger patients only exceptionally, but one tumor presented in a 10-month-old boy (57). Myofibroblastomas are encountered in men, as frequently as in women.

Most patients present with a solitary, slow-growing, painless, mobile mass. The tumors may enlarge over the course of years. Rare tumors demonstrate rapid enlargement, and associated *peau d'orange* (orange peel-like) change of the skin has been described in a 65-year-old man (58). The vast majority of tumors are unilateral. Rare examples of bilateral myofibroblastomas have been reported in males (59). Two of the lesions described by Toker et al (60) as "benign spindle cell breast tumors" in men were probably myofibroblastomas. One patient had two myofibroblastomas in his left breast, which were treated by simple mastectomy, and 17 years later he underwent a right mastectomy, which disclosed six additional foci. Concurrent gynecomastia is reported in some patients.

Mammographically, the tumors are oval, circumscribed, hyperdense or isodense, and lack microcalcifications (61). Ultrasonography demonstrates an oval, parallel, isoechoic mass with internal vascularity (62), findings which may suggest the diagnosis of fibroadenoma.

The mean maximum extent of the tumors is approximately 2 cm; most are smaller than 4 cm and range from 0.9 (55) to 16 (63) cm. An attempt at NCB in one case (64) was not successful because the tumor was "stony hard," although the excised tumor was not calcified or ossified. Cystic degeneration, necrosis, and hemorrhage have not been reported.

The classic myofibroblastoma is devoid of mammary ducts and lobules. The border of the tumor is usually circumscribed. Some examples incorporate adipocytes or glandular tissue into the periphery of the mass, a phenomenon that indicates invasion of surrounding parenchyma. Two distinctive histologic features are bundles of slender, bipolar, uniform spindle cells typically arranged in short fascicles, and intervening broad bands of ropy or hyalinized collagen **(Fig. 20.8)**. The spindle cells have bland, ovoid nuclei with dispersed chromatin and small nucleoli. Nuclear grooves

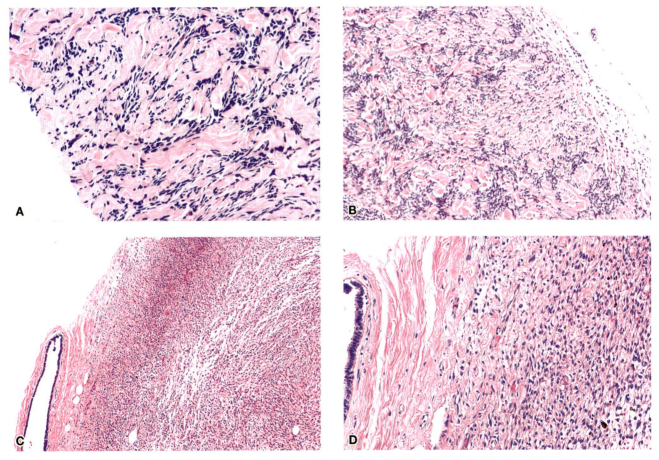

FIGURE 20.8 Myofibroblastoma. A: This needle core biopsy (NCB) shows the characteristic fascicles of myofibroblasts and intervening bands of collagen. **B:** The excised tumor has a circumscribed border. **C, D:** A less collagenous example of myofibroblastoma shows nondescript spindle cells abutting a benign duct.

may be present. The cytoplasm is typically pale and eosinophilic, and cell borders are indistinct. Mitotic figures are sparse or undetectable. Multinucleated cells are uncommon, and pleomorphic nuclei, which are believed to represent a degenerative phenomenon, are encountered only rarely (65). Nuclear palisading can create Verocay-like bodies, which can resemble schwannoma (66,67). Rarely, adipocytes are dispersed separately or in small groups throughout the tumor, and some myofibroblastomas have foci of leiomyomatous or cartilaginous differentiation (68-70). Most tumors contain many mast cells, and a perivascular lymphoplasmacytic infiltrate can be seen.

Several variants of myofibroblastoma have been described based on histopathologic features. A single pattern may dominate in a tumor, or several patterns may be mixed. In the *collagenized* or *fibrous myofibroblastoma*, the spindle cells are distributed in collagenous stroma **(Fig. 20.9)**. The broad, deeply eosinophilic fibrous bands that are so prominent in a classic myofibroblastoma are absent or greatly reduced in number. Irregular slit-like spaces are formed between tumor cells. The stroma is reminiscent of PASH, and some have a fascicular structure.

The *epithelioid variant* of myofibroblastoma features medium to large polygonal or epithelioid cells arranged in alveolar groups **(Fig. 20.10)**. Nuclei are round to oval and may be eccentrically located. Mild to moderate nuclear pleomorphism can be seen, and scattered binucleated and multinucleated cells are not uncommon (67,71). Mitotic activity is absent or minimal. The term *epithelioid myofibroblastoma* is used arbitrarily for tumors in which more than 50% of the lesion has this histologic pattern. The lesional cells in an epithelioid myofibroblastoma with sclerotic stroma can have a linear growth pattern that resembles invasive lobular carcinoma **(Fig. 20.11)** (72). In contrast to invasive carcinoma, epithelioid myofibroblastoma usually has well-circumscribed borders. Rare tumors composed of large cells with abundant glassy cytoplasm and vesicular nuclei have been referred to as a *"deciduoid-like" variant* (73).

A *cellular variant* of myofibroblastoma features a dense proliferation of spindle-shaped neoplastic myofibroblasts. Collagenous bands may be absent in parts of the lesion. These tumors tend to have infiltrative borders. Rarely, cellular and collagenous or fibrous growth patterns are combined in a single tumor.

The *infiltrative variant* of myofibroblastoma is characterized by invasive growth **(Fig. 20.12)**. One finds bundles of relatively evenly dispersed spindle, ovoid, and epithelioid cells embedded in collagenous stroma interspersed with fat, mammary stroma, ducts, and lobules. The classic and other foregoing variants of myofibroblastoma do not demonstrate either the abundance or the diffuse distribution of mammary tissues seen in the infiltrative types of myofibroblastoma.

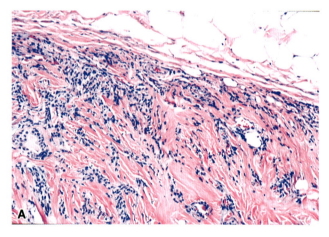

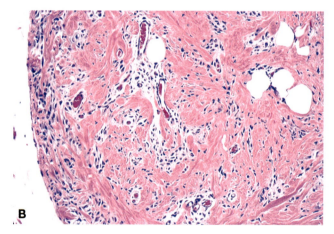

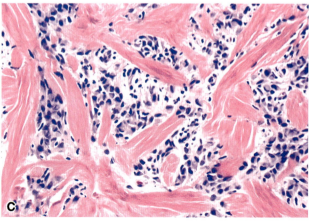

FIGURE 20.9 Myofibroblastoma, Collagenized. A: Bundles of myofibroblasts are distributed between prominent bands of collagen. The tumor has a circumscribed border. Note adipocytes entrapped within the tumor. **B, C:** Another tumor consists of dense collagen bands and epithelioid myofibroblasts.

MESENCHYMAL LESIONS 385

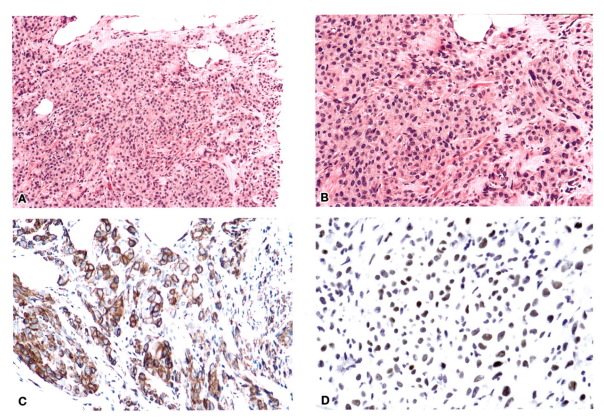

FIGURE 20.10 **Myofibroblastoma, Epithelioid. A, B:** Epithelioid myofibroblasts form alveolar clusters and bundles in this hypercellular needle core biopsy (NCB). This appearance could be mistaken for invasive carcinoma. **C:** The cells are strongly immunoreactive for smooth muscle actin. **D:** The epithelioid myofibroblasts demonstrate reactivity for estrogen receptor.

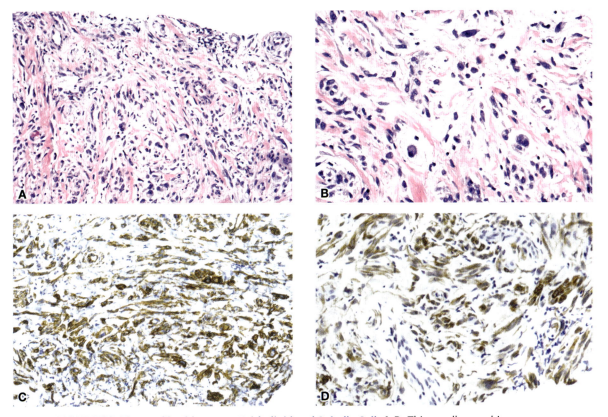

FIGURE 20.11 **Myofibroblastoma, Epithelioid and Spindle Cell. A-D:** This needle core biopsy (NCB) is from a spindle and epithelioid myofibroblastoma with myxoid stroma. The tumor was strongly reactive for CD34 **(C)** and desmin **(D)**.

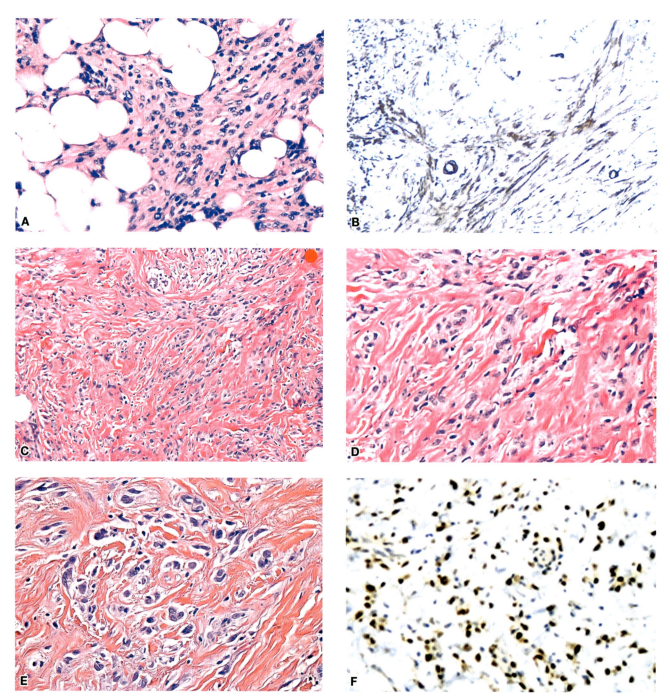

FIGURE 20.12 Myofibroblastoma, Infiltrating. A, B: Tumor cells in fat might be mistaken for infiltrating carcinoma in this needle core biopsy (NCB). The tumor cells are strongly immunoreactive for smooth muscle actin (**B**). **C-F:** This tumor with infiltrating epithelioid cells, small nucleoli, and apparent dyscohesion (**E**) was initially mistaken for invasive lobular carcinoma. The lesional cells were strongly estrogen receptor (ER)-positive (**F**). Immunoreactivity for actin, CD34, and desmin supported the final diagnosis of myofibroblastoma.

Certain infiltrative myofibroblastomas exhibit a tendency for the neoplastic myofibroblasts to be oriented around blood vessels.

Myxoid myofibroblastomas consist of sparse spindle cells distributed in myxoid stroma **(Fig. 20.13)**. This variety of myofibroblastoma often exhibits an infiltrative manner of growth. Certain tumors classified as nodular mucinosis may represent myxoid myofibroblastomas. Magro et al (74) described a myofibroblastoma with extensive myxedematous stromal change.

Rarely, myofibroblastomas contain abundant fat suggestive of a lipomatous element. The term *lipomatous myofibroblastoma* has been suggested for this type of lesion **(Fig. 20.14)** (75,76).

MESENCHYMAL LESIONS 387

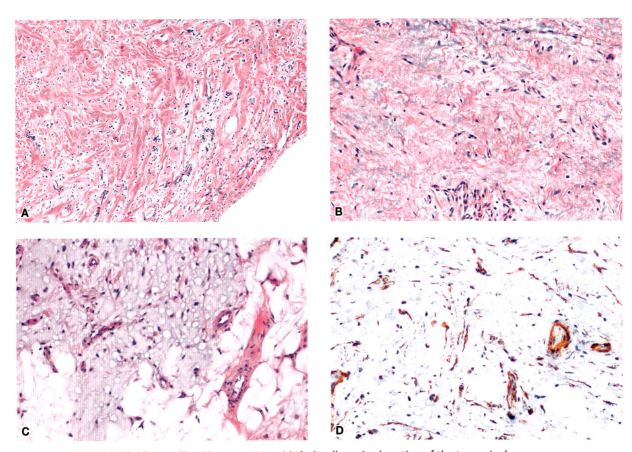

FIGURE 20.13 **Myofibroblastoma, Myxoid. A:** A collagenized portion of the tumor is shown. **B:** Basophilic myxoid material is evident in the tumor. **C:** Fully developed myxoid myofibroblastoma invades fat. **D:** The invasive myxoid portion of the tumor is immunoreactive for CD34.

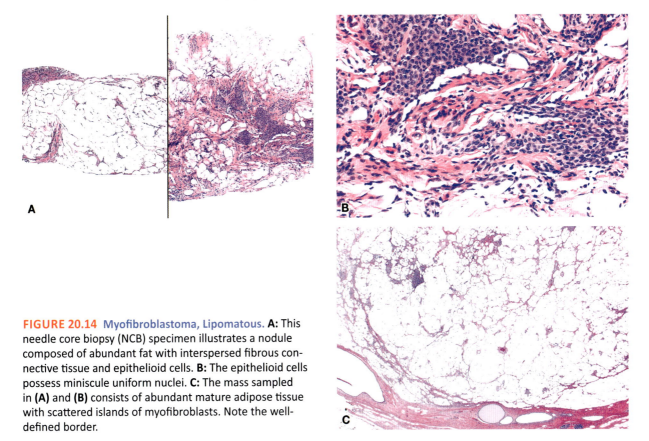

FIGURE 20.14 **Myofibroblastoma, Lipomatous. A:** This needle core biopsy (NCB) specimen illustrates a nodule composed of abundant fat with interspersed fibrous connective tissue and epithelioid cells. **B:** The epithelioid cells possess miniscule uniform nuclei. **C:** The mass sampled in **(A)** and **(B)** consists of abundant mature adipose tissue with scattered islands of myofibroblasts. Note the well-defined border.

Most myofibroblastomas, including the epithelioid variety, are diffusely immunoreactive for CD34 and vimentin, and variably so for desmin, calponin, SMA, muscle actin, CD10, BCL2, and CD99. Uncommon examples show absent or only focal CD34, especially in NCB samples (77). The tumors do not stain for cytokeratin or factor VIII, and stain for S-100 protein only rarely and weakly. Myofibroblasts with smooth muscle differentiation are strongly immunoreactive for desmin and variably reactive for actin, SMA, and h-caldesmon. The myofibroblasts typically stain for ER and PR, and about one-half stain for androgen receptor (AR), although the reactivity can be variable.

About 90% of myofibroblastomas show loss of Rb expression, owing to recurrent 13q14 deletions involving *RB1* and *FKHR* (*FOXO1*) (78). This can be demonstrated by IHC or FISH. Myofibroblastoma belongs to the "13q family of tumors," a group of tumors with overlapping histologic, IHC, and molecular features. Spindle cell lipoma, another member of the 13q family of tumors, commonly occurs in males and can be circumscribed, similar to myofibroblastoma (67,79-82). These tumors have more abundant adipose tissue, less cellularity, and less fascicular architecture than myofibroblastomas. It has been suggested that these two tumors may be variants of the same entity (83). Ibrahim and Shousha reported a case with intermixed, distinct regions of spindle cell lipoma within a myofibroblastoma (84).

Myofibroblastoma must be considered in the differential diagnosis of benign or low-grade mammary spindle cell tumors. Nodular fasciitis and fibromatosis, which also contain myofibroblasts, tend to be stellate infiltrative lesions. Plump myoid cells and the inflammatory reaction of fasciitis are not seen in a myofibroblastoma. Fibromatosis exhibits abundant collagen and spindle cells arranged in broad bands rather than in short fascicles. SFT is "patterness" rather than fascicular and is positive for STAT6.

The epithelioid variant of myofibroblastoma can mimic an invasive carcinoma including pleomorphic lobular carcinoma and apocrine carcinoma (67,71,85). The distinction can be particularly problematic in an NCB. Morphologic features that suggest epithelioid myofibroblastoma include a well-circumscribed, pushing border; absent or minimal mitotic activity; associated spindle cells with typical myofibroblastic morphology; lack of glandular elements within the tumor; and dense collagenized stroma.

Complete excision provides adequate treatment for virtually all patients, although large lesions in men have necessitated mastectomies. Reexcision may be considered if a myofibroblastoma is present at the margin of an excision. Recurrences have not been reported after follow-up periods of 3 to 126 months after complete excision.

Solitary Fibrous Tumor

Solitary fibrous tumor (SFT, originally termed *hemangiopericytoma*) is an uncommon neoplasm in the breast with low malignant potential. Fewer than 60 cases of the breast and axilla have been reported. Hoda et al (86)

listed clinical and pathologic features of 58 cases reported in the literature. Patient ages ranged from 5 days to 88 years. Eleven (19%) cases were diagnosed as malignant. Patients presented with enlarging painless masses, which occurred in left and right breasts with equal frequency. The masses had been present for a few weeks or months, but symptomatic periods as long as 1 year have been noted (87). The masses were described as irregular and firm. SFTs originating from extramammary sites have metastasized to the breast, and one SFT of the pectoralis major presented as a breast mass (88).

Mammography reveals a dense mass without calcifications, and sonography demonstrates a solid hypoechogenic mass with heterogeneous internal echoes and posterior enhancement. MRI findings may include a well-defined oval lesion with low signal intensity on T1, heterogeneous high signal on T2, rapid enhancement, and washout (89). The maximum extent ranges from 1 (90) to 20 (91) cm, and the average size is 6.5 cm.

The histologic features of mammary SFTs duplicate those of examples arising in other sites. The tumor consists of regions of variable cellularity distributed in a haphazard or "patternless" fashion **(Fig. 20.15)**. The round, oval, or spindle-shaped tumor cells form sheets, bands, and trabeculae around vascular spaces. The cells possess uniform bland nuclei, and mitotic figures are infrequent. The blood vessels vary in caliber and typically display a branching or "staghorn" configuration. Fibrosis is variably present around vessels at the tumor's periphery. Necrosis rarely occurs in mammary SFTs. Histologic findings suggesting an aggressive nature include an infiltrative border, cytologic atypia, and mitotic activity (92).

The tumor cells typically express STAT6 (93), as well as CD34, vimentin, CD99, and BCL2. Diffuse, strong, nuclear STAT6 expression results from an intrachromosomal rearrangement on chromosome 12 that leads to formation of the *NAB2-STAT6* oncogene. The proximity of these genes on 12q13 makes it difficult to identify the fusion gene using FISH; however, STAT6 can reliably be detected by IHC. Other benign spindle cell tumors have been reported to exhibit only weak cytoplasmic expression of STAT6 (83). SFTs do not stain for keratin. Endothelial cells lining the capillaries are immunoreactive for CD34 and CD31.

The differential diagnosis of SFT mainly centers on malignant tumors. Leiomyosarcoma and UPS may have vascular areas that resemble SFT. These sarcomas have readily identifiable mitotic figures and exhibit other specific structural features. Metastatic sarcomatoid renal cell carcinoma may mimic SFT. Staining for STAT6 may be useful in problematic cases.

Reported follow-up varies from less than 12 months to 23 years. Most patients have been treated by breast-conserving surgery, with mastectomy being reserved for larger tumors (median and mean size 9.0 cm) (86). Axillary lymph node metastasis has not been documented. One patient with SFT of the axilla developed recurrent disease 122 months after initial presentation, and went on to undergo forequarter amputation and radiation therapy (86).

MESENCHYMAL LESIONS **389**

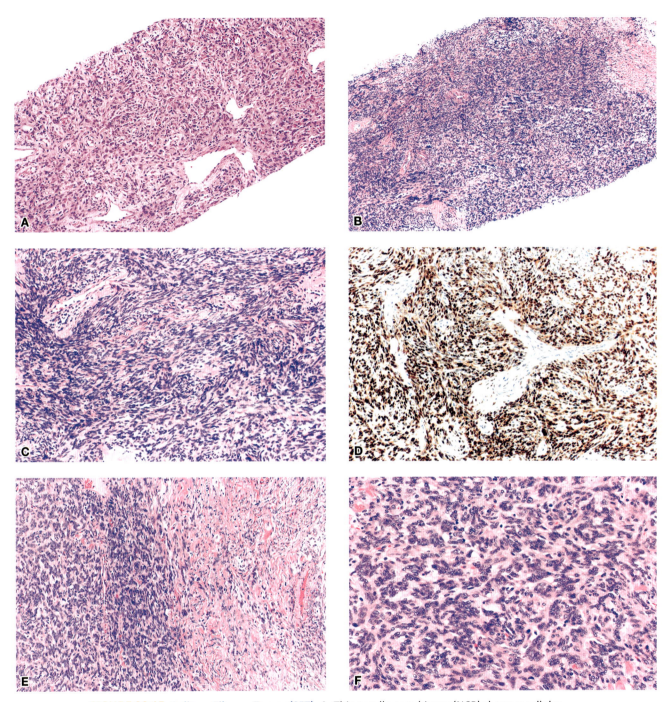

FIGURE 20.15 Solitary Fibrous Tumor (SFT). A: This needle core biopsy (NCB) shows a cellular tumor of plump spindle cells interspersed with characteristic dilated, irregular vessels. **B:** The NCB from another SFT shows a well-defined mass. **C:** Long spindle cells, collagen, and thick-walled blood vessels compose the mass shown in **(B)**. **D:** An immunostain for STAT6 is shown. **E, F:** The excision specimen from the mass shown in **(B)** to **(D)** displays regions of variable cellularity and aggregates of small, uniform tumor cells with bland nuclei.

One patient treated with a modified radical mastectomy for a 5.5-cm SFT (apparently confined to the breast) succumbed to metastatic disease involving bone, brain, lungs, pleura, skin, and liver 14 months after diagnosis (94). The modified Demicco et al (95) model has been demonstrated to accurately risk stratify these tumors (86). In general, mammary SFTs that lack high-grade features such as necrosis or numerous mitoses should be considered low-grade neoplasms. Treatment can be conservative, with emphasis on wide local excision rather than mastectomy—if an adequate margin can be achieved with an acceptable cosmetic result. Axillary dissection is not indicated.

Dermatofibrosarcoma Protuberans

Dermatofibrosarcoma protuberans (DFSP) is a locally aggressive cutaneous neoplasm that can arise in the skin of breast and axilla. Uncommon examples of DFSP might seem to involve the breast parenchyma; however, pathologists should think carefully before rendering a diagnosis of DFSP for a deep-seated mammary tumor.

The age of most patients with DFSP falls within the range of 25 to 50 years, with a mean age of 39.4 years (96). Approximately 90% of reported tumors arose in women. The presenting symptom in almost every case is a mass, which can be present for months to decades (97). Patients with long-standing tumors may report recent rapid enlargement, and some may endure pain or skin ulceration (96-98). Several cases have arisen in the setting of prior chest wall irradiation (99). Clinical examination may suggest a diagnosis of fibroadenoma, benign skin appendage tumor, or epidermal cyst.

Mammography demonstrates a well-defined, dense mass attached to the skin or in the subcutis, with neither calcifications nor fat. On ultrasonography, the masses typically appear circumscribed, oval, and parallel to the skin surface, although some have ill-defined margins (100). Doppler studies demonstrate high vascularity (101). MRI usually shows isointensity on T1-weighted images and hyperintensity on T2-weighted images (100,102,103).

Like DFSP arising in other sites, the lesion in the breast is composed of closely packed, uniform spindle cells arranged in a storiform ("whirligig") pattern **(Fig. 20.16)**. The lesional cells possess oval, variably elongated nuclei and scant faintly eosinophilic or amphophilic cytoplasm. Mitotic figures are usually inconspicuous and number about 2 to 3 per 10 HPF (104). Collagen composes the intercellular matrix in less cellular regions, and one can also find myxoid stroma (96,104,105), especially in recurrent tumors. The neoplastic cells interdigitate with fat lobules in a "lace-like" or "honeycomb" pattern. The tumor may encase but not destroy skin appendages and mammary ducts.

DFSPs are reactive for CD34 in all reported cases, and all but a few stained for vimentin. Stains for S-100, actin, desmin, and CD31 have been consistently negative. Like DFSPs arising at other sites, those involving the breast possess a characteristic t(17;22)(q22;q13) translocation resulting in the oncogenic fusion product *COL1A1-PDGFB*. This fusion gene is demonstrable by FISH, karyotyping, and quantitative polymerase chain reaction (PCR) (106,107) and most commonly resides on a supernumerary ring chromosome with other genetic material from chromosomes 17, 22, and others. Dickson et al described an alternative translocation resulting in a *COL6A3-PDGFD* fusion, which is not seen in the usual cases of extramammary DFSPs (108). Six of 20 mammary DFSPs were found to harbor the novel fusion, and they resembled conventional DFSPs in all essential respects. Importantly, this alternate variant is not detected by usual PCR- or FISH-based assays for DFSP.

DFSPs can rarely spawn sarcoma, mostly fibrosarcoma. The sarcoma cells in this setting can demonstrate the fusion gene characteristic of DFSP. Fibrosarcoma exhibits a characteristic herringbone pattern, cellular atypia, and mitotic activity of 5 to 10 figures per 10 HPF (97,107). The fibrosarcoma population often displays reduced or absent staining for CD34. Myxoid stroma has been noted in most DFSPs harboring fibrosarcoma. Kim et al described a myxoid liposarcoma that arose from DFSP (107).

DFSPs do not metastasize but frequently recur if not adequately excised. The neoplastic stromal cells tend to penetrate into surrounding tissue, and this phenomenon makes it imperative to remove wide margins of grossly uninvolved tissue. Intraoperative evaluation of margins using frozen sections can be used to define the extent of the surgery. Some experts advocate for Mohs micrographic surgery (109). Lymph node excision is not necessary in the absence of clinical suspicion. Most recurrences become apparent within a few years but can come to attention in as few as 6 months and as long as 26 years (110). There is no established benefit of radiation. Imatinib mesylate, an inhibitor of the platelet-derived growth factor receptor-associated tyrosine kinase,

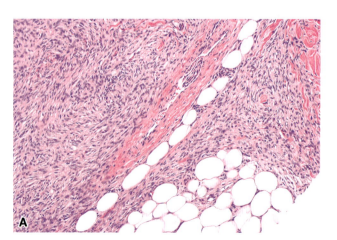
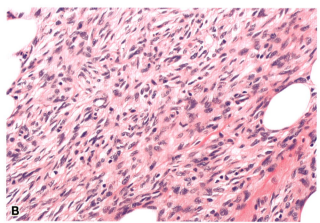

FIGURE 20.16 Dermatofibrosarcoma Protuberans. A, B: This needle core biopsy (NCB) shows spindle cells in a storiform pattern infiltrating between dermal collagen and subcutaneous adipocytes.

has demonstrated clinical activity in advanced extramammary DFSPs and may offer a therapeutic option for problematic breast tumors.

Fibrosarcoma arising from DFSP requires treatment appropriate for a sarcoma, including adjuvant radiation (97,107).

NEURAL

Neural neoplasms occur in the breast rarely. Benign nerve sheath tumors in the breast which have been reported include schwannomas ("neurilemomas") and neurofibromas. Many of these tumors occupy the mammary subcutaneous tissue (111); however, parenchymal lesions have also been described, and one schwannoma originating in the chest wall presented as a mass in the breast (112). The age range at diagnosis is 6 to 83 years, with most patients in their fourth to sixth decade. Although most patients have been female, benign neural neoplasms have arisen in the male breast (113,114). The literature includes a few cases of primary mammary malignant peripheral nerve sheath tumors (115).

Schwannoma

Mammary schwannomas account for less than 3% of all schwannomas (116). Two publications (116,117) list clinical and pathologic findings of 23 cases. A typical schwannoma presents as a painless, well-defined mass, which has grown slowly (112,118) or remained stable for as long as 25 years (119). Two reports (118,120) illustrate exophytic tumors. The outer quadrants, especially the upper outer quadrant, seem to be favored sites, but reports describe examples in all regions of the breast. One report (121) describes a patient with two schwannomas of the right breast.

Mammography demonstrates a well-defined mass. Using sonography, the mass appears hypoechoic and exhibits posterior enhancement. The MRI characteristics resemble those of other benign lesions. The tumors usually span a few centimeters. One asymptomatic 7-mm schwannoma was detected by mammography (122), and a long-standing exophytic schwannoma spanned 15 cm (118). Cystic degeneration, which develops rarely, can create a multicystic mass (123).

Microscopic examination discloses the typical wavy spindle cells growing in bundles. Palisading of nuclei gives rise to the Antoni A pattern **(Fig. 20.17)**; less cellular areas containing thick-walled blood vessels represent the Antoni B pattern. One can observe thrombi, hyalinized blood vessels, cells with atypical nuclei, and xanthomatous areas.

Benign peripheral nerve sheath tumors stain for S-100. Schwannomas tend to demonstrate intense homogeneous staining, whereas neurofibromas display heterogeneous positivity for this marker. Staining for SOX-10 demonstrates similar results.

The differential diagnosis includes other spindle cell tumors such as fibroadenoma, phyllodes tumor, fibromatosis, myofibroblastoma, and metaplastic carcinoma. The diagnosis of schwannoma is suggested when an NCB sample demonstrates palisading spindle cells (123), but a limited specimen may not demonstrate this finding, which can also be seen in myofibroblastomas. The diagnosis of a benign peripheral nerve sheath tumor is supported by the absence of glandular elements, lack of mitotic activity, a positive IHC stain for S-100, and the absence of immunostaining for actin. Complete excision provides adequate therapy.

Neurofibroma

Mammary neurofibroma commonly involves the nipple-areolar region (124,125). The clinical appearance of cutaneous tumors ranges from large pedunculated masses to small nodules that mimic accessory nipples. Neurofibroma is less commonly situated within the breast parenchyma. Multiple parenchymal neurofibromas in a single breast have been reported (126). Neurofibromas can cause breast enlargement mimicking gynecomastia in prepubertal boys (113). Patients with von Recklinghausen disease (NF1) develop neurofibromas in the mammary subcutaneous tissues and in the breast. Massive neurofibromatosis of the breast is uncommon.

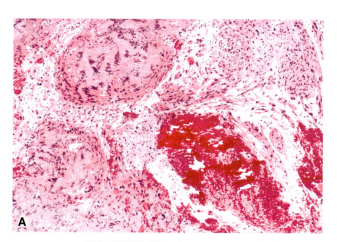
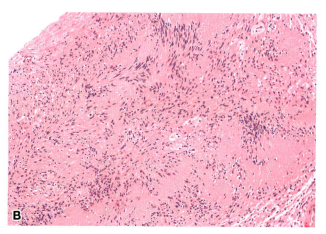

FIGURE 20.17 Schwannoma. A: The lesion demonstrates the Antoni A pattern. Hemorrhage marks the site of a recent needle core biopsy (NCB). **B:** Another example of schwannoma in an NCB.

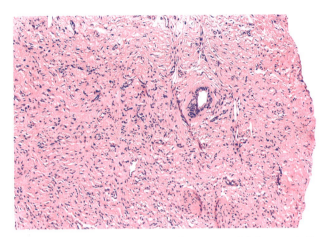

FIGURE 20.18 Neurofibroma. This tumor of delicate spindle cells with slender wavy nuclei incorporates a benign breast duct.

Patients with NF1 are at increased risk for developing mammary carcinoma; therefore, the appearance of a new breast mass in this setting should prompt appropriate evaluation.

Mammogram, ultrasound, and MRI findings are similar to those of schwannoma. Regions of cystic degeneration or accumulation of myxoid ground substances can give rise to hyperintense regions on T2-weighted images (126).

The pathologic characteristics of neurofibromas of the breast are similar to those of neurofibromas found in other organs: delicate spindle cells with wavy, hyperchromatic nuclei with pointed ends **(Fig. 20.18)**. The extracellular matrix consists of ropy collagen often described as resembling "shredded carrots" (127) or myxoid material. IHC reveals variable staining for S-100 (128). On NCB, the differential diagnosis may include traumatic neurofibroma, a reactive proliferation associated with an injured nerve **(Fig. 20.19)**.

Excision of the mass is curative.

Granular Cell Tumor

Granular cell tumors are derived from Schwann cells of peripheral nerves. These tumors occur throughout the body (most commonly in the tongue) and approximately 5% arise in the breast (129). NCB represents an accurate method for rendering a diagnosis of granular cell tumor of the breast (GCTB). Among the cases collated by Brown et al (129), correct diagnosis was made in all NCB specimens. GCTBs are rarely malignant; however, these tumors can mimic carcinoma clinically, radiologically, and histologically.

GCTB typically affects women between the ages of 30 and 50 years, but it has been described in adolescents and elderly women. Patient ages range from 14 to 77 years. About 10% of GCTBs occur in males. In several studies, the majority of patients have been African American. Papalas et al (130) reported a younger mean age at presentation for African Americans (41 years) than for Caucasians (54 years).

Most patients present with a firm painless mass. Left and right breasts are affected equally. GCTB may arise in any part of the breast including axillary tail and subcutis. Superficial lesions may cause skin retraction, and nipple inversion has been reported with subareolar tumors. In one woman, hyperplastic skin and underlying nests of tumor cells created a polypoid mass likened to a mulberry (131). Large and deep tumors may involve the pectoral fascia, pectoral muscle, and ribs (132). GCTB usually occurs as a solitary mass, but instances of multiple and bilateral tumors have been reported (133,134). GCTB as large as 9 cm has been reported, but the typical example spans 2 cm or less. Patients who have multiple granular cell tumors at various sites may have one or more lesions in the breast (130,133,135). Brown et al (129) reported the clinical, radiologic, and pathologic details of 91 cases of GCTB.

On mammography, GCTB typically forms a stellate mass, but circumscribed lesions occasionally occur (134,136). The mass usually has a dense core and lacks calcifications.

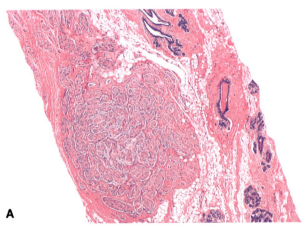
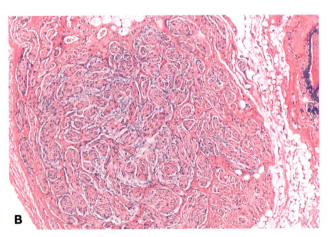

FIGURE 20.19 Traumatic Neuroma. **A, B:** Needle core biopsy (NCB) of a mass in this patient with a history of reduction mammaplasty shows a nodular proliferation of nerve components. Small bundles of axons, Schwann cells, and perineural cells are arrayed haphazardly within a myxoid matrix in this example.

MESENCHYMAL LESIONS 393

Ultrasound often shows a solid mass with indistinct margins and posterior shadowing suggestive of carcinoma. One unique feature is their anisotropic effect, similar to that seen on sonographic examination of tendons, because of their internal fibrillary composition (137). On T2-weighted MRI, most GCTBs show a signal intensity equal to or slightly higher than glandular tissue, whereas T1-weighted sequences show a low signal intensity (138).

The histologic and IHC features of GCTB duplicate those of extramammary granular cell tumors. The tumor consists of compact nests or sheets of cells containing eosinophilic cytoplasmic granules **(Fig. 20.20)**. The lesional cells vary from polygonal to spindled, and the cell borders appear well defined. The nuclei are round to oval with open chromatin and prominent nucleoli. In some cases, moderate nuclear pleomorphism, multinucleated cells, and rare mitoses may be found. These features should not be interpreted as evidence of malignancy. Granules usually fill the cytoplasm; in some lesions, the cytoplasm displays vacuolization and clearing. The cytoplasmic granules are periodic acid-Schiff (PAS)-positive and diastase-resistant. Variable amounts of collagenous stroma are present. The neoplastic cells may surround ducts and lobules and incorporate them into the mass, and these cells may penetrate into lobules. When the

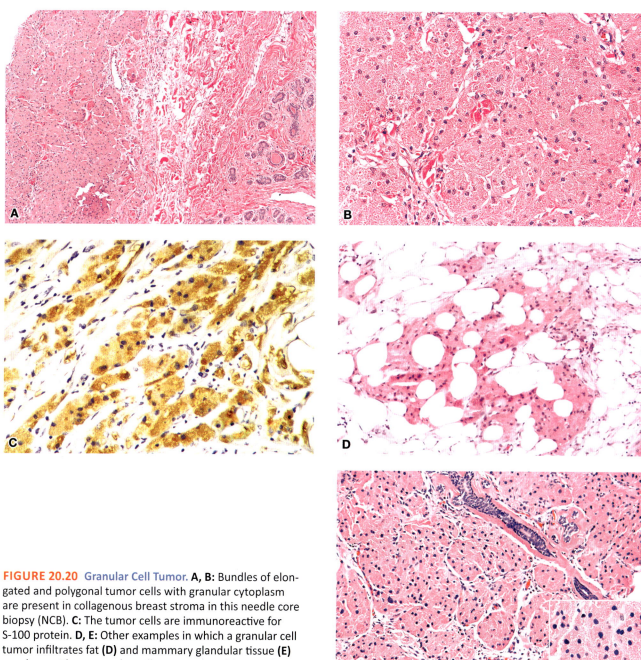

FIGURE 20.20 Granular Cell Tumor. A, B: Bundles of elongated and polygonal tumor cells with granular cytoplasm are present in collagenous breast stroma in this needle core biopsy (NCB). **C:** The tumor cells are immunoreactive for S-100 protein. **D, E:** Other examples in which a granular cell tumor infiltrates fat **(D)** and mammary glandular tissue **(E)** are shown. These granular cell tumors resemble apocrine carcinoma.

neoplastic cells invade the dermis, the overlying epidermis may demonstrate pseudoepitheliomatous hyperplasia (131,132).

GCTB typically stains for S-100 protein, carcinoembryonic antigen, AR, and vimentin. GCTB does not stain for cytokeratin, GCDFP-15, ER, PR, and myoglobin. The cytoplasmic granules in these tumors are Luxol fast blue-positive, an observation that suggests the presence of myelin.

The differential diagnosis of GCTB includes histiocytic lesions, mammary carcinoma, and metastatic neoplasms. The superficial resemblance to histiocytes can lead to confusion with a granulomatous inflammatory reaction or a histiocytic tumor. GCTB does not stain for histiocyte markers such as α1-antitrypsin, α1-antichymotrypsin, and muramidase, but reactivity for CD68 (KP-1, a marker of lysosomal activity) has been described (139).

GCTB can resemble an invasive apocrine carcinoma. The presence of carcinoma in situ as well as cytologic pleomorphism usually serves to identify apocrine carcinoma. IHC can be useful. Apocrine carcinomas stain for epithelial markers such as cytokeratin, and often epithelial membrane antigen (EMA) and AR; and are negative for vimentin. Positivity for S-100 does not entirely rule out carcinoma. GCTB must also be distinguished from metastatic neoplasms which have oncocytic or clear cell features such as renal carcinoma and melanoma.

GCTB is treated by wide excision. Local recurrence may occur after incomplete excision, but it is sometimes difficult to distinguish recurrences from metachronous lesions. Most patients with positive or close margins do not experience recurrence.

Fewer than 1% of all granular cell tumors, including mammary lesions, are malignant. Criteria of malignancy proposed for extramammary granular cell tumors include a size more than 5 cm, necrosis, spindling of tumor cells, nuclear pleomorphism, vesicular chromatin, prominent nucleoli, high nuclear-to-cytoplasmic ratio, increased mitotic activity (>2 mitoses per 10 HPF), and elevated Ki67 index.

Both locoregional and metastatic spread from GCTB have been described (92). Metastases in the breast and axillary lymph nodes from extramammary granular cell tumors have also been reported (140,141).

SMOOTH MUSCLE

Leiomyoma

Most leiomyomas of the breast arise from smooth muscle in the nipple and areola (142). Parenchymal leiomyomas almost certainly arise either from smooth muscle metaplasia of myoepithelial cells or myofibroblasts, or from vascular smooth muscle. The diagnosis of leiomyoma should be restricted to lesions composed entirely of smooth muscle. One should exclude fibroadenomas and sclerosing adenosis with myoid metaplasia (myoid "hamartoma"), for example, from this category.

Leiomyomas of the nipple and breast parenchyma are rare. The literature contains approximately 50 reports of leiomyomas in each location (143-148). The age of patients ranges from the third to the eighth decade. Approximately one-third of leiomyomas of the nipple arise in men, but they are seldom intraparenchymal (149).

Patients with leiomyomas of the nipple frequently report pain or discomfort. The duration of symptoms ranges from a few weeks to more than two decades. Leiomyomas involving the nipple may cause nipple erosion (143). One tumor situated immediately superior to the nipple was described as "cauliflower-shaped" (150), and another growing beneath the nipple caused nipple inversion (151). A 31-year-old woman presented with bilateral nipple leiomyomas (152), and a 61-year-old man developed a leiomyoma of the nipple in the setting of spironolactone-induced gynecomastia (153). Intraparenchymal leiomyomas usually present as palpable, solitary masses, and approximately one-half are painful. There is no predilection as to the location of parenchymal lesions. One report describes a 38-year-old woman with four synchronous parenchymal leiomyomas (154). Multiple breast leiomyomas may raise the possibility of hereditary leiomyomatosis and renal cell carcinoma, a syndrome attributed to germline *FH* mutation (155).

Mammographic studies of parenchymal leiomyomas typically reveal smoothly contoured, high-density masses without calcifications. Sonography and MRI disclose findings consistent with a benign tumor. The radiologic findings of nipple leiomyomas and parenchymal leiomyomas appear similar (143,156). Tumors as large as a "small grapefruit" and another spanning 13.8 cm have been reported (146), but most leiomyomas are smaller than 5 cm.

Microscopically, leiomyomas are typically circumscribed and consist of interlacing fascicles of bland cigar-shaped spindle cells with eosinophilic cytoplasm **(Fig. 20.21)**. Mild degenerative atypia may be seen. An epithelioid variant of mammary parenchymal leiomyoma was described by Roncaroli et al (157). Leiomyomas stain for vimentin, desmin, SMA, h-caldesmon, ER, and PR.

When examining an NCB, several other lesions must be considered in the differential diagnosis of leiomyoma. Leiomyosarcoma represents the neoplasm most likely to cause diagnostic confusion. Leiomyomas do not exhibit the cytologic atypia, mitotic activity, necrosis, or infiltration of parenchyma which characterize leiomyosarcoma. Differentiation from hypertrophic scar or keloid is aided by history of previous trauma or procedure. Special stains such as Masson trichrome may help to distinguish collagen from smooth muscle. Other lesions in the differential diagnosis include myofibroblastoma, fibromatosis, PASH, and low-grade spindle cell metaplastic carcinoma (158).

Complete excision is usually recommended. This may necessitate removing the nipple. Treatment with carbon dioxide laser (159) and ultrasound-guided microwave ablation (160) have been applied with apparent success. Local recurrence has been reported (142,161).

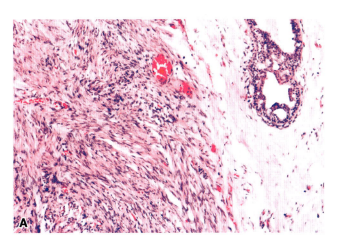
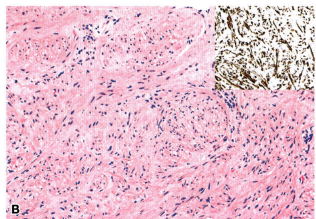

FIGURE 20.21 **Leiomyoma. A:** There is a suggestion of palisading in the arrangement of the smooth muscle cells in this circumscribed tumor. An adjacent duct shows micropapillary ductal hyperplasia. **B:** A nipple leiomyoma showing bundles of lesional cells with cigar-shaped nuclei and without atypia. Inset shows cytoplasmic immunoreactivity for caldesmon.

Leiomyosarcoma

Leiomyosarcoma accounts for fewer than 10% of sarcomas of the breast. Three publications (162-164) tabulated several reports published before 2017. Like leiomyoma, leiomyosarcoma most likely originates from blood vessels or the smooth muscle of the nipple-areolar complex. One leiomyosarcoma may have arisen in an ectopic areola (165). A leiomyosarcoma of uncertain origin diagnosed by NCB presented as bilateral mammary masses (166).

More than 90% of patients have been female (167). The age at diagnosis ranges from 18 to 86 years, and the mean age is approximately 53. Patients present with a mass measuring less than 1 to 23 cm and averaging approximately 5.5 cm. Almost one-half of the tumors are in or near the nipple-areolar complex. The tumors are circumscribed and firm. Fixation to the skin and ulceration can occur. Patients rarely report pain. Cases of radiation-associated leiomyosarcoma of the breast have been described (168,169).

Imaging reveals a dense, lobulated mass with a defined border. Calcifications are infrequent.

Microscopy reveals interlacing bundles of fusiform cells with the blunt-end nuclei characteristic of smooth muscle tumors **(Fig. 20.22)**. Epithelioid cells may be present. Malignant features include nuclear hyperchromasia, pleomorphism, and multinucleated giant cells. Mitotic figures range from 2 to 50 per 10 HPF and average 12 per 10 HPF. Areas of degeneration exhibit nuclear pyknosis and necrosis. Areas of stromal fibrosis with a pattern that resembles PASH may be present. The border is infiltrative. Mammary ducts and lobules can become incorporated into the neoplasm. This finding may lead one to consider diagnoses such as metaplastic carcinoma and phyllodes tumor. Uncommon histologic findings include metaplastic bone and cartilage, rhabdomyoblastic features, and osteoclast-like giant cells.

The malignant cells usually stain for desmin, SMA, and vimentin. Reactivity for h-caldesmon has been reported. Up to 40% of leiomyosarcomas stain for keratin and/or EMA (170),

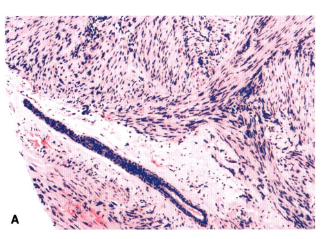
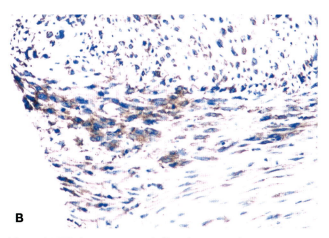

FIGURE 20.22 **Leiomyosarcoma. A:** A needle core biopsy (NCB) shows sarcoma infiltrating around a duct. **B:** The sarcoma is immunoreactive for smooth muscle actin.

the significance of which remains uncertain. Apart from one reportedly ER-positive tumor (171), leiomyosarcomas are negative for ER, PR, and human epidermal growth factor receptor 2 (HER2).

The tumors show complex karyotypes, including deletions of chromosomes 13q and 10q—findings present in 75% of leiomyosarcomas of the uterus and deep soft tissues—and 16q and 1p (172).

The combination of mitotic activity and ominous histologic features such as hypercellularity, cytologic atypia, and necrosis suggests the diagnosis of leiomyosarcoma, although definitive criteria are yet to be established. Long et al described an "atypical leiomyoma" in a breast excision showing infiltrative growth, mild nuclear atypia, up to 3 mitoses per 10 HPF, and a Ki67 index of about 5% (145). This proposed nomenclature was likened to the uterine smooth muscle tumor of uncertain malignant potential (STUMP). The "atypical leiomyoma" did not recur in nearly 9 years of follow-up.

The publication by Rane et al (164) lists the treatment and follow-up of most reported cases. Primary treatment consisted of mastectomy in approximately 75% of the patients. Approximately one-half of the patients treated with excision developed recurrences. Axillary nodal metastases have been reported in rare cases (173,174), but routine axillary lymph node sampling is not required. Irradiation and chemotherapy have been used in selected circumstances.

Among the nearly 50 reported cases of mammary leiomyosarcoma, approximately 20% have proved to be fatal. The outcome has not correlated well with mitotic rate in the primary tumor. Fatalities occurred in cases with at least 2 or 3 mitoses per 10 HPF. Late recurrences and death from disease have occurred 15 and 20 years after initial diagnoses.

LIPOMATOUS

Lipoma

Lipomas of the breast usually affect women (and men) between the ages of 40 and 60 years (175). Many are located in the subcutaneous fat. Lipomas typically present as painless solitary masses spanning a few centimeters, but examples as large as 50 cm have been reported (176). Slow growth of the tumor over many years is typical. In one woman, the mass grew from 2 to 32 cm over 30 years (177). Multiple lipomas may be encountered.

Mammograms sometimes disclose a radiolucent homogeneous mass with a distinct border or capsule (178). The tumor may be inapparent in a fatty breast. Fat necrosis within a lipoma may present as a spiculated lesion on mammography, and skin ulceration may develop in association with large tumors (176).

Microscopy of a lipoma reveals mature adipose tissue essentially devoid of glandular elements. A pseudocapsule may not be appreciable on NCB. The diagnosis of lipoma can be suggested by a mass with appropriate imaging characteristics and mature fat in the NCB specimen. Lipomas can exhibit several variant patterns, which are described below.

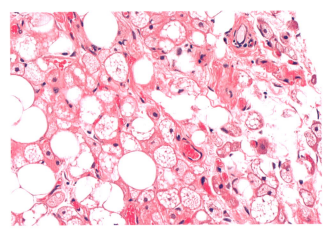

FIGURE 20.23 **Hibernoma.** Brown fat is present in a tumor from the axillary tail of the breast.

Hibernomas are composed of "brown" fat. In the breast region, hibernomas occur in the axillary tail or axilla (179) **(Fig. 20.23)**. They consist of multivacuolated adipocytes containing small, central nuclei without atypia or mitoses. The cytoplasm varies from pale to deeply eosinophilic and granular. Univacuolar adipocytes are usually present. The stroma can show myxoid change or consist of spindle cells with ropy collagen and interspersed mast cells. Small blood vessels traverse the mass. *Osteolipomas* consist entirely of fat with isolated foci of osseous calcification **(Fig. 20.24A)**. *Fibrolipomas* are well-circumscribed tumors composed of mature adipose tissue and collagenous stroma with prominent fibroblasts. Microscopically, the lesion may blend with glandular parenchyma. *Myolipomas* consist of fat, smooth muscle, and fibrous connective tissue. *Chondrolipoma* is composed of sharply defined islands of hyaline cartilage distributed in mature fat **(Fig. 20.24B)** (180,181). Parenthetically, benign chondroid metaplasia can be encountered in myofibroblastomas of the breast.

Spindle cell lipomas rarely occur in the breast (178,182). One example presented as a 3.3-cm palpable mass with imaging features suggestive of hamartoma (182). Biopsy reveals lipomatous tissue mixed with spindly myofibroblasts and variably collagenous stroma. CD10 and CD34 immunoreactivity can be demonstrated in the spindle cell component; desmin and Rb are negative. Spindle cell lipoma is one of the 13q family of tumors along with myofibroblastoma.

Angiolipomas similar to those of subcutaneous tissue can arise in the breast. Several cases have been described in men (183,184). Typical angiolipomas occur as solitary masses, which span 2 cm or less. Imaging characteristics are variable. Histology reveals mature adipose tissue separated by capillary channels which form lobulated aggregates at the perimeter of the lesion and contain fibrin thrombi **(Fig. 20.25)**. Mild cytologic atypia can be seen **(Fig. 20.26)**. Eighty percent of angiolipomas harbor mutations in *PRKD2* (185).

All varieties of lipoma are adequately treated with excision.

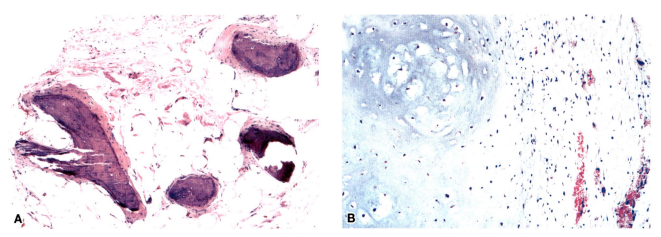

FIGURE 20.24 Osteolipoma and Chondrolipoma. A: Mature bone is evident in this needle core biopsy specimen from an osteolipoma. **B:** The presence of mature hyaline cartilage characterizes this chondrolipoma.

Liposarcoma

Liposarcomas account for fewer than 10% of mammary sarcomas (186,187). Primary mammary liposarcomas are far less common than malignant phyllodes tumors with liposarcomatous differentiation, and the two tumors cannot always be distinguished on NCB. The ages of patients range from the teens to 90 years, with a mean age of 49. Male patients have been described (188,189), though some tumors may have arisen in the pectoralis muscle. The presenting symptom is a mass occasionally accompanied by pain. One woman was pregnant at the

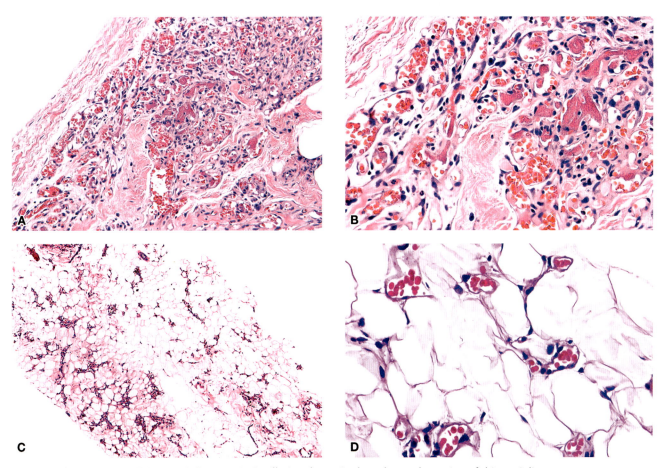

FIGURE 20.25 Angiolipoma. A: Capillaries cluster in the subcapsular region of this angiolipoma. **B:** The endothelial cells appear flat and they contain small, bland nuclei. Fibrin thrombi occlude several vessels. **C, D:** Capillaries are dispersed in fat in this needle core biopsy (NCB).

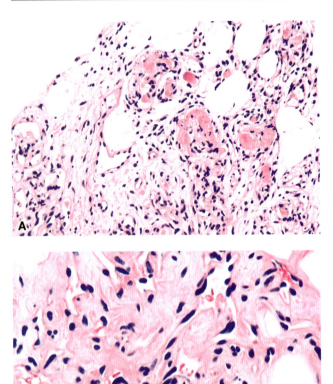
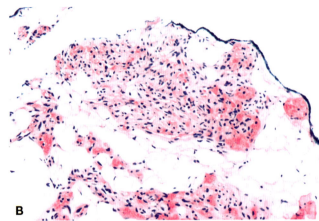

FIGURE 20.26 Angiolipoma With Atypia. **A:** This needle core biopsy (NCB) displays a compact area of capillary proliferation. Some cells have hyperchromatic nuclei. Microthrombi characteristics of angiolipoma are present. **B:** The excised tumor extended to a margin. **C:** This part of the excised tumor resembles the NCB specimen. Prominent hyperchromatic nuclei are shown.

time of diagnosis, and a few came to attention during the postpartum period (190). Twenty-one months following resection of a myxoid liposarcoma from the thigh of a 66-year-old woman, an NCB disclosed a solitary mammary metastasis (191).

The tumor is typically firm and circumscribed, and the overlying skin is unaffected. A few liposarcomas form ill-defined masses. Imaging demonstrates a mass that may appear well defined and smoothly outlined. The presence of cystic and solid components may give rise to a complex echo pattern. Liposarcomas span 2 to 40 cm and average approximately 8 cm. Necrosis and cavitation can occur.

The histologic features of liposarcoma in the breast are like those of liposarcoma arising in the extremities or trunk. Among published reports, 14 (41%) were myxoid **(Fig. 20.27A)**, 9 (26%) were well differentiated, 7 (21%) were pleomorphic **(Fig. 20.27B,C)**, and 4 (12%) were poorly differentiated. The well-differentiated liposarcomas include several examples of sclerosing or fibrous liposarcomas. Well-differentiated liposarcomas of the breast that are easily resectable (eg, without chest wall involvement) may be designated atypical lipomatous tumors.

IHC yields results seen in liposarcomas at other sites. The malignant cells do not stain for epithelial markers in most cases and typically stain for S-100. Limited data show that TRPS1 is highly expressed in mammary liposarcoma, liposarcomatous components of malignant phyllodes tumors, and extramammary liposarcoma (192).

Well-differentiated and dedifferentiated liposarcomas show amplification of *MDM2* and/or *CDK4* (193). Staining for these proteins can help differentiate liposarcoma from lipoma or phyllodes tumor (194,195). Myxoid liposarcomas show *DDIT3* (formerly *CHOP*) rearrangements (196).

Nandipati et al (190) tabulated the treatment and outcome of many reported cases of mammary liposarcoma. Treatment often consisted of mastectomy; wide excision constituted the primary surgery in a few cases. Axillary lymph node metastases have not been reported. Systemic chemotherapy and irradiation have been used for palliative purposes. With follow-up intervals ranging from less than 1 to 20 years, approximately 70% of patients have remained recurrence-free, 6% were alive with systemic recurrence, and 24% died of metastatic liposarcoma. Systemic recurrences and deaths due to disease usually occurred within 2 years of diagnosis and were limited to patients with pleomorphic or high-grade liposarcomas. The size of the tumor did not predict patient outcomes.

MESENCHYMAL LESIONS 399

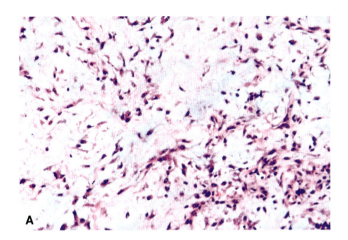
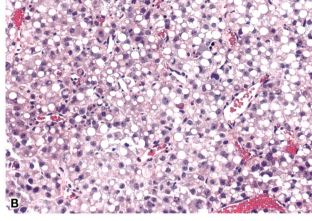
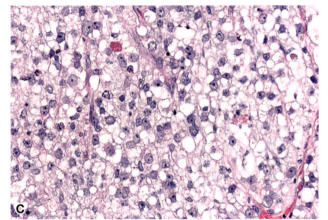

FIGURE 20.27 Liposarcoma. A: This myxoid liposarcoma exhibits the characteristic network of capillaries. **B:** The tumor in this needle core biopsy (NCB) shows the nuclear features of a pleomorphic liposarcoma. **C:** The excision specimen of the mass shown in **(B)** illustrates the presence of abundant cytoplasmic vacuoles of varying sizes.

VASCULAR

Hemangioma

Hemangiomas are benign vascular tumors, which occur in the breasts of women ranging from 18 months to 82 years of age and only rarely affect men (197). Palpable hemangiomas typically create well-defined, firm masses, but a substantial number of hemangiomas are nonpalpable and evident only on radiologic imaging.

Mammography of a hemangioma usually demonstrates a well-defined lobulated mass, which may have calcifications (198,199). Ultrasonography reveals a hypoechoic, lobulated, well-defined nodule oriented parallel to the skin surface. On MRI, hemangiomas are isointense on T1-weighted images and hyperintense on T2, with an early and diffuse enhancement pattern (200,201). Multiple mammary hemangiomas were demonstrated by MRI in the breast of a 41-year-old woman with Kasabach-Merritt syndrome (202).

The histopathologic spectrum of benign vascular lesions is broad, and the chief concern is differentiation from angiosarcoma. They can be classified as parenchymal or non-parenchymal depending on involvement of the mammary glandular tissue. Variants of hemangioma are described below.

Perilobular hemangioma is usually an incidental microscopic finding or a source of MRI enhancement (203). It typically measures less than 4 mm. Perilobular hemangiomas were found in 1.3% of mastectomies performed for carcinoma (204), 4.5% of excisions showing benign conditions, and 11% of breasts sampled in forensic autopsies (205). Multiple perilobular hemangiomas may occur in one or both breasts. "Perilobular" hemangiomas are not always limited to a perilobular distribution. The typical lesion consists of a compact collection of delicate, non-anastomosing blood vessels, varying in caliber from capillaries to cavernous channels **(Fig. 20.28)**. The endothelial cells are flat and inconspicuous without cytologic atypia. Rarely, perilobular hemangiomas exhibit isolated endothelial cell atypia. The latter finding is of no known clinical significance. Perilobular hemangiomas do not require treatment and do not progress to more advanced lesions.

Cavernous hemangioma is the most common form of mammary hemangioma. The lesion is typically described as a circumscribed mass spanning up to 2 cm, but larger examples have been reported (197,206,207). Microscopy reveals dilated vessels congested with red blood cells **(Fig. 20.29)**. There are few, if any, anastomosing vessels. The endothelial nuclei are inconspicuous and flat. The vessels are supported

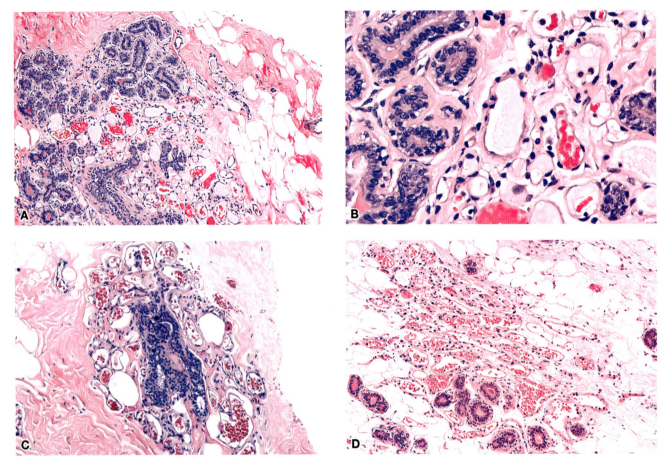

FIGURE 20.28 Perilobular Hemangioma. A, B: This vascular lesion occupying the intralobular stroma was an incidental finding in a needle core biopsy (NCB) obtained to sample nearby calcifications. **C:** The hemangioma in this NCB is centered on a duct. **D:** Hemangioma within perilobular adipose tissue.

by fibrous stroma, which tends to be more prominent toward the center of the tumor. Stromal calcification may occur. There is variability in the degree of circumscription. In many cavernous hemangiomas, the vascular channels become smaller at the periphery of the tumor and drift into fat. This pattern mimics the appearance of the periphery of some well-differentiated angiosarcomas.

Capillary hemangiomas consist of a compact collection of blood vessels of capillary dimensions. The mean size is 1.0 cm. Many are detected by mammography. Most cutaneous hemangiomas are of this type. Capillary hemangiomas often appear cellular and well circumscribed. Fibrous septa frequently divide capillary hemangiomas into segments resulting in a lobulated structure that superficially resembles

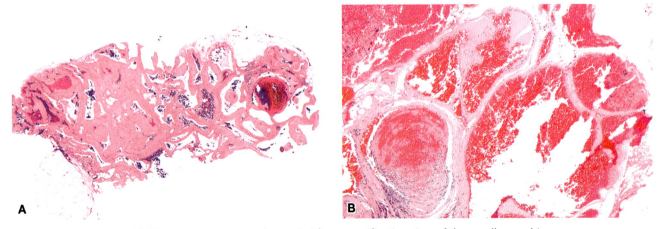

FIGURE 20.29 Cavernous Hemangioma. A: A low-magnification view of the needle core biopsy (NCB) is shown. Dilated vascular spaces are evident, some congested with red blood cells. **B:** A blood clot (lower left) has formed in one of the cavernous vascular channels.

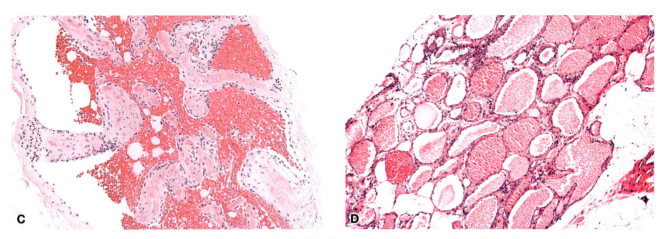

FIGURE 20.29 (*continued*) **C:** Flat endothelial cells with small, oval, bland nuclei line the channels of the cavernous hemangioma in another NCB. **D:** Numerous congested round and oval vascular channels can be seen.

a pyogenic granuloma **(Fig. 20.30)**. The lining endothelial cells are bland but may have hyperchromatic nuclei.

Several *venous hemangiomas* of the breast have been reported (208). The mean patient age is 40 years and all presented with a palpable tumor. One patient reported that the mass had been present for 13 years; another patient became aware of the lesion after trauma to the breast. It is not known whether these lesions are neoplasms or malformations. Venous hemangiomas are histologically diverse. Most have dilated venous channels of varying caliber, with smooth muscle walls of varying structural completeness **(Fig. 20.31)**, an impression confirmed by trichrome stain or SMA IHC. Red blood cells are present in the lumina of some vascular spaces; other spaces are empty or contain fluid.

Complex hemangiomas consist of a combination of the foregoing types, appearing as dilated vascular channels of varying sizes and compact, dense aggregates of capillaries. Some complex hemangiomas have conspicuous, anastomosing vascular channels **(Fig. 20.32)**.

Some additional findings may be encountered in hemangiomas. A "feeding" vessel can sometimes be observed at the periphery. These nonneoplastic vessels often display sinuous configurations and malformed or incomplete muscular layers in their walls. A "feeding" vessel is unlikely to be sampled in an NCB. Extramedullary hematopoiesis (EMH) in vascular channels should be distinguished from stromal lymphocytic reaction. Among mammary vascular lesions, EMH occurs almost exclusively in hemangiomas. Hemorrhage and infarction can occur in all types of hemangiomas, especially those subjected to NCB. These phenomena should not be confused with hemorrhagic necrosis which results in the formation of "blood lakes" characteristically found in high-grade angiosarcomas. Calcification rarely occurs in thrombi, sometimes associated with papillary endothelial hyperplasia (PEH). Mast cells are frequently present individually or in small clusters.

The Ki67 immunostain may be a useful adjunct in the diagnosis of the mammary hemangiomas. Nuclear

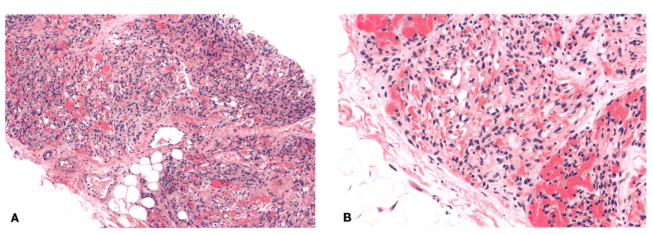

FIGURE 20.30 **Capillary Hemangioma. A, B:** A proliferation of capillaries is present in this needle core biopsy (NCB).

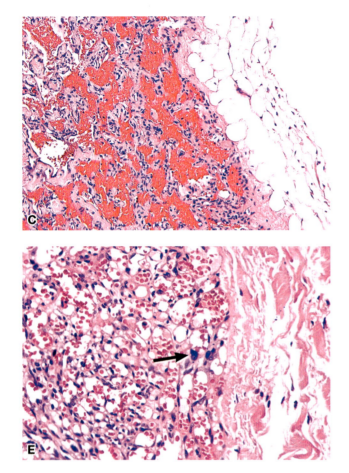

Ki67-labeling index in mammary hemangiomas is very low and rarely exceeds 5%, but it may be higher in organizing thrombi or adjacent to a biopsy site. The Ki67 of mammary angiosarcomas typically exceeds 20% even in low-grade tumors; however, the distribution of labeling may not be uniform. A robust Ki67-labeling index on an NCB from a mammary vascular lesion would strongly favor angiosarcoma. Sparse (<2%) labeling in an NCB can assist in making a diagnosis of hemangioma in the context of appropriate clinical and histologic findings.

FIGURE 20.30 (*continued*) **C, D:** Congested anastomosing capillaries can be seen in another NCB **(C)** and in the excised 5-mm tumor **(D)**. **E:** This NCB shows the circumscribed border of the tumor. A few endothelial cells have prominent hyperchromatic nuclei (arrows).

Hemangiomas with mild nuclear enlargement or mild pleomorphism, anastomosing vascular channels, and microscopically invasive borders were once classified as *"atypical" hemangiomas* **(Fig. 20.33)** (203). Additional follow-up has not borne out concerns that such hemangiomas are borderline or low-grade variants of angiosarcoma or that they predispose to the development of angiosarcoma (209,210). Consequently, the designation of "atypical" is no longer warranted in most cases, and the tumors should be classified simply as *hemangiomas* of one type or another. The

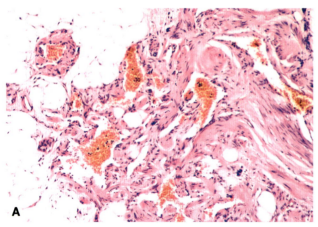
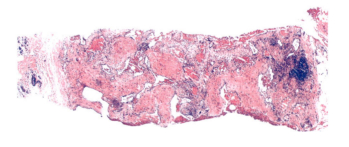

FIGURE 20.31 Venous Hemangioma. A: The lesion shown in this needle core biopsy (NCB) consists of vascular structures of various sizes with mural smooth muscle. **B:** Another NCB contains a smoothly contoured discrete vascular tumor within the mammary parenchyma.

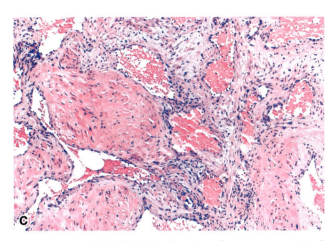
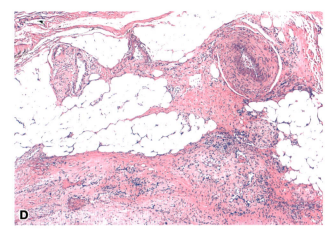

FIGURE 20.31 (*continued*) **C:** Disorganized collagen and smooth muscle compose the walls of the neoplastic blood vessels. **D:** The excision specimen from the mass shown in **(B)** and **(C)** contains residual hemangioma (lower) and a "feeding" vessel (upper right).

designation "atypical" should be reserved for those uncommon hemangiomas with cytologic atypia or proliferative activity on NCB.

Complete excision is usually necessary for an accurate diagnosis of a vascular lesion in the breast. When NCB removes most or all of a histologically benign lesion and a clip has been left at the biopsy site, follow-up by mammography can be an alternative to excision. Excision of the tissue surrounding the biopsy site is indicated if it seems that a substantial portion of the lesion remains in place. Reexcision may not be necessary if only a few peripheral capillaries extend to the margin of a specimen that is clearly a hemangioma. It is often not possible to recognize residual hemangioma in the granulation tissue of a healing biopsy site. No patient with any of the foregoing types of hemangiomas has been reported to have a recurrence after excision in a mean follow-up of 44 months.

Angiomatosis

Angiomatosis is a proliferation of thin-walled vessels permeating mammary tissue (211). The term represents a descriptive compromise because these tumors often consist of both hemangiomatous and lymphangiomatous channels. Angiomatosis should be distinguished from multiple perilobular hemangiomas, a condition sometimes referred to as *hemangiomatosis*. Whereas perilobular hemangiomas retain a localized structure, angiomatosis consists of larger, irregularly shaped channels growing in a seemingly infiltrative manner, belying its benign nature.

The literature contains about 20 well-documented cases (211-213). The mean patient age is 35.4 years; the lesion rarely affects children. The upper outer quadrant seems to be a favored site. Most patients present with a slowly enlarging, well-defined palpable mass. A minority are discovered by imaging findings, including subtle MRI enhancement (213).

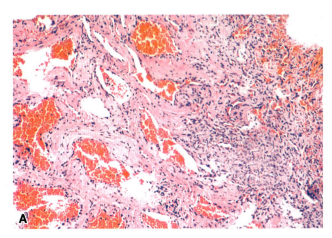
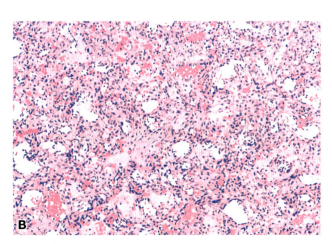

FIGURE 20.32 **Complex Hemangioma. A:** Vessels on the left have a cavernous appearance, whereas a cellular capillary network is evident on the right. **B:** This image depicts another hemangioma in which cellular fibrous stroma is distributed between capillaries.

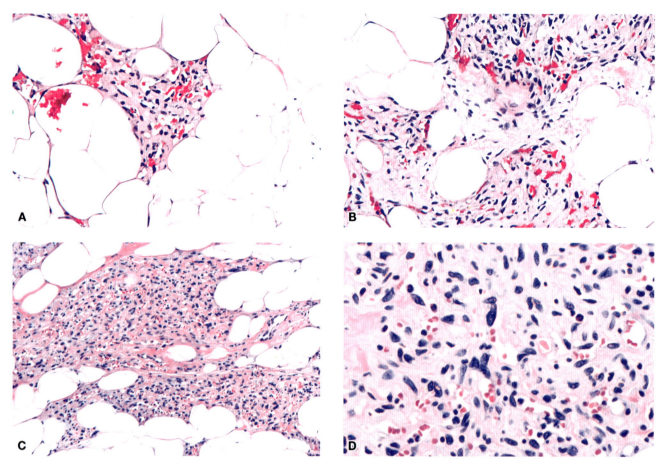

FIGURE 20.33 "Atypical" Hemangioma. A: This needle core biopsy (NCB) shows capillary vessels in fat. B: A more compact portion of the same specimen is depicted. C, D: The excised tumor has an invasive growth pattern. Endothelial cell nuclei in the anastomosing capillary channels are modestly pleomorphic and hyperchromatic. Mitotic figures were not identified.

Angiomatosis lacks the microscopic circumscription that typifies other benign vascular lesions. The lesion is composed of anastomosing, large vascular channels extending diffusely in the breast parenchyma. The lesion surrounds and displaces ducts and lobules but does not invade the lobular stroma. The vessels are lined by flat inconspicuous endothelium and supported by sparse mural tissue virtually devoid of smooth muscle **(Fig. 20.34)**. The vascular structures consist predominantly of hemangiomatous erythrocyte-containing channels, lymphangiomatous "empty" channels accompanied by lymphoid aggregates, or a mixture of the two.

The distinction between angiomatosis and low-grade angiosarcoma may be difficult, especially in an NCB. The vascular channels in angiomatosis are distributed uniformly throughout the tumor. In contrast, even the most well-differentiated angiosarcoma is heterogeneous, showing numerous aggregated

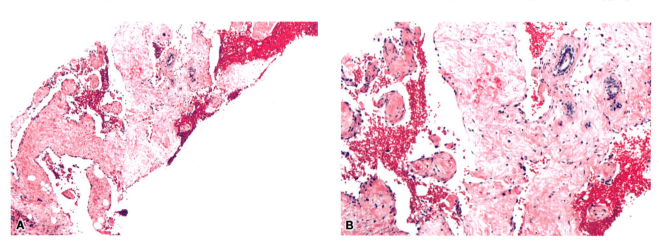

FIGURE 20.34 Angiomatosis. A, B: This needle core biopsy (NCB) reveals anastomosing dilated vascular spaces in fibrous breast stroma, which contains small ducts.

vessels in some regions, and sparse widely separated vessels elsewhere. The vascular structures of angiomatosis tend not to diminish in caliber at the periphery, whereas malignant capillaries of angiosarcoma merge with the surrounding tissue at the periphery. The vascular proliferation in angiomatosis surrounds but does not invade lobules; however, in angiosarcomas, the vascular channels grow into and destroy lobules. Finally, endothelial nuclei are histologically bland in angiomatosis. Prominent, hyperchromatic endothelial nuclei are found in angiosarcomas, even when papillary endothelial proliferation is absent. Mitoses are not found in angiomatosis, and the lesion has a very low Ki67-labeling index.

Angiomatosis of the breast is comparable to similar lesions that arise at other sites. Mastectomy may be necessary to control a bulky lesion, but less extensive surgery is preferable whenever possible. Recurrences can develop after long intervals (211,212).

Papillary Endothelial Hyperplasia

This reactive vascular lesion (also known as Masson lesion) represents a form of organizing thrombus. It can arise in an indigenous vessel or in the neoplastic vessel of a hemangioma. Guilbert et al (214) collected 4 cases from 14,542 breast NCBs, a frequency of 0.03%. Seventy-one percent of cases in the largest series (215) were subcutaneous. Some have been reported in the fibrous capsules associated with breast implants (216,217).

Microscopy of PEH demonstrates widely anastomosing vascular spaces and branching papillary fronds **(Fig. 20.35)**. PEH is crucial to differentiate from the complex anastomosing vessels of angiosarcoma (214). PEH usually spans less than 3.0 cm, smaller than most angiosarcomas. PEH has a noninfiltrative pushing border; angiosarcomas infiltrate the surrounding tissue. PEH can exhibit rare mitoses and necrosis (215), but findings such as solid growth, tufting of endothelial cells, pleomorphism, spindle cells, atypical mitotic figures, and cytologic atypia are highly suggestive of angiosarcoma. Radiation-related cytologic atypia may be seen in PEH in that particular setting (218).

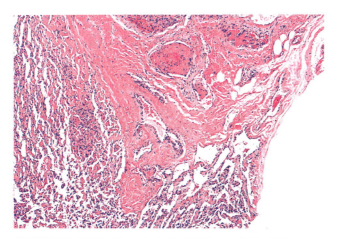

FIGURE 20.35 Papillary Endothelial Hyperplasia. This proliferation of widely anastomosing vascular spaces among branching papillary fronds of collagenous stroma should not be mistaken for angiosarcoma.

Excision serves as adequate treatment. Recurrences were not reported in the largest series (215), in a median follow-up of 1.5 years. Excision may not be needed if the NCB findings and clinical features establish a secure diagnosis of PEH.

Atypical Vascular Lesion

Benign cutaneous vascular lesions can arise in the field of radiation either postmastectomy or after breast conservation. Known in earlier days by a variety of names, these vascular lesions are now referred to by the term proposed by Fineberg and Rosen (219), *atypical vascular lesions* (AVLs).

AVLs have developed in women between the ages of 29 and 91 years. The mean age is 57.8 years, approximately 10 years younger than patients with postirradiation angiosarcomas. AVLs typically develop 2 to 5 years after radiotherapy, but intervals as long as 27 years have been reported. Up to half of affected patients develop multiple synchronous or metachronous lesions (219,220). The lesions present as one or more pink or brown papules in the skin of the breast, axilla, or chest wall. Plaques, vesicles, and cystic examples have also been reported. The aggregate lesion usually spans 5 mm or less. Only rarely do AVLs develop in the breast parenchyma. Thus, most AVLs are not sampled by NCB and are instead observed in a punch biopsy or a superficial excision.

Histologic examination reveals a localized, wedge-shaped proliferation of dilated, anastomosing vascular channels centered in the papillary and reticular dermis and lined by a single layer of endothelial cells **(Fig. 20.36)**. The overlying epidermis appears normal or mildly acanthotic. The superficial vascular channels often appear ectatic, whereas those in the deeper dermis are minute and compressed. There are two types of AVLs: lymphatic and vascular.

Lymphatic AVLs, the more common type, usually form a circumscribed collection of ectatic, thin-walled vessels lined by flat or slightly protuberant (hobnail) endothelial cells within the superficial dermis. In a minority of cases, the vessels grow in a serpiginous or infiltrative manner and extend into the deep dermis or subcutis. The neoplastic vessels can surround preexisting vessels or skin adnexa. The vascular spaces usually appear empty, but occasionally lymphocytes can be found in the nearby stroma or in the vascular lumina. Tufts of stroma typically project into the vascular lumina.

Vascular AVLs consist of irregular collections of capillaries in the dermis and are surrounded by pericytes. In certain respects, vascular AVLs resemble capillary hemangiomas, although the former lack the lobular pattern characteristic of the latter. The vessels in the vascular type of AVL usually do not intercommunicate in the manner of an angiosarcoma. The stroma often contains lymphocytes, mast cells, and plasma cells. Hemorrhage and hemosiderin deposition occur frequently. The background stromal cells in all types of AVLs often display cellular atypia characteristic of radiation damage.

Bland endothelial cells line the vessels of both types of AVLs. The nuclei can appear slightly hyperchromatic or hobnailed but do not demonstrate enlargement, angulation of contours, or prominence of nucleoli. Stratification

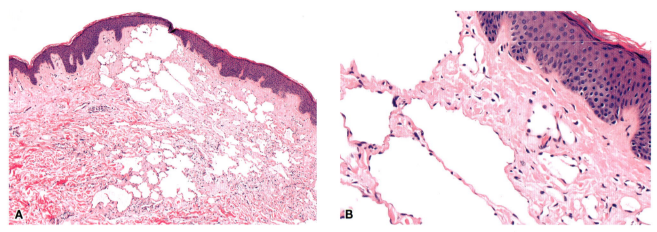

FIGURE 20.36 **Atypical Vascular Lesion. A, B:** Irregular, thin-walled vascular channels containing a few erythrocytes occupy the superficial regions of the dermis in this punch biopsy specimen. Some vascular channels contain erythrocytes; others appear devoid of cells.

of endothelial cells is absent. Mitotic figures are rarely seen; their presence increases the suspicion of low-grade angiosarcoma.

The endothelial cells of the lymphatic type of AVL stain for CD31 and D2-40, and they may stain for CD34. Those of the vascular type of AVL stain for CD31 and CD34 and are bordered by SMA-positive pericytes, but do not typically stain for D2-40 (220). Reactivity for factor VIII–related antigen has been described, but the endothelial cells do not stain for Ki67. Santi et al (221) demonstrated IHC staining for p53 in 9 of 10 AVLs and alterations in the *TP53* gene in 10 of 12 AVLs.

The differential diagnosis of AVL includes postirradiation angiosarcomas. There are no strict differentiating criteria on NCB. AVLs tend to occur earlier and to form smaller masses than angiosarcomas. Large nuclei, prominent nucleoli, vascular complexity, and extension into subcutaneous tissue are not common in AVL. None of the AVLs from 48 patients showed evidence of the amplification of *MYC* characteristic of postirradiation angiosarcomas (222-226), and only one case displayed immunoreactivity for MYC, which was seen in just a few cells (226). Two studies suggested that IHC for H3K27me3 (227) or Prox-1 (226) may help in this differential.

Excision represents adequate treatment for AVL. Fineberg and Rosen (219) did not find evidence that AVLs evolved into angiosarcoma in patients who had been followed up for as long as 10 years; however, local recurrences of AVLs were reported in this publication and others. There are no reports of metastasis or death because of AVL alone.

Uncommon examples of AVLs show focal cytologic atypia or rare mitotic figures associated with otherwise entirely bland, typical AVLs. The study of Gengler et al (228) includes 10 patients who had AVLs with "atypical" features: focal nuclear hyperchromasia of endothelial cells, prominence of nucleoli, or an infiltrative pattern of growth. None of the patients developed an angiosarcoma despite incomplete excision in two cases. Patton et al (220) noted "significant cytologic atypia" in 4 of the 10 vascular-type AVLs in their study. One patient developed angiosarcoma, and one developed additional AVLs with atypical features.

It has been suggested that the diagnosis of AVL not be rendered on limited biopsy material; but rather a description of "atypical vascular proliferation" with final categorization deferred to the evaluation of the excision (229).

Primary Angiosarcoma

Angiosarcoma is the most common mammary sarcoma. It arises in the breast more often than in any other organ. It occurs in two forms: primary (sporadic) and secondary (postirradiation). Although these forms exhibit many common features, they differ in certain clinical, histologic, molecular, and therapeutic respects.

Primary angiosarcoma afflicts women almost exclusively. Fewer than 10 instances of angiosarcoma in men have been reported (230-232). The age at diagnosis ranges from the teens to the 10th decade with a mean age of 34 (233). Several patients have been pregnant at the time of diagnosis, an observation that reflects the relative youth of women with sporadic angiosarcoma. Two reports (234,235) described angiosarcomas associated with breast implants, and a third depicted an angiosarcoma involving the site of cosmetic silicone injection (236). The literature contains several reports of synchronous or metachronous presentations of mammary angiosarcoma and carcinoma. Primary angiosarcomas have been reported in a small number of patients carrying *BRCA* mutations (237), but there are no established genetic associations.

Sporadic angiosarcoma typically presents as a painless mass. Patients usually report the presence of symptoms for only a short time. Blue or purple discoloration of the skin reflecting hemorrhage accompanies large or superficial tumors. Blistering has been noted. Large angiosarcomas can present as fungating masses. The left and right breasts are involved with equal frequency. Concurrent bilateral angiosarcomas are uncommon (238) and are usually evidence of metastatic spread.

Primary breast angiosarcoma is usually not visualized by screening mammography (239), potentially because of the relative youth and breast density of these patients (240). MRI can help to determine the extent of the tumor (241) and

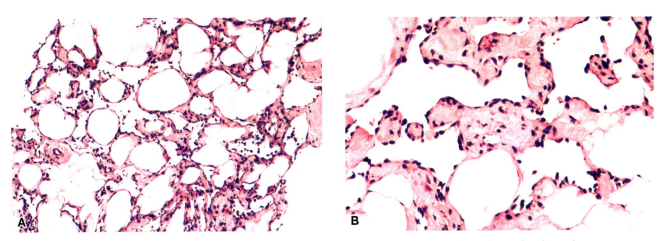

FIGURE 20.37 Angiosarcoma, Low-Grade. A, B: Open, empty irregularly shaped vascular channels are distributed diffusely in this needle core biopsy (NCB). The endothelial layer is flat, and the endothelial nuclei appear slightly prominent.

shows a T2 hyperintense enhancing mass with rapid initial uptake and washout kinetics (239,241,242).

The size of tumors ranges from 0.7 to 25 cm and averages between 5.5 and 7.0 cm. Few angiosarcomas are smaller than 3 cm. There is no significant difference in the average size of high- and low-grade lesions (243).

Three histologic grades of the primary tumor have been described. These patterns, which reflect the degree of differentiation of the tumor, correlate with prognosis (231,233). *Low-grade* (type I) tumors are composed of open, anastomosing vascular channels that proliferate diffusely in mammary tissue **(Fig. 20.37)**. Infiltration into lobules is characterized by the spread of the vascular channels within the intralobular stroma, which leads to separation and atrophy of the lobular units **(Fig. 20.38)**. Endothelial cells are distributed in a flat single-cell layer around the vascular

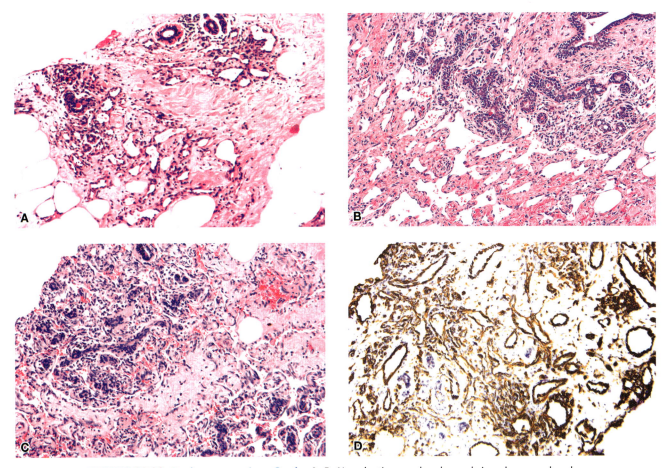

FIGURE 20.38 Angiosarcoma, Low-Grade. A, B: Neoplastic vascular channels invade around and into lobules in these needle core biopsy (NCB) specimens. **C, D:** Angiosarcoma has disrupted the lobules in this NCB. In **(D)**, the neoplastic vessels are reactive for CD31.

spaces. Some prominent, hyperchromatic endothelial nuclei may be found. Endothelial cells often have inconspicuous nuclei. Papillary formations are absent or infrequent. Mitotic figures are rare, and the Ki67-labeling index averages 25% in low-grade angiosarcomas (244). If mitotic figures are encountered with regularity in a low-grade area in a biopsy, high-grade areas are likely to be present elsewhere in the tumor. The vascular lumina are usually large, open, and anastomosing in low-grade angiosarcomas. Red blood cells are typically few, but vessels in occasional lesions are congested.

Several unusual structural variants of low-grade angiosarcoma may be difficult to recognize in an NCB. One variant is composed predominantly of capillary-like vascular spaces; another consists of narrow vascular channels without a conspicuous anastomosing structure. In a third pattern, the neoplastic vessels are dispersed in the stroma in a pattern that may be mistaken for PASH. Finally, diffusely infiltrating low-grade angiosarcoma composed predominantly of spindle cells may be mistaken for an angiolipoma.

The amount of stroma in low-grade angiosarcomas varies to a considerable degree. In most instances, little stroma is formed, and the lesion consists largely of vascular channels. A minority of low-grade angiosarcomas have diffuse collagenous stroma. Despite their denser appearance, these lesions qualify as low-grade tumors if there is no endothelial proliferation and mitoses are sparse.

Intermediate-grade (type II) angiosarcomas are distinguished from low-grade tumors by more pronounced cellular proliferation. The proliferative foci usually consist of buds or papillary fronds of endothelial cells which project into vascular lumina **(Fig. 20.39)**. Less often, the cellular areas feature polygonal and spindle cells, or there are foci that combine spindle cell and papillary elements. Infrequent mitoses may be found. Some spindle cell foci resemble Kaposi sarcoma. Ki67-labeling is most evident in the cellular areas, whereas the remainder of the tumor exhibits labeling similar to that found in low-grade angiosarcoma. The mean Ki67-labeling index is about 40% in cellular areas (244).

Low-grade components are variability present in intermediate- and high-grade lesions and sometimes comprise the bulk of the tumor. This is particularly true for type II or intermediate-grade angiosarcomas. At least 75% of intermediate-grade angiosarcomas contain low-grade elements. Transitions to the intermediate-grade foci occur abruptly.

High-grade (type III) angiosarcoma exhibits the characteristic histologic features usually attributed to angiosarcomas. Part of the lesion may be composed of low- and intermediate-grade elements; however, more than half of the tumor has high-grade malignant features. These features include prominent endothelial tufting and solid papillary formations which contain cytologically malignant endothelial cells and conspicuous solid and spindle cell areas **(Fig. 20.40)**. Mitoses are readily identified. Typically,

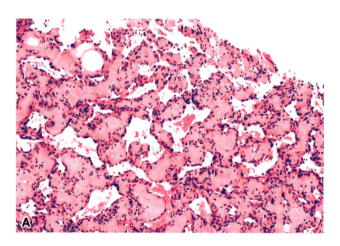

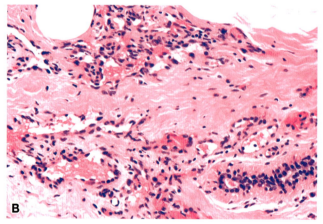

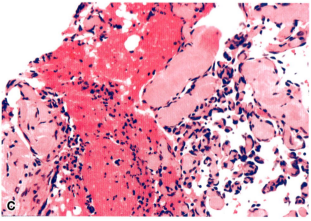

FIGURE 20.39 Angiosarcoma, Intermediate-Grade.
A, B: This needle core biopsy specimen shows a low-grade area with fibrous stroma between anastomosing vascular channels. **C:** This region of the specimen shows focal intermediate-grade papillary endothelial growth and thrombosis.

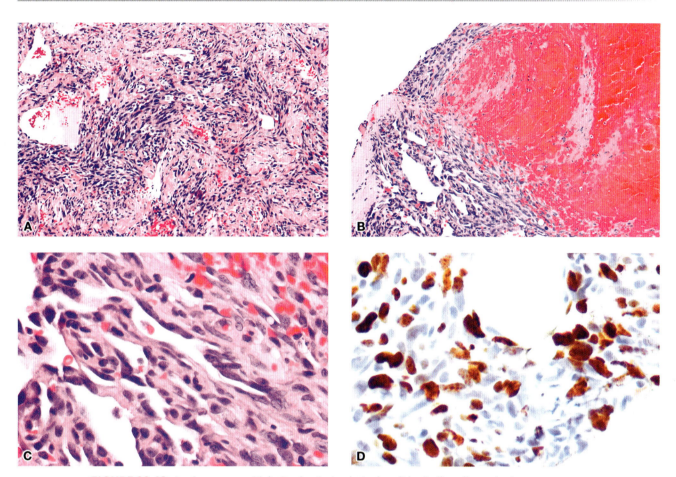

FIGURE 20.40 **Angiosarcoma, High-Grade. A:** A relatively solid spindle cell area is shown. **B:** Hemorrhage forms a blood lake in another needle core biopsy (NCB). **C:** The tumor cell nuclei appear hyperchromatic. **D:** Many nuclei are reactive for Ki67.

Ki67-labeling is found in 45% or more of the tumor cells in high-grade angiosarcoma. Areas of hemorrhage, often accompanied by necrosis, have been referred to as *blood lakes*. Only high-grade angiosarcomas demonstrate necrosis and "blood lakes."

With few exceptions, angiosarcomas have infiltrative borders composed of well-formed or low-grade vascular channels. In some cases, the peripheral vascular component is so orderly that the neoplastic vessels are either structurally indistinguishable from existing capillaries in the normal breast or those in an angiolipoma.

Epitheloid angiosarcoma **(Fig. 20.41)** is an uncommon high-grade variant. The lesion consists predominantly of large, polygonal or rounded epithelioid endothelial cells lining slit-like spaces and containing abundant amphophilic or eosinophilic cytoplasm and large vesicular nuclei. The tumor may be mistaken for mammary adenocarcinoma because of the epithelioid appearance of the lesional cells. IHC for epithelial and vascular proteins may assist in distinguishing the two lesions, although weak or focal keratin expression can be seen in epithelioid angiosarcoma (232,245).

Of note, a two-tier grading system for primary angiosarcoma of the breast has recently been proposed by Kuba et al (246). However, the clinical utility and prognostic value of this "simpler" system of grading will have to be duplicated and stand the test of time (247).

Because of intratumor heterogeneity, it is not possible to definitively classify a tumor as low-grade angiosarcoma unless it has been excised and generously sampled. The tendency for peripheral portions of an intermediate- or high-grade angiosarcoma to have a low-grade morphology is likely to lead to an erroneous diagnosis based on NCB or a superficial biopsy.

Two studies of mammary angiosarcomas reported more intense staining for factor VIII–related antigens in well-differentiated than in poorly differentiated portions of the tumor (248). Angiosarcomas also exhibit reactivity for CD31 and CD34, markers useful for distinguishing epithelioid angiosarcoma from carcinoma and other neoplasms. Epithelioid angiosarcomas typically stain for CD31, but reactivity for CD34 varies. Reactivity for D2-40 has been reported in most angiosarcomas (249). Although angiosarcomas usually do not stain for keratin, three reports (232,243,245), including two describing epithelioid angiosarcomas (232,245), noted staining for keratin in three cases. Angiosarcomas do not stain for ER or PR, and the few tested do not show evidence of *HER2* overexpression. Unlike extramammary angiosarcomas that are enriched for *TP53* mutations, primary

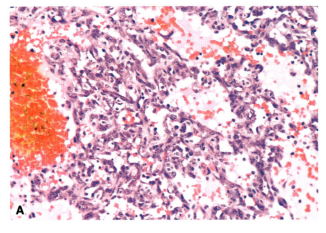
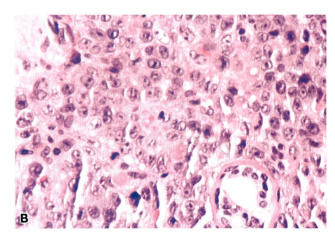
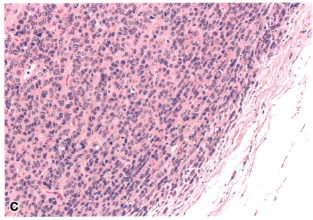

FIGURE 20.41 Angiosarcoma, High-Grade, Epithelioid.
A: This angiosarcoma arose in the breast 4 years after conservative surgery and radiotherapy. **B:** The neoplastic cells in this high-grade postirradiation angiosarcoma demonstrate an epithelioid appearance. The cells possess the characteristic vesicular nuclei and prominent nucleoli. **C:** This epithelioid angiosarcoma could be mistaken for poorly differentiated carcinoma.

breast angiosarcomas frequently demonstrate activating mutations in *KDR* and *PIK3CA* (250,251), of potential diagnostic and therapeutic significance (252).

It is not difficult to distinguish a high-grade angiosarcoma from a hemangioma, but problems may be encountered with low-grade and intermediate-grade tumors on NCB. Some general guidelines are helpful in these situations. Hemangiomas are rarely more than 2 cm, and few angiosarcomas measure less than 3 cm. Most hemangiomas have well-circumscribed borders, whereas angiosarcomas have infiltrative margins. Many hemangiomas are divided into lobules or nodules by fibrous septa, a feature not seen in angiosarcomas. Hemangiomas usually consist of isolated, largely unconnected vascular channels. Anastomosing vascular spaces may be found in hemangiomas; however, except in angiomatosis, the anastomoses are not as numerous or as serpiginous as those in angiosarcomas. The vascular proliferation in angiosarcomas invades into and expands native mammary lobules, whereas the vessels in hemangiomas tend to surround lobules and ducts. A thick-walled, nonneoplastic "feeding" blood vessel is sometimes found at the periphery of hemangiomas; this feature is not present in angiosarcomas. The Ki67-labeling index of hemangiomas is substantially lower than that of angiosarcomas (244).

In 1981, Donnell et al (233) studied 40 patients with mammary angiosarcoma treated by mastectomy and found that the grade of the tumor was the most important prognostic factor. Most patients with low-grade lesions remained disease-free, whereas virtually all those with high-grade tumors died of recurrent angiosarcoma within 5 years. A later study of 87 patients confirmed the correlation between the tumor grade and prognosis (231), as did a study of 226 women in the SEER database (253). Despite the relatively favorable prognosis of low-grade angiosarcoma, patients with these tumors can develop local and systemic recurrences (231,233). A patient who initially has a low-grade angiosarcoma may develop intermediate- or high-grade recurrences. Conversely, recurrences and metastases that originate from high-grade sarcomas can be composed in part or entirely of low-grade components.

A review by Kaklamanos et al (254) summarized treatment and survival data from 10 major series including mammary angiosarcomas. Total mastectomy is the recommended primary surgical therapy. Unless there is a clinically apparent nodal abnormality, axillary dissection is not indicated because metastases involve these lymph nodes in fewer than 10% of cases. Radical mastectomy is not appropriate unless the tumor is close to or involves the deep fascia. Rarely, a solitary and relatively smaller lesion might be encompassed by excision.

The role of radiation in the treatment of mammary angiosarcoma has not been determined nor has the use of adjuvant systemic chemotherapy (255). Data suggest that adjuvant radiation does not confer a survival benefit for patients with localized disease (253), but this approach may have a role in tumors refractory to other forms of therapy.

Postirradiation Angiosarcoma

Postirradiation angiosarcomas can arise either in the skin of the chest wall after mastectomy or in the breast parenchyma after partial mastectomy. Other sarcoma subtypes, including UPS, leiomyosarcoma, and fibrosarcoma, can also arise in this setting albeit less commonly (256,257). An analysis of SEER data (2) revealed that women with breast carcinoma who undergo irradiation experience a relative risk of 15.9 for the development of angiosarcoma at all sites compared with nonirradiated patients. When considering only angiosarcoma of the breast or chest wall, the comparable relative risk is 59.3. Angiosarcoma of the irradiated breast is an infrequent complication of breast conservation therapy. The incidence averages approximately 0.1%. A publication by Abbott and Palmieri (258) lists selected clinical details of 237 cases. In almost every case, radiation was delivered using an external beam, but one angiosarcoma arose in the breast of a 74-year-old woman 4 years after receiving MammoSite balloon brachytherapy (259).

The interval between irradiation and the diagnosis of angiosarcoma ranges from 1 to more than 24 years, but most cases come to attention within 6 years after radiotherapy (260). The latent period tends to be shorter than that for other types of radiation-associated sarcoma and appears inversely related to the patient's age at the time of treatment for breast carcinoma (261). Billings et al (262) reported that for each 1-year increase in age, the latency period decreases by 0.5 month. Studies have not discovered a relationship between the radiation dose, the use of a radiation boost, or the presence of postirradiation edema and the development of radiation-related angiosarcoma.

With few exceptions, women with postirradiation angiosarcoma have been older than 50 when treated for mammary carcinoma. In one study (260), the median age at diagnosis of angiosarcoma was 70.6 years, and the range was 46.2 to 87.2 years. A meta-analysis of 184 published cases (258) yielded a median age of 70 and a range of 36 to 92. A 98-year-old woman developed an epithelioid angiosarcoma 5 years after radiation treatment for an invasive ductal carcinoma (263).

In contrast to primary angiosarcoma, postirradiation sarcoma presents most often with skin changes rather than a mass. The tumors usually involve the skin overlying the site of the prior carcinoma and can present as palpable skin or subcutaneous nodules, plaques, or papules. Some cause edema, skin thickening, vesicles, dimpling, or *peau d'orange* change, and others clinically mimic a hematoma. Multiple nodules are common, and when numerous can cover the entire breast. The formation of an exophytic mass has been described (264). In certain patients, the skin changes may be subtle. Many patients who present with angiosarcoma in the skin will also have parenchymal involvement.

Imaging studies in patients with postirradiation angiosarcomas do not demonstrate distinctive findings. Posttreatment changes such as skin thickening and architectural distortion may obscure the sarcoma on mammography or ultrasonography (even after lesional skin changes are clinically observed) (265). MRI is the most sensitive modality for the disease (266). Findings can include an enhancing cutaneous or parenchymal mass, parenchymal non-mass enhancement, and cutaneous nodularity or thickening (240).

Certain histologic features of postirradiation angiosarcoma differ from those of angiosarcomas not associated with radiotherapy (219) **(Fig. 20.42)**. High-grade areas, found in the majority of postirradiation angiosarcoma cases, consist of compact epithelioid or spindle cell foci, which may contain extravasated red blood cells or slit-like, erythrocyte-containing spaces. Hemorrhage resulting in the formation of blood lakes is typically distributed in these cellular foci. In contrast to sporadic angiosarcomas, in which nuclear grade frequently parallels structural differentiation, the malignant cells in postirradiation angiosarcoma typically have high-grade nuclei, dark chromatin, prominent nucleoli, and mitotic figures. The mitotic rate varies from less than 1 to 35 mitotic figures per HPF with a mean of 9 per HPF. Unusual histologic variants of cutaneous angiosarcoma include perithelial, storiform, cavernous, and epidermotropic patterns (267).

Like their sporadic counterparts, postirradiation angiosarcomas typically stain for vimentin, CD31, CD34, and factor VIII. Epithelioid angiosarcomas can stain for keratin (245,263,268). Sheu et al (269) reported strong nuclear staining for NOTCH1, previously observed in 77% of angiosarcomas of various organs, including epithelioid and solid variants (270). The tumors do not stain for ER or PR. Genetic studies implicate overexpression of *MYC* in the development of postirradiation mammary angiosarcomas. Of the 115 cases studied by 4 groups (222-224,271), 103 showed evidence of amplification of the *MYC* gene or overexpression of the MYC protein. In contrast, none of the 25 sporadic mammary angiosarcomas (224-226) or 53 AVLs (224,226,272) exhibited amplification or overexpression. Co-amplification with *FLT4* can be seen (222,225).

The prognosis of angiosarcoma arising in the breast after radiotherapy does not seem to differ substantially from that of primary sporadic angiosarcoma. A meta-analysis based on 151 cases (258) demonstrated a median overall survival

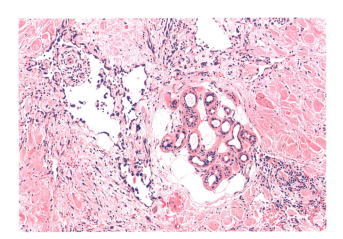

FIGURE 20.42 Postirradiation Angiosarcoma. Anastomosing spaces with markedly atypical endothelium surround a benign lobule. Erythrocytes extravasate from these poorly formed vessels into the surrounding stroma.

of 18 months for patients with postirradiation angiosarcoma; however, studies from single institutions report higher median overall survival values. The largest single-institution study (273) includes 95 patients followed up for a median of 10.8 years. Local recurrences occurred in 48% and distant metastases in 27% of the patients. Tumor size, tumor grade, and *MYC* amplification have been associated with worse prognosis (271,274).

As is the case with sporadic angiosarcomas, surgery constitutes the primary treatment of postirradiation angiosarcomas. The surgical procedure is most often a mastectomy, but surgery does not always control the disease. Several studies report recurrences within a year of excision even when the margins are free of the angiosarcoma. The high rate of local recurrence has led several investigators to conclude that many postirradiation angiosarcomas involve the irradiated tissue in a discontinuous, multifocal manner. Based on this belief, some advocate excision of all irradiated skin. Two patients in the series of Seinen et al (275) underwent mastectomy and excision of all irradiated tissue, and 12 of the 33 patients in the study of Morgan et al (276) were treated similarly. The authors of the latter study reported: "Although this did not universally prevent recurrence, we found that patients who did not undergo resection of all irradiated breast skin trended toward a worse median [local relapse-free survival] (10.0 vs 80.8 months) and [overall survival] (29 months vs not achieved)." Further studies will define the value of this approach.

Because angiosarcomas spread to lymph nodes uncommonly, lymph node excision is not usually undertaken. Radiation therapy has not usually played a role in the treatment of postirradiation angiosarcomas, although it has been used in certain settings. Adjuvant chemotherapy has demonstrated a trend toward improved recurrence-free survival in high-grade tumors (274). Therapies targeted to the vascular endothelial growth factor (VEGF) receptor or c-kit may hold promise.

OTHER MESENCHYMAL TUMORS

Hamartoma

Robbins Basic Pathology defines hamartoma as "a disorganized but benign-appearing [tumor] composed of cells indigenous to the particular site" (277). Mammary tumors that fit this concept usually consist of disordered glands and stroma. Those composed of glands and fat have been referred to as *adenolipomas*, or *adenohibernomas* in the case of brown fat (278), as well as hamartomas.

Hamartomas represent approximately 4% of benign breast lesions (279). These neoplasms typically occur in premenopausal women, but they have been described in teenagers and in women in their ninth decade. The mean age ranges from 38 to 50 years. An association with pregnancy has been noted in some cases. Reviews by Sevim et al (280) and Alran et al (281) list clinical and pathologic findings of hamartomas.

Approximately 50% of hamartomas present as palpable painless masses; screening mammography detects the remainder. A few patients have presented with two ipsilateral hamartomas (279). Some patients report slow growth over years, whereas others describe rapid enlargement. Large hamartomas may present as unilateral macromastia or asymmetry (282). Multiple and bilateral hamartomas and "hamartoma-like lesions" have been described in patients with Cowden syndrome; however, most patients with mammary hamartomas do not have the syndrome. One publication describes a hamartoma arising in axillary breast tissue (283).

Mammography may reveal a well-circumscribed oval mass surrounded by a narrow lucent zone, an appearance which has been described as "breast within a breast" (284). Some palpable tumors are mammographically occult. Predominantly fatty tumors may have the appearance of lipomas, whereas those with abundant glandular tissue appear dense. Calcifications may be present. Ultrasonography reveals a mixed pattern of echogenic and lucent regions. On MRI, hamartomas have been described as oval or irregular masses, or non-mass lesions with homogeneous enhancement (281).

Microscopically, the lesion consists of intermixed breast glandular tissue and stroma bounded by a pseudocapsule of compressed breast parenchyma **(Fig. 20.43)**. The glandular tissue usually consists of ducts and lobules, although the lobules may be larger or more disorganized than normal. The stroma usually predominates, varies widely from collagenous to adipose, and frequently demonstrates PASH (285). Because they lack a distinctive microscopic appearance, hamartomas may be misinterpreted as normal breast on NCB, especially if clinical and imaging features are not taken into account (281). Positivity for CD34, HMGA2, and PR may distinguish tumoral fibroblasts from normal breast stroma (281).

The most important differential diagnoses are normal breast and phyllodes tumor. Hamartomas are adequately treated by excision but may recur if incompletely excised (285).

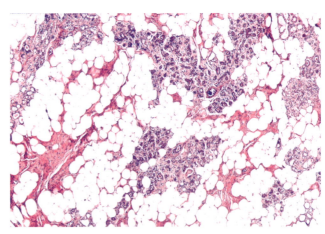

FIGURE 20.43 Hamartoma. Haphazard aggregates of acini are distributed in a circumscribed mass of fibroadipose tissue.

The so-called *myoid (leiomyomatous) hamartoma* does not represent a hamartoma as defined earlier. The lesion most often develops as a mass-forming type of sclerosing adenosis with smooth muscle metaplasia of the myoepithelial cell component (286). Adequate sampling reveals foci of sclerosing adenosis in almost all myoid "hamartomas." Most such lesions would be better classified as adenosis tumors or PASH with myoid metaplasia.

Myxoma and Angiomyxoma

Myxoma and angiomyxoma are uncommon benign neoplasms consisting of stromal cells within abundant myxoid extracellular material. They are likely underrecognized because of the lack of uniform nomenclature. A minority (<10%) are associated with the Carney complex (287,288). Both syndromic and sporadic myxomas and angiomyxomas may exhibit inactivation of the tumor suppressor *PRKAR1A*.

Microscopy of myxoma reveals a well-defined mass within the breast surrounded by a delicate pseudocapsule. The tumor consists of hypocellular myxoid tissue containing round, stellate, or spindle-shaped mesenchymal cells. The latter possess oval nuclei, small nucleoli, and pale cytoplasm. The lesional cells may form dendrite-like processes. The myxoid matrix stains with Alcian blue at pH 2.5 and does not react with PAS. The stroma may also contain collagen fibers, blood vessels, mast cells, and lymphocytes. Ducts and lobules are absent.

Angiomyxomas tend to be superficial, multilobular, and unencapsulated yet circumscribed. The myxoid matrix is imbued with prominent spindled fibroblasts and thin-walled vessels, and it can entrap mammary ducts and lobules. Most lesional cells are positive for CD34 and negative for S-100, SMA, desmin, cytokeratin, p63, and MUC4 (287). In one study, two-thirds of angiomyxomas showed loss of PRKAR1A expression (287).

Other myxoid breast lesions in the differential diagnosis include myxoid fibroadenoma, nodular mucinosis, nodular fasciitis, and mucocele-like lesion. Magro and colleagues (288) tabulated morphologic and IHC attributes that could help resolve these diagnoses.

Excision is generally curative. Diagnosis may allow recognition of the Carney complex in some patients.

Extraskeletal Osteosarcoma and Chondrosarcoma

Malignant tumors with features of extraskeletal osteosarcoma or chondrosarcoma occasionally arise in the breast. Some authors (289) suggest that essentially all mammary malignancies with osseous or chondroid features represent either matrix-producing metaplastic carcinomas or phyllodes tumors with massive stromal overgrowth. Preliminary data have demonstrated molecular overlap between osteosarcomas and metaplastic carcinomas with osseous differentiation (290). Irrespective of the pathogenesis of these tumors, the literature describes their clinical and pathologic features.

Publications by Silver and Tavassoli (291), Trihia et al (292), Pasta et al (293), and Yin et al (187) list many cases. The ages of patients range from 16 to 96 years. The mean age of patients with osteosarcoma is 62.5 years; the mean age of patients with chondrosarcoma is 57.0 years. Incidence in the male breast has been described (291,294). The presenting symptom is a mass typically described as circumscribed and freely movable. Fixation to the skin or chest wall and ulceration of skin occur in some cases. Rapid growth of a previously unchanging mass or new onset of pain may prompt the patient to seek medical care. Osteosarcoma has developed in the breast following breast conservation therapy, and both osteosarcoma and chondrosarcoma have arisen following postmastectomy irradiation (295). Sarcomas arising in the chest wall (296) and metastases from extramammary sarcomas (297) can present as mammary tumors.

Mammography reveals a dense mass, which can be either ill-defined or well-defined and even suggest the diagnosis of fibroadenoma. Tumors in which the osteosarcomatous component dominates appear heavily calcified and may be positive on skeletal scintigraphy (298). Digital tomosynthesis of an osteosarcoma showed "sunburst" calcifications (a pattern often associated with bone-producing soft tissue tumors) (299). Chondrosarcomatous tumors appear hyperdense and may contain calcifications. Findings suggestive of hemorrhage, necrosis, and bone formation may be seen on MRI (300). The tumors have measured 1.4 to 25 cm, with a mean size of 5.3 cm.

Although the diagnosis of a mammary osteo- or chondrosarcoma may be suggested by the clinical findings and NCB (293,298), thorough examination of the excised tumor is necessary to ensure an accurate diagnosis. Histologic characteristics of the resected tumor duplicate their conventional skeletal counterparts, and they may demonstrate a spectrum of patterns (**Fig. 20.44**). The tumors have in common a prominent component of high-grade spindle cell sarcoma. Multinucleate osteoclastic giant cells are usually present in areas of bone formation. Rarely, giant cells may be associated with hemorrhagic cysts. Chondroid differentiation rarely occurs without osseous components and can demonstrate low-grade, high-grade, mesenchymal, and other patterns.

IHC for cytokeratins, myoepithelial proteins, and molecules found in myocytes are negative. Lack of reactivity for cytokeratin and myoepithelial markers is essential to rule out metaplastic carcinoma. Areas with cartilaginous differentiation can be immunoreactive for EMA or S-100. Nuclear expression of SATB2 can confirm osteoblastic differentiation but is not specific for osteosarcoma (301). In a study by Wang et al (192), TRPS1 was highly expressed in all three breast primary osteosarcomas and all four chondrosarcomas, whereas in only 56% and 28% of extramammary osteosarcomas and chondrosarcomas, respectively. None of the cases studied have expressed ER, PR, or HER2.

The series of patients studied by Silver and Tavassoli (291) provides the most detailed analysis of the treatment and outcome of patients with mammary osteosarcomas.

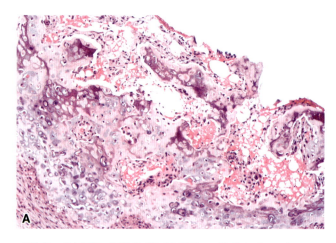
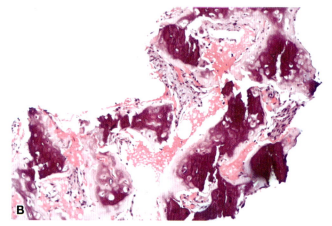
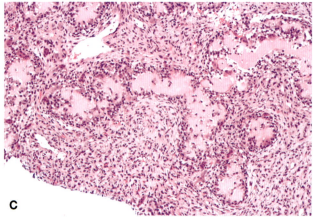

FIGURE 20.44 Osteochondrosarcoma. A: This needle core biopsy (NCB) shows malignant cartilage with ossification. Cytokeratin immunostains did not support epithelial differentiation. **B:** This part of the NCB contains trabeculae of bone. **C:** Another area in the specimen consists of high-grade spindle cell sarcoma and osteoid.

Complete excision with negative margins is needed to forestall local recurrence. Axillary staging is not necessary unless clinical evaluation indicates otherwise. Metastases usually appear within a year of diagnosis, and death ensues within 2 years thereafter. Using the Kaplan-Meier method, the probability of overall survival is 38% at 5 years and 10% at 10 years (291). Patients with osteosarcomas smaller than 4.6 cm had a higher likelihood for survival than patients with larger tumors, and patients with the fibroblastic type of osteosarcoma had better prognosis than patients with the osteoclastic or osteoblastic subtypes. Follow-up provided in other reports supports these observations. Irradiation and chemotherapy have been administered in several cases, but the variability of these treatments precludes secure conclusions regarding their efficacy.

Undifferentiated Pleomorphic Sarcoma

UPS represents a type of sarcoma lacking morphologic, IHC, and genetic evidence indicative of a specific cellular lineage. As such, it is a diagnosis of exclusion that should be considered only after detailed investigation. Although rare in general, UPS accounts for 36% of the 240 breast sarcomas in the studies tabulated by Adem et al (302) and 22% of the 562 mammary sarcomas in the SEER 18 data set (187). Most tumors classified earlier as fibrosarcoma or "malignant fibrous histiocytoma" would now be considered UPS, subtypes of fibrosarcoma, malignant phyllodes tumor, or other types of sarcoma.

The majority of patients have been women, but tumors of male breast have been reported (303). Jeong et al (304) described the case of a 76-year-old man in whom a tumor classified as an "atypical spindle cell lesion" recurred after 1 year as UPS. The age at diagnosis ranges from 15 to 94 years and averages 52 years. The initial symptom is an enlarging breast mass. Reported symptomatic intervals vary from 1 month to 17 years. The tumors are usually solitary, but multiple tumors have been described. The overlying skin can exhibit dimpling, induration, ecchymosis, or ulceration. Rarely, patients give a history of antecedent trauma. In several case reports, irradiation for breast carcinoma preceded sarcoma (305).

Radiology does not demonstrate distinctive findings. Mammograms reveal a homogeneous mass with regular or irregular margins. The mean size is 7.5 cm (91).

The microscopic hallmark of UPS is the *storiform* growth pattern—in which oval or spindle-shaped cells are arranged in a pinwheel pattern **(Fig. 20.45)**. Capillaries or minute blood vessels may be found at the centers of the storiform collections. Multinucleate giant cells with bizarre nuclei, myxoid change, and a chronic inflammatory cell infiltrate are variably present. Low-grade tumors have little mitotic activity, minimal pleomorphism, and scant or no necrosis. Easily identified mitoses, generally numbering more than 3 per HPF, prominent cellular pleomorphism, and necrosis

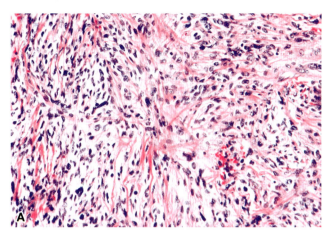 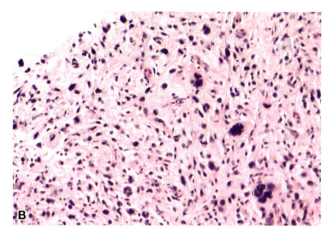

FIGURE 20.45 **Undifferentiated Pleomorphic Sarcoma. A:** The spindle cell tumor has a typical storiform structure. No epithelial differentiation was detected. **B:** This needle core biopsy (NCB) from another tumor shows multinucleate giant cells.

characterize high-grade UPS. Cellularity alone is not a reliable criterion for distinguishing between low- and high-grade tumors.

IHC serves only to exclude other diagnoses. The malignant cells are reactive for vimentin; occasionally for actin, CD68, S-100, or SMA; and rarely for cytokeratin. All pathologic and clinical features must be given careful consideration when a tumor with storiform growth displays cytokeratin reactivity. Such lesions usually represent metaplastic carcinomas. One tumor displayed "rare focal" expression of ER and PR (303). Another tumor with focal melan-A staining underwent whole-exome sequencing, FISH, and reverse transcription polymerase chain reaction (RT-PCR), which revealed no common melanoma driver mutations, ultraviolet (UV)-associated mutational signatures, nor common clear cell sarcoma translocations; but one *TP53* missense mutation (306).

Many patients with UPS have been treated with mastectomy, but wide local excision is becoming common. Local recurrences have developed after local excision and mastectomy. Rare examples of UPS have metastasized to axillary lymph nodes (307); however, axillary dissection is not indicated unless needed to obtain adequate margin or whenever clinical findings suggest nodal metastases. Chemotherapy used for soft tissue sarcomas of other sites is sometimes administered, although data regarding chemosensitivity of breast sarcomas are lacking.

Recurrence and death due to disease have been reported in approximately 25% of patients (303). Local recurrence is common among low-grade tumors. Metastases usually originate from high-grade tumors. Metastases and deaths most commonly occur within 3 years and rarely more than 5 years after diagnoses. The most frequent sites of metastases are the lungs and bones (308).

Other Sarcomas

Other sarcomas described in the breast include *rhabdomyosarcoma* (309), *malignant peripheral nerve sheath tumor* (115), *primitive neuroectodermal tumor* (PNET) (310), *alveolar soft part sarcoma* (311), *synovial sarcoma* (312), *myofibroblastic sarcoma* (313), *Kaposi sarcoma* (314), and follicular dendritic cell sarcoma (erstwhile "follicular dendritic cell tumor") (315).

REFERENCES

1. Zelek L, Llombart-Cussac A, Terrier P, et al. Prognostic factors in primary breast sarcomas: a series of patients with long-term follow-up. *J Clin Oncol*. 2003;21:2583-2588.
2. Huang J, Mackillop WJ. Increased risk of soft tissue sarcoma after radiotherapy in women with breast carcinoma. *Cancer*. 2001;92:172-180.
3. Mery CM, George S, Bertagnolli MM, et al. Secondary sarcomas after radiotherapy for breast cancer: sustained risk and poor survival. *Cancer*. 2009;115:4055-4063.
4. Yap J, Chuba PJ, Thomas R, et al. Sarcoma as a second malignancy after treatment for breast cancer. *Int J Radiat Oncol Biol Phys*. 2002;52:1231-1237.
5. Vuitch MF, Rosen PP, Erlandson RA. Pseudoangiomatous hyperplasia of mammary stroma. *Hum Pathol*. 1986;17:185-191.
6. Asioli S, Eusebi V, Gaetano L, et al. The pre-lymphatic pathway, the rooths of the lymphatic system in breast tissue: a 3D study. *Virchows Arch*. 2008;453:401-406.
7. Ibrahim RE, Sciotto CG, Weidner N. Pseudoangiomatous hyperplasia of mammary stroma. Some observations regarding its clinicopathologic spectrum. *Cancer*. 1989;63:1154-1160.
8. Degnim AC, Frost MH, Radisky DC, et al. Pseudoangiomatous stromal hyperplasia and breast cancer risk. *Ann Surg Oncol*. 2010;17:3269-3277.
9. Cohen MA, Morris EA, Rosen PP, et al. Pseudoangiomatous stromal hyperplasia: mammographic, sonographic, and clinical patterns. *Radiology*. 1996;198:117-120.
10. Mercado CL, Naidrich SA, Hamele-Bena D, et al. Pseudoangiomatous stromal hyperplasia of the breast: sonographic features with histopathologic correlation. *Breast J*. 2004;10:427-432.
11. Speer ME, Yoon EC, Berg WA, et al. Pseudoangiomatous stromal hyperplasia: radiologic-pathologic correlation. *J Breast Imaging*. 2023;5:67-72.
12. Bowman E, Oprea G, Okoli J, et al. Pseudoangiomatous stromal hyperplasia (PASH) of the breast: a series of 24 patients. *Breast J*. 2012;18:242-247.
13. Ferreira M, Albarracin CT, Resetkova E. Pseudoangiomatous stromal hyperplasia tumor: a clinical, radiologic and pathological study of 26 cases. *Mod Pathol*. 2008;21:201-207.
14. Shehata BM, Fishman I, Collings MH, et al. Pseudoangiomatous stromal hyperplasia of the breast in pediatric patients: an underrecognized entity. *Pediatr Dev Pathol*. 2009;12:450-454.
15. Singh KA, Lewis MM, Runge RL, et al. Pseudoangiomatous stromal hyperplasia. A case for bilateral mastectomy in a 12-year-old girl. *Breast J*. 2007;13:603-606.
16. Milanezi MF, Saggioro FP, Zanati SG, et al. Pseudoangiomatous hyperplasia of mammary stroma associated with gynaecomastia. *J Clin Pathol*. 1998;51:204-206.
17. Pizem J, Velikonja M, Matjasic A, et al. Pseudoangiomatous stromal hyperplasia with multinucleated stromal giant cells is neither exceptional in gynecomastia nor characteristic of neurofibromatosis type 1. *Virchows Arch*. 2015;466:465-472.
18. Badve S, Sloane JP. Pseudoangiomatous hyperplasia of male breast. *Histopathology*. 1995;26:463-466.
19. Mizutou A, Nakashima K, Moriya T. Large pseudoangiomatous stromal hyperplasia complicated with gynecomastia and lobular differentiation in a male breast. *Springerplus*. 2015;4:282.

20. Vega RM, Pechman D, Ergonul B, et al. Bilateral pseudoangiomatous stromal hyperplasia tumors in axillary male gynecomastia: report of a case. *Surg Today*. 2015;45:105-109.
21. Iancu D, Nochomovitz LE. Pseudoangiomatous stromal hyperplasia: presentation as a mass in the female nipple. *Breast J*. 2001;7:263-265.
22. Jordan AC, Jaffer S, Mercer SE. Massive nodular pseudoangiomatous stromal hyperplasia (PASH) of the breast arising simultaneously in the axilla and vulva. *Int J Surg Pathol*. 2011;19:113-116.
23. Almohawes E, Khoumais N, Arafah M. Pseudoangiomatous stromal hyperplasia of the breast: a case report of a 12-year-old girl. *Radiol Case Rep*. 2015;10:1-4.
24. Krawczyk N, Fehm T, Ruckhaberle E, et al. Bilateral diffuse Pseudoangiomatous Stromal Hyperplasia (PASH) causing gigantomastia in a 33-year-old pregnant woman: case report. *Breast Care (Basel)*. 2016;11:356-358.
25. Damiani S, Eusebi V. Gynecomastia in type-1 neurofibromatosis with features of pseudoangiomatous stromal hyperplasia with giant cells. Report of two cases. *Virchows Arch*. 2001;438:513-516.
26. Ozerdem U, Wells J, Hoda SA. Hyaline globules in mammary myofibroblastoma: a case report. *Int J Surg Pathol*. 2015;23:89-91.
27. Noda Y, Nishimae A, Sawai Y, et al. Atypical pseudoangiomatous stromal hyperplasia showing rapid growth of the breast: report of a case. *Pathol Int*. 2019;69:300-305.
28. Celliers L, Wong DD, Bourke A. Pseudoangiomatous stromal hyperplasia: a study of the mammographic and sonographic features. *Clin Radiol*. 2010;65:145-149.
29. Gresik CM, Godellas C, Aranha GV, et al. Pseudoangiomatous stromal hyperplasia of the breast: a contemporary approach to its clinical and radiologic features and ideal management. *Surgery*. 2010;148:752-757; discussion 757-758.
30. Pruthi S, Reynolds C, Johnson RE, et al. Tamoxifen in the management of pseudoangiomatous stromal hyperplasia. *Breast J*. 2001;7:434-439.
31. Seltzer MH, Kintiroglou M. Pseudoangiomatous hyperplasia and response to tamoxifen therapy. *Breast J*. 2003;9:344.
32. Rosen PP, Ernsberger D. Mammary fibromatosis. A benign spindle-cell tumor with significant risk for local recurrence. *Cancer*. 1989;63:1363-1369.
33. Abraham SC, Reynolds C, Lee JH, et al. Fibromatosis of the breast and mutations involving the APC/beta-catenin pathway. *Hum Pathol*. 2002;33:39-46.
34. Caulfield RH, Maleki-Tabrizi A, Birch J, et al. An unusual case of fibromatosis of the axilla. *Breast J*. 2008;14:110-112.
35. Brown CS, Jeffrey B, Korentager R, et al. Desmoid tumors of the bilateral breasts in a patient without Gardner syndrome: a case report and review of literature. *Ann Plast Surg*. 2012;69:220-222.
36. Balzer BL, Weiss SW. Do biomaterials cause implant-associated mesenchymal tumors of the breast? Analysis of 8 new cases and review of the literature. *Hum Pathol*. 2009;40:1564-1570.
37. Matrai Z, Toth L, Gulyas G, et al. A desmoid tumor associated with a ruptured silicone breast implant. *Plast Reconstr Surg*. 2011;127:1e-4e.
38. Plaza MJ, Yepes M. Breast fibromatosis response to tamoxifen: dynamic MRI findings and review of the current treatment options. *J Radiol Case Rep*. 2012;6:16-23.
39. Silva S, Lage P, Cabral F, et al. Bilateral breast fibromatosis after silicone prosthetics in a patient with classic familial adenomatous polyposis: a case report. *Oncol Lett*. 2018;16:1449-1454.
40. Kim T, Jung EA, Song JY, et al. Prevalence of the CTNNB1 mutation genotype in surgically resected fibromatosis of the breast. *Histopathology*. 2012;60:347-356.
41. Neuman HB, Brogi E, Ebrahim A, et al. Desmoid tumors (fibromatoses) of the breast: a 25-year experience. *Ann Surg Oncol*. 2008;15:274-280.
42. Pettinato G, Manivel JC, Gould EW, et al. Inclusion body fibromatosis of the breast. Two cases with immunohistochemical and ultrastructural findings. *Am J Clin Pathol*. 1994;101:714-718.
43. Lacroix-Triki M, Geyer FC, Lambros MB, et al. β-catenin/Wnt signalling pathway in fibromatosis, metaplastic carcinomas and phyllodes tumours of the breast. *Mod Pathol*. 2010;23:1438-1448.
44. Norkowski E, Masliah-Planchon J, Le Guellec S, et al. Lower rate of CTNNB1 mutations and higher rate of APC mutations in desmoid fibromatosis of the breast: a series of 134 tumors. *Am J Surg Pathol*. 2020;44:1266-1273.
45. Goto K, Ishikawa M, Aizawa D, et al. Nuclear β-catenin immunoexpression in scars. *J Cutan Pathol*. 2021;48:18-23.
46. Kuba MG, Lester SC, Giess CS, et al. Fibromatosis of the breast: diagnostic accuracy of core needle biopsy. *Am J Clin Pathol*. 2017;148:243-250.
47. Duazo-Cassin L, Le Guellec S, Lusque A, et al. Breast desmoid tumor management in France: toward a new strategy. *Breast Cancer Res Treat*. 2019;176:329-335.
48. Brown V, Carty NJ. A case of nodular fasciitis of the breast and review of the literature. *Breast*. 2005;14:384-387.
49. Samardzic D, Chetlen A, Malysz J. Nodular fasciitis in the axillary tail of the breast. *J Radiol Case Rep*. 2014;8:16-26.
50. Maly B, Maly A. Nodular fasciitis of the breast: report of a case initially diagnosed by fine needle aspiration cytology. *Acta Cytol*. 2001;45:794-796.
51. Squillaci S, Tallarigo F, Patarino R, et al. Nodular fasciitis of the male breast: a case report. *Int J Surg Pathol*. 2007;15:69-72.
52. Iwatani T, Kawabata H, Miura D, et al. Nodular fasciitis of the breast. *Breast Cancer*. 2012;19:180-182.
53. Cloutier JM, Kunder CA, Charville GW, et al. Nodular fasciitis of the breast: clinicopathologic and molecular characterization with identification of novel USP6 fusion partners. *Mod Pathol*. 2021;34:1865-1875.
54. Erickson-Johnson MR, Chou MM, Evers BR, et al. Nodular fasciitis: a novel model of transient neoplasia induced by MYH9-USP6 gene fusion. *Lab Invest*. 2011;91:1427-1433.
55. Hamele-Bena D, Cranor ML, Sciotto C, et al. Uncommon presentation of mammary myofibroblastoma. *Mod Pathol*. 1996;9:786-790.
56. Magro G, Bisceglia M, Michal M, et al. Spindle cell lipoma-like tumor, solitary fibrous tumor and myofibroblastoma of the breast: a clinico-pathological analysis of 13 cases in favor of a unifying histogenetic concept. *Virchows Arch*. 2002;440:249-260.
57. Soyer T, Ayva S, Senyucel MF, et al. Myofibroblastoma of breast in a male infant. *Fetal Pediatr Pathol*. 2012;31:164-168.
58. Abeysekara AM, Siriwardana HP, Abbas KF, et al. An unusually large myofibroblastoma in a breast: a case report. *J Med Case Rep*. 2008;2:157.
59. Viswanathan K, Cheng E, Linver MN, et al. Bilateral multiple mammary myofibroblastomas in an adult male. *Int J Surg Pathol*. 2018;26:242-244.
60. Toker C, Tang CK, Whitely JF, et al. Benign spindle cell breast tumor. *Cancer*. 1981;48:1615-1622.
61. Lee EJ, Chang YW, Jin YM, et al. Multimodality images of myofibroblastoma in the male breast: a case report and a review of the literature. *Clin Imaging*. 2018;51:300-306.
62. Laasri K, Marrakchi S, Halfi IM, et al. Male breast myofibroblastoma: imaging features and ultrasound-guided core biopsy diagnosis. *Radiol Case Rep*. 2023;18:830-834.
63. Kataria K, Srivastava A, Singh L, et al. Giant myofibroblastoma of the male breast: a case report and literature review. *Malays J Med Sci*. 2012;19:74-76.
64. Bharathi K, Chandrasekar VA, Hemanathan G, et al. Myofibroblastoma of female breast masquerading as scirrhous malignancy—a rare case report with review of literature. *J Clin Diagn Res*. 2014;8:ND10-ND11.
65. Magro G, Amico P, Gurrera A. Myxoid myofibroblastoma of the breast with atypical cells: a potential diagnostic pitfall. *Virchows Arch*. 2007;450:483-485.
66. Akiya M, Osako T, Morizono H, et al. Myofibroblastoma of the breast showing rare palisaded morphology and uncommon desmin- and CD34-negative immunophenotype: a case report. *Pathol Int*. 2021;71:548-555.
67. Magro G, Foschini MP, Eusebi V. Palisaded myofibroblastoma of the breast: a tumor closely mimicking schwannoma: report of 2 cases. *Hum Pathol*. 2013;44:1941-1946.
68. D'Alfonso TM, Scognamiglio T. Myofibroblastoma with chondroid metaplasia. *Breast J*. 2013;19:549-551.
69. D'Alfonso TM, Subramaniyam S, Ginter PS, et al. Characterization of the leiomyomatous variant of myofibroblastoma: a rare subset distinct from other smooth muscle tumors of the breast. *Hum Pathol*. 2016;58:54-61.
70. Strait AM, Bridge JA, Iafrate AJ, et al. Mammary-type myofibroblastoma with leiomyomatous differentiation: a rare variant with potential pitfalls. *Int J Surg Pathol*. 2022;30:200-206.
71. Magro G. Epithelioid-cell myofibroblastoma of the breast: expanding the morphologic spectrum. *Am J Surg Pathol*. 2009;33:1085-1092.
72. Arafah MA, Ginter PS, D'Alfonso TM, et al. Epithelioid mammary myofibroblastoma mimicking invasive lobular carcinoma. *Int J Surg Pathol*. 2015;23:284-288.
73. Magro G, Gangemi P, Greco P. Deciduoid-like myofibroblastoma of the breast: a potential pitfall of malignancy. *Histopathology*. 2008;52:652-654.
74. Magro G, Salvatorelli L, Spadola S, et al. Mammary myofibroblastoma with extensive myxoedematous stromal changes: a potential diagnostic pitfall. *Pathol Res Pract*. 2014;210:1106-1111.
75. Magro G, Longo FR, Salvatorelli L, et al. Lipomatous myofibroblastoma of the breast: case report with diagnostic and histogenetic considerations. *Pathologica*. 2014;106:36-40.
76. Magro G, Michal M, Vasquez E, et al. Lipomatous myofibroblastoma: a potential diagnostic pitfall in the spectrum of the spindle cell lesions of the breast. *Virchows Arch*. 2000;437:540-544.
77. D'Alfonso TM, Subramaniyam S, Ginter PS, et al. Characterization of CD34-deficient myofibroblastomas of the breast. *Breast J*. 2018;24:55-61.
78. Chen BJ, Marino-Enriquez A, Fletcher CD, et al. Loss of retinoblastoma protein expression in spindle cell/pleomorphic lipomas and cytogenetically related tumors: an immunohistochemical study with diagnostic implications. *Am J Surg Pathol*. 2012;36:1119-1128.
79. Fritchie KJ, Carver P, Sun Y, et al. Solitary fibrous tumor: is there a molecular relationship with cellular angiofibroma, spindle cell lipoma, and mammary-type myofibroblastoma? *Am J Clin Pathol*. 2012;137:963-970.
80. Magro G, Righi A, Casorzo L, et al. Mammary and vaginal myofibroblastomas are genetically related lesions: fluorescence in situ hybridization analysis shows deletion of 13q14 region. *Hum Pathol*. 2012;43:1887-1893.
81. Pauwels P, Sciot R, Croiset F, et al. Myofibroblastoma of the breast: genetic link with spindle cell lipoma. *J Pathol*. 2000;191:282-285.
82. Trepant AL, Sibille C, Frunza AM, et al. Myofibroblastoma of the breast with smooth muscle differentiation showing deletion of 13q14 region: report of a case. *Pathol Res Pract*. 2014;210:389-391.
83. Magro G, Angelico G, Righi A, et al. Utility of STAT6 and 13q14 deletion in the classification of the benign spindle cell stromal tumors of the breast. *Hum Pathol*. 2018;81:55-64.
84. Ibrahim HA, Shousha S. Myofibroblastoma of the female breast with admixed but distinct foci of spindle cell lipoma: a case report. *Case Rep Pathol*. 2013;2013:738014.
85. Wahbah MM, Gilcrease MZ, Wu Y. Lipomatous variant of myofibroblastoma with epithelioid features: a rare and diagnostically challenging breast lesion. *Ann Diagn Pathol*. 2011;15:454-458.

86. Hoda RS, Duckworth LA, Gilmore HL, et al. Solitary fibrous tumor of breast and axilla. *Int J Surg Pathol*. 2023. (in press).
87. Koukourakis G, Filopoulos E, Kapatou K, et al. Hemangiopericytoma of the breast: a case report and a review of the literature. *Case Rep Oncol Med*. 2015;2015:210643.
88. Dragoumis D, Desiris K, Kyropoulou A, et al. Hemangiopericytoma/solitary fibrous tumor of pectoralis major muscle mimicking a breast mass. *Int J Surg Case Rep*. 2013;4:338-341.
89. Park BN, Woo OH, Kim C, et al. Recurrent solitary fibrous tumor of the breast: magnetic resonance imaging and pathologic findings. *Breast J*. 2018;24:1064-1065.
90. Mittal KR, Gerald W, True LD. Hemangiopericytoma of breast: report of a case with ultrastructural and immunohistochemical findings. *Hum Pathol*. 1986;17:1181-1183.
91. Callery CD, Rosen PP, Kinne DW. Sarcoma of the breast. A study of 32 patients with reappraisal of classification and therapy. *Ann Surg*. 1985;201:527-532.
92. Yang LH, Dai SD, Li QC, et al. Malignant solitary fibrous tumor of breast: a rare case report. *Int J Clin Exp Pathol*. 2014;7:4461-4466.
93. Cheah AL, Billings SD, Goldblum JR, et al. STAT6 rabbit monoclonal antibody is a robust diagnostic tool for the distinction of solitary fibrous tumour from its mimics. *Pathology*. 2014;46:389-395.
94. Ruhland B, Dittmer C, Thill M, et al. Metastasized hemangiopericytoma of the breast: a rare case. *Arch Gynecol Obstet*. 2009;280:491-494.
95. Demicco EG, Wagner MJ, Maki RG, et al. Risk assessment in solitary fibrous tumors: validation and refinement of a risk stratification model. *Mod Pathol*. 2017;30:1433-1442.
96. Roy AD, Nishant K, Joshi D. Painful late recurrence of dermatofibrosarcoma protuberans of breast in a Centurion female. *J Clin Diagn Res*. 2013;7:2278-2279.
97. Kim MS, Kim KS, Han HY, et al. Fibrosarcomatous transformation in dermatofibrosarcoma protuberans of the breast—a case report. *J Clin Ultrasound*. 2009;37:420-423.
98. Bishnoi A, De D, Parsad D, et al. Dermatofibrosarcoma protuberans—a rare lesion on breast. *Breast J*. 2018;24:664-665.
99. Lin CT, Chang SC, Chen TM, et al. Postradiation dermatofibrosarcoma protuberans: case report and literature review. *Acta Chir Belg*. 2015;115:87-90.
100. Liu SZ, Ho TL, Hsu SM, et al. Imaging of dermatofibrosarcoma protuberans of breast. *Breast J*. 2010;16:541-543.
101. Pernicone E, Fabrega-Foster K. Breast imaging findings in dermatofibrosarcoma protuberans: a case report and review of literature. *Cureus*. 2022;14:e30175.
102. Lee HJ, Kim MJ, Choi J, et al. Dermatofibrosarcoma protuberans arising on the skin of the breast. *Breast J*. 2011;17:93-95.
103. Lee SJ, Mahoney MC, Shaughnessy E. Dermatofibrosarcoma protuberans of the breast: imaging features and review of the literature. *AJR Am J Roentgenol*. 2009;193:W64-W69.
104. Tsang AK, Wong FC, Ng PW, et al. Fine needle aspiration cytology of dermatofibrosarcoma protuberans in the breast: a case report. *Pathology*. 2005;37:84-86.
105. Sin FN, Wong KW. Dermatofibrosarcoma protuberans of the breast: a case report. *Clin Imaging*. 2011;35:398-400.
106. Ahmed AA, Ostlie D, Fraser JD, et al. Dermatofibrosarcoma protuberans in the breast of a 2-year-old girl. *Ann Diagn Pathol*. 2010;14:279-283.
107. Kim T, Choi YL, Park HY, et al. Dermatofibrosarcoma protuberans of the breast skin. *Pathol Int*. 2010;60:784-786.
108. Dickson BC, Hornick JL, Fletcher CDM, et al. Dermatofibrosarcoma protuberans with a novel COL6A3-PDGFD fusion gene and apparent predilection for breast. *Genes Chromosomes Cancer*. 2018;57:437-445.
109. Saiag P, Grob JJ, Lebbe C, et al. Diagnosis and treatment of dermatofibrosarcoma protuberans. European consensus-based interdisciplinary guideline. *Eur J Cancer*. 2015;51:2604-2608.
110. Swan MC, Banwell PE, Hollowood K, et al. Late recurrence of dermatofibrosarcoma protuberans in the female breast: a case report. *Br J Plast Surg*. 2005;58:84-87.
111. Fujii T, Yajima R, Morita H, et al. A rare case of anterior chest wall schwannoma masquerading as a breast tumor. *Int Surg*. 2014;99:196-199.
112. Datta S, Pal A, Maiti M, et al. Rare case of chest wall schwannoma with destruction of rib, masquerading as a breast mass. *J Clin Diagn Res*. 2014;8:FD01-FD02.
113. Cho YR, Jones S, Gosain AK. Neurofibromatosis: a cause of prepubertal gynecomastia. *Plast Reconstr Surg*. 2008;121:34e-40e.
114. Yadav KK, Poudel N, Acharya K, et al. Right breast schwannoma in a male: a rare case report. *Int J Surg Case Rep*. 2022;99:107667.
115. Tahir M, Zedan M, Bellamkonda V, et al. Primary malignant peripheral nerve sheath tumor of the breast: a rare case report and review of literature. *Cureus*. 2022;14:e31586.
116. Bellezza G, Lombardi T, Panzarola P, et al. Schwannoma of the breast: a case report and review of the literature. *Tumori*. 2007;93:308-311.
117. Uchida N, Yokoo H, Kuwano H. Schwannoma of the breast: report of a case. *Surg Today*. 2005;35:238-242.
118. Thejaswini M, Padmaja K, Srinivasamurthy V, et al. Solitary intramammary schwannoma mimicking phyllodes tumor: cytological clues in the diagnosis. *J Cytol*. 2012;29:258-260.
119. Salihoglu A, Esatoglu SN, Eskazan AE, et al. Breast schwannoma in a patient with diffuse large B-cell lymphoma: a case report. *J Med Case Rep*. 2012;6:423.
120. Lee EK, Kook SH, Kwag HJ, et al. Schwannoma of the breast showing massive exophytic growth: a case report. *Breast*. 2006;15:562-566.
121. Galant C, Mazy S, Berliere M, et al. Two schwannomas presenting as lumps in the same breast. *Diagn Cytopathol*. 1997;16:281-284.
122. Gultekin SH, Cody HS 3rd, Hoda SA. Schwannoma of the breast. *South Med J*. 1996;89:238-239.
123. Casey P, Stephens M, Kirby RM. A rare cystic breast lump—schwannoma of the breast. *Breast J*. 2012;18:491-492.
124. Bongiorno MR, Doukaki S, Arico M. Neurofibromatosis of the nipple-areolar area: a case series. *J Med Case Rep*. 2010;4:22.
125. Friedrich RE, Hagel C. Appendices of the nipple and areola of the breast in Neurofibromatosis type 1 patients are neurofibromas. *Anticancer Res*. 2010;30:1815-1817.
126. Gokalp G, Hakyemez B, Kizilkaya E, et al. Myxoid neurofibromas of the breast: mammographical, sonographical and MRI appearances. *Br J Radiol*. 2007;80:e234-e237.
127. Cheng E, Viswanathan K, Hoda S. Solitary neurofibroma of the breast, and "The Man From Istanbul" syndrome. *Int J Surg Pathol*. 2018;26:153-154.
128. Hero E, Carey M, Hero I, et al. Bilateral neurofibromas of the nipple-areolar complex: a case report and approach to diagnosis. *Case Rep Pathol*. 2018;2018:6702561.
129. Brown AC, Audisio RA, Regitnig P. Granular cell tumour of the breast. *Surg Oncol*. 2011;20:97-105.
130. Papalas JA, Wylie JD, Dash RC. Recurrence risk and margin status in granular cell tumors of the breast: a clinicopathologic study of 13 patients. *Arch Pathol Lab Med*. 2011;135:890-895.
131. Desimone RA, Ginter PS, Chen YT. Granular cell tumor of the breast eliciting exuberant pseudoepitheliomatous hyperplasia. *Int J Surg Pathol*. 2014;22:156-157.
132. Coates SJ, Mitchell K, Olorunnipa OB, et al. An unusual breast lesion: granular cell tumor of the breast with extensive chest wall invasion. *J Surg Oncol*. 2014;110:345-347.
133. Adeniran A, Al-Ahmadie H, Mahoney MC, et al. Granular cell tumor of the breast: a series of 17 cases and review of the literature. *Breast J*. 2004;10:528-531.
134. Gibbons D, Leitch M, Coscia J, et al. Fine needle aspiration cytology and histologic findings of granular cell tumor of the breast: review of 19 cases with clinical/radiologic correlation. *Breast J*. 2000;6:27-30.
135. Patel HB, Leibman AJ. Granular cell tumor in a male breast: mammographic, sonographic, and pathologic features. *J Clin Ultrasound*. 2013;41:119-121.
136. Matrai Z, Langmar Z, Szabo E, et al. Granular cell tumour of the breast: case series and review of the literature. *Eur J Gynaecol Oncol*. 2010;31:636-640.
137. Stavros AT. *Breast Ultrasound*. 1st ed. Lippincott Williams & Wilkins; 2004.
138. Scaranelo AM, Bukhanov K, Crystal P, et al. Granular cell tumour of the breast: MRI findings and review of the literature. *Br J Radiol*. 2007;80:970-974.
139. Rekhi B, Jambhekar NA. Morphologic spectrum, immunohistochemical analysis, and clinical features of a series of granular cell tumors of soft tissues: a study from a tertiary referral cancer center. *Ann Diagn Pathol*. 2010;14:162-167.
140. Chen J, Wang L, Xu J, et al. Malignant granular cell tumor with breast metastasis: a case report and review of the literature. *Oncol Lett*. 2012;4:63-66.
141. Mir F, Alnajar H, Rohra P, et al. Metastatic granular cell tumor to the breast diagnosed by fine needle aspiration cytology: a case report with review of the literature. *Diagn Cytopathol*. 2019;47:226-229.
142. Nascimento AG, Karas M, Rosen PP, et al. Leiomyoma of the nipple. *Am J Surg Pathol*. 1979;3:151-154.
143. Cho HJ, Kim SH, Kang BJ, et al. Leiomyoma of the nipple diagnosed by MRI. *Acta Radiol Short Rep*. 2012;1:arsr.2012.120025.
144. Granic M, Stefanovic-Radovic M, Zdravkovic D, et al. Intraparenchymal leiomyoma of the breast. *Arch Iran Med*. 2015;18:608-612.
145. Long M, Hu XL, Zhao G, et al. Intraparenchymal breast leiomyoma and atypical leiomyoma. *BMC Women's Health*. 2022;22:119.
146. Minami S, Matsuo S, Azuma T, et al. Parenchymal leiomyoma of the breast: a case report with special reference to magnetic resonance imaging findings and an update review of literature. *Breast Cancer*. 2011;18:231-236.
147. Thakur V, Kumar S, Aggarwal D, et al. Leiomyoma cutis of breast. *Breast J*. 2020;26:1853-1854.
148. Zhong E, Swistel A, Viswanathan K, et al. Leiomyoma of the nipple: a common neoplasm in an uncommon location. *Breast J*. 2020;26:529-530.
149. Strader LA, Galan K, Tenofsky PL. Intraparenchymal leiomyoma of the male breast. *Breast J*. 2013;19:675-676.
150. Pavlidis L, Vakirlis E, Spyropoulou GA, et al. A 35-year-old woman presenting with an unusual post-traumatic leiomyoma of the nipple: a case report. *J Med Case Rep*. 2013;7:49.
151. Wang H, Luo B, Li F. Nipple inversion caused by a breast leiomyoma. *Breast J*. 2012;18:376-377.
152. Deveci U, Kapakli MS, Altintoprak F, et al. Bilateral nipple leiomyoma. *Case Rep Surg*. 2013;2013:475215.
153. Nakamura S, Hashimoto Y, Takeda K, et al. Two cases of male nipple leiomyoma: idiopathic leiomyoma and gynecomastia-associated leiomyoma. *Am J Dermatopathol*. 2012;34:287-291.
154. Alawad AA. Multiple parenchymal leiomyomas of the breast in a Sudanese female. *Breast Dis*. 2014;34:165-167.
155. Carter CS, Skala SL, Chinnaiyan AM, et al. Immunohistochemical characterization of fumarate hydratase (FH) and succinate dehydrogenase (SDH) in

155. cutaneous leiomyomas for detection of familial cancer syndromes. *Am J Surg Pathol.* 2017;41:801-809.

156. Brandao RG, Elias S, Pinto Nazario AC, et al. Leiomyoma of the breast parenchyma: a case report and review of the literature. *Sao Paulo Med J.* 2018;136:177-181.

157. Roncaroli F, Rossi R, Severi B, et al. Epithelioid leiomyoma of the breast with granular cell change: a case report. *Hum Pathol.* 1993;24:1260-1263.

158. Vecchio GM, Cavaliere A, Cartaginese F, et al. Intraparenchymal leiomyoma of the breast: report of a case with emphasis on needle core biopsy-based diagnosis. *Pathologica.* 2013;105:122-127.

159. Lopez V, Lopez I, Alcacer J, et al. Successful treatment of leiomyoma of the nipple with carbon dioxide laser. *Actas Dermosifiliogr.* 2013;104:928-930.

160. Zhang S, Wang L, Yang J, et al. Ultrasound-guided microwave ablation for giant breast leiomyoma: a case report. *Front Oncol.* 2023;13:1095891.

161. Boscaino A, Ferrara G, Orabona P, et al. Smooth muscle tumors of the breast: clinicopathologic features of two cases. *Tumori.* 1994;80:241-245.

162. Amberger M, Park T, Petersen B, et al. Primary breast leiomyosarcoma with metastases to the lung in a young adult: case report and literature review. *Int J Surg Case Rep.* 2018;47:34-37.

163. Fujita N, Kimura R, Yamamura J, et al. Leiomyosarcoma of the breast: a case report and review of the literature about therapeutic management. *Breast.* 2011;20:389-393.

164. Rane SU, Batra C, Saikia UN. Primary leiomyosarcoma of breast in an adolescent girl: a case report and review of the literature. *Case Rep Pathol.* 2012;2012:491984.

165. Alessi E, Sala F. Leiomyosarcoma in ectopic areola. *Am J Dermatopathol.* 1992;14:165-169.

166. Vasan N, Saglam O, Killelea BK. Metastatic leiomyosarcoma presenting as bilateral, multifocal breast masses. *BMJ Case Rep.* 2012;2012:bcr2012007188.

167. Cheikh TE, Hamza K, Hicham B, et al. Leiomyosarcoma of the male breast: case report. *Ann Med Surg (Lond).* 2021;67:102495.

168. Liu Y, Wang J, Su R, et al. Postoperative radiotherapy-induced leiomyosarcoma in breast cancer: a case report and literature review. *Breast Cancer.* 2020;27:780-784.

169. Zhang W, Qu X, Fang Y. Recurrent radiation-associated leiomyosarcoma after postoperative radiotherapy for breast invasive ductal carcinoma: a case report and literature review. *Ann Palliat Med.* 2021;10:8467-8473.

170. Heim-Hall J, Yohe SL. Application of immunohistochemistry to soft tissue neoplasms. *Arch Pathol Lab Med.* 2008;132:476-489.

171. Testori A, Meroni S, Voulaz E, et al. Primary breast leiomyosarcoma and synchronous homolateral lung cancer: a case report. *J Thorac Dis.* 2017;9:E1054-E1059.

172. Beck AH, Lee CH, Witten DM, et al. Discovery of molecular subtypes in leiomyosarcoma through integrative molecular profiling. *Oncogene.* 2010;29:845-854.

173. Agrawal P, Garg N, Pandey BB. Primary leiomyosarcoma of the breast: a rare case report. *Arch Breast Cancer.* 2015;2:100-103.

174. Naveed S, Panjwani G, Qari H, et al. Primary leiomyosarcoma of the breast with axillary nodal metastasis: a case report and review of literature. *World J Med Surg Case Rep.* 2016;5:9-13.

175. Groh O, In't Hof K. Giant lipoma of the male breast: case report and review of literature. *Eur J Plast Surg.* 2012;35:407-409.

176. Schmidt J, Schelling M, Lerf B, et al. Giant lipoma of the breast. *Breast J.* 2009;15:107-108.

177. Li YF, Lv MH, Chen LF, et al. Giant lipoma of the breast: a case report and review of the literature. *Clin Breast Cancer.* 2011;11:420-422.

178. Pui MH, Movson IJ. Fatty tissue breast lesions. *Clin Imaging.* 2003;27:150-155.

179. Riley MP, Karamchandani DM. Mammary hibernoma: a rare entity. *Arch Pathol Lab Med.* 2015;139:1565-1567.

180. Banev SG, Filipovski VA. Chondrolipoma of the breast—case report and a review of literature. *Breast.* 2006;15:425-426.

181. Shintaku M, Yamamoto Y, Nono F, et al. Chondrolipoma of the breast as a rare variant of myofibroblastoma: an immunohistochemical study of two cases. *Virchows Arch.* 2017;471:531-535.

182. Jaffar R, Zaheer S, Vasenwala SM, et al. Spindle cell lipoma breast. *Indian J Pathol Microbiol.* 2008;51:234-236.

183. Dilege E, Bozkurt E, Kulle CB, et al. A rare tumor of the male breast "angiolipoma" case report and review of literature. *Ann Ital Chir.* 2022;11:S2239253X22036945.

184. Noel JC, Van Geertruyden J, Engohan-Aloghe C. Angiolipoma of the breast in a male: a case report and review of the literature. *Int J Surg Pathol.* 2011;19:813-816.

185. Hofvander J, Arbajian E, Stenkula KG, et al. Frequent low-level mutations of protein kinase D2 in angiolipoma. *J Pathol.* 2017;241:578-582.

186. Briski LM, Jorns JM. Primary breast atypical lipomatous tumor/well-differentiated liposarcoma and dedifferentiated liposarcoma. *Arch Pathol Lab Med.* 2018;142:268-274.

187. Yin M, Mackley HB, Drabick JJ, et al. Primary female breast sarcoma: clinicopathological features, treatment and prognosis. *Sci Rep.* 2016;6:31497.

188. Giselle HP, Mariana CB, Cintia F, et al. Liposarcoma of the chest wall mimicking a breast mass in a man: a case report. *Radiol Case Rep.* 2021;16:3400-3405.

189. Singh BK, Pol MM, Toshib GA, et al. Pleomorphic liposarcoma of the male breast: lessons from a rare malignancy during COVID-19 pandemic. *BMJ Case Rep.* 2021;14:e244056.

190. Nandipati KC, Nerkar H, Satterfield J, et al. Pleomorphic liposarcoma of the breast mimicking breast abscess in a 19-year-old postpartum female: a case report and review of the literature. *Breast J.* 2010;16:537-540.

191. Yokouchi M, Nagano S, Kijima Y, et al. Solitary breast metastasis from myxoid liposarcoma. *BMC Cancer.* 2014;14:482.

192. Wang J, Wang WL, Sun H, et al. Expression of TRPS1 in phyllodes tumor and sarcoma of the breast. *Hum Pathol.* 2022;121:73-80.

193. Kanojia D, Nagata Y, Garg M, et al. Genomic landscape of liposarcoma. *Oncotarget.* 2015;6:42429-42444.

194. Inyang A, Thomas DG, Jorns J. Heterologous liposarcomatous differentiation in malignant phyllodes tumor is histologically similar but immunohistochemically and molecularly distinct from well-differentiated liposarcoma of soft tissue. *Breast J.* 2016;22:282-286.

195. Lyle PL, Bridge JA, Simpson JF, et al. Liposarcomatous differentiation in malignant phyllodes tumours is unassociated with MDM2 or CDK4 amplification. *Histopathology.* 2016;68:1040-1045.

196. Panagopoulos I, Hoglund M, Mertens F, et al. Fusion of the EWS and CHOP genes in myxoid liposarcoma. *Oncogene.* 1996;12:489-494.

197. Vourtsi A, Zervoudis S, Pafiti A, et al. Male breast hemangioma—a rare entity: a case report and review of the literature. *Breast J.* 2006;12:260-262.

198. Glazebrook KN, Morton MJ, Reynolds C. Vascular tumors of the breast: mammographic, sonographic, and MRI appearances. *AJR Am J Roentgenol.* 2005;184:331-338.

199. Mesurolle B, Sygal V, Lalonde L, et al. Sonographic and mammographic appearances of breast hemangioma. *AJR Am J Roentgenol.* 2008;191:W17-W22.

200. Aslan O, Oktay A, Serin G, et al. Breast hemangioma evaluation with magnetic resonance imaging: a rare case report. *Eur J Breast Health.* 2022;18:190-194.

201. Lafci O, Oztekin PS, Kosar PN. Cavernous hemangioma of the breast: radiologic and pathologic findings. *Breast J.* 2020;26:531-533.

202. Courcoutsakis NA, Hill SC, Chow CK, et al. Breast hemangiomas in a patient with Kasabach-Merritt syndrome: imaging findings. *AJR Am J Roentgenol.* 1997;169:1397-1399.

203. Jozefczyk MA, Rosen PP. Vascular tumors of the breast. II. Perilobular hemangiomas and hemangiomas. *Am J Surg Pathol.* 1985;9:491-503.

204. Rosen PP, Ridolfi RL. The perilobular hemangioma. A benign microscopic vascular lesion of the breast. *Am J Clin Pathol.* 1977;68:21-23.

205. Lesueur GC, Brown RW, Bhathal PS. Incidence of perilobular hemangioma in the female breast. *Arch Pathol Lab Med.* 1983;107:308-310.

206. Gopal SV, Nayak P, Dharanipragada K, et al. Breast hemangioma simulating an inflammatory carcinoma. *Breast J.* 2005;11:498-499.

207. Tuan HX, Duc NM, Huy NA, et al. Giant breast cavernous hemangioma. *Radiol Case Rep.* 2023;18:697-700.

208. Rosen PP, Jozefczyk MA, Boram LH. Vascular tumors of the breast. IV. The venous hemangioma. *Am J Surg Pathol.* 1985;9:659-665.

209. Hoda SA, Cranor ML, Rosen PP. Hemangiomas of the breast with atypical histological features. Further analysis of histological subtypes confirming their benign character. *Am J Surg Pathol.* 1992;16:553-560.

210. Zhang H, Han M, Varma K, et al. Follow-up outcomes of benign vascular lesions of breast diagnosed on core needle biopsy: a study of 117 cases. *Breast J.* 2019;25:401-407.

211. Rosen PP. Vascular tumors of the breast. III. Angiomatosis. *Am J Surg Pathol.* 1985;9:652-658.

212. Ginter PS, McIntire PJ, Irshaid L, et al. Angiomatosis of the breast: a clinicopathological and immunophenotypical characterisation of seven cases. *J Clin Pathol.* 2019;72:597-602.

213. Mekhail Y, Prather A, Hanna C, et al. Focal angiomatosis of the breast with MRI and histologic features. *Radiol Case Rep.* 2017;12:219-222.

214. Guilbert MC, Frost EP, Brock JE, et al. Distinguishing papillary endothelial hyperplasia and angiosarcoma on core needle biopsy of the breast: the importance of clinical and radiologic correlation. *Breast J.* 2018;24:487-492.

215. Branton PA, Lininger R, Tavassoli FA. Papillary endothelial hyperplasia of the breast: the great impostor for angiosarcoma: a clinicopathologic review of 17 cases. *Int J Surg Pathol.* 2003;11:83-87.

216. Klonk I, Povoski SP, Tozbikian G, et al. Masson's tumor of the reconstructed breast. *Radiol Case Rep.* 2023;18:1748-1753.

217. Lorente-Ramos RM, Azpeitia Arman J, Martinez Izquierdo MA, et al. Papillary endothelial hyperplasia (Masson's tumor) developed in the capsule of the implant in a breast cancer patient treated with mastectomy and radiation therapy. *J Clin Ultrasound.* 2020;48:222-226.

218. Khazai L, Chau A, Hoover S, et al. Papillary endothelial hyperplasia arising in the irradiated breast: a diagnostic dilemma. *Pathol Res Pract.* 2016;212:604-607.

219. Fineberg S, Rosen PP. Cutaneous angiosarcoma and atypical vascular lesions of the skin and breast after radiation therapy for breast carcinoma. *Am J Clin Pathol.* 1994;102:757-763.

220. Patton KT, Deyrup AT, Weiss SW. Atypical vascular lesions after surgery and radiation of the breast: a clinicopathologic study of 32 cases analyzing histologic heterogeneity and association with angiosarcoma. *Am J Surg Pathol.* 2008;32:943-950.

221. Santi R, Cetica V, Franchi A, et al. Tumour suppressor gene TP53 mutations in atypical vascular lesions of breast skin following radiotherapy. *Histopathology.* 2011;58:455-466.

222. Cornejo KM, Deng A, Wu H, et al. The utility of MYC and FLT4 in the diagnosis and treatment of postradiation atypical vascular lesion and angiosarcoma of the breast. *Hum Pathol.* 2015;46:868-875.

223. Fernandez AP, Sun Y, Tubbs RR, et al. FISH for MYC amplification and anti-MYC immunohistochemistry: useful diagnostic tools in the assessment of secondary angiosarcoma and atypical vascular proliferations. *J Cutan Pathol.* 2012;39:234-242.

224. Ginter PS, Mosquera JM, MacDonald TY, et al. Diagnostic utility of MYC amplification and anti-MYC immunohistochemistry in atypical vascular lesions, primary or radiation-induced mammary angiosarcomas, and primary angiosarcomas of other sites. *Hum Pathol.* 2014;45:709-716.

225. Guo T, Zhang L, Chang NE, et al. Consistent MYC and FLT4 gene amplification in radiation-induced angiosarcoma but not in other radiation-associated atypical vascular lesions. *Genes Chromosomes Cancer.* 2011;50:25-33.

226. Mentzel T, Schildhaus HU, Palmedo G, et al. Postradiation cutaneous angiosarcoma after treatment of breast carcinoma is characterized by MYC amplification in contrast to atypical vascular lesions after radiotherapy and control cases: clinicopathological, immunohistochemical and molecular analysis of 66 cases. *Mod Pathol.* 2012;25:75-85.

227. Mentzel T, Kiss K. Reduced H3K27me3 expression in radiation-associated angiosarcoma of the breast. *Virchows Arch.* 2018;472:361-368.

228. Gengler C, Coindre JM, Leroux A, et al. Vascular proliferations of the skin after radiation therapy for breast cancer: clinicopathologic analysis of a series in favor of a benign process: a study from the French Sarcoma Group. *Cancer.* 2007;109:1584-1598.

229. Baker GM, Schnitt SJ. Vascular lesions of the breast. *Semin Diagn Pathol.* 2017;34:410-419.

230. da Silva BB, Eulalio Filho WMN, Costa PVL, et al. A rare case of primary breast angiosarcoma in a male: a case report. *BMC Cancer.* 2018;18:978.

231. Rosen PP, Kimmel M, Ernsberger D. Mammary angiosarcoma. The prognostic significance of tumor differentiation. *Cancer.* 1988;62:2145-2151.

232. Wang ZS, Zhan N, Xiong CL, et al. Primary epithelioid angiosarcoma of the male breast: report of a case. *Surg Today.* 2007;37:782-786.

233. Donnell RM, Rosen PP, Lieberman PH, et al. Angiosarcoma and other vascular tumors of the breast. *Am J Surg Pathol.* 1981;5:629-642.

234. Cuesta-Mejias T, de Leon-Bojorge B, Abel de la Pena J, et al. [Breast angiosarcoma in a patient with multiple surgical procedures and breast implant. Report of a case]. *Ginecol Obstet Mex.* 2002;70:76-81.

235. Kotton DN, Muse VV, Nishino M. Case records of the Massachusetts General Hospital. Case 2-2012. A 63-year-old woman with dyspnea and rapidly progressive respiratory failure. *N Engl J Med.* 2012;366:259-269.

236. Takenaka M, Tanaka M, Isobe M, et al. Angiosarcoma of the breast with silicone granuloma: a case report. *Kurume Med J.* 2009;56:33-37.

237. West JG, Weitzel JN, Tao ML, et al. BRCA mutations and the risk of angiosarcoma after breast cancer treatment. *Clin Breast Cancer.* 2008;8:533-537.

238. Ooe Y, Terakawa H, Kawashima H, et al. Bilateral primary angiosarcoma of the breast: a case report. *J Med Case Rep.* 2023;17:60.

239. Yang WT, Hennessy BT, Dryden MJ, et al. Mammary angiosarcomas: imaging findings in 24 patients. *Radiology.* 2007;242:725-734.

240. Bentley H, Roberts J, Hayes M, et al. The role of imaging in the diagnosis of primary and secondary breast angiosarcoma: twenty-five-year experience of a provincial cancer institution. *Clin Breast Cancer.* 2023;23:e45-e53.

241. Glazebrook KN, Magut MJ, Reynolds C. Angiosarcoma of the breast. *AJR Am J Roentgenol.* 2008;190:533-538.

242. Darre T, Djiwa T, N'Timon B, et al. Breast primary angiosarcoma: a clinicopathologic and imaging study of a series cases. *Breast Cancer (Auckl).* 2022;16:11782234221086726.

243. Nascimento AF, Raut CP, Fletcher CD. Primary angiosarcoma of the breast: clinicopathologic analysis of 49 cases, suggesting that grade is not prognostic. *Am J Surg Pathol.* 2008;32:1896-1904.

244. Shin SJ, Lesser M, Rosen PP. Hemangiomas and angiosarcomas of the breast: diagnostic utility of cell cycle markers with emphasis on Ki-67. *Arch Pathol Lab Med.* 2007;131:538-544.

245. Wang L, Lao IW, Yu L, et al. Primary breast angiosarcoma: a retrospective study of 36 cases from a single Chinese medical institute with clinicopathologic and radiologic correlations. *Breast J.* 2017;23:282-291.

246. Kuba MG, Dermawan JK, Xu B, et al. Histopathologic grading is of prognostic significance in primary angiosarcoma of breast: proposal of a simplified 2-tier grading system. *Am J Surg Pathol.* 2023;47:307-317.

247. Hoda SA, Hoda RS. "Time shall unfold...": the clinical value of grading mammary angiosarcoma. *Am J Surg Pathol.* 2023;47:279-280.

248. Guarda LA, Ordonez NG, Smith JL, Jr., et al. Immunoperoxidase localization of factor VIII in angiosarcomas. *Arch Pathol Lab Med.* 1982;106:515-516.

249. *Churchill's Illustrated Medical Dictionary.* Churchill Livingstone; 1989.

250. Beca F, Krings G, Chen YY, et al. Primary mammary angiosarcomas harbor frequent mutations in KDR and PIK3CA and show evidence of distinct pathogenesis. *Mod Pathol.* 2020;33:1518-1526.

251. Painter CA, Jain E, Tomson BN, et al. The Angiosarcoma Project: enabling genomic and clinical discoveries in a rare cancer through patient-partnered research. *Nat Med.* 2020;26:181-187.

252. Antonescu CR, Yoshida A, Guo T, et al. KDR activating mutations in human angiosarcomas are sensitive to specific kinase inhibitors. *Cancer Res.* 2009;69:7175-7179.

253. Pandey M, Sutton GR, Giri S, et al. Grade and prognosis in localized primary angiosarcoma. *Clin Breast Cancer.* 2015;15:266-269.

254. Kaklamanos IG, Birbas K, Syrigos KN, et al. Breast angiosarcoma that is not related to radiation exposure: a comprehensive review of the literature. *Surg Today.* 2011;41:163-168.

255. Gutkin PM, Ganjoo KN, Lohman M, et al. Angiosarcoma of the breast: management and outcomes. *Am J Clin Oncol.* 2020;43:820-825.

256. Hoshina H, Kubouchi K, Tsutsumi Y, et al. Radiation-induced fibrosarcoma after breast-conserving therapy for breast cancer: a case report and literature review. *Surg Case Rep.* 2023;9:50.

257. Kokkali S, Moreno JD, Klijanienko J, et al. Clinical and molecular insights of radiation-induced breast sarcomas: is there hope on the horizon for effective treatment of this aggressive disease? *Int J Mol Sci.* 2022;23:4125.

258. Abbott R, Palmieri C. Angiosarcoma of the breast following surgery and radiotherapy for breast cancer. *Nat Clin Pract Oncol.* 2008;5:727-736.

259. Andrews S, Wilcoxon R, Benda J, et al. Angiosarcoma following MammoSite partial breast irradiation. *Breast Cancer Res Treat.* 2010;124:279-282.

260. Vorburger SA, Xing Y, Hunt KK, et al. Angiosarcoma of the breast. *Cancer.* 2005;104:2682-2688.

261. Strobbe LJ, Peterse HL, van Tinteren H, et al. Angiosarcoma of the breast after conservation therapy for invasive cancer, the incidence and outcome. An unforseen sequela. *Breast Cancer Res Treat.* 1998;47:101-109.

262. Billings SD, McKenney JK, Folpe AL, et al. Cutaneous angiosarcoma following breast-conserving surgery and radiation: an analysis of 27 cases. *Am J Surg Pathol.* 2004;28:781-788.

263. Mobini N. Cutaneous epithelioid angiosarcoma: a neoplasm with potential pitfalls in diagnosis. *J Cutan Pathol.* 2009;36:362-369.

264. Poellinger A, Landt S, Diekmann F, et al. Rapid growth of an exophytic angiosarcoma of the breast. *Breast J.* 2006;12:80-82.

265. Chesebro AL, Chikarmane SA, Gombos EC, et al. Radiation-associated angiosarcoma of the breast: what the radiologist needs to know. *AJR Am J Roentgenol.* 2016;207:217-225.

266. Salminen SH, Sampo MM, Bohling TO, et al. Radiation-associated angiosarcoma of the breast: analysis of diagnostic tools in a registry-based population. *Acta Radiol.* 2022;63:22-27.

267. Liu YC, Fung MA. Angiosarcoma with pseudoepidermotropism in a patient with breast cancer: a mimic of epidermotropic metastatic adenocarcinoma. *Am J Dermatopathol.* 2011;33:400-402.

268. Seo IS, Min KW. Postirradiation epithelioid angiosarcoma of the breast: a case report with immunohistochemical and electron microscopic study. *Ultrastruct Pathol.* 2003;27:197-203.

269. Sheu TG, Hunt KK, Middleton LP. MYC and NOTCH1-positive postradiation cutaneous angiosarcoma of the breast. *Breast J.* 2021;27:264-267.

270. Kluk MJ, Ashworth T, Wang H, et al. Gauging NOTCH1 activation in cancer using immunohistochemistry. *PLoS One.* 2013;8:e67306.

271. Kuba MG, Xu B, D'Angelo SP, et al. The impact of MYC gene amplification on the clinicopathological features and prognosis of radiation-associated angiosarcomas of the breast. *Histopathology.* 2021;79:836-846.

272. Fraga-Guedes C, Andre S, Mastropasqua MG, et al. Angiosarcoma and atypical vascular lesions of the breast: diagnostic and prognostic role of MYC gene amplification and protein expression. *Breast Cancer Res Treat.* 2015;151:131-140.

273. Torres KE, Ravi V, Kin K, et al. Long-term outcomes in patients with radiation-associated angiosarcomas of the breast following surgery and radiotherapy for breast cancer. *Ann Surg Oncol.* 2013;20:1267-1274.

274. Abdou Y, Elkhanany A, Attwood K, et al. Primary and secondary breast angiosarcoma: single center report and a meta-analysis. *Breast Cancer Res Treat.* 2019;178:523-533.

275. Seinen JM, Styring E, Verstappen V, et al. Radiation-associated angiosarcoma after breast cancer: high recurrence rate and poor survival despite surgical treatment with R0 resection. *Ann Surg Oncol.* 2012;19:2700-2706.

276. Morgan EA, Kozono DE, Wang Q, et al. Cutaneous radiation-associated angiosarcoma of the breast: poor prognosis in a rare secondary malignancy. *Ann Surg Oncol.* 2012;19:3801-3808.

277. Kumar V, Abbas AK, Aster JC. *Robbins Basic Pathology.* 10th ed. Elsevier; 2018.

278. Kapucuoglu N, Percinel S, Angelone A. Adenofibroma of the breast. *Virchows Arch.* 2008;452:351-352.

279. Herbert M, Sandbank J, Liokumovich P, et al. Breast hamartomas: clinicopathological and immunohistochemical studies of 24 cases. *Histopathology.* 2002;41:30-34.

280. Sevim Y, Kocaay AF, Eker T, et al. Breast hamartoma: a clinicopathologic analysis of 27 cases and a literature review. *Clinics (Sao Paulo).* 2014;69:515-523.

281. Alran L, Chamming's F, Auriol-Leizagoyen S, et al. Breast hamartoma: reassessment of an under-recognised breast lesion. *Histopathology.* 2022;80:304-313.

282. Birrell AL, Warren LR, Birrell SN. Misdiagnosis of massive breast asymmetry: giant hamartoma. *ANZ J Surg.* 2012;82:941-942.

283. Desai A, Ramesar K, Allan S, et al. Breast hamartoma arising in axillary ectopic breast tissue. *Breast J.* 2010;16:433-434.

284. Paraskevopoulos JA, Hosking SW, Stephenson T. Breast within a breast: a review of breast hamartomas. *Br J Clin Pract.* 1990;44:30-32.

285. Tse GM, Law BK, Ma TK, et al. Hamartoma of the breast: a clinicopathological review. *J Clin Pathol.* 2002;55:951-954.

286. Stafyla V, Kotsifopoulos N, Grigoriadis K, et al. Myoid hamartoma of the breast: a case report and review of the literature. *Breast J.* 2007;13:85-87.

287. Baranov E, Alston ELJ, Lester SC, et al. Angiomyxoma of the breast: a clinicopathologic analysis of 40 cases. *Am J Surg Pathol.* 2023;47:296-306.

288. Magro G, Cavanaugh B, Palazzo J. Clinico-pathological features of breast myxoma: report of a case with histogenetic considerations. *Virchows Arch.* 2010;456:581-586.

289. Rakha EA, Tan PH, Shaaban A, et al. Do primary mammary osteosarcoma and chondrosarcoma exist? A review of a large multi-institutional series of malignant matrix-producing breast tumours. *Breast*. 2013;22:13-18.

290. Neville G, Fletcher CD, Dillon D, et al. Are metaplastic carcinomas with osseous differentiation and primary osteosarcomas of the breast one and the same? (abstract 117) in "abstracts from USCAP 2021: Breast pathology". *Mod Pathol*. 2021;34(suppl 2):134-135.

291. Silver SA, Tavassoli FA. Primary osteogenic sarcoma of the breast: a clinicopathologic analysis of 50 cases. *Am J Surg Pathol*. 1998;22:925-933.

292. Trihia H, Valavanis C, Markidou S, et al. Primary osteogenic sarcoma of the breast: cytomorphologic study of 3 cases with histologic correlation. *Acta Cytol*. 2007;51:443-450.

293. Pasta V, Sottile D, Urciuoli P, et al. Rare chondrosarcoma of the breast treated with quadrantectomy instead of mastectomy: a case report. *Oncol Lett*. 2015;9:1116-1120.

294. Badyal RK, Kataria AS, Kaur M. Primary chondrosarcoma of male breast: a rare case. *Indian J Surg*. 2012;74:418-419.

295. Bartlett H, Elghobashy M, Deshmukh N, et al. Radiation-associated primary osteosarcoma of the breast. *Pathobiology*. 2020;87:322-326.

296. Tounsi N, Zemni I, Abdelwahed N, et al. Costal chondrosarcoma mimicking a breast cancer: case report and review of literature. *Int J Surg Case Rep*. 2019;56:37-39.

297. Lubana SS, Bashir T, Tuli SS, et al. Breast metastasis of extraskeletal myxoid chondrosarcoma: a case report. *Am J Case Rep*. 2015;16:406-414.

298. Krishnamurthy A. Primary breast osteosarcoma: a diagnostic challenge. *Indian J Nucl Med*. 2015;30:39-41.

299. Bennett DL, Merenda G, Schnepp S, et al. Primary breast osteosarcoma mimicking calcified fibroadenoma on screening digital breast tomosynthesis mammogram. *Radiol Case Rep*. 2017;12:648-652.

300. Mujtaba B, Nassar SM, Aslam R, et al. Primary osteosarcoma of the breast: pathophysiology and imaging review. *Curr Probl Diagn Radiol*. 2020;49:116-123.

301. Conner JR, Hornick JL. SATB2 is a novel marker of osteoblastic differentiation in bone and soft tissue tumours. *Histopathology*. 2013;63:36-49.

302. Adem C, Reynolds C, Ingle JN, et al. Primary breast sarcoma: clinicopathologic series from the Mayo Clinic and review of the literature. *Br J Cancer*. 2004;91:237-241.

303. Hartel PH, Bratthauer G, Hartel JV, et al. Primary malignant fibrous histiocytoma (myxofibrosarcoma/pleomorphic sarcoma not otherwise specified) of the breast: clinicopathologic study of 19 cases. *Ann Diagn Pathol*. 2011;15:407-413.

304. Jeong YJ, Oh HK, Bong JG. Undifferentiated pleomorphic sarcoma of the male breast causing diagnostic challenges. *J Breast Cancer*. 2011;14:241-246.

305. Komaei I, Guccione F, Sarra F, et al. Radiation-induced undifferentiated pleomorphic sarcoma of the breast: a rare but serious complication following breast-conserving therapy. A case report and literature review. *G Chir*. 2019;40:544-550.

306. Gambichler T, Horny K, Mentzel T, et al. Undifferentiated pleomorphic sarcoma of the breast with neoplastic fever: case report and genomic characterization. *J Cancer Res Clin Oncol*. 2023;149:1465-1471.

307. Hu Y, Li X, Deng Y, et al. Primary malignant fibrous histiocytoma of the breast: a case report and review of 38 Chinese cases. *Clin Breast Cancer*. 2012;12:382-385.

308. Yamazaki H, Shimizu S, Yoshida T, et al. A case of undifferentiated pleomorphic sarcoma of the breast with lung and bone metastases. *Int J Surg Case Rep*. 2018;51:143-146.

309. Li DL, Zhou RJ, Yang WT, et al. Rhabdomyosarcoma of the breast: a clinicopathologic study and review of the literature. *Chin Med J (Engl)*. 2012;125:2618-2622.

310. Shohdy KS, Attia H, Mahmoud N, et al. Primary primitive neuroectodermal tumor of the breast: analysis of clinical outcomes of twenty-one patients. *Breast J*. 2020;26:1893-1894.

311. Wu J, Brinker DA, Haas M, et al. Primary alveolar soft part sarcoma (ASPS) of the breast: report of a deceptive case with xanthomatous features confirmed by TFE3 immunohistochemistry and electron microscopy. *Int J Surg Pathol*. 2005;13:81-85.

312. Yoshitani K, Kido A, Honoki K, et al. Pelvic metastasis of breast synovial sarcoma. *J Orthop Sci*. 2009;14:219-223.

313. Lucin K, Mustac E, Jonjic N. Breast sarcoma showing myofibroblastic differentiation. *Virchows Arch*. 2003;443:222-224.

314. Hamed KA, Muller KE, Nawab RA. Kaposi's sarcoma of the breast. *AIDS Patient Care STDS*. 2000;14:85-88.

315. Hanfee AR, Ghazi KR, Ashfaq Z, et al. Primary follicular dendritic cell sarcoma of breast: 2 further cases with review of the literature. *Int J Surg Pathol*. 2022;30:55-62.

21

Lymphoid and Hematopoietic Tumors

ALIYAH R. SOHANI AND JUDITH A. FERRY

LYMPHOMAS OF THE BREAST

Primary lymphoma of the breast is defined as lymphoma involving one or both breasts with or without ipsilateral axillary lymph node involvement, without evidence of disease elsewhere at presentation, in a patient without a prior history of lymphoma (1). Some authorities also accept cases with more distant lymph node or bone marrow involvement, so long as clinically, the primary or major manifestation of the lymphoma is the breast (2). The breast is a very uncommon primary site for lymphoma, accounting for 0.1% to 0.15% (2-5) of all malignant neoplasms of the breast, for 0.34% to 0.85% of all non-Hodgkin lymphomas (2,4,6-8), and for less than 2% of all extranodal non-Hodgkin lymphomas (2).

Establishing a diagnosis based on a needle biopsy specimen presents special challenges in the diagnosis of lymphoma. For high-grade lymphomas with obvious cytologic atypia, needle biopsies are often adequate to establish a diagnosis. For low-grade lymphomas such as follicular lymphoma and extranodal marginal zone lymphoma of mucosa-associated lymphoid tissue (MALT lymphoma) that often have features overlapping with those of reactive, chronic inflammatory lymphoid proliferations, establishing a diagnosis on a needle biopsy may be difficult. In such instances, ancillary studies play a key role in diagnosis. Obtaining a larger specimen may also be required.

Clinical Features

Most patients are middle-aged to elderly women, although occasionally younger females and rarely males are affected (1,3-6,8-23). They typically present with a palpable breast mass, with or without ipsilateral axillary lymphadenopathy (4,6,15,17,20,21,23). A few patients have had the lymphoma detected by mammography; lymphomas detected initially by routine mammography are typically low-grade lymphomas (4,10,11,13). Constitutional symptoms are uncommon, being found in 0% (6,13,15,17,24) to 4% (19) of patients in different series. In some series, right-sided lymphoma was more common than left-sided lymphoma (23,25). Approximately 10% of primary breast lymphomas are bilateral (1,3,5,7,8,16,17,19,22-24,26). A few patients have a history of autoimmune disease, diabetes mellitus, mastitis (2,4,5,15), or human immunodeficiency virus (HIV) infection (27). However, most patients have no underlying illness, and specific factors predisposing to lymphoma of the breast are not identified (8,21,26). On physical examination, patients usually have discrete, mobile masses. The overlying skin is involved infrequently; it may be thickened (20), erythematous, or inflamed (3,28), mimicking inflammatory carcinoma. Skin retraction and nipple discharge are virtually never found. The proportion of cases with ipsilateral axillary lymphadenopathy varies widely among series from 11% (10) to about 50%.

Pathologic Features and Clinicopathologic Correlates

The specimen obtained must yield sufficient tissue to firmly establish a diagnosis (29). Excision is not required if a smaller biopsy is diagnostic. A diagnosis of lymphoma may be established by fine needle aspiration biopsy, but tissue for histopathology or at least a cell block is typically required to establish a complete diagnosis with subclassification (30). In most series, diffuse large B-cell lymphoma is the most common type, accounting for approximately 60% of cases (3-7,12,13,17,18,21,31,32). The remainder are mainly low-grade lymphomas (MALT lymphoma or follicular lymphoma). Burkitt lymphoma is uncommon. T-cell lymphoma is very rare (11,21). The breast is rarely involved by post-transplant lymphoproliferative disorders, which are usually high-grade B-lineage lymphomas (33).

Diffuse Large B-cell Lymphoma

Diffuse large B-cell lymphoma affects women (and a few men) across a wide age range (4,12,15,19,22,29), with a median age in the sixth decade (32). Lesions range from 1 to 20 cm in greatest dimension, with a median size of 4 to 5 cm. A few patients have diffuse breast enlargement (7,8,15,17,19,22,32). The tumors have been described as discrete, hard, rubbery (16), soft, or fleshy masses (3) that are sometimes rapidly enlarging (1,16,28).

The lymphomas are composed of a diffuse infiltrate of large lymphoid cells. Histologic and immunophenotypic features overlap with those seen in other sites **(Table 21.1)** (3,18,21,34). The lymphomas are CD45[+], CD20[+], with rare CD5[+] cases (22) and a relatively high Ki67 proliferation index (60%-95% in one series) (22). Most cases have a nongerminal center B-cell (non-GCB) immunophenotype (CD10[−],

TABLE 21.1
Hematolymphoid Neoplasms of the Breast: Principal Features

Type of Neoplasm	Patients Affected	Histology	Usual Immunophenotype of Neoplastic Cells	Genetic Features	Clinical Behavior
Diffuse large B-cell lymphoma	Adults, females >> males, broad age range; few pregnant	Diffuse proliferation of large lymphoid cells; CB more common than IB	CD45$^+$, CD20$^+$, CD10 usually−, BCL6$^{+/-}$, BCL2 and MUM1/IRF4 usually +, Ki67 high; EBV$^-$; non-GC > GC	Clonal *IGH*; *MYD88* L265P and *CD79B* mutations leading to NFκB pathway activation; *BCL6*, *BCL2*, *MYC* translocations rare to absent	Aggressive; CNS, opposite breast: common sites of relapse; best outcomes with R-CHOP or R-CHOP-like chemo +/− RT
Extranodal marginal zone lymphoma (MALT lymphoma)	Middle-aged and older adults; females >> males	Marginal zone B cells; plasma cells: few to many; reactive follicles may be present +/− follicular colonization. LELs not prominent. Rarely, amyloid deposition	CD45$^+$, CD20$^+$, CD5$^-$, CD10$^-$, CD23$^-$, CD43$^{+/-}$, BCL2$^{+/-}$, cyclin D1$^-$, cIg$^{+/-}$; Ki67 low except in reactive follicles	Clonal *IGH*; Rare *MALT1* rearrangements; minority of cases: trisomy 3, 12, and/or 18	Good prognosis. Localized extranodal relapses may occur. Few have large cell transformation. Few die of lymphoma.
Follicular lymphoma (FL)	Middle-aged and older women	Ill-defined follicles occupied by centrocytes and variable # of centroblasts; sclerosis is common	CD45$^+$, CD20$^+$, CD10$^+$, BCL6$^+$, CD5$^-$, CD23$^-$, CD43$^-$, BCL2$^+$, cyclin D1$^-$, sIg$^+$, occasionally BCL2$^-$	Translocation of *BCL2* with *IGH* [t(14;18)] in most cases. *EZH2* mutations in a subset of cases.	Prognosis less good than MALT lymphoma. Behavior similar to nodal FL
Burkitt lymphoma	Adolescent to middle-aged females, few older women, some pregnant or lactating	Diffuse infiltrate of medium-sized round cells, many mitoses, starry sky pattern	CD45$^+$, CD20$^+$, CD10$^+$, BCL6$^+$, BCL2$^-$, Ki67 ~100%[a]	Translocation of *MYC* with *IGH* [t(8;14)], less often with *IGK* or *IGL*; Endemic: EBV$^+$; sporadic or immunodeficiency-associated: EBV$^{-/+a}$	Very aggressive; disease is often widespread.
Mantle cell lymphoma	Middle-aged and older adults	Diffuse infiltrate of small to medium-sized centrocyte-like or blast-like cells; some cases with prominent nucleoli or pleomorphic nuclei	CD45$^+$, CD20$^+$, CD5$^+$, CD10$^+$, CD23$^-$, cyclin D1$^+$, SOX11$^+$	Translocation of *CCND1* with *IGH* [t(11;14)]; *TP53* mutations, LOH, or both confer a worse prognosis	Typically widespread disease, including bone marrow, blood, nodal, and other extranodal sites (GI tract and Waldeyer ring most common)
B- and T-lymphoblastic lymphoma/leukemia	Mostly adolescents and young adults, often with concurrent acute lymphoblastic leukemia involving bone marrow and/or blood	Diffuse infiltrate of small to medium-sized cells with oval or irregular nuclei, fine chromatin, small nucleoli, and scant cytoplasm	B-lineage: CD19$^+$, CD20$^-$/weak, CD10$^+$, TdT^{+a} T-lineage: Variable expression of T-cell markers, but often CD3$^+$, CD7$^+$, CD4$^+$/CD8$^+$ (double$^+$), CD1a$^+$, TdT^{+a}	Variable	Aggressive disease with relatively good prognosis depending on underlying genetic abnormalities, if optimally treated

TABLE 21.1
Hematolymphoid Neoplasms of the Breast: Principal Features (*continued*)

Type of Neoplasm	Patients Affected	Histology	Usual Immunophenotype of Neoplastic Cells	Genetic Features	Clinical Behavior
Breast implant-associated anaplastic large cell lymphoma (BIA-ALCL)	Women with textured (saline or silicone) implants, for cosmetic purposes or following mastectomy; lymphoma occurs years after implant; effusion rather than discrete mass	Large atypical, pleomorphic cells in a background of fibrosis, debris, and sometimes chronic inflammation	$CD30^+$, $ALK1^-$, $CD45^{-/+}$, $CD4^{+/-}$, $CD43^{+/-}$, $CD3^{-/+}$, $CD5^{-/+}$, $CD8^-$, $EMA^{+/-}$, $TIA1^{+/-}$, granzyme B +/−, EBV^-, $HHV8^-$	JAK/STAT pathway activating mutations, somatic and germline *TP53* mutations, PD-L1 amplification *TRG*: clonal, *IGH*: polyclonal No *ALK*, *DUSP22*, or *TP63* rearrangements seen in systemic or primary cutaneous ALCL	Very good prognosis in absence of a discrete mass or spread beyond breast
Classic Hodgkin lymphoma (CHL)	Rare; breast involvement virtually always secondary to lymph nodal disease	Reed-Sternberg cells and variants in a reactive background	$CD15^+$, $CD30^+$, $CD45^-$, weakly $PAX5^+$, $CD20^-$, $CD3^-$, $ALK1^-$	Variable including JAK/STAT and NFκB pathway activating mutations, PD-L1/PD-L2 copy number gains	Outcome likely similar to other CHL of same stage
Plasmacytoma	Rare; usually in setting of plasma cell myeloma; rarely isolated	Sheets of mature and/or immature plasma cells	$CD138^+$, $MUM1^+$, cIg^+, $EMA^{+/-}$, $CD45^{-/+}$, keratin$^-$	Variable abnormalities, including dup(1q); *TP53* LOH and/or mutations; *KRAS*, *NRAS*, and *MYC* abnormalities; and *IGH* rearrangements with various partners, including *CCND1*	Relatively poor in setting of myeloma, especially with adverse prognostic genetic abnormalities

CB, centroblastic; cIg, monotypic cytoplasmic immunoglobulin; CNS, central nervous system; EBV, Epstein-Barr virus; GC, germinal center immunophenotype; GI, gastrointestinal; IB, immunoblastic; *IGH*, immunoglobulin heavy chain gene; *IGK*, immunoglobulin kappa light chain gene; *IGL*, immunoglobulin lambda light chain gene; JAK/STAT, Janus kinase/signal transducer and activator of transcription; LELs, lymphoepithelial lesions; LOH, loss of heterozygosity; MALT, mucosa-associated lymphoid tissue; NFκB, nuclear factor kappa B; non-GC, nongerminal center immunophenotype; R-CHOP, rituximab, cyclophosphamide, Adriamycin, vincristine, prednisone; chemo: chemotherapy; RT, radiation therapy; sIg, monotypic surface immunoglobulin; *TRG*, T-cell receptor γ gene.

[a]Based in part on data on same types of lymphoma in other sites.

$BCL6^+$, $MUM1/IRF4^+$, or $CD10^-$, $BCL6^-$) **(Fig. 21.1)**, while a few have a germinal center B-cell (GCB) phenotype ($CD10^+$, $BCL6^+$ or $CD10^-$, $BCL6^+$, $MUM1/IRF4^-$) (21,29). In recent large series, 77% of the cases (32) and 95% of the cases (35) had a non-GCB immunophenotype. Immunohistochemical staining for p50 and p65 has shown nuclear localization of p50 in a minority, suggesting nuclear factor kappa B (NFκB) activation in a subset of cases (34). In situ hybridization for Epstein-Barr virus (EBV) using a probe for EBV-encoded small RNAs (EBER) is typically negative

(22), although rare cases of EBV^+ large B-cell lymphoma arising adjacent to breast implants have been reported (see the section on Lymphomas of the Breast in Association With Implants). As is true of other nongerminal center/activated B-cell type diffuse large B-cell lymphomas, primary breast diffuse large B-cell lymphomas often have mutations of *MYD88* (*MYD88* L265) and *CD79B*, resulting in activation of the NFκB pathway, contributing to lymphomagenesis (36). Translocations of *BCL6*, *BCL2*, and *MYC* are absent or rare (36).

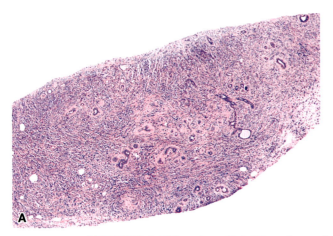
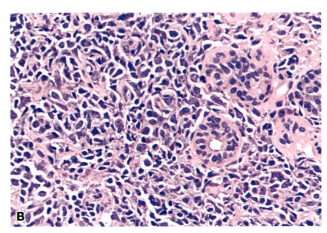

FIGURE 21.1 **Diffuse Large B-Cell Lymphoma. A:** This needle core biopsy shows a dense, diffuse infiltrate of lymphoid cells. **B:** High magnification shows closely packed large atypical lymphoid cells surrounding lobular glands.

Extranodal Marginal Zone Lymphoma of Mucosa-Associated Lymphoid Tissue

MALT lymphoma affects mainly middle-aged and older women and rarely men (2-4,6,10,25,31,37,38), with a median age of 68 years in one large series (39). Patients with MALT lymphoma of the breast typically have no recognized factors predisposing to lymphoma. Patients present with a lesion that is typically unilateral and that may be detected by physical examination or by mammography. Constitutional symptoms are almost never present (39).

The lymphomas range from less than 1 to 20 cm, with a median size of approximately 3 cm (3,6,10,31,37-39). Their histologic features are similar to those of MALT lymphomas in other sites. The lymphomas have a vaguely nodular to diffuse appearance on low-power microscopic examination. They are composed of small- to medium-sized cells with slightly irregular nuclei and a scant-to-abundant quantity of pale cytoplasm. Reactive follicles, sometimes with follicular colonization (infiltration and partial-to-complete replacement by neoplastic marginal zone cells), and plasmacytic differentiation, sometimes accompanied by Dutcher bodies (intranuclear protrusions of cytoplasm containing immunoglobulin), are found in some cases. Mitotic activity is low, except in residual reactive follicles **(Fig. 21.2)**. Necrosis and sclerosis are typically absent. Well-formed lymphoepithelial lesions are found less often than in MALT lymphomas involving some other sites (4,10,21,34). Rare MALT lymphomas with plasmacytic differentiation are associated with localized deposition of amyloid (3,40).

The neoplastic cells are typically $CD45^+$, $CD20^+$, $CD5^-$, $CD10^-$, $CD23^-$, $CD43^{+/-}$, $BCL2^{+/-}$, and cyclin $D1^-$, with monotypic cytoplasmic immunoglobulin in those cases with plasmacytic differentiation (5,25,37). The Ki67 proliferation index is low. If there are remnants of reactive follicles, the germinal center cells are usually $CD10^+$, $BCL6^+$, and $BCL2^-$, with a high Ki67 proliferation index. Markers of follicular dendritic cells (CD21, CD23) typically show underlying follicular dendritic meshworks, which are often expanded and disrupted. The presence of follicular dendritic cell meshworks tends to correlate with a vaguely nodular growth pattern in MALT lymphomas.

The pathogenesis underlying the development of MALT lymphoma of the breast is not well understood. Genetic defects seen in MALT lymphomas arising at other sites are uncommon in the breast: chromosomal translocations that involve the *MALT1* gene, including t(11;18) involving *API2* and *MALT1*, and t(14;18) involving *IGH* and *MALT1*, are rare, as are trisomies of chromosomes 3, 12, and 18 (34,41,42). The absence of nuclear p50 and p65 expression is reported, which suggests lack of NFκB activation, a pathway commonly implicated in MALT lymphoma at other sites (34,43). In one case series, MALT lymphoma of the breast did not share the distinct histopathologic or immunophenotypic features of primary cutaneous marginal zone lymphoma (44,45).

Follicular Lymphoma

Follicular lymphoma mainly affects middle-aged and older women (6,10,31), and rarely men (39). Patients present with lesions that are unilateral in approximately 95% of the cases, typically unaccompanied by constitutional symptoms (39). The tumors appear to range from less than 1 to 9 cm, with a median size of about 2 to 3 cm (6,10,31,39). Histologic and immunophenotypic features are similar to those of nodal follicular lymphomas. The lymphomas are sometimes associated with sclerosis. Follicular lymphomas of all grades (1-2, 3A, and 3B) have been reported **(Fig. 21.3)** (10,11,15,17). Neoplastic follicles are typically $CD45^+$, $CD20^+$, $CD10^+$, $CD5^-$, $CD23^-$, $CD43^-$, $BCL2^+$ or $BCL2^-$, and cyclin $D1^-$.

Burkitt Lymphoma

Burkitt lymphoma occurs in one of three clinical settings: endemic Burkitt lymphoma, occurring mainly in equatorial Africa, where malaria is endemic; sporadic Burkitt lymphoma, occurring worldwide in individuals without immunodeficiency; and immunodeficiency-associated Burkitt lymphoma, occurring in immunodeficient individuals. The

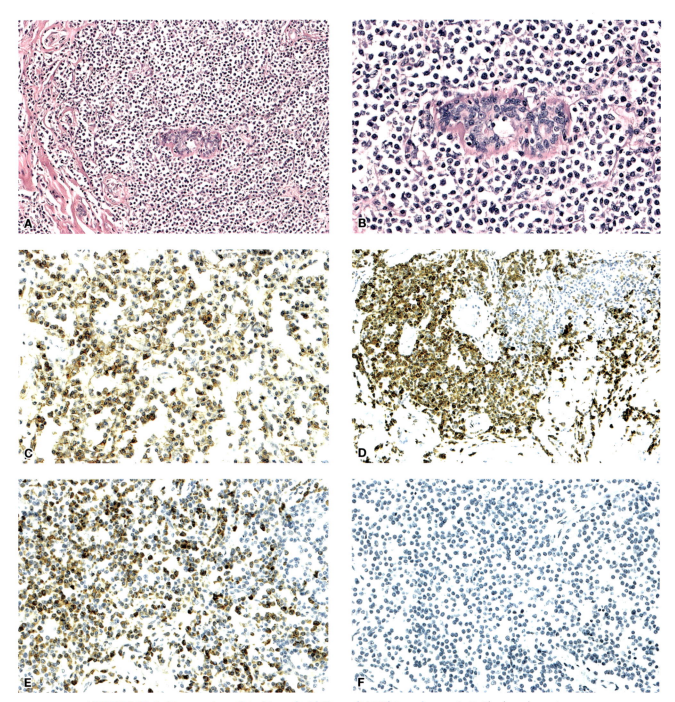

FIGURE 21.2 Mucosa-Associated Lymphoid Tissue (MALT) Lymphoma. A, B: The lymphomatous infiltrate around a mammary duct consists of small cells with clear cytoplasm and scattered plasma cells. **C:** The tumor cells are reactive for CD43. **D:** Immunoreactivity for CD79a is shown. **E:** Immunoreactivity for kappa is shown. **F:** There was no reactivity for lambda.

most common cause of immunodeficiency in the third scenario is HIV infection (46). The breast can be affected in any of these clinical settings.

Burkitt lymphoma affects mainly young to middle-aged females (4,17,18,47); some have been pregnant or postpartum at the time of diagnosis (4,17,18). Cases of endemic Burkitt lymphoma resulting in dramatic, bilateral mammary enlargement in African females who were sometimes pregnant or lactating were recognized by Burkitt and Wright (48). Premenarchal girls are rarely affected (49).

Burkitt lymphoma is typically composed of a dense, diffuse proliferation of uniform, medium-sized cells with round nuclei, clumped chromatin, several nucleoli, and scant to moderate cytoplasm that is deeply basophilic on a Giemsa stain. The proliferation is highly cellular with minimal intervening stroma. The mitotic rate is very high, and there is abundant apoptotic debris. Burkitt lymphoma has many interspersed pale tingible body macrophages containing apoptotic debris in a background of darkly stained neoplastic cells, creating the characteristic starry sky pattern **(Fig. 21.4)** (46).

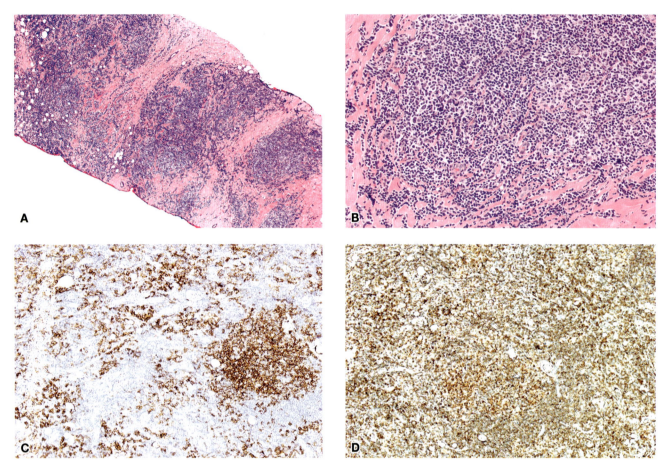

FIGURE 21.3 **Follicular Lymphoma, Follicular, and Diffuse Pattern, Grade 1 to 2 of 3. A:** The needle core biopsy shows ill-defined follicles and a patchy interfollicular lymphoid infiltrate. **B:** High magnification shows one poorly delineated follicle composed of centrocytes and occasional centroblasts in a background of small lymphocytes. **C:** The atypical cells were also CD20+ and BCL6+ (not shown); CD10 highlights atypical cells in a follicular and diffuse pattern. **D:** The atypical B cells coexpress BCL2.

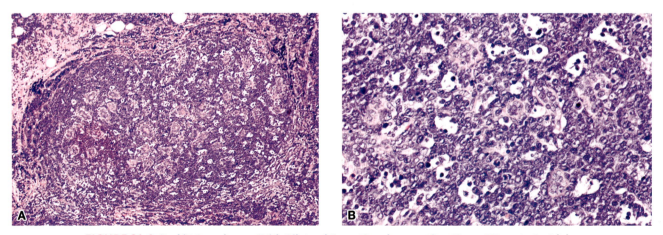

FIGURE 21.4 **Burkitt Lymphoma, With Bilateral Breast Involvement in a Young Woman. A:** A lobule is surrounded and infiltrated by a dense infiltrate of deeply basophilic, atypical lymphoid cells, with scattered tingible body macrophages creating a "starry sky" pattern. **B:** High magnification shows numerous medium-sized lymphoid cells with occasional distinct nucleoli, as well as frequent mitoses and scattered tingible body macrophages.

Burkitt lymphoma also has a characteristic immunophenotype: the neoplastic cells are uniformly CD20+, CD10+, BCL6+, BCL2−, monotypic surface immunoglobulin (IgM)+, with virtually all cells positive for Ki67 (proliferation). The underlying genetic event is a translocation involving *MYC* on chromosome 8 and *IGH* on chromosome 14 and less often the gene for κ or λ light chain rather than the *IGH*. The neoplastic cells almost always harbor EBV in endemic cases; sporadic and immunodeficiency-associated Burkitt lymphoma are each EBV-associated in about one-third of cases (46).

Other Systemic B-Cell Lymphomas

Other B-cell lymphomas involve the breast less frequently, typically in the setting of disseminated disease with involvement of bone marrow, blood, nodal, and/or other extranodal sites. These comprise both aggressive neoplasms, such as mantle cell lymphoma **(Fig. 21.5)** and B-lymphoblastic lymphoma **(Fig. 21.6)**, as well as indolent leukemic lymphomas, such as small lymphocytic lymphoma/chronic lymphocytic leukemia and hairy cell leukemia **(Table 21.1)** (50,51). Their

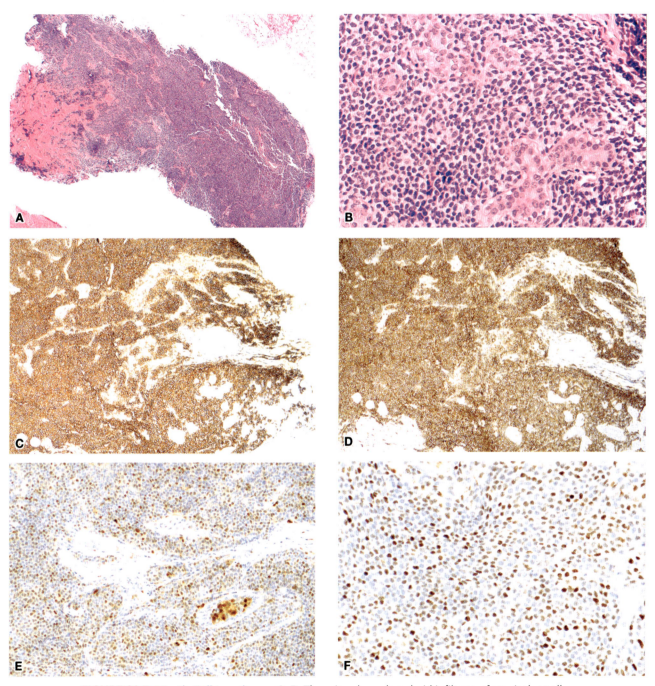

FIGURE 21.5 Mantle Cell Lymphoma. A, B: There is a dense lymphoid infiltrate of atypical, small to medium-sized cells with dispersed chromatin surrounding breast glandular tissue. **C:** There is a marked predominance of CD20+ B cells. **D:** B cells aberrantly coexpress CD5. **E:** B cells show diffuse nuclear positivity for cyclin D1, indicative of an underlying *CCND1* rearrangement. **F:** B cells show diffuse nuclear expression of SOX11, a transcription factor upregulated in mantle cell lymphoma.

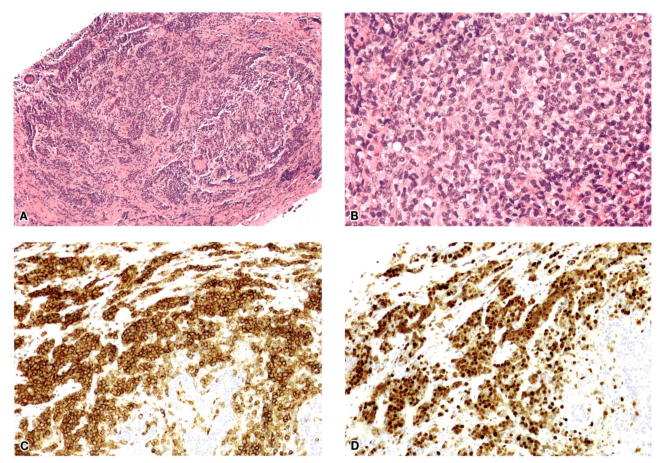

FIGURE 21.6 **B-Lymphoblastic Lymphoma. A:** On low magnification, there are infiltrative collections of atypical cells involving terminal duct lobular units. The pattern of infiltration mimics carcinoma. **B:** On high magnification, the atypical infiltrate consists of medium-sized to large mononuclear cells with irregular to folded nuclei and occasional prominent nucleoli. **C, D:** By immunohistochemistry, the mononuclear cells are strongly positive for CD10 (**C**), and TdT (**D**), as well as CD19 (not shown), consistent with B lymphoblasts.

distinction from one another and from the B-cell lymphomas discussed previously is important to ensure institution of appropriate therapy. Their correct diagnosis often relies on careful correlation with clinical history and other prior or concurrent pathology specimens (51).

T-Cell Lymphomas

Primary breast lymphoma of T-lineage is rare, accounting for only about 2% to 3% of the cases (4,16,21). Breast implant-associated anaplastic large cell lymphoma (ALCL) is a distinct entity (see the section on Lymphomas of the Breast in Association With Implants). Other T-cell lymphomas arise sporadically; they include ALK+ ALCL, peripheral T-cell lymphoma, not otherwise specified, including both CD4+ and CD8+ cases, subcutaneous panniculitis-like T-cell lymphoma, and T-lymphoblastic lymphoma (4,21,31,52-57). T-cell lymphomas involving the breast in the setting of widespread disease are more common than primary T-lineage breast lymphoma (57). These secondary lymphomas are also of a variety of types (52). Cases of adult T-cell leukemia/lymphoma occurring in patients from areas endemic for human T-lymphotropic virus-1 (HTLV1) infection, involving the breasts unilaterally and bilaterally, have been reported **(Fig. 21.7)** (57).

Hodgkin Lymphoma

Rare cases of Hodgkin lymphoma, most often nodular sclerosis classic Hodgkin lymphoma, have involved the breast at the time of presentation or at relapse (21,58-60). Typically, Hodgkin lymphoma involves the breast in the setting of concurrent lymph node involvement, and sometimes widespread disease. Relapse in the form of isolated breast involvement is very rare but has been described (60). Primary Hodgkin lymphoma of the breast is vanishingly rare, and when breast involvement occurs, it is generally secondary (21). There are very rare instances in which Hodgkin lymphoma presents first in the breast (59). Breast involvement is usually unilateral but occasionally bilateral (58).

LYMPHOID AND HEMATOPOIETIC TUMORS 429

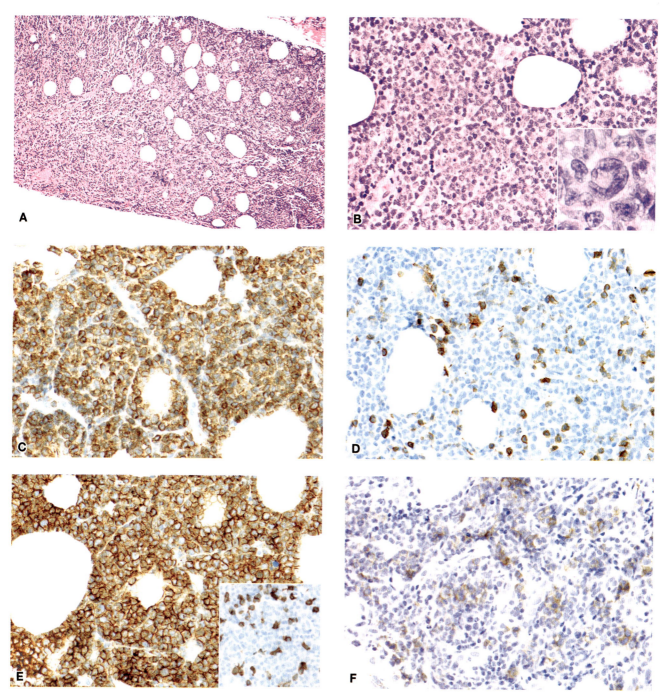

FIGURE 21.7 **Adult T-Cell Leukemia/Lymphoma, HTLV1-Associated.** This echogenic breast mass arose in the upper outer quadrant of a woman from the Caribbean, a region endemic for HTLV1 infection **A, B:** Microscopic examination shows a dense infiltrate of large lymphoid cells with oval to irregular nuclei and dispersed chromatin, including frequent anaplastic forms (**B, inset**). **C:** The neoplastic cells are strongly, diffusely positive for CD3. **D:** A stain for CD5 is negative on the neoplastic cell and positive in benign, small T cells, reflecting aberrant loss of CD5, a pan-T-cell antigen. CD7 was similarly negative (not shown). **E:** The lymphoma cells are positive for CD4 and negative for CD8 (**inset**). **F:** CD25 shows positive staining in a subset of lymphoma cells, an antigen characteristic of T regulatory cells and this type of lymphoma. Confirmation of HTLV1 infection would be undertaken by serology or PCR. HTLV1, human T-lymphotropic virus-1; PCR, polymerase chain reaction.

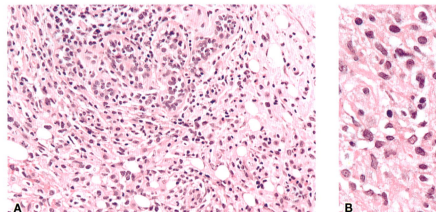
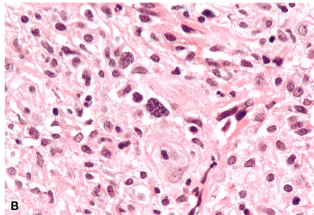

FIGURE 21.8 **Hodgkin Lymphoma. A, B:** Breast involvement in a patient with a diagnosis previously established in a cervical lymph node. Large atypical cells are present in small numbers in a background of sclerosis with scattered reactive cells.

As in other sites, Hodgkin lymphoma in the breast takes the form of a mixed infiltrate of reactive cells in varying proportions (lymphocytes, histiocytes, eosinophils, plasma cells, and/or neutrophils) with scattered large atypical uninucleate, binucleated, or multinucleated Reed-Sternberg cells and variants with large oval or irregular nuclei, inclusion-like reddish nucleoli, paranucleolar haloes, and scant to moderate quantity of pale cytoplasm **(Fig. 21.8)**. The neoplastic cells are typically $CD15^+$, $CD30^+$, weakly $PAX5^+$, $CD20^-$, $CD3^-$, and $ALK1^-$. Because of the rarity of Hodgkin lymphoma involving the breast, the diagnosis should be made with extreme caution, particularly in the absence of concurrent lymph nodal involvement by Hodgkin lymphoma or in the absence of a history of Hodgkin lymphoma.

Lymphomas of the Breast in Association With Implants

Lymphoma has rarely arisen adjacent to breast implants used for both cosmetic purposes and reconstruction after mastectomy for carcinoma (31,51,57,61-65). In contrast to the marked preponderance of B-cell lymphomas among breast lymphomas, the most common type of lymphoma arising in patients with implants is a site-specific form of ALK-negative ALCL termed breast implant-associated ALCL (BIA-ALCL) (65).

This lymphoma represents a small proportion of all breast lymphomas, accounting for only 2% of cases in each of two large series of lymphoma involving the breast (21,31). Risk estimates range from 1 in 3,000 to 1 in 30,000 individuals with breast implants. Although the overall risk of development of BIA-ALCL is low, it is significantly higher than that of primary ALCL of the breast in the general population with a reported odds ratio of 18.2 and relative risk of 67.6 to 400-fold in different studies (47,65-67). This risk is attributable to the surface area and degree of roughness of the implant surface, with essentially all cases developing in the setting of macro-textured implants, rather than smooth-surfaced implants (65,66). The implant fillings have been of saline and silicone types; however, even saline-filled implants typically have a silicone capsule, leading to speculation about a role for silicone or its breakdown products in the pathogenesis of lymphoma through an immunologic mechanism that is enhanced in macro-textured implants (61,62,65,68-72). A role for periprosthetic bacterial biofilm with bacterial lipopolysaccharide-induced immunologic responses has also been postulated (65).

Affected patients are adult women, including rare cases in transgender women, with a median age of 50 years (range 21 to >80 years) (65). The interval from insertion of the implant to diagnosis of lymphoma ranges from 2 to 32 years, with a median of approximately 10 years based on several larger series (31,47,56,61,65,72-79). Most patients present with a unilateral swelling related to a fluid collection (effusion or "seroma") developing between the implant and the fibrous capsule surrounding the implant, without a discrete mass (31,51,61-63,65,73-77,79). The effusion may be of high volume, up to 700 mL (65). A minority of patients, about 10% to 30%, have a discrete mass, with disease not confined by the fibrous capsule around the implant (65,72). Patients usually present with localized disease (61,62,75).

Microscopic examination reveals large, atypical, pleomorphic, mitotically active cells with oval or indented nuclei, prominent nucleoli, and moderately abundant cytoplasm often accompanied by a mixed inflammatory infiltrate composed of lymphocytes, plasma cells, histiocytes, and sometimes eosinophils, neutrophils, and giant cells. The neoplastic cells typically form a thin, discontinuous layer along the inner aspect of the fibrous capsule, sometimes with nodular foci of more abundant tumor cells, present in a background of necrotic debris or fibrinoid material ("in situ BIA-ALCL" or "seroma BIA-ALCL") **(Fig. 21.9)** (62). The infrequent higher tumor stages are characterized by invasion of the fibrous capsule through to surrounding breast parenchyma, soft tissue, or overlying skin by clusters of tumor cells or a discrete mass lesion ("tumor BIA-ALCL") (51,56,65,73,77).

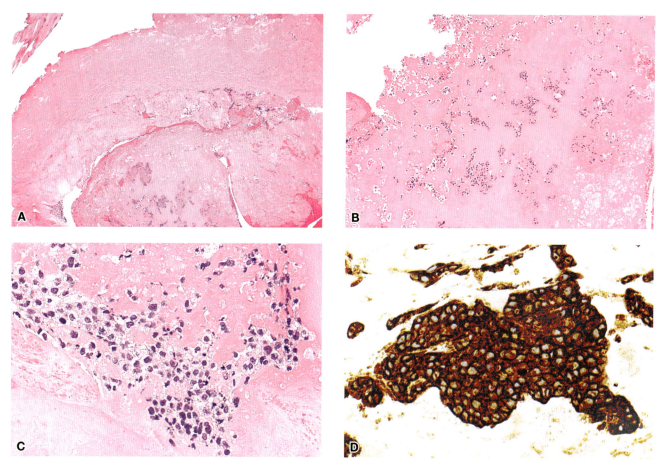

FIGURE 21.9 **Breast Implant-Associated Anaplastic Large Cell Lymphoma. A:** Low magnification shows a hypocellular fibrous pseudocapsule (top of image) overlying an area with hyaline material with a few clusters of cells. **B:** Clusters of atypical cells are scattered in a background of hyalinized collagen and amorphous debris. **C:** High magnification shows large atypical cells with oval and irregular nuclei in a background of debris. **D:** The large atypical cells are intensely positive for CD30.

Cytologic examination of fluid from the effusion may reveal large numbers of neoplastic cells with the features described previously **(Fig. 21.10)**. The effusion fluid may be used for cell block preparation for immunohistochemistry, as well as additional ancillary studies, including flow cytometry and molecular genetic analysis (80).

BIA-ALCL is, by definition, CD30$^+$ and ALK$^-$, and typically CD45$^{+/-}$ and EMA$^+$, with variable expression of T-cell antigens. CD4, CD43, and cytotoxic granule proteins (eg, TIA1 and granzyme B) are usually positive, whereas CD3, CD5, CD7, and CD8 are often negative. EBV and human herpes virus 8 (HHV8) are absent (51,61-63,73,74,76-80). The Ki67 proliferation index is high (77). Clonal rearrangement of the T-cell receptor γ chain gene (*TRG*) can typically be demonstrated, whereas clonal B cells are not found (61,62,73,74,77,80). There is Janus kinase/signal transducer and activator of transcription (JAK-STAT). pathway activation, as evidenced by expression of pSTAT by immunohistochemistry in essentially all cases (81,82). JAK-STAT pathway mutations are common; *JAK1* and *STAT3* are most commonly affected (81-83). Mutations of epigenetic modifiers are present in most cases; the most commonly affected are *KMT2C* and *KMT2D* (84). PI3K signaling pathway mutations are found in a minority of cases (84). Copy number aberrations (CNA) are found in nearly all cases. They include gains of chromosomes 2, 9p, 12p, and 21 and losses of 4q, 8p, 15, 16, and 20. Regions of CNA encompass genes involved in the JAK-STAT pathway and epigenetic regulators (84). Losses at chromosome 20q13.13 were found in 66% of cases in one study, an abnormality not found in ALCL involving the breast unassociated with an implant (67).

Patients presenting with the classic picture of BIA-ALCL associated with an effusion without a discrete mass and with disease confined by the capsule appear to have an excellent prognosis. Implant removal with total capsulectomy, with close follow-up to monitor for recurrence, constitutes sufficient therapy for these patients with a 5-year overall survival of nearly 100% (65,85). Patients with tumors that have penetrated beyond the fibrous capsule to form a discrete mass and those with regional nodal involvement or more distant spread have more aggressive disease, requiring systemic chemoimmunotherapy, with deaths reported in some cases (65,72,73,78).

Establishing a diagnosis may be problematic. The manner of presentation can lead to a clinical impression of

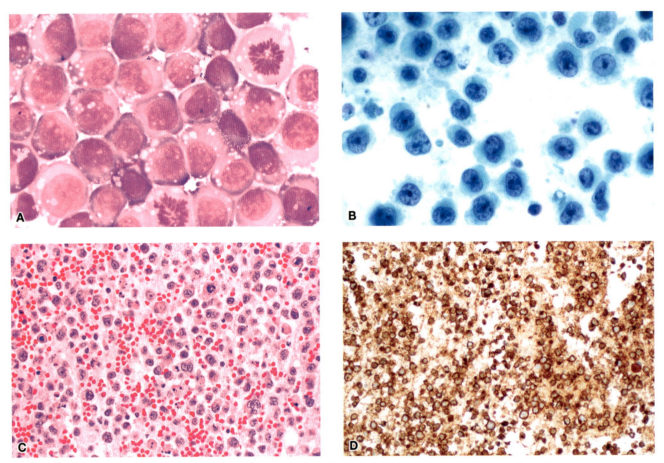

FIGURE 21.10 Cytologic Features of Breast Implant-Associated Anaplastic Large Cell Lymphoma.
A, B: Cytologic evaluation on Giemsa (**A**) and Papanicolaou (**B**) stains of fluid from a periprosthetic effusion sample demonstrates a population of large atypical cells with irregular nuclei, prominent nucleoli, conspicuous mitotic activity, and abundant cytoplasm with frequent cytoplasmic vacuoles. **C:** Similar cytologic features are seen on an H&E-stained cell block specimen. **D:** A CD30 stain of the cell block shows strong and uniform CD30 expression. H&E, hematoxylin and eosin.

inflammation, infection, or leaking implant. The associated inflammation may obscure the neoplastic population. The neoplastic lymphoid cells may be mistaken for carcinoma, particularly in women previously treated for breast carcinoma. Familiarity with the rare occurrence of BIA-ALCL will assist the pathologist in establishing a diagnosis.

Lymphomas other than BIA-ALCL have only rarely been reported in association with breast implants, including both B- and T-cell neoplasms (68-71). Among these, cases of EBV+ large B-cell lymphoma, including diffuse large B-cell lymphoma associated with chronic inflammation and fibrin-associated large B-cell lymphoma, have shown morphologic overlap with BIA-ALCL exhibited by clusters of tumor cells present within the inner layer of a thick, sclerotic capsule and associated benign chronic inflammation, adding to the differential diagnosis listed previously and underscoring the need for thorough pathologic evaluation with appropriate ancillary testing, including EBER in situ hybridization (86-89). In the largest reported series, all patients were exposed to textured implants, suggesting a pathogenetic role for both EBV and textured implants in the development of this lymphoma (86).

Differential Diagnosis of Mammary Lymphoma

The diagnosis of lymphoma of the breast is almost never suspected preoperatively. The clinical impression is typically carcinoma but may also be fibroadenoma or phyllodes tumor (28). On average, lymphoma forms a larger mass than carcinoma, with lymphomas having a mean or median diameter of about 4 cm (23,32). Occasionally, lymphomas can present with a clinical picture that mimics inflammatory carcinoma (90) or mastitis (91,92). Evaluation of histologic and immunophenotypic features, in conjunction with familiarity of the range of types of lymphoma that can involve the breast, typically allows a diagnosis to be established. In particular, lymphocytic mastitis secondary to diabetes, autoimmune disease, or other immune conditions can usually be distinguished from low-grade lymphoma on the basis of its multifocal, discontinuous perilobular, periductal, and/or perivascular distribution, characteristic background sclerosis, lack of cytologic atypia and cellular monomorphism, and absence of clonal B cells or plasma cells (**Fig. 21.11**).

LYMPHOID AND HEMATOPOIETIC TUMORS   **433**

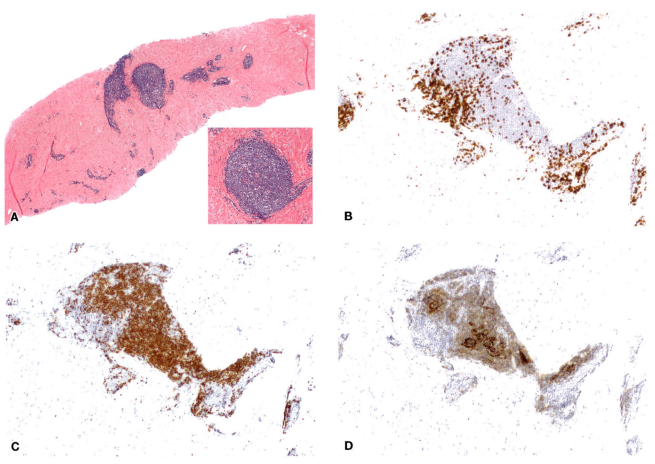

FIGURE 21.11 Lymphocytic Mastitis. A: There is a discontinuous perilobular and periductal infiltrate of small lymphocytes with bland nuclear features and scant cytoplasm (**inset**). Note the dense background sclerosis. **B-D:** Immunohistochemical stains show CD3$^+$ T cells (**B**) admixed with more numerous CD20$^+$ small B cells (**C**), which are encompassed by CD21$^+$ follicular dendritic cell aggregates (**D**).

PLASMA CELL NEOPLASMS

Breast involvement by a plasmacytoma is much less common than involvement by lymphoma and usually occurs in patients with plasma cell (multiple) myeloma. Patients are mostly middle-aged and older women (93-98), with rare cases affecting the male breast (97). Patients present with painless or painful nodules within the breast; usually, the nodules are multiple and bilateral (96). Plasmacytoma of the breast rarely presents as an isolated lesion, which usually (78,99), but not always, progresses to myeloma (100-102). The histologic and immunophenotypic features of the breast lesions in plasma cell myeloma and solitary plasmacytoma are similar (see **Table 21.1 and Fig. 21.12**). Plasma cell myeloma may be associated with a number of cytogenetic abnormalities that have both prognostic and therapeutic implications. For example, tumors with a *CCND1::IGH* rearrangement have shown sensitivity to the BCL2 inhibitor, venetoclax, in combination with standard therapy (103). The same rearrangement is also seen in mantle cell lymphoma; however, plasmacytic differentiation or monotypic cytoplasmic light chain expression is vanishingly rare in the latter.

MYELOID SARCOMA

Myeloid sarcoma is a mass-forming neoplasm composed of myeloid blasts, with or without maturation, occurring at a site other than the bone marrow (104,105). Myeloid sarcoma involving the breast is rare. It can occur in the breast as an isolated finding in a patient with no history of a myeloid neoplasm; this accounts for a minority of the cases (106,107). It is more commonly found in a patient with concurrent acute myeloid leukemia (AML) or concurrent myeloid sarcoma in other sites or as a relapse of AML in a patient previously treated for AML (107-111). Myeloid sarcoma may also arise in patients with other myeloid neoplasms such as myelodysplastic or myeloproliferative neoplasms (107). When myeloid sarcomas occur in this setting, they may represent the first sign of progression to AML or blast crisis.

Irrespective of the clinical scenario, myeloid sarcoma of the breast shows a marked female preponderance, with men accounting for only about 5% of patients (109). Patients are affected over a wide age range; many are adolescents or young adults (109). Patients present with a mass lesion or

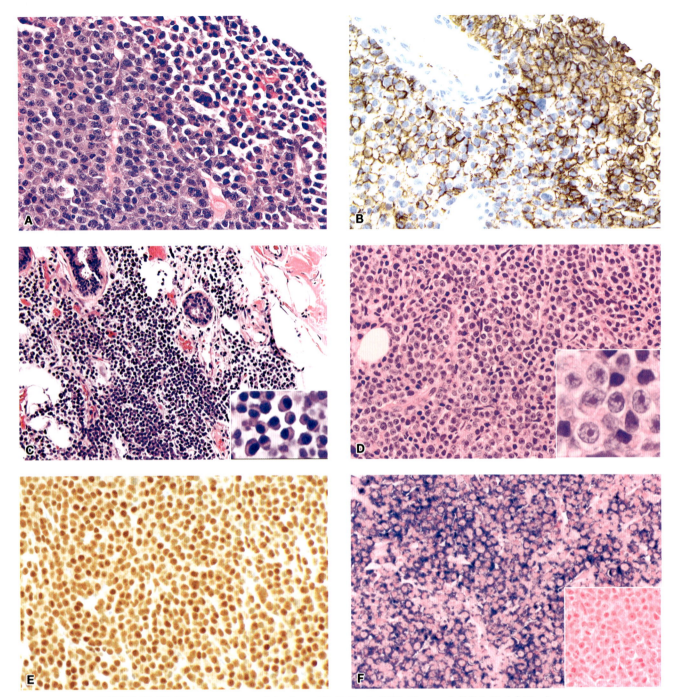

FIGURE 21.12 Plasmacytomas of the Breast in Patients With Plasma Cell (Multiple) Myeloma.
A: Numerous mature to slightly immature plasma cells are present. **B:** Plasma cells are CD138⁺.
C: The plasma cells infiltrate breast glandular tissue. The inset shows detail. **D:** A different patient whose plasma cell myeloma showed plasmablastic morphology with dispersed chromatin, prominent nucleoli, and more subtle plasmacytic differentiation with occasional cells showing slightly eccentric nuclei (**inset**). **E:** The neoplastic cells are MUM1⁺. **F:** Neoplastic cells are lambda-restricted with no staining for kappa (**inset**) by RNA in situ hybridization.

swelling of the breast unassociated with nipple discharge or retraction of overlying skin. Lesions are usually unilateral but may be bilateral (109,111). Most are in the range of 1 to 6 cm (105-108,110,111). Concurrent ipsilateral axillary lymph node involvement is common (107,109,111). Among patients with sites of extramedullary disease other than the breast, including disease occurring before, concurrent with, or after the diagnosis of myeloid sarcoma of the breast, the most common sites are skin and subcutaneous tissue, female genital tract, central nervous system, and lymph nodes (axillary and non-axillary) (109).

Outcome has been variable. Patients who present with isolated breast myeloid sarcoma appear to have a favorable outcome, particularly if they receive systemic chemotherapy (106,107). Those patients with widespread disease have a guarded prognosis (105-107), although outcome is strongly dependent on the underlying molecular genetic and cytogenetic abnormalities of the associated AML.

Myeloid sarcomas are composed of primitive myeloid and/or monocytic cells. In a subset of cases, there is some maturation of the neoplastic clone to more mature myeloid forms. On microscopic examination, the tumors usually have a diffuse pattern, although typically with sparing of mammary epithelial structures. In some instances, the neoplastic cells infiltrate stroma and mimic carcinoma. This occurs when a string of single cells takes on a linear appearance or surrounds nonneoplastic ducts and lobules in a layered, "targetoid" pattern. Mitoses are usually easily found (106,107,110). The neoplastic cells are discohesive, with round, oval, irregular or reniform, medium-sized nuclei with finely dispersed chromatin and variably prominent nucleoli. The cytoplasm ranges from scant in primitive cells to moderately abundant, sometimes with a distinct eosinophilic color owing to the presence of granules, if there is some maturation of the blasts **(Fig. 21.13)**. There may be admixed eosinophils and their precursors **(Fig. 21.13E,F)**.

With immunohistochemistry, the neoplastic cells are usually positive for myeloperoxidase, lysozyme, CD117, and CD43. CD45 (leukocyte common antigen) is often expressed but may be weak. Myeloid sarcomas composed exclusively of monocytes and their precursors (monoblastic sarcoma) are typically CD68$^+$, lysozyme$^+$, PU.1$^+$, and IRF8$^+$, but are negative for myeloperoxidase and often negative for CD34 and

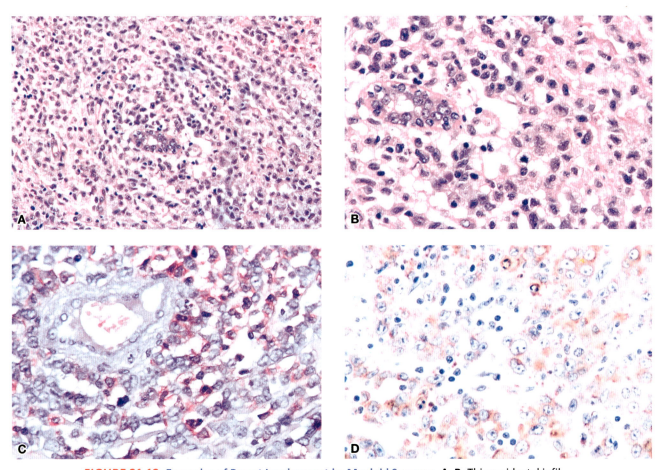

FIGURE 21.13 Examples of Breast Involvement by Myeloid Sarcoma. A, B: This periductal infiltrate of undifferentiated granulocytic cells could be mistaken for carcinoma. **C:** A few tumor cells are reactive (red) with naphthol AS-D chloroacetate esterase stain. Undifferentiated cells are not stained. **D:** Many primitive cells are positive for lysozyme (muramidase) by immunohistochemistry.

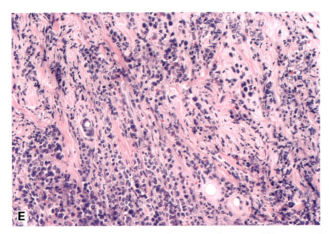
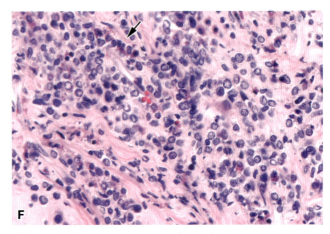

FIGURE 21.13 (*continued*) **E, F:** A different patient with myeloid sarcoma concurrently involving the parotid gland (not shown) and breast containing a dense infiltrate of primitive-appearing, medium-sized cells with dispersed chromatin and small prominent nucleoli. Note the admixed eosinophil precursors forming small clusters in areas (arrow), a morphologic clue to the subsequently identified in(16)/*CBFB::MYH11* FISH abnormality characteristically associated with eosinophilia. FISH, fluorescence in situ hybridization.

CD117. Tumor cells are negative for CD20, CD3, and keratins. In a few cases, there may be expression of one or more lymphoid antigens, such as TdT, CD79a, or PAX5; a broad panel of immunohistochemical stains, including myeloid and monocytic markers, will help avoid misinterpretation of such cases as lymphoblastic lymphoma (106,107,110).

The main entity in the differential diagnosis of myeloid sarcoma is lymphoma, especially diffuse large B-cell lymphoma. On routinely stained sections, large lymphoid cells typically have slightly larger nuclei, with either more vesicular or more coarsely clumped chromatin, and less delicate nuclear membranes than the neoplastic cells of myeloid sarcoma. Differentiation into recognizable maturing myeloid elements, when present, helps to identify a neoplasm as myeloid sarcoma. Immunophenotyping with an appropriate panel of lymphoid and myeloid antigens will confirm the diagnosis.

When myeloid sarcoma grows in a linear or targetoid pattern, it can mimic carcinoma, particularly lobular carcinoma. The presence of in situ carcinoma makes myeloid sarcoma less likely (107). Areas with cohesive neoplastic cells and the formation of tubules or lumina support carcinoma. A history of a myeloid neoplasm should prompt consideration of myeloid sarcoma. Of note, a small subset of patients treated for breast carcinoma with chemotherapy develop therapy-related AML, so a history of carcinoma does not exclude the possibility of AML/myeloid sarcoma.

The differential diagnosis also includes extramedullary hematopoiesis, or myeloid metaplasia, which rarely involves the breast, usually in association with an underlying hematologic disorder. Breast masses formed by extramedullary hematopoiesis are rare but have been reported in middle-aged and elderly female patients, most of whom carry a diagnosis of a myeloproliferative neoplasm, most often primary myelofibrosis. Extramedullary hematopoiesis also occurs rarely in the breast in women with no prior hematologic disorder (112–116). Microscopic examination reveals a diffuse infiltrate of mature and maturing hematopoietic cells, including megakaryocytes **(Fig. 21.14)**. There is a variable admixture of cells of myeloid and erythroid lines, with predominance of myeloid elements described in some cases. In patients with primary myelofibrosis, the megakaryocytes are often large, hyperchromatic, and atypical or even bizarre (116,117). The presence of more than one cell line, full maturation, and fewer blasts exclude myeloid sarcoma.

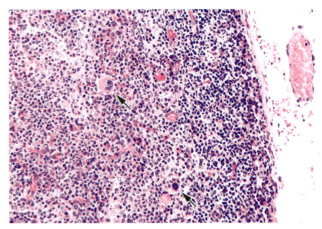

FIGURE 21.14 Intramammary Lymph Node With Extramedullary Hematopoiesis. Megakaryocytes (**arrows**) are evident in this intramammary lymph node from a patient with myelofibrosis.

HISTIOCYTIC PROLIFERATIONS OF THE BREAST

Rosai-Dorfman Disease

Rosai-Dorfman disease (formerly, sinus histiocytosis with massive lymphadenopathy) is an uncommon disorder of unknown etiology that typically presents with lymphadenopathy and less often with extranodal involvement. Breast involvement by Rosai-Dorfman disease is very unusual. Most patients with Rosai-Dorfman disease involving the breast are adults, with rare occurrence during adolescence. Patients range from 15 to 84 years of age, with a median age in the early 50s at presentation (118-121). There is a marked female preponderance, with a male to female ratio of about 1:10 (119,121,122). Patients usually present with a firm, painless, ill-defined, or irregular breast mass (118,120). In rare instances, retraction and inflammation of skin overlying the lesion has been described (118). The lesions range in size from 1 to 6.5 cm (median, 3 cm) (119). They are usually single and unilateral, but a few cases with multifocal or bilateral breast involvement are described (118-120,122). Most patients have Rosai-Dorfman disease confined to the breast, but a minority have axillary lymph node involvement (118,123), or more widespread disease (118). Patients with bilateral breast involvement appear more likely to have spread of Rosai-Dorfman disease beyond the breast than those with unilateral involvement (118,120).

Microscopic examination of the lesions reveals a dense infiltrate of lymphocytes, plasma cells, histiocytes, and sometimes lymphoid follicles. The histiocytes are distinctive in appearance: they are large with large oval nuclei, open chromatin, distinct nucleoli, and abundant cytoplasm. Some of these large histiocytes show emperipolesis, which may be translated as "inside round about wandering," in which intact cells, usually lymphocytes, but sometimes plasma cells, red blood cells, and neutrophils, are present within the cytoplasm. A clear halo may surround the engulfed cells. Although the large nuclei of the histiocytes give them an atypical appearance, mitoses and necrosis are absent. Eosinophils are very infrequent. Abscess formation and granulomas are absent. In lymph nodes, the large histiocytes are mainly confined to expanded sinuses (sinus histiocytosis with massive lymphadenopathy). Emperipolesis may be more difficult to identify in extranodal sites than in lymph nodes. Examination of touch preps may help with identification of emperipolesis. Extranodal lesions may be associated with fibrosis, which may be prominent and band-like. The alternating cellular inflammatory areas and paucicellular fibrofatty areas may yield a "checkerboard" appearance at low power. The distinctive histiocytes are positive for S-100 and for histiocytic markers such as CD68 and PU.1, and are negative for CD1a and langerin. The S-100 stain can be helpful in highlighting cells with emperipolesis (**Fig. 21.15**) (118-120,122,123). The histiocyte nuclei are additionally positive for OCT2 and cyclin D1, indicative of mitogen-activated protein kinase (MAPK) pathway upregulation, and mutations involving MAPK pathway genes have been identified in a subset of cases (124). Unlike other histiocytoses, *BRAF* mutations are rare. The plasma cells in Rosai-Dorfman disease are polytypic for immunoglobulin light chains and often show a high immunoglobulin G4 (IgG4)-to-immunoglobulin G (IgG) ratio, a localized characteristic immunologic response that is not indicative of systemic IgG4-related disease.

When follow-up is available, patients have typically been alive and well (119,121). The breast lesions may persist for months to years if not excised, however (121,123). Recurrence after excision has also been reported (121,123). Rare patients with disease involving the breast and other sites at presentation have had persistent or progressive disease. One death caused by widespread Rosai-Dorfman disease that involved the breast has been reported (118).

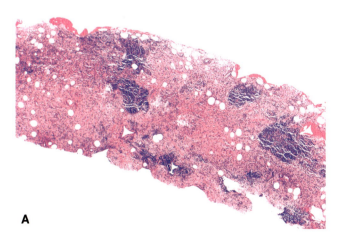
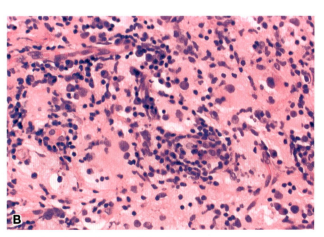

FIGURE 21.15 **Rosai-Dorfman Disease. A:** Low magnification shows dense cellular foci containing lymphoplasmacytic infiltrates and intervening paucicellular fibrofatty areas, yielding a "checkerboard"-like appearance. **B:** The distinctive histiocytes have round nuclei, small prominent nucleoli, and copious amounts of cytoplasm. Many appear to contain small lymphocytes and plasma cells, reflective of emperipolesis.

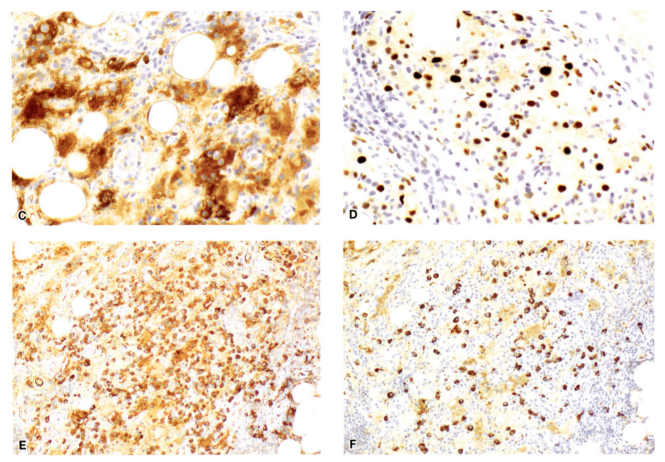

FIGURE 21.15 (*continued*) **C:** An S-100 immunohistochemical stain shows strong nuclear and cytoplasmic staining of the histiocytes with absent staining of the intracytoplasmic inflammatory cells. **D:** The histiocytes also show strong nuclear staining for OCT2 and cyclin D1 (not shown), consistent with MAP kinase pathway upregulation. **E, F:** Numerous IgG$^+$ plasma cells are present (**E**), many of which are positive for IgG4 (**F**). Ig, immunoglobulin; MAP, mitogen-activated protein.

Erdheim-Chester Disease

Erdheim-Chester disease is a rare non-Langerhans cell histiocytosis characterized by xanthomatous features. Nearly all cases show involvement of long bones of the lower extremities associated with characteristic radiographic features. About half of the patients have extraskeletal involvement that may include skin, orbit, lung, and other sites. Breast involvement is very rare, but when it occurs, it can take the form of mass lesions clinically mimicking carcinoma. Histologic examination shows CD68$^+$ xanthomatous histiocytes, scattered Touton-type giant cells, admixed lymphocytes, and fibrosis (125).

Langerhans Cell Histiocytosis

Langerhans cell histiocytosis is a clonal proliferation of Langerhans cells that affects children more than adults and can present as unifocal or multifocal disease in one of three clinical patterns: (1) unifocal disease (previously referred to as eosinophilic granuloma), (2) multifocal disease (formerly referred to as Hand-Schüller-Christian disease), or (3) multifocal disease with disseminated or visceral involvement (formerly called Letterer-Siwe disease) (126). Breast involvement by Langerhans cell histiocytosis is rare. Biopsy shows an infiltrate of large Langerhans cells with large pale nuclei with longitudinal or complex folds and moderately abundant pale cytoplasm. The Langerhans cells are CD1a$^+$, S-100$^+$, langerin$^+$, and in a subset, BRAF V600E$^+$ (126,127). There is a background inflammatory cell infiltrate of eosinophils and small lymphocytes. Langerhans cell histiocytosis is rarely found in association with Hodgkin or non-Hodgkin lymphoma. A case of follicular lymphoma involving the breast with nodules of Langerhans cells present within the lymphoma has been reported (128).

INTRAMAMMARY LYMPH NODES

The differential diagnosis of lymphoid tissue obtained in a biopsy specimen includes intramammary lymph nodes that may be single or multiple. Differentiating an intramammary lymph node from a lymphoid infiltrate involving the breast parenchyma itself is important, and can occasionally be difficult, particularly on a small biopsy. The area with the lymphoid infiltrate should be examined for evidence of an underlying lymph node, such as a discrete capsule or patent sinuses, confirming the presence of a lymph node, whereas finding the infiltrate in continuity with ducts or lobules indicates breast parenchymal involvement. Mammographic examination usually reveals a well-circumscribed mass that may have a lucent center and a peripheral notch corresponding to the hilus of the lymph node (129). Lymph nodes measuring 3 to 15 mm have been described (130,131). Lymph nodes larger than 1 cm are considered abnormal (131) and warrant further investigation. Enlargement of intramammary lymph nodes may be caused by lymphoid hyperplasia, including sinus histiocytosis, involvement by or reaction to inflammatory conditions, HIV-associated lymphadenopathy, and neoplasms such as metastatic tumor or lymphoma (132-135). Reactive lymph nodes sampled by fine needle aspiration show a range of findings. Some show a polymorphous admixture of germinal center cells, small lymphocytes, plasma cells, and immunoblasts, whereas others may show mainly small lymphocytes with some plasma cells and few immunoblasts (131). Flow cytometry shows a mixture of phenotypically normal T cells and polytypic B cells in such cases.

A number of studies have focused on involvement of intramammary lymph nodes by breast carcinoma. In one study of 1,655 retrospectively reviewed mammograms from patients with breast carcinoma, 16 (0.9%) had metastatic carcinoma in an intramammary lymph node detected radiologically (136). All lymph nodes with carcinoma were larger than 1.0 cm, and one had calcifications. Predictors of intramammary nodal metastases are tumor size greater than 1 cm, high-grade tumor, and positive axillary lymph nodes (137). Rampaul et al (138) studied completion mastectomy specimens from 157 women who were not candidates for conservation therapy after wide local excision for invasive carcinoma because of findings such as extensive intraductal carcinoma or multifocal invasion. Intramammary lymph nodes were found in 44 of 70 (63%) women with negative axillary lymph nodes. Ten (14%) had a positive intramammary lymph node and were consequently converted from stage I to stage II.

Shen et al (139) reported that the presence of metastatic carcinoma in an intramammary lymph node was usually associated with concurrent axillary nodal metastases. However, 2 (5%) of the 36 patients with positive intramammary lymph nodes had negative axillary lymph nodes. In another review, 71% of patients with a positive intramammary lymph node had a positive axillary sentinel node (140). The presence of metastatic carcinoma in an intramammary lymph node has been associated with a significantly less favorable prognosis when compared with patients with a negative intramammary lymph node (139). Nassar et al (137) found that the presence of positive intramammary lymph nodes was a predictor of poor prognosis in univariate analysis, but it was not an independent prognostic factor in multivariate analysis. For the minority of patients with a positive intramammary lymph node and negative axillary sentinel lymph node, completion

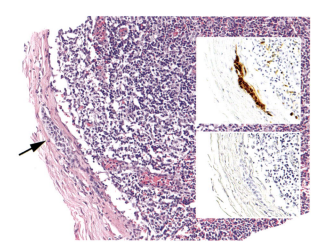

FIGURE 21.16 Intramammary Lymph Node With Nevus Cell Aggregate. The capsule of the lymph node contains an elongate aggregate of cytologically bland, cohesive cells (arrow) that are positive for S-100 (inset, upper right) and negative for cytokeratin (inset, lower right).

axillary lymph node dissection is almost always negative for carcinoma (140). Therefore, full axillary dissection may not be warranted in patients with a negative sentinel node, despite intramammary lymph nodal involvement.

The distinction between breast carcinoma with a dense lymphoid infiltrate and metastatic carcinoma in an intramammary lymph node is sometimes difficult and may not always be made with confidence in a needle core biopsy sample. This issue can arise in the breast proper and in the axillary region. The presence of a capsule and sinusoidal structure is the best evidence of a lymph node. Germinal centers suggest a lymph node, but they are present rarely at sites of extranodal carcinoma. Intramammary lymph nodes are rarely the site of metastasis from a carcinoma arising outside the breast (141).

Nevus cell aggregates that occur in the capsule **(Fig. 21.16)** or rarely in the parenchyma of axillary or intramammary lymph nodes may be mistakenly interpreted as metastatic carcinoma (142,143). This possibility should be considered when examining a needle core biopsy sample from a mammary parenchymal lymph node.

TISSUE PROCESSING AND ANCILLARY STUDIES

Several different types of specimens may be submitted for pathologic evaluation, and, depending on the quantity of tissue, triage for routine processing and ancillary studies varies. When a relatively large amount of tissue is obtained and there is clinical suspicion for lymphoma (an uncommon scenario), tissue should be submitted fresh to the Pathology Laboratory. A frozen section should be performed, and if the features are suspicious for lymphoma, separate tissue samples should be fixed for routine sections, submitted for flow cytometry and, particularly if features suggest a high-grade lymphoma, submitted for cytogenetic analysis. However, ensuring that ample tissue remains for routinely stained sections is paramount.

In most cases in which only needle core biopsies are obtained, tissue should be fixed entirely for routine sections. If the needle cores are large, multiple, and submitted fresh, triaging a portion of tissue for flow cytometry can be considered if lymphoma is known to be a concern. Alternatively, if there is preprocedural suspicion for lymphoma, a separate pass can be performed to obtain freshly aspirated material for flow cytometry to aid in establishing a diagnosis.

In most cases, there is no prebiopsy suspicion for lymphoma, and material is not obtained for flow cytometry or cytogenetics. In such cases, particularly for low-grade lymphomas, a differential diagnosis of lymphoma and a reactive lymphoid infiltrate may remain, even after careful study of hematoxylin and eosin (H&E)- and immunohistochemical stained sections. Sending paraffin-embedded tissue for molecular genetic studies to evaluate clonality using polymerase chain reaction (PCR) may be useful in these cases. For high-grade lymphomas in which the differential diagnosis includes entities such as diffuse large B-cell lymphoma, Burkitt lymphoma, and others, sending paraffin sections for fluorescence in situ hybridization (FISH) to investigate for the presence of rearrangements involving *MYC*, *BCL2*, and *BCL6* can be helpful. FISH can also be helpful in investigating the presence of an *IGH::BCL2* rearrangement in follicular lymphoma, a *CCND1::IGH* rearrangement in mantle cell lymphoma, or to investigate for characteristic abnormalities in AML or plasma cell neoplasms. Multigene next-generation sequencing (NGS) panels are becoming increasingly used to identify druggable targets in AML (eg, *FLT3*, *IDH1*, and *IDH2* mutations) and lymphoma (eg, *MYD88* mutations in DLBCL, *EZH2* mutations in follicular lymphoma).

REFERENCES

1. Wiseman C, Liao K. Primary lymphoma of the breast. *Cancer.* 1972;29:1705-1712.
2. Hugh J, Jackson F, Hanson J, et al. Primary breast lymphoma—an immunohistologic study of 20 new cases. *Cancer.* 1990;66:2602-2611.
3. Lamovec J, Jancar J. Primary malignant lymphoma of the breast—lymphoma of the mucosa-associated lymphoid tissue. *Cancer.* 1987;60:3033-3041.
4. Domchek SM, Hecht JL, Fleming MD, et al. Lymphomas of the breast: primary and secondary involvement. *Cancer.* 2002;94:6-13.
5. Farinha P, Andre S, Cabecadas J, et al. High frequency of MALT lymphoma in a series of 14 cases of primary breast lymphoma. *Appl Immunohistochem Mol Morphol.* 2002;10:115-120.
6. Cabras MG, Amichetti M, Nagliati M, et al. Primary non-Hodgkin's lymphoma of the breast: a report of 11 cases. *Haematologica.* 2004;89:1527-1528.
7. Lin Y, Guo XM, Shen KW, et al. Primary breast lymphoma: long-term treatment outcome and prognosis. *Leuk Lymphoma.* 2006;47:2102-2109.
8. Vigliotti ML, Dell'olio M, La Sala A, et al. Primary breast lymphoma: outcome of 7 patients and a review of the literature. *Leuk Lymphoma.* 2005;46:1321-1327.
9. Liu M, Hsieh C, Wang A, et al. Primary breast lymphoma: a pooled analysis of prognostic factors and survival in 93 cases. *Ann Saudi Med.* 2005;25:288-293.
10. Mattia A, Ferry J, Harris N. Breast lymphoma: a B-cell spectrum including the low grade B-cell lymphoma of mucosa associated lymphoid tissue. *Am J Surg Pathol.* 1993;17:574-587.
11. Wang LA, Harris NL, Ferry JA. Lymphoma of the breast and the role of mammography in the detection of low-grade lymphomas. *Mod Pathol.* 2004;17:276A.
12. Lin YC, Tsai CH, Wu JS, et al. Clinicopathologic features and treatment outcome of non-Hodgkin lymphoma of the breast—a review of 42 primary and secondary cases in Taiwanese patients. *Leuk Lymphoma.* 2009;50:918-924.
13. Lyons J, Myles J, Pohlman B, et al. Treatment and prognosis of primary breast lymphoma—a review of 13 cases. *Am J Clin Oncol.* 2000;23:334-336.
14. Aviles A, Delgado S, Nambo MJ. Primary breast lymphoma: results of a controlled clinical trial. *Oncology.* 2005;69:256-260.

15. Fruchart C, Denoux Y, Chasle J, et al. High grade primary breast lymphoma: is it a different clinical entity? *Breast Cancer Res Treat.* 2005;93:191-198.
16. Uesato M, Miyazawa Y, Gunji Y, et al. Primary non-Hodgkin's lymphoma of the breast: report of a case with special reference to 380 cases in the Japanese literature. *Breast Cancer (Tokyo, Japan).* 2005;12:154-158.
17. Vignot S, Ledoussal V, Nodiot P, et al. Non-Hodgkin's lymphoma of the breast: a report of 19 cases and a review of the literature. *Clin Lymphoma.* 2005;6:37-42.
18. Ribrag V, Bibeau F, El Weshi A, et al. Primary breast lymphoma: a report of 20 cases. *Br J Haematol.* 2001;115:253-256.
19. Ryan G, Martinelli G, Kuper-Hommel M, et al. Primary diffuse large B-cell lymphoma of the breast: prognostic factors and outcomes of a study by the International Extranodal Lymphoma Study Group. *Ann Oncol.* 2008;19:233-241.
20. Sabate JM, Gomez A, Torrubia S, et al. Lymphoma of the breast: clinical and radiologic features with pathologic correlation in 28 patients. *Breast J.* 2002;8:294-304.
21. Talwalkar SS, Miranda RN, Valbuena JR, et al. Lymphomas involving the breast: a study of 106 cases comparing localized and disseminated neoplasms. *Am J Surg Pathol.* 2008;32:1299-1309.
22. Yoshida S, Nakamura N, Sasaki Y, et al. Primary breast diffuse large B-cell lymphoma shows a non-germinal center B-cell phenotype. *Mod Pathol.* 2005;18:398-405.
23. Brustein S, Filippa DA, Kimmel M, et al. Malignant lymphoma of the breast: a study of 53 patients. *Ann Surg.* 1987;205:144-150.
24. Pisani F, Romano A, Anticoli Borza P, et al. Diffuse large B-cell lymphoma involving the breast: a report of four cases. *J Exp Clin Cancer Res.* 2006;25:277-281.
25. Liguori G, Cantile M, Cerrone M, et al. Breast MALT lymphomas: a clinicopathological and cytogenetic study of 9 cases. *Oncol Rep.* 2012;28:1211-1216.
26. Aozasa K, Ohsawa M, Saeki K, et al. Malignant lymphoma of the breast: immunologic type and association with lymphocytic mastopathy. *Am J Clin Pathol.* 1992;97:699-704.
27. Chanan-Khan A, Holkova B, Goldenberg AS, et al. Non-Hodgkin's lymphoma presenting as a breast mass in patients with HIV infection: a report of three cases. *Leuk Lymphoma.* 2005;46:1189-1193.
28. Jeon H, Akagi T, Hoshida Y, et al. Primary non-Hodgkin's malignant lymphoma of the breast. *Cancer.* 1992;70:2451-2459.
29. Aviv A, Tadmor T, Polliack A. Primary diffuse large B-cell lymphoma of the breast: looking at pathogenesis, clinical issues and therapeutic options. *Ann Oncol.* 2013;24:2236-2244.
30. Arora S, Gupta N, Srinivasan R, et al. Non-Hodgkin's lymphoma presenting as breast masses: a series of 10 cases diagnosed on FNAC. *Diagn Cytopathol.* 2011;41:53-59.
31. Gualco G, Bacchi CE. B-cell and T-cell lymphomas of the breast: clinical, pathological features of 53 cases. *Int J Surg Pathol.* 2008;16:407-413.
32. Aviles A, Neri N, Nambo MJ. The role of genotype in 104 cases of diffuse large B-cell lymphoma primary of breast. *Am J Clin Oncol.* 2012;35:126-129.
33. Law MF, Chan HN, Leung C, et al. Burkitt-like post-transplant lymphoproliferative disorder (PTLD) presenting with breast mass in a renal transplant recipient: a report of a rare case. *Ann Hematol.* 2014;93:2083-2085.
34. Talwalkar SS, Valbuena JR, Abruzzo LV, et al. MALT1 gene rearrangements and NF-kB activation involving p65 and p50 are absent or rare in primary MALT lymphomas of the breast. *Mod Pathol.* 2006;19:1402-1408.
35. Yhim HY, Kim JS, Kang HJ, et al. Matched-pair analysis comparing the outcomes of primary breast and nodal diffuse large B-cell lymphoma in patients treated with rituximab plus chemotherapy. *Int J Cancer.* 2012;131:235-243.
36. Taniguchi K, Takata K, Chuang SS, et al. Frequent MYD88 L265P and CD79B mutations in primary breast diffuse large B-cell lymphoma. *Am J Surg Pathol.* 2016;40:324-334.
37. Duman BB, Sahin B, Guvenc B, et al. Lymphoma of the breast in a male patient. *Med Oncol.* 2011;28(suppl 1):S490-S493.
38. Ghetu D, Membrez V, Bregy A, et al. Expect the unexpected: primary breast MALT lymphoma. *Arch Gynecol Obstet.* 2011;284:1323-1324.
39. Martinelli G, Ryan G, Seymour JF, et al. Primary follicular and marginal-zone lymphoma of the breast: clinical features, prognostic factors and outcome: a study by the International Extranodal Lymphoma Study Group. *Ann Oncol.* 2009;20:1993-1999.
40. Kambouchner M, Godmer P, Guillevin L, et al. Low grade marginal zone B-cell lymphoma of the breast associated with localised amyloidosis and corpora amylacea in a woman with long standing primary Sjogren's syndrome. *J Clin Pathol.* 2003;56:74-77.
41. Joao C, Farinha P, da Silva MG, et al. Cytogenetic abnormalities in MALT lymphomas and their precursor lesions from different organs: a fluorescence in situ hybridization (FISH) study. *Histopathology.* 2007;50:217-224.
42. Mulligan S, Hu P, Murphy A, et al. Variations in MALT1 gene disruptions detected by FISH in 109 MALT lymphomas occurring in different primary sites. *J Assoc Genet Technol.* 2011;37:76-79.
43. Cheuk W, Delabie J, Ott G, et al. Extranodal marginal zone lymphoma of mucosa-associated lymphoid tissue. In: *WHO Classification of Tumours. Haematolymphoid Tumours.* 5th ed. International Agency for Research on Cancer; 2023 (in press).
44. Yan M, Wang J, Gadde R, et al. Breast MALT lymphoma: a clinical, histomorphologic, and immunophenotypic evaluation. *Int J Surg Pathol.* 2023. doi:10.1177/10668969231152585

45. Geyer J, Willemze R. Primary cutaneous marginal zone lymphoma. In: *WHO Classification of Tumours. Haematolymphoid Tumours.* 5th ed. International Agency for Research on Cancer; 2023 (in press).
46. Sayed S, Leoncini L, Siebert R, et al. Burkitt lymphoma. In: *WHO Classification of Tumours. Haematolymphoid Tumours.* 5th ed. International Agency for Research on Cancer; 2023 (in press).
47. de Jong D, Vasmel WL, de Boer JP, et al. Anaplastic large-cell lymphoma in women with breast implants. *JAMA.* 2008;300:2030-2035.
48. Burkitt D, Wright D. *Burkitt's Lymphoma.* 1st ed. E & S Livingstone; 1970.
49. Lingohr P, Eidt S, Rheinwalt KP. A 12-year-old girl presenting with bilateral gigantic Burkitt's lymphoma of the breast. *Arch Gynecol Obstet.* 2009;279:743-746.
50. Alsadi A, Lin D, Alnajar H, et al. Hematologic malignancies discovered on investigation of breast abnormalities. *South Med J.* 2017;110:614-620.
51. Farkash EA, Ferry JA, Harris NL, et al. Rare lymphoid malignancies of the breast: a report of two cases illustrating potential diagnostic pitfalls. *J Hematop.* 2009;2:237-244.
52. Kebudi A, Coban A, Yetkin G, et al. Primary T-lymphoma of the breast with bilateral involvement, unusual presentation. *Int J Clin Pract.* 2005;59(suppl 147):95-98.
53. Vakiani E, Savage DG, Pile-Spellman E, et al. T-cell lymphoblastic lymphoma presenting as bilateral multinodular breast masses: a case report and review of the literature. *Am J Hematol.* 2005;80:216-222.
54. Aguilera NS, Tavassoli FA, Chu WS, et al. T-cell lymphoma presenting in the breast: a histologic, immunophenotypic and molecular genetic study of four cases. *Mod Pathol.* 2000;13:599-605.
55. Briggs JH, Algan O, Stea B. Primary T-cell lymphoma of the breast: a case report. *Cancer Invest.* 2003;21:68-72.
56. Popplewell L, Thomas SH, Huang Q, et al. Primary anaplastic large-cell lymphoma associated with breast implants. *Leuk Lymphoma.* 2011;52:1481-1487.
57. Gualco G, Chioato L, Harrington WJ Jr, et al. Primary and secondary T-cell lymphomas of the breast: clinico-pathologic features of 11 cases. *Appl Immunohistochem Mol Morphol.* 2009;17:301-306.
58. Ergul N, Guner SI, Sager S, et al. Bilateral breast involvement of Hodgkin lymphoma revealed by FDG PET/CT. *Med Oncol.* 2012;29:1105-1108.
59. Hoimes CJ, Selbst MK, Shafi NQ, et al. Hodgkin's lymphoma of the breast. *J Clin Oncol.* 2010;28:e11-e13.
60. Park J, Rizzo M, Jackson S, et al. Reed–Sternberg cells in breast FNA of a patient with left breast mass. *Diagn Cytopathol.* 2010;38:663-668.
61. Roden AC, Macon WR, Keeney GL, et al. Seroma-associated primary anaplastic large-cell lymphoma adjacent to breast implants: an indolent T-cell lymphoproliferative disorder. *Mod Pathol.* 2008;21:455-463.
62. Wong AK, Lopategui J, Clancy S, et al. Anaplastic large cell lymphoma associated with a breast implant capsule: a case report and review of the literature. *Am J Surg Pathol.* 2008;32:1265-1268.
63. Miranda RN, Lin L, Talwalkar SS, et al. Anaplastic large cell lymphoma involving the breast: a clinicopathologic study of 6 cases and review of the literature. *Arch Pathol Lab Med.* 2009;133:1383-1390.
64. Keech JA Jr, Creech BJ. Anaplastic T-cell lymphoma in proximity to a saline-filled breast implant. *Plast Reconstr Surg.* 1997;100:554-555.
65. Miranda R, Ott G, Schmitt F, et al. Breast implant-associated anaplastic large cell lymphoma. In: *WHO Classification of Tumours. Haematolymphoid Tumours.* 5th ed. International Agency for Research on Cancer; 2023 (in press).
66. Doren EL, Miranda RN, Selber JC, et al. U.S. Epidemiology of Breast Implant-Associated Anaplastic Large Cell Lymphoma. *Plast Reconstr Surg.* 2017;139:1042-1050.
67. Los-de Vries GT, de Boer M, van Dijk E, et al. Chromosome 20 loss is characteristic of breast implant-associated anaplastic large cell lymphoma. *Blood.* 2020;136:2927-2932.
68. Cook PD, Osborne BM, Connor RL, et al. Follicular lymphoma adjacent to foreign body granulomatous inflammation and fibrosis surrounding silicone breast prosthesis. *Am J Surg Pathol.* 1995;19:712-717.
69. Duvic M, Moore D, Menter A, et al. Cutaneous T-cell lymphoma in association with silicone breast implants. *J Am Acad Dermatol.* 1995;32:939-942.
70. Kraemer DM, Tony HP, Gattenlohner S, et al. Lymphoplasmacytic lymphoma in a patient with leaking silicone implant. *Haematologica.* 2004;89:ELT01.
71. Sendagorta E, Ledo A. Sezary syndrome in association with silicone breast implant. *J Am Acad Dermatol.* 1995;33:1060-1061.
72. Miranda RN, Aladily TN, Prince HM, et al. Breast implant-associated anaplastic large-cell lymphoma: long-term follow-up of 60 patients. *J Clin Oncol.* 2014;32:114-120.
73. Aladily TN, Medeiros LJ, Amin MB, et al. Anaplastic large cell lymphoma associated with breast implants: a report of 13 cases. *Am J Surg Pathol.* 2012;36:1000-1008.
74. Gaudet G, Friedberg JW, Weng A, et al. Breast lymphoma associated with breast implants: two case-reports and a review of the literature. *Leuk Lymphoma.* 2002;43:115-119.
75. Newman MK, Zemmel NJ, Bandak AZ, et al. Primary breast lymphoma in a patient with silicone breast implants: a case report and review of the literature. *J Plast Reconstr Aesthet Surg.* 2008;61:822-825.
76. Olack B, Gupta R, Brooks GS. Anaplastic large cell lymphoma arising in a saline breast implant capsule after tissue expander breast reconstruction. *Ann Plast Surg.* 2007;59:56-57.

77. Sahoo S, Rosen PP, Feddersen RM, et al. Anaplastic large cell lymphoma arising in a silicone breast implant capsule: a case report and review of the literature. *Arch Pathol Lab Med.* 2003;127:e115-e118.
78. Carty MJ, Pribaz JJ, Antin JH, et al. A patient death attributable to implant-related primary anaplastic large cell lymphoma of the breast. *Plast Reconstr Surg.* 2011;128:e112-e118.
79. Taylor KO, Webster HR, Prince HM. Anaplastic large cell lymphoma and breast implants: five Australian cases. *Plast Reconstr Surg.* 2012;129:e610-e617.
80. Jaffe ES, Ashar BS, Clemens MW, et al. Best practices guideline for the pathologic diagnosis of breast implant-associated anaplastic large-cell lymphoma. *J Clin Oncol.* 2020;38:1102-1111.
81. Letourneau A, Maerevoet M, Milowich D, et al. Dual JAK1 and STAT3 mutations in a breast implant-associated anaplastic large cell lymphoma. *Virchows Arch.* 2018;473:505-511.
82. Oishi N, Brody GS, Ketterling RP, et al. Genetic subtyping of breast implant-associated anaplastic large cell lymphoma. *Blood.* 2018;132:544-547.
83. Blombery P, Thompson ER, Jones K, et al. Whole exome sequencing reveals activating JAK1 and STAT3 mutations in breast implant-associated anaplastic large cell lymphoma anaplastic large cell lymphoma. *Haematologica.* 2016;101:e387-e390.
84. Laurent C, Nicolae A, Laurent C, et al. Gene alterations in epigenetic modifiers and JAK-STAT signaling are frequent in breast implant-associated ALCL. *Blood.* 2020;135:360-370.
85. Clemens MW, Medeiros LJ, Butler CE, et al. Complete surgical excision is essential for the management of patients with breast implant-associated anaplastic large-cell lymphoma. *J Clin Oncol.* 2016;34:160-168.
86. Medeiros LJ, Marques-Piubelli ML, Sangiorgio VFI, et al. Epstein-Barr-virus-positive large B-cell lymphoma associated with breast implants: an analysis of eight patients suggesting a possible pathogenetic relationship. *Mod Pathol.* 2021;34:2154-2167.
87. Mescam L, Camus V, Schiano JM, et al. EBV+ diffuse large B-cell lymphoma associated with chronic inflammation expands the spectrum of breast implant-related lymphomas. *Blood.* 2020;135:2004-2009.
88. Khoo C, McTigue C, Hunter-Smith DJ, Walker P. EBV positive fibrin/chronic inflammation associated diffuse large B-cell lymphoma: an incidental finding associated with a breast implant. *Pathology.* 2021;53:673-675.
89. Morgan S, Tremblay-LeMay R, Lipa JE, et al. Breast implant-associated EBV-positive diffuse large B-cell lymphoma: two case reports and literature review. *Pathol Res Pract.* 2021;226:153589.
90. Anne N, Pallapothu R. Lymphoma of the breast: a mimic of inflammatory breast cancer. *World J Surg Oncol.* 2011;9:125.
91. Antoniou SA, Antoniou GA, Makridis C, et al. Bilateral primary breast lymphoma masquerading as lactating mastitis. *Eur J Obstet Gynecol Reprod Biol.* 2010;152:111-112.
92. Sun LM, Huang EY, Meng FY, et al. Primary breast lymphoma clinically mimicking acute mastitis: a case report. *Tumori.* 2011;97:233-235.
93. Pasquini E, Rinaldi P, Nicolini M, et al. Breast involvement in immunolymphoproliferative disorders: report of two cases of multiple myeloma of the breast. *Ann Oncol.* 2000;11:1353-1359.
94. Ross JS, King TM, Spector JI, et al. Plasmacytoma of the breast: an unusual case of recurrent myeloma. *Arch Intern Med.* 1987;147:1838-1840.
95. Kumar PV, Vasei M, Daneshbod Y, et al. Breast myeloma: a report of 3 cases with fine needle aspiration cytologic findings. *Acta Cytol.* 2005;49:445-448.
96. Escobar PF, Patrick RJ, Hicks D, et al. Myeloma of the breast. *Breast J.* 2006;12:387-388.
97. Daneshbod Y, Bagheri MH, Zakernia M, et al. Multiple myeloma recurrence presenting as bilateral breast masses. *Breast J.* 2007;13:310-311.
98. Fayyaz A, Ghani UF. Multiple breast masses in a case of multiple myeloma. *J Coll Physicians Surg Pak.* 2009;19:529-530.
99. Ben-Yehuda A, Steiner-Saltz D, Libson E, et al. Plasmacytoma of the breast: unusual initial presentation of myeloma: report of two cases and review of the literature. *Blut.* 1989;58:169-170.
100. Innes J, Newall J. Myelomatosis. *Lancet.* 1961;1:239-245.
101. Proctor NS, Rippey JJ, Shulman G, et al. Extramedullary plasmacytoma of the breast. *J Pathol.* 1975;116:97-100.
102. Cao S, Kang HG, Liu YX, et al. Synchronous infiltrating ductal carcinoma and primary extramedullary plasmacytoma of the breast. *World J Surg Oncol.* 2009;7:43.
103. Kumar SK, Harrison SJ, Cavo M, et al. Venetoclax or placebo in combination with bortezomib and dexamethasone in patients with relapsed or refractory multiple myeloma (BELLINI): a randomised, double-blind, multicentre, phase 3 trial. *Lancet Oncol.* 2020;21:1630-1642.
104. Chen W, Medeiros LJ. Myeloid sarcoma. In: *WHO Classification Tumours. Haematolymphoid Tumours.* 5th ed. International Agency for Research on Cancer; 2023 (in press).
105. Jelic-Puskaric B, Ostojic-Kolonic S, Planinc-Peraica A, et al. Myeloid sarcoma involving the breast. *Coll Antropol.* 2010;34:641-644.
106. Azim HA Jr, Gigli F, Pruneri G, et al. Extramedullary myeloid sarcoma of the breast. *J Clin Oncol.* 2008;26:4041-4043.
107. Valbuena JR, Admirand JH, Gualco G, et al. Myeloid sarcoma involving the breast. *Arch Pathol Lab Med.* 2005;129:32-38.
108. Choschzick M, Bacher U, Ayuk F, et al. Immunohistochemistry and molecular analyses in myeloid sarcoma of the breast in a patient with relapse of NPM1-mutated and FLT3-mutated AML after allogeneic stem cell transplantation. *J Clin Pathol.* 2010;63:558-561.

109. Cunningham I. A clinical review of breast involvement in acute leukemia. *Leuk Lymphoma*. 2006;47:2517-2526.
110. Lim HS, Park MH, Heo SH, et al. Myeloid sarcoma of the breast mimicking hamartoma on sonography. *J Ultrasound Med*. 2008;27:1777-1780.
111. Toumeh A, Phinney R, Kobalka P, et al. Bilateral myeloid sarcoma of the breast and cerebrospinal fluid as a relapse of acute myeloid leukemia after stem-cell transplantation: a case report. *J Clin Oncol*. 2012;30:e199-e201.
112. Brooks JJ, Krugman DT, Damjanov I. Myeloid metaplasia presenting as a breast mass. *Am J Surg Pathol*. 1980;4:281-285.
113. Glew RH, Haese WH, McIntyre PA. Myeloid metaplasia with myelofibrosis: the clinical spectrum of extramedullary hematopoiesis and tumor formation. *Johns Hopkins Med J*. 1973;132:253-270.
114. Martinelli G, Santini D, Bazzocchi F, et al. Myeloid metaplasia of the breast: a lesion which clinically mimics carcinoma. *Virchows Arch A Pathol Anat Histopathol*. 1983;401:203-207.
115. Zonderland HM, Michiels JJ, ten Kate FJ. Case report: mammographic and sonographic demonstration of extramedullary haematopoiesis of the breast. *Clin Radiol*. 1991;44:64-65.
116. Cufer T, Bracko M. Myeloid metaplasia of the breast. *Ann Oncol*. 2001;12:267-270.
117. Al-Nafussi A, Al-Okati D, Alsewan M. Extramedullary haematopoietic tumour of the breast: a case report in a woman with secondary myelofibrosis following essential thrombocythaemia. *Histopathol*. 2004;44:625-626.
118. Green I, Dorfman RF, Rosai J. Breast involvement by extranodal Rosai–Dorfman disease: report of seven cases. *Am J Surg Pathol*. 1997;21:664-668.
119. Morkowski JJ, Nguyen CV, Lin P, et al. Rosai–Dorfman disease confined to the breast. *Ann Diagn Pathol*. 2010;14:81-87.
120. Bansal P, Chakraborti S, Krishnanand G, et al. Rosai–Dorfman disease of the breast in a male: a case report. *Acta Cytol*. 2010;54:349-352.
121. Wu YC, Hsieh TC, Kao CH, et al. A mimic of breast lymphoma: extranodal Rosai–Dorfman disease. *Am J Med Sci*. 2010;339:282-284.
122. Baladandapani P, Hu Y, Kapoor K, et al. Rosai–Dorfman disease presenting as multiple breast masses in an otherwise asymptomatic male patient. *Clin Radiol*. 2012;67:393-395.
123. Tenny SO, McGinness M, Zhang D, et al. Rosai–Dorfman disease presenting as a breast mass and enlarged axillary lymph node mimicking malignancy: a case report and review of the literature. *Breast J*. 2011;17:516-520.
124. Elbaz Younes I, Sokol L, Zhang L. Rosai–Dorfman disease between proliferation and neoplasia. *Cancers (Basel)*. 2022;14:5271.
125. Provenzano E, Barter SJ, Wright PA, et al. Erdheim–Chester disease presenting as bilateral clinically malignant breast masses. *Am J Surg Pathol*. 2010;34:584-588.
126. Picarsic J, Demicco EG, Jacques TS, et al. Langerhans cell histiocytosis. In: *WHO Classification of Tumours. Haematolymphoid Tumours*. 5th ed. International Agency for Research on Cancer; 2023 (in press).
127. Roden AC, Hu X, Kip S, et al. BRAF V600E expression in Langerhans cell histiocytosis: clinical and immunohistochemical study on 25 pulmonary and 54 extrapulmonary cases. *Am J Surg Pathol*. 2014;38:548-551.
128. Adu-Poku K, Thomas DW, Khan MK, et al. Langerhans cell histiocytosis in sequential discordant lymphoma. *J Clin Pathol*. 2005;58:104-106.
129. Kopans DB, Meyer JE, Murphy GF. Benign lymph nodes associated with dermatitis presenting as breast masses. *Radiology*. 1980;137:15-19.
130. McSweeney MB, Egan RL. Prognosis of breast cancer related to intramammary lymph nodes. *Recent Results Cancer Res*. 1984;90:166-172.
131. Vigliar E, Cozzolino I, Fernandez LV, et al. Fine-needle cytology and flow cytometry assessment of reactive and lymphoproliferative processes of the breast. *Acta Cytol*. 2012;56:130-138.
132. Arnaout AH, Shousha S, Metaxas N, et al. Intramammarytuberculous lymphadenitis. *Histopathology*. 1990;17:91-93.
133. Kinoshita T, Yashiro N, Yoshigi J, et al. Inflammatory intramammary lymph node mimicking the malignant lesion in dynamic MRI: a case report. *Clin Imaging*. 2002;26:258-262.
134. Konstantinopoulos PA, Dezube BJ, March D, et al. HIV-associated intramammary lymphadenopathy. *Breast J*. 2007;13:192-195.
135. Lindfors KK, Kopans DB, Googe PB, et al. Breast cancer metastasis to intramammary lymph nodes. *AJR Am J Roentgenol*. 1986;146:133-136.
136. Gunhan-Bilgen I, Memis A, Ustun EE. Metastatic intramammary lymph nodes: mammographic and ultrasonographic features. *Eur J Radiol*. 2001;40:24-29.
137. Nassar A, Cohen C, Cotsonis G, et al. Significance of intramammary lymph nodes in the staging of breast cancer: correlation with tumor characteristics and outcome. *Breast J*. 2008;14:147-152.
138. Rampaul RS, Dale OT, Mitchell M, et al. Incidence of intramammary nodes in completion mastectomy specimens after axillary node sampling: implications for breast conserving surgery. *Breast (Edinburgh, Scotland)*. 2008;17:195-198.
139. Shen J, Hunt KK, Mirza NQ, et al. Intramammary lymph node metastases are an independent predictor of poor outcome in patients with breast carcinoma. *Cancer*. 2004;101:1330-1337.
140. Diaz R, Degnim AC, Boughey JC, et al. A positive intramammary lymph node does not mandate a complete axillary node dissection. *Am J Surg*. 2012;203:151-155.
141. Maffini F, Bozzini A, Casadio C, et al. Ovarian serous papillary carcinoma, metastatic to intramammary lymph-node mimic a primary breast carcinoma on RX mammography. *Breast J*. 2012;18:484-485.
142. Biddle DA, Evans HL, Kemp BL, et al. Intraparenchymal nevus cell aggregates in lymph nodes: a possible diagnostic pitfall with malignant melanoma and carcinoma. *Am J Surg Pathol*. 2003;27:673-681.
143. Ridolfi RL, Rosen PP, Thaler H. Nevus cell aggregates associated with lymph nodes: estimated frequency and clinical significance. *Cancer*. 1977;39:164-171.

Metastases From Nonmammary Malignant Neoplasms

ELAINE W. ZHONG AND SYED A. HODA

INTRODUCTION

The preoperative clinical workup of an apparently healthy patient with a breast mass can be cursory and is unlikely to exclude a metastasis from a clinically inapparent (ie, "occult") nonmammary malignant neoplasm (NMMN). Even if a history of a previously treated NMMN is known to the clinician when a needle core biopsy (NCB) is obtained, this information may not be conveyed to the pathologist. Thus, when faced with a mammary neoplasm that has unusual clinical, radiologic, or histologic features, it is important to consider metastasis in the differential diagnosis.

CLINICAL FEATURES

Metastases from NMMN in the breast are rare and account for less than 1% of all mammary malignant neoplasms in clinical series (1,2), and less than 1% to 5% of autopsies of patients who die as a result of NMMN (3,4). Such tumors are vastly more common in females. The interval between initial diagnosis of an NMMN and mammary metastases is usually about 2 years—but it can vary from a few weeks to several years. In approximately one-third of the cases, the metastasis in the breast is the first presentation of the NMMN. Typically, there have already been metastases at other sites, or the tumors are detected at various sites synchronously (1,5).

Metastatic foci in breast often present initially as solitary masses (1). Upon disease progression, such tumors can become multiple and bilateral (5). Metastases have been described in the ipsilateral axillary lymph nodes in a substantial proportion of patients with metastases in the breast (1).

Hematologic and lymphoid neoplasms involving the breast are sometimes listed under the rubric of breast "metastases," but they are best regarded as either primary breast neoplasms or as a manifestation of a systemic condition, depending upon the extent of organ involvement. If hematopoietic and lymphoid neoplasms are excluded, the most common NMMNs that secondarily involve the breast include cutaneous melanoma and carcinomas of the lung, ovary, stomach, and kidney. Metastasis from the contralateral breast is a diagnostic consideration when there is bilateral involvement (or history thereof), the histologic appearances of the tumors in the breasts are similar, and there is no evidence of in situ carcinoma in the contralateral breast. In the pediatric population, lymphoma and rhabdomyosarcoma are the most common sources of NMMN in the breast.

IMAGING FEATURES

On *mammography*, metastatic tumors tend to present as discrete, solitary, or multiple round masses without spiculation (5). As a result, metastatic tumors cannot be distinguished radiologically from circumscribed primary breast carcinomas (PBCs), particularly those of the papillary, medullary, or mucinous types. Calcific deposits are uncommon in metastases from NMMN but may occur in metastatic müllerian (tubal, ovarian, or peritoneal) carcinomas (6,7). *Ultrasonography* typically shows the lesions to be hypoechoic without spiculations (1,8). Radiologic techniques such as *MRI* (magnetic resonance imaging) and *FDG-PET/CT* (fluorodeoxyglucose-positron emission tomography/computed tomography) have also detected metastases in the breast from carcinoma of the thyroid (9), ovary (10), and soft tissue liposarcoma (11). In the latter two instances, the diagnosis of a metastatic NMMN was confirmed by NCB.

HISTOPATHOLOGIC EVALUATION

The histopathologic appearance of NMMN in the breast is seldom specifically indicative of the site of origin. A notable exception is pigmented metastatic melanoma, although pigmented melanocytic differentiation can occur in metaplastic mammary carcinoma (12). Melanoma arising in the breast is usually a form of metaplastic carcinoma, and it may therefore express cytokeratin. Non-cytokeratin expressing primary melanoma of the breast is neurogenic in origin (and obviously cytokeratin-negative). Nonetheless, primary melanocytic lesions of the breast are exceedingly less common than metastatic melanocytic neoplasms.

Among the metastatic carcinomas in the breast that are most likely to be mistaken for a breast primary are those arising in the lung, ovary, müllerian system, and bowel. Included in this group are mucinous, signet ring cell, clear cell, and poorly differentiated non-small-cell carcinomas of various organs, as well as malignant melanoma (13). Some types of breast tumors such as small cell, adenoid cystic, and mucoepidermoid carcinomas can occur in other organs, and appropriate clinical workup is prudent in these cases. Metastatic neuroendocrine carcinomas of various organs generally share histologic features with primary mammary carcinoma (14).

Histopathologic evaluation of the limited material obtained in NCB samples is unlikely to provide all of the information that would help to distinguish between a primary and a metastatic tumor. The presence of in situ carcinoma that is histologically similar to the invasive lesion evidences a PBC. On the other hand, the absence of in situ carcinoma in association with invasive carcinoma is supportive (but not diagnostic) of metastatis rather than a PBC. Metastatic tumor often surrounds and displaces histologically unremarkable breast glandular parenchyma. This phenomenon is less frequent in primary mammary ductal carcinoma, but it is encountered in invasive lobular carcinoma. The latter typically shows little or no associated ductal hyperplasia. A peripheral lymphocytic infiltrate and stromal reaction are not unusual at the site of metastatic tumors in the breast as well as in PBCs. The finding of more than two grossly evident tumor nodules should lead one to consider metastatic tumors, especially if the histologic pattern is unusual. Lymphovascular tumor emboli may result from metastases in the breast as well as from PBCs. Diffuse lymphatic spread of metastatic tumor within the breast can occur and rarely produces the clinical appearance of inflammatory carcinoma (15,16).

An unusual histologic pattern and clinical information about a prior neoplasm are the best clues for identifying a metastatic tumor in the breast. It is important to be sensitive to histopathologic patterns and cytologic features that are not typical for breast carcinoma, including glands with necrosis for colonic primaries, intranuclear inclusions for melanoma, and clear cells for renal carcinoma (17).

COMMON SOURCES OF NMMN INVOLVING THE BREAST

Carcinoma of the Lung and Mesothelioma

Non-small-cell carcinoma of the lung is among the most common NMMNs to metastasize to the breast (18-21). Pulmonary adenocarcinoma has diverse histologic appearances; some of which resemble mammary carcinoma **(Fig. 22.1)**.

Knowledge of any synchronous or metachronous carcinoma of the lung as well as comparative histopathologic review of the concurrent or prior lung tumor is vital aid in this circumstance (22).

About 75% of pulmonary carcinomas are positive for thyroid transcription factor (TTF1). Although TTF1 immunoreactivity has been reported in mammary carcinomas, the main factor influencing the purported prevalence of TTF1 expression in tumors other than those of pulmonary and thyroid origin is the type of clone used. It has been reported that clone SPT24 (Leica/Novocastra) is more sensitive but less specific than clone 8G7G3/1 (DakoCytomation) (23). Napsin A can further support lung primary (24).

Small-cell carcinoma can be primary or metastatic in the breast. The diagnosis of primary small-cell carcinoma of the breast is supported by the concurrent presence of a conventional ductal type of invasive and/or in situ carcinoma. The diagnosis of metastatic small-cell carcinoma in the breast from another organ including the lung can be rendered by the exclusion of a mammary primary and comparative histopathologic review of the nonmammary primary tumor. Metastatic small carcinoma, like most metastatic carcinomas, is more often multifocal and multicentric. When present, diffuse expression of estrogen receptor (ER) or androgen receptor (AR), seen in 30% and 15% of breast small-cell carcinomas, respectively, and typically absent in the lung counterpart, strongly favors breast origin (25). Notably, TTF1 may be expressed in small-cell carcinoma of any organ. Massively parallel sequencing (MPS) has demonstrated a high rate of *TP53* mutation and variable loss of *RB1* in both breast and lung small-cell carcinomas; however, the breast tumors more commonly harbor *PIK3CA* mutations (26).

An exceedingly rare source of metastatic tumor in the breast is *mesothelioma*, especially the epithelioid variant which may mimic a mammary primary. Immunoreactivity for D2-40 (podoplanin) and calretinin strongly favors mesothelioma over carcinoma (27). Other stains that are

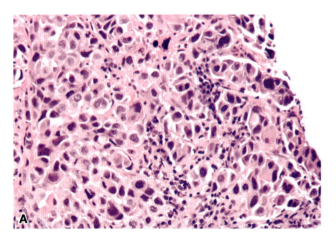
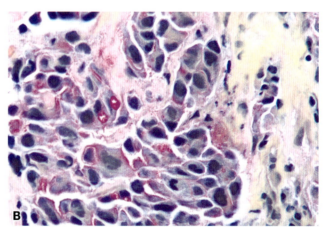

FIGURE 22.1 Metastatic Pulmonary Adenocarcinoma. A: Adenocarcinoma in a needle core biopsy specimen of the breast. Without a clinical history of pulmonary carcinoma, this tumor might be interpreted as mammary carcinoma. **B:** Intracytoplasmic mucin appears magenta with the mucicarmine stain. A histologically similar adenocarcinoma of lung had been previously diagnosed and treated.

helpful to evaluate for the diagnosis of mesothelioma include claudin-4, CD15, and MOC-31 (27-30).

Malignant Melanoma

Metastatic malignant melanoma presenting clinically as a breast tumor may be difficult to recognize if the primary (cutaneous or ocular) lesion is occult or if the pathologist is uninformed of the clinical history **(Fig. 22.2)** (31). Metastatic melanoma has been reported in the male breast, and it may also involve axillary lymph nodes (1). As stated earlier, exceedingly rare examples of metaplastic mammary carcinoma display melanocytic differentiation (12).

Gastrointestinal Neoplasms

Adenocarcinomas originating in the gastrointestinal tract, especially in the colon and rectum, are rarely the source of metastatic carcinoma in the breast, despite their relatively higher prevalence (32-34). In this setting, nuclear immunoreactivity for CDX2 is supportive of the diagnosis of metastatic colorectal adenocarcinoma **(Fig. 22.3)** (35-37).

Neuroendocrine ("carcinoid") tumors of the gastrointestinal tract are a surprisingly frequent source of metastases in one or both breasts (14,38,39). Without knowledge of an extramammary primary, a metastatic neuroendocrine tumor in the breast can be mistaken for a mammary carcinoma with neuroendocrine differentiation (40) or for invasive lobular carcinoma. Neuroendocrine markers including synaptophysin, chromogranin, CD56, and INSM1 can be strongly, diffusely positive in either scenario. Expression of extramammary site-specific markers such as CDX2 and absent or only weak expression of ER and progesterone receptor (PR) support a metastasis (41,42).

Neoplasms of Gynecologic Organs

Metastatic müllerian (ie, tubo-ovarian or peritoneal) carcinomas to the breast have generally been serous rather than mucinous. Serous carcinomas of müllerian origin usually display a papillary appearance with abundant psammoma bodies **(Fig. 22.4)**. The typical immunoprofile of these neoplasms is CK7(+), CK20(−), CA125(+), WT1(+), and PAX8(+). The final diagnosis depends on clinical and radiologic correlation (6,43-45). Clinically occult serous carcinomas of tubal origin can present with axillary lymph nodal involvement (46). Metastatic endometrial carcinoma with a solid growth pattern may mimic poorly differentiated or solid papillary mammary carcinoma **(Fig. 22.5)** (47).

The immunostain for WT1 (Wilms tumor suppressor gene 1), a nuclear marker associated with müllerian serous papillary carcinomas (43,48,49), is positive in a minority of mammary carcinomas including rare cases of invasive micropapillary carcinoma (18,50,51). This is of interest because of the reported upregulation of the *WT1* gene in breast carcinomas (52), and the observation that higher WT1 messenger ribonucleic acid (mRNA) levels were associated with a relatively poor prognosis in some (but not all) analyses (53).

Cytoplasmic reactivity for WT1 in breast carcinomas noted in some reports (51,54) may be related to the antibody used or altered WT1 phosphorylation and should not be considered to be a positive result (55). Because the majority of müllerian carcinomas are CA125-positive, and WT1 is negative in most mammary carcinomas, nuclear reactivity for WT1 and cytoplasmic reactivity for CA125 strongly favor metastatic müllerian carcinoma over primary mammary carcinoma (18,56).

PAX8 is a key transcription factor for organogenesis of the thyroid gland, kidney, and müllerian system. Nonaka et al (57) studied 124 ovarian carcinomas (84 serous papillary, 18 endometrioid, 12 mucinous, 10 clear cells) and 243 invasive breast carcinomas (178 ductal, 65 lobular) by immunostaining for PAX8 and WT1 in tissue microarrays. PAX8 reactivity was found in 108 of 124 ovarian carcinomas (87.1%), whereas WT1 expression was observed in 78 of 124 ovarian carcinomas (62.9%). All mammary carcinomas were negative for PAX8, but WT1 expression was seen in 5 of 243 cases (2.1%). In this study, PAX8 was found to be a useful marker in the differential diagnosis of ovarian and breast carcinomas, and superior to WT1 for the diagnosis of all types of nonmucinous ovarian carcinomas, especially clear cell and endometrioid types wherein WT1 expression is generally negative or only focal.

UNCOMMON SOURCES OF BREAST METASTASES

Metastatic medullary carcinoma of the thyroid gland growing in the breast with a pattern of invasive lobular carcinoma has been described (58). Papillary and follicular carcinomas of the thyroid gland may rarely metastasize to the breast (59). Papillary carcinoma of the thyroid and lung can produce cystic papillary metastases that mimic primary papillary carcinoma of the breast. Metastatic tall cell variant of papillary thyroid carcinoma overlaps morphologically with tall cell carcinoma with reversed polarity, a rare primary breast tumor with recurrent *IDH2* p.R172 mutation (60-62). Thyroid carcinoma will be immunoreactive for TTF1 and thyroglobulin, two markers typically not expressed in mammary carcinoma (63,64).

Among sarcomas metastatic to the breast, solitary fibrous tumor (erstwhile hemangiopericytoma), pleomorphic sarcoma (formerly malignant fibrous histiocytoma), and liposarcoma may be difficult to distinguish from primary mammary sarcomas (including malignant phyllodes tumors) and spindle cell metaplastic mammary carcinomas (11,65). Leiomyosarcomas metastatic to the breast, originating in gynecologic organs, have been reported **(Fig. 22.6)** (1).

Instances of mammary metastases of extremely uncommon tumors, such as esthesioneuroblastoma, have been recorded (66). Mammary metastases from various other small, blue, round cell tumors such as medulloblastoma, rhabdomyosarcoma, and neuroblastoma can occur in children and adults **(Fig. 22.7)** (67-70).

At least one case of tumor-to-tumor metastasis (specifically a renal cell carcinoma metastatic to invasive ductal carcinoma) has been reported in the breast (71). This "collision tumor" was evident only on the excisional biopsy.

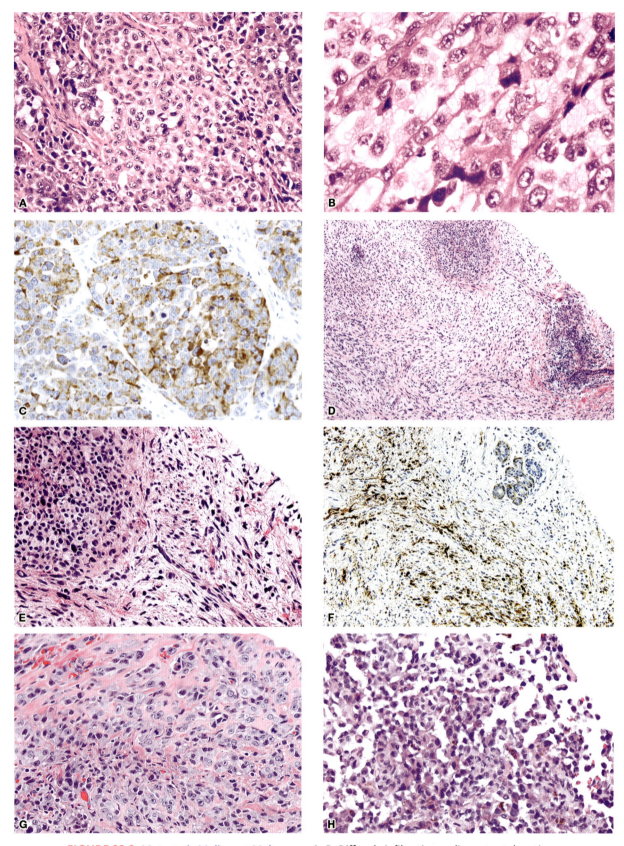

FIGURE 22.2 Metastatic Malignant Melanoma. A, B: Diffusely infiltrating malignant cytokeratin-negative (not shown) cells with an epithelioid appearance. **C:** The tumor cells are immunoreactive for HMB-45. **D-F:** Metastatic spindle and epithelioid melanoma in another needle core breast biopsy sample. The spindle cell component is reactive for S-100 protein **(F)**. There was no reactivity for HMB-45 or Melan-A (not shown). **G, H:** Histopathologic diversity of metastatic melanoma is evident in two additional needle core biopsy specimens of the breast. The melanoma cells appear epithelioid and relatively cohesive in **(G)** and are discohesive and pigmented in **(H)**.

METASTASES FROM NONMAMMARY MALIGNANT NEOPLASMS 447

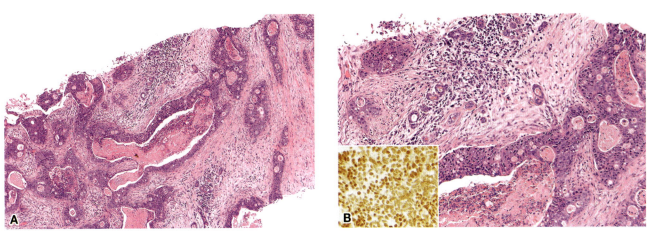

FIGURE 22.3 Metastatic Adenocarcinoma in a Patient With a Known Primary Tumor of Sigmoid Colon. A, B: This needle core biopsy of the breast shows adenocarcinoma. A cluster of native benign inactive breast glands is evident (top center). The tumor cells are immunoreactive with CDX2 (inset in **B**)—a result that supports the diagnosis of metastatic colonic carcinoma. (Courtesy of Drs S. Titi and A. Ahmad.)

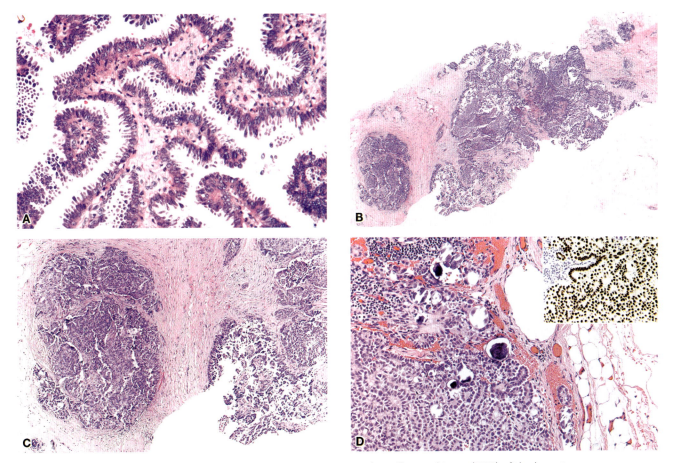

FIGURE 22.4 Metastatic Ovarian Carcinoma. A: Part of needle core biopsy (NCB) of the breast with metastatic papillary serous ovarian carcinoma. **B, C:** This NCB sample of the breast shows metastatic poorly differentiated ovarian carcinoma with a solid architecture that resembles mammary carcinoma. **D:** This biopsy of an axillary lymph node shows metastatic papillary serous carcinoma of the ovary with calcifications. PAX8 positivity is shown in inset.

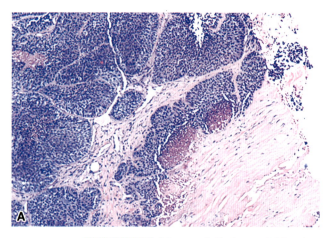
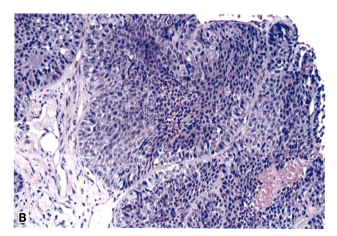

FIGURE 22.5 Metastatic Endometrial Carcinoma. **A, B:** The solid growth pattern divided into alveolar nests in this needle core biopsy of metastatic endometrial carcinoma resembles the structure of solid papillary mammary carcinoma.

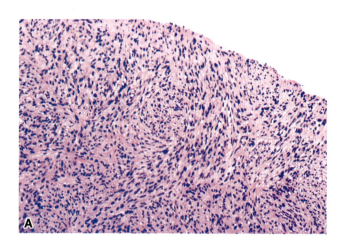
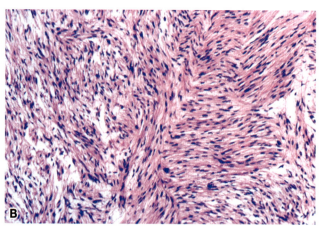

FIGURE 22.6 Metastatic Leiomyosarcoma. **A:** This needle core biopsy shows a dense tumor composed of interlacing spindle cells with eosinophilic cytoplasm. The tumor cells were immunoreactive for smooth muscle actin (not shown). **B:** The source of the metastasis was a primary leiomyosarcoma of the groin which had been resected 1 year earlier.

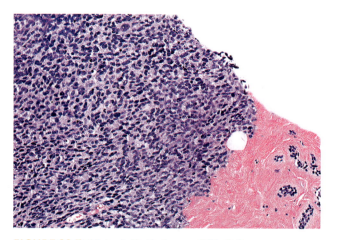

FIGURE 22.7 Metastatic Embryonal Rhabdomyosarcoma. The needle core biopsy specimen showing a small blue round cell tumor is from a breast mass in a female child. The patient had a history of embryonal rhabdomyosarcoma.

The initial NCB showed only ductal carcinoma in situ—illustrating the sampling issues inherent with this technique.

OCCULT PRIMARY NEOPLASMS

A review of records over a 92-year period at Royal London Hospital revealed that about one-third of metastatic NMMN originated from an occult primary tumor (19). A surprising proportion of occult lung tumors that have presented with breast metastases have been small-cell carcinomas. Other sites of occult neoplasms include the kidney, stomach, and ovary and tube, as well as the intestinal neuroendocrine system (erstwhile "carcinoid" tumors) (38,72).

METASTATIC PROSTATIC CARCINOMA

When a breast mass is discovered in a man known to have prostate carcinoma, comparative histopathologic review of

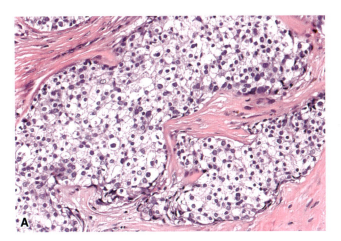 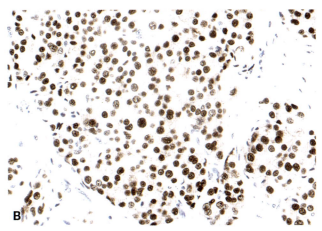

FIGURE 22.8 Metastatic Prostatic Carcinoma. The primary tumor was diagnosed 1 year ago. The patient presented with elevated serum prostate-specific antigen (PSA), bone metastases, and the breast tumor shown here. **A:** The metastatic carcinoma showed prominent clear cell features, which were focally present in the primary prostatic tumor. **B:** Strong diffuse nuclear immunoreactivity for androgen receptor (AR) is shown. The carcinoma displayed cytoplasmic reactivity for PSA (not shown).

the two tumors is essential **(Fig. 22.8)**. Stains for prostate-specific antigen (PSA), prostate acid phosphatase (PsAP), prostate specific membrane antigen (PSMA), and NKX3.1 should be performed in equivocal cases (73,74). Since PSA has been detected by immunostaining in breast carcinomas from men and women, a positive result is not by itself diagnostic of metastatic prostate carcinoma (75). ER and AR immunoreactivity may not be helpful in this regard, because prostate carcinomas can be ER(+) and AR(+) (76) (see Table 22.1). GATA3 expression was documented in 2 of 95 prostatic adenocarcinomas in one study (77), but the expression, if any, of gross cystic disease fluid protein-15 (GCDFP-15) in prostate carcinoma remains to be determined.

A "collision" tumor consisting of metastatic prostatic carcinoma in a primary solid papillary carcinoma of the male breast has been described (78).

LATE PRESENTATION OF METASTATIC NMMN IN THE BREAST

Previously diagnosed neoplasms that have given rise to breast metastases later in the clinical course of the disease include malignant melanoma, sarcoma, lung carcinoma, intestinal "carcinoid," bladder (urothelial) carcinoma, renal (clear cell and sarcomatoid) carcinoma **(Fig. 22.9)**, and ovarian carcinoma (5,79-81). Metastases have been found in the breast as long as 16 years after the diagnosis of the primary neoplasm (1).

AXILLARY LYMPH NODE METASTASES FROM NMMN

Metastatic carcinoma in axillary lymph nodes without an apparent ipsilateral or contralateral breast primary is a

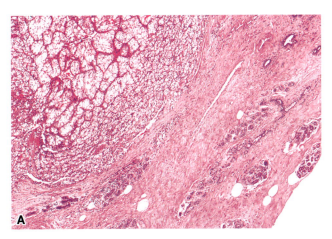 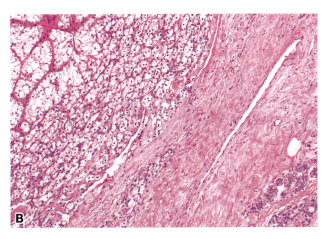

FIGURE 22.9 Metastatic Renal Carcinoma. A: A needle core biopsy of the breast showing metastatic renal clear cell carcinoma in a patient with a remote history of histologically similar renal carcinoma. **B:** The tumor shows an alveolar structure and cytoplasmic clearing that resemble mammary apocrine carcinoma with clear cell change.

well-recognized clinical scenario. An occult mammary primary should be the primary consideration in the differential diagnosis, and initial evaluation should be guided by this concept. Mammography, ultrasound, and MRI examinations are helpful in this regard. Apocrine carcinomas of the breast have a predilection to present either as occult mammary primaries or axillary nodal metastases. Most of these tumors are CK(+), ER(−), PR (−), AR(+), and HER2(−). This immunoprofile can distinguish apocrine carcinoma from metastatic melanoma, which it can resemble. The axillary region is also a common primary site of cutaneous adnexal carcinoma with apocrine differentiation. The differential diagnosis of primary apocrine carcinoma of the breast arising in the axillary tail can be difficult if not impossible to resolve by morphologic, immunohistochemical, or even molecular analysis (82).

Axillary nodal involvement by metastatic NMMN is usually accompanied by coincidental metastatic spread to one or both breasts (1). However, NMMN may involve axillary lymph nodes without clinically evident metastases in either breast. Delair (1) studied 85 patients with breast and/or axillary lymph node metastatic NMMN. Axillary involvement alone occurred in 6/85 (7%) cases, with the most frequent primary lesion being cutaneous malignant melanoma. The authors did not indicate how many of the primary lesions were contiguous to the axillary metastasis. Other NMMNs with axillary nodal involvement in the absence of breast metastases include serous papillary ovarian carcinoma (83), large cell neuroendocrine carcinoma of the lung (84), and squamous cell carcinoma of the tonsil (85).

Benign inclusions of nevoid nature and of the glandular and squamous types can simulate metastatic NMMN. See *Rosen's Breast Pathology* 5th edition (p.1366-1376) for a detailed review of such inclusions.

"IMPLANTATION METASTASES" IN THE BREAST

The development of secondary tumor deposit along the healing biopsy tract of a needle biopsy procedure has been called "implantation metastasis." Several cases have been reported in the breast. In some instances, the track of the fine needle aspiration (FNA) biopsy procedure traversed breast tissues *en route* to and from the targeted lesion in the lung.

In one such case, a 57-year-old woman developed an "implant metastasis" in the breast 3 months after a CT-guided FNA of the ipsilateral lung with a 20-gauge needle. The tumor deposit involved breast tissue as well as skin (86). In another notable case, a 52-year-old woman developed an "implant metastasis" in the skin and subcutaneous tissue of the breast 4 months after a CT-guided FNA of the ipsilateral lung with a 22-gauge needle (87) **(Fig. 22.10)**.

An unusual case of "implantation metastasis" was reported in a 38-year-old woman who had been treated by skin-sparing mastectomy for microinvasive carcinoma associated with high-grade ductal carcinoma in situ (88). The ipsilateral breast underwent immediate autologous reconstruction. Three years later, Paget disease of the skin occurred at the puncture site of the original NCB site.

An implantation metastasis can mimic PBC. The clinical history, a comparative review of the primary and secondary tumors, and immunohistochemical studies will usually clarify the diagnosis.

USE OF IMMUNOSTAINS IN THE DIAGNOSIS OF METASTASES IN THE BREAST

Typically, a panel of immunostains ought to be employed in this setting as no single marker is completely sensitive or specific **(Table 22.1)**. The use of several immunostains has been discussed in the foregoing.

USE OF IMMUNOSTAINS TO SUPPORT PRIMARY BREAST CARCINOMA

It is occasionally necessary to use immunohistochemistry as an adjunct to histopathology to help establish a carcinoma located in the breast (or elsewhere) as a PBC. ER-positivity can be observed in approximately 75% of PBC, and positivity for both ER and PR is encountered in around 65% of PBC. Notably, non-breast carcinomas (particularly those of müllerian, skin adnexal, and lung origin) can also be ER-positive. PBC is characteristically immunoreactive for CK7 and negative for CK20. Positivity for mammaglobin, GCDFP-15 (BRST-2), and GATA3 also support PBC. Most triple-negative breast carcinomas (TNBC) are negative for both mammaglobin and GCDFP-15; SOX-10 and TRPS1 can be positive in this setting.

Mammaglobin is an epithelial intracytoplasmic secretory glycoprotein of mammary epithelial cells. Mammary carcinomas of all grades may be positive for mammaglobin, whereas normal epithelial cells are typically not immunoreactive. The sensitivity of mammaglobin for breast carcinoma is around 77%, but it lacks the specificity of GCDFP-15 (89,90). Carcinomas of cutaneous adnexal glands as well as salivary glands may also be mammaglobin-positive.

GCDFP-15 (BRST-2) is a secretory product of mammary cells that can be demonstrated via immunostains in mammary and extramammary apocrine epithelia. Only rare cells in normal breast epithelial glands are positive for GCDFP-15. Up to 70% of breast carcinomas are positive for GCDFP-15 (89,90). Rare examples of pulmonary adenocarcinoma (approximately 5%) can be positive for GCDFP-15 (91).

GATA3, a transcription factor that mainly regulates differentiation of mammary and urothelial epithelia, can be useful in confirming mammary origin of a tumor. Immunohistochemical expression of GATA3 can be found in more than 90% of mammary carcinomas, including about 70% of those that are triple-negative (92,93). GATA3 is as sensitive for PBC as mammaglobin and GCDFP-15. GATA3 immunoreactivity is encountered in the majority of urothelial

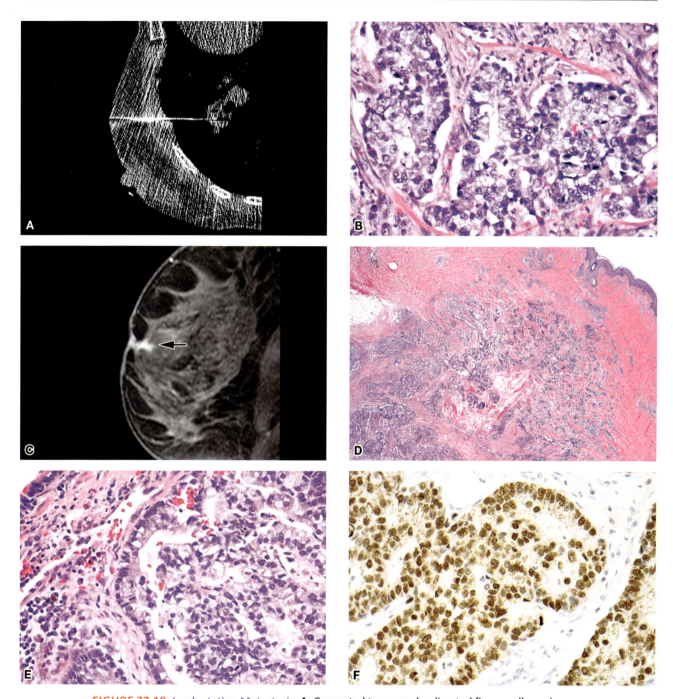

FIGURE 22.10 Implantation Metastasis. A: Computed tomography-directed fine needle aspiration (FNA) of the right lung shows passage of the needle through the right breast and anterior chest wall. Cytologic examination of the FNA showed malignant cells (not shown). **B:** The subsequent lobectomy showed adenocarcinoma of the lung. **C:** Contrast-enhanced magnetic resonance imaging (MRI) of the "tumor in the breast," 14 months after the FNA, shows a superficial tumor mass. **D, E:** Implantation metastasis in the skin and subcutaneous tissue of the breast. The tumor is similar to the previously diagnosed adenocarcinoma of the lung (seen in **B**) and is positive for thyroid transcription factor-1 **(F)**.

TABLE 22.1

Immunohistochemical Approach to Establish Possible Primary Site of a Suspected Metastatic Malignant Neoplasms in the Breast

To Determine...	Diagnosis	Marker
Basic lineage	Carcinoma	Cytokeratins
	Lymphoma	CD45
	Melanoma	A103, MITF, S100, SOX10
	Sarcoma[a]	Vimentin
Type of carcinoma	Adenocarcinoma	CK7, CK20
	Germ cell	PLAP, OCT4, AFP, β-HCG
	Hepatocellular	HepPar1, pCEA, CD10, CD13
	Renal cell	RCC, CD10, PAX2, PAX8
	Squamous cell	CK5/6, p40, p63
	Neuroendocrine	Chromogranin, Synaptophysin, INSM1
	Urothelial	GATA3
Site	Colorectal	CDX2, CK7(−), CK20(+)
	Lung	TTF1, Napsin A, CK7(+), CK20(−)
	Ovary and tube	ER, CA125, WT1, PAX2, PAX8
	Pancreatobiliary	CDX2, CK7(+), CK20(+), SMAD4 inactivation
	Prostate	NKX3.1[b], PSA, PsAP, PSMA
	Thyroid	PAX8, TTF1, thyroglobulin

AFP, alpha fetoprotein; β-HCG, beta human chorionic gonadotrophin; ca, carcinoma; CK, cytokeratin; ER, estrogen receptor; MITF, microphthalmic transcription factor; pCEA, polyclonal carcinoembryonic antigen; PLAP, placental alkaline phosphatase; PSA, prostate-specific antigen; PsAP, prostate acid phosphatase; PSMA, prostate specific membrane antigen; RCC, renal cell carcinoma; TTF1, thyroid transcription factor-1; WT1, Wilms tumor-1.

[a]In tumors negative for carcinoma, lymphoma, and melanoma markers, and with appropriate histologic appearance. [b]NKX3.1 can be positive in lobular carcinoma and ER(-)/AR(+) breast carcinomas.

References: Beauchamp K, Moran B, O'Brien T, et al. Carcinoma of unknown primary: an update for histopathologists. *Cancer Metastasis Rev.* 2023. doi:10.1007/s10555-023-10101-6; Cimino-Mathews A. Novel uses of immunohistochemistry in breast pathology: interpretation and pitfalls. *Mod Pathol.* 2021;34(suppl 1): 62-77; Kim KW, Krajewski KM, Jagannathan JP, et al. Cancer of unknown primary sites: what radiologists need to know and what oncologists want to know. *AJR Am J Roentgenol.* 2013;200:484-492.

carcinomas, and it has also been reported in cutaneous basal cell carcinomas as well as trophoblastic and yolk sac tumors.

SOX-10 (Sry-related HMg-Box gene 10) is a key nuclear transcription factor in the differentiation of neural crest progenitor cells to melanocytes and is widely utilized as a melanoma marker. SOX-10 also marks normal mammary (and salivary gland) myoepithelial cells and is a useful breast lineage marker in TNBC, wherein the sensitivity of usual breast lineage markers is reduced. In the latter regard, SOX-10 is complementary to GATA3 (94).

Another useful marker in TNBC is *TRPS1* (transcriptional repressor GATA binding 1, formerly trichorhinophalangeal syndrome type 1), a GATA transcription factor and regulator of epithelial-mesenchymal transition. TRPS1 is highly expressed in TNBC that are negative for GATA3 and/or SOX-10, and it is generally negative in urothelial

carcinoma and melanoma (95,96). Special subtypes of TNBC such as acinic cell carcinoma, adenoid cystic carcinoma, and neuroendocrine carcinoma may be TRPS1-negative (96). Matrix G1a protein (MGP) is another emerging breast marker (97).

MANAGEMENT

The distinction between a primary breast tumor and a metastasis in the breast is critical for appropriate management. A multidisciplinary integrated approach among pathologists, oncologists, surgeons, and radiologists is important (98). It is vital that comparative histopathologic review of the primary nonmammary and mammary tumors be performed whenever possible. When an occult extramammary neoplasm presents with a breast metastasis, the diagnostic workup of the patient will be largely influenced by morphologic features of the tumor that may suggest one or more particular primary sites. Advances in immunohistochemistry and molecular techniques can enable the identification of the primary site, facilitating site-specific therapy.

In most cases, mastectomy is not appropriate for metastatic tumor in the breast, but it may be performed to obtain local control of bulky, ulcerated, multifocal, necrotic, or otherwise highly symptomatic lesions. Wide excision can be supplemented by radiation therapy to the breast for appropriately selected neoplasms, and axillary dissection should be performed if the lymph nodes therein are involved. Emphasis should necessarily be placed on systemic treatment appropriate to the primary lesion. Metastatic involvement of the breast is a manifestation of generalized metastases in virtually all cases, and the prognosis depends on the clinical characteristics of the particular primary neoplasm. Median survival was 15 months after the diagnosis of breast or axillary metastases in 55 patients in one series (1).

MOLECULAR TESTING

MPS is a useful tool to define the relationship, clonality, and intratumoral genetic heterogeneity between the primary malignant neoplasms and metastatic deposits in patients with multiple primary neoplasms and synchronous metastases (99). The increasing sensitivity of MPS facilitates analysis of small NCB or even circulating cell-free DNA, in the metastatic setting. Complex, bioinformatics-based classifiers using MPS findings in conjunction with immunohistochemical analysis to clarify primary disease site are under development (100).

Techniques for the *molecular profiling* of tumors, utilizing various platforms including RT-PCR, cDNA microarray, microRNA profiling, and methylome profiling, have become increasingly available in recent years. When a metastatic NMMN is suspected, the aim of such profiling is to reliably establish the primary site, thus enabling site-specific therapy. The latter, when initiated on the basis of either immunohistochemistry or molecular profiling, can be more effective than empiric chemotherapy (101).

REFERENCES

1. DeLair DF, Corben AD, Catalano JP, et al. Non-mammary metastases to the breast and axilla: a study of 85 cases. *Mod Pathol.* 2013;26:343-349.
2. Picasso R, Pistoia F, Zaottini F, et al. Breast metastases: updates on epidemiology and radiologic findings. *Cureus.* 2020;12:e12258.
3. Abrams HL, Spiro R, Goldstein N. Metastases in carcinoma; analysis of 1000 autopsied cases. *Cancer.* 1950;3:74-85.
4. Di Bonito L, Luchi M, Giarelli L, et al. Metastatic tumors to the female breast. An autopsy study of 12 cases. *Pathol Res Pract.* 1991;187:432-436.
5. Toombs BD, Kalisher L. Metastatic disease to the breast: clinical, pathologic, and radiographic features. *AJR Am J Roentgenol.* 1977;129:673-676.
6. Recine MA, Deavers MT, Middleton LP, et al. Serous carcinoma of the ovary and peritoneum with metastases to the breast and axillary lymph nodes: a potential pitfall. *Am J Surg Pathol.* 2004;28:1646-1651.
7. Goldstein NS, Uzieblo A. WT1 immunoreactivity in uterine papillary serous carcinomas is different from ovarian serous carcinomas. *Am J Clin Pathol.* 2002;117:541-545.
8. Mun SH, Ko EY, Han BK, et al. Breast metastases from extramammary malignancies: typical and atypical ultrasound features. *Korean J Radiol.* 2014;15:20-28.
9. Formicola F, Riccardi A, Vigliar E, et al. Multimetastatic medullary thyroid carcinoma to the breast: PET/CT—mammographic-US and MR findings. *Breast J.* 2014;20:653-654.
10. Gayer G, Ben-Haim S. Ovarian carcinoma metastasis to breast: role of PET/CT. *Isr Med Assoc J.* 2013;15:784.
11. Yokouchi M, Nagano S, Kijima Y, et al. Solitary breast metastasis from myxoid liposarcoma. *BMC Cancer.* 2014;14:482.
12. Ruffolo EF, Koerner FC, Maluf HM. Metaplastic carcinoma of the breast with melanocytic differentiation. *Mod Pathol.* 1997;10:592-596.
13. Boutis AL, Andreadis C, Patakiouta F, et al. Gastric signet-ring adenocarcinoma presenting with breast metastasis. *World J Gastroenterol.* 2006;12:2958-2961.
14. Perry KD, Reynolds C, Rosen DG, et al. Metastatic neuroendocrine tumour in the breast: a potential mimic of in-situ and invasive mammary carcinoma. *Histopathology.* 2011;59:619-630.
15. Njiaju UO, Truica CI. Metastatic prostatic adenocarcinoma mimicking inflammatory breast carcinoma: a case report. *Clin Breast Cancer.* 2010;10:E3-E5.
16. Ninan J, Naik V, George GM. "Inflammatory breast cancer" due to metastatic adenocarcinoma of lung. *BMJ Case Rep.* 2016;2016:bcr2016215857.
17. Lee AHS, Hodi Z, Soomro I, et al. Histological clues to the diagnosis of metastasis to the breast from extramammary malignancies. *Histopathology.* 2020;77:303-313.
18. Lee AH. The histological diagnosis of metastases to the breast from extramammary malignancies. *J Clin Pathol.* 2007;60:1333-1341.
19. Georgiannos SN, Chin J, Goode AW, et al. Secondary neoplasms of the breast: a survey of the 20th Century. *Cancer.* 2001;92:2259-2266.
20. Hsu W, Sheen-Chen SM, Wang JL, et al. Squamous cell lung carcinoma metastatic to the breast. *Anticancer Res.* 2008;28:1299-1301.
21. Wang B, Jiang Y, Li SY, et al. Breast metastases from primary lung cancer: a retrospective case series on clinical, ultrasonographic, and immunohistochemical features. *Transl Lung Cancer Res.* 2021;10:3226-3235.
22. Mirrielees JA, Kapur JH, Szalucki LM, et al. Metastasis of primary lung carcinoma to the breast: a systematic review of the literature. *J Surg Res.* 2014;188:419-431.
23. Masood S, Davis C, Kubik MJ. Changing the term "breast tumor resembling the tall cell variant of papillary thyroid carcinoma" to "tall cell variant of papillary breast carcinoma". *Adv Anat Pathol.* 2012;19:108-110.
24. Turner BM, Cagle PT, Sainz IM, et al. Napsin A, a new marker for lung adenocarcinoma, is complementary and more sensitive and specific than thyroid transcription factor 1 in the differential diagnosis of primary pulmonary carcinoma: evaluation of 1674 cases by tissue microarray. *Arch Pathol Lab Med.* 2012;136:163-171.
25. Uccella S, Finzi G, Sessa F, et al. On the endless dilemma of neuroendocrine neoplasms of the breast: a journey through concepts and entities. *Endocr Pathol.* 2020;31:321-329.
26. McCullar B, Pandey M, Yaghmour G, et al. Genomic landscape of small cell carcinoma of the breast contrasted to small cell carcinoma of the lung. *Breast Cancer Res Treat.* 2016;158:195-202.
27. Ordóñez NG. Immunohistochemical diagnosis of epithelioid mesothelioma: an update. *Arch Pathol Lab Med.* 2005;129:1407-1414.
28. Hyun TS, Barnes M, Tabatabai ZL. The diagnostic utility of D2-40, calretinin, CK5/6, desmin and MOC-31 in the differentiation of mesothelioma from adenocarcinoma in pleural effusion cytology. *Acta Cytol.* 2012;56:527-532.
29. Mohammad T, Garratt J, Torlakovic E, et al. Utility of a CEA, CD15, calretinin, and CK5/6 panel for distinguishing between mesotheliomas and pulmonary adenocarcinomas in clinical practice. *Am J Surg Pathol.* 2012;36:1503-1508.
30. Ordóñez NG. Application of immunohistochemistry in the diagnosis of epithelioid mesothelioma: a review and update. *Hum Pathol.* 2013;44:1-19.
31. Ravdel L, Robinson WA, Lewis K, et al. Metastatic melanoma in the breast: a report of 27 cases. *J Surg Oncol.* 2006;94:101-104.
32. Ho YY, Lee WK. Metastasis to the breast from an adenocarcinoma of the colon. *J Clin Ultrasound.* 2009;37:239-241.
33. Noh KT, Oh B, Sung SH, et al. Metastasis to the breast from colonic adenocarcinoma. *J Korean Surg Soc.* 2011;81(suppl 1):S43-S46.
34. Alexander HR, Turnbull AD, Rosen PP. Isolated breast metastases from gastrointestinal carcinomas: report of two cases. *J Surg Oncol.* 1989;42:264-266.
35. Ahmad A, Baiden-Amissah K, Oyegade A, et al. Primary sigmoid adenocarcinoma metastasis to the breast in a 28-year-old female: a case study and a review of literature. *Korean J Pathol.* 2014;48:58-61.
36. Werling RW, Yaziji H, Bacchi CE, et al. CDX2, a highly sensitive and specific marker of adenocarcinoma of intestinal origin: an immunohistochemical survey of 476 primary and metastatic carcinomas. *Am J Surg Pathol.* 2003;27:303-310.
37. Koyama T, Sekine S, Taniguchi H, et al. Hepatocyte nuclear factor 4A expression discriminates gastric involvement by metastatic breast carcinomas from primary gastric adenocarcinomas. *Hum Pathol.* 2011;42:1777-1784.
38. Geyer HL, Viney J, Karlin N. Metastatic carcinoid presenting as a breast lesion. *Curr Oncol.* 2010;17:73-77.
39. Upalakalin JN, Collins LC, Tawa N, et al. Carcinoid tumors in the breast. *Am J Surg.* 2006;191:799-805.
40. Mosunjac MB, Kochhar R, Mosunjac MI, et al. Primary small bowel carcinoid tumor with bilateral breast metastases: report of 2 cases with different clinical presentations. *Arch Pathol Lab Med.* 2004;128:292-297.
41. Mohanty SK, Kim SA, DeLair DF, et al. Comparison of metastatic neuroendocrine neoplasms to the breast and primary invasive mammary carcinomas with neuroendocrine differentiation. *Mod Pathol.* 2016;29:788-798.

42. Pareja F, D'Alfonso TM. Neuroendocrine neoplasms of the breast: a review focused on the updated World Health Organization (WHO) 5th Edition morphologic classification. *Breast J.* 2020;26:1160-1167.

43. Abehsera D, Hernández A, Santisteban J, et al. Ovarian serous cystadenocarcinoma metastasising to the breast. *J Obstet Gynaecol.* 2013;33:215-216.

44. Laury AR, Perets R, Piao H, et al. A comprehensive analysis of PAX8 expression in human epithelial tumors. *Am J Surg Pathol.* 2011;35:816-826.

45. Akturk G, Guray Durak M, Cakir Y, et al. Metastatic ovarian serous carcinoma of the breast. *Breast J.* 2017;23:362-364.

46. Atallah C, Altinel G, Fu L, et al. Axillary metastasis from an occult tubal serous carcinoma in a patient with ipsilateral breast carcinoma: a potential diagnostic pitfall. *Case Rep Pathol.* 2014;2014:534034.

47. Moore DH, Wilson DK, Hurteau JA, et al. Gynecologic cancers metastatic to the breast. *J Am Coll Surg.* 1998;187:178-181.

48. Hedley C, Sriraksa R, Showeil R, et al. The frequency and significance of WT-1 expression in serous endometrial carcinoma. *Hum Pathol.* 2014;45:1879-1884.

49. Tornos C, Soslow R, Chen S, et al. Expression of WT1, CA 125, and GCDFP-15 as useful markers in the differential diagnosis of primary ovarian carcinomas versus metastatic breast cancer to the ovary. *Am J Surg Pathol.* 2005;29:1482-1489.

50. Lee AH, Paish EC, Marchio C, et al. The expression of Wilms' tumour-1 and Ca125 in invasive micropapillary carcinoma of the breast. *Histopathology.* 2007;51:824-828.

51. Provenzano E, Byrne DJ, Russell PA, et al. Differential expression of immunohistochemical markers in primary lung and breast cancers enriched for triple-negative tumours. *Histopathology.* 2016;68:367-377.

52. Loeb DM, Evron E, Patel CB, et al. Wilms' tumor suppressor gene (WT1) is expressed in primary breast tumors despite tumor-specific promoter methylation. *Cancer Res.* 2001;61:921-925.

53. Zhang Y, Yan WT, Yang ZY, et al. The role of WT1 in breast cancer: clinical implications, biological effects and molecular mechanism. *Int J Biol Sci.* 2020;16:1474-1480.

54. Duhig EE, Kalpakos L, Yang IA, et al. Mesothelial markers in high-grade breast carcinoma. *Histopathology.* 2011;59:957-964.

55. Niksic M, Slight J, Sanford JR, et al. The Wilms' tumour protein (WT1) shuttles between nucleus and cytoplasm and is present in functional polysomes. *Hum Mol Genet.* 2004;13:463-471.

56. Domfeh AB, Carley AL, Striebel JM, et al. WT1 immunoreactivity in breast carcinoma: selective expression in pure and mixed mucinous subtypes. *Mod Pathol.* 2008;21:1217-1223.

57. Nonaka D, Chiriboga L, Soslow RA. Expression of pax8 as a useful marker in distinguishing ovarian carcinomas from mammary carcinomas. *Am J Surg Pathol.* 2008;32:1566-1571.

58. Ali SZ, Teichberg S, Attie JN, et al. Medullary thyroid carcinoma metastatic to breast masquerading as infiltrating lobular carcinoma. *Ann Clin Lab Sci.* 1994;24:441-447.

59. Loureiro MM, Leite VH, Boavida JM, et al. An unusual case of papillary carcinoma of the thyroid with cutaneous and breast metastases only. *Eur J Endocrinol.* 1997;137:267-269.

60. Chiang S, Weigelt B, Wen HC, et al. IDH2 mutations define a unique subtype of breast cancer with altered nuclear polarity. *Cancer Res.* 2016;76:7118-7129.

61. Fiche M, Cassagnau E, Aillet G, et al. [Breast metastasis from a "tall cell variant" of papillary thyroid carcinoma]. *Ann Pathol.* 1998;18:130-132.

62. Zhong E, Scognamiglio T, D'Alfonso T, et al. Breast tumor resembling the tall cell variant of papillary thyroid carcinoma: molecular characterization by next-generation sequencing and histopathological comparison with tall cell papillary carcinoma of thyroid. *Int J Surg Pathol.* 2019;27:134-141.

63. Bisceglia M, Galliani C, Rosai J. TTF-1 expression in breast carcinoma-the chosen clone matters. *Am J Surg Pathol.* 2011;35:1087-1088.

64. Robens J, Goldstein L, Gown AM, et al. Thyroid transcription factor-1 expression in breast carcinomas. *Am J Surg Pathol.* 2010;34:1881-1885.

65. Ruhland B, Dittmer C, Thill M, et al. Metastasized hemangiopericytoma of the breast: a rare case. *Arch Gynecol Obstet.* 2009;280:491-494.

66. Larbcharoensub N, Kanoksil W, Cheewaruangroj W, et al. Esthesioneuroblastoma metastasis to the breast: a case report and review of the literature. *Oncol Lett.* 2014;8:1505-1508.

67. Jung SP, Lee Y, Han KM, et al. Breast metastasis from rhabdomyosarcoma of the anus in an adolescent female. *J Breast Cancer.* 2013;16:345-348.

68. Lamovec J, Pogaènik A. Metastatic medulloblastoma to the breast. *Virchows Arch.* 2001;439:201-205.

69. Merced C, Rubio IT, Rodriguez J, et al. Breast metastasis from rhabdomyosarcoma of the nasal septum in a pregnant adult woman. *Breast J.* 2011;17:420-421.

70. Yaren A, Guclu A, Sen N, et al. Breast metastasis in a pregnant woman with alveolar rhabdomyosarcoma of the upper extremity. *Eur J Obstet Gynecol Reprod Biol.* 2008;140:131-133.

71. Chen TD, Lee LY. A case of renal cell carcinoma metastasizing to invasive ductal breast carcinoma. *J Formos Med Assoc.* 2014;113:133-136.

72. La Rosa S, Casnedi S, Maragliano R, et al. Breast metastasis as the first clinical manifestation of ileal neuroendocrine tumor. A challenging diagnosis with relevant clinical implications. *Endocr Pathol.* 2015;26:145-151.

73. Green LK, Klima M. The use of immunohistochemistry in metastatic prostatic adenocarcinoma to the breast. *Hum Pathol.* 1991;22:242-246.

74. Gurel B, Ali TZ, Montgomery EA, et al. NKX3.1 as a marker of prostatic origin in metastatic tumors. *Am J Surg Pathol.* 2010;34:1097-1105.

75. Kraus TS, Cohen C, Siddiqui MT. Prostate-specific antigen and hormone receptor expression in male and female breast carcinoma. *Diagn Pathol.* 2010;5:63.

76. Asgari M, Morakabati A. Estrogen receptor beta expression in prostate adenocarcinoma. *Diagn Pathol.* 2011;6:61.

77. Miettinen M, McCue PA, Sarlomo-Rikala M, et al. GATA3: a multispecific but potentially useful marker in surgical pathology: a systematic analysis of 2500 epithelial and nonepithelial tumors. *Am J Surg Pathol.* 2014;38:13-22.

78. Sahoo S, Smith RE, Potz JL, et al. Metastatic prostatic adenocarcinoma within a primary solid papillary carcinoma of the male breast. *Arch Pathol Lab Med.* 2001;125:1101-1103.

79. Belton AL, Stull MA, Grant T, et al. Mammographic and sonographic findings in metastatic transitional cell carcinoma of the breast. *AJR Am J Roentgenol.* 1997;168:511-512.

80. Ding GT, Hwang JS, Tan PH. Sarcomatoid renal cell carcinoma metastatic to the breast: report of a case with diagnosis on fine needle aspiration cytology. *Acta Cytol.* 2007;51:451-455.

81. Vassalli L, Ferrari VD, Simoncini E, et al. Solitary breast metastases from a renal cell carcinoma. *Breast Cancer Res Treat.* 2001;68:29-31.

82. Libertini M, Oneda E, Di Biasi B, et al. Cutaneous adnexal carcinoma with apocrine differentiation: a challenging diagnosis and personalized treatment with mTOR inhibitor in a very rare disease. *Case Rep Oncol.* 2020;13:1091-1096.

83. Sibio S, Sammartino P, Accarpio F, et al. Axillary lymph node metastasis as first presentation of peritoneal carcinomatosis from serous papillary ovarian cancer: case report and review of the literature. *Eur J Gynaecol Oncol.* 2014;35:170-173.

84. Terada T. Pathologic diagnosis of large cell neuroendocrine carcinoma of the lung in an axillary lymph node: a case report with immunohistochemical and molecular genetic studies. *Int J Clin Exp Pathol.* 2013;6:1177-1179.

85. Cheng CY, Su TF, Lin YH, et al. Rare axillary metastasis from squamous cell carcinoma of the tonsil. *Clin Nucl Med.* 2013;38:e304-e305.

86. Sacchini V, Galimberti V, Marchini S, et al. Percutaneous transthoracic needle aspiration biopsy: a case report of implantation metastasis. *Eur J Surg Oncol.* 1989;15:179-183.

87. Schreiner AM, Jones JG, Swistel AJ, et al. Transthoracic fine needle aspiration resulting in implantation metastasis in the superficial tissues of the breast. *Cytopathology.* 2013;24:58-60.

88. Calvillo KZ, Guo L, Brostrom V, et al. Recurrence of breast carcinoma as Paget disease of the skin at a prior core needle biopsy site: case report and review of the literature. *Int J Surg Case Rep.* 2015;15:152-156.

89. Bhargava R, Beriwal S, Dabbs DJ. Mammaglobin vs GCDFP-15: an immunohistologic validation survey for sensitivity and specificity. *Am J Clin Pathol.* 2007;127:103-113.

90. Lewis GH, Subhawong AP, Nassar H, et al. Relationship between molecular subtype of invasive breast carcinoma and expression of gross cystic disease fluid protein 15 and mammaglobin. *Am J Clin Pathol.* 2011;135:587-591.

91. Striebel JM, Dacic S, Yousem SA. Gross cystic disease fluid protein-(GCDFP-15): expression in primary lung adenocarcinoma. *Am J Surg Pathol.* 2008;32:426-432.

92. Cimino-Mathews A, Subhawong AP, Illei PB, et al. GATA3 expression in breast carcinoma: utility in triple-negative, sarcomatoid, and metastatic carcinomas. *Hum Pathol.* 2013;44:1341-1349.

93. Clark BZ, Beriwal S, Dabbs DJ, et al. Semiquantitative GATA-3 immunoreactivity in breast, bladder, gynecologic tract, and other cytokeratin 7-positive carcinomas. *Am J Clin Pathol.* 2014;142:64-71.

94. Tozbikian GH, Zynger DL. A combination of GATA3 and SOX10 is useful for the diagnosis of metastatic triple-negative breast cancer. *Hum Pathol.* 2019;85:221-227.

95. Ai D, Yao J, Yang F, et al. TRPS1: a highly sensitive and specific marker for breast carcinoma, especially for triple-negative breast cancer. *Mod Pathol.* 2021;34:710-719.

96. Yoon EC, Wang G, Parkinson B, et al. TRPS1, GATA3, and SOX10 expression in triple-negative breast carcinoma. *Hum Pathol.* 2022;

97. Du T, Pan L, Zheng C, et al. Matrix Gla protein (MGP), GATA3, and TRPS1: a novel diagnostic panel to determine breast origin. *Breast Cancer Res.* 2022; 24:70. doi: 10.1186/s13058-022-01569-1.

98. Abbas J, Wienke A, Spielmann RP, et al. Intramammary metastases: comparison of mammographic and ultrasound features. *Eur J Radiol.* 2013;82:1423-1430.

99. De Mattos-Arruda L, Bidard FC, Won HH, et al. Establishing the origin of metastatic deposits in the setting of multiple primary malignancies: the role of massively parallel sequencing. *Mol Oncol.* 2014;8:150-158.

100. Varghese AM, Arora A, Capanu M, et al. Clinical and molecular characterization of patients with cancer of unknown primary in the modern era. *Ann Oncol.* 2017;28:3015-3021.

101. Kim KW, Krajewski KM, Jagannathan JP, et al. Cancer of unknown primary sites: what radiologists need to know and what oncologists want to know. *AJR Am J Roentgenol.* 2013;200:484-492.

23

Pathologic Effects of Therapy

ELAINE W. ZHONG AND SYED A. HODA

INTRODUCTION

Nonsurgical regional and systemic therapies are increasingly being used to treat patients with invasive breast carcinoma. Radiation therapy after breast-conserving surgery is standard of care for most patients with invasive and in situ breast carcinoma, and the indications for neoadjuvant chemotherapy are expanding. Recognition of the effects of these procedures on benign and malignant breast histology is essential for evaluation of therapeutic response as well as prevention of overinterpretation of findings in subsequent specimens.

IRRADIATION

Radiation and Breast-Conserving Therapy

Irradiation of the breast most commonly occurs as a component of breast-conserving therapy for breast carcinoma. A small percentage of patients treated with breast-conserving therapy (re)develop carcinoma in the treated breast. Recurrences most often occur 2 to 6 years after the completion of breast-conserving treatment and typically occur near the site of prior mass, whereas new primary carcinomas tend to develop more than 10 years following treatment and most often involve tissue distant from the excision site (1). Imaging studies often disclose parenchymal distortion, scarring, organized fat necrosis, and scattered coarse calcifications in the treated breast. Cases exhibiting a new mass, a suspicious area of enhancement on magnetic resonance imaging (MRI), a change in the features of a postoperative scar, or the appearance of pleomorphic calcifications warrant a biopsy to investigate the possibility of recurrent carcinoma.

The histologic alterations associated with irradiation of native benign mammary tissue are most obvious in terminal duct lobular units and are less pronounced in larger ducts (Figs. 23.1-23.3) (Table 23.1) (2,3). The changes include collagenization of intralobular stroma, thickening of periacinar and periductular basement membranes, atrophy of acinar and ductular epithelium, cytologic atypia of epithelial cells, and relative prominence of acinar myoepithelial cells. The latter seem to be preserved to a greater extent than the epithelial cells (4). Apocrine epithelium is susceptible to developing severe cytologic atypia after radiotherapy, especially in hyperplastic foci. When evaluating a posttreatment biopsy, it is useful to examine the pretreatment specimen for evidence of apocrine metaplasia. Atypical fibroblasts can be found in a minority of cases (Fig. 23.4).

In any one patient, most of the glandular tissue responds in a relatively uniform fashion if the entire breast has been irradiated; however, one can observe substantial variation in the severity of changes from one patient to another. The changes occasionally may be so slight as to be virtually indistinguishable from physiologic atrophy. In one study,

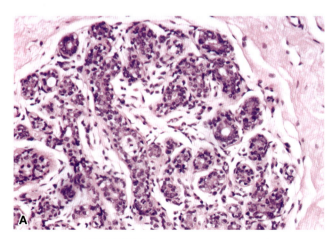 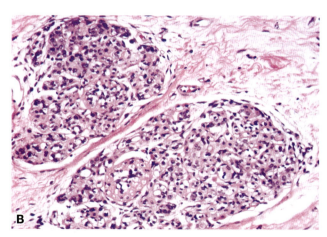

FIGURE 23.1 Radiation Atrophy of Lobules. A: This image depicts a normal lobule in the breast of a 35-year-old woman before the start of radiotherapy for invasive ductal carcinoma. **B:** A needle core biopsy was performed 3 years after irradiation. The posttreatment lobules exhibit moderate radiation atrophy, thickening of basement membranes, atrophy of epithelial cells, and clearing of the cytoplasm of the myoepithelial cells.

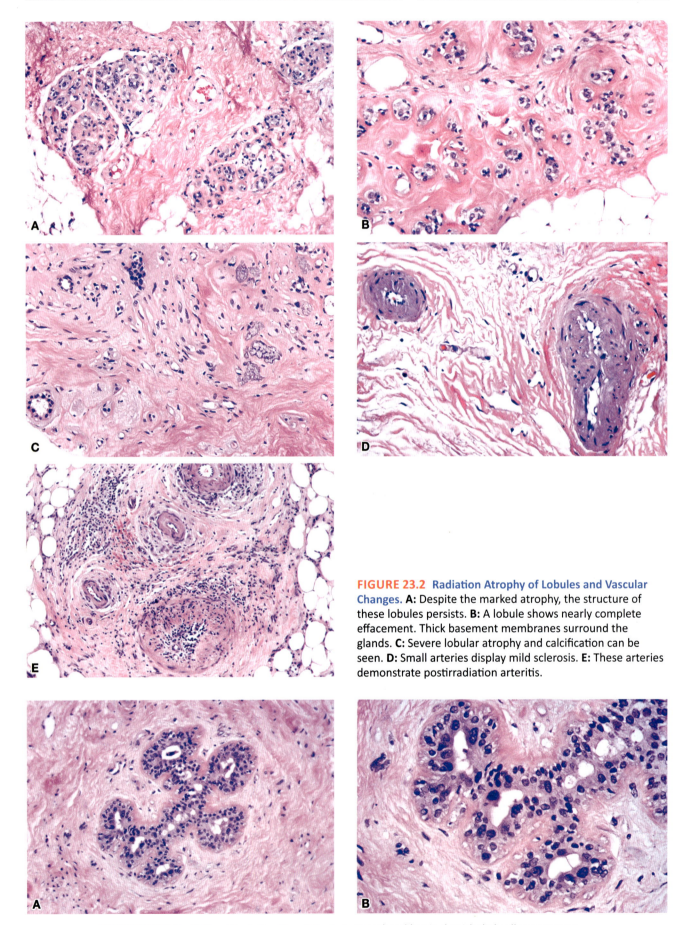

FIGURE 23.2 **Radiation Atrophy of Lobules and Vascular Changes. A:** Despite the marked atrophy, the structure of these lobules persists. **B:** A lobule shows nearly complete effacement. Thick basement membranes surround the glands. **C:** Severe lobular atrophy and calcification can be seen. **D:** Small arteries display mild sclerosis. **E:** These arteries demonstrate postirradiation arteritis.

FIGURE 23.3 **Radiation Atypia in a Small Duct. A, B:** Isolated luminal epithelial cells possess enlarged hyperchromatic nuclei. The basement membrane appears thick.

TABLE 23.1
Pathologic Effects of Radiation on Breast Carcinoma and Native Breast Tissue

Effects on breast carcinoma
- Persistent carcinomas remain intact, and affected glands may appear filled or expanded.
- More pronounced nuclear atypia, giant cells, abnormal mitoses
- Tumor necrosis

Effects on nonneoplastic breast tissue
- Gland atrophy, most pronounced in terminal duct lobular units
- Collagenization of intralobular stroma
- Thickened glandular basement membrane
- Epithelial cytologic atypia, most pronounced in apocrine metaplasia
- Myoepithelial prominence
- Endothelial atypia
- Arterial sclerosis, fragmentation of elastic layer, myointimal hyperplasia
- Myofibroblastic prominence and atypia
- Changes are permanent.

differences in histologic radiation effects among individual patients did not correlate with the radiation dose, patient age, posttreatment interval, or the use of adjuvant chemotherapy (2). Once established, the effects of irradiation do not regress. After studying 120 breast specimens obtained at intervals ranging from less than 1 year to more than 6 years after radiotherapy, Moore et al (3) did not observe significant variation in the appearance of the radiation-related alterations.

When a radioactive implant or an external "boost" has been used, histologic changes in the adjacent area may be relatively more severe than those in the distant regions of the breast. Epithelial atypia may occur in larger ducts and it may be superimposed on existing hyperplasia or apocrine metaplasia **(Fig. 23.5)**. Fat necrosis and atypia of stromal

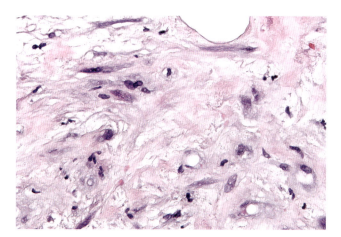

FIGURE 23.4 Radiation Atypia of Stromal Fibroblasts. Seven months after the completion of partial breast irradiation, this patient underwent a needle core biopsy to evaluate the presence of cutaneous erythema. Several fibroblasts appear enlarged and they contain large, pleomorphic nuclei.

fibroblasts are more common in proximity to such areas (5,6). Radiation-induced vascular changes, which may not ordinarily be seen after external radiotherapy, can be seen in this setting. Small- and medium-sized arteries may show sclerosis, fragmentation of elastica, endothelial atypia, and myointimal proliferation leading to narrowing of the vascular lumina. Prominent, cytologically atypical endothelial cells are also apparent in capillaries.

In situ lobular and ductal carcinomas persisting after radiation therapy are largely intact; consequently, the affected lobules and ducts appear filled and, often, expanded by the neoplastic cell population. Frequently, little or no microscopic change attributable to treatment is evident when pre- and postirradiation samples of in situ carcinoma are compared **(Figs. 23.6 and 23.7)**; however, greater cytologic atypia after treatment is encountered in a minority of cases **(Fig. 23.8)**. In one study (7), the grade of the pretreatment ductal carcinoma in situ (DCIS) matched that of the recurrent DCIS in 95 (84%) of 113 cases. Recurrent invasive carcinomas also resemble their pretreatment counterparts in their histologic type, grade, and receptor expression **(Fig. 23.9)** (8). Irradiated invasive carcinoma cells occasionally contain multiple hyperchromatic nuclei or display focal necrosis not evident in the pretreatment tissue. These findings suggest that the cells represent residual carcinoma showing radiation effect.

Differentiating irradiated glandular tissue from carcinoma can pose diagnostic problems, especially when examining needle core biopsy (NCB) specimens. The cytologic atypia produced by irradiation resembles the atypia seen in high-grade carcinoma cells, and the glandular atrophy and scarring seen after surgery and irradiation can give rise to irregular clusters of atypical cells that resemble invasive carcinoma. Comparison of the features of a posttreatment biopsy sample with the pretreatment tumor and nontumor tissue will usually help to clarify the nature of the atypical epithelial cells. Evidence of cellular proliferation—stratification of cells, filling of glandular lumina, distention of glands, and mitotic figures—especially if associated with necrosis supports the diagnosis of carcinoma. Attention to the presence of apocrine metaplasia in the native glandular tissue will also help to avoid mistaking irradiated benign glandular cells for carcinoma cells. Staining for myoepithelial cells will usually allow one to recognize foci of invasive carcinoma, but irradiated myoepithelial cells sometimes fail to stain for the usual myoepithelial markers (4). As always, one must integrate the immunohistochemical findings with those evident on hematoxylin and eosin (H&E)-stained sections.

Therapeutic or adjuvant irradiation of the breast does not seem to significantly increase the risk of contralateral breast carcinoma (9), but it has been associated with increased risk for the development of carcinomas of the esophagus and lung (10,11). Locoregional irradiation for breast carcinoma also leads to an increased risk for acute myeloid leukemia, which is enhanced by chemotherapy (12). The incidence of such neoplasms appears to be low. Approximately 160 such cases developed in a cohort of 33,763 women irradiated for breast carcinoma (10). The relationship between breast irradiation and the development of vascular lesions is discussed in Chapter 20.

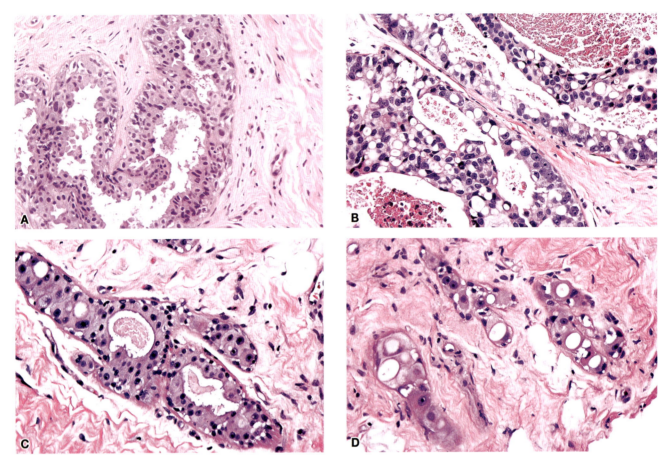

FIGURE 23.5 Radiation Atypia in Apocrine Duct Hyperplasia. A: Scattered cells in the hyperplastic apocrine epithelium have pleomorphic, hyperchromatic nuclei. Note the even nuclear chromatin and absence of nucleoli in the atypical nuclei. **B:** Ductal carcinoma in situ in this needle core biopsy specimen taken prior to irradiation displays signet ring cells and necrotic debris. **C, D:** The specimen from a needle core biopsy taken following radiation treatment of the patient shown in **(B)** demonstrates atypical apocrine hyperplasia in a duct **(C)** and in atrophic lobules **(D)**.

Radiation and Hodgkin Lymphoma

The breasts may be secondarily exposed to radiation during diagnostic procedures such as mammography (13) or in the course of irradiation administered to another organ, such as mediastinal radiotherapy for Hodgkin lymphoma (14-16). The radiation exposure in these situations has been associated with an increased risk for the development of breast carcinoma (15,17,18). Wendland et al (19) reported

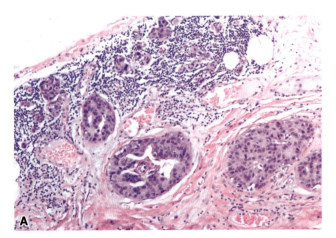
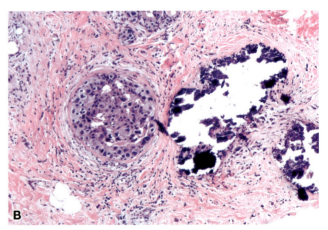

FIGURE 23.6 Recurrent Ductal Carcinoma In Situ (DCIS) After Radiotherapy. A: This needle core biopsy specimen obtained before treatment contains DCIS. **B:** The needle core biopsy specimen taken 4 years after irradiation shows DCIS similar to that in **(A)**.

PATHOLOGIC EFFECTS OF THERAPY 459

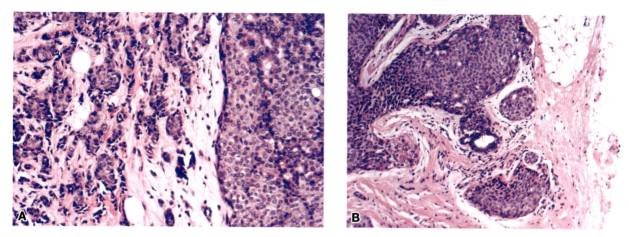

FIGURE 23.7 **Recurrent Carcinoma After Radiotherapy. A:** This image illustrates in situ and invasive poorly differentiated breast carcinoma in a specimen collected before radiotherapy. **B:** This specimen from a needle core biopsy performed 1 year after radiotherapy shows ductal carcinoma in situ identical to that on the right in **(A)**.

that the standard incidence ratio (SIR) for breast carcinoma among Hodgkin lymphoma patients who received radiotherapy was 3.17 when compared to the general population, and Schaapveld et al (20) recorded an SIR of 4.7. Girls irradiated between the ages of 9 and 16 years face an especially high likelihood of developing breast carcinoma compared with those irradiated in later adolescence or early adulthood (18,21). This suggests greater susceptibility to breast carcinoma when radiation exposure is near puberty. Postirradiation breast carcinoma also occurs

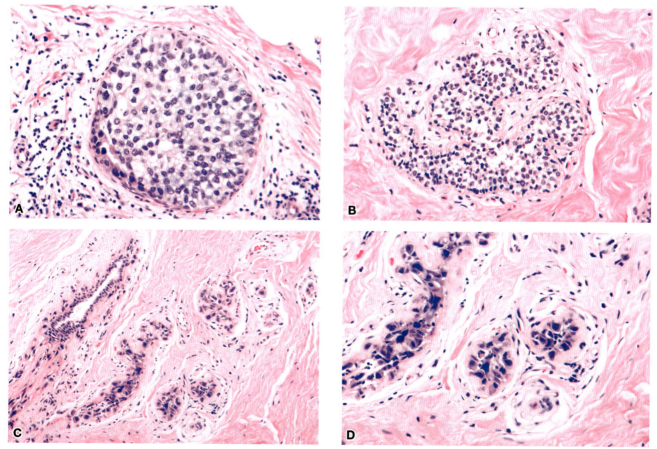

FIGURE 23.8 **Radiation Atypia in Terminal Ducts With Atypical Lobular Hyperplasia (ALH). A, B:** Tissue excised prior to irradiation shows ductal carcinoma in situ in **(A)** and ALH (23) in **(B)**. **C, D:** A needle core biopsy performed 2 years later revealed marked cytologic atypia in these terminal ducts. The atypical cells probably represent foci of ALH like those shown in **(B)**.

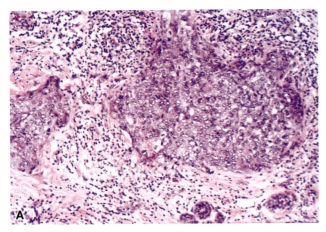 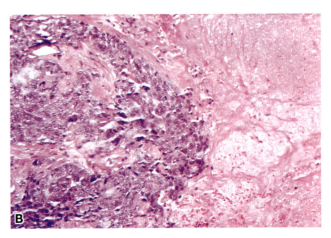

FIGURE 23.9 **Recurrent Infiltrating Carcinoma. A:** This untreated, poorly differentiated invasive breast carcinoma has a prominent lymphocytic reaction. **B:** One year after lumpectomy and radiotherapy, the recurrent, partially necrotic carcinoma lacks a lymphocytic reaction but otherwise looks similar to the pretreatment tumor.

rarely in men (22). The cumulative probability of developing breast carcinoma by 50 years of age in Hodgkin lymphoma patients has been reported to be about 35%, comparable with *BRCA* gene mutation carriers (21,23). Recent data from the National Cancer Institute's Surveillance, Epidemiology, and End Results (SEER) database (15) included 257 patients who developed 321 breast carcinomas after radiotherapy for Hodgkin lymphoma. The median age at the time of diagnosis of Hodgkin lymphoma was 22 years. The median age at the time of diagnosis of breast carcinoma was 43 years, younger than patients with sporadic breast carcinoma, and the median interval was 20 years. The frequency of bilaterality was 21.8%; 50% of contralateral tumors were metachronous. Axillary lymph node metastases occurred in 43% of the invasive carcinomas for which axillary lymph nodes were examined.

Patients who received supradiaphragmatic radiotherapy for the treatment of Hodgkin lymphoma are candidates for radiologic surveillance for breast carcinoma. Mammography and breast MRI are recommended for patients who received 10 Gy or greater chest radiation, at least annually up to age 60 (17). In the absence of randomized controlled clinical trials, the efficacy of various imaging techniques has not been established for this situation. Mammography is reported to have high sensitivity for detecting carcinomas in the breasts of women irradiated for Hodgkin lymphoma, especially when calcifications are present (24,25). In young high-risk women, MRI is superior to mammography for detecting invasive carcinoma within dense breast tissue.

Nearly all breast carcinomas detected in this setting have been invasive ductal carcinomas of no special type; however, special types such as mucinous carcinoma and medullary carcinoma have been encountered rarely, as have invasive lobular carcinomas (22,26). Approximately 15% are DCIS. The carcinomas are more likely to be bilateral, and both synchronous and metachronous bilateral carcinomas have been reported (26,27). Carcinomas arising after irradiation for Hodgkin lymphoma are significantly more likely to be high-grade and triple-negative relative to sporadic breast carcinomas, although the majority are estrogen receptor (ER)-positive (15,28,29).

Mastectomy (without adjuvant irradiation) represents the most common primary surgical treatment of patients in this setting. Deutsch et al (30) described 12 patients successfully treated with lumpectomy and radiation with "good to excellent cosmetic results" and "no significant acute adverse reactions and no late sequelae" after a median follow-up of 46 months. In another cohort (31), three patients underwent lumpectomy, of whom two received adjuvant radiation, and two patients who were felt to be at higher risk for locoregional failure received chest wall irradiation following mastectomy. None experienced complications of radiation in a median follow-up of 63.4 months.

CHEMOTHERAPY

Treatment-related histologic changes may be seen in mammary carcinomas and nonneoplastic mammary tissues following neoadjuvant chemotherapy. Previously, neoadjuvant chemotherapy was mostly used to treat locally advanced breast carcinomas, but its usage has broadened to include the treatment of earlier stages of breast carcinoma (32).

Mammography may suggest a response in patients treated with neoadjuvant chemotherapy, but this procedure is not reliable for predicting the pathologic response to the treatment. Yeh et al (33) reported that concordance with pathology findings regarding chemotherapy response was 19%, 26%, 35%, and 71% for clinical examination, mammography, sonography, and MRI, respectively. Positron emission tomography (PET) appears to be a specific but less sensitive method for identifying patients with complete pathologic responses early in the course of chemotherapy treatment (34).

Nonneoplastic breast parenchyma can show histologic changes following chemotherapy. The glandular elements undergo diffuse atrophy causing a reduction in the size of existing lobules, loss of acinar luminal cells, shrinkage of the acini, and condensation of the basement membrane **(Fig. 23.10)** (35-37).

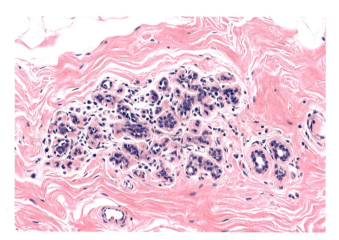

FIGURE 23.10 Chemotherapy Effect Involving a Normal Terminal Duct Lobular Unit. This specimen comes from a 34-year-old woman treated with neoadjuvant chemotherapy. The acini have small calibers, and their lumina appear inconspicuous. The basement membranes are thickened.

Cytologic atypia may be seen in ductal and lobular epithelial cells **(Fig. 23.11)**; however, in many cases, these changes are not specifically attributable to chemotherapy. Comparison with a pretreatment specimen is particularly helpful in this situation.

The changes induced in invasive carcinoma cells are more pronounced, and they often correlate with the extent of clinical response **(Table 23.2)**. The greatest alterations are usually found in patients who clinically appear to have complete resolution of their carcinomas (38). The most noticeable changes are a decrease in tumor cellularity accompanied by chronic inflammation, histiocyte accumulation, stromal fibrosis, and elastosis **(Figs. 23.12 and 23.13)**. Rajan et al (38) observed a decrease in median tumor cellularity from 40% in pretreatment core biopsy specimens to 10% in samples resected after neoadjuvant chemotherapy. There was considerable variation in change in cellularity among clinical response categories. Many tumors had a pronounced decrease in cellularity but only minimal reduction in size.

In the most favorable situation, no residual carcinoma is detected on pathologic evaluation, an occurrence reported in 13% (39) and 27.1% (40) of cases in cohorts with mixed subtypes of carcinoma. Breast carcinoma cohorts that are enriched for certain subtypes and treatments can show much higher rates of pathologic complete response (pCR). For example, the pCR rate of human epidermal growth factor receptor 2 (HER2)-positive breast carcinomas treated with trastuzumab and chemotherapy was 65% in the study by Buzdar et al (41). If the breast of a patient who has a complete histologic and clinical response is examined histologically soon after treatment, residual degenerated and infarcted necrotic invasive carcinoma may be recognized by the loss of normal staining properties and decreased architectural detail. With time, the degenerated invasive carcinoma is absorbed. Healed sites of previous infiltrating carcinoma (benign "tumor bed") may be appreciated because of architectural distortion characterized by fibrosis, stromal edema, increased vascularity composed largely of thin-walled vessels, and a chronic inflammatory cell infiltrate **(Fig. 23.13) (Table 23.3)** (37).

Residual invasive carcinoma cells can appear morphologically unaltered after neoadjuvant chemotherapy, but in most cases they exhibit cytologic changes attributable to the treatment (37,39,42,43). The alterations may appear more pronounced after combined chemoradiotherapy than following treatment with the same agents individually. The invasive carcinoma cells usually appear enlarged. They possess increased amounts of cytoplasm, which often contains vacuoles or eosinophilic granules (35). Cell borders are typically well defined, and the cells tend to shrink from the stroma **(Fig. 23.12)** (43). The cells contain large, hyperchromatic, and pleomorphic nuclei. Multinucleated tumor giant cells and abnormal mitotic figures may be encountered in cases treated with taxanes (44). The altered carcinoma cells can mimic histiocytes, especially when present individually, but they retain immunohistochemical reactivity for cytokeratin (CK) and epithelial membrane antigen (EMA). Occasionally, the residual invasive carcinoma cells appear smaller

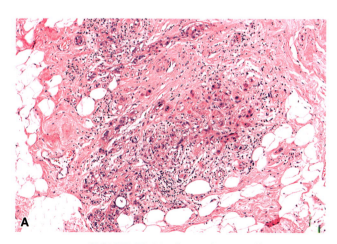
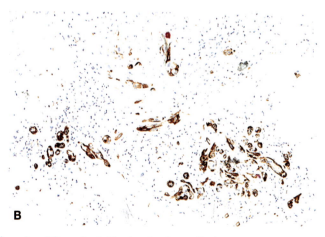

FIGURE 23.11 Chemotherapy Effect Involving Sclerosing Adenosis. A: The benign focus displays squamous metaplasia, therapy-related atypia, and inflammation mimicking invasive carcinoma. **B:** Smooth muscle myosin heavy chain demonstrates the presence of myoepithelial cells.

TABLE 23.2
Histopathologic Features of Breast Status Post Neoadjuvant Chemotherapy

- Effects in cases with partial response vary according to the degree of clinical response.
- Decreased tumor cellularity
- Decreased tumor gland formation, altered nuclear grade, reduced mitoses
- Fibrosis, lymphohistiocytic infiltrate, hemosiderin deposition
- Atrophy of native breast glandular tissue, smaller lobules and acini, condensed basement membrane

See Table 23.3 for effects in cases with complete response.

than those in the pretreatment specimen. Such cells contain scant eosinophilic cytoplasm and small collapsed nuclei.

The effect of adjuvant chemotherapy on the grade of carcinoma is variable. An analysis of 348 cases found that the grade of pretreatment carcinoma matched that of the posttreatment carcinoma in 85% of cases (45). Others (37) reported that nuclear grade was increased in 32% of cases. In the majority of cases, it is feasible (and clinically desirable) to determine histologic grade in residual carcinoma after neoadjuvant chemotherapy.

The effect of chemotherapy on tumor cell proliferation as measured with the Ki67 antibody or mitotic counts is likewise variable. Most patients receiving neoadjuvant chemotherapy show a reduction in Ki67, and there is some evidence of greater reductions in patients who respond to treatment (46). In patients who do not achieve pCR, Ki67 in the residual tumor is a strong predictor of outcome and may help triage patients to additional therapy (47,48). The International Ki67 in Breast Cancer working group suggests that assessment of Ki67 in serial biopsies during short-term (2-4 weeks) or long-term (>3 months) neoadjuvant *endocrine* therapy can determine whether a patient is likely to benefit from ongoing treatment. However, there is insufficient evidence to support the use of Ki67 to determine neoadjuvant *chemo*therapy benefit. It is strongly recommended that all samples for Ki67 immunohistochemistry (IHC) be taken by NCB, including close to or at the time of surgery for the posttreatment measurement, to minimize differences in fixation time from the pretreatment NCB, which may artifactually lower the index (49).

Changes in hormone receptor and HER2 status before and after neoadjuvant chemotherapy are occasionally observed. Mohan et al (50) examined breast carcinomas from 303 patients and observed a loss in ER or progesterone receptor (PR) in 1% of the cases. HER2 immunohistochemical status changed in 5% of cases: 12 tumors became negative,

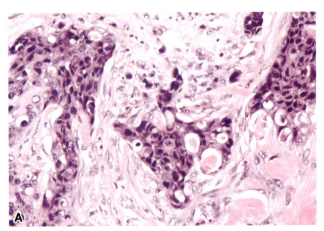

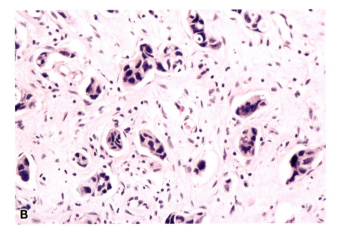

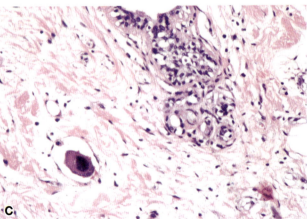

FIGURE 23.12 Chemotherapy Effect. A: The patient with this poorly differentiated invasive breast carcinoma received neoadjuvant chemotherapy. **B:** The needle core biopsy sample obtained after the patient experienced a partial clinical response contains small nests of carcinoma cells with pleomorphic hyperchromatic nuclei within collagenous stroma. Shrinkage of the clusters of carcinoma cells has created an appearance that mimics lymphatic invasion. **C:** A markedly enlarged hyperchromatic cell in a lymphatic space near an atrophic lobule is shown. The cytologic changes in the carcinoma are largely attributable to the chemotherapy.

PATHOLOGIC EFFECTS OF THERAPY

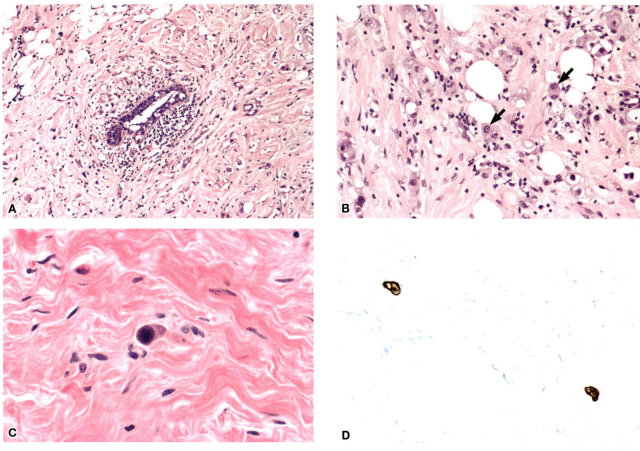

FIGURE 23.13 Chemotherapy Effect in the Breast. A, B: This needle core biopsy sample was obtained after a partial clinical response to chemotherapy. Isolated residual carcinoma cells (arrows) accompanied by scattered lymphocytes are dispersed in the fibrotic stroma. **C, D:** Rare dispersed tumor cells remaining after chemotherapy, which may be difficult to detect in hematoxylin and eosin (H&E)-stained sections, can be highlighted using a cytokeratin stain (**D**). **E:** Complete disappearance of carcinoma following chemotherapy. Reparative changes, histiocytes, lymphocytes, and fibrous tissue have taken the place of carcinoma cells.

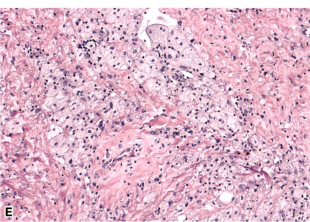

TABLE 23.3
Histopathologic Features of "Tumor Bed" Status Post Neoadjuvant Chemotherapy

- Fibrosis
- Elastosis
- Lymphohistiocytic infiltrate
- Hemosiderin deposition
- Capillary proliferation
- Stromal edema

Note: These changes may exist with or without residual invasive carcinoma.

whereas 3 tumors became positive. Loss of hormone receptor status in HER2-negative tumors was associated with worse disease-free and overall survival.

In a minority of instances, the residual carcinoma found after neoadjuvant chemotherapy consists only of DCIS, lymphatic tumor emboli, or both **(Fig. 23.14)**. Sharkey et al (37) reported finding "unusually prominent intraductal and/or intralymphatic tumor" in 40% of specimens obtained after preoperative doxorubicin/cyclophosphamide administration. Residual DCIS sometimes demonstrates marked cellular enlargement and extreme nuclear pleomorphism **(Fig. 23.15)**.

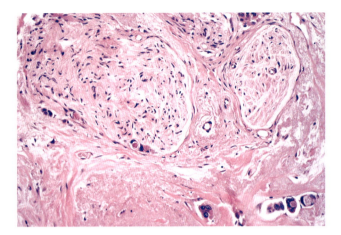

FIGURE 23.14 Chemotherapy Effect Involving Lymphatic Tumor Emboli. The clusters of carcinoma cells in a nerve and in lymphatic channels show cytologic changes related to chemotherapy. The patient had a complete clinical response, and this was the extent of the histologically detectable residual carcinoma.

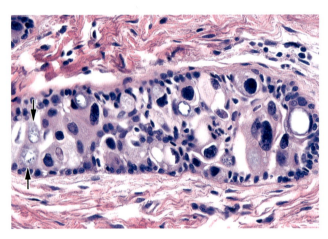

FIGURE 23.15 Chemotherapy Effect Involving Ductal Carcinoma In Situ. Neoplastic ductal cells showing marked nuclear pleomorphism overlie a layer of prominent myoepithelial cells. Intracellular mucin vacuoles are evident (arrows).

These bizarre cells can form confluent collections overlying a layer of easily recognized myoepithelial cells, or they can persist as individual cells and small clusters scattered among benign cells in the epithelium of ducts and lobules. Rabban et al (51) observed intralymphatic carcinoma in the breasts of 11 of 146 (7.5%) patients treated with neoadjuvant chemotherapy. In six of these patients (4%), the only residual carcinoma was within the lymphatic vessels.

Chemotherapy effects in axillary nodal metastases are similar to those affecting the primary tumor. Metastatic carcinoma can disappear completely, leaving behind only areas of scarring and lymphohistiocytic infiltration, fat necrosis, or calcifications, reminiscent of "tumor bed" in the breast tissue **(Fig. 23.16)** (35,37,52,53). Minute clusters of carcinoma cells may remain embedded in regions of fibrosis and chronic inflammation. Immunohistochemical staining for CK will facilitate the detection of residual micrometastases and/or isolated tumor cells. The uninvolved lymphoid tissue may show lymphocyte depletion (37) or extramedullary hematopoiesis **(Fig. 23.17)** (54).

pCR is an important prognostic indicator as well as a primary endpoint for clinical trials. It is therefore essential that assessment of pathologic response to neoadjuvant chemotherapy on the excision or mastectomy specimen be done accurately and systematically. Several approaches have been proposed, including the Miller-Payne grading system (55) and the Residual Cancer Burden system (56,57). Review of the prior pretreatment NCB sample is essential for assessing change in neoplastic cellularity. Key findings to report in excisional biopsy/mastectomy are summarized in **Table 23.4**.

Although the findings present in a pretreatment NCB specimen do not predict a patient's response to neoadjuvant chemotherapy in most circumstances, one can make a few general statements. For example, tumors with high nuclear grade respond better to neoadjuvant chemotherapy than those with intermediate or low nuclear grade (45). The use of anti-HER2 therapy often leads to pCR of HER2-amplified carcinomas (41). Invasive lobular carcinoma rarely achieves

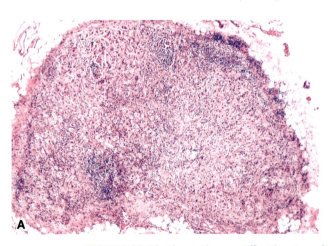
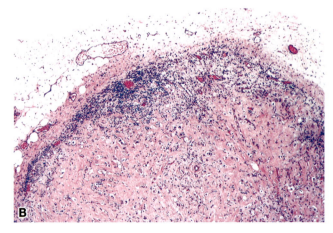

FIGURE 23.16 Chemotherapy Effect in a Lymph Node With Metastatic Carcinoma. A: Before chemotherapy, carcinoma diffusely involved a lymph node. **B:** After chemotherapy, the tumor is largely necrotic, and the background tissue shows fibrosis and lymphoid atrophy.

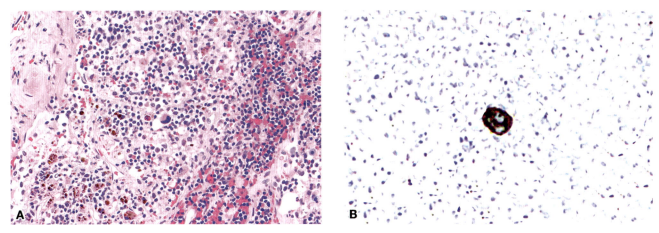

FIGURE 23.17 **Extramedullary Hematopoiesis Within a Lymph Node After Chemotherapy. A:** A megakaryocyte with an unsegmented nucleus is conspicuous in the center of the field, not to be confused with a tumor cell. **B:** CD61 staining confirms the lineage of this cell.

pCR when treated with neoadjuvant chemotherapy **(Fig. 23.18)** (45,58). Pu et al (59) reported that 80% of patients with pCRs had tumor necrosis in their NCB samples, whereas only 17% of nonresponders demonstrated the same finding. In one study (60), pretreatment Ki67 and apoptotic indices were not predictive of response to neoadjuvant chemotherapy.

The histologic changes associated with various forms of immunotherapy are yet to be characterized.

ABLATION METHODS

The use of several, largely investigational, techniques to ablate unresected carcinomas in the breast, including interstitial laser therapy, radiofrequency ablation (RFA), microwave ablation, high-intensity focused ultrasound (HIFU) ablation, cryoablation, and irreversible electroporation, has been studied (61). Except for HIFU, these procedures use a

TABLE 23.4

Essential Elements of Breast Carcinoma Reporting Status Post Neoadjuvant Chemotherapy (NACT)[a]

Residual invasive carcinoma	present/absent
Focality of residual invasive carcinoma	single circumscribed/multiple scattered
Extent of invasive carcinoma, if single/circumscribed	___ mm
Extent of invasive carcinoma, if multiple/scattered, range	___-___ mm
Lymphovascular involvement in breast	present/suspicious/absent
Lymphatic tumor emboli in dermis	present/suspicious/absent/not applicable
Residual in situ carcinoma	present/absent
Response in breast carcinoma	not evident/probable/definite
Response in "negative" lymph node(s)	not evident/probable/definite (#)
Response in positive lymph node(s)	not evident/probable/definite (#)
Core biopsy site changes in tumor bed	not evident/probable/definite
Core biopsy site changes in lymph node(s)	not evident/probable/definite
Primary tumor bed area	___ mm × ___ mm (macro/microscopic)
Overall cancer cellularity (% of tumor bed)	___%
Percentage of cancer that is in situ disease	___%
Number of positive lymph nodes	
Extent of largest metastasis in lymph node	>2 mm /<2 mm /isolated tumor cells (#)
Reduction in cancer cellularity vis-à-vis pre-NACT sample	___ mm ___%
Tumor bed, final margin status	negative/positive/(multi)focally involves ___

[a]For use in excisions/mastectomies.
Note: "Tumor bed", in this context, implies extent of residual viable invasive carcinoma (with or without therapy-related changes).

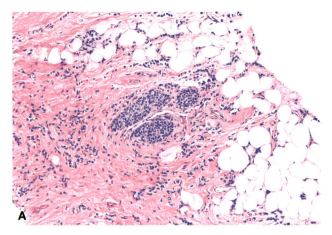 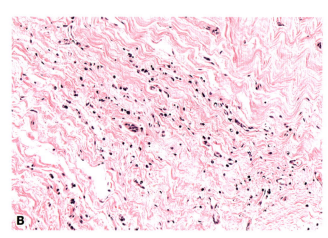

FIGURE 23.18 Chemotherapy Effect in Lobular Carcinoma. A: Pretreatment biopsy demonstrates lobular carcinoma in situ and invasive lobular carcinoma, both classic type. **B:** The mastectomy specimen status post neoadjuvant chemotherapy contains multiple dispersed foci of residual invasive lobular carcinoma within a fibrotic tumor bed.

probe placed in the lesion to ablate (ie, remove mainly by vaporizing) it. The most commonly used therapies heat the target tissue using electromagnetic (interstitial laser therapy, RFA, and microwave ablation) or sonic (HIFU) energy; cryoablation freezes it; and electroporation opens nanoscale pores in cell membranes. Histologic changes associated with these procedures appear limited to the target and the immediately surrounding tissue.

See Bloom et al (62), Izzo et al (63), and Knuttel et al (64) for detailed evaluation of carcinomas after laser ablation, RFA, and HIFU. With cryoablation, the affected tissue displays coagulative necrosis surrounded by a zone of fat necrosis and scar formation (65,66).

REFERENCES

1. Chansakul T, Lai KC, Slanetz PJ. The postconservation breast: part 2, imaging findings of tumor recurrence and other long-term sequelae. *AJR Am J Roentgenol*. 2012;198:331-343.
2. Schnitt SJ, Connolly JL, Harris JR, et al. Radiation-induced changes in the breast. *Hum Pathol*. 1984;15:545-550.
3. Moore GH, Schiller JE, Moore GK. Radiation-induced histopathologic changes of the breast: the effects of time. *Am J Surg Pathol*. 2004;28:47-53.
4. Anderson K, Williams EM, Kaplan J, et al. Utility of immunohistochemical markers in irradiated breast tissue: an analysis of the role of myoepithelial markers, p53, and Ki-67. *Am J Surg Pathol*. 2014;38:1128-1137.
5. Piroth MD, Fischedick K, Wein B, et al. Fat necrosis and parenchymal scarring after breast-conserving surgery and radiotherapy with an intraoperative electron or fractionated, percutaneous boost: a retrospective comparison. Breast *Cancer*. 2014;21:409-414.
6. Rivera R, Smith-Bronstein V, Villegas-Mendez S, et al. Mammographic findings after intraoperative radiotherapy of the breast. *Radiol Res Pract*. 2012;2012:758371.
7. Millis RR, Pinder SE, Ryder K, et al. Grade of recurrent in situ and invasive carcinoma following treatment of pure ductal carcinoma in situ of the breast. *Br J Cancer*. 2004;90:1538-1542.
8. Sigal-Zafrani B, Bollet MA, Antoni G, et al. Are ipsilateral breast tumour invasive recurrences in young (< or =40 years) women more aggressive than their primary tumours? *Br J Cancer*. 2007;97:1046-1052.
9. Obedian E, Fischer DB, Haffty BG. Second malignancies after treatment of early-stage breast cancer: lumpectomy and radiation therapy versus mastectomy. *J Clin Oncol*. 2000;18:2406-2412.
10. Roychoudhuri R, Evans H, Robinson D, et al. Radiation-induced malignancies following radiotherapy for breast cancer. *Br J Cancer*. 2004;91:868-872.
11. Zablotska LB, Neugut AI. Lung carcinoma after radiation therapy in women treated with lumpectomy or mastectomy for primary breast carcinoma. *Cancer*. 2003;97:1404-1411.
12. Curtis RE, Boice JD Jr, Stovall M, et al. Risk of leukemia after chemotherapy and radiation treatment for breast cancer. *N Engl J Med*. 1992;326:1745-1751.
13. Yaffe MJ, Mainprize JG. Risk of radiation-induced breast cancer from mammographic screening. *Radiology*. 2011;258:98-105.
14. Bhatia S, Robison LL, Oberlin O, et al. Breast cancer and other second neoplasms after childhood Hodgkin's disease. *N Engl J Med*. 1996;334:745-751.
15. Wong SM, Ajjamada L, Weiss AC, et al. Clinicopathologic features of breast cancers diagnosed in women treated with prior radiation therapy for Hodgkin lymphoma: results from a population-based cohort. *Cancer*. 2022;128:1365-1372.
16. Yahalom J, Petrek JA, Biddinger PW, et al. Breast cancer in patients irradiated for Hodgkin's disease: a clinical and pathologic analysis of 45 events in 37 patients. *J Clin Oncol*. 1992;10:1674-1681.
17. Mulder RL, Hudson MM, Bhatia S, et al. Updated breast cancer surveillance recommendations for female survivors of childhood, adolescent, and young adult cancer from the International Guideline Harmonization Group. *J Clin Oncol*. 2020;38:4194-4207.
18. Swerdlow AJ, Cooke R, Bates A, et al. Breast cancer risk after supradiaphragmatic radiotherapy for Hodgkin's lymphoma in England and Wales: a National Cohort Study. *J Clin Oncol*. 2012;30:2745-2752.
19. Wendland MM, Tsodikov A, Glenn MJ, et al. Time interval to the development of breast carcinoma after treatment for Hodgkin disease. *Cancer*. 2004;101:1275-1282.
20. Schaapveld M, Aleman BM, van Eggermond AM, et al. Second cancer risk up to 40 years after treatment for Hodgkin's lymphoma. *N Engl J Med*. 2015;373:2499-2511.
21. Schellong G, Riepenhausen M, Ehlert K, et al. Breast cancer in young women after treatment for Hodgkin's disease during childhood or adolescence—an observational study with up to 33-year follow-up. *Dtsch Ärztebl Int*. 2014;111:3-9.
22. Ninkovic S, Azanjac G, Knezevic M, et al. Lobular breast cancer in a male patient with a previous history of irradiation due to Hodgkin's disease. *Breast Care (Basel)*. 2012;7:315-318.
23. Moskowitz CS, Chou JF, Wolden SL, et al. Breast cancer after chest radiation therapy for childhood cancer. *J Clin Oncol*. 2014;32:2217-2223.
24. Diller L, Medeiros Nancarrow C, Shaffer K, et al. Breast cancer screening in women previously treated for Hodgkin's disease: a prospective cohort study. *J Clin Oncol*. 2002;20:2085-2091.
25. Howell SJ, Searle C, Goode V, et al. The UK national breast cancer screening programme for survivors of Hodgkin lymphoma detects breast cancer at an early stage. *Br J Cancer*. 2009;101:582-588.
26. Cutuli B, Kanoun S, Tunon De Lara C, et al. Breast cancer occurred after Hodgkin's disease: clinico-pathological features, treatments and outcome: analysis of 214 cases. *Crit Rev Oncol Hematol*. 2012;81:29-37.
27. Cutuli B, Borel C, Dhermain F, et al. Breast cancer occurred after treatment for Hodgkin's disease: analysis of 133 cases. *Radiother Oncol*. 2001;59:247-255.
28. Elkin EB, Klem ML, Gonzales AM, et al. Characteristics and outcomes of breast cancer in women with and without a history of radiation for Hodgkin's lymphoma: a multi-institutional, matched cohort study. *J Clin Oncol*. 2011;29:2466-2473.
29. Horst KC, Hancock SL, Ognibene G, et al. Histologic subtypes of breast cancer following radiotherapy for Hodgkin lymphoma. *Ann Oncol*. 2014;25:848-851.
30. Deutsch M, Gerszten K, Bloomer WD, et al. Lumpectomy and breast irradiation for breast cancer arising after previous radiotherapy for Hodgkin's disease or lymphoma. *Am J Clin Oncol*. 2001;24:33-34.
31. Alm El-Din MA, Hughes KS, Raad RA, et al. Clinical outcome of breast cancer occurring after treatment for Hodgkin lymphoma: case-control analysis. *Radiat Oncol*. 2009;4:19.
32. Thompson AM, Moulder-Thompson SL. Neoadjuvant treatment of breast cancer. *Ann Oncol*. 2012;23(suppl 10):x231-x236.

33. Yeh E, Slanetz P, Kopans DB, et al. Prospective comparison of mammography, sonography, and MRI in patients undergoing neoadjuvant chemotherapy for palpable breast cancer. *AJR Am J Roentgenol.* 2005;184:868-877.
34. Tateishi U, Miyake M, Nagaoka T, et al. Neoadjuvant chemotherapy in breast cancer: prediction of pathologic response with PET/CT and dynamic contrast-enhanced MR imaging—prospective assessment. *Radiology.* 2012;263:53-63.
35. Aktepe F, Kapucuoğlu N, Pak I. The effects of chemotherapy on breast cancer tissue in locally advanced breast cancer. *Histopathology.* 1996;29:63-67.
36. Kennedy S, Merino MJ, Swain SM, et al. The effects of hormonal and chemotherapy on tumoral and nonneoplastic breast tissue. *Hum Pathol.* 1990;21:192-198.
37. Sharkey FE, Addington SL, Fowler LJ, et al. Effects of preoperative chemotherapy on the morphology of resectable breast carcinoma. *Mod Pathol.* 1996;9:893-900.
38. Rajan R, Poniecka A, Smith TL, et al. Change in tumor cellularity of breast carcinoma after neoadjuvant chemotherapy as a variable in the pathologic assessment of response. *Cancer.* 2004;100:1365-1373.
39. Frierson HF Jr, Fechner RE. Histologic grade of locally advanced infiltrating ductal carcinoma after treatment with induction chemotherapy. *Am J Clin Pathol.* 1994;102:154-157.
40. Vasudevan D, Jayalakshmy PS, Kumar S, et al. Assessment of pathological response of breast carcinoma in modified radical mastectomy specimens after neoadjuvant chemotherapy. *Int J Breast Cancer.* 2015;2015:536145.
41. Buzdar AU, Ibrahim NK, Francis D, et al. Significantly higher pathologic complete remission rate after neoadjuvant therapy with trastuzumab, paclitaxel, and epirubicin chemotherapy: results of a randomized trial in human epidermal growth factor receptor 2-positive operable breast cancer. *J Clin Oncol.* 2005;23:3676-3685.
42. McCready DR, Hortobagyi GN, Kau SW, et al. The prognostic significance of lymph node metastases after preoperative chemotherapy for locally advanced breast cancer. *Arch Surg.* 1989;124:21-25.
43. Sahoo S, Lester SC. Pathology of breast carcinomas after neoadjuvant chemotherapy: an overview with recommendations on specimen processing and reporting. *Arch Pathol Lab Med.* 2009;133:633-642.
44. Zombori T, Cserni G. Patterns of regression in breast cancer after primary systemic treatment. *Pathol Oncol Res.* 2019;25:1153-1161.
45. Fisher ER, Wang J, Bryant J, et al. Pathobiology of preoperative chemotherapy: findings from the National Surgical Adjuvant Breast and Bowel (NSABP) protocol B-18. *Cancer.* 2002;95:681-695.
46. Assersohn L, Salter J, Powles TJ, et al. Studies of the potential utility of Ki67 as a predictive molecular marker of clinical response in primary breast cancer. *Breast Cancer Res Treat.* 2003;82:113-123.
47. Jones RL, Salter J, A'Hern R, et al. The prognostic significance of Ki67 before and after neoadjuvant chemotherapy in breast cancer. *Breast Cancer Res Treat.* 2009;116:53-68.
48. von Minckwitz G, Schmitt WD, Loibl S, et al. Ki67 measured after neoadjuvant chemotherapy for primary breast cancer. *Clin Cancer Res.* 2013;19:4521-4531.
49. Nielsen TO, Leung SCY, Rimm DL, et al. Assessment of Ki67 in breast cancer: updated recommendations from the International Ki67 in Breast Cancer Working Group. *J Natl Cancer Inst.* 2021;113:808-819.
50. Mohan SC, Walcott-Sapp S, Lee MK, et al. Alterations in breast cancer biomarkers following neoadjuvant therapy. *Ann Surg Oncol.* 2021;28: 5907-5917.
51. Rabban JT, Glidden D, Kwan ML, et al. Pure and predominantly pure intralymphatic breast carcinoma after neoadjuvant chemotherapy: an unusual and adverse pattern of residual disease. *Am J Surg Pathol.* 2009;33:256-263.
52. Brown AS, Hunt KK, Shen J, et al. Histologic changes associated with false-negative sentinel lymph nodes after preoperative chemotherapy in patients with confirmed lymph node-positive breast cancer before treatment. *Cancer.* 2010;116:2878-2883.
53. Pinder SE, Provenzano E, Earl H, et al. Laboratory handling and histology reporting of breast specimens from patients who have received neoadjuvant chemotherapy. *Histopathology.* 2007;50:409-417.
54. Prieto-Granada C, Setia N, Otis CN. Lymph node extramedullary hematopoiesis in breast cancer patients receiving neoadjuvant therapy: a potential diagnostic pitfall. *Int J Surg Pathol.* 2013;21:264-266.
55. Ogston KN, Miller ID, Payne S, et al. A new histological grading system to assess response of breast cancers to primary chemotherapy: prognostic significance and survival. *Breast.* 2003;12:320-327.
56. Symmans WF, Peintinger F, Hatzis C, et al. Measurement of residual breast cancer burden to predict survival after neoadjuvant chemotherapy. *J Clin Oncol.* 2007;25:4414-4422.
57. Symmans WF, Wei C, Gould R, et al. Long-term prognostic risk after neoadjuvant chemotherapy associated with residual cancer burden and breast cancer subtype. *J Clin Oncol.* 2017;35:1049-1060.
58. Cristofanilli M, Gonzalez-Angulo A, Sneige N, et al. Invasive lobular carcinoma classic type: response to primary chemotherapy and survival outcomes. *J Clin Oncol.* 2005;23:41-48.
59. Pu RT, Schott AF, Sturtz DE, et al. Pathologic features of breast cancer associated with complete response to neoadjuvant chemotherapy: importance of tumor necrosis. *Am J Surg Pathol.* 2005;29:354-358.
60. Burcombe R, Wilson GD, Dowsett M, et al. Evaluation of Ki-67 proliferation and apoptotic index before, during and after neoadjuvant chemotherapy for primary breast cancer. *Breast Cancer Res.* 2006;8:R31.
61. Fornage BD, Hwang RF. Current status of imaging-guided percutaneous ablation of breast cancer. *AJR Am J Roentgenol.* 2014;203:442-448.
62. Bloom KJ, Dowlat K, Assad L. Pathologic changes after interstitial laser therapy of infiltrating breast carcinoma. *Am J Surg.* 2001;182:384-388.
63. Izzo F, Thomas R, Delrio P, et al. Radiofrequency ablation in patients with primary breast carcinoma: a pilot study in 26 patients. *Cancer.* 2001;92:2036-2044.
64. Knuttel FM, Waaijer L, Merckel LG, et al. Histopathology of breast cancer after magnetic resonance-guided high-intensity focused ultrasound and radiofrequency ablation. *Histopathology.* 2016;69:250-259.
65. Roubidoux MA, Sabel MS, Bailey JE, et al. Small (< 2.0-cm) breast cancers: mammographic and US findings at US-guided cryoablation—initial experience. *Radiology.* 2004;233:857-867.
66. Simmons RM, Ballman KV, Cox C, et al. A phase II trial exploring the success of cryoablation therapy in the treatment of invasive breast carcinoma: results from ACOSOG (alliance) Z1072. *Ann Surg Oncol.* 2016;23:2438-2445.

24

Men and Children

ELAINE W. ZHONG AND SYED A. HODA

BREAST LESIONS IN MALES

Lesions of the breast are rare in men. They have much in common with their female counterparts, which are discussed in greater detail elsewhere in this book. Differences in anatomy and endocrine activity are discussed below where appropriate.

Male breast lesions are sampled with fine needle aspiration (FNA) more often than with needle core biopsy (NCB). A pathology group servicing several community hospitals in the Netherlands received only 26 NCB specimens of the male breast between 1993 and the end of 2002, or 2.6 specimens per year (1). Between 2011 and 2013, 539 men underwent mammographic evaluation of a breast mass at a center in Norway (2); FNA was performed in 62% of patients and NCB in 2.2%. The sensitivity of FNA in male breast lesions is between 95.8% (3) and 100% (4).

Notably, transgender[†] men (female-to-male) pursuing testosterone therapy for gender affirmation can have breast findings resembling those of cisgender[‡] men, depending on the duration of therapy. These include lobular atrophy, gynecomastoid change, and decreased rates of fibrocystic change (FCC), fibroadenoma (FA), pseudoangiomatous stromal hyperplasia (PASH), and papilloma compared with cisgender women (5).

Gynecomastia

Gynecomastia is the most common clinical and pathologic abnormality in the breast of males. Preoperative evaluation aims to distinguish gynecomastia from the comparatively rare male breast carcinoma.

Etiology

Gynecomastia is benign enlargement of the breast resulting from imbalance of estrogens and androgens via various mechanisms. Prepubertal gynecomastia is uncommon, except as a transient phenomenon in newborn male infants exposed to maternal estrogens in utero. Approximately 30% to 40% of pubertal males develop physiologic gynecomastia, which usually regresses spontaneously in a few months. Adult males can develop gynecomastia secondary

to systemic disorders (eg, hyperthyroidism, hepatic cirrhosis, chronic renal failure, chronic pulmonary disease, and hypogonadism), exogenous hormones (eg, estrogens, androgens, anabolic steroids), and other drugs (eg, finasteride, digitalis, cimetidine, spironolactone, marijuana (6,7), tricyclic antidepressants, 3-hydroxy-3-methyl-glutaryl-CoA acetyl reductase inhibitors for the control of cholesterol level (8,9), imatinib mesylate for the treatment of chronic myeloid leukemia or gastrointestinal stromal tumors (10,11), and antiretroviral therapy for HIV (12,13)). Gynecomastia secondary to paraneoplastic hormone production has been reported in patients with pulmonary carcinoma and testicular germ cell tumors (14). An association with Klinefelter syndrome has been documented (15).

Clinical Features

In a recent study (2), the mean age of men with mammographic diagnosis of gynecomastia was 55 years (median age 60 years; range 15-91). Symptoms include breast enlargement or a palpable, ill-defined mass in the central and subareolar breast. Mass-forming gynecomastia spans 2 to 6 cm clinically, but it can be larger. Lesions of recent onset may be tender or painful. Gynecomastia is usually bilateral and synchronous, but asynchronous lesions can occur. Unilateral gynecomastia is more likely to produce a discrete mass. Nipple alterations are uncommon. Invasive carcinoma arising in gynecomastia usually manifests as a localized, asymmetric area of firmness.

Imaging Studies

Mammographically, gynecomastia has three different appearances, approximately corresponding to the different histologic phases (vide infra) (16). In the *nodular* phase, it appears as a fan-shaped subareolar density; this is the most common mammographic pattern and correlates with the florid histologic phase. The *dendritic* phase is characterized by a "flame-shaped" subareolar density with prominent radial extensions and correlates histologically with the onset of stromal fibrosis. The *diffuse* phase is characterized by heterogeneous breast density, with a combination of nodular and dendritic patterns (17); the latter is typically seen in transgender females undergoing gender-affirming hormonal therapy (16). The combined use of mammography and ultrasonography is considered the optimal approach to rule out carcinoma in a patient who presents with clinical findings of gynecomastia (18-20).

[†]*Transgender* refers to one whose gender identity and expression differ from the biologic sex assigned at birth.

[‡]*Cisgender* refers to one whose gender identity and expression match the biologic sex assigned at birth.

468

Microscopic Pathology

The histologic changes of gynecomastia are similar regardless of its etiology. *Florid gynecomastia* is common in the first year of onset. The ducts are lined by micropapillary and/or flat usual ductal epithelial hyperplasia **(Fig. 24.1)**. Scattered epithelial mitoses may be encountered. Coexisting myoepithelial hyperplasia is common. The periductal stroma shows increased cellularity, prominent vascularity, edema, and a mild chronic inflammatory cell infiltrate. *Intermediate gynecomastia* shows both florid and fibrous components, and tends to be present for 6 months or less **(Fig. 24.2)**. *Fibrous (inactive) gynecomastia* is usually seen in long-standing lesions (12 months or longer). The epithelial proliferation is less conspicuous than in the florid phase; the stroma is more collagenous with less edema, reduced vascularity, and inconspicuous inflammation **(Fig. 24.3)**. PASH can be present in any phase of gynecomastia, but it is more pronounced in the active and intermediate stages. Gynecomastia-like hyperplasia sometimes occurs in the breast of adolescent females.

Additional epithelial changes include lobule formation **(Fig. 24.4)**, squamous metaplasia, and apocrine metaplasia. Atypical ductal hyperplasia (ADH) occurs in 0.4% to 5.4% of gynecomastia (21,22) and morphologically resembles ADH in the female breast **(Fig. 24.5)**. Ducts with ADH (and also ducts with ductal carcinoma in situ [DCIS]) usually lack the periductal fibrosis and increased stromal vascularity characteristic of gynecomastia.

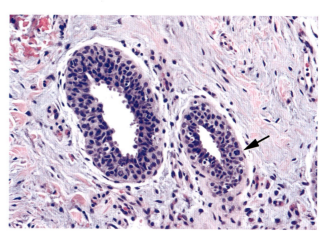

FIGURE 24.2 Gynecomastia, Intermediate. An intermediate phase lesion with compact epithelial and myoepithelial hyperplasia. An epithelial mitotic figure is present (arrow). Note the periductal edema and hypervascularity.

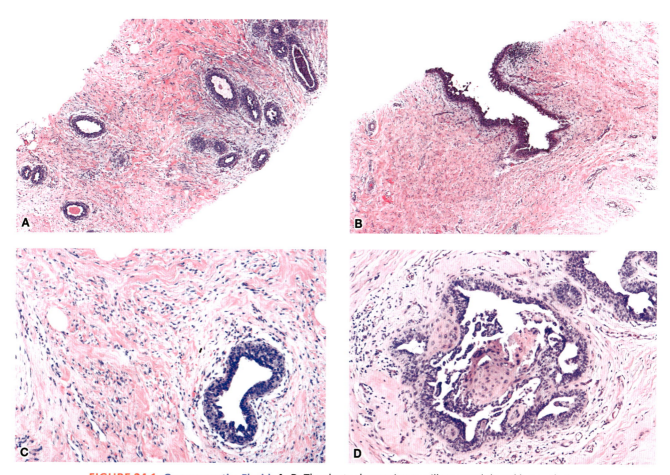

FIGURE 24.1 Gynecomastia, Florid. A, B: The ducts show micropapillary usual ductal hyperplasia. The periductal stroma has increased cellularity and prominent vascularity. **C:** Pseudoangiomatous hyperplasia of the stroma surrounds a duct with myoepithelial hyperplasia. **D:** Florid gynecomastia with squamous metaplasia in hyperplastic duct epithelium. Note mild periductal inflammation.

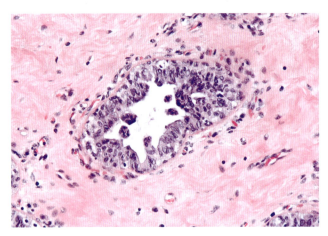

FIGURE 24.3 Gynecomastia, Inactive. This focus features micropapillary epithelial hyperplasia and a mild increase in periductal vascularity. The periductal stroma is collagenized.

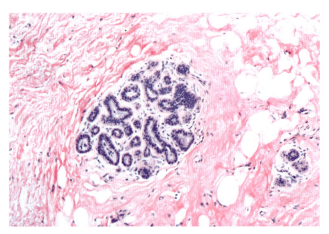

FIGURE 24.4 Gynecomastia. Lobule formation in a male breast.

Immunohistochemistry

The epithelium of gynecomastia consists of three cell layers (23) **(Fig. 24.6)**. The myoepithelial cells express CK5, CK14, and p63 but are negative for estrogen receptor (ER), progesterone receptor (PR), and androgen receptor (AR). The intermediate layer consists of cuboidal or columnar ductal cells immunoreactive for ER, PR, and AR but negative for CK5 and CK14. The epithelium lining the ductal lumen consists of flattened cells that are reactive for CK5, and CK14, but only weakly positive for ER, PR, and AR. The use of immunohistochemical stains for ER and CK5/6 may be helpful to document foci of ADH in the background of gynecomastia (see also Chapter 8).

Treatment and Prognosis

Early gynecomastia sometimes may regress when the underlying conditions are treated, or the inciting drugs are discontinued, but in most cases breast enlargement persists. Most patients with gynecomastia receive no specific treatment. The use of radiation (24) and tamoxifen (25) to prevent gynecomastia in men with prostatic carcinoma treated with bicalutamide is a subject of debate. Multiple studies have shown tamoxifen to be a safe and effective treatment for idiopathic gynecomastia (26,27), though randomized controlled trials are lacking. Surgical excision of gynecomastia is indicated clinically only to exclude carcinoma, but sometimes it is performed for cosmetic reasons. Recurrence is common if the underlying cause is not identified and treated. Ultrasound-assisted liposuction may be considered in overweight or obese men, when adipose tissue is thought to contribute to the mass (28). Liposuction can result in epithelial displacement that mimics invasive carcinoma (29). A conservative approach is adopted in children with gynecomastia, as the lesions usually resolve without treatment. In a study of men younger than 21 years who underwent surgery for gynecomastia (15), the average age at the time of the procedure was 16.2 years, and most patients were overweight or obese. Although carcinoma may rarely arise in conjunction with gynecomastia (22), gynecomastia is not associated with an increased risk of subsequent mammary carcinoma (30,31).

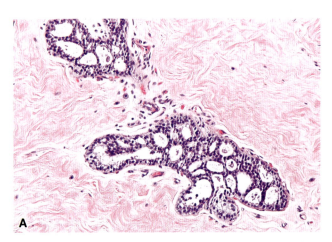
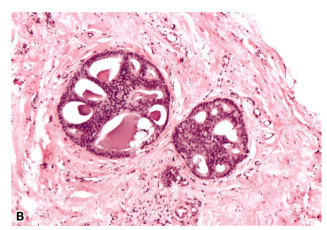

FIGURE 24.5 Gynecomastia With Atypical Duct Hyperplasia. A: The proliferation is almost entirely epithelial with a minimal myoepithelial component. **B:** Atypical cribriform duct hyperplasia.

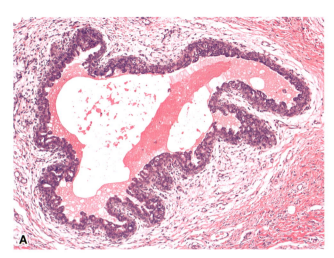 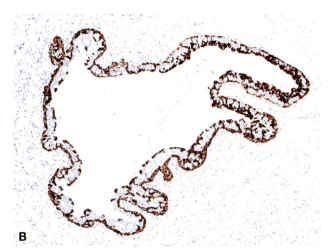

FIGURE 24.6 "Three-Layer" Epithelium in Gynecomastia. **A, B:** The peripheral myoepithelial cells are immunoreactive for CK5. The intermediate cell layer, composed of vertically oriented cuboidal to columnar cells, is negative for CK5. The flattened cells forming the inner luminal layer are reactive for CK5.

Intraductal Papilloma

Intraductal papillomas can occur at any age, including in adolescence (32). Bloody nipple discharge is a common presenting symptom. Large or cystic lesions may be palpable. The mammographic and sonographic appearance of papillomas of the male breast does not differ significantly from that of similar tumors in females (17,32).

Papillomas of the male breast are histologically similar to those occurring in females. Multiple papillomas can occur. Adenomyoepithelioma has also been reported (33). Because papillary carcinomas are relatively more common in the male breast than papillomas, careful evaluation of the epithelial component is required to rule out atypia or carcinoma (see also discussion in Chapters 4 and 11). The absence of myoepithelium in the fibrovascular cores of a papillary lesion supports the diagnosis of papillary carcinoma but does not distinguish between papillary DCIS, encapsulated papillary carcinoma (EPC), and invasive papillary carcinoma. CK5/6 immunostain highlights the myoepithelium and also decorates usual ductal hyperplasia (UDH) with a characteristic "mosaic" or "checkerboard" pattern, whereas atypical and neoplastic ductal epithelium is usually CK5/6-negative.

The need for surgical excision of papillomas without atypia diagnosed at NCB with radiologic and pathologic concordant findings in females remains a subject of investigation (see also Chapter 4). Papillary lesions in the breast of males, including papillomas without epithelial atypia, usually undergo surgical excision to rule out papillary carcinoma.

Fibroepithelial Lesions

The age of men with FAs in one series (34) ranged from 37 to 71 years; a 20-year-old man had a benign (low-grade) phyllodes tumor (PT). A 15-year-old boy with unilateral gynecomastia reportedly had a 7-cm benign fibroepithelial tumor (36). Bilateral FAs were described in a 66-year-old man under treatment with leuprolide for prostatic adenocarcinoma (37).

Fibroepithelial lesions (FELs) in men usually arise in the context of gynecomastia (34,35,37), particularly in patients treated with estrogens or antiandrogen therapy, which can result in lobule formation. Other drugs associated with FA and/or fibroadenomatoid alterations include spironolactone, methyldopa, and chlordiazepoxide (34). Increasingly, FAs are encountered in transgender patients in the course of gender reassignment surgical excision of breast tissue (38-41).

The morphology of FELs in men resembles that in females. Some lesions clinically regarded as FAs may just represent nodular foci of gynecomastia or associated PASH (42).

The treatment of PTs in men is similar to that in females. Most PTs in men are clinically benign. One breast mass in a 62-year-old man, diagnosed as a spindle cell tumor on NCB, was treated with neoadjuvant chemotherapy to facilitate resection from the underlying pectoralis major muscle; the postmastectomy diagnosis was malignant phyllodes, and the patient received adjuvant radiotherapy (43).

Proliferative Fibrocystic Changes

Proliferative FCCs in the male breast are extremely rare. Most men with proliferative FCCs were under 50 years of age at the time of diagnosis (44,45). At least two men were described as karyotypically and phenotypically normal (44,46). Hormonal imbalance is usually the predisposing factor.

Proliferative FCCs in men include apocrine cysts, papillary apocrine metaplasia, UDH, and duct stasis with mastitis. The microscopic features in some lesions can resemble those of juvenile papillomatosis (JP) (47).

FCCs without epithelial atypia do not require surgical treatment, but excision of a mass-forming lesion might be considered. The diagnosis of FCCs in the male breast should prompt the assessment of systemic metabolic and/or hormonal imbalances, as well as evaluation of the use of hormones and drugs with hormonal side effects.

Carcinoma of the Male Breast

The standardized incidence rate of breast carcinoma in men is 0.4 per 100,000 person-years (48), and it is highest in men aged 85 years or older (49). A rise in the incidence of breast carcinoma in males has been observed in recent decades across all racial and ethnic groups (50,51), likely owing to an increase in obesity (52). In a comparative analysis of the National Cancer Database (53), 80% of men with breast carcinoma were non-Hispanic White. Race and ethnicity did not affect patient survival.

Etiology

Hormonal imbalance (eg, testicular dysfunction, hyperprolactinemia, prolonged estrogen or anabolic steroid treatment, hepatic insufficiency, etc.) is one of the most common predisposing factors for male breast carcinoma. The association with prostatic carcinoma is partly because of hormonal treatment but may also reflect a genetic predisposition (54,55). Most men with familial breast carcinoma are *BRCA2* germline mutation carriers; *BRCA1* germline mutations are less common (56,57). The mean age at diagnosis in men with *BRCA2*-associated breast carcinoma is 59 years, and about 25% have prostate carcinoma and/or contralateral breast carcinoma. Human epidermal growth factor receptor 2 (HER2) positivity in male breast carcinoma is significantly associated with *BRCA2* germline mutation carrier status (57). Klinefelter syndrome is also a predisposing genetic condition. Men with prior diagnosis of breast carcinoma have a 30-fold increased risk of developing a contralateral breast carcinoma; the risk is 110-fold higher if breast carcinoma was diagnosed before the age of 50 years (58). Exposure to radiation, high environmental temperatures, and certain chemicals for motor vehicle maintenance have also been implicated as possible risk factors (59-61). Gynecomastia is neither a predisposing factor nor a morphologic precursor of breast carcinoma.

Clinical Features

The median age at diagnosis of invasive carcinoma is 68 years (50), but carcinoma can occur at any age, including rare cases in boys. Men with breast carcinoma are 5 to 10 years older than women with the same disease (51,62-64). Younger men have significantly more HER2-positive carcinomas (50). The median age of men with DCIS is 58 to 65 years (65,66). The most common presenting symptom is a painless retroareolar mass. The mean duration of symptoms prior to clinical consultation ranges between 6 months and 1 year. Synchronous bilateral carcinomas are uncommon.

Imaging Studies

Mammography and ultrasonography of invasive carcinoma typically reveal a mass with irregular margins (17). Concurrent gynecomastia may occasionally obscure a carcinoma, but ultrasonography usually distinguishes the two lesions. Microcalcifications are detected in 10% to 30% of male breast carcinomas, including DCIS, EPC, and invasive carcinoma. The magnetic resonance imaging (MRI) findings of breast carcinomas in males resemble those of similar tumors in females. At present, there are no guidelines recommending radiographic screening for men, even in individuals with known genetic predisposition (67).

Microscopic Pathology

Approximately 65% to 85% of carcinomas in men are *invasive ductal carcinomas*, and most are moderately or poorly differentiated (50,57,68-74) **(Fig. 24.7)**. Apocrine differentiation can be present. A small percentage of invasive carcinomas have tubular, cribriform, mucinous, micropapillary, secretory, and adenoid cystic morphology. In a series of men with familial breast carcinoma, invasive micropapillary morphology showed a trend for association with *BRCA2* germline mutation status (56). Kornegoor et al described that 25% of 134 male breast carcinomas had a central fibrotic focus

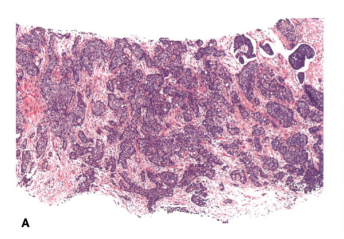
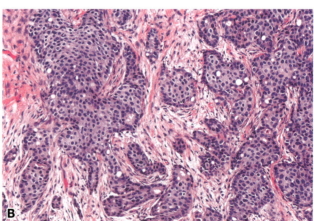

FIGURE 24.7 Invasive Carcinoma. A, B: The patient was an 85-year-old man with a palpable tumor. The needle core biopsy specimen reveals **(A)** invasive breast carcinoma, moderately differentiated. Gland formation is evident **(B)**. The invasive carcinoma was positive for estrogen receptor (ER) in 95% of the cells (not shown).

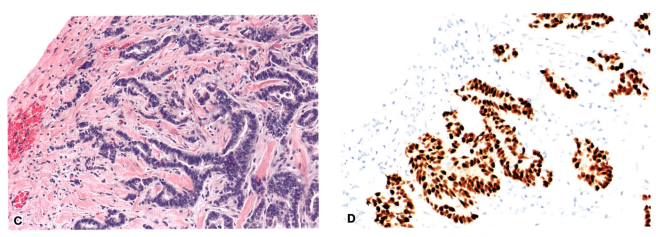

FIGURE 24.7 (*continued*) **C, D:** Invasive breast carcinoma, moderately differentiated, in a 71-year-old man. ER **(D)** is diffusely positive.

associated with overexpression of hypoxia-inducible factor 1α (HIF-1α) (75).

Carcinomas with papillary morphology constitute 3% to 5% of all breast carcinomas in men and are relatively more common in males than in females (72). These span the clinicopathologic spectrum, with papillary DCIS being the most common type, followed by solid papillary carcinoma (SPC) (33). The diagnosis of papillary lesions of the male breast in NCB samples relies on the same histologic and immunohistochemical criteria used to evaluate papillary proliferations of the female breast (see Chapters 4 and 11). In many cases, the NCB sample of SPC yields only detached papillary fragments of carcinoma devoid of myoepithelium **(Fig. 24.8)**. In the absence of stromal desmoplasia or reactive changes,

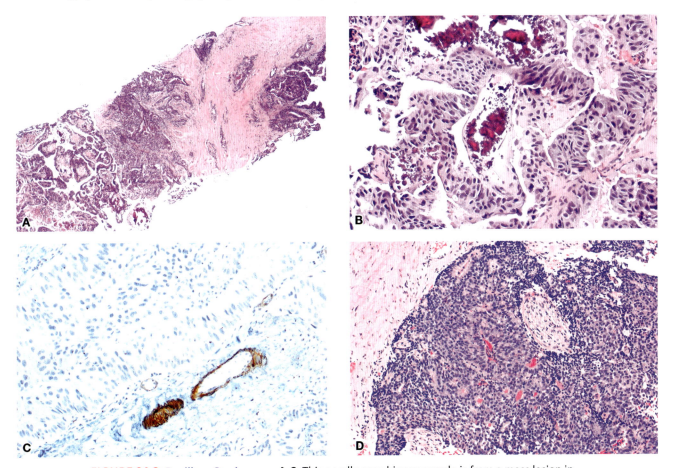

FIGURE 24.8 Papillary Carcinomas. A-C: This needle core biopsy sample is from a mass lesion in the breast of a 67-year-old man. **A:** Cystic papillary carcinoma is shown at both ends of the sample with invasive carcinoma in the center. **B:** Part of the papillary carcinoma in **(A)** with calcifications. **C:** Actin reactivity is absent from the papillary carcinoma. Only vascular structures are actin-positive. **D:** A needle core biopsy from an 82-year-old man shows noninvasive papillary carcinoma without definite stromal invasion.

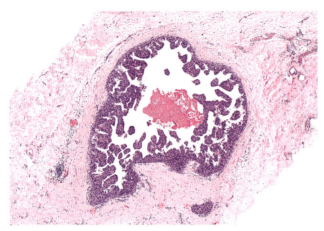

FIGURE 24.9 Ductal Carcinoma In Situ (DCIS). A needle core biopsy from an 86-year-old man with bloody nipple discharge shows micropapillary-type DCIS.

the absence of myoepithelium around a low-grade papillary carcinoma should not be interpreted as evidence of stromal invasion. In these cases, the assessment of stromal invasion requires examination of the entire tumor and of its interface with the surrounding stroma.

Other special subtypes are rarer. Lobular carcinoma is seldom seen because of the absence of native lobules; however, examples of invasive pleomorphic lobular carcinoma (68,76,77) and E-cadherin-negative histiocytoid lobular carcinoma (78) are reported (see Chapter 19). Secretory carcinoma in men harbors the characteristic *ETV6-NTRK3* gene fusion (79). Mucinous carcinoma (64,70,72,80), carcinoma with osteoclast-like giant cells (70), and invasive micropapillary carcinoma (64,80,81) have also been seen in men.

DCIS accounts for 6% (72) to 13% (82) of breast carcinomas in males and morphologically duplicates the appearance of DCIS in women **(Fig. 24.9)**. Cribriform and papillary architecture are the most common (66); solid DCIS with comedo-necrosis and micropapillary DCIS are rare. Most intraductal micropapillary epithelial proliferations occurring in the male breast are hyperplastic, especially in the context of gynecomastia. Calcifications are more common in DCIS than in hyperplastic epithelium. Intraepidermal adenocarcinoma (Paget disease of the nipple) can also occur (83).

Immunohistochemistry

Approximately 90% of invasive carcinomas in the male breast are ER-positive (80,84,85). AR is expressed in 65% (58) to 97% (68) of the cases. HER2-positive invasive carcinoma is rare but represents approximately 10% of familial cases (56), and it is significantly associated with *BRCA2* germline mutation carrier status (57). Triple-negative breast carcinoma is exceedingly rare in men. GATA3, mammaglobin, and gross cystic disease fluid protein (GCDFP) 15 are expressed in the majority of cases (86).

Differential Diagnosis in Needle Core Biopsy Material

In men, the differential diagnosis of primary mammary carcinoma includes *metastases from an extramammary site*, such as the lung, thyroid, kidney, and prostate; metastatic melanoma can also simulate breast carcinoma (87). Accurate clinical information is critical. Metastatic disease often involves both breasts, but it can be unilateral and unifocal. The identification of DCIS favors a primary mammary carcinoma. Morphologically, metastatic prostate carcinoma can closely resemble invasive ductal carcinoma of the breast and EPC. Tubular, mucinous, and micropapillary morphology and intracellular mucin are uncommon in prostate carcinoma. Most metastatic prostatic adenocarcinomas express AR, but they can also express ER, and immunohistochemical stains for these markers are not always contributory. Most primary prostate carcinomas express prostate-specific antigen (PSA), prostate-specific associated protein (PSAP), racemase, and ETS-related gene (ERG), but these antigens may be reduced in the metastases. PSA is also expressed in breast carcinomas from men and women. Prostatic carcinoma treated with hormonal therapy can acquire poorly differentiated and/or neuroendocrine morphology, and/or lose immunoreactivity for AR and prostatic markers **(Fig. 24.10)**. For these reasons, the diagnosis of primary mammary carcinoma with triple-negative immunophenotype in a man with a long-standing history of prostate carcinoma should be rendered with extreme caution. GATA3 is a nuclear antigen expressed in most breast carcinoma in females but only in less than 7% of prostate carcinomas (88). The utility of GCDFP-15 in the differential diagnosis of mammary versus prostatic carcinoma has not yet been studied (see also Chapter 22).

Molecular Characteristics

Data on the molecular biology of male breast carcinoma are limited, but they support that it is distinct from female breast cancer. *PIK3CA* and *GATA3* are the most frequently mutated genes; alterations of *TP53* are significantly less common

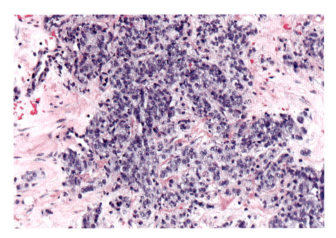

FIGURE 24.10 Metastatic Prostatic Carcinoma. This needle core biopsy sample is from a rapidly growing mass in the breast of an 85-year-old man with a long-standing history of prostatic carcinoma metastatic to bone treated with antiandrogen therapy. The patient developed rapidly progressive hormone-refractory metastatic disease. The carcinoma involving the breast was negative for estrogen receptor (ER), progesterone receptor (PR), and human epidermal growth factor receptor 2 (HER2), and focally positive for prostate-specific antigen (PSA) (not shown).

than in females (56,81,89). A study of hormone receptor-positive male breast carcinoma with 21-gene breast recurrence score (RS) results demonstrated a higher frequency of RS greater than or equal to 31 (12.4% vs 7.4%, though the average RS was similar) and higher expression of ER, proliferation, and invasion gene groups compared with female controls (64). RS was shown to be predictive of mortality in men but at a much lower score (up to RS 21) than in women (90). A lower frequency of copy number changes has been reported in Klinefelter syndrome (89).

Treatment and Prognosis

Men tend to present with higher-stage disease than women. In one study (72), 42% of males had lymph node (LN) metastases at diagnosis. Sentinel lymph node (SLN) biopsy is used to assess axillary LN status in clinically node-negative patients. Most men with DCIS and invasive carcinoma undergo mastectomy. Postsurgical radiation therapy in men is associated with significantly improved local relapse-free survival (RFS) (91) but not overall survival (OS) (92). Distant metastasis occurs in 5% to 6% of patients (93).

Treatment recommendations for men with breast carcinoma follow the guidelines established for female patients with carcinoma of similar tumor-node-metastasis (TNM) staging and include adjuvant hormonal therapy and chemotherapy (94). In men, tamoxifen treatment appears to be more beneficial than treatment with aromatase inhibitors (95), conferring a reduction in recurrence risk comparable to that seen in women (96). Nevertheless, the high incidence in men of side effects such as hair loss, impotence, decreased libido, and mood disorders perhaps explains the low rate of compliance with tamoxifen (97). HER2-targeted therapy is prescribed if the carcinoma is HER2-positive.

The prognosis of male breast carcinoma is related to stage at diagnosis and receptor status. Earlier studies reported similar prognosis in male and female patients with the same stage of disease, but more recent series have documented significantly lower OS for males compared with stage-matched women (53,72,98). The results remained the same after adjusting for age, comorbidity score, race, grade, and ER/PR status among other factors (53). The OS of men with node-negative disease was also significantly lower than that for women (6.1 vs 14.6 years, respectively). In another series, disease-specific survival for all male patients was 75.2% at 5 years and 52.5% at 10 years (72).

BREAST LESIONS IN CHILDREN AND ADOLESCENTS

Mass-forming lesions in the breast of children and adolescents are rare, vary according to age (99), and most are benign. Transient bilateral breast swelling in the newborn is secondary to maternal hormones. Bilateral breast enlargement in a child usually indicates a systemic hormonal imbalance. Most breast lesions in children under 18 years of age develop around the time of puberty: the most common are gynecomastia in boys and FAs in girls. Accessory breast tissue, supernumerary nipples, and inflammatory lesions, such as mastitis and fat necrosis, are also more common in the 10 to 15 years age group. Juvenile hypertrophy and JP occur mainly in adolescent girls and young women. Primary mammary fibromatosis and metastatic alveolar rhabdomyosarcoma also can involve the breast of teenage girls.

Sonographic examination is the preferred technique for evaluation of a mass in the breast of a child or adolescent. Most solid masses identified on ultrasound in the breast of adolescent girls are FAs (100). Mammography is less accurate because of the high density of glandular and stromal tissue; it also entails exposure to some radiation.

Most benign mass-forming lesions occurring in the breast in the first two decades of life are not associated with an increased risk of subsequent breast carcinoma. All such lesions should be managed extremely conservatively to spare the developing breast bud. That said, close clinical follow-up to monitor for local recurrence is prudent.

Juvenile Papillomatosis

Clinical Features

JP usually presents in women younger than 30 years and is uncommon prior to puberty (101,102). There is no specific data on the incidence of JP in adolescents. JP rarely occurs in young men (47). The reported frequency of family history for breast carcinoma in patients with JP was similar to (103) or higher (104) than the reported frequency in patients with mammary carcinoma. JP typically presents as a solitary, firm, discrete unilateral tumor that clinically mimics an FA (102). Bilateral lesions are rare.

Imaging Studies

Information on the imaging findings of JP is limited. Sonographically, JP presents as an ill-defined or discrete heterogeneous, hypoechoic mass with multiple cysts (105). Mammographically, JP tends to present as a localized area of increased density not as well defined as an FA. By MRI, JP can be a mass-forming lesion with a complex solid and cystic pattern, multiple small cysts on T2-weighted images, and continuous or clumped enhancement (105,106).

Microscopic Pathology

JP consists of nodular proliferative FCCs, with cysts and florid ductal hyperplasia. Cribriform or micropapillary ADH (occasionally with necrosis) can be found. In one series, atypia was present in 40% of JP cases, and intraductal necrosis was seen in 15% of the cases (104). Apocrine metaplasia is common. Other findings include sclerosing adenosis, lobular hyperplasia, fibroadenomatoid hyperplasia, and dense stromal sclerosis **(Fig. 24.11)**.

A definitive diagnosis of JP requires evaluation of the entire lesion. JP can be suspected when the imaging findings are suggestive of FA and an NCB sample shows proliferative FCCs. The differential diagnosis of JP in NCB material includes florid FCCs, papilloma, complex FA, and complex sclerosing lesion.

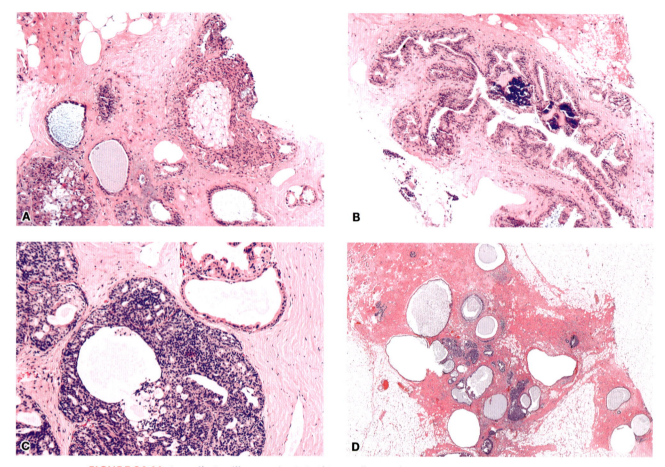

FIGURE 24.11 Juvenile Papillomatosis. A-C: This needle core biopsy specimen is from a 2-cm breast tumor in an 18-year-old girl. The diagnostic features are cysts, cystic and papillary apocrine metaplasia, duct hyperplasia, and stasis with accumulation of histiocytes. Calcifications are present in the papillary epithelium in **(B)**. **D:** This sampling from a 19-year-old girl displays a localized collection of proliferative and fibrocystic changes including florid ductal hyperplasia, apocrine metaplasia, sclerosing adenosis, cysts, and pseudoangiomatous stromal hyperplasia.

Molecular Characteristics

Massively parallel sequencing of 10 cases of JP identified mutations in *PIK3CA* in 5 patients, *AKT1* in 2 patients, and *MET*, *FGFR3*, *PTEN*, *ATM*, *NF1*, and *GNAS* in individual patients (107). Whole-exome sequencing of one JP with coexisting DCIS and invasive carcinoma of NST identified a shared *PIK3CA* E542K mutation in all three, supporting clonal relatedness (108).

Treatment and Prognosis

Based on the limited available data, at least in a subset of cases, JP serves as a substrate from which DCIS and invasive carcinoma develop (108,109). Nevertheless, in the absence of cytologic atypia, surgical excision of a lesion suggestive of JP does not appear to be required in cases with radiologic-pathologic concordant findings, and the decision to excise will depend on clinical evaluation and patient preference. If no carcinoma or atypia is identified in JP in a surgical excision specimen, no further treatment is necessary. Local recurrence is rare.

Papilloma

Most young patients with papillomas are female, ranging between 15 and 25 years of age. Young males are rarely affected. The most frequent presenting symptom is a retroareolar and/or subareolar mass. Nipple discharge or bleeding is rare. Sonographic examination is the preferred method of preoperative evaluation in children and adolescents. It usually shows a papillary mass within an anechoic or hypoechoic cystic cavity. Microscopically, papillomas in children and adolescents resemble their adult counterparts (see Chapter 4) **(Fig. 24.12)**.

There are no specific guidelines for management of pediatric patients with papilloma without atypia, but most patients continue to undergo excisional biopsy. Papillomas do not appear to predispose children and young women to develop subsequent breast carcinoma.

"Juvenile" Atypical Ductal Hyperplasia

"Juvenile" ADH (ADH in young women) was first described in females with mean age of 21 years (range 18-26) (110).

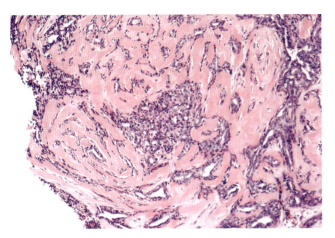

FIGURE 24.12 Sclerosing Papilloma. This needle core biopsy specimen from a breast tumor in a 19-year-old girl shows areas of dense sclerosis with epithelium compressed into slender cords.

Rarely, ADH occurs in the breast of an adolescent male, usually in the context of gynecomastia. Neither lobular hyperplasia (typical or atypical) nor lobular carcinoma in situ has been reported in this population.

Juvenile ADH usually constitutes an incidental finding. The morphology of juvenile ADH is similar to that of ADH in adult females but is somewhat less developed **(Figs. 24.13 and 24.14)**.

The identification of ADH in an NCB sample should prompt follow-up excision. In the absence of a more serious lesion in the surgical excision specimen, the clinical significance of juvenile ADH has not been fully evaluated in studies with long-term follow-up. One 24-year-old with a small focus of ADH on NCB opted for observation, and she developed no lesions of concern in 6 years of clinical and ultrasound follow-up (111).

Gynecomastia

See the discussion of gynecomastia at the beginning of this chapter.

Fibroepithelial Lesions

FELs, especially FAs, are the most common tumors in the breast of adolescent females. The median age at diagnosis in two series was 14 years (112) and 16 years (113). Most FELs occur after menarche. In one series (113), the mean age of patients with usual/adult-type FAs was 17 years, and the mean age of patients with juvenile FAs was 15 years. The mean age at menarche of patients with either lesion was 12 years, but the mean time from menarche to diagnosis was 72 months for adult-type FAs and 36 months for juvenile FAs. FELs tend to be relatively more common in African-American girls.

Fibroadenoma

FAs usually present as a discrete, rubbery, ovoid, and mobile mass. Pain and nipple discharge are exceedingly rare. An infarcted FA is usually asymptomatic; rarely it is painful or may cause bloody discharge. Ultrasound examination is the most common imaging modality. It reveals a solid and hypoechoic lobulated mass, with smooth and circumscribed edges. FAs account for at least 75% of all solid masses in the breasts of adolescent females (100). FAs in young females can reach a considerable size and show relatively rapid growth. The mean size of FAs (any type) was 2.9 cm in one series (113) and 3.6 cm in another (112). FAs have a benign clinical course, independent of size (112,113).

Usual FAs constitute 30% (76) to 40% (75) of all FAs in young females. "Juvenile" FAs (characterized by florid epithelial hyperplasia, hypercellular and pericanalicular stroma, and often rapid growth) are not exclusive to adolescents and constitute approximately half (112) to two-thirds (113) of FAs in adolescents. Epithelial hyperplasia is detected in 18% of usual FAs and in 30% juvenile FAs (113).

A substantial mitotic rate can be found in FAs in adolescents, especially in juvenile FAs (112,113); this finding needs to be interpreted with caution in the absence of other features of PT (see Chapter 7). In one series of patients under 18 years, the mean mitotic rate was 1.3 per 10 high-power fields (HPFs) in usual FAs, 1.8 per 10 HPFs in juvenile FAs, 3.1 per 10 HPFs in benign PTs, 10 per 10 HPFs in borderline PTs, and 17 per 10 HPFs in malignant PTs (113).

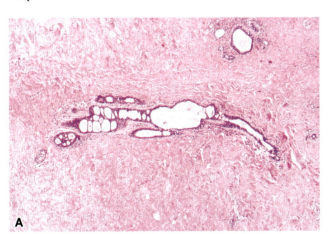
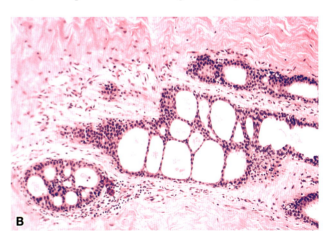

FIGURE 24.13 Juvenile Atypical Ductal Hyperplasia. A, B: This specimen was obtained from a reduction mammoplasty performed for juvenile hypertrophy in a 23-year-old woman. Cribriform hyperplasia is a focal abnormality in the duct. Note the broad expanse of collagenous stroma.

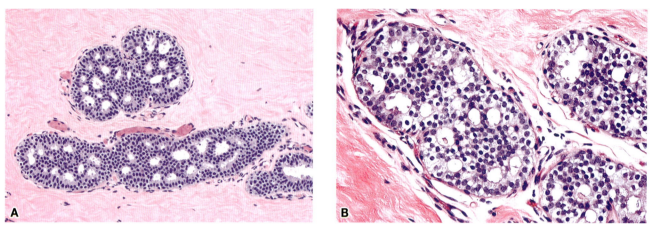

FIGURE 24.14 Juvenile Atypical Ductal Hyperplasia, Male. A: This specimen is from a 14-year-old boy who presented with bilateral breast enlargement. The stroma lacks the cellularity of gynecomastia. **B:** Atypical cribriform ductal hyperplasia in a 19-year-old boy with bilateral breast enlargement.

The diagnosis of a classic FA is generally straightforward, but some lesions may show hypercellular stroma, raising the differential diagnosis of benign PT **(Figs. 24.15 and 24.16)**. Complex FAs may raise the differential diagnosis of JP; the elongated ducts characteristic of FA are typically absent in JP. The term "cellular FA" could be used in NCB specimens to signify a stroma-rich FA. Such tumors may await definitive diagnosis at excision.

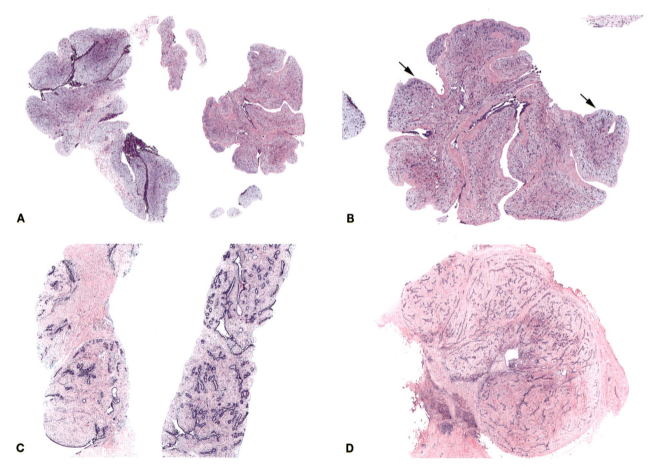

FIGURE 24.15 Benign Fibroepithelial Lesions, Excisions Yielded Fibroadenomas (FAs). A, B: Needle core biopsy (NCB) from a breast mass in a 17-year-old girl. Surgical excision yielded a 3.3-cm juvenile FA (not shown). **A:** Multiple detached fragments of fibroadenomatous stroma with a few elongated ducts. **B:** The stroma shows increased cellularity and slight condensation under the basement membrane layer (arrows). The epithelium of these fragments has been stripped. **C, D:** Right breast mass in a 19-year-old girl. **C:** NCB demonstrated a well-circumscribed lesion with homogeneously cellular stroma, without notable atypia or mitoses. **D:** Excision of the lesion in **(C)** revealed a 1.2-cm FA with biopsy site changes, adjacent to a 1.2-cm benign phyllodes tumor (not shown).

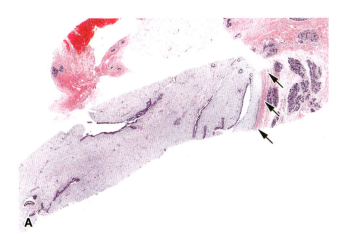
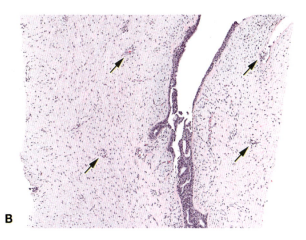
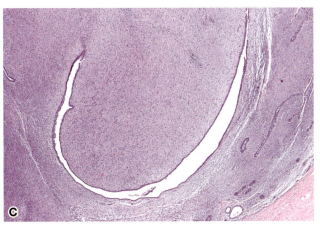

FIGURE 24.16 **Benign Fibroepithelial Lesion, Excision Yielded a Benign Phyllodes Tumor. A, B:** This needle core biopsy specimen was obtained from a breast mass in a 19-year-old girl. **A:** The stroma is expanded and shows slightly increased cellularity. Elongated and clefted ducts are shown. The interface with the adjacent breast parenchyma is focally represented (arrows). **B:** A magnified view shows slight periductal condensation of the stroma, with minimally enlarged stromal nuclei and increased vascularity (arrows). **C:** The surgical excision specimen yielded a benign phyllodes tumor.

Phyllodes Tumor

PTs present clinically as mass lesions, often with rapid growth. PTs in children and adolescents have the same histologic characteristics as comparable tumors in adults (see Chapter 7) **(Fig. 24.17)**. Most PTs in children follow a benign clinical course after excision (112,113), but rare instances of local recurrence and malignant tumors with systemic metastases are reported.

Pseudoangiomatous Stromal Hyperplasia

PASH is often present in the stroma of pediatric FELs, in gynecomastia, and in adolescent macromastia. It can also present as a discrete tumor indistinguishable clinically from FA in girls and in the breast of pubertal boys with gynecomastia (114). Surgical excision of a breast mass yielding only PASH at NCB depends on the clinical and radiologic characteristics of the lesion. Peripheral and/or incomplete sampling of a PT is a possible consideration in some cases (see Chapter 20 for a detailed discussion of PASH).

Carcinoma in Children and Adolescents

Primary carcinoma of the breast is extremely unusual in children and adolescents, and accounts for less than 1% of all pediatric breast lesions (99). Most patients are females, with an average age of about 13 years. The presenting symptom is usually a mass. Prior irradiation is a predisposing factor in some instances.

The most common histologic type in this age group is secretory carcinoma (>80%) (99,115,116) **(Fig. 24.18)** followed by invasive ductal carcinoma NST. Poorly differentiated and pleomorphic carcinoma, adenoid cystic carcinoma (ACC) (117-119), and DCIS are also reported (120-122). The aforementioned carcinomas are morphologically similar to carcinomas of the same type occurring in adults. A secretory carcinoma in a 9-year-old girl showed the characteristic

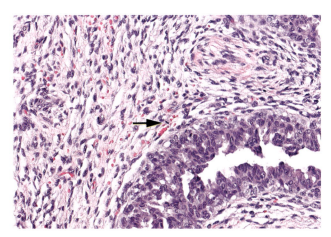

FIGURE 24.17 **Borderline Phyllodes Tumor.** This 14.5-cm mass from a 13-year-old girl exhibits marked stromal hypercellularity and modest stromal cell atypia and heterogeneity. The mitotic rate is up to 9 mitoses per 10 high-power fields (arrow). No stromal overgrowth or tumoral necrosis is present.

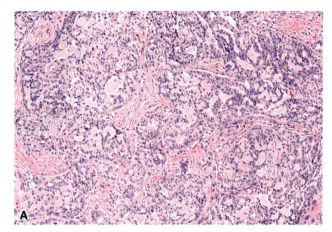
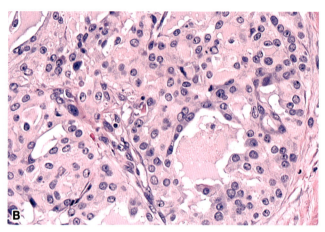

FIGURE 24.18 **Secretory Carcinoma. A, B:** This secretory carcinoma from the breast of a 16-year-old girl shows the characteristic vacuolated, lacelike, low-grade appearance (**B**) and harbored the diagnostic *ETV6-NTRK3* fusion gene. The tumor recurred locally and developed distant metastases.

ETV6-NTRK3 fusion gene and reportedly was ER-positive (116). No examples of ACC with solid and basaloid morphology have yet been reported.

Primary breast carcinoma with small-cell morphology is exceedingly rare in children. The differential diagnosis includes high-grade lymphoma, embryonal rhabdomyosarcoma, and primitive neuroectodermal tumor (PNET). Immunoreactivity for CK is usually detectable, and the cells are not reactive with markers for lymphoma (CD45) or rhabdomyosarcoma (myogenin, MyoD1).

Nonepithelial Malignant Neoplasms

Primary mammary sarcoma is exceedingly uncommon in children and adults. Rare cases of primary mammary angiosarcoma have been identified in the second decade of life (123,124). Metastases from sarcomas arising at other sites have also been reported. In particular, alveolar-type rhabdomyosarcoma tends to metastasize to the breast in adolescent girls (125), with most tumors originating in the extremities or buttocks. Systemic diseases such as lymphoma or leukemia can involve the breast (126). For further discussion of these topics, see relevant chapters elsewhere in this volume.

REFERENCES

1. Westenend PJ. Core needle biopsy in male breast lesions. *J Clin Pathol*. 2003;56:863-865.
2. Tangerud A, Potapenko I, Skjerven HK, et al. Radiologic evaluation of lumps in the male breast. *Acta Radiol*. 2016;57:809-814.
3. Hoda RS, Arpin Iii RN, Gottumukkala RV, et al. Diagnostic value of fine-needle aspiration in male breast lesions. *Acta Cytol*. 2019;63:319-327.
4. Wauters CA, Kooistra BW, de Kievit-van der Heijden IM, et al. Is cytology useful in the diagnostic workup of male breast lesions? A retrospective study over a 16-year period and review of the recent literature. *Acta Cytol*. 2010;54:259-264.
5. Baker GM, Guzman-Arocho YD, Bret-Mounet VC, et al. Testosterone therapy and breast histopathological features in transgender individuals. *Mod Pathol*. 2021;34:85-94.
6. Mieritz MG, Christiansen P, Jensen MB, et al. Gynaecomastia in 786 adult men: clinical and biochemical findings. *Eur J Endocrinol*. 2017;176:555-566.
7. Harmon J, Aliapoulios MA. Gynecomastia in marihuana users. *N Engl J Med*. 1972;287:936.
8. Oteri A, Catania MA, Travaglini R, et al. Gynecomastia possibly induced by rosuvastatin. *Pharmacotherapy*. 2008;28:549-551.
9. Roberto G, Biagi C, Montanaro N, et al. Statin-associated gynecomastia: evidence coming from the Italian spontaneous ADR reporting database and literature. *Eur J Clin Pharmacol*. 2012;68:1007-1011.
10. Liu H, Liao G, Yan Z. Gynecomastia during imatinib mesylate treatment for gastrointestinal stromal tumor: a rare adverse event. *BMC Gastroenterol*. 2011;11:116.
11. Tanriverdi O, Unubol M, Taskin F, et al. Imatinib-associated bilateral gynecomastia and unilateral testicular hydrocele in male patient with metastatic gastrointestinal stromal tumor: a literature review. *J Oncol Pharm Pract*. 2012;18:303-310.
12. Pantanowitz L, Sen S, Crisi GM, et al. Spectrum of breast disease encountered in HIV-positive patients at a community teaching hospital. *Breast*. 2011;20:303-308.
13. Schininà V, Busi Rizzi E, Zaccarelli M, et al. Gynecomastia in male HIV patients MRI and US findings. *Clin Imaging*. 2002;26:309-313.
14. Coen P, Kulin H, Ballantine T, et al. An aromatase-producing sex-cord tumor resulting in prepubertal gynecomastia. *N Engl J Med*. 1991;324:317-322.
15. Koshy JC, Goldberg JS, Wolfswinkel EM, et al. Breast cancer incidence in adolescent males undergoing subcutaneous mastectomy for gynecomastia: is pathologic examination justified? A retrospective and literature review. *Plast Reconstr Surg*. 2011;127:1-7.
16. Billa E, Kanakis GA, Goulis DG. Imaging in gynecomastia. *Andrology*. 2021;9:1444-1456.
17. Nguyen C, Kettler MD, Swirsky ME, et al. Male breast disease: pictorial review with radiologic-pathologic correlation. *Radiographics*. 2013;33:763-779.
18. Iuanow E, Kettler M, Slanetz PJ. Spectrum of disease in the male breast. *AJR Am J Roentgenol*. 2011;196:W247-W259.
19. Munoz Carrasco R, Alvarez Benito M, Munoz Gomariz E, et al. Mammography and ultrasound in the evaluation of male breast disease. *Eur Radiol*. 2010;20:2797-2805.
20. Rahmani S, Turton P, Shaaban A, et al. Overview of gynecomastia in the modern era and the Leeds Gynaecomastia Investigation algorithm. *Breast J*. 2011;17:246-255.
21. Lapid O, Jolink F, Meijer SL. Pathological findings in gynecomastia: analysis of 5113 breasts. *Ann Plast Surg*. 2015;74:163-166.
22. Wells JM, Liu Y, Ginter PS, et al. Elucidating encounters of atypical ductal hyperplasia arising in gynaecomastia. *Histopathology*. 2015;66:398-408.
23. Kornegoor R, Verschuur-Maes AH, Buerger H, et al. The 3-layered ductal epithelium in gynecomastia. *Am J Surg Pathol*. 2012;36:762-768.
24. Van Poppel H, Tyrrell CJ, Haustermans K, et al. Efficacy and tolerability of radiotherapy as treatment for bicalutamide-induced gynaecomastia and breast pain in prostate cancer. *Eur Urol*. 2005;47:587-592.
25. Fradet Y, Egerdie B, Andersen M, et al. Tamoxifen as prophylaxis for prevention of gynaecomastia and breast pain associated with bicalutamide 150 mg monotherapy in patients with prostate cancer: a randomised, placebo-controlled, dose-response study. *Eur Urol*. 2007;52:106-114.
26. Lapid O, van Wingerden JJ, Perlemuter L. Tamoxifen therapy for the management of pubertal gynecomastia: a systematic review. *J Pediatr Endocrinol Metab*. 2013;26:803-807.
27. Mannu GS, Sudul M, Bettencourt-Silva JH, et al. Role of tamoxifen in idiopathic gynecomastia: a 10-year prospective cohort study. *Breast J*. 2018;24:1043-1045.
28. Li CC, Fu JP, Chang SC, et al. Surgical treatment of gynecomastia: complications and outcomes. *Ann Plast Surg*. 2012;69:510-515.
29. McLaughlin CS, Petrey C, Grant S, et al. Displaced epithelium after liposuction for gynecomastia. *Int J Surg Pathol*. 2011;19:510-513.

30. Coopey SB, Kartal K, Li C, et al. Atypical ductal hyperplasia in men with gynecomastia: what is their breast cancer risk? *Breast Cancer Res Treat.* 2019;175:1-4.
31. Olsson H, Bladstrom A, Alm P. Male gynecomastia and risk for malignant tumours—a cohort study. *BMC Cancer.* 2002;2:26.
32. Durkin ET, Warner TF, Nichol PF. Enlarging unilateral breast mass in an adolescent male: an unusual presentation of intraductal papilloma. *J Pediatr Surg.* 2011;46:e33-e35.
33. Zhong E, Cheng E, Goldfischer M, et al. Papillary lesions of the male breast: a study of 117 cases and brief review of the literature demonstrate a broad clinicopathologic spectrum. *Am J Surg Pathol.* 2020;44:68-76.
34. Ansah-Boateng Y, Tavassoli FA. Fibroadenoma and cystosarcoma phyllodes of the male breast. *Mod Pathol.* 1992;5:114-116.
35. Gupta P, Foshee S, Garcia-Morales F, et al. Fibroadenoma in male breast: case report and literature review. *Breast Dis.* 2011;33:45-48.
36. Hilton DA, Jameson JS, Furness PN. A cellular fibroadenoma resembling a benign phyllodes tumour in a young male with gynaecomastia. *Histopathology.* 1991;18:476-477.
37. Shin SJ, Rosen PP. Bilateral presentation of fibroadenoma with digital fibroma-like inclusions in the male breast. *Arch Pathol Lab Med.* 2007;131:1126-1129.
38. de Faria LL, Brasil ST, Endo E, et al. Breast fibroadenoma in transgender woman. *Breast J.* 2020;26:293-294.
39. Kanhai RC, Hage JJ, Bloemena E, et al. Mammary fibroadenoma in a male-to-female transsexual. *Histopathology.* 1999;35:183-185.
40. Lemmo G, Garcea N, Corsello S, et al. Breast fibroadenoma in a male-to-female transsexual patient after hormonal treatment. *Eur J Surg Suppl.* 2003;(588):69-71.
41. Torous VF, Schnitt SJ. Histopathologic findings in breast surgical specimens from patients undergoing female-to-male gender reassignment surgery. *Mod Pathol.* 2019;32:346-353.
42. Bowman E, Oprea G, Okoli J, et al. Pseudoangiomatous stromal hyperplasia (PASH) of the breast: a series of 24 patients. *Breast J.* 2012;18:242-247.
43. Khalid IB, Parvaiz MA, Sarwar A, et al. A leafy surprise: case report of male breast malignant phyllodes. *Int J Surg Case Rep.* 2021;88:106536.
44. Banik S, Hale R. Fibrocystic disease in the male breast. *Histopathology.* 1988;12:214-216.
45. Robertson KE, Kazmi SA, Jordan LB. Female-type fibrocystic disease with papillary hyperplasia in a male breast. *J Clin Pathol.* 2010;63:88-89.
46. McClure J, Banerjee SS, Sandilands DG. Female type cystic hyperplasia in a male breast. *Postgrad Med J.* 1985;61:441-443.
47. Sund BS, Topstad TK, Nesland JM. A case of juvenile papillomatosis of the male breast. *Cancer.* 1992;70:126-128.
48. Miao H, Verkooijen HM, Chia KS, et al. Incidence and outcome of male breast cancer: an international population-based study. *J Clin Oncol.* 2011;29:4381-4386.
49. Hodgson NC, Button JH, Franceschi D, et al. Male breast cancer: is the incidence increasing? *Ann Surg Oncol.* 2004;11:751-755.
50. Chavez-Macgregor M, Clarke CA, Lichtensztajn D, et al. Male breast cancer according to tumor subtype and race: a population-based study. *Cancer.* 2013;119:1611-1617.
51. Giordano SH, Cohen DS, Buzdar AU, et al. Breast carcinoma in men: a population-based study. *Cancer.* 2004;101:51-57.
52. Keinan-Boker L, Levine H, Leiba A, et al. Adolescent obesity and adult male breast cancer in a cohort of 1,382,093 men. *Int J Cancer.* 2018;142:910-918.
53. Elimimian EB, Elson L, Li H, et al. Male breast cancer: a comparative analysis from the National Cancer Database. *World J Mens Health.* 2021;39:506-515.
54. Kiluk JV, Lee MC, Park CK, et al. Male breast cancer: management and follow-up recommendations. *Breast J.* 2011;17:503-509.
55. Leibowitz SB, Garber JE, Fox EA, et al. Males with diagnoses of both breast cancer and prostate cancer. *Breast J.* 2003;9:208-212.
56. Deb S, Jene N, Kconfab Investigators, Fox SB. Genotypic and phenotypic analysis of familial male breast cancer shows under representation of the HER2 and basal subtypes in BRCA-associated carcinomas. *BMC Cancer.* 2012;12:510.
57. Ottini L, Silvestri V, Rizzolo P, et al. Clinical and pathologic characteristics of BRCA-positive and BRCA-negative male breast cancer patients: results from a collaborative multicenter study in Italy. *Breast Cancer Res Treat.* 2012;134:411-418.
58. Auvinen A, Curtis RE, Ron E. Risk of subsequent cancer following breast cancer in men. *J Natl Cancer Inst.* 2002;94:1330-1332.
59. Cocco P, Figgs L, Dosemeci M, et al. Case-control study of occupational exposures and male breast cancer. *Occup Environ Med.* 1998;55:599-604.
60. Rosenbaum PF, Vena JE, Zielezny MA, et al. Occupational exposures associated with male breast cancer. *Am J Epidemiol.* 1994;139:30-36.
61. Villeneuve S, Cyr D, Lynge E, et al. Occupation and occupational exposure to endocrine disrupting chemicals in male breast cancer: a case-control study in Europe. *Occup Environ Med.* 2010;67:837-844.
62. Anderson WF, Jatoi I, Tse J, et al. Male breast cancer: a population-based comparison with female breast cancer. *J Clin Oncol.* 2010;28:232-239.
63. Leone J, Zwenger AO, Leone BA, et al. Overall survival of men and women with breast cancer according to tumor subtype: a population-based study. *Am J Clin Oncol.* 2019;42:215-220.
64. Massarweh SA, Sledge GW, Miller DP, et al. Molecular characterization and mortality from breast cancer in men. *J Clin Oncol.* 2018;36:1396-1404.

65. Cutuli B, Lacroze M, Dilhuydy JM, et al. Male breast cancer: results of the treatments and prognostic factors in 397 cases. *Eur J Cancer.* 1995;31A:1960-1964.
66. Hittmair AP, Lininger RA, Tavassoli FA. Ductal carcinoma in situ (DCIS) in the male breast: a morphologic study of 84 cases of pure DCIS and 30 cases of DCIS associated with invasive carcinoma—a preliminary report. *Cancer.* 1998;83:2139-2149.
67. Woods RW, Salkowski LR, Elezaby M, et al. Image-based screening for men at high risk for breast cancer: benefits and drawbacks. *Clin Imaging.* 2020;60:84-89.
68. Cardoso F, Bartlett JMS, Slaets L, et al. Characterization of male breast cancer: results of the EORTC 10085/TBCRC/BIG/NABCG International Male Breast Cancer Program. *Ann Oncol.* 2018;29:405-417.
69. Arslan UY, Oksuzoglu B, Ozdemir N, et al. Outcome of non-metastatic male breast cancer: 118 patients. *Med Oncol.* 2012;29:554-560.
70. Burga AM, Fadare O, Lininger RA, et al. Invasive carcinomas of the male breast: a morphologic study of the distribution of histologic subtypes and metastatic patterns in 778 cases. *Virchows Arch.* 2006;449:507-512.
71. Kornegoor R, Verschuur-Maes AH, Buerger H, et al. Molecular subtyping of male breast cancer by immunohistochemistry. *Mod Pathol.* 2012;25:398-404.
72. Nahleh ZA, Srikantiah R, Safa M, et al. Male breast cancer in the veterans affairs population: a comparative analysis. *Cancer.* 2007;109:1471-1477.
73. Nilsson C, Johansson I, Ahlin C, et al. Molecular subtyping of male breast cancer using alternative definitions and its prognostic impact. *Acta Oncol.* 2013;52:102-109.
74. Tural D, Selçukbiricik F, Aydoğan F, et al. Male breast cancers behave differently in elderly patients. *Jpn J Clin Oncol.* 2013;43:22-27.
75. Kornegoor R, Verschuur-Maes AH, Buerger H, et al. Fibrotic focus and hypoxia in male breast cancer. *Mod Pathol.* 2012;25:1397-1404.
76. Maly B, Maly A, Pappo I, et al. Pleomorphic variant of invasive lobular carcinoma of the male breast. *Virchows Arch.* 2005;446:344-345.
77. Rohini B, Singh PA, Vatsala M, et al. Pleomorphic lobular carcinoma in a male breast: a rare occurrence. *Patholog Res Int.* 2010;2010:871369.
78. Hutchinson CB. Geradts J. Histiocytoid carcinoma of the male breast. *Ann Diagn Pathol.* 2011;15:190-193.
79. Diallo R, Schaefer KL, Bankfalvi A, et al. Secretory carcinoma of the breast: a distinct variant of invasive ductal carcinoma assessed by comparative genomic hybridization and immunohistochemistry. *Hum Pathol.* 2003;34:1299-1305.
80. Shaaban AM, Ball GR, Brannan RA, et al. A comparative biomarker study of 514 matched cases of male and female breast cancer reveals gender-specific biological differences. *Breast Cancer Res Treat.* 2012;133:949-958.
81. Piscuoglio S, Ng CK, Murray MP, et al. The genomic landscape of male breast cancers. *Clin Cancer Res.* 2016;22:4045-4056.
82. Flynn LW, Park J, Patil SM, et al. Sentinel lymph node biopsy is successful and accurate in male breast carcinoma. *J Am Coll Surg.* 2008;206:616-621.
83. Adams SJ, Kanthan R. Paget's disease of the male breast in the 21st century: a systematic review. *Breast.* 2016;29:14-23.
84. Greif JM, Pezzi CM, Klimberg VS, et al. Gender differences in breast cancer: analysis of 13,000 breast cancers in men from the National Cancer Data Base. *Ann Surg Oncol.* 2012;19:3199-3204.
85. Ottini L, Rizzolo P, Zanna I, et al. BRCA1/BRCA2 mutation status and clinical-pathologic features of 108 male breast cancer cases from Tuscany: a population-based study in central Italy. *Breast Cancer Res Treat.* 2009;116:577-586.
86. Kornegoor R, Verschuur-Maes AH, Buerger H, et al. Immunophenotyping of male breast cancer. *Histopathology.* 2012;61:1145-1155.
87. DeLair DF, Corben AD, Catalano JP, et al. Non-mammary metastases to the breast and axilla: a study of 85 cases. *Mod Pathol.* 2013;26:343-349.
88. Miettinen M, McCue PA, Sarlomo-Rikala M, et al. GATA3: a multispecific but potentially useful marker in surgical pathology: a systematic analysis of 2500 epithelial and nonepithelial tumors. *Am J Surg Pathol.* 2014;38:13-22.
89. Moelans CB, de Ligt J, van der Groep P, et al. The molecular genetic make-up of male breast cancer. *Endocr Relat Cancer.* 2019;26:779-794.
90. Wang F, Reid S, Zheng W, et al. Sex disparity observed for Oncotype DX breast recurrence score in predicting mortality among patients with early stage ER-positive breast cancer. *Clin Cancer Res.* 2020;26:101-109.
91. Yu E, Suzuki H, Younus J, et al. The impact of post-mastectomy radiation therapy on male breast cancer patients—a case series. *Int J Radiat Oncol Biol Phys.* 2012;82:696-700.
92. Bateni SB, Perry LM, Zhao X, et al. The role of radiation therapy in addition to lumpectomy and hormone therapy in men 70 years of age and older with early breast cancer: a NCDB analysis. *Ann Surg Oncol.* 2021;28:2463-2471.
93. Gucalp A, Traina TA, Eisner JR, et al. Male breast cancer: a disease distinct from female breast cancer. *Breast Cancer Res Treat.* 2019;173:37-48.
94. Cardoso F, Kyriakides S, Ohno S, et al. Early breast cancer: ESMO clinical practice guidelines for diagnosis, treatment and follow-up. *Ann Oncol.* 2019;30:1194-1220.
95. Eggemann H, Ignatov A, Smith BJ, et al. Adjuvant therapy with tamoxifen compared to aromatase inhibitors for 257 male breast cancer patients. *Breast Cancer Res Treat.* 2013;137:465-470.
96. Giordano SH, Perkins GH, Broglio K, et al. Adjuvant systemic therapy for male breast carcinoma. *Cancer.* 2005;104:2359-2364.
97. Wibowo E, Pollock PA, Hollis N, et al. Tamoxifen in men: a review of adverse events. *Andrology.* 2016;4:776-788.

98. Liu N, Johnson KJ, Ma CX. Male breast cancer: an updated surveillance, epidemiology, and end results data analysis. *Clin Breast Cancer*. 2018;18:e997-e1002.

99. Mareti E, Vatopoulou A, Spyropoulou GA, et al. Breast disorders in adolescence: a review of the literature. *Breast Care (Basel)*. 2021;16:149-155.

100. Sanchez R, Ladino-Torres MF, Bernat JA, et al. Breast fibroadenomas in the pediatric population: common and uncommon sonographic findings. *Pediatr Radiol*. 2010;40:1681-1689.

101. Rosen PP, Cantrell B, Mullen DL, et al. Juvenile papillomatosis (Swiss cheese disease) of the breast. *Am J Surg Pathol*. 1980;4:3-12.

102. Rosen PP, Holmes G, Lesser ML, et al. Juvenile papillomatosis and breast carcinoma. *Cancer*. 1985;55:1345-1352.

103. Rosen PP, Lyngholm B, Kinne DW, et al. Juvenile papillomatosis of the breast and family history of breast carcinoma. *Cancer*. 1982;49:2591-2595.

104. Rosen PP, Kimmel M. Juvenile papillomatosis of the breast. A follow-up study of 41 patients having biopsies before 1979. *Am J Clin Pathol*. 1990;93:599-603.

105. Sabate JM, Clotet M, Torrubia S, et al. Radiologic evaluation of breast disorders related to pregnancy and lactation. *Radiographics*. 2007;27(suppl 1):S101-S124.

106. Durur-Subasi I, Alper F, Akcay MN, et al. Magnetic resonance imaging findings of breast juvenile papillomatosis. *Jpn J Radiol*. 2013;31:419-423.

107. Guillet C, Rechsteiner M, Bellini E, et al. Juvenile papillomatosis of the breast (Swiss cheese disease) has frequent associations with PIK3CA and/or AKT1 mutations. *Hum Pathol*. 2020;98:64-73.

108. D'Alfonso TM, Pareja F, Da Cruz Paula A, et al. Whole-exome sequencing analysis of juvenile papillomatosis and coexisting breast carcinoma. *J Pathol Clin Res*. 2021;7:113-120.

109. Viswanathan K, McMillen B, Cheng E, et al. Juvenile papillomatosis (Swiss-cheese disease) of breast in an adult male with sequential diagnoses of ipsilateral intraductal, invasive, and widely metastatic carcinoma: a case report and review of the disease in males. *Int J Surg Pathol*. 2017;25:536-542.

110. Eliasen CA, Cranor ML, Rosen PP. Atypical duct hyperplasia of the breast in young females. *Am J Surg Pathol*. 1992;16:246-251.

111. Johnson D, Pyke CM, Norris DL, et al. Atypical ductal hyperplasia of the breast in young women: two case reports. *Asian J Surg*. 2003;26:37-39.

112. Tay TK, Chang KT, Thike AA, et al. Paediatric fibroepithelial lesions revisited: pathological insights. *J Clin Pathol*. 2015;68:633-641.

113. Ross DS, Giri DD, Akram MM, et al. Fibroepithelial lesions in the breast of adolescent females: a clinicopathological study of 54 cases. *Breast J*. 2017;23:182-192.

114. Shehata BM, Fishman I, Collings MH, et al. Pseudoangiomatous stromal hyperplasia of the breast in pediatric patients: an underrecognized entity. *Pediatr Dev Pathol*. 2009;12:450-454.

115. Cabello C, Alvarenga M, Alvarenga CA, et al. Case report and review of the literature: secretory breast cancer in a 13-year-old boy—10 years of follow up. *Breast Cancer Res Treat*. 2012;133:813-820.

116. Yorozuya K, Takahashi E, Kousaka J, et al. A case of estrogen receptor positive secretory carcinoma in a 9-year-old girl with ETV6-NTRK3 fusion gene. *Jpn J Clin Oncol*. 2012;42:208-211.

117. Delanote S, Van den Broecke R, Schelfhout VR, et al. Adenoid cystic carcinoma of the breast in a 19-year-old girl. *Breast*. 2003;12:75-77.

118. Miliauskas JR, Leong AS. Adenoid cystic carcinoma in a juvenile male breast. *Pathology*. 1991;23:298-301.

119. Tang P, Yang S, Zhong X, et al. Breast adenoid cystic carcinoma in a 19-year-old man: a case report and review of the literature. *World J Surg Oncol*. 2015;13:19.

120. Chang HL, Kish JB, Smith BL, et al. A 16-year-old male with gynecomastia and ductal carcinoma in situ. *Pediatr Surg Int*. 2008;24:1251-1253.

121. Sato T, Muto I, Hasegawa M, et al. Ductal carcinoma in situ with isolated tumor cells in the sentinel lymph node in a 17-year-old adolescent girl. *Breast Cancer*. 2013;20:271-274.

122. Wadie GM, Banever GT, Moriarty KP, et al. Ductal carcinoma in situ in a 16-year-old adolescent boy with gynecomastia: a case report. *J Pediatr Surg*. 2005;40:1349-1353.

123. van Geel AN, den Bakker MA. Bilateral angiosarcoma of the breast in a fourteen-year-old child. *Rare Tumors*. 2009;1:e38.

124. Yang WT, Hennessy BT, Dryden MJ, et al. Mammary angiosarcomas: imaging findings in 24 patients. *Radiology*. 2007;242:725-734.

125. D'Angelo P, Carli M, Ferrari A, et al. Breast metastases in children and adolescents with rhabdomyosarcoma: experience of the Italian Soft Tissue Sarcoma Committee. *Pediatr Blood Cancer*. 2010;55:1306-1309.

126. Edison MN, O'Dell MC, Letter HP, et al. Juvenile myelomonocytic leukemia presenting as bilateral breast masses. *Pediatr Radiol*. 2017;47:104-107.

25

Pathologic Changes and Clinical Complications Associated With Needling Procedures

ELAINE W. ZHONG AND SYED A. HODA

INTRODUCTION

The objective of a needle core biopsy (NCB) procedure is adequate sampling of the target lesion. An efficacious NCB sampling may remove a portion, or all, of the target. The latter is almost always either a nonpalpable radiologically detected (mammographic, sonographic, or magnetic resonance–detected) lesion or a discrete mass. The procedure inevitably results in disruption of lesional and/or perilesional tissue. NCB-induced tissue disruption varies widely and depends mainly upon the gauge of needle used and the volume of sample obtained. In recent years, the trend is toward obtaining bulkier sampling by utilizing larger gauge needles and procuring multiple samples, which results in greater tissue damage (1). Such damage is evident in the subsequently performed excision and is the main topic of this chapter **(Table 25.1)**. Other needling procedures such as fine needle aspirations (FNAs), needle localization procedures, and even liposuctions can cause similar disruption (2-4).

Automated NCB procedures that are typically used for targeting masses are more frequently associated with epithelial displacement than vacuum-assisted NCB procedures (5).

TABLE 25.1

Histologic Artifacts Following Needle Core Biopsy of Breast

Displacement of benign/neoplastic epithelia along needle track[a]

Displacement of benign/neoplastic epithelia into lymphovascular channels[a]

Displacement of benign/neoplastic epithelia to regional lymph nodes[a]

Displacement of epidermis into breast tissue

Intralesional hemorrhage and infarction[a]

Reactive spindle cell proliferation at healing needle core biopsy site

Epidermal inclusion cyst along healing needle core biopsy track

Reactive changes of metallic clip markers, "plugs," or "pellets"

[a]Particularly in papillary lesions.

The latter are generally used for targeting radiographically detected lesions and are more common. In the automated procedure, the needle is pushed into the target, and the sample is then directly acquired. In the vacuum-assisted procedure, the tissue sample is drawn into a suction chamber and sliced off with a rotating cutter. Direct mechanical sampling causes relatively more trauma to the lesional epithelium than vacuum-assisted acquisition.

RADIOLOGIC AND HISTOPATHOLOGIC CHANGES IN THE BREAST CAUSED BY NEEDLE CORE BIOPSY

Long-standing or significant effects of the NCB procedure on perilesional tissue, beyond that of hemorrhage, organizing fat necrosis, and subsequent scarring, are usually not apparent in imaging studies. In 24 patients studied by Kaye et al (6), follow-up mammography performed 6 months after stereotactic 14-gauge biopsy revealed no mammographically detectable architectural distortion attributable to the procedure. In two instances, there were fewer calcifications in postbiopsy mammograms, and a 6-mm fibroadenoma contained a 3-mm defect. Lamm and Jackman (7) reported the formation of a "small" (mean size: 8 mm) mammographic density in 6 to 8 months at the biopsy site when larger (11-gauge) needles were utilized. These as well as multiple other reports indicate that, in general, the performance of NCBs does not inflict notable effects on subsequent radiographic (including ultrasound, mammographic, and magnetic resonance imaging [MRI]) studies.

Nonetheless, **procedural trauma-induced changes** in and around the NCB site can affect the histopathologic interpretation of the subsequently performed excisional biopsy—an observation noted almost three decades ago (8,9). Evidence of previous NCB track (or, less accurately, "tract"), for example, hemorrhage, granulation tissue formation, and fibroplasia, should be sought in excisional biopsies, as evidence that the target lesion has been sampled (8,9). The presence of fresh blood or hemosiderin (depending upon the time interval between the procedures) within the lumina of glands and stroma in the vicinity of the target is a frequent manifestation of prior needling procedures, including needle-localizing techniques **(Fig. 25.1)**. Fragments

483

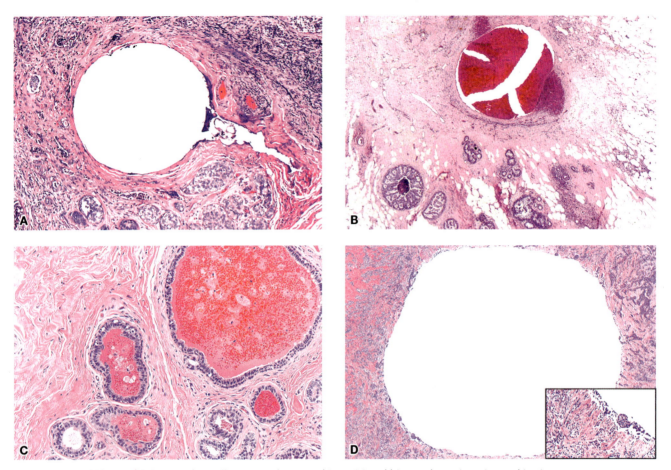

FIGURE 25.1 **Site of Needling Procedure. A:** This excisional biopsy shows invasive and in situ lobular carcinoma as well as changes following a radiologic needle localization procedure that was performed less than an hour prior to the excision. The absence of reactive inflammatory changes is notable. **B:** An excisional biopsy specimen showing ductal carcinoma in situ in which the needle core biopsy had been performed 1 week previously. Note reactive fibroplasia around the circular defect caused by the core biopsy sampling. **C:** Fresh intraductal hemorrhage is present in this excisional biopsy in the vicinity of the site of a needle core biopsy. **D:** In vitro procurement of tumor tissue with a 4 mm punch. Note lack of reactive changes.

of epidermis may be dislodged into breast tissue by the needle if a cutaneous incision was not made before inserting the needle. An epidermal inclusion cyst may form from the displaced skin epithelium (10) **(Fig. 25.2)**. Considerable diagnostic difficulties can ensue as a result of displacement of neoplastic or non-neoplastic epithelium along the healing biopsy track (vide infra) (11,12).

The healing NCB site initially develops granulation tissue (ie, proliferating fibroblasts and capillaries amid inflammatory cells) and eventually forms a *scar*. The maturity of the scar depends on the time interval between the initial NCB and the subsequent excisional procedure. In some cases, the reactive process displays exuberant myofibroblastic or histiocytic hyperplasia with mitotic activity (13) to a degree that it forms a "pseudotumor" (14) or appears "pseudosarcomatous" (15), similar to those reported in the prostate and thyroid after NCBs. Such post-NCB spindle cell nodules can be mistaken for a de novo mesenchymal lesion (eg, fibromatosis) **(Fig. 25.3)**. Subtle histopathologic evidence of organizing fat necrosis can be present in such cases. Association with a healing biopsy track and comparative histopathologic review with findings in the NCB can be helpful in rendering the appropriate diagnoses. In the NCB sample itself, a peculiar artifact can be induced by the vacuum and suction process applied during mammotome biopsies, resulting in spherules or whorls of fibrous tissue (16).

The foregoing post-NCB changes, as well as those induced by clip or seed placement (vide infra), can assist in the localization of "tumor beds" and sentinel lymph nodes (SLNs) after neoadjuvant chemotherapy—because both can be difficult to assess macroscopically and/or microscopically, especially in cases wherein there is complete pathologic remission **(Fig. 25.4)**.

NCB-induced infarction (ie, ischemic necrosis) in a benign proliferative epithelial lesion can be mistaken for a de novo process, particularly in a cystic papillary neoplasm

PATHOLOGIC CHANGES AND CLINICAL COMPLICATIONS ASSOCIATED WITH NEEDLING PROCEDURES

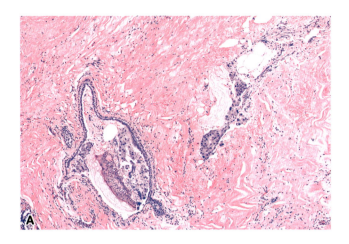

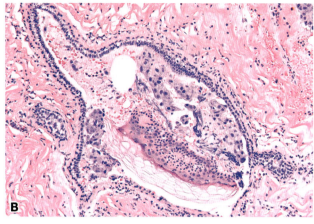

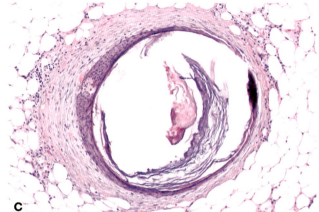

FIGURE 25.2 Displacement of Skin Into Breast Tissue.
A, B: A recently detached fragment of epidermis and clusters of hyperplastic apocrine epithelium are present in a duct near a needle biopsy site. Displaced apocrine epithelium is present in the biopsy track **(A)**. **C:** Another excisional biopsy specimen in which displaced epidermis has formed a cyst and become encapsulated amid reactive fibroplasia. The needle core biopsy had been performed approximately 3 weeks previously.

(Fig. 25.5). Such an infarct can be recognized by its association with a linear needle track leading to a wedge-shaped necrotic process. Organization of hemorrhage with fibroplasia can entrap portions of the benign epithelia and may simulate invasive carcinoma either within the lesion or at its periphery. In these cases, eliciting a history of a previous needling procedure may help prevent an incorrect interpretation.

Biopsy Clips

It is routine practice to place a **clip at the site of a targeted lesion** after the performance of an NCB. Clip placement primarily serves to localize the site of the lesion by spatially guiding the subsequent surgical procedure and helps optimize the volume of tissue excised. Other advantages of clip placement are listed in **Table 25.2**.

A wide variety of clips are commercially available, including those that are composed principally of stainless steel, ceramic, or titanium **(Fig. 25.6)**. Clips have to be removed at the time of gross pathologic evaluation to enable complete inspection of the specimen, document their presence, and ensure that the subsequently prepared tissue block does not inadvertently contain the clip. The latter

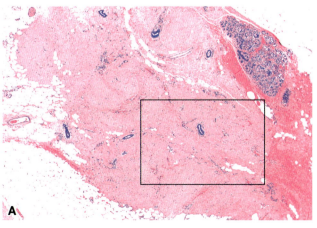

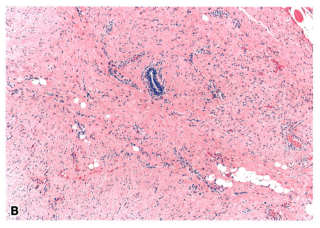

FIGURE 25.3 Postbiopsy Spindle Cell Nodule. A, B: Pseudotumoral proliferation of myofibroblasts and vessels 8 weeks after needle core biopsy.

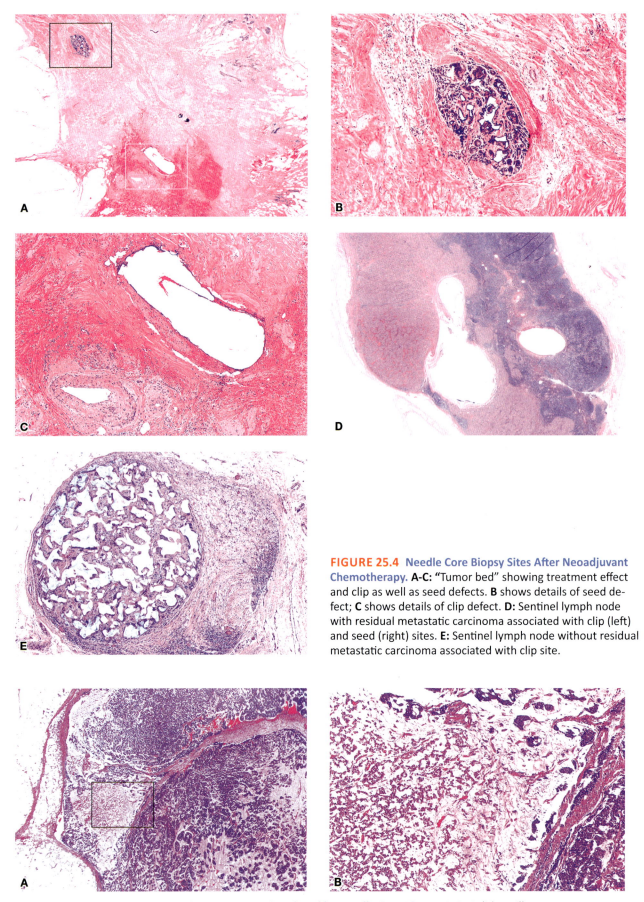

FIGURE 25.4 Needle Core Biopsy Sites After Neoadjuvant Chemotherapy. A-C: "Tumor bed" showing treatment effect and clip as well as seed defects. **B** shows details of seed defect; **C** shows details of clip defect. **D:** Sentinel lymph node with residual metastatic carcinoma associated with clip (left) and seed (right) sites. **E:** Sentinel lymph node without residual metastatic carcinoma associated with clip site.

FIGURE 25.5 Iatrogenic Tumor Necrosis Induced by Needle Core Biopsy. A, B: Solid papillary carcinoma with mucinous features showing a linear disruption associated with wedge-shaped necrosis on postbiopsy excision.

TABLE 25.2
Advantages of Clip Placement After Needle Core Biopsy of Breast

When surgical excision follows soon after needle core biopsy

Helpful at surgery in localizing lesions
Confirm excision of the target lesion on specimen imaging.
Guide pathologists in identifying target area during gross examination of specimen.
Mark separate targets by use of multiple clips of different shapes.

When there is follow-up after needle core biopsy

Identifiable on sequential imaging examination
Helpful in determining progression (or regression) of lesions over time
Indicate location of antecedent tumor even when there is complete pathologic response.

References: Corsi F, Sorrentino L, Sartani A, et al. Localization of nonpalpable breast lesions with sonographically visible clip: optimizing tailored resection and clear margins. *Am J Surg*. 2015;209:950-958; Samimi M, Bonneau C, Lebas P, et al. Mastectomies after vacuum core biopsy procedure for microcalcification clusters: value of clip. *Eur J Radiol*. 2009;69:296-299; Thomassin-Naggara I, Lalonde L, David J, et al. A plea for the biopsy marker: how, why and why not clipping after breast biopsy? *Breast Cancer Res Treat*. 2012;132:881-893; Uematsu T, Kasami M, Takahashi K, et al. Clip placement after an 11-gauge vacuum-assisted stereotactic breast biopsy: correlation between breast thickness and clip movement. *Breast Cancer*. 2012;19:30-36.

circumstance could potentially damage the microtome during sectioning of the tissue block and also compromise the quality of histologic sections. Minute sharp hooks serve to anchor some types of clips into the soft tissues, and the process of clip removal should be undertaken with caution to avoid damage to breast tissue.

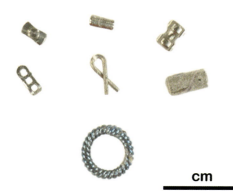

FIGURE 25.6 Commonly Used Commercially Available Clips and Seeds. These clips are utilized to mark the site of a targeted lesion after the performance of a needle core biopsy. "Extraction" of the clips at the time of gross examination of the subsequently performed excisional biopsy may cause damage to lesional tissue. It is important that the presence of one or more clips be documented in the excisional biopsy by the pathologist. Specimen radiography is helpful in localizing the clip(s) in most cases.

Diligent efforts at the time of gross examination may be required to find the clip within the specimen. These efforts include specimen radiography and serial "thin" (approximately 2 mm) sectioning. Rarely, despite a concerted effort, the clip cannot be found in the excisional biopsy or mastectomy, and the most likely explanation is loss incurred either through the intraoperative use of a suction device with a larger aperture (most clips span 2-3 mm) or through inattentive specimen procurement, transport, or handling (17,18).

Various types of **bioresorbable embedding material** such as bovine collagen (Avitene), polylactic acid/polyglycolic acid (PGA) pellets, starch pellets, PGA pads, and polyethylene glycol (PEG) hydrogel are embedded, deployed with, or interwoven into the clip at the biopsy site to prevent displacement ("migration") of the clip and improve hemostasis by filling the newly created cavity (19). These materials can also improve long-term sonographic detectability of the clip site (20). Each embedding material has a distinctive histologic appearance **(Fig. 25.7)**, and some of these may be mistaken by the uninitiated for amyloid, osteoid, other foreign material, or even a mass lesion (21-23). Although these materials do not typically elicit a reactive tissue response, occasionally a prominent fibroinflammatory reaction might be evident.

Wire/Seed Localization

Before the advent of "seed" placement, **radiographic wire localization immediately before surgical resection** was the accepted standard of care for preoperative localization of nonpalpable breast lesions. This procedure can fail owing to mislocalization of the wire; subsequent inadvertent wire displacement (during patient transfer, surgical positioning, or postprocedure mammography); and, rarely, breakage of the wire. Another limitation of wire localization is the need for same-day scheduling of the two procedures to reduce the risk of wire migration. Various nonwire ("wireless") preoperative localization techniques have the potential to mitigate these limitations, resulting in greater patient satisfaction, better coordination between specialties, ease of excision, potential improvement in attainment of negative surgical margins, reduction in re-excision rates, and enhanced cosmesis (24-26). In current practice, "seed" placement has supplanted wire localization. ^{125}I radioactive seed localization (RSL) utilizes a titanium "seed" about the size of a sesame seed **(Fig. 25.8)** that is inserted through a hollow needle under imaging guidance and its position confirmed using mammography. The seed is then localized intraoperatively with a handheld probe. Because the signal emitted from the seed is different from the signal emitted from ^{99m}Tc, used for SLN identification, both the tumor and lymph nodes can be removed simultaneously. Other nonwire localization techniques include radar reflectors (SAVI SCOUT), magnetic seed markers (Magseed), and radio-frequency identification (RFID) tags (LOCalizer). The preoperative placement of any of these devices has the potential to inflict tissue damage similar to that caused by other needling procedures.

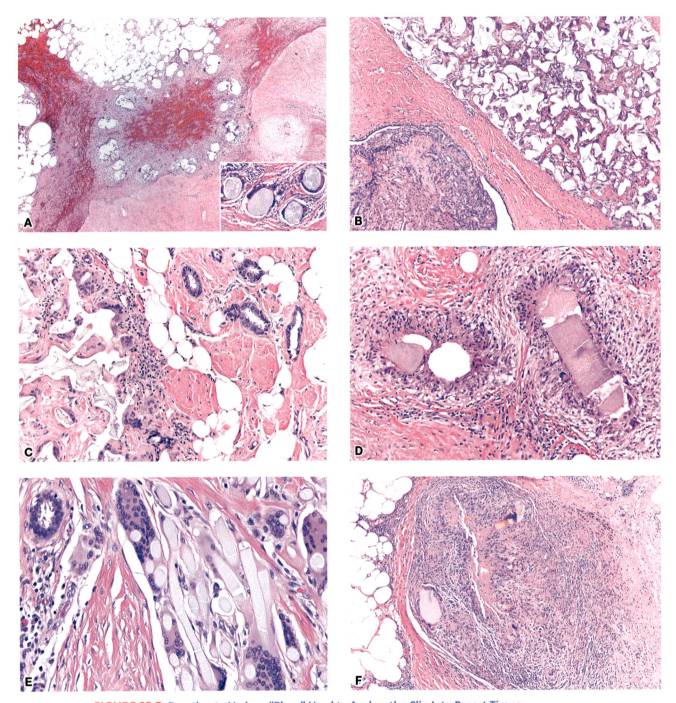

FIGURE 25.7 Reaction to Various "Plugs" Used to Anchor the Clip Into Breast Tissue.
A-F: Various embedding materials have distinctive histologic appearances. Some of these "plugs" may be mistaken by the uninitiated for amyloid, osteoid, or other foreign material. All figures show various degrees of giant cell reaction against the "plug." Inset in **A** shows detail at the healing needle core biopsy site. A pronounced inflammatory reaction is evident in **D-F.**

Displaced Epithelium Within Breast Tissue

Tissue disruption may result in displacement of lesional epithelial cells into the healing needle track and into stroma in the lesional area. This can produce a pattern that simulates invasive carcinoma (2,27,28) **(Figs. 25.9 and 25.10)**. Youngson et al (8,9) were among the first to report finding displaced epithelium in excisional biopsies of breast with various types of lesions after the performance of NCBs. The average interval between the needling procedure and excisional biopsy was 10 days. Fragments of benign or malignant epithelium were present within lymphovascular channels in seven cases, six of which also had stromal displacement. One of these women, who had extensive intraductal carcinoma associated with stromal displacement and lymphovascular tumor emboli in the breast, also had clusters

PATHOLOGIC CHANGES AND CLINICAL COMPLICATIONS ASSOCIATED WITH NEEDLING PROCEDURES 489

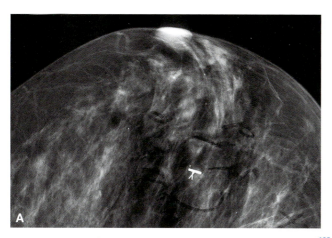
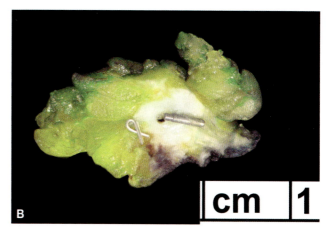

FIGURE 25.8 Preoperative Localization With ^{125}I Radioactive Seed. A: The preoperative mammogram is shown with the "seed" and "clip" in place. **B:** Cut section of the subsequently performed excisional biopsy shows the "seed" and "clip." The clip is associated with hemorrhage. The placement of these foreign devices is achieved via needling procedures, which have the potential to traumatize lesional tissue.

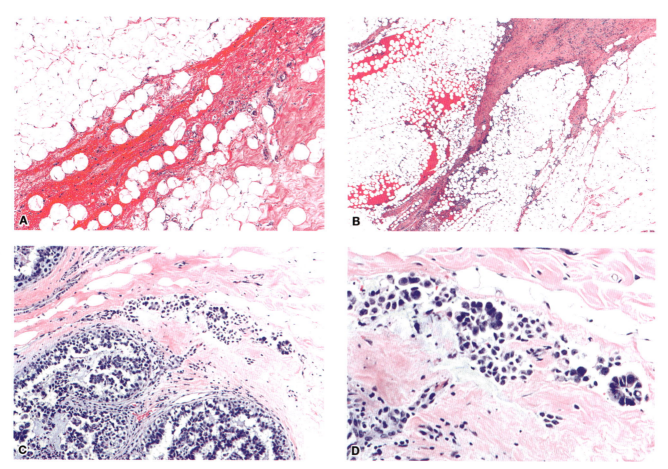

FIGURE 25.9 Needle Tracks in Postbiopsy Excisions. A: Fresh hemorrhage in the track of a guide wire placed 2 hours before surgery. **B:** Healing needle track 2 weeks status post needle core biopsy. **C, D:** Displaced fragments of intraductal carcinoma are shown in the stroma near the site of a needle core biopsy procedure performed 7 days previously. Note the absence of reactive changes in the stroma and the well-preserved cytologic appearance of the displaced tumor cells.

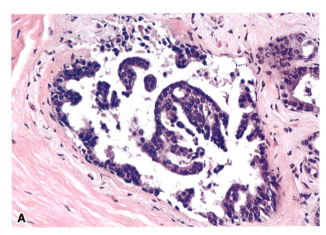 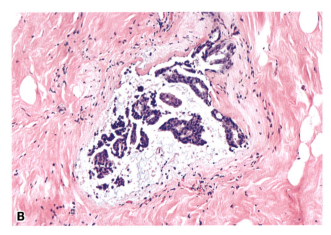

FIGURE 25.10 Disruption of Intraductal Carcinoma in Postbiopsy Excision. A: Portions of the intraductal carcinoma have been dislodged from the basement membrane and are displaced into the duct lumen after a needle core biopsy procedure. **B:** Another area in the specimen shown in **A** with severe disruption of intraductal carcinoma. The detached epithelial fragments have remained within the confines of the basement membrane.

of carcinoma cells in the subcapsular sinuses of two axillary lymph nodes. Hoorntje et al (29) reported finding displaced carcinoma cells in 11 of 22 (50%) needle tracks after 14-gauge needle biopsy procedures. Prospectively, these authors found displaced carcinoma in 7 of 11 (64%) needle tracks examined 7 to 35 days (median interval, 25 days) after 14-gauge needle biopsy.

Displacement of benign or carcinomatous epithelium is suggested by the finding of isolated clusters of epithelium in minuscule spaces within the healing biopsy track—usually in a linear distribution. Depending on the time elapsed since the procedure, the displaced epithelium is accompanied by hemorrhage, hemosiderin-laden macrophages, fat necrosis, an inflammatory cell infiltrate or granulation tissue, and scarring **(Fig. 25.11)**. Displaced epithelium that is not in the immediate vicinity of the biopsy site may not be accompanied by any significant degree of stromal reaction. This may lead to the mistaken diagnosis of invasive carcinoma even in a benign lesion. It is not unusual to find fragments of displaced epithelium within lumina of benign glands. Rarely, portions of intraductal carcinoma that are entirely dislodged into the lumen of an atrophic duct may simulate lymphatic invasion.

Immunostains for confirming the presence of epithelial displacement can be helpful if myoepithelial cells can be demonstrated via p63, p40, myosin, DOG1, etc., around the extralesional epithelial cells **(Fig. 25.12)**—provided myoepithelial cells are also immunohistochemically detectable in the target lesion sampled by the NCB. However, failure to detect myoepithelial cells in association with the

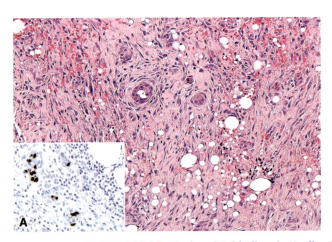 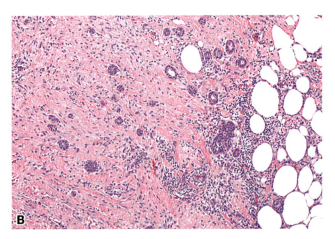

FIGURE 25.11 Displaced Epithelium in Healing Postbiopsy Scars. A: This patient underwent a needle core biopsy procedure that showed a sclerosing papilloma. This image is from the subsequent excisional biopsy specimen performed 1 week after the needle biopsy procedure. Myoepithelial cells display nuclear p63 reactivity (inset) around some displaced epithelial cell fragments. **B:** Displaced epithelial fragments in fibrous scar tissue at the site of a needle core biopsy performed 3 weeks previously.

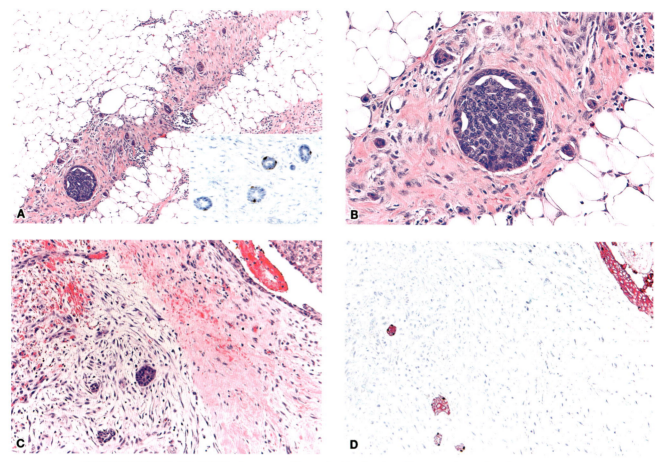

FIGURE 25.12 Epithelial Displacement Along the Healing Needle Core Biopsy (NCB) Track.
A, B: Clusters of disrupted epithelial cells appear along the linear healing biopsy track in an excisional biopsy specimen. Myoepithelial cells display nuclear p63 reactivity (inset in **A**) around some displaced epithelial cell clusters. **C, D:** Displaced in situ carcinomatous epithelia amid granulation tissue following NCB (**C**). Cytokeratin (CK)/p63 staining shows myoepithelial cells accompanying displaced epithelia (CK: red, p63: brown).

extralesional epithelium is not by itself diagnostic of invasive carcinoma, because displaced epithelial cells derived from a benign lesion may not adhere to myoepithelial cells. When myoepithelial marker–positive cells can be demonstrated as evidence of epithelial displacement, they are usually associated with a minor proportion of the displaced epithelial clusters. Epithelial displacement can also be difficult to distinguish from lymphovascular channel involvement **(Fig. 25.13)** when intraductal carcinoma is present and epithelial clusters are devoid of myoepithelial cells.

The identification of unequivocal lymphovascular channel invasion by carcinoma cells can be facilitated by the use of immunostains for endothelial cells (30,31). These markers include CD31, D2-40 (podoplanin), ETS-related gene (ERG), and factor VIII. Notably, CD31, D2-40, and factor VIII are immunoreactive in the cytoplasm of the endothelial cells; however, these three markers either show cross-reactivity with other cell types or display background stromal reactivity. ERG marks endothelial cell nuclei and does not cross-react with nuclei of other cell types; however, nuclear immunoreactivity may be difficult to visualize in minute lymphovascular channels. D2-40 is purportedly reactive in the cytoplasm of *lymphatic endothelial* cells, whereas the other markers are regarded as *pan-endothelial*. As always, immunostains should be interpreted with caution, as the results can be misleading when "floaters" or artifactually displaced malignant cells fortuitously occupy the lumen of a vascular channel.

The **frequency of epithelial displacement** in the needle track has been substantially reduced since the introduction of vacuum-assisted stereotactic biopsy (32), possibly because the device allows multiple specimens to be collected in a single needle pass (33). Nonetheless, epithelial displacement following NCBs remains a ubiquitous diagnostic problem, particularly when papillary lesions are targeted (27,34,35). Lee et al (2) drew attention to epithelial displacement in granulation tissue adjacent to a benign papillary tumor simulating invasive carcinoma. Others have encountered the same problem around noninvasive papillary carcinomas that were excised after an NCB (27,34).

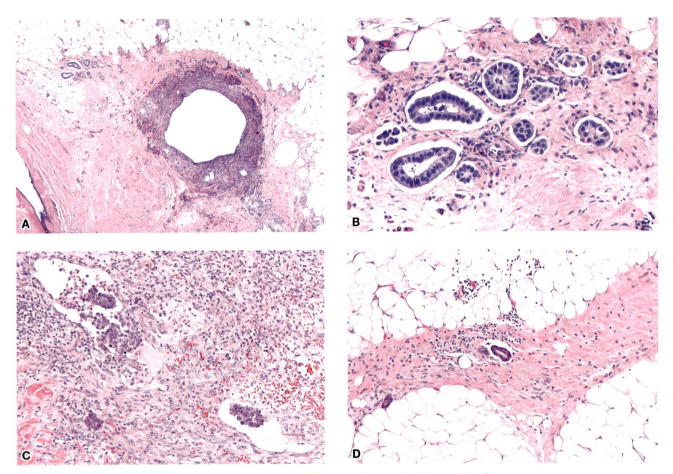

FIGURE 25.13 Epithelial Disruption Simulating Lymphovascular Channel Involvement.
A: Hyperplastic epithelial clusters have been dislodged and simulate carcinomatous involvement within lymphovascular channels (upper left). **B:** Magnified view of displaced epithelium in **A**. **C:** Another excisional biopsy in which the displaced epithelial fragments are in lacunae in granulation tissue. The needle core biopsy had been performed 1 week previously. **D:** Another example of disrupted epithelial clusters simulating lymphovascular channel involvement. The needle core biopsy had been performed 4 weeks previously.

The **long-term viability of displaced epithelium** at the biopsy site in the breast, whether benign or malignant, is uncertain. Diaz et al (36) found epithelial displacement in 32% of excisions performed after an NCB procedure. Displacement was less frequent after vacuum-assisted biopsy than when an automated gun device was used. The observation that the incidence of detectable epithelial displacement was inversely related to the post-NCB interval led investigators to conclude that displaced epithelium underwent degenerative changes in some instances (33,36). Such changes can be seen histologically as squamous metaplasia (occasionally even mimicking low-grade adenosquamous carcinoma), pyknotic nuclei, shrunken eosinophilic cytoplasm, or vesicular cytoplasm (37).

Local recurrence arising from carcinomatous epithelial displacement is a concern after breast conservation surgery, particularly in patients who do not receive radiotherapy. Tumor seeding of the dermis overlying the breast was reported by Stolier et al (38), leading to local recurrence at the biopsy site in one case. Chao et al (39) described two patients who had subcutaneous recurrence of carcinoma in an NCB track 12 and 17 months postbiopsy. A third patient was found to have cutaneous involvement in a mastectomy.

Thurfjell et al (40) studied 303 consecutive women with nonpalpable carcinomas treated by excision. The majority had undergone a preoperative NCB procedure (71%) and postoperative radiotherapy (82%). Overall, 33 (11%) of the women developed local recurrence after median follow-up of 5.4 years. On the basis of the location of the recurrence and the position of the needle track, it was considered likely that recurrences were attributable to epithelial displacement in three women who did not receive radiotherapy. Chen et al (41) investigated the role of epithelial displacement in local recurrence by comparing women who underwent NCB before excision and those who had a needle localization biopsy as the diagnostic procedure. In a series of 551 consecutive patients treated with conservation surgery and radiotherapy, the frequency of local recurrence after a mean follow-up of 4.9 years in the NCB group (2.3%) was not significantly different from the needle localization group (5.4%).

Excising the skin puncture site with an "adequate margin" of skin at the time of breast conservation surgery reduces the risk of local recurrence in the skin (42,43). However, it is not always practical or cosmetically sustainable to excise the skin or the entire parenchymal biopsy track, and it has been suggested that in most cases postoperative radiotherapy can be relied on to eliminate displaced carcinoma cells (29,33).

Retraction artifact around clusters or nests of displaced carcinoma cells can simulate lymphovascular channel involvement in NCBs, as it does in excisional biopsies. In general, the established diagnostic criteria for identifying lymphovascular involvement are helpful in both types of specimens. These criteria include: presence of carcinoma within endothelial-lined space, nonconformance of the shape of the carcinoma cluster to the contour of the space, and presence of other veins or arteries in the immediate vicinity (44). It has been suggested that retraction around tumor cells after NCB may not be a "random artifactual phenomenon" when it is associated with an invasive carcinoma exhibiting micropapillary architectural features, and in this setting these findings have "a significant association with nodal metastasis" (45). It is notable that displaced epithelial clusters along the healing biopsy track often display micropapillary features (with a "doughnut"-like appearance).

Parenthetically, a significant degree of retraction artifact occurs much more often around invasive carcinoma than around in situ carcinoma—and this observation may be helpful in situations wherein the differential diagnosis lies between invasive carcinoma and in situ carcinoma. In this particular context, the finding of retraction artifact has been termed as "the pathologist's friend" (46).

Displaced Epithelium Within Lymphovascular Spaces and Axillary Lymph Nodes

Displaced carcinomatous epithelium in lymphovascular spaces is sometimes indistinguishable from intrinsic lymphovascular invasion (8,9) **(Fig. 25.14)**, although displaced epithelial clusters are typically larger than bona fide tumor emboli. The significance of carcinomatous lymphovascular emboli in the setting of epithelial displacement remains uncertain. Until unequivocal evidence to the contrary comes to the fore, the finding of lymphovascular tumor emboli can be considered as a risk factor for the transport of carcinoma cells to axillary lymph nodes even when conventional stromal invasion cannot be identified. Carter et al (47) introduced the term "benign transport" to describe instances that they concluded were iatrogenic displacement of breast epithelium to axillary lymph nodes. It was suggested that benign transport could be recognized by the absence of reactive changes indicative of tumor growth at the site of carcinomatous nodal involvement and the concurrence of foamy histiocytes. Such cells were considered to lack native metastatic capacity and be unlikely to implicate a risk for widespread disease.

At present, there is no objective method for determining with certainty whether a deposit of epithelial cells in an SLN has resulted from biologically dictated lymphovascular channel invasion or from the iatrogenic phenomenon of epithelial displacement. Some studies have shown that the nuclei of breast carcinoma cells metastatic to lymph nodes are larger or similar in size to the nuclei of the primary breast carcinoma cells (48). Based on this hypothesis, a study by van Deurzen (49) found the nuclear size of isolated tumor cells in SLNs of 16 patients with breast carcinoma to be significantly smaller than the nuclear size of the corresponding

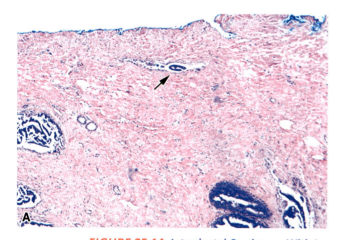
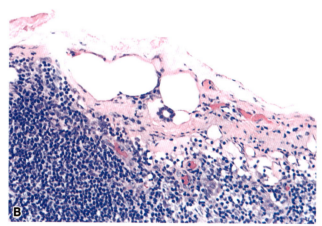

FIGURE 25.14 Intraductal Carcinoma With Lymphatic Tumor Emboli and Lymph Node Metastasis. A, B: This excisional biopsy specimen is from a procedure performed 8 days after a needle core biopsy sampling of mammographically detected calcifications revealed intraductal carcinoma. There is a U-shaped group of carcinoma cells in the lymphatic space near the upper border of the tissue (arrow). Ducts with disrupted ductal carcinoma in situ (DCIS) are depicted on the left, and intact micropapillary DCIS is shown on the right. **B:** Isolated tumor cells that formed a ring in the subcapsular sinus of a lymph node obtained in an axillary lymph node dissection performed because lymphatic tumor emboli were demonstrated in the excisional biopsy specimen shown in **A**.

primary carcinoma and concluded that "some of these deposits could represent benign epithelium or degenerated malignant cells lacking outgrowth potential."

Rarely, displaced clusters of carcinoma cells can be present within lymphovascular channels in NCBs that show only ductal carcinoma in situ (DCIS) **(Fig. 25.15)**. In the series reported by Koo et al (50), epithelial displacement was found in 3.2% (7 of 218) of DCIS cases on NCBs. The diagnosis of true lymphovascular invasion by carcinoma cells in NCBs can be questioned when invasive carcinoma cannot be identified in the NCB or in the subsequently performed excisional biopsy. In Koo's series, the phenomenon of displaced clusters of carcinoma cells in lymphovascular channels was encountered with biopsies acquired utilizing "automated" rather than "vacuum-assisted" techniques.

The **clinical significance of displaced carcinoma cells in regional lymph nodes**, sentinel or otherwise, remains uncertain (51-55). The indeterminate nature of these findings was highlighted some years back by Carter and Page (51), who stated that they "look forward to the future development of laboratory assays that will correctly differentiate small lymph node deposits that are truly metastatic… from those minimal deposits that are unlikely to have any significant impact on the patient and those deposits that have been benignly transported to the lymph node as a cleanup-mechanism by the lymphatic system." Each case requires careful scrutiny that takes into consideration the histologic and immunohistochemical appearances of the primary tumor and epithelial "microdeposits" in the lymph node and the presence or absence of epithelial displacement at the primary site.

The MIRROR (Micrometastases and Isolated Tumor Cells: Relevant and Robust or Rubbish?) trial showed that adjuvant therapy significantly improved disease-free survival in patients with isolated tumor cells as well as micrometastases in early breast carcinoma versus those who were not treated (56); thus, it is imperative, at a minimum, that the biologic implication of finding minute deposits of carcinoma cells in the lymph node in this setting be unequivocally established.

Molecular techniques may be helpful to differentiate displaced benign cells in lymph nodes from true nodal metastases. Gene transcription analysis of The Cancer Genome Atlas data has demonstrated widespread cancer type–specific differences between primary cancers and paired metastases, including genes with functional roles in metastasis such as *EPL3*, *MYCNOS*, and *FOXF2*—differences that should not exist in cells that are displaced (57). Comparative genomic hybridization, massively parallel sequencing, and transcriptome or methylome profiling of the tumor microenvironment may also help establish the benign, in situ, or invasive nature of epithelial clusters in stroma or lymph nodes (58-61).

MAJOR CLINICAL COMPLICATIONS OF NEEDLE CORE BIOPSIES

The incidence of major clinical complications after the performance of NCB is low. These complications are relatively uncommon—given the ubiquity of the technique (62) **(Table 25.3)**.

Pneumothorax is the most life-threatening complication of NCB of the breast, and the risk is greatest when the target lesion lies close to the chest wall. Inadvertent entry into the pleural space can be averted by real-time radiologic monitoring of the procedure and by angling the needle parallel to, rather than toward, the chest wall.

Compression upon completion of the procedure usually suffices to prevent **hematoma** formation. Use of anticoagulants and antithrombotics, including aspirin, may increase the likelihood of postprocedural hematoma. In this setting, the procedure should be performed with caution, and any manipulation of therapy should be carefully monitored (63,64).

Rare cases of **infection** have been reported to follow NCBs. These infections have been of the acute necrotizing (65), necrotizing fasciitis (66), and recurrent (67) types.

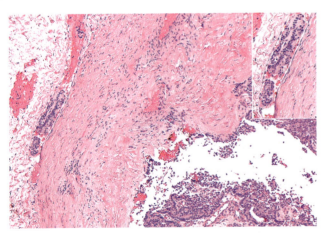

FIGURE 25.15 Displaced Epithelial Clusters of Carcinoma Cells in a Lymphovascular Channel in a Needle Core Biopsy. The needle core biopsy and the excision showed only intraductal papillary carcinoma. Inset shows detail of displaced epithelial clusters within a lymphovascular channel (left).

TABLE 25.3
Major Clinical Complications Following Needle Core Biopsy of Breast

Syncope
Significant hematoma
Infection
Necrotizing fasciitis
Milk fistula (in pregnant/lactating women)
Embolia cutis medicamentosa (Nicolau syndrome)
Pseudoaneurysm
Pneumothorax
Implantation metastasis

Direct injury to intramammary blood vessels in the course of the NCB can induce pseudoaneurysm formation (68), development of arteriovenous fistulas (69,70), and significant arterial bleeding to a degree that requires emergent embolization (71).

NCB procedures of the breast are preceded by cutaneous infiltration by local anesthesia. All usual, typically minor, complications that can attend such local injections can occur in this setting; however, a remarkable case of **Nicolau syndrome** (embolia cutis medicamentosa) has been reported in this setting (72,73). This rare syndrome, presumably because of vasospasm caused by sympathetic overstimulation, occurs at an injection site and is manifested by macular rash that progresses rapidly to hemorrhagic necrosis of skin and underlying tissues.

NEEDLE CORE BIOPSIES AND RATE OF DISTANT METASTASES

Experimental evidence raises the possibility that NCBs might increase the rate of distant metastases, at least in the mouse model, by creating an immunosuppressive tumor microenvironment and upregulating key epithelial-mesenchymal transition genes that enable the release of circulating tumor cells (74,75). Sennerstam et al (76) demonstrated a higher rate of distant metastasis (but not local recurrence) following breast NCB compared to FNA in a strictly matched patient cohort, presumably because of greater tissue disruption and injury. However, these diagnostic procedures were performed in the 1970s and 1990s, and a similar matched comparison using current techniques is yet to be performed. Additional studies to understand the biologic traits leading to metastases associated with NCB procedures need to be conducted.

REFERENCES

1. Meeuwis C, Veltman J, van Hall HN, et al. MR-guided breast biopsy at 3T: diagnostic yield of large core needle biopsy compared with vacuum-assisted biopsy. *Eur Radiol*. 2012;22:341-349.
2. Lee KC, Chan JK, Ho LC. Histologic changes in the breast after fine-needle aspiration. *Am J Surg Pathol*. 1994;18:1039-1047.
3. McLaughlin CS, Petrey C, Grant S, et al. Displaced epithelium after liposuction for gynecomastia. *Int J Surg Pathol*. 2011;19:510-513.
4. Michalopoulos NV, Zagouri F, Sergentanis TN, et al. Needle tract seeding after vacuum-assisted breast biopsy. *Acta Radiol*. 2008;49:267-270.
5. Liberman L. Clinical management issues in percutaneous core breast biopsy. *Radiol Clin North Am*. 2000;38:791-807.
6. Kaye MD, Vicinanza-Adami CA, Sullivan ML. Mammographic findings after stereotaxic biopsy of the breast performed with large-core needles. *Radiology*. 1994;192:149-151.
7. Lamm RL, Jackman RJ. Mammographic abnormalities caused by percutaneous stereotactic biopsy of histologically benign lesions evident on follow-up mammograms. *AJR Am J Roentgenol*. 2000;174:753-756.
8. Youngson BJ, Cranor M, Rosen PP. Epithelial displacement in surgical breast specimens following needling procedures. *Am J Surg Pathol*. 1994;18:896-903.
9. Youngson BJ, Liberman L, Rosen PP. Displacement of carcinomatous epithelium in surgical breast specimens following stereotaxic core biopsy. *Am J Clin Pathol*. 1995;103:598-602.
10. Davies JD, Nonni A, D'Costa HF. Mammary epidermoid inclusion cysts after wide-core needle biopsies. *Histopathology*. 1997;31:549-551.
11. Liebens F, Cariy B, Cusumano P, et al. Breast cancer seeding associated with core needle biopsies: a systematic review. *Maturitas*. 2009;62:113-123.
12. Phelan S, O'Doherty A, Hill A, et al. Epithelial displacement during breast needle core biopsy causes diagnostic difficulties in subsequent surgical excision specimens. *J Clin Pathol*. 2007;60:373-376.
13. Gobbi H, Tse G, Page DL, et al. Reactive spindle cell nodules of the breast after core biopsy or fine-needle aspiration. *Am J Clin Pathol*. 2000;113:288-294.

14. Sciallis AP, Chen B, Folpe AL. Cellular spindled histiocytic pseudotumor complicating mammary fat necrosis: a potential diagnostic pitfall. *Am J Surg Pathol*. 2012;36:1571-1578.
15. Garijo MF, Val-Bernal JF, Vega A, et al. Postoperative spindle cell nodule of the breast: pseudosarcomatous myofibroblastic proliferation following endosurgery. *Pathol Int*. 2008;58:787-791.
16. Crisi GM, Pantanowitz L, Otis CN. Images in pathology. Mammotome footprints: histologic artefacts in the era of stereotactic vacuum mammotome biopsy. *Int J Surg Pathol*. 2006;14:221-222.
17. Bourke AG, Peter P, Jose CL. The disappearing clip: an unusual complication in MRI biopsy. *BMJ Case Rep*. 2014;2014:bcr2014204092.
18. Calhoun K, Giuliano A, Brenner RJ. Intraoperative loss of core biopsy clips: clinical implications. *AJR Am J Roentgenol*. 2008;190:W196-W200.
19. Portnow LH, Thornton CM, Milch HS, et al. Biopsy marker standardization: what's in a name?. *AJR Am J Roentgenol*. 2019;212:1400-1405.
20. Sakamoto N, Fukuma E, Tsunoda Y, et al. Evaluation of the dislocation and long-term sonographic detectability of a hydrogel-based breast biopsy site marker. *Breast Cancer*. 2018;25:575-582.
21. Alatassi H, Pile NS, Chagpar AB, et al. Breast biopsy marker masquerading as a mass lesion. *Breast J*. 2005;11:504-505.
22. Gombos EC, Esserman LE, Odzer-Umlas SL, et al. Collagen plug metallic marker clip: mammographic and histopathologic appearance. *Breast J*. 2005;11:292-293.
23. Guarda LA, Tran TA. The pathology of breast biopsy site marking devices. *Am J Surg Pathol*. 2005;29:814-819.
24. Da Silva M, Porembka J, Mokdad AA, et al. Bracketed radioactive seed localization vs bracketed wire-localization in breast surgery. *Breast J*. 2018;24:161-166.
25. Garzotto F, Comoretto RI, Michieletto S, et al. Preoperative non-palpable breast lesion localization, innovative techniques and clinical outcomes in surgical practice: a systematic review and meta-analysis. *Breast*. 2021;58:93-105.
26. Sharek D, Zuley ML, Zhang JY, et al. Radioactive seed localization versus wire localization for lumpectomies: a comparison of outcomes. *AJR Am J Roentgenol*. 2015;204:872-877.
27. Nagi C, Bleiweiss I, Jaffer S. Epithelial displacement in breast lesions: a papillary phenomenon. *Arch Pathol Lab Med*. 2005;129:1465-1469.
28. Usami S, Moriya T, Kasajima A, et al. Pathological aspects of core needle biopsy for non-palpable breast lesions. *Breast Cancer*. 2005;12:272-278.
29. Hoorntje LE, Schipper ME, Kaya A, et al. Tumour cell displacement after 14G breast biopsy. *Eur J Surg Oncol*. 2004;30:520-525.
30. Gujam FJ, Going JJ, Mohammed ZM, et al. Immunohistochemical detection improves the prognostic value of lymphatic and blood vessel invasion in primary ductal breast cancer. *BMC Cancer*. 2014;14:676.
31. Kim S, Park HK, Jung HY, et al. ERG immunohistochemistry as an endothelial marker for assessing lymphovascular invasion. *Korean J Pathol*. 2013;47:355-364.
32. Liberman L. Impact of image-guided core biopsy on the clinical management of breast disease. In: Rosen PP, ed. *Breast Pathology: Diagnosis by Needle Core Biopsy*. 2nd ed. Lippincott Williams & Wilkins; 2006:314-324.
33. Loughran CF, Keeling CR. Seeding of tumour cells following breast biopsy: a literature review. *Br J Radiol*. 2011;84:869-874.
34. Douglas-Jones AG, Verghese A. Diagnostic difficulty arising from displaced epithelium after core biopsy in intracystic papillary lesions of the breast. *J Clin Pathol*. 2002;55:780-783.
35. Layfield LJ, Frazier S, Schanzmeyer E. Histomorphologic features of biopsy sites following excisional and core needle biopsies of the breast. *Breast J*. 2015;21:370-376.
36. Diaz LK, Wiley EL, Venta LA. Are malignant cells displaced by large-gauge needle core biopsy of the breast?. *AJR Am J Roentgenol*. 1999;173:1303-1313.
37. Nayak A, Bleiweiss IJ. Iatrogenically false positive sentinel lymph nodes in breast cancer: methods of recognition and evaluation. *Semin Diagn Pathol*. 2018;35:228-235.
38. Stolier A, Skinner J, Levine EA. A prospective study of seeding of the skin after core biopsy of the breast. *Am J Surg*. 2000;180:104-107.
39. Chao C, Torosian MH, Boraas MC, et al. Local recurrence of breast cancer in the stereotactic core needle biopsy site: case reports and review of the literature. *Breast J*. 2001;7:124-127.
40. Thurfjell MG, Jansson T, Nordgren H, et al. Local breast cancer recurrence caused by mammographically guided punctures. *Acta Radiol*. 2011;41:435-440.
41. Chen AM, Haffty BG, Lee CH. Local recurrence of breast cancer after breast conservation therapy in patients examined by means of stereotactic core-needle biopsy. *Radiology*. 2002;225:707-712.
42. Kwo S, Grotting JC. Does stereotactic core needle biopsy increase the risk of local recurrence of invasive breast cancer?. *Breast J*. 2006;12:191-193.
43. Uriburu JL, Vuoto HD, Cogorno L, et al. Local recurrence of breast cancer after skin-sparing mastectomy following core needle biopsy: case reports and review of the literature. *Breast J*. 2006;12:194-198.
44. Rosen PP. Tumor emboli in intramammary lymphatics in breast carcinoma: pathologic criteria for diagnosis and clinical significance. *Pathol Annu*. 1983;18 Pt 2:215-232.
45. Acs G, Paragh G, Chuang ST, et al. The presence of micropapillary features and retraction artifact in core needle biopsy material predicts lymph node metastasis in breast carcinoma. *Am J Surg Pathol*. 2009;33:202-210.

46. Irie J, Manucha V, Ioffe OB, et al. Artefact as the pathologist's friend: peritumoral retraction in in situ and infiltrating duct carcinoma of the breast. *Int J Surg Pathol.* 2007;15:53-59.
47. Carter BA, Jensen RA, Simpson JF, et al. Benign transport of breast epithelium into axillary lymph nodes after biopsy. *Am J Clin Pathol.* 2000;113:259-265.
48. Van der Linden HC, Baak JP, Smeulders AW, et al. Morphometry of breast cancer. I. Comparison of the primary tumours and the axillary lymph node metastases. *Pathol Res Pract.* 1986;181:236-242.
49. van Deurzen CH, Bult P, de Boer M, et al. Morphometry of isolated tumor cells in breast cancer sentinel lymph nodes: metastases or displacement?. *Am J Surg Pathol.* 2009;33:106-110.
50. Koo JS, Jung WH, Kim H. Epithelial displacement into the lymphovascular space can be seen in breast core needle biopsy specimens. *Am J Clin Pathol.* 2010;133:781-787.
51. Page DL. Sentinel lymph node histopathology in breast cancer: minimal disease versus artifact. *J Clin Oncol.* 2006;24:1978-1979.
52. Meijnen P, Oldenburg HS, Loo CE, et al. Risk of invasion and axillary lymph node metastasis in ductal carcinoma in situ diagnosed by core-needle biopsy. *Br J Surg.* 2007;94:952-956.
53. Newman EL, Kahn A, Diehl KM, et al. Does the method of biopsy affect the incidence of sentinel lymph node metastases?. *Breast J.* 2006;12:53-57.
54. Rosser RJ. A point of view: trauma is the cause of occult micrometastatic breast cancer in sentinel axillary lymph nodes. *Breast J.* 2000;6:209-212.
55. Tille JC, Loubeyre P, Bodmer A, et al. Isolated tumor cells in sentinel lymph nodes of invasive breast cancer: cell displacement or metastasis? *Breast J.* 2014;20:502-507.
56. Maaskant-Braat AJ, van de Poll-Franse LV, Voogd AC, et al. Sentinel node micrometastases in breast cancer do not affect prognosis: a population-based study. *Breast Cancer Res Treat.* 2011;127:195-203.
57. Chen F, Zhang Y, Varambally S, et al. Molecular correlates of metastasis by systematic pan-cancer analysis across the cancer genome atlas. *Mol Cancer Res.* 2019;17:476-487.
58. Cowell CF, Weigelt B, Sakr RA, et al. Progression from ductal carcinoma in situ to invasive breast cancer: revisited. *Mol Oncol.* 2013;7:859-869.
59. Trinh A, Gil Del Alcazar CR, Shukla SA, et al. Genomic alterations during the in situ to invasive ductal breast carcinoma transition shaped by the immune system. *Mol Cancer Res.* 2021;19:623-635.
60. Weigelt B, Peterse JL, van't Veer LJ. Breast cancer metastasis: markers and models. *Nat Rev Cancer.* 2005;5:591-602.

61. Xu H, Lien T, Bergholtz H, et al. Multi-omics marker analysis enables early prediction of breast tumor progression. *Front Genet.* 2021;12:670749.
62. Mahoney MC, Ingram AD. Breast emergencies: types, imaging features, and management. *AJR Am J Roentgenol.* 2014;202:W390-W399.
63. Chetlen AL, Kasales C, Mack J, et al. Hematoma formation during breast core needle biopsy in women taking antithrombotic therapy. *AJR Am J Roentgenol.* 2013;201:215-222.
64. Somerville P, Seifert PJ, Destounis SV, et al. Anticoagulation and bleeding risk after core needle biopsy. *AJR Am J Roentgenol.* 2008;191:1194-1197.
65. Roque DR, MacLaughlan S, Tejada-Berges T. Necrotizing infection of the breast after core needle biopsy. *Breast J.* 2013;19:201-202.
66. Flandrin A, Rouleau C, Azar CC, et al. First report of a necrotising fasciitis of the breast following a core needle biopsy. *Breast J.* 2009;15:199-201.
67. Kasprowicz N, Bauerschmitz GJ, Schonherr A, et al. Recurrent mastitis after core needle biopsy: case report of an unusual complication after core needle biopsy of a phyllodes tumor. *Breast Care (Basel).* 2012;7:240-244.
68. Swain B, Castelhano R, Litton K, et al. Core needle biopsy causing a pseudoaneurysm in the breast. *Ann R Coll Surg Engl.* 2022;104:e21-e24.
69. Gregg A, Leddy R, Lewis M, et al. Acquired arteriovenous fistula of the breast following ultrasound guided biopsy of invasive ductal carcinoma. *J Clin Imaging Sci.* 2013;3:38.
70. Haider MH, Satpathy A, Abou-Samra W. Iatrogenic arteriovenous fistula of the breast as a complication of core needle biopsy. *Ann R Coll Surg Engl.* 2014;96:e20-e22.
71. Fischman AM, Epelboym Y, Siegelbaum RH, et al. Emergent embolization of arterial bleeding after vacuum-assisted breast biopsy. *Cardiovasc Intervent Radiol.* 2012;35:194-197.
72. Garcia-Vilanova-Comas A, Fuster-Diana C, Cubells-Parrilla M, et al. Nicolau syndrome after lidocaine injection and cold application: a rare complication of breast core needle biopsy. *Int J Dermatol.* 2011;50:78-80.
73. Tabor D, Bertram CG, Williams AJK, et al. Nicolau syndrome (embolia cutis medicamentosa): a rare and poorly recognized iatrogenic cause of cutaneous thrombotic vasculopathy. *Am J Dermatopathol.* 2018;40:212-215.
74. Fu Y, Guo F, Chen H, et al. Core needle biopsy promotes lung metastasis of breast cancer: an experimental study. *Mol Clin Oncol.* 2019;10:253-260.
75. Mathenge EG, Dean CA, Clements D, et al. Core needle biopsy of breast cancer tumors increases distant metastases in a mouse model. *Neoplasia.* 2014;16:950-960.
76. Sennerstam RB, Franzen BSH, Wiksell HOT, et al. Core-needle biopsy of breast cancer is associated with a higher rate of distant metastases 5 to 15 years after diagnosis than FNA biopsy. *Cancer Cytopathol.* 2017;125:748-756.

Processing, Examining, and Reporting of Needle Core Biopsy Specimens

26

RAZA S. HODA AND SYED A. HODA

INTRODUCTION

The performance of a needle core biopsy (NCB) procedure for a *palpable* breast lesion is currently considered the appropriate initial step in its evaluation. NCB of *nonpalpable* radiologically detected breast lesions, under the guidance of various imaging techniques, that is, ultrasound (US), stereotactic guidance, or magnetic resonance imaging (MRI), is becoming increasingly common around the world (1,2). *Concordance between clinical, imaging, and pathologic findings must be ensured—for any combination of guidance and needle types used.*

BIOPSY TECHNIQUES AND SIZE OF NEEDLES

Fine needle aspiration (FNA) provides cells for cytologic examination. NCB provides tissue for histopathologic evaluation. These two techniques can, in theory, be guided by mammographic/tomosynthesis, US, or MRI guidance. However, in practice, FNA is almost always performed only under US guidance. NCB is performed under US, mammographic/tomosynthesis, or MRI guidance **(Table 26.1)**.

In current practice, FNA cytology procedures of breast are becoming increasingly uncommon. The high rate of inadequate and false-negative diagnoses and lower accuracy rates have reduced the use of FNA as the first-line approach to the diagnoses of palpable breast lesions. FNA retains utility in draining simple cysts ("cyst aspiration") and in triaging cases in certain settings (including wherever resources for NCB are not readily available); however, the practice of FNA without appropriate technical expertise and interpretative skills is of negligible value **(Table 26.2)**.

It is notable that the diameter (gauge or bore) of the needle is inversely proportional to the number of needle gauge (eg, 7-gauge needle is *larger* than 14-gauge needle). By convention, a fine needle is defined as a gauge of ≥ 22 (the latter corresponds to an outer diameter of ≤ 0.7 mm). FNA typically utilizes a 25-gauge needle (outer diameter of 0.5 mm) **(Table 26.3)**.

NCB is generally performed with a relatively larger-gauge needle, usually ranging from 20 gauge to 14 gauge (an outer diameter of 0.9-2.1 mm and an inner diameter of 0.6-1.6 mm). Two main types of NCBs are in use: cutting (spring-loaded) type and vacuum-assisted (VA) type. In recent years, multiple percutaneous image–guided NCB systems have been developed. One device that has the potential to completely remove the target lesion uses *radiofrequency* to remove the target in toto by using a "bucket," for example, *BLES* (Breast Lesion Excision System, Medtronic). Devices designed to optimize sampling by using a thinner needle after in vivo

---

TABLE 26.1

Fine Needle Aspiration (FNA) and Needle Core Biopsy: Sampling Options Per Imaging Guidance

Image Guidance	FNA[a]	C(SL)-NCB	VA-NCB
Ultrasound	([a])	(+)	(+)
Stereotactic[b]	(−)	(−)	(+)
MRI	(−)	(−)	(+)

C(SL)-NCB, cutting (spring-loaded) needle core biopsy; FNA, fine needle aspiration; MRI, magnetic resonance imaging; NCB, needle core biopsy; VA-NCB, vacuum-assisted needle core biopsy.

[a]FNA should be performed and interpreted only by those with expertise.
[b]Mammographic/tomosynthesis.

TABLE 26.2

Fine Needle Aspiration (FNA): Advantages and Disadvantages

Advantages:
Rapid
Minimal resources needed
Low cost
Aspiration may be therapeutic in draining simple cysts[a], seromas, hematomas, and abscesses.

Disadvantages:
Need technical and diagnostic expertise.
Inability to distinguish between various proliferative lesions
Inability to distinguish between invasive and in situ carcinoma
May not provide adequate tissue for biomarker testing

[a]Complex and complicated cysts are best sampled via needle core biopsy (if FNA is used, the aspirated fluid ought to be submitted for cytopathologic examination). Aspirated abscess fluid should be submitted for microbiologic studies also.

TABLE 26.3

Size (Gauge) of Commonly Used Needles and Corresponding Outer and Inner Diameters

Needle Size (Gauge)	Inner Diameter (mm)	Outer Diameter (mm)
27[a]	0.2	0.4
20	0.6	0.9
16	1.1	1.6
14	1.6	2.1
12	2.1	2.7
9	3.0	3.7
7[a]	3.8	4.6

mm, millimeter.

[a]Uncommonly used for needle core biopsy; 14-gauge needle is by far the most popular size for ultrasound-guided needle core biopsy; 27-gauge needles are typically used to administer local anesthetic. Largest needle used in most settings is 9 gauge (and is typically utilized for stereotactic- and magnetic resonance imaging [MRI]-guided needle core biopsies). A fine needle is defined as one with a gauge of ≥22.

TABLE 26.4

Features of Cutting (Spring-Loaded) Needle Core Biopsy, Typically Ultrasound Guided[a]

Most commonly used approach for NCB worldwide
Biopsy device uses a cutting (spring-loaded) gun that "fires" upon deployment.
Size range of needle used: 18- to 12-gauge
Most common size of needle used: 14-gauge
Multiple tissue samples (cores) are obtained.
Multiple samples entail multiple needle insertions.
Use of coaxial needle is an option for place holding.
Number of cores obtained: variable, typically 3-5
Typical length of cores: 10 to >20 mm
Low (~2%) mean false-negative rate
"Firing" is accompanied by a snapping sound (not unlike that produced by a stapler).

mm, millimeter; NCB, needle core biopsy.

[a]"Tru-Cut," a manual NCB device, is an alternative to cutting (spring-loaded) device.

freezing ("stabilizing") of the tissue, that is, *cryobiopsy*, have been developed (3). Mega-sized NCB devices (eg, *ABBI*: Advanced Breast Biopsy Instrument; U.S. Surgical Corp) that utilize extremely large-gauge needles (with a diameter of up to 20 mm!) have met with limited success (4).

The *cutting* (*non-VA, spring-loaded gun*) NCB is typically used for sampling breast masses using 14-gauge needles. Needles of wider bore are used less often. The cutting NCB system is a simple, but noisy, guillotine-type device. Drawbacks of the system include the need for multiple insertions if a larger volume of tissue is to be obtained and procurement of relatively small artifact-prone specimens. Yet, the procedure is relatively inexpensive and typically takes approximately 15 minutes (**Table 26.4**).

Vacuum-assisted needle core biopsy (VA-NCB) is the method of choice to sample suspicious calcifications without an accompanying palpable mass and for investigating lesions considered suspicious on breast US or MRI (**Table 26.5**). This technique utilizes larger (7-12 gauge) needles than those used in cutting-type biopsy instruments. An inner rotating cutting cannula is advanced into the target where it cuts a core of tissue. Vacuum delivers the sampled tissue through the needle into the collection chamber. Multiple biopsies are taken by rotating the needle without the need for multiple insertions. VA-NCB yields specimens with minimum artifact. The procedure typically takes 30 to 60 minutes to perform—depending upon which guidance (stereotactic, US, or MRI) system is utilized—and is relatively more expensive (5,6).

US-guided NCBs are usually performed for solid masses or complex cystic lesions. US guidance is particularly helpful for patients with mammary implants (**Table 26.6**).

Stereotactic guidance is typically used for NCB performed to investigate suspicious calcifications detected on mammograms (**Table 26.7**). *MRI-guided NCBs* are useful for lesions that are not detectable on clinical examination or mammographic and US evaluation. MRI-directed NCBs have a high sensitivity but poor specificity and require sophisticated and specialized equipment and the use of contrast media (**Table 26.8**) (7,8).

The number of cores removed for optimal sampling should depend on the nature of the targeted lesion (ie, calcifications, mass, etc), the particular imaging technique employed for guidance (US, stereotactic, MRI), and the size of the needle used (**Figs. 26.1 and 26.2**). An interdisciplinary

TABLE 26.5

Features of Vacuum-Assisted Needle Core Biopsy

Relatively common approach for NCB
VA-NCB can be performed under mammographic/tomo-syntheses, US, or MRI guidance.
Multiple samples can be obtained without removing the needle.
Typically, 6 or more samples are obtained with a 12- or 9-gauge needle.
Size range of needle used: 14-7 gauge
Approximately 1 g or 1 cm^3 of tissue is usually removed per procedure.
Smaller lesions (<1 cm) may be completely removed via VA-NCB.
Extremely low false-negative rate
Procedure time: relatively short, includes setup, targeting, and table time

MRI, magnetic resonance imaging; NCB, needle core biopsy; US, ultrasound; VA-NCB, vacuum-assisted needle core biopsy.

TABLE 26.6

Stereotactic[a] (Mammographic/Tomographic) Guidance for Needle Core Biopsy

Optimal choice for lesions evident only on mammography (lesions without ultrasound correlate)
Typical target: calcification, architectural distortion, relatively small (<1 cm) mass
Needs special equipment and facility.
Range of needle size used: 12 to 8 gauge (most commonly used: 12 and 9 gauge)

On mammogram: fat appears darker, "fibroglandular" tissue looks lighter, and calcifications are white. Mammography guidance can also be provided by digital tomosynthesis. The latter provides images of slim sections and allows for accurate targeting, with reduced exposure to ionizing radiation.

[a]*Stereotaxis*, from Greek, *stereo*: two, *taxis*: order. The term refers to the two oblique projections providing dual (*stereo*) views. A "spiculated" lesion is one with spikes (sharp pointed lines) radiating from a mass.

TABLE 26.8

MRI Guidance for Needle Core Biopsy

Best choice for lesions evident on MRI[a]
Equipment is not readily available.
Need special facilities: ie, MRI suite
Safe and accurate
Not particularly amenable to superficial and deep lesions
Time consuming (~1 hr) and complicated procedure
Contraindications include gadolinium allergy, renal disease, and implants considered unsafe
Expensive procedure

MRI, magnetic resonance imaging. Patterns of MRI enhancement: mass-like and nonmass; of distribution: focal, segmental, diffuse; of edges: circumscribed and spiculated; of internal patterns; and of "kinetics": rate of contrast uptake and exit; etc reflect vascularity in a lesion and correlate poorly with pathologic findings. However, *nonmass enhancement* (NME) is most often associated with cystic apocrine hyperplasia, *linear clumped enhancement* with ductal carcinoma in situ (DCIS); and *larger irregular pattern of enhancement with appropriate kinetics* is suspicious for invasive carcinoma.

[a]Approximately 50% of MRI-detected lesions may have a corresponding "correlate" on "targeted" ("second look") ultrasound (US) examination. Such targeted US examinations reduce the need for MRI-guided sampling.

group recommended at least 20 cores with 11-gauge needles for VA-stereotactic breast biopsy (9) and at least 24 cores with 11-gauge needles for MRI-guided NCBs (10). For US-guided VA-NCB, another consensus paper recommended the removal of at least 10 cores with an 11-gauge needle and at least 6 cores with 8-gauge needles (11). Preibsch et al (12) have devised a matrix that facilitates the implementation of German recommendations vis-à-vis required number of VA-NCBs to be taken for different needle sizes. In summary, the authors calculated that the required minimum number of cores obtained to conform to German guidelines is 20, 14, 9, and 5 for 11-, 9-, 8-, and 7-gauge needle sizes, respectively. The German guidelines recommend a sample number of at least 12 cores with 10-gauge needle for stereotactic VA-NCB (12). Of note, 14-gauge needles (one of the least invasive needles that can be used for NCB purposes) are typically used in handheld US-guided VA-NCB. As stated earlier, counterintuitively, a smaller-gauge needle indicates larger needle diameter, for example, a 27-gauge

TABLE 26.7

Ultrasound Guidance for Needle Core Biopsy

Optimal choice for lesions evident on US
US is relatively more available.
Can be performed anywhere (even on bedside)
No ionizing radiation
Most common needle size used: 14-gauge
Real-time check of needle placement
Few contraindications
Typical duration of procedure: <20 min, including setup

US, ultrasound.

needle has an inner diameter of 0.2 mm, and a 7-gauge needle has an inner diameter of 3.8 mm.

TISSUE FIXATION

Ischemic time is the duration between the time of acquisition (ie, loss of blood supply) to the time when the biopsied sample is placed into fixative. The ischemic time can be measured in seconds for most NCBs; however, it does not typically exceed 15 minutes even when specimen radiography is performed. Prolonged ischemic time (>60 minutes) should be documented because an extended ischemic period can affect the results of tests that utilize protein, mRNA, and DNA (more so for the former two). Refrigeration of the specimen is *not* a substitute for its prompt formalin fixation.

As soon as possible after procurement, the NCB specimen should be placed in 10% *neutral buffered formalin* (13,14). Prompt formalin fixation preserves cytologic and architectural details and ensures optimal immunohistochemical (IHC) staining, although delayed tissue fixation has been shown to impair human epidermal growth factor receptor 2 (HER2) protein expression (14). *Bouin fixative* is known to degrade DNA and reduces immunoreactivity for estrogen receptor (ER) and progesterone receptor (PR). *Alcohol fixative* can interfere with ER, PR, and HER2 testing.

Fixation time is defined as the time from the sample being placed into fixative to commencement of tissue processing. "Cross-linking" occurs during the fixation period, and this process inhibits deterioration. The fixation time should

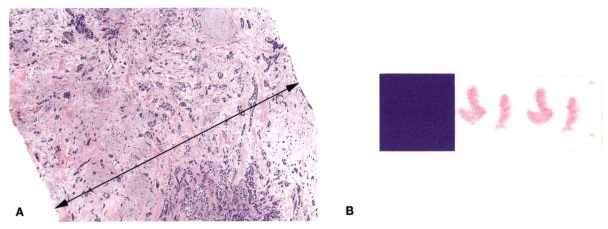

FIGURE 26.1 Microscopic and Macroscopic Appearance of a Needle Core Biopsy. A: Needles are available in a wide variety of outer diameters. The latter are indicated by various "gauges." Smaller gauge numbers of needles indicate larger outer diameters. The double-headed arrow corresponds to the *inner* diameter of the needle (eg, the 14-gauge needle has an inner diameter of 1.6 mm). Needle wire gauge (G) scale is derived from the Birmingham Wire Gauge system. **B:** Macroscopic appearance of a glass slide with sections prepared from a core biopsy procedure utilizing a 9-gauge needle.

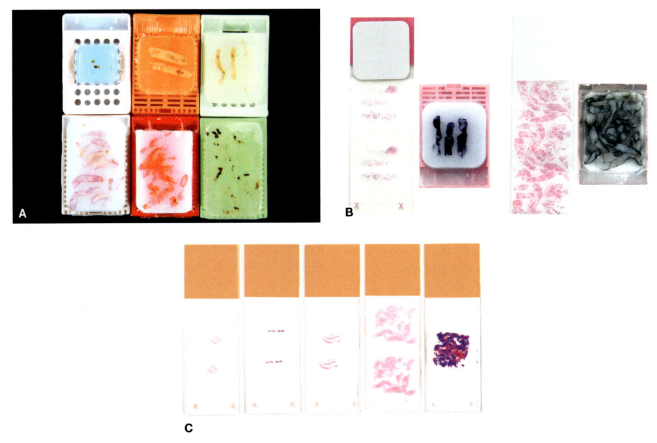

FIGURE 26.2 Demonstration of the Wide Array of Dimensions of Needle Core Biopsy (NCB) Specimens in a Random Set of Tissue Blocks. A: Note the minuscule dimension of the NCB specimen in the tissue block on the top left and the numerous tightly packed NCB specimens in the green tissue block on the bottom right. The bottom row demonstrates haphazard placement of NCB samples in three tissue blocks rather than the orderly arrays of NCB in the top row. **B:** Two sets of tissue blocks and slides are depicted. The set on the left shows an array of NCBs embedded in an orderly manner in the paraffin block. The linear arrangement of the core biopsies in the corresponding glass slide facilitates efficient microscopic review. The set on the right shows tissue block overly packed in a disorderly manner with numerous NCB samples. Microscopic examination of the corresponding glass slide can be unnecessarily time consuming. A minute lesion could be missed in such a slide. **C:** Glass slides with NCBs using various gauge needles. Note wide variation in width of core biopsies. The last slide on the right shows a hematoxylin and eosin (H&E)-stained section obtained after improper, crowded, and haphazardly aggregated placement of multiple cores in the tissue block.

be at least 6 hours and not more than 72 hours before tissue processing starts. Underfixation (<6 hours) and overfixation (>72 hours) can lead to suboptimal histology, false-negative results on IHC, and problems in performing other ancillary tests. Short fixation time results in poor preservation of antigens for IHC. Prolonged fixation time results in alterations of proteins in the tissue. Extended periods of fixation may also result in the radiographic disappearance of calcifications (15).

The American Society of Clinical Oncology-College of American Pathologists (ASCO-CAP) practice guidelines recommend a minimum of 6 hours of formalin fixation for breast tissue specimens including NCBs (16,17), although some reports have suggested that shorter fixation time for NCB has no negative impact on the histopathologic quality as well as the reliability of IHC—at least for ER and Ki67 testing, if not for all others (18-21). For 14-gauge handheld US-guided NCBs (with an inner diameter of 1.6 mm) that are typically used for palpable lumps, there is increasing literature supporting the use of accelerated processing (including that which is microwave assisted), with less than 6 hours of formalin fixation (20,21).

Decalcification of NCB specimens may be necessary for some highly calcified specimens; however, every attempt must be made to separately process any noncalcified portions of the specimen and minimize time in decalcifying solution. Immunostains performed on decalcified tissue ought to be interpreted with caution.

Three decalcification methods, that is, utilizing acetic acid, hydrochloric/formic acid, and EDTA, are commonly used for specimens (including NCBs) containing bone. Of these, EDTA has been shown *not* to affect IHC testing, and only seldom effect in situ hybridization testing. Hydrochloric/formic acid has the potential to alter ER and PR results. In situ hybridization testing may fail following decalcification with acetic acid and hydrochloric/formic acid (22,23).

REQUISITION FORM

The requisition form submitted with the NCB specimen should include the following information: patient name, age, and gender; laterality of the specimen; sampled site(s); indication for the procedure; and clinical diagnosis. The name of the submitting physician and the date and time of the procedure must also be provided. The specimen container must be labeled with patient and specimen identification information. The latter must match the identifying information on the accompanying requisition form.

Basic clinical and imaging information that should ideally accompany NCB specimens is listed in **Table 26.9**. The sampled site is generally indicated by a clock-face designation and distance from nipple (eg, right breast, 2N4), indicating that the specimen was taken from the upper-inner quadrant of right breast at the 2 o'clock position from a site 4 cm from the center of the nipple. Multiple palpable as well as impalpable lesions may be simultaneously sampled via

TABLE 26.9
Clinical and Imaging Information to Accompany Needle Core Biopsy Specimens
PALPABLE MASS
Location
Size
Shape
Margins
Density
Associated calcifications
Other features
IMAGING ABNORMALITY
BI-RADS Category
Mammographic calcification/architectural distortion/ asymmetry:
Location
Morphology
Distribution
Associated features
Ultrasound/MRI abnormality:
Location
Morphology
Distribution
Associated features
BI-RADS, Breast Imaging-Reporting and Data System; MRI, magnetic resonance imaging.

NCB, safely and efficiently, and this practice favorably influences management (24,25).

The pathologic findings in any previously performed breast biopsy procedure must be conveyed in the requisition form. Relevant history of treatment (eg, surgery, radiation, hormone modulation therapy, or chemotherapy) that could affect the histopathology of the breast should be provided **(Fig. 26.3)**. Information regarding any known systemic disease that may affect the breast (eg, neoplasm at another site, diabetes mellitus, sarcoidosis, vasculitis, etc) should be noted. Family history of breast or ovarian carcinoma, or of *BRCA1* or *BRCA2* mutations, should be included. Ideally, the instrument (cutting or VA) type utilized to procure NCB specimens should be stated. The imaging modality used for guidance to the target (eg, stereotactic, US, or MRI) ought also to be included. The ischemic time, that is, the time between specimen procurement and its placement in fixative, must be recorded in the requisition form (26).

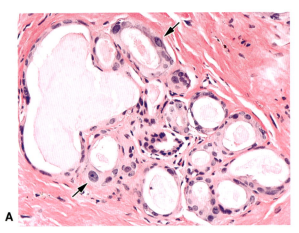
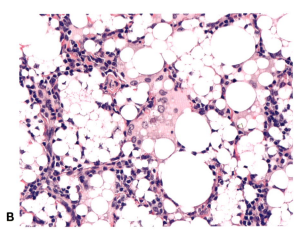

FIGURE 26.3 Significance of Clinical Information in Diagnosis of Needle Core Biopsy (NCB) Specimens. **A:** This focus of apocrine metaplasia in an NCB shows scattered, isolated enlarged nuclei with prominent nucleoli (arrows) indicative of radiation effect. Clinical history of radiation was not provided, and a diagnosis of atypical hyperplasia had been rendered. **B:** The presence of foreign material represented by clear vacuoles of varying size with associated histiocytic infiltrate is diagnostic of leaked mammary implant contents. A clinical history of implant placement was not provided, and a diagnosis of organizing fat necrosis had been made.

GROSS EXAMINATION AND DESCRIPTION

A gross description should be recorded for each specimen with documentation of the number of cores, the range (and *aggregate* extent) of their lengths, as well as any other notable feature (eg, color). The entire specimen, including any accompanying blood clot, must be processed for histologic evaluation. The bottom surface of the lid of the specimen container should be examined for tissue that may be stuck to it. If the material in a sample is too abundant to be placed in one tissue cassette (ie, >10.0 cm in aggregate length), the cores should be separated into groups of approximately equal number and size **(Fig. 26.2B)**. In general, no more than three (ideally two) intact cores should be placed in one cassette. The number of cassettes/blocks corresponding to each sample should be recorded, and each cassette/block should be labeled with a unique identifier. Formalin fixation causes minimal shrinking of NCB samples (the shrinkage effect has been estimated to be 7% for 16-gauge Tru-Cut biopsy samples from the liver) (27).

Dipping of NCB specimens in dyes that are routinely available, such as methylene blue or eosin, increases the visibility of the embedded tissue in the paraffin block **(Fig. 26.4)**. Inking of cores at the time of gross examination has been proposed as a simple, inexpensive, and effective way to reduce the possibility of specimen mix-up during tissue processing in the laboratory **(Fig. 26.5)**. All cores from a patient are inked with a single color. The next set of cores from another patient is inked with a different color, and so on. The color of ink used for a case should be noted in the gross description. Three discrepancies were discovered in a study of 1,000 core biopsies that were inked sequentially with six different colors. In one instance, the error was related to switching of a tissue block. In another case, the error was related to incorrect labeling, and in a third, the error was typographic (28). Of course, no laboratory procedure can guard against the misidentification of specimens in the radiology clinics where NCB samples are usually obtained.

Some pathology and radiology departments weigh the NCB specimens as an objective measure of the volume sampled. In this regard, it must be kept in mind that tissue weight is proportional to tissue volume only if tissue density (ie, weight divided by volume) is constant. Mammary tissue density, of course, is variable and depends upon the ratio of fibrous, glandular, and adipose tissue in any sampling. Of note, typically the 14-gauge needle collects 40 mg of tissue in each sample, the 11-gauge needle obtains 100 mg, and the 8-gauge needle acquires at least 250 mg.

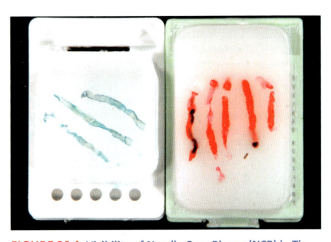

FIGURE 26.4 Visibility of Needle Core Biopsy (NCB) in Tissue Blocks. Dipping the NCBs in methylene blue (left) or eosin (right) renders the samples more readily visible in the tissue block. This is helpful to the histotechnologist when cutting histologic sections.

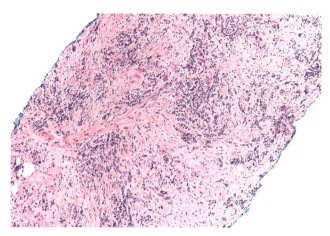

FIGURE 26.5 Inked Needle Core Biopsy Specimens. This sample was stained with blue ink after gross examination. The ink is visible in the resultant histologic sections (hematoxylin and eosin [H&E]).

In general, tissue from NCB acquired for diagnostic purposes should *not* be taken for research studies until slides are prepared from that material. Harvesting of tissue for research should use formalin-fixed, paraffin-embedded NCB tissue rather than "fresh" tissue—to verify the disease process, if any, in it.

SPECIMEN PROCESSING

Routine methods of paraffin embedding, sectioning, and hematoxylin and eosin (H&E) staining can be used for NCB specimens from the breast. A "fast-track" method for rapid processing of such specimens has been described (29). However, compliance with regulatory processing standards and achievement of optimal histologic and IHC staining should be ensured before the adoption of this technique (30). See section on Tissue Fixation.

The NCB samples must be embedded in a manner that positions them at approximately the same plane in the paraffin block. Histologic sections should be 4- to 5-μm thick. The evaluation of multiple levels (at least two "interval" levels, 50 μm apart) for NCB is standard practice in most pathology laboratories. Sectioning at lesser intervals is appropriate for samples obtained with smaller needles. Evaluation of three "levels" reportedly maximizes the chances of visualizing microcalcifications in NCB samples (31). Examination of a minimum of five levels has been recommended to ensure maximum sensitivity for detecting "atypical foci" (32) and of six levels to ensure "accurate" diagnosis (33).

At the Cleveland Clinic, two H&E-stained "levels," typically with one section on each slide (ribbon of tissue sections if core volume allows), are prepared from each tissue block with NCB material. The first slide is taken when the microtome knife reaches the tissue, and the second slide is taken when the knife reaches the first full-face section of tissue. At Weill-Cornell, two H&E-stained slides are also prepared from each block. The deeper of the two levels is cut at full face (typically ~25% into the block). In this manner, approximately 75% of the tissue volume is saved to obtain subsequent H&E-stained levels, as well as biomarker and molecular testing if needed.

Of note, the 14-gauge needle that yields a 1.6-mm inner diameter core of tissue can be used to produce at least 300 slides when cut at 4 μm (the typical thickness of histologic sections in most laboratories). In pragmatic terms, the number of slides prepared is much less important than the depth of the tissue blocks from where the sections are obtained. Be that as it may, one section from an NCB from a mass-forming lesion and an MRI-detected lesion (even taken at the surface of the tissue block) is diagnostic in the great majority of cases (34,35). NCB taken for calcifications usually requires more levels for identification thereof (15% require two additional levels, and 10% need even more levels) (31). It should also be remembered that the point of such NCBs is not the identification of calcifications per se, but that of the lesion that is harboring calcifications.

The value of obtaining multiple levels for NCB performed to investigate mammographically detected calcifications has been well established (see later) **(Fig. 26.6)**; however, the routine examination of levels for NCB taken for lesions other than calcifications is of limited value. Lee et al (34)

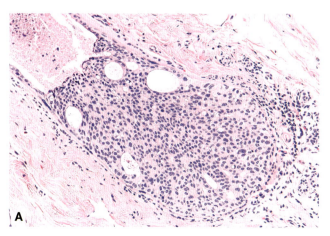
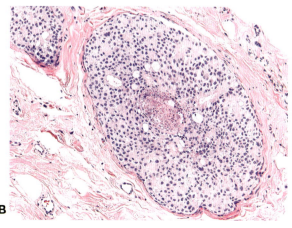

FIGURE 26.6 Facilitating a Pathologic Diagnosis via Examination of "Deeper" Levels. A, B: The initial section shows a focus of epithelial proliferation initially interpreted as atypical ductal hyperplasia (ADH) **(A)**, and the deeper level shows overt ductal carcinoma in situ (DCIS) **(B)**.

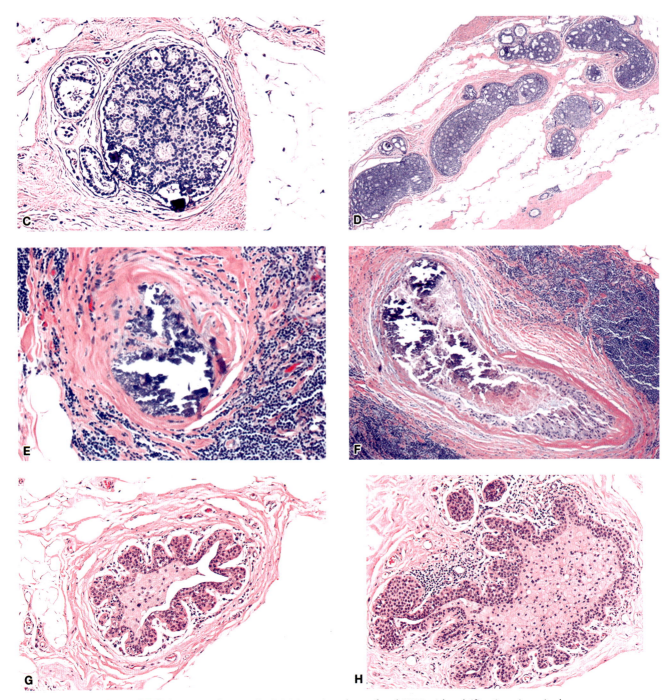

FIGURE 26.6 (*continued*) **C, D:** The initial section shows focal ADH with calcifications in a single duct (**C**), and the deeper level shows unequivocal DCIS in multiple ducts (**D**). **E, F:** The initial section shows dense calcification amid densely sclerotic tissue associated with marked lymphocytic infiltration (**E**), and the deeper level shows rare degenerating, highly atypical ductal epithelial cells that are highly suspicious for high-grade DCIS (**F**). **G, H:** In this case, the initial section was diagnosed as focal atypical lobular hyperplasia in a terminal duct lobular unit (**G**), and the deeper level shows unequivocal lobular carcinoma in situ (**H**).

demonstrated that the diagnosis after examining three levels was different from that in the initial level in 4 of 272 (1.5%) NCBs taken for reasons other than calcification and 13 of 103 (13%) NCBs taken to investigate calcifications.

It is important not to exhaust the NCB tissue in preparing the initial histologic sections so that material is preserved for ancillary studies that may be necessary to establish or refine a diagnosis. If laboratory resources allow, intervening sections cut between the various stained levels can be mounted unstained on labeled slides and saved for possible IHC or other ancillary studies. Such a protocol saves tissue, time, and effort that may be subsequently spent in the retrieval and processing of tissue blocks; however, it is prudent for an appropriate multi-tissue IHC "sausage control" to be placed on

IMAGING MODALITIES

Findings on various imaging modalities in a particular case should be stated in the requisition. NCBs are being increasingly performed under some form of image guidance; thus, pathologists ought to be acquainted with the fundamentals of breast imaging and reporting. Imaging techniques commonly employed to study the breast include mammography (including digital mammography), US, MRI, and positron emission tomography (PET). The ACR *BI-RADS* (*American College of Radiology's Breast Imaging-Reporting and Data System*) is used in reporting findings on mammography and has also been applied to the reporting of findings on other imaging modalities (**Table 26.10**).

NCB can be performed under stereotactic image (ie, mammographic) guidance. *Stereotactic NCB* is generally used for calcifications, masses, and architectural distortion. Mammography using low-dose ionizing radiation can detect masses, architectural distortion, or calcifications. For a mammographically detected *mass* (or lesion causing architectural distortion), the radiology report usually states its density, shape, and borders. On mammography, a mass suspicious for malignancy may be dense and irregular with spiculated edges. For mammographically detected abnormal *calcifications*, the radiology report usually describes their morphology and distribution. Calcifications suspicious for malignancy may be linear ("casting type"), branching, and/or pleomorphic. The key classic mammographic findings and the most common corresponding histopathologic findings are listed in **Table 26.11**. *Digital breast tomosynthesis* is an evolving, enhanced three-dimensional mammographic technique that increases lesional visibility by detecting subtle changes in the texture of parenchyma.

such slides. One new H&E-stained recut slide should always be prepared whenever unstained slides are made at a second sitting for IHC (36).

The *specimen radiograph* corresponding to the NCB specimen, particularly in cases wherein the target lesion is calcification, should be available for review, either electronically or via the film (or print thereof) physically accompanying the specimen. A brief description of the abnormality seen in the specimen radiograph should be a part of the gross description.

US imaging utilizes high-frequency sound waves to detect lesions through varying echo patterns. It is useful for determining the size and shape of masses and identifying cysts. The echogenicity of a lesion vis-à-vis that of subcutaneous adipose tissue and the orientation of the lesion in relation to the skin of the breast are usually reported in US reports. US is often employed to further study lesions identified on mammography and MRI. A US-guided biopsy procedure is relatively simple and quick to perform. On US examination, an *anechoic target* (ie, one with no internal shadow) typically indicates a cyst; a *hyperechoic target* (one with increased shadow, ie, those that appear lighter) indicates a fatty lesion; a *hypoechoic target* (those with lesser shadow, ie, appear darker) indicates a solid neoplasm; an *isoechoic target* (same as background adipose tissue) is indicative of fatty lesion, *posterior shadowing* (white echoes behind the lesion) are more often encountered in malignancy, "taller than wide" (lesions nonparallel to skin surface) are more often malignant, and "wider than tall" (lesions parallel to skin surface, following planes of tissue) are typically benign.

MRI screening is based on the premise that neoplasms incite neovascularity, which results in locally increased blood flow and permeability. MRI-guided biopsies are performed for lesions that cannot be identified by other methods. Injection of contrast (intravenous gadolinium) leads to enhanced and accelerated deposition of contrast in the region of the tumor ("wash-in") and accelerated loss of contrast ("washout"). MRI can evaluate lesional morphology (shape and border) and the kinetics of contrast enhancement (initial and delayed). On MRI, a lesion suspicious for carcinoma may be

---

TABLE 26.10

BI-RADS (Breast Imaging-Reporting and Data System) Categories: Clinical Implications

Category	Management	Likelihood of Malignancy
0, Incomplete	Need additional evaluation	—
1, Negative	Routine	0
2, Benign	Routine	0
3, Probably benign	Surveillance (short interval follow-up)	<2%
4, Suspicious		
4A, Low suspicion	Biopsy or close surveillance	2%-10%
4B, Moderate suspicion	Biopsy	10%-50%
4C, High suspicion	Biopsy	50%-95%
5, Highly suspicious	Biopsy[a]	>95%
6, Biopsy-proven malignancy	Multidisciplinary approach	—

[a]Excision should be performed if NCB is negative.

TABLE 26.11

Classic Mammographic Findings and Most Common Corresponding Pathology Findings

	Common Benign Finding	Common Malignant Finding
Architectural distortion	Radial scar	Invasive lobular carcinoma
	Postprocedure scar	DCIS
	Fat necrosis	
Asymmetry	Postprocedure scar	Invasive lobular carcinoma
Calcifications[a]	Columnar cell change	DCIS
	Sclerosing adenosis	LCIS variants
	Fibroadenoma	Invasive carcinoma
	Cysts	
	Fat necrosis	
	Postprocedure scar	
	Hemosiderin deposition	
Circumscribed mass	Fibroadenoma	Mucinous carcinoma
	Cyst	Papillary carcinoma
	Nodular adenosis	Typical triple-negative carcinoma
Ill-defined mass	Fibroadenomatoid change	Invasive lobular carcinoma
	PASH	
Spiculated mass	Radial scar	Invasive ductal carcinoma
	Postsurgical scar	
	Fibromatosis	

DCIS/LCIS, ductal/lobular carcinoma in situ; PASH, pseudoangiomatous stromal hyperplasia.

[a]Minimum extent of calcifications evident on mammography: 0.05-0.1 mm. Five distinct deposits of calcification in a cluster are considered as "group."

irregular in outline with rim enhancement and can exhibit characteristic kinetics. MRI of the breast has diagnostic and screening applications (eg, evaluation of occult tumor, extent of tumor, multifocality, multicentricity, response to neoadjuvant chemotherapy, recurrence, and in the screening of high-risk women). In a study of 445 MRI-guided biopsies, all performed on high-risk patients, 79% were benign (37). The technique requires sophisticated equipment, including open-coil MRI and MRI-compatible needles.

PET screening of the breast assesses the level of glycolysis in tissues after injecting a patient with a radiotracer with an unstable nucleus. PET scans of the breast have been used in a limited fashion with mixed results for screening in high-risk patients, for evaluating recurrences, and for evaluating response to chemotherapy or hormonal therapy.

The concordance of the clinical impression, imaging results, and pathologic findings is often referred to as the "triple test." It is important to ensure that the clinical and radiographic findings are consistent with the pathologic findings on NCB. Re-biopsy with NCB or an excisional biopsy is usually recommended for discordant cases (ie, cases that fail the "triple test").

The histopathologic diagnosis ought to be based entirely on the microscopic appearance of the sampled tissue in the NCB specimen. The results of a pathologic interpretation that is not consistent with the clinical impression should be discussed with the submitting radiologist or responsible

clinician to ensure that the sample is representative of the lesion. Documentation of this discussion should be kept with the records. The repeated procurement of minuscule or otherwise inadequate samples (eg, blood only) ought to be discussed with the appropriate clinician.

CALCIFICATIONS

NCB specimens derived from a target with calcifications, as demonstrated by mammography, should undergo specimen radiography immediately after the procedure, and the presence of calcifications in the sampling should be confirmed. This process makes it possible to identify and segregate the NCB samples containing calcifications from those without before submission to the laboratory. The cores with and without calcifications from each biopsy site can then be placed in fixative in separately labeled containers. Alternatively, the two sets of cores can be placed into separate tissue cassettes, differentiated by color and/or label, and submitted in a single container. The method chosen to separate specimens before submission to the pathology laboratory should be standardized within a given institution. The practice of separating the specimens with and without calcifications is useful for correlation with the specimen radiograph. The diagnostic yield has been reported to be higher in the segregated cores containing calcifications, although equally careful attention must be paid to samples with and without calcifications. A commercially available "tray" has been devised to facilitate radiology-pathology correlation mainly by allowing the usually fragile cores to maintain their orientation and integrity **(Fig. 26.7)**. Calcifications can be visualized in x-ray images of paraffin blocks, and they remain detectable in this condition for an indefinite period.

Calcifications greater than 1 mm (>1,000 μm) or those with "popcorn" configuration are seldom associated with malignancy (as these take several years to materialize). Some of the classic radiologic descriptors of calcifications, and the corresponding usual histopathologic correlates, are listed in **Table 26.12**.

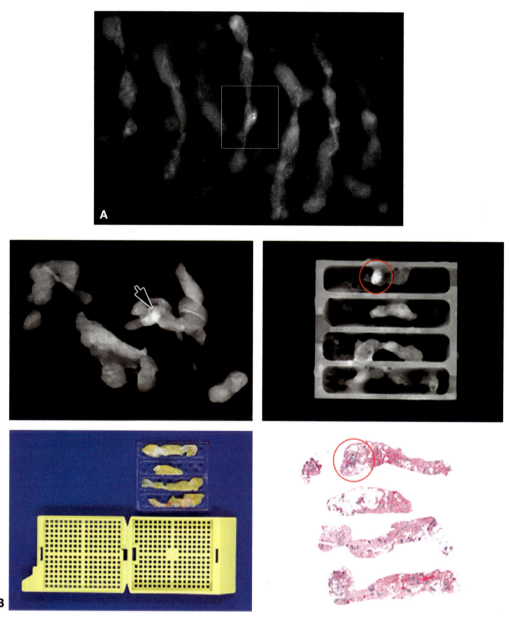

FIGURE 26.7 Radiograph of a Breast Needle Core Biopsy (NCB) Specimen. A: This NCB specimen radiograph shows a solitary focus of calcification in one (center) of several samples. Optimally, the radiologist should select the samples with calcifications and submit them separately from those without calcifications. **B:** Radiologic-pathologic correlation in an NCB specimen. A commercially available "tray" can facilitate radiology-pathology correlation mainly by allowing the usually fragile biopsy tissue to maintain its orientation and integrity. A set of NCB samples in a specimen radiograph. The arrow indicates the suspicious lesion (upper left). The individual core biopsy samples have been placed into one of the four separate slots in the "tray." This radiograph of the tray indicates the location of the lesional tissue (upper right, circle). The tray fits into a standard tissue cassette for histologic processing. The biopsies are embedded into the tissue block with the same orientation as in the "tray" (lower left). The corresponding histologic slides have the tissue samples with similar orientation, allowing ready radiologic-pathologic comparison of the circled calcifications and density (lower right). (Courtesy of Dr O. Tawfik; Gallagher R, Schafer G, Redick M, et al. Microcalcifications of the breast: a mammographic-histologic correlation study using a newly designed Path/Rad Tissue Tray. *Ann Diagn Pathol*. 2012;16:196-201.)

TABLE 26.12
Some Classic Radiologic Descriptors of Calcifications and Usual Pathologic Correlates

Descriptors	Usual Pathologic Correlate
"Egg-shell"	Fat necrosis ("oil cyst")
"Linear branching"	DCIS
"Milk of calcium"	Cysts (called "milk" because the white fluid level changes with position)
"Popcorn"	Sclerotic fibroadenoma
"Pleomorphic"	Typical of malignancy, fine deposits are more suspicious than coarse
"Rod-like"	Duct ectasia
"Tea-cupping"	Same as "milk of calcium"
"Tram-track"	Arterial calcifications

DCIS, ductal carcinoma in situ.

Calcifications that are less than 100 μm (0.1 mm) in maximum dimension are unlikely to be radiographically evident (38). Consequently, histologically detected calcifications of minuscule proportions cannot be assumed to represent the calcifications seen in a clinical mammogram. Whenever an NCB procedure is performed for calcifications, the pathology report should specify whether calcific deposits are microscopically evident and the type of breast tissue in which they are located **(Fig. 26.8)**.

One possible explanation for the occasional lack of histologic visualization of calcification in NCB obtained for mammographically detected microcalcification is their loss during histologic sectioning. This may occur either because of discarding of shavings containing calcifications in the microtome or "fracturing" of the calcifications when they are hit by the microtome blade, resulting in ejection ("chipping") of shattered calcific debris, in the course of preparation of levels **(Fig. 26.9)**. Radiography of histologic shavings has provided evidence for both eventualities (39,40). "Chipping" occurs more often with larger deposits of calcification (such as those in sclerotic fibroadenomas) rather than with

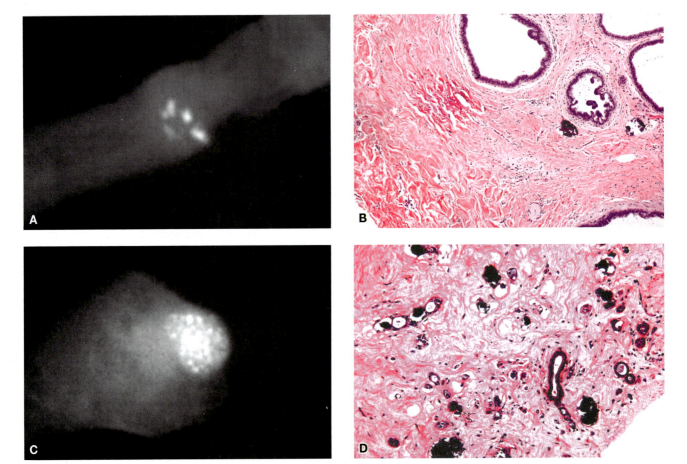

FIGURE 26.8 Radiology-Pathology Correlation of Needle Core Biopsy Samples With Calcium Phosphate Deposition. **A, B:** Stromal calcifications. **C, D:** Sclerosing adenosis.

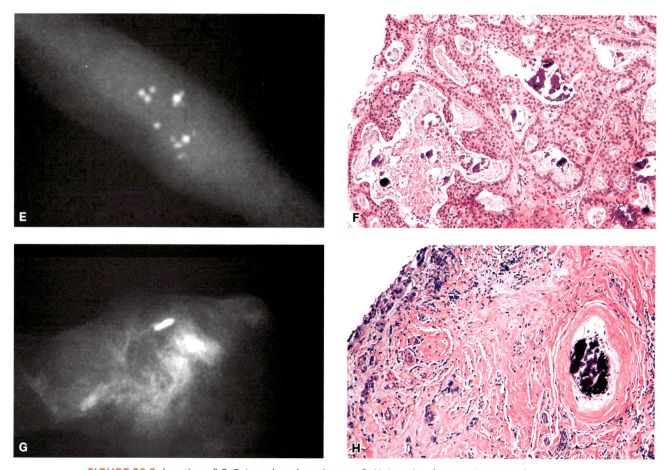

FIGURE 26.8 (*continued*) **E, F:** Intraductal carcinoma. **G, H:** Invasive duct carcinoma with a sclerotic and calcified duct.

microcalcifications. Other explanations for "missing" calcification are inadequate sampling, mislabeling of samples, and failure to recognize calcium deposits in histologic sections. This is more likely to occur with calcium oxalate than with calcium phosphate calcifications.

If calcifications are described in the radiograph of the NCB and none are histologically evident initially, the slides should be examined for calcium oxalate ("weddellite") crystals. These crystals do not stain with the H&E stain but are birefringent with polarized light (41). Calcium oxalate crystals are usually located in cysts lined by apocrine epithelium and may rarely elicit a foreign body–type giant cell reaction in the cyst or in the periductal stroma. Less common types of calcifications are shown in **Figure 26.10**.

Correlation with imaging findings is crucial to the reporting of NCB specimens, as exemplified even by the seemingly innocuous finding of histologically unremarkable adipose tissue—an instance that may represent fatty breast parenchyma, a lipoma, or a missed target. It must also be kept in mind that several non-calcium elements in breast tissue can radiologically simulate microcalcifications. In this context, *suture material* from prior surgical procedure is commonly encountered. *Tattoo pigment* used for cutaneous adornments or tissue marking for targeting of radiation therapy can simulate calcifications, including when the pigment is carried into intramammary lymphatic channels distant from the source. Hemosiderin (from hemorrhage at an earlier date) has been known to simulate calcifications. Injection of material into breast tissue, such as gold (injected into breast tissue for therapeutic use) and various substances (particularly those used to "lace" or "cut" recreational drugs), can also radiographically mimic calcifications.

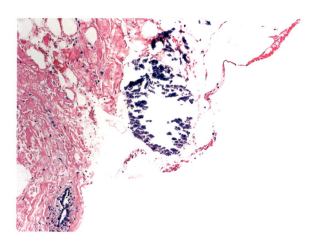

FIGURE 26.9 Displacement of Calcifications. An entire focus of calcification has become dislodged. A definitive diagnosis is not possible in such a situation.

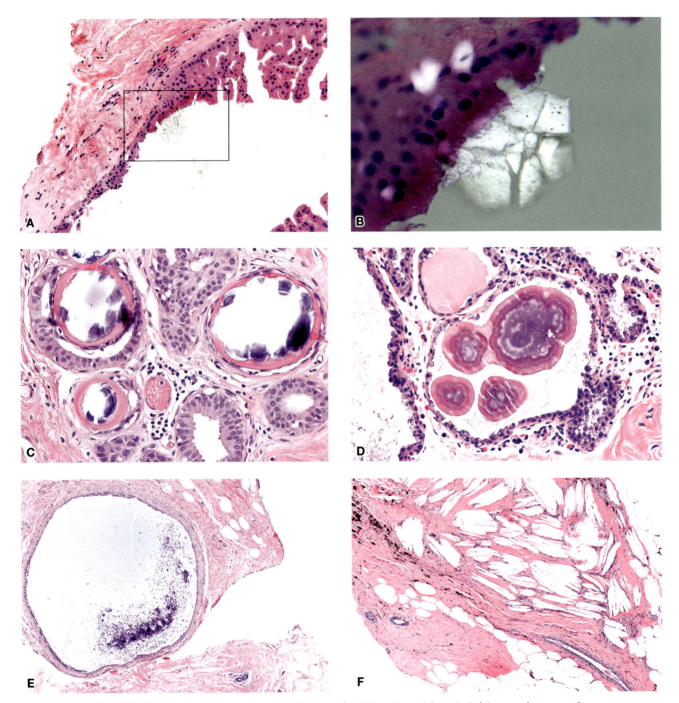

FIGURE 26.10 Less Common Types and Forms of Calcium Deposition. A: Calcium oxalate crystals are barely visible in a focus of cystic papillary apocrine hyperplasia on routine light microscopy (hematoxylin and eosin [H&E]). **B:** The birefringent calcium oxalate crystals are readily demonstrated by polarizing microscopy (H&E). **C:** "Ossifying" type of calcification in ducts with columnar cell change. **D:** "Liesegang" rings with calcifications amid pregnancy-like change. **E:** A cystically dilated duct with luminal fine "powdery" calcifications. The corresponding mammogram showed calcifications of the so-called milk of calcium type. **F:** A cluster of cholesterol crystals that formed a mass lesion (so-called cholesteroloma).

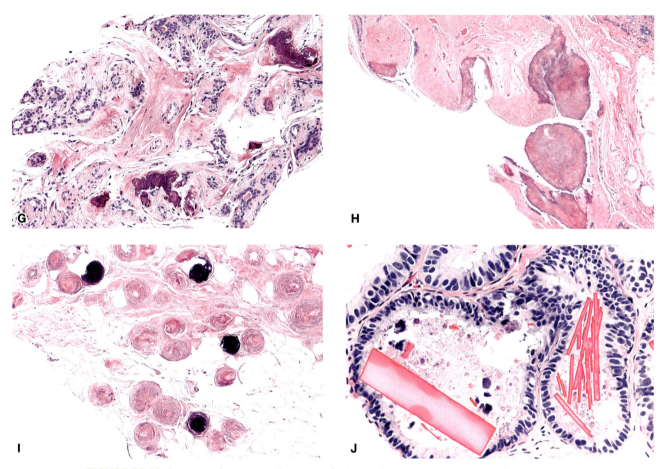

FIGURE 26.10 (*continued*) **G:** Unusual pattern of calcium deposition in stroma in otherwise unremarkable breast tissue. This patient with chronic renal failure had hypercalcemia (with so-called metastatic depositions of calcium). Multiple amyloid stains were negative. **H:** Calcium deposition on dense fibrous tissue—possibly a senescent fibroadenoma. **I:** An unusual pattern of calcium deposition on minute stromal fibrous nodules (most likely representing obliterated lobules) in an elderly woman. There was no history of radiation treatment or chemotherapy. Various amyloid stains were negative. **J:** Rectangular crystals in cystically dilated ducts. Note concomitant intraductal deposits of calcium phosphate.

Occasionally, calcifications are not identified in the routine slides prepared from NCB that had targeted calcifications. In such cases, the source of the specimen should be verified. This step should be followed by review of the specimen radiograph (which should always be available for review). In most cases, radiography of the tissue block(s) can identify calcifications that have not yet been sectioned. The choice of obtaining additional "serials" (continuous sections), "levels" (sections at thinner intervals), or "deepers" (sections at thicker intervals) depends upon the thickness of the core biopsies and imaging findings in each case. Initially, at least two "levels" should be obtained from those tissue blocks that exhibit readily evident calcifications on radiography. It should be kept in mind that the definitions of "serials," "levels," and "deepers" vary between laboratories. It may be helpful in some cases to discuss requests for additional sections with the histotechnologist to optimize slide preparation. In certain cases, for example, those in which minuscule calcifications are evident on specimen radiographs and none are identified in the initially prepared slides, it is prudent to save the intervening sections between the H&E-stained "levels." Such intervening sections would then be available for H&E staining in case the "levels" are noncontributory. In exceptionally rare cases, calcifications within cysts ("milk of calcium") can be irretrievably lost. This can happen by mechanical drainage of the contents when the cyst is sectioned either at the time of biopsy or at the time of microtome sectioning in the laboratory. Occasionally, the "missing" calcifications are found in the stroma (amid fibroelastic tissue) or within arterial vessels (in the pattern of Monckeberg medial sclerosis, named after Johann Georg Monckeberg, German pathologist, 1877-1925). Calcifications can rarely appear as minuscule "vesicles" within the stroma of some sclerotic fibroadenomas.

Well-prepared and optimally stained H&E-stained sections are crucial for the rendering of correct interpretation. A definitive diagnosis may not be possible on slides that are not "full face" or are present in multiple minute fragments **(Fig. 26.11)**. Additional slides ("serials," "levels," or "deepers," as appropriate) prepared in such cases may occasionally be helpful.

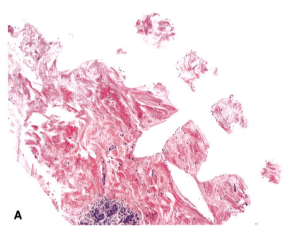
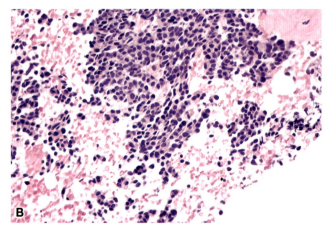

FIGURE 26.11 **Artifactual Defects in Tissue. A:** Tight packing of the tissue cassette with needle core biopsy (NCB) specimens may result in the "grid" of the cassette causing artifactual geometric defects in the samples. When such a case is encountered, a "full-face" deeper level should be obtained to visualize all of the tissue in the block. Furthermore, the practice of overstuffing cassettes should be discontinued. Overly tight foam ("sponges") used in cassettes, to hold NCB in place and prevent them from being lost during processing, may result in a similar appearance of the tissue section. **B:** NCB showing extreme fragmentation of the sampled tissue with proliferative epithelial cells. Additional "deeper" levels are occasionally but not always helpful in such cases.

FROZEN SECTION EXAMINATION

In general, frozen section examination (FSE) should not be performed on NCB samples regardless of whether they were obtained from radiographically detected nonpalpable breast lesions or palpable tumors. This recommendation is based on the following observations: (a) interpretation of diagnostically difficult lesions is compromised by frozen section artifact, increasing the risk of misdiagnosis and (b) significant portions of the diagnostic tissue may be exhausted in the process of preparing the frozen section slide. Despite the foregoing counterarguments, a recent study of FSE of 59 cases of US-guided NCB of breast found no false-positive and two false-negative results, with the sensitivity, specificity, positive predictive value (PPV), and negative predictive value (NPV) of this technique being 95%, 100%, 100%, and 90%, respectively, in this series (42).

In practice, FSE of an NCB specimen from a nonpalpable breast tumor is clinically warranted only in rare and emergency situations. Optimally, a request for an FSE on an NCB specimen should be discussed with the responsible pathologist preoperatively. FSE is a particularly inappropriate method for rendering a diagnosis if nonsurgical ablation of a tumor or neoadjuvant chemotherapy is being immediately considered. It is imperative to reach a diagnosis with "permanent" H&E-stained sections before these forms of treatment, which could radically alter the histology of the target lesion (or even eliminate it), are initiated.

TOUCH IMPRINT CYTOLOGY

Touch imprint cytology (TIC) of an NCB specimen is a technique that provides a cytologic diagnosis without the risks of tissue loss attendant on preparing an FSE (43,44). However, this procedure substitutes the limitations of cytology preparation for those of frozen sections. Imprints are subject to drying artifacts and other distortions that may present substantial pitfalls.

The TIC is prepared by either "touching" (ie, gently compressing) or "rolling" the NCB specimen on glass slides. Air-dried slides are suitable for the Diff-Quik stain. Alcohol-fixed slides may be utilized for either H&E or Papanicolaou stains. TIC has the potential of improving patient management in "one-stop" breast clinics by providing a prompt diagnosis. Kulkarni et al (45) reported a 95% adequacy rate and 55% malignant rate in 819 cases in a recent series from such a setting. This method of evaluating NCB may also be of value in the immediate assessment of specimen adequacy, thus reducing the number of insufficient specimens. The interpretation of low-grade carcinoma and fibroadenoma in a TIC preparation may be particularly challenging. Consequently, it is recommended that TIC of NCB specimens be undertaken only by pathologists or cytologists who examine this type of material with sufficient frequency to maintain a high level of proficiency and work in close collaboration with radiologists and surgeons who routinely perform the NCB procedure. TIC can provide same-day diagnosis (46).

"Core wash cytology" examination utilizes cells taken from the fixative fluid in which the NCB is placed. The "core wash" is subjected to liquid-based preparation and then stained by the routine Papanicolaou method. This technique has been successfully employed for the immediate diagnosis of NCBs, and in a series of 30 cases it was found to have better morphology and fewer insufficient diagnoses than TIC (6.6% vs 13.3%) (47). Core wash cytology entails diagnostic risks similar to TIC.

THE PATHOLOGY REPORT

The pathology report of an NCB specimen should render the diagnosis in a concise and clinically meaningful manner. A detailed microscopic description of the histologic findings is not necessary if the specific diagnosis is clearly stated. For example, it is sufficient to report "fibroadenoma" without listing the microscopic characteristics. On occasions, microscopic details may be added to the diagnosis to convey additional clinically significant information, as for example, in the diagnosis: "fibroadenoma with cellular stroma; recommend excision to rule out phyllodes tumor." When a carcinoma is diagnosed, the presence or absence of invasion must be stated if this can be ascertained.

In Situ Carcinoma

For in situ carcinoma, the diagnosis should state the type (ductal or lobular), nuclear grade, and the presence of luminal necrosis and calcification. In cases of ductal carcinoma in situ (DCIS), the architectural pattern, such as solid, cribriform, and micropapillary, should be mentioned. A high degree of concordance in the classification of DCIS has been found between NCBs and the subsequent excisions. Jackman et al (48) found "comedo" DCIS in 91% of excisions after a diagnosis of similar DCIS in NCBs, and in 15% of excisions following the diagnosis of "noncomedo" DCIS in NCBs. Approximately 25% of DCIS diagnosed on NCB is upgraded to invasive ductal carcinoma on excision.

Invasive Carcinoma

The most important histologic factors that determine the prognosis of invasive breast carcinoma are tumor size, lymph node involvement, and histologic grade. Only one of these three factors, histologic grade, can be reliably assessed in NCB material.

The determination of *tumor size* on NCB is unreliable because the samples are taken randomly and may not represent their maximum extent. In one study, NCBs underestimated tumor size in 79% of the cases (49), and in another report tumor size determined from an NCB was "upstaged" in 72% of the cases upon assessment of size in the subsequent excision (50). However, it may be useful to routinely include the largest single histologically contiguous extent of invasive carcinoma in a single core in an NCB. This information is particularly significant whenever little or no residual invasive carcinoma is identified in the subsequent excision. In this regard, the extent of invasive carcinoma should *not* be added to the extent of invasive carcinoma on excision. Stereotactic VA-NCB usually removes a "substantial" quantity of tissue, and complete extirpation of the tumor may occur in 20% of nonpalpable invasive carcinomas (51-53).

If the size of invasive carcinoma is not routinely provided prospectively, then it is important to document it retrospectively whenever no residual invasive carcinoma is identified upon excision (ie, the invasive size should be reported in an addendum to the NCB report, and this information must be included in the excisional biopsy report).

The *diagnosis of invasive carcinoma* should describe the type of tumor (ductal, lobular, or special type, eg, tubular or mucinous), coexisting in situ carcinoma, presence of lymphovascular invasion, and any significant benign proliferative lesions. Information may be limited for microinvasive carcinoma. The nuclear grade of invasive tumor cells should be reported in each case (54). The presence of in situ carcinoma supports the primary mammary origin of invasive carcinoma, and this information may be clinically relevant. However, the determination of extensive intraductal component (>25% of tumor mass composed of DCIS and extension of DCIS beyond the invasive carcinoma) is not possible in an NCB specimen.

E-cadherin immunostaining should be employed in those circumstances when there is difficulty in distinguishing ductal from lobular carcinoma. This applies to in situ as well as invasive lesions (55). The cytoplasmic membranes of tumor cells are immunoreactive for E-cadherin in virtually all ductal lesions and display weak, interrupted, or absent reactivity in lobular carcinomas. p120 immunostaining may also be helpful in distinguishing ductal and lobular carcinomas (including its pleomorphic and apocrine-pleomorphic variants) (56-58). p120 immunostain (similar to E-cadherin) is localized on the cytoplasmic membrane in ductal carcinoma (and ductal benign) cells and appears within the cytoplasm in lobular carcinoma cells.

The *nuclear and histologic grade* (both on a three-tier scale) can be reported for an NCB specimen of invasive carcinoma. Underestimation of grading occurs in about 20% to 33% of NCB cases (59,60); however, the agreement rate of up to 84% has been reported for high-grade breast carcinomas (grade 3), the type of carcinoma most likely to benefit from neoadjuvant chemotherapy (61).

Evaluation of the *mitotic count* in NCB samples has been considered unreliable in some studies (62). Underscoring of mitotic activity, especially if fewer than four cores are available for examination, is likely (63); however, it has been shown that grading in the Nottingham system is rendered more reliable by reducing the threshold for mitotic scoring by one-half (64).

The assessment of *lymphovascular involvement* (LVI) by tumor cells in NCBs is not reliable because of the limited samples obtained and the potential for retraction artifact. A sensitivity of only 8% and PPV of 87% for LVI were reported in one study (61). Adherence to established histologic criteria for LVI (ie, location of LVI away from tumor, presence of endothelial cells around tumor, difference between the shape of tumor embolus and the space within which it lies) and confirmatory immunostains for endothelial cells such as CD31, D2-40, or WT1 may be helpful in confirming the presence of LVI (65,66).

Nonneoplastic Tissue

It is unfortunate that some pathologists routinely resist the reporting of benign inactive breast tissue as "normal" even if it is the only histopathologic finding and yield to the temptation of using the all-encompassing rubric of "fibrocystic changes." The use of the latter term as a diagnosis without specifying the elements of those changes is clinically unhelpful. The report should state the *specific* fibrocystic changes that are present, such as sclerosing adenosis and ductal hyperplasia. In the absence of fibrocystic changes, a diagnosis of breast tissue with physiologic changes can be offered (eg, atrophy) depending on the findings that are present. *Prominent* stromal findings, such as pseudoangiomatous stromal hyperplasia (PASH), should be reported. In sum, only potentially "actionable" findings (eg, radial scar) and those which in all likelihood explain the clinical presentation (eg, lymphocytic mastopathy in a case presenting with a mass) or imaging appearance (eg, cystic apocrine hyperplasia in a case of nonmass enhancement on MRI).

STANDARDIZED REPORTING

Standardized forms listing the most common diagnoses are a useful method for reporting breast pathology findings in routine cases. Such a checklist is an efficient way to record the diagnosis in a comprehensive manner and for the development of a database. The major drawback of formatted diagnoses is the rigidity of the report, which tends to give equal weightage to all components and presents the histologic findings in an inflexible sequence. In a particular case, certain diagnoses may require emphasis by being given priority in the report as well as by additional commentary. If the preformatted report does not offer sufficient latitude to rearrange the diagnostic components whenever necessary, the pathologist should have the option to issue a nonstructured diagnosis. This is especially important if critical information cannot be conveyed by amplifying the formatted text with comments.

In the United Kingdom, a scoring system (category classification) has been adopted for reporting NCB specimens (67). All NCB samples of the breast are classified as B1 to B5, with the assigned designation appearing prominently in each report. B1 is normal or inadequate (eg, fibrosis), B2 is benign (eg, sclerosing adenosis), B3 is benign with uncertain malignant potential (eg, atypical hyperplasia), B4 is suspicious (eg, minimal diagnostic tissue or crushed/distorted tissue), and B5 is positive (eg, in situ or invasive carcinoma). In general, an excisional biopsy might not be performed unless clinically indicated for categories B1 and B2, but local excision would follow for categories B3 to B5 (68). Although the system may appear "restrictive," it helps "concentrate the mind of the pathologist when writing a report" (51). A microscopic description or comments may be added at the pathologists' discretion. In one study, the B4 category was shown to have a high PPV: 74.2% (range: 62.5%-90.6%); the PPV of B5 category was more than 99%, and the PPV of B3 category was reported to be 19.1% (69).

ROLE OF THE NEEDLE CORE BIOPSY PATHOLOGY REPORT IN PATIENT CARE

The role of the pathologist in the interpretation of NCB is not only "limited to diagnosis," but it also has a "critical role in accurately applying histologic criteria and diagnostic terminology to guide risk stratification and appropriate patient management" (70).

The NCB procedure is highly accurate for the diagnosis of most breast lesions with a PPV for the diagnosis of invasive carcinoma of 98% to 99.8% (71). The pathologic diagnosis made on NCBs can be, and often is, a key determinant in planning optimal management. Nonetheless, it cannot be relied upon to provide comprehensive data equal to that which can be obtained from excisional biopsies. In a series of 1,168 NCBs, there was complete histologic agreement with the diagnosis rendered on the subsequent excisions in 83% of the cases (72). Consideration must be given to the potential limitations of NCB diagnosis in the planning of treatment plans. In a series of 952 consecutive cases, the overall false-negative rate of NCBs was 9.1%, based on the results of a standard radiology follow-up protocol for all patients (73). The pathology report for an NCB must be integrated with the clinical history, physical examination, and radiographic findings to plan the management of an individual patient.

The diagnosis rendered on NCB obviously applies only to information available from that sample. Final characterization of the lesion must be based on the composite pathologic data from NCB and subsequent excisions. It is therefore essential that the pathologist entrusted with the responsibility of diagnosing the subsequent specimen has slides available from the NCB. It is substandard practice for a patient to undergo an excision for a lesion diagnosed in another institution on an NCB specimen without prior review of the relevant slides at the hospital where the surgical procedure is to be performed (74). It is the responsibility of the surgeon in these cases to ensure that such a review occurs.

Some diagnoses of NCB specimens could qualify for the designation of "critical." An example of this would be the unexpected diagnosis of carcinoma in an NCB specimen from a mass in a young woman which was clinically presumed to be a fibroadenoma. It has been proposed that a list of such "critical" diagnoses for various organ systems and types of biopsies should be customized for each institution (75).

RECOMMENDATIONS FOR MANAGEMENT IN THE ERA OF DE-ESCALATION

NCBs that yield either "nondefinitive" or "high-risk" lesions are encountered in around 10% of cases. A variable proportion of these cases, approximately 10% to 33% or even higher, are "upgraded" to (ie, subsequently diagnosed as) malignant on excisional biopsy. The upgrade rate varies with clinical findings, type of lesion, quality of imaging studies, instrument utilized, volume of lesion sampled, radiologists' experience, and pathologists' expertise, among other factors. For context, approximately 25% of cases diagnosed as DCIS on NCB are diagnosed as invasive carcinoma upon excision.

The "nondefinitive" lesions include, but are not limited to, fibroepithelial tumors and papillary tumors—and typically require excision for definitive classification.

The category of lesions that are widely regarded as being "high risk" had traditionally undergone excision upon being diagnosed on NCB. Such "high-risk" lesions include atypical ductal hyperplasia (ADH), radial scars, and flat epithelial atypia (FEA) among others. These lesions are not uniformly "high risk." As most recent "upgrade" studies have demonstrated, FEA may actually be a particularly "low-risk" entity (76-78). The reported upgrade rate of "high-risk" lesions diagnosed on NCB to a more significant lesion on excisional biopsy has seemingly lowered over recent years. This reduction can be attributable to more reliable imaging studies and ampler sampling—leading to greater likelihood of attaining radiology-pathology concordance (**Table 26.13**). The lowering of upgrade rates has led to more such cases being managed by surveillance rather than excision.

However, such "de-escalation" of management can be challenging in certain situations: (a) in some "high-risk" cases, for example, lobular carcinoma in situ (LCIS), excisional biopsy does not mitigate the long-term risk for invasive carcinoma to either breast; (b) some proactive patients have considerable anxiety regarding living with "high-risk" lesions without "doing something about it"; (c) there is the valid concern regarding noncompliance with long-term high-quality surveillance in resource-poor settings; (d) some studies continue to show an unacceptably high risk of "upgrade" for some "high-risk" lesions (76,77); and finally

(e) it is also difficult to overcome firmly held opinions among surgeons and clinicians (and pathologists!)—beliefs that are often conveyed to patients.

Be that as it may, the weight of the evidence increasingly suggests that excision is not always necessary for some "high-risk" lesions (78-80). Surveillance may be feasible in many asymptomatic and radiology-pathology concordant lesions in whom reliable follow-up can be ensured. Indeed, there are several ongoing clinical trials, for example, Comparison of Operative versus Monitoring and Endocrine Therapy (COMET) of active surveillance for cases histopathologically proven to be low-grade DCIS (81). The management of "high-risk" lesions diagnosed on NCB is highly dependent on imaging correlation and multidisciplinary input (see **Table 26.14**).

Forward-thinking surgeons and clinicians ought to discuss not only the recent remarkable advances in imaging techniques and biopsy methodologies but also the relatively low upgrade rate as reported in most well-conducted contemporary studies of some "high-risk" lesions. Patients should also be made aware of the usual and unusual complications of surgery and of the potential of volume loss and consequent adverse cosmetic outcome in some cases.

TABLE 26.13

"High-Risk" Lesions Diagnosed on Needle Core Biopsy: Management Is Highly Dependent on Imaging Correlation and Multidisciplinary Input

Lesion	Typical Management
ADH	Excise (upgrade rate of 15%-20%)
	Close surveillance seldom an option[a], only after multidisciplinary input
ALH	Close surveillance after multidisciplinary input
	Excise in rad-path discordant cases, or if otherwise indicated.
FEA	Surveillance after imaging correlation
	Prudent to ensure removal of bulk (>90%) of targeted calcifications
	Excise rarely, eg, those with ADH, or those who border on DCIS.
LCIS, classic	Surveillance in screen-detected cases after multidisciplinary input
	Excise in rad-path discordant cases (mass, suspicious calcifications, etc).
LCIS, variants[b]	Excise. Surveillance is seldom, if ever, an option.
	Close surveillance is a consideration only after multidisciplinary input.
Papillary lesion	Excise. Surveillance in screen-detected cases after imaging correlation.
	Excision for symptomatic, palpable, larger, and atypical lesions
Radial scar[c]	Surveillance in selected cases after imaging correlation, ie, in asymptomatic incidental, "smaller," well-sampled radial scars
	Excise for "larger" (ie, >1 cm) lesions or those associated with ADH.

ADH, atypical ductal hyperplasia; ALH, atypical lobular hyperplasia; DCIS, ductal carcinoma in situ; FEA, flat epithelial atypia/atypical columnar cell hyperplasia; LCIS, lobular carcinoma in situ; rad-path, radiology-pathology.

[a]May be an option in radiology-pathology concordant cases with 2-3 foci of ADH in vacuum-assisted needle core biopsy (VA-NCB) (with removal of 50%-90% of calcifications).
[b]Variant LCIS: florid, pleomorphic, and pleomorphic apocrine types.
[c]Radiology-pathology concordance can be challenging for radial scars (radial sclerosing lesions) because both spicule formation and architectural distortion are commonly present in invasive ductal carcinoma as well.

TABLE 26.14

"High-Risk" Lesions Diagnosed on Needle Core Biopsy: Upgrade Rate to a More Significant Lesion on Excisional Biopsy[a]

Lesion	Historical Upgrade Rate		Recent Studies[b]
	Mean (%)	Range (%)	Mean (%)
ADH	20	2 to >50	14
ALH	9	0-67	<5
C-LCIS	18	5-60	5
FEA	3	1.5-20	0-<2
Mucocele-like lesion[c]	<5	0-5	<5
Papillary lesion[d]	<10	5-31	<3
Radial scar	10	0-25	1

ADH, atypical ductal hyperplasia; ALH, atypical lobular hyperplasia; C-LCIS, classic lobular carcinoma in situ; FEA, flat epithelial atypia/atypical columnar cell hyperplasia.

[a]Based on combined data from the literature.
[b]Based on review of recent larger, well-conducted studies with radiology-pathology concordance.
[c]Mucocele-like lesion without atypia.
[d]Papillary lesion without atypia.

In sum, a multidisciplinary approach to the management of each "high-risk" case diagnosed on NCB with involvement of the surgeon, radiologist, oncologist, and pathologist is desirable. In most cases, consensus regarding the need for excision versus surveillance can be achieved after review of clinical, imaging, and pathology findings. In particular, the choice of surveillance versus excisional biopsy (or even bilateral mastectomy) for LCIS and atypical lobular hyperplasia (ALH) should be made with patient involvement after due consideration of personal and family history, "informed" preference, and other factors. Such a "consensus" method would be no different from the current approach, in most settings, to the management of breast carcinoma.

REFERENCES

1. Iwase T, Takahashi K, Gomi N, et al. Present state of and problems with needle core biopsy for non-palpable breast lesions. *Breast Cancer.* 2006;13:32-37.
2. Bick U, Trimboli RM, Athanasiou A, et al. Image-guided breast biopsy and localisation: recommendations for information to women and referring physicians by the European Society of Breast Imaging. *Insights Imaging.* 2020;11:12. doi:10.1186/s13244-019-0803-x
3. Sanderink WBG, Laarhuis BI, Strobbe LJA, et al. A systematic review on the use of the breast lesion excision system in breast disease. *Insights Imaging.* 2019;10:49. doi:10.1186/s13244-019-0737-3
4. Smathers RL. Advanced breast biopsy instrumentation device: percentages of lesion and surrounding tissue removed. *AJR Am J Roentgenol.* 2000;175:801-803.
5. Park HL, Kim LS. The current role of vacuum assisted breast biopsy system in breast disease. *J Breast Cancer.* 2011;14:1-7.
6. Park HL, Hong J. Vacuum-assisted breast biopsy for breast cancer. *Gland Surg.* 2014;3:120-127.
7. Plantade R. Interventional radiology: the corner-stone of breast management. *Diagn Interv Imaging.* 2013;94:575-591.
8. Ginter PS, Winant AJ, Hoda SA. Cystic apocrine hyperplasia is the most common finding in MRI detected breast lesions. *J Clin Pathol.* 2014;67:182-186.
9. Heywang-Köbrunner SH, Schreer I, Decker T, et al. Interdisciplinary consensus on the use and technique of vacuum-assisted stereotactic breast biopsy. *Eur J Radiol.* 2003;47:232-236.
10. Heywang-Köbrunner SH, Sinnatamby R, Lebeau A, et al. Interdisciplinary consensus on the uses and technique of MR-guided vacuum-assisted breast biopsy (VAB): results of a European consensus meeting. *Eur J Radiol.* 2009;72:289-294.

11. Hahn M, Krainick-Strobel U, Toellner T, et al. Interdisciplinary consensus recommendations for the use of vacuum-assisted breast biopsy under sonographic guidance: first update 2012. *Ultraschall Med.* 2012;33:366-371.
12. Preibsch H, Baur A, Wietek BM, et al. Vacuum-assisted breast biopsy with 7-gauge, 8-gauge, 9-gauge, 10-gauge, and 11-gauge needles: how many specimens are necessary? *Acta Radiol.* 2015;56:1078-1084.
13. Thavarajah R, Mudimbaimannar VK, Elizabeth J, et al. Chemical and physical basics of routine formaldehyde fixation. *J Oral Maxillofac Pathol.* 2012;16:400-405.
14. Lee AH, Key HP, Bell JA, et al. The effect of delay in fixation on HER2 expression in invasive carcinoma of the breast assessed with immunohistochemistry and in situ hybridization. *J Clin Pathol.* 2014;67:573-575.
15. Moritz JD, Luftner-Nagel S, Westerhof JP, et al. Microcalcifications in breast core biopsy specimens: disappearance at radiography after storage in formaldehyde. *Radiology.* 1996;200:361-363.
16. Hammond ME, Hayes DF, Dowsett M, et al. ASCO-CAP guideline recommendations for immunohistochemical testing of estrogen and progesterone receptors in breast cancer. *J Clin Oncol.* 2010;28:2784-2795.
17. Wolff AC, Hammond MEH, Allison KH, et al.. Human epidermal growth factor receptor 2 testing in breast cancer: American Society of Clinical Oncology/College of American Pathologists clinical practice guideline focused update. *J Clin Oncol.* 2018;36:2105-2122.
18. Sujoy V, Nadji M, Morales AR. Brief formalin fixation and rapid tissue processing do not affect the sensitivity of ER immunohistochemistry of breast core biopsies. *Am J Clin Pathol.* 2014;141:522-526.
19. Kalkman S, Bulte JP, Halilovic A, et al. Brief fixation does not hamper the reliability of Ki67 analysis in breast cancer core-needle biopsies: a double-centre study. *Histopathology.* 2015;66:380-387.
20. Halilovic A, Bulte J, Jacobs Y, et al. Brief fixation enables same-day breast cancer diagnosis with reliable assessment of hormone receptors, E-cadherin and HER2/neu. *J Clin Pathol.* 2017;70:781-786.
21. Bulte JP, Halilovic A, Burgers LJM, et al. Accelerated tissue processing with minimal formalin fixation time for 9-gauge vacuum-assisted breast biopsy specimens. *Am J Clin Pathol.* 2020;153:58-65.
22. van Es SC, van der Vegt B, Bensch F, et al. Decalcification of breast cancer bone metastases with EDTA does not affect ER, PR, and HER2 results. *Am J Surg Pathol.* 2019;43:1355-1360.
23. Washburn E, Tang X, Caruso C, et al. Effect of EDTA decalcification on estrogen receptor and progesterone receptor immunohistochemistry and HER2/neu fluorescence *in situ* hybridization in breast carcinoma. *Hum Pathol.* 2021;117:108-114.
24. Liberman L, Dershaw DD, Rosen PP, et al. Core needle biopsy of synchronous ipsilateral breast lesions: impact on treatment. *AJR Am J Roentgenol.* 1996;166:1429-1432.
25. Senn Bahls E, Dupont Lampert V, Oelschlegel C, et al. Multitarget stereotactic core-needle breast biopsy (MSBB)—an effective and safe diagnostic intervention for non-palpable breast lesions: a large prospective single institution study. *Breast.* 2006;15:339-346.

26. Wolff AC, Hammond ME, Schwartz JN, et al. ASCO-CAP guideline recommendations for human epidermal growth factor receptor 2 testing in breast cancer. *J Clin Oncol*. 2007;25:118-145.
27. Riley TR III, Ruggiero FM. The effect of processing on liver biopsy core size. *Dig Dis Sci*. 2008;53:2775-2777.
28. Renshaw AA, Kish R, Gould EW. The value of inking breast cores to reduce specimen mix up. *Am J Clin Pathol*. 2007;127:271-272.
29. Ragazzini T, Magrini E, Cucci MC, et al. The fast-track biopsy: description of a rapid histology and immunohistochemistry method for evaluation of preoperative breast core biopsies. *Int J Surg Pathol*. 2005;13:247-252.
30. Yaziji H, Taylor CR. Begin at the beginning, with the tissue! The key message underlying the ASCO/CAP Task-force Guideline Recommendations for HER2 testing. *Appl Immunohistochem Mol Morphol*. 2007;15:239-241.
31. Grimes MM, Karageorge LS, Hogge JP. Does exhaustive search for microcalcifications improve diagnostic yield in stereotactic core needle breast biopsies? *Mod Pathol*. 2001;14:350-353.
32. Renshaw A. Adequate histologic sampling of breast core needle biopsies. *Arch Pathol Lab Med*. 2001;125:1055-1057.
33. Kumaraswamy V, Carder PJ. Examination of breast needle core biopsy specimens performed for screen-detected microcalcification. *J Clin Pathol*. 2007;60:681-684.
34. Lee AH, Villena Salinas NM, Hodi Z, Rakha EA, Ellis IO. The value of examination of multiple levels of mammary needle core biopsy specimens taken for investigation of lesions other than calcification. *J Clin Pathol*. 2012;65:1097-1099.
35. Cornea V, Jaffer S, Bleiweiss IJ, Nagi C. Adequate histologic sampling of breast magnetic resonance imaging-guided core needle biopsy. *Arch Pathol Lab Med*. 2009;133:1961-1964.
36. Hoda SA, Rosen PP. Contemporaneous H&E sections should be standard practice in diagnostic immunopathology. *Am J Surg Pathol*. 2007;31:1627.
37. Manion E, Brock JE, Raza S, et al. MRI-guided breast needle core biopsies: pathologic features of newly diagnosed malignancies. *Breast J*. 2014;20:453-460.
38. Dahlstrom JE, Sutton S, Jain S. Histologic-radiologic correlation of mammographically detected microcalcification in stereotactic core biopsies. *Am J Surg Pathol*. 1998;22:256-259.
39. Winston JS, Geradts J, Liu DF, et al. Microtome shaving radiography: demonstration of loss of mammographic microcalcifications during histologic sectioning. *Breast J*. 2004;10:200-203.
40. Friedman PD, Sanders LM, Menendez C, et al. Retrieval of lost microcalcifications during stereotactic vacuum-assisted core biopsy. *AJR Am J Roentgenol*. 2003;180:275-280.
41. Tornos C, Silva E, el-Naggar A, et al. Calcium oxalate crystals in breast biopsies: the missing microcalcifications. *Am J Surg Pathol*. 1990;14:961-968.
42. Brunner AH, Sagmeister T, Kremer J, et al. The accuracy of frozen section analysis in ultrasound-guided core needle biopsy of breast lesion. *BMC Cancer*. 2009;9:341.
43. Carmichael AR, Berresford A, Sami A, et al. Imprint cytology of needle core-biopsy specimens of breast lesion: is it best of both worlds? *Breast*. 2004;13:232-234.
44. Kass R, Henry-Tillman RS, Nurko J, et al. Touch preparation of breast core needle specimens is a new method for same-day diagnosis. *Am J Surg*. 2003;186:737-742.
45. Kulkarni D, Irvine T, Reves RJ. The use of core biopsy imprint cytology in the 'one-stop' breast clinic. *Eur J Surg Oncol*. 2009;35:1037-1040.
46. Schulz-Wendtland R, Fasching PA, Bani MR, et al. Touch imprint cytology and stereotactically-guided core needle biopsy of suspicious breast lesions: 15-year follow-up. *Geburtshilfe Frauenheilkd*. 2016;76:59-64.
47. Wauters CA, Sanders-Eras CT, Kooistra BW, et al. Modified core wash cytology procedure for the immediate diagnosis of core needle biopsies of breast lesions. *Cancer Cytopathol*. 2009;117:333-337.
48. Jackman RJ, Nowels KW, Shepard MJ, et al. Stereotaxic large-core needle biopsy of 450 nonpalpable breast lesions with surgical correlation in lesions with cancer or atypical hyperplasia. *Radiology*. 1994;193:91-95.
49. Sharifi S, Peterson M, Baum J. Assessment of pathologic prognostic factors in breast core needle biopsies. *Mod Pathol*. 1999;12:941-945.
50. Lara JF, Abellar RG, Singh NV. Benefits and pitfalls of tumor size and/or volume determination on core needle biopsy in invasive breast cancer: a year of experience from a community hospital. *Mod Pathol*. 2005;18(Suppl 1):39A.
51. Shousha S. Issues in the interpretation of breast core biopsies. *Int J Surg Pathol*. 2003;11:167-176.
52. Ozerdem U, Hoda SA. Correlation of maximum breast carcinoma dimension on needle core biopsy and subsequent excisional biopsy: a retrospective study of 50 non-palpable imaging-detected cases. *Pathol Res Pract*. 2014;210:603-605.
53. Varma S, Ozerdem U, Hoda SA. Complexities and challenges in the pathologic assessment of size (T) of invasive breast carcinoma. *Adv Anat Pathol*. 2014;21:420-432.
54. Hoda SA, Harigopal M, Harris GC, et al. Expert opinion: what should be included in reports of needle core biopsies of breast? *Histopathology*. 2003;43:87-90.
55. Goldstein NS, Bassi D, Watts JC, et al. E-cadherin reactivity of 95 noninvasive ductal and lobular lesions of the breast: implications for the interpretation of problematic lesions. *Am J Clin Pathol*. 2001;115:534-542.
56. Dabbs DJ, Bhargava R, Chivkula M. Lobular versus ductal breast neoplasms: the diagnostic utility of p120 catenin. *Am J Surg Pathol*. 2007;31:427-437.
57. Chivukula M, Haynik DM, Brufsky A, et al. Pleomorphic lobular carcinoma in situ (PLCIS) on breast core needle biopsies: clinical significance and immunoprofile. *Am J Surg Pathol*. 2008;32:1721-1726.
58. Zhong E, Solomon JP, Cheng E, et al. Apocrine variant of pleomorphic lobular carcinoma in situ: further clinical, histopathologic, immunohistochemical, and molecular characterization of an emerging entity. *Am J Surg Pathol*. 2020;44:1092-1103.
59. Knuttel FM, Menezes GL, van Diest PJ, et al. Meta-analysis of the concordance of histological grade of breast cancer between core needle biopsy and surgical excision specimen. *Br J Surg*. 2016;103:644-655.
60. Petrau C, Clatot F, Cornic M, et al. Reliability of prognostic and predictive factors evaluated by needle core biopsies of large breast invasive tumors. *Am J Clin Pathol*. 2015;144:555-562.
61. Harris GC, Denley HE, Pinder SE, et al. Correlation of histologic prognostic factors in core biopsies and therapeutic excisions of invasive breast carcinoma. *Am J Surg Pathol*. 2003;27:11-15.
62. Dhaliwal CA, Graham C, Loane J. Grading of breast cancer on needle core biopsy: does a reduction in mitotic count threshold improve agreement with grade on excised specimens? *J Clin Pathol*. 2014;67:1106-1108.
63. McIlhenny C, Doughty JC, George WD, et al. Optimum number of core biopsies for accurate assessment of histologic grade in breast cancer. *Br J Surg*. 2002;89:84-85.
64. Lee AH, Rakha EA, Hodi Z, et al. Re-audit of revised method for assessing the mitotic component of histological grade in needle core biopsies of invasive carcinoma of the breast. *Histopathology*. 2012;60:1166-1167.
65. Rosen PP. Tumor emboli in intramammary lymphatics in breast carcinoma: pathologic criteria for diagnosis and clinical significance. *Pathol Annu*. 1983;18(pt 2):215-232.
66. Hoda SA, Hoda RS, Merlin S, et al. Issues relating to lymphovascular invasion in breast carcinoma. *Adv Anat Pathol*. 2006;13:308-315.
67. Ellis IO, Humphrey S, Mitchell M, et al. Best practice no. 179: guidelines for breast needle core biopsy handling and reporting in breast screening assessment. *J Clin Pathol*. 2004;57:897-902.
68. Reefy S, Osman H, Chao C, et al. Surgical excision for B3 breast lesions diagnosed by vacuum-assisted core biopsy. *Anticancer Res*. 2010;30:2287-2290.
69. El-Sayed ME, Rakha EA, Reed J, et al. Predictive value of needle core biopsy diagnoses of lesions of uncertain malignant potential (B3) in abnormalities detected by mammographic screening. *Histopathology*. 2008;53:650-657.
70. Calhoun BC, Collins LC. Recommendations for excision following core needle biopsy of the breast: a contemporary evaluation of the literature. *Histopathology*. 2016;68:138-151.
71. Liberman L, Dershaw D, Rosen PP. Stereotaxic core biopsy of breast carcinoma: accuracy at predicting invasion. *Radiology*. 1995;194:379-381.
72. Crowe JP, Rim A, Patrick RJ, et al. Does core needle breast biopsy accurately reflect breast pathology? *Surgery*. 2003;134:523-528.
73. Shah VL, Raju U, Chitale D, et al. False-negative core needle biopsies of the breast: an analysis of clinical, radiologic, and pathologic findings in 27 consecutive cases of missed breast cancer. *Cancer*. 2003;97:1824-1831.
74. Rosen PP. Review of 'outside' pathology before treatment should be mandatory. *Am J Surg Pathol*. 2002;26:1235-1236.
75. Huang EC, Kuo FC, Fletcher CD, et al. Critical diagnoses in surgical pathology: a retrospective single-institution study to monitor guidelines for communication of urgent results. *Am J Surg Pathol*. 2009;33:1098-1102.
76. Willers N, Neven P, Floris G, et al. The upgrade risk of B3 lesions to (pre)invasive breast cancer after diagnosis on core needle or vacuum assisted biopsy. A Belgian national cohort study. *Clin Breast Cancer*. 2023;S1526-8209(23)00075-7.
77. Jani C, Lotz M, Keates S, et al. Management of lobular neoplasia diagnosed by core biopsy. *Breast J*. 2023;2023:8185446. doi:10.1155/2023/8185446
78. Warwar S, Kulkarni S. Selective surgical excision of high-risk lesions. *Surgery*. 2023;174: 125-128. doi:10.1016/j.surg.2023.02.028. Epub ahead of print. 37059651.
79. Lilly AJ, Johnson M, Kuzmiak CM, et al. MRI-guided core needle biopsy of the breast: radiology-pathology correlation and impact on clinical management. *Ann Diagn Pathol*. 2020;48:151563. doi:10.1016/j.anndiagpath.2020.151563
80. Harbhajanka A, Gilmore HL, Calhoun BC. High-risk and selected benign breast lesions diagnosed on core needle biopsy: evidence for and against immediate surgical excision. *Mod Pathol*. 2022;35:1500-1508.
81. Hwang ES, Hyslop T, Lynch T, et al. The COMET (Comparison of Operative versus Monitoring and Endocrine Therapy) trial: a phase III randomised controlled clinical trial for low-risk ductal carcinoma in situ. *BMJ Open*. 2019;9(3):e026797. doi:10.1136/bmjopen-2018-026797

27

Biomarker, Molecular, and Other Ancillary Testing

ELAINE W. ZHONG AND SYED A. HODA

INTRODUCTION

Advances in biomarker (ie, biological marker) and molecular testing have reinforced the understanding that breast carcinoma is not a single disease, but a broad range of diseases with diverse biology, natural history, and therapeutic response. The biomarker tests discussed herein refine traditional morphologic classification of breast carcinoma into predictive and prognostic subclasses, providing opportunities for targeted first-line treatment as well as treatment options for relapsed or refractory disease (1-3). New biomarkers are continually emerging, and these tests are being increasingly, if not exclusively, performed on needle core biopsy (NCB) samplings.

Gene expression profiling is based on the relative patterns of expression of genes. Of the several gene classifiers that have been reported, the so-called "intrinsic system" has garnered the most interest and following. This system divides breast carcinoma into four main groups, which broadly correspond to immunohistochemistry (IHC) findings for estrogen receptor (ER), progesterone receptor (PR), human epidermal growth factor receptor 2 (HER2), and the proliferation marker Ki67 **(Table 27.1)**. The largest group (constituting ~60% of invasive breast carcinomas) is the *luminal A*, which comprises tumors that are low-grade, ER-positive, PR-positive, and HER2-negative with a low proliferation rate. Each of the other three groups constitutes approximately 15% of all invasive carcinomas. The *luminal B* group is typically ER-positive, PR-positive, and HER2-positive or HER2-negative, with a high proliferation rate.

The *HER2*(*-enriched*) group is ER-negative, PR-negative, and (as the name implies) HER2-positive. The *basal-like* group is negative for ER, PR, and HER2. The latter group is so named because its transcriptomic profile duplicates that of normal myoepithelial (ie, *basal*) cells. Other systems of molecular taxonomy have been described (4-7). Although molecular subtyping is not essential for diagnosis, gene expression data provide important prognostic and predictive information (vide infra).

ER and HER2 are both prognostic (ie, foretell the likely clinical outcome) and predictive (ie, predict response to treatment). ER-positive invasive carcinomas (~70% of all breast carcinomas) can be treated by selective estrogen receptor modulators (SERMs) or aromatase inhibitors (AIs). Prognostic molecular assays such as Oncotype Dx are validated only for ER-positive carcinomas. HER2-positive carcinomas can potentially be managed by HER2-targeted therapies (eg, trastuzumab, pertuzumab, lapatinib, and neratinib). The development of antibody-drug conjugates (ADCs) has further expanded anti-HER2 therapy.

Current College of American Pathologists (CAP) regulatory guidelines dictate that when ancillary IHC testing is performed, the pathology report should specify the antibody clone, the general form of detection, and the scoring system used. Deviations from standard processing or antigen retrieval techniques should be noted. Appropriate negative and positive controls should be used and documented.

The concordance rate between ancillary test results performed on NCB and excisional biopsy samples has been established to be acceptable (8). In general, when hormone receptors are positive on NCB, they are seldom negative on excisional biopsy specimen, and vice versa (9). Testing for biomarkers on the initial NCB, prior to definitive surgery, is critical for planning management, including consideration of neoadjuvant chemotherapy.

TESTING FOR ESTROGEN, PROGESTERONE AND ANDROGEN RECEPTORS

At present, almost all clinical testing for ER and PR is performed using IHC. The optimal procedures for tissue handling, testing conditions, quality assurance, and so on, have been outlined elsewhere (10,11). Antibodies should have well-established specificity and sensitivity. For ER, these

---

TABLE 27.1

Gene Expression Profiling of Breast Carcinoma: Surrogate Immunohistochemical Classification

	%	ER	PR	HER2	Ki67
Luminal A	~60	+	+	−	↓
Luminal B	~15	+	+	−/+	↑
HER2-enriched	~15	−	−	+	↑↑
Basal-like	~15	−	−	−	↑↑

ER, estrogen receptor; HER2; human epidermal growth factor receptor 2; PR, progesterone receptor.

antibodies include 1D5, 6F11, and SP1. For PR, these include 1294, 1A6, and 312. PR expression is a surrogate for a functional ER pathway, but the predictive role of PR independent of ER is not well established (12). Commercially available mRNA-based assays, discussed later in this chapter, also provide quantitative measures of ER and PR expression, with good concordance with IHC. However, there are currently no data that these assays can predict response to endocrine therapy (1).

The American Society of Clinical Oncology (ASCO)-CAP recommendation is that the percentage (*proportion*) of carcinoma cells showing nuclear staining as well as the average *intensity* of staining (strong, intermediate, or weak) should be reported. An interpretation (ie, "positive" or "negative") should also be offered. The carcinoma is considered ER- or PR-positive if >1% of tumor cell nuclei stain regardless of intensity **(Fig. 27.1)**. This threshold for positivity applies to invasive as well as in situ carcinomas. Some laboratories report ER and PR using the "H" score or the "Allred score" (13) **(Tables 27.2 and 27.3)**.

Using currently available IHC techniques and antibodies, about 95% of breast carcinomas are unequivocally reported as either hormone receptor–positive or hormone receptor–negative. Nevertheless, presently available antibodies for ER (and PR) are highly sensitive, and there is concern that carcinomas reported as "low-positive" (staining in 1%-10% of nuclei, regardless of intensity) for ER should be classified as triple-negative because these patients could benefit from treatments tailored toward the latter group. Indeed, there is growing evidence that low ER-positive carcinomas have morphology, gene expression profiling, and chemotherapy response closer to triple-negative (basal-like) carcinomas than to luminal A carcinomas (14-16). ASCO-CAP recommends that a comment be included referencing the limited data on the most appropriate treatment for patients with ER-low tumors (10). Of note, the term "low-positive" does *not* apply to *PR* staining of 1% to 10% of nuclei, per ASCO-CAP guidelines (10).

The androgen receptor (AR) is a potential therapeutic target for triple-negative breast carcinomas (TNBCs) and apocrine breast carcinomas. Biologically, AR interacts with the phosphatidylinositol-3-kinase/mammalian target of rapamycin (PI3K/mTOR), phosphate and tensin homolog (PTEN),

TABLE 27.2
The H (Histochemical)-Score System for Quantifying Immunostaining

Obtaining the H-Score	
1. Record percentage of cells staining.	0–100
2. Record staining intensity factor: 0: negative, 1: weak, 2: moderate, 3: strong.	0–3
3. *Multiply* percentage of cells staining by the staining intensity factor to obtain the H (histochemical)-score.	Range: 0–300

Interpreting the H-Score	
0–50	Negative
51–100	Weak-positive (1+)
101–200	Moderate-positive (2+)
201–300	Strong-positive (3+)

Based on Snead DR, Bell JA, Dixon AR, et al. Methodology of immunohistological detection of oestrogen receptor in human breast carcinoma in formalin-fixed, paraffin-embedded tissue: a comparison with frozen section methodology. *Histopathology.* 1993;23:233-238.

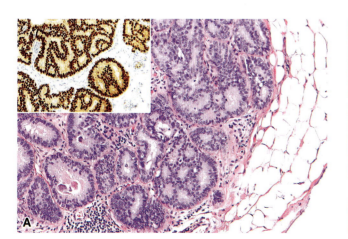 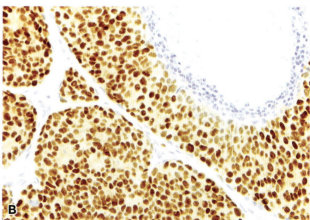

FIGURE 27.1 Estrogen receptor (ER) Immunohistochemistry on Needle Core Biopsies. A: Ductal carcinoma in situ (DCIS) of the cribriform type with intermediate grade nuclei with diffuse (almost 100%) and strong immunoreactivity for ER (inset). **B:** ER immunostaining of DCIS of the cribriform type with intermediate grade nuclei and central necrosis shows diffuse (~95%) and strong immunoreactivity. Note lack of ER immunoreactivity in the necrotic cells (upper right).

TABLE 27.3

The Allred Scoring System for Quantifying Immunostaining of ER and PR

This method yields the *sum* of the estimated proportion and intensity of positive tumor cells.

Obtaining the Allred Score

1. Score proportion of "positive" cell nuclei from 0 to 5.
   0: total negativity in tumor cell nuclei
   1: <1% positive cell nuclei
   2: 1%–10% positive cell nuclei
   3: 33% positive cell nuclei
   4: 66% positive cell nuclei
   5: 100% positive cell nuclei
2. Score intensity of staining from 0 to 3.
   0: no staining in tumor cells
   1: weak staining
   2: intermediate staining
   3: strong staining
3. Add proportion score and intensity score to obtain the Allred score.
   Total score could range from 0 to 8.

Interpreting the Allred Score

A score of >2 (ie, ≥3) has been adjudged the minimum score for defining ER-positive breast carcinoma.

ER, estrogen receptor; PR, progesterone receptor.

Based on Ellredge RM, Allred DC. Clinical aspects of estrogen and progesterone receptors. In: Harris JR, Lippman ME, Morrow M, et al, eds. *Diseases of the Breast*. Lippincott Williams & Wilkins; 2004:603-617; Allred DC, Harvey JM, Berardo M, et al. Prognostic and predictive factors in breast cancer by immunohistochemical analysis. *Mod Pathol*. 1998;11:155-168.

and other pathways to support oncogenesis (17). About 12% of TNBC are AR-positive by IHC. AR antagonists such as bicalutamide and enzalutamide have shown promise in these tumors (18,19). Guidelines for IHC and assessment of AR are lacking at this time.

Three practical caveats deserve iteration with regard to hormone receptor testing by IHC. First, positive and negative internal "controls" must not be overlooked. Ideally, hormone receptor immunoreactivity in normal breast glandular tissue should be confirmed. The complete absence of immunoreactivity for ER and PR (in all neoplastic and nonneoplastic breast tissue, and in control tissue) is most likely due to technical failure. This finding may also be the result of loss of immunogenicity of tissue being tested because of improper fixation. In such situations, the use of vimentin or another ubiquitous antibody is helpful to assess the "immunocompetence" of the tissue. Second, the status of receptors cannot be reliably calculated if only a minute amount of carcinoma is present. Lastly, optimal testing for prognostic markers depends on an NCB sample that is representative of the whole tumor. In tumors that show heterogeneity of grade, multifocality, or multicentricity, retesting on appropriately selected tumor tissue from excised specimens is typically indicated.

Testing for ER is routinely performed on all ductal carcinoma in situ (DCIS) and reported in a manner similar to that for invasive carcinoma, whereas testing for PR is generally considered optional in DCIS.

TESTING FOR HUMAN EPIDERMAL GROWTH FACTOR RECEPTOR 2 (HER2)

The use of targeted HER2 treatment in patients with breast carcinoma relies on reliable determination of HER2 status on tumor tissue. Approximately 15% of invasive breast carcinomas are HER2-positive, mostly because of amplification of the tyrosine kinase receptor *ERBB2*. A variety of technologies exist to assess HER2 status (20), through the detection of either protein expression or gene amplification. The former is detectable by IHC and the latter by various in situ hybridization (ISH) techniques.

Almost all laboratories in the United States follow the ASCO-CAP guidelines for HER2 testing: IHC for initial HER2 testing and fluorescence in situ hybridization (FISH) testing for cases with equivocal result (an IHC score of 2+), as only about 15% to 30% of these tumors show *ERBB2* amplification. Some laboratories use FISH as the only technique for HER2 testing, and some use both testing methodologies concurrently (to prevent false-negative results, 4% in one series) (21). HER2 assessment on NCB specimens is generally considered reliable—provided ASCO-CAP-compliant fixation and processing times (22). The 2015 UK guidelines for HER2 testing (23, p. 94) state that "there is insufficient data to define the amount of invasive tumour tissue in core biopsy sufficient for analysis; however, this can be left to the reporting pathologist's discretion." It seems reasonable to report HER2 results even when a microinvasive (<1 mm) carcinoma is either unequivocally negative or unequivocally positive. Reporting 1+ or 2+ (equivocal) results in this setting can be clinically vexing, because further testing via ISH is seldom possible.

Currently, there are four reporting categories for HER2 testing by IHC: negative (0), low (1+), equivocal (2+), and positive (3+) **(Table 27.4** and **Fig. 27.2)**. Only membranous staining of invasive tumor cells is scored. One exception is invasive micropapillary carcinoma, in which incomplete basolateral "cuplike" staining should be scored as 2+ (24). In most instances, HER2 protein overexpression and gene amplification are strongly correlated. Tumors with heterogeneous HER2 staining can be interpreted as positive if qualitatively 3+ staining is present in >10% of the sample; however, it is worth including a comment that there is a HER2-negative component.

With the development and U.S. Food and Drug Administration (FDA) approval of many HER2-targeted ADCs (eg, ado-trastuzumab emtansine [T-DM1], fam-trastuzumab deruxtecan [T-DXd]), there has been increased interest in the "HER2-low" subset of breast carcinomas. These are defined as tumors with HER2 IHC scores of 1+ or 2+ without *ERBB2* gene amplification and comprise about half of all breast carcinomas (25,26). These tumors generally do not

BIOMARKER, MOLECULAR, AND OTHER ANCILLARY TESTING

TABLE 27.4
ASCO-CAP Scoring System for Quantifying Immunostaining of HER2

Score, Interpretation	Criteria
0, negative	No staining observed, or incomplete faint/barely perceptible membrane staining in ≤10% of carcinoma cells
1+, negative (low)	Incomplete faint/barely perceptible membrane staining in >10% of carcinoma cells
2+, equivocal	Weak to moderate complete membrane staining in >10% of carcinoma cells
3+, positive	Complete intense circumferential membrane staining in >10% of carcinoma cells

ASCO, American Society of Clinical Oncology; CAP, College of American Pathologists; HER2; human epidermal growth factor receptor 2.

Based on Wolff AC, Hammond EH, Allison KH, et al. Human epidermal growth factor receptor 2 testing in breast cancer: American Society of Clinical Oncology/College of American Pathologists clinical practice guideline focused update. *J Clin Oncol*. 2018;36:2105-2122.

respond to conventional HER2-targeted therapy; however, they may respond to ADCs (27,28). Hence, it is now essential to distinguish between 0 and 1+ HER2 IHC.

FISH is currently considered the "gold standard" for determining HER2 status. Other ISH assays include chromogenic ISH (CISH) and silver ISH (SISH). The latter two techniques are comparable to FISH and offer the advantage of being permanent, and thus available for retrospective review (29-31). FISH, CISH, and SISH techniques can all be performed on NCB material. ISH assays for HER2 can use either two (dual) probes or a single probe. One of the two probes used in the former, and the only probe in the latter, is for the HER2 locus on the long arm of chromosome 17. The second probe in the dual-probe test is a chromosome enumerator probe 17 (CEP17) that controls for polysomy 17. The criteria for reporting of dual-probe ISH testing appear in **Table 27.5**. Currently, mRNA-based assays for HER2 such as Oncotype Dx are not recommended for therapeutic use (11).

Another emerging category of HER2-driven tumors is those with activating mutations. Approximately 3% of breast carcinomas, and 8% of invasive lobular carcinomas, harbor activating *ERBB2* mutations. These are typically negative by HER2 IHC and ISH. Early clinical evidence suggests that these tumors are resistant to conventional anti-HER2 therapy but respond to the pan-HER inhibitor neratinib (32,33). HER2-activating mutations are considered an emerging biomarker by NCCN (34).

The 2018 ASCO-CAP guidelines for HER2 testing recommend that "if the initial HER2 test result in a core needle biopsy is negative, a new HER2 test **may** (*emphasis added*) be ordered on the excision specimen" (11). Lack of concordance between HER2 status on NCB and surgical specimens is usually attributable to intratumoral heterogeneity or levels of gene amplification close to the cutoff for defining positivity (35). Loss of ER and PR expression following endocrine therapy and loss of HER2 expression following anti-HER2 therapy may occur. Certain circumstances in which ER, PR, and HER2 testing should be repeated on excisional biopsy specimens are listed in **Table 27.6**.

DETERMINATION OF PROLIFERATION RATE

The proliferation rate of a carcinoma can be immunohistochemically assessed by Ki67 (MIB1). Ki67 is expressed in the G1, S, G2, and M phases of the cell cycle. The utilization of Ki67 in breast pathology practice varies. Carcinomas with higher proliferation rate are generally more aggressive and

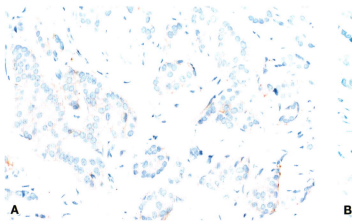
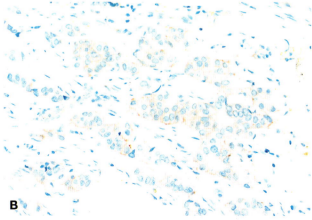

FIGURE 27.2 HER2 Immunohistochemistry and FISH on Needle Core Biopsies. A: Faint, barely detectable staining in rare cells is scored as HER2 0. **B:** Weak, incomplete membrane staining in HER2 1+.

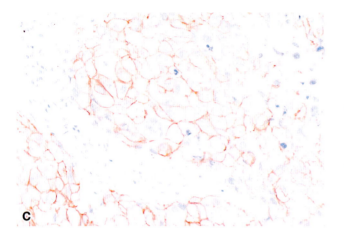
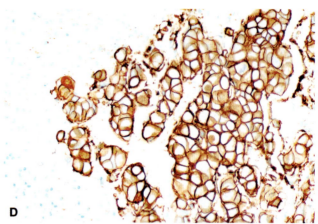
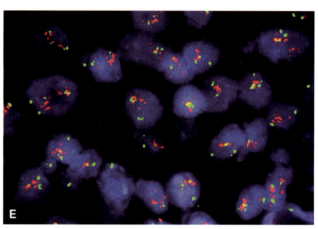

FIGURE 27.2 (*continued*) **C:** HER2 2+ staining is complete and diffuse but lacking the intensity needed for unequivocal positivity. **D:** Positive (3+) HER2 immunoreactivity that is complete intense circumferential membrane staining in >10% (almost 100%) of cells in this invasive ductal carcinoma. **E:** Dual-probe HER2 FISH. Numerous red signals indicate amplification of *ERBB2*. FISH, fluorescence in situ hybridization; HER2; human epidermal growth factor receptor 2.

TABLE 27.5

ASCO-CAP Dual-Probe HER2 In Situ Hybridization (ISH) Guidelines

Group	HER2/CEP17 Ratio	Average HER2 Copy Number (Signals per Cell)	Interpretation[a]
1	≥2.0	≥4.0	Positive
2	≥2.0	<4.0	Positive[b]
3	<2.0	≥6.0	Positive[b]
4	<2.0	≥4.0 and <6.0	Equivocal[c]
5	<2.0	<4.0	Negative

ASCO, American Society of Clinical Oncology; CAP, College of American Pathologists; CEP17, chromosome enumerator probe 17; HER2; human epidermal growth factor receptor 2; IHC, immunohistochemistry.

[a]Interpretations are for tumors that are 2+ by HER2 IHC.
[b]Recount ISH by an additional observer blinded to the previous result. If count remains in the same category, diagnosis is HER2-positive.
[c]Recount ISH by an additional observer blinded to the previous result. If count remains in the same category, diagnosis is HER2-negative with a comment.

Based on Wolff AC, Hammond EH, Allison KH, et al. Human epidermal growth factor receptor 2 testing in breast cancer: American Society of Clinical Oncology/College of American Pathologists clinical practice guideline focused update. *J Clin Oncol*. 2018;36:2105-2122.

TABLE 27.6

Repeat ER, PR, and HER2 Testing on Excision Following Negative Result on Needle Core Biopsy

1. Suboptimal processing of needle core biopsy (*ie*, extended ischemic time: >1 h, suboptimal fixation: <6 h or >72 h, inappropriate fixative)
2. Minimal diagnostic tissue (eg, <0.1 cm) on needle core biopsy
3. Lower-grade carcinoma on needle core biopsy
4. Unexpected results on needle core biopsy (*eg*, ER-negativity in invasive lobular carcinoma, HER2 3+ in tubular carcinoma)
5. Equivocal (2+) HER2 results on needle core biopsy
6. Postneoadjuvant chemotherapy
7. "If the initial HER2 test result in a core needle biopsy of a primary breast cancer is negative, a new HER2 test *may* (emphasis added) be ordered on the excision specimen."[a]

[a]Hammond ME, Hicks DG. ASCO-CAP HER2 testing clinical practice guideline upcoming modifications: proof that clinical practice guidelines are living documents. *Arch Pathol Lab Med*. 2015;139:970-971.

ER, estrogen receptor; HER2, human epidermal growth factor receptor 2; PR, progesterone receptor.

BIOMARKER, MOLECULAR, AND OTHER ANCILLARY TESTING

more responsive to chemotherapy. High Ki67 can identify poor responders to anastrozole inhibitors (36,37) and patients at higher risk of relapse postneoadjuvant therapy (38). The recent FDA approval of CDK4/6 inhibitors (abemaciclib, palbociclib, and ribociclib) imparted additional value to Ki67 assessment. These agents are approved, in conjunction with adjuvant endocrine therapy, for the treatment of ER-positive, HER2-negative breast carcinoma with four or more positive axillary lymph nodes, or 1 to 3 positive nodes and another high-risk factor: (a) high grade, (b) size ≥5 cm, or (c) Ki67 ≥20% (39,40).

The optimal cutoffs, antibodies, and scoring methods for Ki67 have been debated (41). The 2021 Ki67 in Breast Cancer Working Group (42) recommended a standardized visual scoring method and cutoffs of ≤5% and ≥30%, rather than a dichotomous scheme. Clinical decisions should not be made on the basis of a "borderline" rate (43). The difficulties in reliably estimating the proliferation rate in a breast carcinoma are compounded in NCBs. In this regard, intratumoral heterogeneity, interobserver variability, and the presence of tumor-infiltrating lymphocytes are major confounding factors (44).

KEY MOLECULAR TESTS

Gene expression analysis on NCB specimens is directed toward predicting recurrence risk and response to chemotherapy (45). In most cases, adequate RNA and cDNA can be obtained from appropriately processed NCB samples of breast carcinoma (46). These assays are endorsed by multiple authorities for treatment planning in patients (women and men) with early-stage, hormone receptor–positive invasive breast carcinoma (34,47,48). Most significantly, Oncotype Dx is included in the AJCC 8th edition prognostic staging system (49).

Oncotype Dx (Genomic Health) (50) is a quantitative reverse transcription polymerase chain reaction (qRT-PCR)-based assay that includes a panel of 21 genes (16 carcinoma-related genes and 5 housekeeping control genes). The output is a recurrence score (RS): a number from 0 to 100 which estimates the likelihood of recurrence as low (<18), intermediate (18-30), or high (>31). The report also includes results for ER, PR, and HER2 gene expression ("quantitative single gene scores"). Patients with low RS can be treated with endocrine therapy without chemotherapy (50). TAILORx demonstrated that patients >50 years of age with ER-positive, HER2-negative, node-negative breast carcinoma with RS <26 can safely forego chemotherapy (51). RxPONDER expanded the utility for Oncotype Dx to patients with up to three positive lymph nodes (52). The assay requires at least 5% tumor cellularity and 500 ng of tumor RNA; therefore, microinvasive carcinomas are insufficient (50). Akashi-Tanaka et al (53) found that half of NCBs submitted for Oncotype Dx yielded insufficient RNA for testing. However, the remaining specimens were "highly predictive" of response to neoadjuvant endocrine therapy.

MammaPrint (Agendia) is a 70-gene DNA microarray-based assay (31) and the first FDA-cleared breast cancer recurrence assay. The output is a binary low- or high-risk category (poor or good response to chemotherapy, respectively) (54). According to the MINDACT study, 46% of patients with high clinical risk can be spared chemotherapy based on low genomic risk according to MammaPrint (55).

Other commercially available assays include **Prosigna/PAM50** (56), **EndoPredict** (57), and the **Breast Cancer Index (BCI)** (58). **Oncotype Dx DCIS** (59) and **DCISionRT** (60) are risk stratification assays for patients with noninvasive disease.

The applications for *gene mutational analysis* in breast carcinoma are currently limited but growing. Sequencing platforms range from single-gene assays to targeted breast carcinoma panels to broad oncology panels such as **MSK-IMPACT**, **Oncomine** (Thermo Fisher), **TruSight Oncology 500** (Illumina), and **FoundationOne CDx** (Foundation Medicine). NCCN guidelines recommend testing for *ESR1* and *PIK3CA* mutations in recurrent, unresectable, or metastatic ER-positive, HER2-negative breast carcinomas; other genomic findings may be "useful in certain circumstances" (34).

Select genetic variants have established clinical significance in breast carcinoma **(Table 27.7)**. *ESR1* mutation is an acquired resistance mechanism seen in 54% of relapsed carcinomas following endocrine therapy (61,62), and it is associated with inferior disease-free and overall survival (63). *PIK3CA* mutations are targetable by the PI3K inhibitor alpelisib, currently approved for hormone receptor–positive, HER2-negative advanced tumors in postmenopausal women (64). Approximately 5% of patients with breast carcinoma carry a deleterious germline mutation in *BRCA1* or *BRCA2*. Germline carriers with *BRCA*-mutated, HER2-negative breast carcinoma are eligible for PARP inhibitor therapy (olaparib, talazoparib) (65,66). Emerging evidence suggests that PARP inhibition may be effective for germline *PALB2* mutations and somatic *BRCA1/2* mutations as well (67).

In patients with advanced disease refractory to multiple lines of therapy, tumor DNA sequencing can open opportunities for clinical trial enrollment. Pathogenic or likely pathogenic variants can be found in 17% of advanced breast carcinomas (68). Mutational analysis can help resolve malignancies of unknown origin in some situations (69). Online knowledge bases, which annotate the clinical significance of somatic variants, are useful resources (70,71).

Molecular alterations associated with specific diagnostic entities of the breast are discussed in their respective chapters.

PD-L1 AND OTHER EMERGING TESTS

Programmed cell death 1 (*PD1*) is a costimulatory receptor present mainly on T cells, which when stimulated by its ligand (**PD-L1**) on carcinoma and immune cells suppresses the antitumor immune response. Immune checkpoint inhibitors are used for PD-L1-positive advanced or metastatic TNBCs to potentiate immune-mediated cancer cell death.

TABLE 27.7
Select Clinically Significant Genetic Alterations in Breast Carcinoma

Gene	Aberration	Significance
AKT1	Activating mutation	PI3K inhibitor, AKT inhibitor (clinical trial)
BRCA1	Loss of function (germline) mutation	PARP inhibitor
BRCA2	Loss of function (germline) mutation	PARP inhibitor
CDH1 (E-cadherin)	Loss of function mutation, loss of expression	ROS1 inhibitor (clinical trial)
ESR1 (estrogen receptor-alpha)	Activating mutation, translocation	Acquired resistance to endocrine therapy in ER-positive aromatase inhibitor–treated metastatic breast carcinoma
ERBB2 (HER2)	Amplification, overexpression Activating mutation	Anti-HER2 therapy Resistance to trastuzumab and lapatinib in HER2-amplified breast carcinoma, alternative HER2-therapy in HER2-negative breast carcinoma (clinical trial)
NTRK	Fusion	TRK inhibitor
PIK3CA	Activating mutation	PI3K inhibitor
PTEN	Loss of function mutation	PI3K inhibitor, PARP inhibitor (clinical trial)
RET	Fusion	RET kinase inhibitor
TP53	Loss of function	Resistance to DNA-damaging chemotherapy, response to paclitaxel, worse outcome in ER-positive breast carcinoma

ER, estrogen receptor; HER2, human epidermal growth factor receptor 2; PI3K, phosphatidylinositol-3-kinase.

The pharmDX kit (Dako Agilent) using the 22C3 PD-L1 antibody predicts benefit from pembrolizumab and is scored using the combined positive scoring (CPS) system (72) **(Fig. 27.3)**. Testing with SP142 (Ventana) for atezolizumab is no longer indicated for breast carcinoma. PD-L1 expression in breast carcinoma is often focal or patchy compared to non-small cell lung carcinoma, for example (73). Moreover, PD-L1 positivity does not consistently correlate with checkpoint inhibitor response in clinical trials (74,75). Accordingly, pembrolizumab was recently approved for high-risk *early*-stage TNBC as neoadjuvant therapy, regardless of PD-L1 expression (75).

Other indications for checkpoint inhibition such as **high tumor mutational burden** or **microsatellite instability** are seldom encountered in breast carcinoma (76). **Tumor-infiltrating lymphocytes** have attracted attention as a potential immunologic biomarker after neoadjuvant chemotherapy and in the setting of immunotherapy (77,78). New biomarkers and assays to triage patients more accurately for immunotherapy are under development.

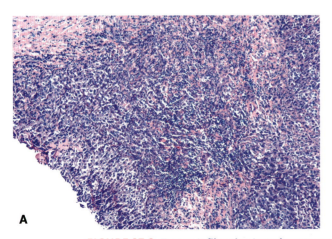
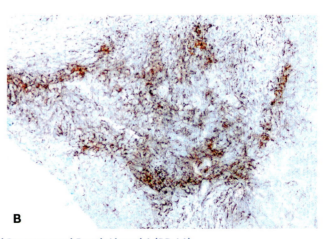

FIGURE 27.3 Tumor-Infiltrating Lymphocytes and Programmed Death Ligand 1 (PD-L1) Immunostain. A: Needle core biopsy specimen showing an invasive ductal carcinoma, high grade with associated prominent tumor-infiltrating immune cells. **B:** PD-L1 immunostain (22C3) shows expression within tumor cells and associated immune cells. Combined positive score: >10.

BIOMARKER, MOLECULAR, AND OTHER ANCILLARY TESTING

"Liquid biopsy" is the sampling of *circulating tumor DNA* (ctDNA) present in the bloodstream. Such samples when analyzed by highly sensitive molecular methods have the potential to facilitate dynamic, minimally invasive disease profiling, monitoring, and screening (79-81). Areas of investigation include detection of acquired *ESR1* mutations (82,83) and *BRCA1/2* reversion mutations (84).

Occasionally, situations arise in which **confirmation of the patient identity** of an NCB sample is desired. **Microsatellite PCR** ("DNA fingerprinting") is among the most discriminatory methods of specimen identification and can be performed on limited formalin-fixed, paraffin-embedded (FFPE) samples (85). The sample DNA is extracted, amplified, and genotyped at a set of highly polymorphic microsatellite loci, and the output is matched to a known patient sample (eg, peripheral blood, cheek swab, or another FFPE sample). This analysis can be performed by laboratories with genetic or forensic testing capabilities. Other IHC and molecular techniques have been utilized for specimen identification (86-89).

REFERENCES

1. Rakha EA, Chmielik E, Schmitt FC, et al. Assessment of predictive biomarkers in breast cancer: challenges and updates. *Pathobiology*. 2022;89:263-277.
2. Rakha EA, Tse GM, Quinn CM. An update on the pathological classification of breast cancer. *Histopathology*. 2023;82:5-16.
3. Wen HY, Collins LC. Breast cancer pathology in the era of genomics. *Hematol Oncol Clin North Am*. 2023;37:33-50.
4. Curtis C, Shah SP, Chin SF, et al. The genomic and transcriptomic architecture of 2,000 breast tumours reveals novel subgroups. *Nature*. 2012;486:346-352.
5. Green AR, Soria D, Powe DG, et al. Nottingham prognostic index plus (NPI+) predicts risk of distant metastases in primary breast cancer. *Breast Cancer Res Treat*. 2016;157:65-75.
6. Nik-Zainal S, Davies H, Staaf J, et al. Landscape of somatic mutations in 560 breast cancer whole-genome sequences. *Nature*. 2016;534:47-54.
7. Perou CM, Sorlie T, Eisen MB, et al. Molecular portraits of human breast tumours. *Nature*. 2000;406:747-752.
8. Chen X, Yuan Y, Gu Z, et al. Accuracy of estrogen receptor, progesterone receptor, and HER2 status between core needle and open excision biopsy in breast cancer: a meta-analysis. *Breast Cancer Res Treat*. 2012;134:957-967.
9. Loubeyre P, Bodmer A, Tille JC, et al. Concordance between core needle biopsy and surgical excision specimens for tumour hormone receptor profiling according to the 2011 St. Gallen Classification, in clinical practice. *Breast J*. 2013;19:605-610.
10. Allison KH, Hammond MEH, Dowsett M, et al. Estrogen and progesterone receptor testing in breast cancer: ASCO/CAP guideline update. *J Clin Oncol*. 2020;38:1346-1366.
11. Wolff AC, Hammond MEH, Allison KH, et al. HER2 testing in breast cancer: American Society of Clinical Oncology/College of American Pathologists clinical practice guideline focused update summary. *J Oncol Pract*. 2018;14:437-441.
12. Early Breast Cancer Trialists' Collaborative Group (EBCTCG); Davies C, Godwin J, Gray R, et al. Relevance of breast cancer hormone receptors and other factors to the efficacy of adjuvant tamoxifen: patient-level meta-analysis of randomised trials. *Lancet*. 2011;378:771-784.
13. Harvey JM, Clark GM, Osborne CK, et al. Estrogen receptor status by immunohistochemistry is superior to the ligand-binding assay for predicting response to adjuvant endocrine therapy in breast cancer. *J Clin Oncol*. 1999;17:1474-81.
14. Gloyeske NC, Dabbs DJ and Bhargava R. Low ER+ breast cancer: Is this a distinct group? *Am J Clin Pathol*. 2014;141:697-701.
15. Iwamoto T, Booser D, Valero V, et al. Estrogen receptor (ER) mRNA and ER-related gene expression in breast cancers that are 1% to 10% ER-positive by immunohistochemistry. *J Clin Oncol*. 2012;30:729-734.
16. Prabhu JS, Korlimarla A, Desai K, et al. A majority of low (1-10%) ER positive breast cancers behave like hormone receptor negative tumors. *J Cancer*. 2014;5:156-165.
17. Gerratana L, Basile D, Buono G, et al. Androgen receptor in triple negative breast cancer: a potential target for the targetless subtype. *Cancer Treat Rev*. 2018;68:102-110.
18. Gucalp A, Tolaney S, Isakoff SJ, et al. Phase II trial of bicalutamide in patients with androgen receptor-positive, estrogen receptor-negative metastatic breast cancer. *Clin Cancer Res*. 2013;19:5505-5512.
19. Walsh EM, Gucalp A, Patil S, et al. Adjuvant enzalutamide for the treatment of early-stage androgen-receptor positive, triple-negative breast cancer: a feasibility study. *Breast Cancer Res Treat*. 2022;195:341-351.

20. Penault-Llorca F, Bilous M, Dowsett M, et al. Emerging technologies for assessing HER2 amplification. *Am J Clin Pathol*. 2009;132:539-548.
21. Kaufman PA, Bloom KJ, Burris H, et al. Assessing the discordance rate between local and central HER2 testing in women with locally determined HER2-negative breast cancer. *Cancer*. 2014;120:2657-2664.
22. Hicks DG, Fitzgibbons P, Hammond E. Core vs breast resection specimen: does it make a difference for HER2 results? *Am J Clin Pathol*. 2015;144:533-535.
23. Rakha EA, Pinder SE, Bartlett JM, et al. Updated UK recommendations for HER2 assessment in breast cancer. *J Clin Pathol*. 2015;68:93-99.
24. Perron M, Wen HY, Hanna MG, et al. HER2 immunohistochemistry in invasive micropapillary breast carcinoma: complete assessment of an incomplete pattern. *Arch Pathol Lab Med*. 2021;145:979-987.
25. Denkert C, Seither F, Schneeweiss A, et al. Clinical and molecular characteristics of HER2-low-positive breast cancer: pooled analysis of individual patient data from four prospective, neoadjuvant clinical trials. *Lancet Oncol*. 2021;22:1151-1161.
26. Gampenrieder SP, Rinnerthaler G, Tinchon C, et al. Landscape of HER2-low metastatic breast cancer (MBC): results from the Austrian AGMT_MBC-Registry. *Breast Cancer Res*. 2021;23:112.
27. Banerji U, van Herpen CML, Saura C, et al. Trastuzumab duocarmazine in locally advanced and metastatic solid tumours and HER2-expressing breast cancer: a phase 1 dose-escalation and dose-expansion study. *Lancet Oncol*. 2019;20:1124-1135.
28. Tozbikian G, Krishnamurthy S, Bui MM, et al. Emerging landscape of targeted therapy of breast cancers with low HER2 protein expression. *Arch Pathol Lab Med*. 2023. doi:10.5858/arpa.2022-0335-RA. Epub ahead of print.
29. Sauter G, Lee J, Bartlett JM, et al. Guidelines for human epidermal growth factor receptor 2 testing: biologic and methodologic considerations. *J Clin Oncol*. 2009;27:1323-1333.
30. Shousha S, Peston D, Amo-Takyi B, et al. Evaluation of automated silver-enhanced in situ hybridization (SISH) for detection of HER2 gene amplification in breast carcinoma excision and core biopsy specimens. *Histopathology*. 2009;54:248-253.
31. van de Vijver MJ, He YD, van't Veer LJ, et al. A gene-expression signature as a predictor of survival in breast cancer. *N Engl J Med*. 2002;347:1999-2009.
32. Bose R, Kavuri SM, Searleman AC, et al. Activating HER2 mutations in HER2 gene amplification negative breast cancer. *Cancer Discov*. 2013;3:224-237.
33. Hyman DM, Piha-Paul SA, Won H, et al. HER kinase inhibition in patients with HER2- and HER3-mutant cancers. *Nature*. 2018;554:189-194.
34. Gradishar WJ, Moran MS, Abraham J, et al. Breast cancer, version 3.2022, NCCN clinical practice guidelines in oncology. *J Natl Compr Canc Netw*. 2022;20:691-722.
35. Lee AH, Key HP, Bell JA, et al. Concordance of HER2 status assessed on needle core biopsy and surgical specimens of invasive carcinoma of the breast. *Histopathology*. 2012;60:880-884.
36. Ellis MJ, Suman VJ, Hoog J, et al. Randomized phase II neoadjuvant comparison between letrozole, anastrozole, and exemestane for postmenopausal women with estrogen receptor-rich stage 2 to 3 breast cancer: clinical and biomarker outcomes and predictive value of the baseline PAM50-based intrinsic subtype-ACOSOG Z1031. *J Clin Oncol*. 2011;29:2342-2349.
37. Yeo B, Dowsett M. Neoadjuvant endocrine therapy: patient selection, treatment duration and surrogate endpoints. *Breast*. 2015;24 Suppl 2:S78-S83.
38. von Minckwitz G, Untch M, Blohmer JU, et al. Definition and impact of pathologic complete response on prognosis after neoadjuvant chemotherapy in various intrinsic breast cancer subtypes. *J Clin Oncol*. 2012;30:1796-1804.
39. Harbeck N, Rastogi P, Martin M, et al. Adjuvant abemaciclib combined with endocrine therapy for high-risk early breast cancer: updated efficacy and Ki-67 analysis from the monarchE study. *Ann Oncol*. 2021;32:1571-1581.
40. Harbeck N, Rastogi P, Shahir A, et al. Letter to the Editor for "Adjuvant abemaciclib combined with endocrine therapy for high-risk early breast cancer: updated efficacy and Ki-67 analysis from the monarchE study". *Ann Oncol*. 2022;33:227-228.
41. Finkelman BS, Zhang H, Hicks DG, et al. The evolution of Ki-67 and breast carcinoma: past observations, present directions, and future considerations. *Cancers (Basel)*. 2023;15.
42. Nielsen TO, Leung SCY, Rimm DL, et al. Assessment of Ki67 in breast cancer: updated recommendations from the international Ki67 in breast cancer working group. *J Natl Cancer Inst*. 2021;113:808-819.
43. Calhoun BC, Collins LC. Recommendations for excision following core needle biopsy of the breast: a contemporary evaluation of the literature. *Histopathology*. 2016;68:138-151.
44. Denkert C, Budczies J, von Minckwitz G, et al. Strategies for developing Ki67 as a useful biomarker in breast cancer. *Breast*. 2015;24 Suppl 2:S67-S72.
45. Mina L, Soule SE, Badve S, et al. Predicting response to primary chemotherapy: gene expression profiling of paraffin-embedded core biopsy tissue. *Breast Cancer Res Treat*. 2007;103:197-208.
46. Symmans WF, Ayers M, Clark EA, et al. Total RNA yield and microarray gene expression profiles from fine-needle aspiration biopsy and core-needle biopsy samples of breast carcinoma. *Cancer*. 2003;97:2960-2971.
47. Andre F, Ismaila N, Allison KH, et al. Biomarkers for adjuvant endocrine and chemotherapy in early-stage breast cancer: ASCO guideline update. *J Clin Oncol*. 2022;40:1816-1837.
48. Burstein HJ, Curigliano G, Thurlimann B, et al. Customizing local and systemic therapies for women with early breast cancer: the St. Gallen International Consensus Guidelines for treatment of early breast cancer 2021. *Ann Oncol*. 2021;32:1216-1235.

49. Amin MB, Edge S, Greene F, et al. *AJCC Cancer Staging Manual*. 8th ed. Springer International Publishing: American Joint Commission on Cancer; 2017.

50. Paik S, Tang G, Shak S, et al. Gene expression and benefit of chemotherapy in women with node-negative, estrogen receptor-positive breast cancer. *J Clin Oncol*. 2006;24:3726-3734.

51. Sparano JA, Gray RJ, Makower DF, et al. Prospective validation of a 21-gene expression assay in breast cancer. *N Engl J Med*. 2015;373:2005-2014.

52. Kalinsky K, Barlow WE, Gralow JR, et al. 21-Gene assay to inform chemotherapy benefit in node-positive breast cancer. *N Engl J Med*. 2021;385:2336-2347.

53. Akashi-Tanaka S, Shimizu C, Ando M, et al. 21-Gene expression profile assay on core needle biopsies predicts responses to neoadjuvant endocrine therapy in breast cancer patients. *Breast*. 2009;18:171-174.

54. Knauer M, Cardoso F, Wesseling J, et al. Identification of a low-risk subgroup of HER-2-positive breast cancer by the 70-gene prognosis signature. *Br J Cancer*. 2010;103:1788-1793.

55. Cardoso F, van't Veer LJ, Bogaerts J, et al. 70-Gene signature as an aid to treatment decisions in early-stage breast cancer. *N Engl J Med*. 2016;375:717-729.

56. Parker JS, Mullins M, Cheang MC, et al. Supervised risk predictor of breast cancer based on intrinsic subtypes. *J Clin Oncol*. 2009;27:1160-1167.

57. Filipits M, Rudas M, Jakesz R, et al. A new molecular predictor of distant recurrence in ER-positive, HER2-negative breast cancer adds independent information to conventional clinical risk factors. *Clin Cancer Res*. 2011;17:6012-6020.

58. Ma XJ, Salunga R, Dahiya S, et al. A five-gene molecular grade index and HOXB13:IL17BR are complementary prognostic factors in early stage breast cancer. *Clin Cancer Res*. 2008;14:2601-2608.

59. Solin LJ, Gray R, Baehner FL, et al. A multigene expression assay to predict local recurrence risk for ductal carcinoma in situ of the breast. *J Natl Cancer Inst*. 2013;105:701-710.

60. Bremer T, Whitworth PW, Patel R, et al. A biological signature for breast ductal carcinoma in situ to predict radiotherapy benefit and assess recurrence risk. *Clin Cancer Res*. 2018;24:5895-5901.

61. Jeselsohn R, Yelensky R, Buchwalter G, et al. Emergence of constitutively active estrogen receptor-alpha mutations in pretreated advanced estrogen receptor-positive breast cancer. *Clin Cancer Res*. 2014;20:1757-1767.

62. Razavi P, Chang MT, Xu G, et al. The genomic landscape of endocrine-resistant advanced breast cancers. *Cancer Cell*. 2018;34:427-438 e6.

63. Dahlgren M, George AM, Brueffer C, et al. Preexisting somatic mutations of estrogen receptor alpha (ESR1) in early-stage primary breast cancer. *JNCI Cancer Spectr*. 2021;5.

64. Andre F, Ciruelos E, Rubovszky G, et al. Alpelisib for PIK3CA-mutated, hormone receptor-positive advanced breast cancer. *N Engl J Med*. 2019;380:1929-1940.

65. Litton JK, Rugo HS, Ettl J, et al. Talazoparib in patients with advanced breast cancer and a germline BRCA mutation. *N Engl J Med*. 2018;379:753-763.

66. Robson M, Im SA, Senkus E, et al. Olaparib for metastatic breast cancer in patients with a germline BRCA mutation. *N Engl J Med*. 2017;377:523-533.

67. Tung NM, Robson ME, Ventz S, et al. TBCRC 048: phase II study of Olaparib for metastatic breast cancer and mutations in homologous recombination-related genes. *J Clin Oncol*. 2020;38:4274-4282.

68. Mandelker D, Zhang L, Kemel Y, et al. Mutation detection in patients with advanced cancer by universal sequencing of cancer-related genes in tumor and normal DNA vs guideline-based germline testing. *JAMA*. 2017;318:825-835.

69. Penson A, Camacho N, Zheng Y, et al. Development of genome-derived tumor type prediction to inform clinical cancer care. *JAMA Oncol*. 2020;6:84-91.

70. Chakravarty D, Gao J, Phillips SM, et al. OncoKB: a precision oncology knowledge base. *JCO Precis Oncol*. 2017;2017.

71. Landrum MJ, Lee JM, Benson M, et al. ClinVar: improving access to variant interpretations and supporting evidence. *Nucleic Acids Res*. 2018;46:D1062-D1067.

72. Cortes J, Cescon DW, Rugo HS, et al. Pembrolizumab plus chemotherapy versus placebo plus chemotherapy for previously untreated locally recurrent inoperable or metastatic triple-negative breast cancer (KEYNOTE-355): a randomised, placebo-controlled, double-blind, phase 3 clinical trial. *Lancet*. 2020;396:1817-1828.

73. Dill EA, Gru AA, Atkins KA, et al. PD-L1 expression and intratumoral heterogeneity across breast cancer subtypes and stages: an assessment of 245 primary and 40 metastatic tumors. *Am J Surg Pathol*. 2017;41:334-342.

74. Mittendorf EA, Zhang H, Barrios CH, et al. Neoadjuvant atezolizumab in combination with sequential nab-paclitaxel and anthracycline-based chemotherapy versus placebo and chemotherapy in patients with early-stage triple-negative breast cancer (IMpassion031): a randomised, double-blind, phase 3 trial. *Lancet*. 2020;396:1090-1100.

75. Schmid P, Cortes J, Pusztai L, et al. Pembrolizumab for early triple-negative breast cancer. *N Engl J Med*. 2020;382:810-821.

76. Le DT, Durham JN, Smith KN, et al. Mismatch repair deficiency predicts response of solid tumors to PD-1 blockade. *Science*. 2017;357:409-413.

77. Dieci MV, Miglietta F, Guarneri V. Immune infiltrates in breast cancer: recent updates and clinical implications. *Cells*. 2021;10.

78. Dieci MV, Radosevic-Robin N, Fineberg S, et al. Update on tumor-infiltrating lymphocytes (TILs) in breast cancer, including recommendations to assess TILs in residual disease after neoadjuvant therapy and in carcinoma in situ: a report of the International Immuno-Oncology Biomarker Working Group on Breast Cancer. *Semin Cancer Biol*. 2018;52:16-25.

79. Garcia-Murillas I, Chopra N, Comino-Mendez I, et al. Assessment of molecular relapse detection in early-stage breast cancer. *JAMA Oncol*. 2019;5:1473-1478.

80. Magbanua MJM, Swigart LB, Wu HT, et al. Circulating tumor DNA in neoadjuvant-treated breast cancer reflects response and survival. *Ann Oncol*. 2021;32:229-239.

81. Radovich M, Jiang G, Hancock BA, et al. Association of circulating tumor DNA and circulating tumor cells after neoadjuvant chemotherapy with disease recurrence in patients with triple-negative breast cancer: preplanned secondary analysis of the BRE12-158 randomized clinical trial. *JAMA Oncol*. 2020;6:1410-1415.

82. Chu D, Paoletti C, Gersch C, et al. ESR1 mutations in circulating plasma tumor DNA from metastatic breast cancer patients. *Clin Cancer Res*. 2016;22:993-999.

83. Fribbens C, O'Leary B, Kilburn L, et al. Plasma ESR1 mutations and the treatment of estrogen receptor-positive advanced breast cancer. *J Clin Oncol*. 2016;34:2961-2968.

84. Weigelt B, Comino-Mendez I, de Bruijn I, et al. Diverse BRCA1 and BRCA2 reversion mutations in circulating cell-free DNA of therapy-resistant breast or ovarian cancer. *Clin Cancer Res*. 2017;23:6708-6720.

85. Gras E, Matias-Guiu X, Catasus L, et al. Application of microsatellite PCR techniques in the identification of mixed up tissue specimens in surgical pathology. *J Clin Pathol*. 2000;53:238-240.

86. Chiang S, Yip S, Betensky RA, et al. Identification of tissue contamination by polymorphic deletion probe fluorescence in situ hybridization. *Am J Surg Pathol*. 2012;36:1464-1471.

87. Ota M, Fukushima H, Akamatsu T, et al. Availability of immunostaining methods for identification of mixed-up tissue specimens. *Am J Clin Pathol*. 1989;92:665-669.

88. Shibata D. Identification of mismatched fixed specimens with a commercially available kit based on the polymerase chain reaction. *Am J Clin Pathol*. 1993;100:666-670.

89. Worsham MJ, Wolman SR, Zarbo RJ. Molecular approaches to identification of tissue contamination in surgical pathology sections. *J Mol Diagn*. 2001;3:11-15.

Index

Note: Page numbers followed by *f* indicate figures; page numbers followed by *t* indicate tables.

A

AAA. *See* Atypical apocrine adenosis
Aberrant E-cadherin staining, 368, 370*f*
ACC. *See* Adenoid cystic carcinoma
Acid-fast bacilli (AFB), 24
ACR BI-RADS (American College of Radiology's Breast Imaging-Reporting and Data System), 505
Actinomycotic abscess, 34
Acute myeloid leukemia (AML), 433
Adenofibromas, 412
Adenoid cystic carcinoma (ACC), 281, 299–308
  clinical features, 299
  differential diagnosis in, 306–308
    adenomyoepithelioma, 307
    collagenous spherulosis, 307, 307*t*
    cribriform ductal carcinoma in situ, 306
    invasive cribriform carcinoma, 306
    metastasis, 308
    microglandular adenosis, high-grade carcinoma arising in, 307
    neuroendocrine features, carcinoma with, 306, 307*f*
    others, 307
    small cell carcinoma, 306
    small tubular proliferations, 307
  histopathologic evaluation, 299–303
    associated lesions, 302–303, 304*f*
    cribriform morphology, 299, 300*f*
    metaplastic alterations, 301
    perineural/lymphovascular invasion, 302, 303*f*
    reticular morphology, 300*f*, 301, 301*f*
    in situ, 302, 303*f*
    solid basaloid morphology, 301, 302*f*
    tubular morphology, 299
  imaging features, 299
  immunohistochemistry, 303–306
    androgen receptor, 305
    basaloid cells, 305
    CD117/KIT, 304–305*f*, 305
    estrogen receptor, 305
    glandular cells, 303, 304–305*f*
    human epidermal growth factor receptor 2, 305
    Ki67, 305
    MYB, 305–306, 306*f*
    progesterone receptor, 305
    SOX10, 305
  molecular testing, 308
  prognosis and management, 308
Adenoid cystic carcinoma in situ, 302, 303*f*
Adenolipomas, 412
Adenomyoepithelioma, 41, 307
Adenomyoepithelioma (AME), 71, 71*f*, 73–74
  atypical, 75–76
    lesions, 79
  benign myoepithelial lesions, 79
  with calcifications, 74, 77*f*
  with collagenous spherulosis, 74, 77*f*
  differential diagnosis of, 79–80
  epithelial/myoepithelial carcinoma, 76–79, 78*f*, 80*f*
  with infarction, 74, 74–75*f*
  mixed tumor (pleomorphic adenoma), 75, 77*f*
  molecular pathology, 80
  with myoepithelial cell (MEC) hyperplasia, 74, 76*f*
  with myoid differentiation, 74, 76*f*
  with sebaceous differentiation, 74, 75*f*
  with squamous differentiation, 74, 75*f*
  squamous metaplasia, 74, 74–75*f*
  variable appearances, 72–73*f*
Adenomyoepitheliosis, 79
Adenosis
  age and incidence, 82
  apocrine adenosis, 88–89, 89*f*
  atypical apocrine adenosis, 88–89, 89–90*f*
  atypical ductal hyperplasia, 92–93, 92*f*
  atypical lobular hyperplasia, 90–92, 91*f*
  blunt duct adenosis, 88, 88*f*
  defined, 82
  differential diagnosis, 93–95, 93–95*f*
  florid adenosis, 84, 87*f*
    in pregnancy, 84, 87*f*
  imaging, 82
  immunohistochemistry, 93
  with invasive pattern, 94–95*f*
  microglandular adenosis (MGA), 96–104
    atypical, 100*f*, 101*t*
    carcinoma in situ associated with, 101*t*
    clinical presentation, 97
    differential diagnosis, 101–102
    ductal carcinoma in situ, 101–102*f*
    imaging, 97
    immunohistochemistry, 98–100
    invasive carcinoma associated with, 101*t*, 103*f*
    microscopic pathology, 97–98, 97*t*
    molecular pathology of, 103–104
    prognosis, 102–103
    treatment, 102–103
  with microinvasive carcinoma, 95*f*
  microscopic pathology, 82–93
  mimics invasive carcinoma, 93*f*
  prognosis, 95
  risk of subsequent carcinoma, 95–96
  sclerosing, 82–84, 83–84*f*
    with apocrine ductal carcinoma in situ, 92, 92*f*
    with calcifications, 84, 86*f*
    with dispersed and compact patterns, 83, 85*f*
    with ductal carcinoma in situ, 92, 92*f*
    in fibroadenoma, 93, 93*f*
    with lobular carcinoma in situ, 90–92, 90–91*f*
    mistaken for carcinoma, 96*f*
    with myoid metaplasia, 83, 85*f*
    with variable appearances, 84, 85–86*f*
  in situ lobular carcinoma, 95*f*
  symptoms, 82
  treatment, 95
  tubular adenosis, 84, 86, 87–88*f*
    with lobular carcinoma in situ, 90–92, 90–91*f*
    with perineural invasion, 86, 88*f*
  types, 82*t*
  variants, 82*t*
Adenosis, papilloma, 43, 43–44*f*
ADH. *See* Atypical ductal hyperplasia
Adult T-cell leukemia/lymphoma, HTLV1-associated, 429*f*
AFB. *See* Acid-fast bacilli
Air-dried slides, 512
AIs. *See* Aromatase inhibitors
Alcian blue methods, 316
Alcohol fixative, 499
Alcohol-fixed slides, 512
ALH. *See* Atypical lobular hyperplasia
ALK (+) histiocytosis, 28
Allred score, 519, 520*t*
α-Methylacyl-CoA racemase (AMACR), 293
Alveolar pattern, of ILC, 365
AME. *See* Adenomyoepithelioma
American Society of Breast Surgeons, 52
The American Society of Clinical Oncology-College of American Pathologists (ASCO-CAP), 152, 501, 519–521, 521*t*, 522*t*
AML. *See* Acute myeloid leukemia

Amyloidoma. *See* Amyloid tumor (AT)
Amyloid tumor (AT), 28, 29*f*
Androgen receptor (AR), 278, 519, 520
Androgen receptor, 293, 305, 518–520, 519*f*, 519*t*, 520*t*
Anechoic target, 505
Angiogenesis, 194, 195*f*
Angiolipoma, 396, 397*f*
  with atypia, 398*f*
Angiomatosis, 403–405, 404*f*
Angiosarcoma, 260
Antigens, 293–294, 293*f*
Apocrine adenosis, 88–89, 89*f*
Apocrine carcinoma, 285–297
  clinical features, 285
  differential diagnosis in, 294–296
    granular cell tumor, 296, 296*f*
    metastasis from an extramammary site, 294, 294*f*
    oncocytic neoplasms, 296
    radiation changes, 295–296, 295*f*
    sclerosing lesion mimics invasive carcinoma, 294–295, 295*f*
    tall cell carcinoma with reversed polarity, 296
  histopathologic evaluation, 285–293
    atypical apocrine proliferations, 285–287, 287*f*
    ductal carcinoma in situ, 287–290, 288–290*f*
    invasive apocrine carcinoma, 290–293, 291–293*f*
    lobular carcinoma in situ, 290, 291*f*
    metaplasia, 285, 286*f*
  immunohistochemistry, 293–294
    androgen receptor, 293
    antigens, 293–294, 293*f*
    cytokeratins, 293–294, 293*f*
    estrogen receptor, 293
    GATA3, 293–294, 293*f*
    gross cystic disease fluid protein 15, 293–294, 293*f*
    human epidermal growth factor receptor 2, 293
    progesterone receptor, 293
  treatment and prognosis, 297
    apocrine ductal carcinoma in situ, 297
    atypical apocrine adenosis, 297
    invasive apocrine carcinoma, 297
Apocrine cytology, secretory carcinoma with, 316*f*
Apocrine ductal carcinoma in situ, 156, 158*f*, 169, 287–290, 288–290*f*, 297
Apocrine lobular carcinoma in situ, 290, 291*f*
Apocrine metaplasia, 12, 12*f*, 285, 286*f*
  papilloma, 45, 45*f*
AR. *See* Androgen receptor
Architectural morphology, 336
Aromatase inhibitors (AIs), 518
Associated lesions, 302–303, 304*f*
Association with implants, lymphomas of the breast in, 430–432, 431*f*, 432*f*
AT. *See* Amyloid tumor
Atypia, apocrine metaplasia with, 287*f*
Atypical apocrine adenosis (AAA), 88–89, 89–90*f*, 285, 287, 297
Atypical apocrine proliferations, 285–287, 287*f*
Atypical columnar cell hyperplasia, 147*f*
Atypical ductal hyperplasia (ADH), 148, 469
  in adenosis, 92–93, 92*f*
  American Society of Breast Surgeons (ASBS) guidelines, 152
  borderline, 143*f*
  chemoprevention of, 153
  clinical implications of, 128*t*
  columnar cell hyperplasia, 142*f*
  cribriform, 141–142*f*
  de-escalation of surgery, 152–153

527

528 INDEX

Atypical ductal hyperplasia (ADH) (*continued*)
diagnosis of, 149–151, 151*t*
excision for, 152
versus LG-DCIS, 150*t*
lobular extension, 141*f*
micropapillary, 139, 141–143*f*
National Cancer Comprehensive Network (NCCN) guidelines, 152
papilloma, 48, 49–50*f*
pathologic features, 150*t*
WHO definition of, 129*t*
Atypical hemangiomas, 402, 404*f*
Atypical lobular hyperplasia (ALH), 332–356, 352–354*f*
in adenosis, 90–92, 91*f*
associated with columnar cell change, 148*f*
classic type, tubular carcinoma, 214, 214*f*
clinical features, 337–338
differential diagnosis, 347–349, 347–350*t*
histopathologic evaluation, 338–343, 338–343*f*
collagenous spherulosis, lobular carcinoma in situ with, 342–343, 343–344*f*
immunohistochemistry, 343–346, 344*t*, 345*f*, 346*f*
microinvasive lobular carcinoma, 349–350, 351*f*
molecular studies, 346–347
needle core biopsy diagnosis of, 353–355
radiologic-pathologic concordance, 355
upgrade rate of variant lobular carcinoma in situ, 354–355
precursor lesion/marker of invasive carcinoma?, 356
prognosis, 350–352
predictors of subsequent invasion, 351–352
terminology of, 332–337, 332–337*f*
treatment, 355–356
Atypical medullary carcinoma, 241
Atypical myoepithelial lesions
management, 79
prognosis, 79
Atypical pregnancy-like hyperplasia, 10, 11*f*
Atypical vascular lesions (AVLs), 405–406, 406*f*
AVLs. *See* Atypical vascular lesions
Axillary lymph node metastases, 449–450
Axillary nodal sarcoidosis, 25–26, 25*f*
Azzopardi effect, 323

B

Bacterial infection
abscess, 34, 34*f*
cystic neutrophilic granulomatous mastitis (CNGM), 36, 36*f*
mycobacterial, 35–36, 35*f*
B- and T-lymphoblastic lymphoma/leukemia, 422*t*
Basal-like carcinomas (BLCs), 246
Basal-like tumors, 203, 204*f*
Basaloid cells, 305
BCI. *See* Breast Cancer Index
Benign myoepithelial lesions
management, 79
prognosis, 79
Benign papillary tumors
collagenous spherulosis
clinical features, 65
with degenerative changes, 66, 67*f*
histologic evaluation, 66, 66*f*
immunohistochemistry, 67
with in situ carcinoma, 67, 67*f*
in papilloma, 66, 66*f*
prognosis, 67
treatment, 67
cystic apocrine metaplasia
with atypia, 60, 60*f*
with calcifications, 59, 60*f*
clinical features, 59
histologic evaluation, 59–61, 59–60*f*
immunohistochemistry, 61
prognosis, 61
treatment, 62
florid papillomatosis
clinical features, 62
differential diagnosis, 63–64
histologic evaluation, 62, 63*f*
imaging studies, 62
immunohistochemistry, 63
prognosis, 64

treatment, 64
intraductal papilloma
clinical features, 41
excision specimen findings, 51
histologic evaluation, 41–48, 42–50*f*
imaging studies, 41
immunohistochemistry, 48–49, 51
needle core biopsy findings, 51
prognosis, 51–52
treatment, 52
radial sclerosing lesions (RSLs)
carcinoma in, 55, 57*f*
clinical features, 52
differential diagnosis, 55
ductal proliferations in, 55, 57*f*
excision specimen findings, 55–57
histologic evaluation, 53–55, 53–54*f*
imaging studies, 52
immunohistochemistry, 55
prognosis, 57–58
treatment, 57
subareolar sclerosing duct hyperplasia (SSDH), 58, 58*f*
syringomatous adenoma of nipple
clinical features, 64
differential diagnosis, 65
imaging studies, 64
immunohistochemistry, 65
microscopic pathology, 64–65, 64*f*
prognosis, 65
treatment, 65
Benign phyllodes tumor (BnPT), 119–120, 120*f*
borderline (low-grade malignant), 120, 121*t*
definition of, 106*t*
differential diagnosis, 116*t*
definition of, 106*t*
differential diagnosis, 116*t*
immunohistochemistry, 123–124
malignant, 120–123, 122*f*, 122*t*
definition of, 106*t*
differential diagnosis, 116*t*
metastatic, 121, 123
recurrent, 121, 123
treatment and prognosis, 124–125
distant metastases, 124
local recurrence, 124
molecular pathology, 124–125
survival, 124
β-catenin, 256, 257*f*, 345
Bilateral carcinoma, 360
Biomarker, 198–199, 198*f*, 199*t*
molecular/ancillary testing, 518–525
androgen receptor, 518–520, 519*f*, 519*t*, 520*t*
breast carcinoma, gene expression profiling of, 518*t*
estrogen receptor, 518–520, 519*f*, 519*t*, 520*t*
human epidermal growth factor receptor 2, 520–521, 521–522*f*, 521*t*, 522*t*
key molecular tests, 523, 524*t*
PD-L1/tests, 523–525, 524*f*
progesterone receptor, 518–520, 519*f*, 519*t*, 520*t*
proliferation rate, determination of, 521–523
Biopsy clips, 485–487, 487*t*, 487*f*, 488*f*
Biopsy techniques/size of needles, 497–499, 497–499*t*, 500*f*
Bioresorbable embedding material, 487
BI-RADS (Breast Imaging-Reporting and Data System) categories, 505*t*
BLCs. *See* Basal-like carcinomas
BLES (Breast Lesion Excision System, Medtronic), 497
Blood vessels
inflammatory lesions of, 28–30, 29*f*
giant cell arteritis, 28–30
lupus mastitis, 30
Blunt duct adenosis, 88, 88*f*
B-lymphoblastic lymphoma, 428*f*
BnPT. *See* Benign phyllodes tumor
BoPT. *See* Borderline (low-grade malignant) phyllodes tumor
Borderline (low-grade malignant) phyllodes tumor (BoPT), 120, 121*t*
definition of, 106*t*
differential diagnosis, 116*t*
Borderline phyllodes tumor, 479*f*

Bouin fixative, 499
BRCA1/BRCA2 mutations, 192, 246, 247*t*, 501, 523
Breast
chemotherapy effect in, 463*f*
density, 1–2
embryology and development, 1
epithelial cells, 3
histiocytic proliferations of, 1–4, 437–438
Erdheim–Chester disease, 438
Langerhans cell histiocytosis, 438
Rosai-Dorfman disease, 437, 437–438*f*
immature, 1, 1*f*
"implantation metastases" in, 450, 451*f*
lactating, uncommon findings in, 7*f*
metaplasia, 12–13, 12*f*
myoepithelial cells, 3, 3*f*
variations in, 3, 4*f*
normal lobules, 1, 2*f*
ochrocytes, 5, 6*f*
physiologic morphology, 4–10
atrophy, 8–9*f*
estrogen and progesterone receptors, 5
follicular phase (days 8-14), 5
lactational hyperplasia, 6, 6*f*
luteal phase (days 15-20), 5
menstrual phase (days 28-2), 5
pregnancy-like change, 7, 9*f*
proliferative phase (days 3-7), 4–5
secretory phase (days 21-27), 5
secretion of milk, 5
immunostains in, use of, 450, 452*t*
Breast Cancer Index (BCI), 523
Breast carcinoma, 310–328
cystic hypersecretory, 318–321
clinical features, 318
differential diagnosis, 320
histopathologic evaluation, 318–320, 319*f*
immunohistochemistry, 320
prognosis and treatment, 320–321
gene expression profiling of, 518*t*
gene mutational analysis, 523
genetic alterations in, 524*t*
glycogen-rich, 326–327
clinical features, 326
differential diagnosis, 327
histopathologic evaluation, 326, 326*f*
immunohistochemistry, 326–327
prognosis and treatment, 327
invasive cribriform, 313–314
clinical features, 313
differential diagnosis, 314
histopathologic evaluation, 313–314, 313*f*, 314*f*
immunohistochemistry, 314
prognosis and treatment, 314
invasive micropapillary, 310–313
clinical features, 310
differential diagnosis, 312–313
histopathologic evaluation, 310–312, 311*f*
prognosis and treatment, 313
ultrastructure and immunohistochemistry, 312
lipid-rich, 327–328
clinical features, 327
differential diagnosis, 328
histochemistry/immunohistochemistry, 328
histopathologic evaluation, 28*f*, 327–328
treatment and prognosis, 328
osteoclast-like giant cells, 321–323
clinical features, 321
differential diagnosis, 322
histopathologic evaluation, 321–322, 321*f*, 322*f*
immunohistochemistry, 322
prognosis and treatment, 322–323
primary histiocytoid, diagnosis of, 21
rare types, 328
secretory, 314–318
clinical features, 315
differential diagnosis, 316
histopathologic evaluation, 315–316, 315–317*f*
immunohistochemistry/molecular studies, 316–318
prognosis and treatment, 318
small cell carcinoma, 323–326
clinical features, 323
differential diagnosis, 325, 325*t*
histopathologic evaluation, 323, 324*f*

immunohistochemistry, 323–325
prognosis and treatment, 325–326
Breast implant-associated anaplastic large cell lymphoma (BIA-ALCL), 423t, 430, 431, 431f, 432
Breast infarct, 16–17
Breast metastases, uncommon sources of, 445–448, 448f
Breast-specific gamma imaging (BSGI), 360
Breast tissue
displaced epithelium within, 488–493, 489–492f
displacement of skin into, 485f
Bridging pattern, 318
BSGI. *See* Breast-specific gamma imaging
Burkitt lymphoma, 422t, 424–427, 426f

C

Capillary hemangiomas, 400–401, 401–402f
Carcinoembryonic antigen (CEA), 317
Carcinoma in situ, papilloma, 48, 50f
Carcinoma, rare types of, 328
Carcinomatous epithelial displacement, local recurrence arising from, 492
Carcinosarcoma, definition of, 106t
Cavernous hemangioma, 399–400, 400–401f
CCH. *See* Columnar cell hyperplasia
CD10, phyllodes tumor, 124
CD117/KIT, 304–305f, 305
CD34, phyllodes tumor, 123
CDH1 gene, 346–347
CEA. *See* Carcinoembryonic antigen
Cellular fibroadenoma, 105t, 107, 109, 109–110f, 110t, 478
Chemotherapy, 460–465, 461–466f, 462t, 463t, 465t
CHH. *See* Cystic hypersecretory hyperplasia
Children and adolescents, carcinoma in, 479–480, 480f
CHL. *See* Classic Hodgkin lymphoma
Chondrolipoma, 396, 397f
Circulating tumor DNA (ctDNA), 525
Classic Hodgkin lymphoma (CHL), 423t
Classic LCIS (C-LCIS), 332, 337–338, 345, 347, 355
Claudin-low tumors, 203
Clear cell DCIS, 156, 158f
Clear cell (change) metaplasia, 12, 12f
Clinical and imaging information, NCB specimens, 501, 501t
CNA. *See* Copy number aberrations
CNGM. *See* Cystic neutrophilic granulomatous mastitis
Collagenized fibrosis, 255
Collagenous spherulosis (CS), 307, 307t
clinical features, 65
with degenerative changes, 66, 67f
with ductal hyperplasia, 137–138, 138f
histologic evaluation, 66, 66f
immunohistochemistry, 67
with in situ carcinoma, 67, 67f
in papilloma, 66, 66f
prognosis, 67
treatment, 67
Columnar cell change
with atypia, 209, 214f
with tubular carcinoma, 209, 213f
Columnar cell hyperplasia (CCH), 144, 145f
with atypia, 146f
histopathologic features of, 145, 145t
with moderate atypia, 146f
Columnar cell lesions
with calcifications, 144, 144f
ductal carcinoma in situ associated with, 147f
histopathologic features of, 145, 145t
hyperplasia, 144, 145f
lobular carcinoma in situ associated with, 148f
with ossifying-type calcifications, 147f
ossifying type of calcifications in, 148f
Rosen triad, 148t
WHO definition of, 129t
Combined positive scoring (CPS) system, 524
Comedo DCIS, 161–162
Comedo necrosis, 165t
Complex fibroadenoma, 105t, 109, 112f
Complex hemangiomas, 401, 403f
Complex sclerosing lesion. *See* Radial sclerosing lesions (RSLs)
Concordant biopsy, 355

Concurrent myeloid sarcoma, 433
Contralateral carcinoma, tubular carcinoma, 209
Copy number aberrations (CNA), 431
Corynebacterium, 36, 36f
Coumadin. *See* Warfarin
Cowden syndrome, 285
CPS system. *See* Combined positive scoring system
Cribriform ductal carcinoma in situ, 161, 162f, 306
Cribriform morphology, 299, 300f
Cryoablation, 114–115
Cryobiopsy, 498
Cryptococcus neoformans, 36, 36f
CS. *See* Collagenous spherulosis
ctDNA. *See* Circulating tumor DNA
Current College of American Pathologists (CAP) regulatory guidelines, 518
Cutaneous myiasis, 38–39
Cutting (non-VA, spring-loaded gun) NCB, 498
Cystic apocrine metaplasia
with atypia, 60, 60f
with calcifications, 59, 60f
clinical features, 59
histologic evaluation, 59–61, 59–60f
immunohistochemistry, 61
prognosis, 61
treatment, 62
Cystic hypersecretory carcinoma, 318–321
clinical features, 318
differential diagnosis, 320
histopathologic evaluation, 318–320, 319f
immunohistochemistry, 320
prognosis and treatment, 320–321
Cystic hypersecretory change, 320
Cystic hypersecretory hyperplasia (CHH), 10, 11f, 320
with atypia, 320
Cystic hypersecretory lesions, 281, 319f
Cystic neutrophilic granulomatous mastitis (CNGM), 25, 36, 36f
Cytokeratins, 293–294, 293f
phyllodes tumor, 123
Cytologically pleomorphic, 336
Cytoplasmic granules, 393

D

DCIS. *See* Ductal carcinoma in situ
DCISionRT, 523
Dendritic phase, 468
Dermatofibrosarcoma protuberans (DFSP), 390–391, 390f
DFSP. *See* Dermatofibrosarcoma protuberans
DH. *See* Ductal hyperplasia
Diabetic mastopathy (DM), 22–24, 23f
lymphocytic lobulitis, 24, 24f
lymphocytic mastitis, 24
sclerosing lymphocytic mastitis, 24
Diffuse large B-cell lymphoma, 421–424, 422–423t, 422t, 424f
Digital breast tomosynthesis, 505
Dimorphic papillary carcinoma, 225, 227f
Discordant biopsy, 355
Displaced epithelium, long-term viability of, 492
DM. *See* Diabetic mastopathy
Ductal carcinoma in situ (DCIS), 71, 147f, 250, 311, 315, 318, 322, 336, 338, 340–343, 347, 474f, 494, 513–515
in adenosis, 92, 92f
apocrine type, 156, 158f, 169
architectural and cytologic features, 155t, 163–164f
associated with columnar cell hyperplasia, 147f
biomarkers in, 173, 173f
classification of, 155t
clear cell type, 156, 158f
clinical implications of, 128t
clinical trials of, 178
comedo, 161–162
cribriform type, 161, 162f
declining rate of recurrence of, 178
differential diagnosis of, 169t
epithelial displacement of, 175
extent of, 172–173
flat micropapillary (clinging) carcinoma, 160f, 161
frequency of, 153
genetic abnormalities, 170, 171t, 176
grading of, 164t, 165f, 170–172
histopathology of, 154–170, 156–157f

lobular cancerization, 154, 155f
Holland classification system of, 172
imaging in, 153–154
intracytoplasmic mucin, 156, 157f
intraoperative consultation (frozen section) diagnosis of, 154, 154f
with invasive ductal carcinoma, 197–198
low-grade *versus* high-grade, 156t
management of, 176–177
Memorial Sloan-Kettering Cancer Center's (MSKCC) Nomogram, 177
microinvasive ductal carcinoma (MiCa), 174–175, 174–175f
micropapillary, 160–161, 160f
necrosis types, 165t
needle core biopsy, 176, 176t
oncotype score, 178
papillary, 167, 230, 231–232f
in radial sclerosing lesions, 169
in sclerosing lesions, 167–169
signet ring cells, 156, 157f
small cell type, 157, 159f
solid type, 161, 163f
spindle cell type, 156, 159f
structure of, 157
triple-negative basal-like, 167
University of Southern California/Van Nuys Prognostic Index (USC/VNPI), 177
in various settings, 170f
with varying degrees of necrosis and calcification, 165–166, 166f
WHO definition of, 129t
Ductal hyperplasia (DH)
atypical, 138–144, 139–140f
American Society of Breast Surgeons (ASBS) guidelines, 152
borderline, 143f
chemoprevention of, 153
columnar cell hyperplasia, 142f
cribriform, 141–142f
de-escalation of surgery, 152–153
diagnosis of, 149–151, 151t
excision for, 152
versus LG-DCIS, 150t
lobular extension, 141f
micropapillary, 139, 141–143f
National Cancer Comprehensive Network (NCCN) guidelines, 152
pathologic features, 150t
clinical features, 128
clinical implications of, 128t
with collagenous spherulosis, 137–138, 138f
columnar cell lesions, 144–149
with calcifications, 144, 144f
ductal carcinoma in situ associated with, 147f
histopathologic features of, 145, 145t
hyperplasia, 144, 145f
lobular carcinoma in situ associated with, 148f
ossifying type of calcifications in, 148f
Rosen triad, 148t
cribriform (fenestrated) growth pattern, 134
florid, 131–133, 132–134f
differential diagnosis of, 136–137, 136f, 137t
with histiocytes, 134, 134f
with necrosis, 134, 134f
with streaming, 131, 133f
histopathology of, 130, 130t
imaging, 129–130
micropapillary, 131, 132f
mild, 131, 131f
moderate, 131, 131–132f
with myoepithelial cells, 135, 135f
papilloma, 43, 43f
usual, 130–137
and breast carcinoma risk, 151–152
Duct ectasia, 18–21, 19–20f
ductitis obliterans, evolution of, 21, 21–22f
without inflammation, 21, 22f
luminal appearances, 19, 20–21f

E

EBER. *See* EBV-encoded small RNAs
EBV. *See* Epstein-Barr virus
EBV-encoded small RNAs (EBER), 423, 432

530 INDEX

E-cadherin immunostaining, 290, 312, 323, 345, 346–347, 351, 365, 368–371, 513
Echinococcal (hydatid) disease, 38, 38*f*
Echinococcus granulosus, 38
Ectopic mammary glandular tissue, 1
EIC. *See* Extensive intraductal component
EMH. *See* Extramedullary hematopoiesis
Encapsulated papillary carcinoma (EPC), 230, 230*f*
EndoPredict (57), 523
Eosinophilic mastitis, 30
EPC. *See* Encapsulated papillary carcinoma
Epidermal Growth Factor Receptor, 261
Epithelial displacement, frequency of, 491
Epithelioid angiosarcoma, 409, 410*f*
Epithelioid myoepithelial hyperplasia, 347
Epstein-Barr virus (EBV), 423, 427
ER. *See* Estrogen receptor
Era of de-escalation, recommendations for management in, 514–516, 515*t*, 516*t*
ERBB2 gene, 328
Erdheim–Chester disease, 14, 16, 438
ESR1 mutation, 523
Estrogen receptor (ER), 5, 278, 293, 305, 312, 518–520, 520*t*
  testing for, 518–520, 519*f*, 519*t*, 520*t*
ETV6-NTRK3 fusion gene, 314, 317, 320
Excisional biopsy with healing marker clip, 30*f*
Extensive intraductal component (EIC), 197–198
Extramedullary hematopoiesis (EMH), 401
Extraskeletal osteosarcoma/chondrosarcoma, 413–414, 414*f*

F

Fat necrosis, 14–16
  calcifications, 14, 16*f*
  causes of, 14
  crown-like structure in, 14, 16*f*
  earlier phases, 14, 15*f*
  Erdheim–Chester disease, 14, 16
  later phases, 14, 15–16*f*
  in male breast, 14
  mammography of, 14
  needle core biopsy, 14, 17*f*
  peculiar form of, 14
FDA. *See* U.S. Food and Drug Administration
FDG-PET/CT (fluorodeoxyglucose-positron emission tomography/computed tomography), 443
FELs. *See* Fibroepithelial lesions
Fibroadenoma, 477–478, 478*f*, 479*f*
  with atypical ductal hyperplasia, 114, 114*f*
  with atypical lobular hyperplasia, 114
  with calcification and ossification, 107, 108*f*
  cellular, 107, 109, 109–110*f*, 110*t*
  clinical presentation, 106–107
  complex, 109, 112*f*
  definition of, 105*t*
  with ductal carcinoma in situ, 114, 114*f*
  growth patterns, 107, 108*f*
  histopathology, 107–112
  imaging, 107
  immunohistochemistry, 114
  infarcted, 109, 111*f*
  juvenile, 112, 113*f*
  with lobular carcinoma in situ, 114, 114*f*
  myxoid, 109, 111–112*f*
  in sclerosing adenosis, 93, 93*f*
  with secretory change, 107, 109*f*
  size, 107
  treatment and prognosis, 114
    excision, 115
    follow-up without excision, 115
    percutaneous forms of, 114
    relative risk, 115
  tubular adenoma, 107, 109
  usual type (adult-type), 107, 108*f*
Fibroadenomatoid change. *See* Sclerosing lobular hyperplasia
Fibroepithelial lesions (FELs), 471, 477–479, 478*f*, 479*f*
  fibroadenoma, 477–478, 478*f*, 479*f*
  phyllodes tumor, 479, 479*f*
  simulating papilloma, 46, 48*f*
Fibroepithelial neoplasms, in adenosis, 93, 93*f*
Fibrolipomas, 396
Fibromatosis, 256, 379–381, 379*f*, 380*f*

Fibrous (inactive) gynecomastia, 469
Fine needle aspiration (FNA), 497, 497*t*
FISH. *See* Fluorescence in situ hybridization
Fixation time, 499–500
FL. *See* Follicular lymphoma
Flat epithelial atypia/atypical columnar cell hyperplasia (FEA/ACCH), 145–146
  histopathologic features of, 145*t*
  WHO definition of, 129*t*
Flat micropapillary (clinging) carcinoma, 160*f*, 161
Florid adenosis, 84, 87*f*
  papilloma, 43, 44*f*
  in pregnancy, 84, 87*f*
Florid ductal hyperplasia, 131–133, 132–134*f*
  differential diagnosis of, 136–137, 136*f*, 137*t*
  with histiocytes, 134, 134*f*
  with necrosis, 134, 134*f*
  with streaming, 131, 133*f*
Florid gynecomastia, 469
Florid LCIS (F-LCIS), 335, 345, 347, 355, 356
Florid papillomatosis
  clinical features, 62
  differential diagnosis, 63–64
  histologic evaluation, 62, 63*f*
  imaging studies, 62
  immunohistochemistry, 63
  prognosis, 64
  treatment, 64
Fluorescence in situ hybridization (FISH), 520, 521
FNA. *See* Fine needle aspiration
Follicular lymphoma (FL), 422*t*, 424, 426*f*
Follicular phase (days 8-14), 5
Foreign material, 282
FoundationOne CDx, 523
Frozen section examination, 512
Fungal infection, 36–37

G

Galactocele, 17–18, 19*f*
Gastrointestinal neoplasms, 445, 447*f*
GATA3, 261–262, 293–294, 293*f*, 449–451
GCDFP-15 (BRST-2), 450
GCT. *See* Granular cell tumor
Gene expression profiling, 518
Germline *CHEK2* mutation, 347
Giant cell arteritis, 28–30
Giant fibroadenoma, 105*t*
Glandular cells, 303, 304–305*f*
Glycogen-rich carcinoma, 326–327, 326*f*
  clinical features, 326
  differential diagnosis, 327
  histopathologic evaluation, 326, 326*f*
  immunohistochemistry, 326–327
  prognosis and treatment, 327
GM. *See* Granulomatous mastitis
Granular cell tumor (GCT), 296, 296*f*, 392–394, 393*f*
Granulomatous lobular mastitis, 24
Granulomatous mastitis (GM), 24–25
  cystic neutrophilic, 25
  differential diagnosis of, 24
  lobular, nonspecific, 24, 25*f*
Gross cystic disease fluid protein 15 (GCDFP-15), 293–294, 293*f*, 317, 449
Gross examination/description, NCB specimens, 502–503, 503*f*, 504*f*
Gynecologic organs, neoplasms of, 445, 447*f*, 448*f*
Gynecomastia, 1, 468–471, 477
  clinical features, 468
  etiology, 468
  imaging studies, 468
  immunohistochemistry, 470, 471*f*
  microscopic pathology, 469, 469*f*, 470*f*
  treatment and prognosis, 470

H

Hamartoma, 105*t*, 106, 107*f*, 412–413, 412*f*
Healing postbiopsy scars, displaced epithelium in, 490*f*
Hemangioma, 399–403, 400–404*f*
Hemangiomatosis, 403
Hemangiopericytoma, 388
Hematoma, 494
Hematoxylin and eosin (H&E)-stained sections, 340
HER2, 123, 203, 518
Herpes simplex, 39

Herpes zoster, 39
Hibernoma, 396, 396*f*
High-grade (type III) angiosarcoma, 408–409, 409*f*
High-grade malignant phyllodes tumor, 253
High tumor mutational burden, 524
Histiocytes, 14
Histiocytoid breast carcinoma
  primary, diagnosis of, 21
Histiocytoid pattern, 327
Histoplasma capsulatum, 36–37
Hodgkin lymphoma, 428–430, 430*f*, 458–460
Holland classification system of DCIS, 172
H (Histochemical)-Score, 519, 519*t*
Human epidermal growth factor receptor 2 (HER2), 272, 278, 293, 305, 312, 345, 472, 518, 520–521, 521–522*f*, 521*t*, 522*t*
Human papillomavirus, 39
Human T-lymphotropic virus-1 (HTLV1) infection, 428
Hyperechoic target, 505
Hyperplastic myoepithelial cells, papilloma, 45, 46*f*
Hypoechoic target, 505

I

IDC. *See* Invasive ductal carcinoma
IgG4-related disease, 27
ILC. *See* Invasive lobular carcinoma
Immature breast, 1, 1*f*
Implant-associated mastitis, 26–27
Implantation metastasis, 451*f*
IMT. *See* Inflammatory myofibroblastic tumor
Indurative mastopathy. *See* Radial sclerosing lesions (RSLs)
Infarction
  breast, 16–17
  papilloma, 46, 47*f*
Infection, 494
  bacterial
    abscess, 34, 34*f*
    cystic neutrophilic granulomatous mastitis (CNGM), 36, 36*f*
    mycobacterial, 35–36, 35*f*
  fungal, 36–37
  parasitic, 37–39, 37–39*f*
  viral, 39
Infiltrating ductal carcinoma with medullary features/ atypical medullary carcinoma, 242
Infiltrating epitheliosis. *See* Radial sclerosing lesions (RSLs)
Inflammatory and reactive lesions
  amyloid tumor (AT), 28, 29*f*
  breast infarct, 16–17
  diabetic mastopathy (DM), 22–24, 23*f*
    lymphocytic lobulitis, 24, 24*f*
    lymphocytic mastitis, 24
    sclerosing lymphocytic mastitis, 24
  duct ectasia, 18–21, 19–20*f*
    ductitis obliterans, evolution of, 21, 21–22*f*
    without inflammation, 21, 22*f*
    luminal appearances, 19, 20–21*f*
  fat necrosis, 14–16
    calcifications, 14, 16*f*
    causes of, 14
    crown-like structure in, 14, 16*f*
    earlier phases, 14, 15*f*
    Erdheim–Chester disease, 14, 16
    later phases, 14, 15–16*f*
    in male breast, 14
    mammography of, 14
    needle core biopsy, 14, 17*f*
    peculiar form of, 14
  galactocele, 17–18, 19*f*
  granulomatous mastitis (GM), 24–25
    cystic neutrophilic, 25
    differential diagnosis of, 24
    lobular, nonspecific, 24, 25*f*
  IgG4-related disease, 27
  implant-associated mastitis, 26–27
  inflammatory myofibroblastic tumor (IMT), 27–28, 27*f*
    ALK (+) histiocytosis, 28
  inflammatory pseudotumor (IPT), 27
  plasma cell mastitis, 22, 22*f*
  sarcoidosis, 25–26, 25*f*
  vasculitis, 28–30, 29*f*

INDEX **531**

giant cell arteritis, 28–30
lupus mastitis, 30
Inflammatory myofibroblastic tumor (IMT), 27–28, 27*f*
ALK (+) histiocytosis, 28
Inflammatory pseudotumor, 27, 257
Infarcted papilloma, 17, 18*f*
Inked needle core biopsy specimens, 503*f*
In situ carcinoma, 513
Intermediate-grade (type II) angiosarcomas, 408, 408*f*
Intermediate gynecomastia, 469
Interval carcinomas, 359
Intracystic papilloma, 41, 42*f*
Intraductal carcinoma, with tubular carcinoma, 209, 213*f*
Intraductal epithelial proliferative lesions, 129*t*
Intraductal papilloma, 471
  clinical features, 41
  excision specimen findings, 51
  histologic evaluation, 41–48, 42–50*f*
  imaging studies, 41
  immunohistochemistry, 48–49, 51
  needle core biopsy findings, 51
  prognosis, 51–52
  treatment, 52
Intraepithelial histiocytes, 347
Intramammary blood vessels, direct injury to, 495
Intramammary lymph nodes, 438–439, 439*f*
Invasive apocrine carcinoma, 290–293, 291–293*f*, 291*f*, 297
Invasive carcinoma, 79, 80*f*, 513
  infarct in, 17, 18*f*
  with mucinous features, 269
Invasive cribriform carcinoma, 306, 313–314, 313*f*, 314*f*
  clinical features, 313
  differential diagnosis, 314
  histopathologic evaluation, 313–314, 313*f*, 314*f*
  immunohistochemistry, 314
  prognosis and treatment, 314
Invasive ductal carcinoma (IDC), 185*f*, 250, 359
  angiogenesis, 194, 195*f*
  biomarkers, 198–199, 198*f*, 199*t*
  changes after neoadjuvant endocrine and chemotherapy, 201, 201*t*, 202*f*
  clinical presentation, 185–186
  concurrent, 183, 183*f*
  ductal carcinoma in situ, 197–198
  extent/size, 186
    and needle core biopsy samples, 187, 187*f*
  frozen section, 185, 185–186*f*
  grading of, 188–192, 188–189*t*, 189–190*f*
  lobular, 183, 183*f*
  lymphovascular involvement, 192–194, 192–194*f*, 193*t*
  management of, 204
  with medullary features, 241
  mitoses, 191*f*
  molecular classification, 201–204, 202–203*t*
  multifocality/multicentricity, 187–188
  myoepithelium, absence of, 195–197, 196–197*f*
  in needle core biopsy specimen, 184, 184*t*
  neoadjuvant chemotherapy, 199–200
  nomenclature, 183–184, 184*t*
  note of caution, 204, 205*f*
  perineural invasion, 195, 195*f*
  prognostic and predictive factors of, 191*t*
  rapid cytologic evaluation, 185
  simulating lobular carcinoma, 183–184, 184*f*
  tumor-infiltrating lymphocytes, 200–201, 200*f*
Invasive lobular carcinoma (ILC), 273, 359–372
  clinical features, 359–360
    bilaterality, 360
    imaging, 359–360
  histopathologic evaluation, 360–368, 361–638*f*, 365*t*
  immunohistochemistry, 368–370, 369*f*, 370*f*, 370*t*
  metastatic lobular carcinoma, 371–372, 371*f*
  molecular studies, 370–371
  prognosis, 372
  treatment, 372
Invasive micropapillary carcinoma, 310–313, 311*f*
  clinical features, 310
  differential diagnosis, 312–313
  histopathologic evaluation, 310–312, 311*f*
  prognosis and treatment, 313

ultrastructure and immunohistochemistry, 312
Invasive micropapillary mucinous carcinoma, 312
Invasive papillary carcinoma, 233–236, 235*f*
IPT. *See* Inflammatory pseudotumor
I radioactive seed localization (RSL), 487, 489*f*
Irradiated glandular epithelium, 295
Irradiation, 455–460
  radiation/breast-conserving therapy, 455–460, 455–460*f*, 457*t*
Ischemic time, 499
Isoechoic target, 505

J

JP. *See* Juvenile papillomatosis
"Juvenile" atypical ductal hyperplasia, 476–477, 477*f*, 478*f*
Juvenile fibroadenoma, 112, 113*f*
  definition of, 105*t*
Juvenile papillomatosis (JP), 475–476, 476*f*
  clinical features, 475
  imaging studies, 475
  microscopic pathology, 475, 476*f*
  molecular characteristics, 476
  treatment and prognosis, 476

K

Kaplan-Meier method, 414
Ki67, 305, 521, 523
  immunostain, 401–402
  phyllodes tumor, 124
  staining, 278
Klinefelter syndrome, 472

L

Lactating/lactational adenoma, 107, 109*f*
  definition of, 105*t*
Lactational hyperplasia, 6, 6*f*
  nonlactating patient, 6*f*
  in nonpregnant patient, 6*f*
  in pregnant patient, 6*f*
Langerhans cell histiocytosis, 438
LCIS. *See* Lobular carcinoma in situ
Leiomyoma, 394, 395*f*
Leiomyosarcoma, 395–396
Less common types/forms of calcium deposition, 510–511*f*
LGASC. *See* Low-grade adenosquamous carcinoma
Lipid-rich carcinoma, 327–328
  clinical features, 327
  differential diagnosis, 328
  histochemistry/immunohistochemistry, 328
  histopathologic evaluation, 327–328, 328*f*
  treatment and prognosis, 328
Lipid-secreting carcinoma, 327
Lipoma, 396, 396–398*f*
Lipomatous, 396–399
  lipoma, 396, 396–398*f*
  liposarcoma, 397–398, 399*f*
Liposarcoma, 397–398, 399*f*
Liquid biopsy, 525
LN. *See* Lobular neoplasia
Lobular carcinoma, 474
  chemotherapy effect in, 466*f*
Lobular carcinoma in situ (LCIS)/atypical lobular hyperplasia (ALH), 332–356
  in adenosis, 90–92, 91*f*
  associated with columnar cell change, 148*f*
  atypical lobular hyperplasia, 352–353, 352–354*f*
  classic type, tubular carcinoma, 214, 214*f*
  clinical features, 337–338
  differential diagnosis, 347–349, 347–350*t*
  histopathologic evaluation, 338–343, 338–343*f*
    collagenous spherulosis, lobular carcinoma in situ with, 342–343, 343–344*f*
  immunohistochemistry, 343–346, 344*t*, 345*f*, 346*f*
  microinvasive lobular carcinoma, 349–350, 351*f*
  molecular studies, 346–347
  needle core biopsy diagnosis of, is excisional biopsy always indicated, 353–355
    radiologic-pathologic concordance, 355
    upgrade rate of variant lobular carcinoma in situ, 354–355
  precursor lesion/marker of invasive carcinoma?, 356
  prognosis, 350–352
    predictors of subsequent invasion, 351–352

terminology of, 332–337, 332–337*f*
  treatment summary, 355–356
Lobular neoplasia (LN), 336
Lobules, normal, 1, 2*f*
Lower-grade intraductal lesions, 129*t*
Low-grade adenosquamous carcinoma (LGASC), 250, 263–266, 264–265*f*
  differential diagnosis of, 266
  histopathologic constituents of, 263–264*t*
  immunoreactivity pattern of, 266
  prognosis and treatment of, 266
Low-grade (type I) tumors, 407, 407*f*
Luminal A group, 518
Luminal B group, 518
Lung/mesothelioma, carcinoma of, 444–445, 444*f*
Lung, non-small-cell carcinoma of, 444
Lupus mastitis, 30
Luteal phase (days 15-20), 5
LVI. *See* Lymphovascular invasion
LVI. *See* Lymphovascular involvement
Lymphatic AVLs, 405
Lymphatic endothelial cells, 491
Lymphatics, definition of, 192
Lymphocytic lobulitis, 24, 24*f*
Lymphocytic mastitis, 24, 433*f*
Lymphocytic mastopathy, 22–24, 23*f*
  lymphocytic lobulitis, 24, 24*f*
  lymphocytic mastitis, 24
  sclerosing lymphocytic mastitis, 24
Lymphoid/hematopoietic tumors, 421–440
  breast, histiocytic proliferations of, 437–438
    Erdheim-Chester disease, 438
    Langerhans cell histiocytosis, 438
    Rosai-Dorfman disease, 437–438*f*
  intramammary lymph nodes, 438–439, 439*f*
  lymphomas of the breast, 421–433
    association with implants, 430–432, 431*f*, 432*f*
    burkitt lymphoma, 424–427, 426*f*
    clinical features, 421
    diffuse large B-cell lymphoma, 421–424, 422–423*t*, 424*f*
    follicular lymphoma, 424, 426*f*
    Hodgkin lymphoma, 428–430, 430*f*
    mammary lymphoma, differential diagnosis of, 432, 433*f*
    mucosa-associated lymphoid tissue, extranodal marginal zone lymphoma of, 424, 425*f*
    pathologic features and clinicopathologic correlates, 421
    systemic B-cell lymphomas, 427–428, 427*f*, 428*f*
    T-cell lymphomas, 428, 429*f*
  myeloid sarcoma, 433–436, 435–436*f*
  plasma cell neoplasms, 433, 434*f*
  tissue processing/ancillary studies, 439–440
Lymphomas of the breast, 421–433
  association with implants, 430–432, 431*f*, 432*f*
  burkitt lymphoma, 424–427, 426*f*
  clinical features, 421
  diffuse large B-cell lymphoma, 421–424, 422–423*t*, 424*f*
  follicular lymphoma, 424, 426*f*
  Hodgkin lymphoma, 428–430, 430*f*
  mammary lymphoma, differential diagnosis of, 432, 433*f*
  mucosa-associated lymphoid tissue, extranodal marginal zone lymphoma of, 424, 425*f*
  pathologic features and clinicopathologic correlates, 421
  systemic B-cell lymphomas, 427–428, 427*f*, 428*f*
  T-cell lymphomas, 428, 429*f*
Lymphovascular invasion (LVI), 290
Lymphovascular involvement (LVI), 513
  invasive ductal carcinoma, 192–194, 192–194*f*, 193*t*
Lymphovascular spaces/axillary lymph nodes, displaced epithelium within, 493–494, 493*f*, 494*f*

M

Magnetic resonance imaging (MRI), 359, 443, 455, 505
Male breast, fat necrosis in, 14
Male breast, carcinoma of, 472–475
  clinical features, 472
  etiology, 472

532 INDEX

Male breast, carcinoma of (*continued*)
  imaging studies, 472
  immunohistochemistry, 474
  microscopic pathology, 472–474, 472–474*f*
  molecular characteristics, 474–475
  needle core biopsy material, differential diagnosis in, 474, 474*f*
  treatment and prognosis, 475
Malignant fibrous histiocytoma, 414
Malignant melanoma, 445, 446*f*
Malignant phyllodes tumor, 120–123, 122*f*, 122*t*
  definition of, 106*t*
  differential diagnosis, 116*t*
  metastatic, 121, 123
  molecular pathology of, 124–125, 125*f*
  recurrent, 121, 123
MALT lymphoma. *See* Mucosa-associated lymphoid tissue lymphoma
Mammaglobin, 450
MammaPrint test, 523
Mammary actinomycosis, 34
Mammary amyloidosis, 28, 29*f*
Mammary cysticercosis, 37
Mammary filariasis, 37, 37*f*
Mammary hamartoma, 106, 107*f*
Mammary hydatid disease, 38, 38*f*
Mammary lobe, structure of, 2
Mammary lymphoma, differential diagnosis of, 432, 433*f*
Mammary ridges, 1
Mammary sarcoidosis, 25–26, 25*f*
Mammary schistosomiasis, 38, 39*f*
Mammary sparganosis, 38, 38*f*
Mammary tuberculosis, 35–36
Mammography, ILC, 359
Mantle cell lymphoma, 422*t*, 427*f*
Massively parallel sequencing (MPS), 444, 453
Mastitis
  granulomatous, 24–25
    cystic neutrophilic, 25
    differential diagnosis of, 24
    lobular, nonspecific, 24, 25*f*
MC. *See* Mucinous carcinoma
MECs. *See* Myoepithelial cells
Medullary carcinoma
  basal-like carcinomas, 248, 248*f*
  BRCA mutations, 246, 247*t*
  clinical presentation, 242
  definition of, 241
  differential diagnosis of, 245, 246*t*
  evolution of, 241*t*
  gross pathology, 242
  histopathology, 242–245, 242*t*, 243–244*f*
  imaging studies, 242
  immunohistochemistry, 245–246
  molecular aspects, 247–248
  needle core biopsy sampling, 245
  prognosis and treatment, 246–247
  triple-negative breast carcinoma, 248, 248*f*
Memorial Sloan-Kettering Cancer Center's (MSKCC) Nomogram, 177, 355
Men/children, 468–480
  and adolescents, breast lesions in, 475–480
    children and adolescents, carcinoma in, 479–480, 480*f*
    fibroepithelial lesions, 477–479, 478*f*, 479*f*
    gynecomastia, 477
    "juvenile" atypical ductal hyperplasia, 476–477, 477*f*, 478*f*
    juvenile papillomatosis, 475–476, 476*f*
    nonepithelial malignant neoplasms, 480
    papilloma, 476, 477*f*
    pseudoangiomatous stromal hyperplasia, 479
  breast lesions in, 468–475
    fibroepithelial lesions, 471
    gynecomastia, 468–471, 469–471*f*
    intraductal papilloma, 471
    male breast, carcinoma of, 472–475, 472–474*f*
    proliferative fibrocystic changes, 471
Menopause, 6
Menstrual cycle, 4–5
Menstrual phase (days 28-2), 5
Mesenchymal lesions, 375–415
  (myo)fibroblastic, 375–391

dermatofibrosarcoma protuberans, 390–391, 390*f*
fibromatosis, 379–381, 379*f*, 380*f*
myofibroblastoma, 383–388, 383–387*f*
nodular fasciitis, 381–382, 382*f*
pseudoangiomatous stromal hyperplasia, 375–379, 376–378*f*
solitary fibrous tumor, 388–389, 389*f*
lipomatous, 396–399
  lipoma, 396, 396–398*f*
  liposarcoma, 397–398, 399*f*
mesenchymal tumors, 412–415
  extraskeletal osteosarcoma/chondrosarcoma, 413–414, 414*f*
  hamartoma, 412–413, 412*f*
  myxoma and angiomyxoma, 413
  other sarcomas, 415
  undifferentiated pleomorphic sarcoma, 414–415, 415*f*
neural, 391–394
  granular cell tumor, 392–394, 393*f*
  neurofibroma, 391–392, 392*f*
  schwannoma, 391, 391*f*
smooth muscle, 394–396
  leiomyoma, 394, 395*f*
  leiomyosarcoma, 395–396
vascular, 399–412
  angiomatosis, 403–405, 404*f*
  atypical vascular lesion, 405–406, 406*f*
  hemangioma, 399–403, 400–404*f*
  papillary endothelial hyperplasia, 405, 405*f*
  postirradiation angiosarcoma, 411–412, 411*f*
  primary angiosarcoma, 406–410, 407–410*f*
Mesenchymal tumors, 412–415
  extraskeletal osteosarcoma/chondrosarcoma, 413–414, 414*f*
  hamartoma, 412–413, 412*f*
  myxoma and angiomyxoma, 413
  other sarcomas, 415
  undifferentiated pleomorphic sarcoma, 414–415, 415*f*
Mesothelioma, 444
Messenger ribonucleic acid (mRNA) levels, 445
Metaplastic alterations, 301
Metaplastic carcinoma, 79, 250–251
  with choriocarcinomatous morphology, 261
  with heterologous elements, 257–260
    acantholytic (pseudoangiosarcomatous) type, 260, 260*f*
    with central zone of necrosis, 259*f*
    matrix-producing type, 258, 258*f*, 259*f*
    mixed tumor (pleomorphic adenoma), 258, 259*f*
    osteocartilaginous metaplasia, 257–258, 258*f*
    with osteoid matrix, 258, 259*f*
  immunohistochemistry of, 261–262
    cytokeratins, 261
    ER, PR, and HER2, 261–262
    matrix components, 262
    myoepithelial antigens, 261
    TRPS1, 262
  low-grade adenosquamous type, 263–266, 264–265*f*
    differential diagnosis of, 266
    histopathologic constituents of, 263–264*t*
    immunoreactivity pattern of, 266
    prognosis and treatment of, 266
  metastatic metaplastic breast carcinoma, 261
  molecular pathology of, 266
  treatment and prognosis of, 262–263
Metaplastic matrix-producing carcinoma, 281
Metaplastic spindle cell carcinoma (MSCC), 250, 251–257
  higher-grade, 252–253, 253*f*
    differential diagnosis, 253–254
  low-grade fibromatosis-like, 254–256, 254–256*f*
    differential diagnosis, 256–257
    versus mammary fibromatosis, 256–257*t*
Metastasis, 308
Metastasis from an extramammary site, 294, 294*f*
Metastatic chondrosarcoma/osteosarcoma, 260
Metastatic clear cell carcinomas, 327
Metastatic embryonal rhabdomyosarcoma, 448*f*
Metastatic endometrial carcinoma, 448*f*
Metastatic leiomyosarcoma, 448*f*
Metastatic malignant melanoma, 446*f*
Metastatic müllerian, 445

Metastatic NMMN in the breast, late presentation of, 449, 449*f*
Metastatic ovarian carcinoma, 447*f*
Metastatic papillary carcinoma, in breast, 238
Metastatic prostatic carcinoma, 448–449, 449*f*, 474*f*
Metastatic pulmonary adenocarcinoma, 444
Metastatic renal carcinoma, 449*f*
MGA. *See* Microglandular adenosis
MiCa. *See* Microinvasive ductal carcinoma
Microglandular adenosis (MGA), 96–104
  atypical, 100*f*, 101*t*
  carcinoma in situ associated with, 101*t*
  clinical presentation, 97
  differential diagnosis, 101–102
  ductal carcinoma in situ, 101–102*f*
  high-grade carcinoma arising in, 307
  imaging, 97
  immunohistochemistry, 98–100
  invasive carcinoma associated with, 101*t*, 103*f*
  microscopic pathology, 97–98, 97*t*
  molecular pathology of, 103–104
  prognosis, 102–103
  treatment, 102–103
  tubular carcinoma, 217, 220–221*f*
Microinvasive ductal carcinoma (MiCa), 174–175, 174–175*f*
Micropapillary DCIS, 160–161, 160*f*
Micropapillary ductal hyperplasia, 131, 132*f*
Micropapillary variant, of MC, 272–273
Microsatellite instability, 524
Microsatellite PCR, 525
Mild ductal hyperplasia, 131, 131*f*
Milk, secretion of, 5
The MIRROR (Micrometastases and Isolated Tumor Cells: Relevant and Robust or Rubbish?) trial, 494
Mitotic count, NCB samples, 513
Mixed invasive micropapillary carcinoma, 310, 311
Mixed ("impure") mucinous carcinoma, 269
Mixed tumor (MT), 75, 77*f*
  differential diagnosis of, 79
Moderate ductal hyperplasia, 131, 131–132*f*
Molecular apocrine group of tumors, 203
MPS. *See* Massively parallel sequencing
MRI. *See* Magnetic resonance imaging
mRNA levels. *See* Messenger ribonucleic acid levels
MSCC. *See* Metaplastic spindle cell carcinoma
MSKCC. *See* Memorial Sloan-Kettering Cancer Center's Nomogram
MSK-IMPACT, 523
MT. *See* Mixed tumor
Mucin-1 (MUC-1), 312
Mucin, 278
Mucinous carcinoma (MC), 79, 258, 269–283
  clinical presentation, 269–278
    histopathology, 270–273, 270–273*f*
    imaging, 269
    mucinous carcinoma, ductal carcinoma in situ in, 273–274, 274*f*
    mucocele-like lesions, 274–278, 275–277*f*, 277*t*
    size, 269–270
  histochemistry/immunohistochemistry, 278
  mucinous carcinoma, molecular pathology of, 283
  mucinous lesions, differential diagnosis of, 278–282, 281*f*
  treatment and prognosis, 282–283
Mucinous cystadenocarcinoma, 281
Mucocele-like lesion, 280
Mucoepidermoid carcinoma, 281
Mucosa-associated lymphoid tissue, extranodal marginal zone lymphoma of, 424, 425*f*
Mucosa-associated lymphoid tissue (MALT lymphoma), 28
Multiple papillomas, 41
MYB, 305–306, 306*f*
Mycobacterium fortuitum, 36
Mycobacterium tuberculosis, 35
Myeloid sarcoma, 433–436, 435–436*f*
Myoepithelial cells (MECs), 71
  immunohistochemical markers for, 71, 74*t*
Myoepithelial hyperplasia, 71, 72*f*
  with adenomyoepithelioma, 74, 76*f*
Myoepithelial lesions
  atypical
    management, 79

INDEX **533**

prognosis, 79
benign
  management, 79
  prognosis, 79
Myoepithelioma, 79
Myoepitheliosis, 79
Myofibroblastic, 375–391
  dermatofibrosarcoma protuberans, 390–391, 390*f*
  fibromatosis, 379–381, 379*f*, 380*f*
  myofibroblastoma, 383–388, 383–387*f*
  nodular fasciitis, 381–382, 382*f*
  pseudoangiomatous stromal hyperplasia, 375–379, 376–378*f*
  solitary fibrous tumor, 388–389, 389*f*
Myofibroblastoma, 257, 383–388, 383–387*f*
Myoid (leiomyomatous) hamartoma, 413
Myoid LCIS, 341
Myolipomas, 396
Myxoid fibroadenoma, 109, 111–112*f*
  definition of, 105*t*
Myxoid stroma, benign/malignant spindle cell lesions with, 281
Myxoma/angiomyxoma, 413

N

N*AB2-STAT6* oncogene, 388
National Cancer Database, 250
National Comprehensive Cancer Network (NCCN) guidelines, 152, 356
NCB. *See* Needle core biopsy
NCCN guidelines. *See* National Comprehensive Cancer Network guidelines
Necrosis, 252
Necrotic cellular debris, 134
Needle core biopsy (NCB), 14, 518, 520, 523
  biopsy techniques/size of needles, 497–499, 497–499*t*, 500*f*
  for breast infarct, 17
  calcifications, 506–512, 507–512*f*, 508*t*
  de-escalation, recommendations for management in the era of, 514–516, 515*t*, 516*t*
  estrogen receptor (ER) immunohistochemistry, 519*f*
  excision following negative result, repeat ER, PR/HER2 testing on, 522
  fat necrosis, invasive carcinoma in, 14, 17*f*
  frozen section examination, 512
  gross examination/description, 502–503, 503*f*, 504*f*
  HER2 immunohistochemistry/FISH, 521–522*f*
  imaging modalities, 505–506, 505*t*, 506*t*
  major clinical complications of, 494–495, 494*t*
  pathology report, 513–514
    invasive carcinoma, 513
    nonneoplastic tissue, 513–514
    in situ carcinoma, 513
  patient care, role of the needle core biopsy pathology report in, 514
  and rate of distant metastases, 495
  requisition form, 501, 501*t*, 502*f*
  specimen processing, 503–505, 503–504*f*
  standardized reporting, 514
  tissue fixation, 499–501
  touch imprint cytology, 512
Needle core biopsy material, differential diagnosis in, 306–308
  adenomyoepithelioma, 307
  collagenous spherulosis, 307, 307*t*
  cribriform ductal carcinoma in situ, 306
  invasive cribriform carcinoma, 306
  metastasis, 308
  microglandular adenosis, high-grade carcinoma arising in, 307
  neuroendocrine features, carcinoma with, 306, 307*f*
  others, 307
  small cell carcinoma, 306
  small tubular proliferations, 307
Needling procedures, pathologic changes/clinical complications associated with, 483–495
  breast caused by needle core biopsy, radiologic/histopathologic changes in, 483–494, 484–486*f*
    biopsy clips, 485–487, 487*t*, 487*f*, 488*f*
    breast tissue, displaced epithelium within, 488–493, 489–492*f*

lymphovascular spaces/axillary lymph nodes, displaced epithelium within, 493–494, 493*f*, 494*f*
    wire/seed localization, 487, 489*f*
  needle core biopsies
    major clinical complications of, 494–495, 494*t*
    and rate of distant metastases, 495
  needle core biopsy of breast, histologic artifacts following, 483*t*
NENs. *See* Neuroendocrine neoplasms
Neoadjuvant chemotherapy, 199–200, 484, 486*f*
Nephrogenic systemic fibrosis, 30
Neural, 391–394
  granular cell tumor, 392–394, 393*f*
  neurofibroma, 391–392, 392*f*
  schwannoma, 391, 391*f*
Neuroendocrine features, carcinoma with, 306, 307*f*
Neuroendocrine neoplasms (NENs), 325
Neurofibroma, 391–392, 392*f*
Next generation sequencing (NGS). *See* Massively parallel sequencing (MPS)
Nicolau syndrome, 495
Nipple adenoma, 256. *See* Florid papillomatosis
Nipple discharge, blood, 17
NMMN. *See* Nonmammary malignant neoplasm
NMMN involving the breast, common sources of, 444–445
  carcinoma of the lung and mesothelioma, 444–445, 444*f*
  gastrointestinal neoplasms, 445, 447*f*
  malignant melanoma, 445, 446*f*
  neoplasms of gynecologic organs, 445, 447*f*, 448*f*
Nodular fasciitis, 257, 381–382, 382*f*
Nodular lactational hyperplasia, 107, 109*f*
Nodular mucinosis, 281
Nodular phase, 468
Nonencapsulated sclerosing lesion. *See* Radial sclerosing lesions
Nonepithelial malignant neoplasms, 480
Noninvasive papillary carcinoma, differential diagnosis of, 225*t*
Nonmammary malignant neoplasm (NMMN), 443–453
  axillary lymph node metastases from, 449–450
  breast
    "implantation metastases" in, 450, 451*f*
    use of immunostains in the diagnosis of metastases in, 450, 452*t*
  breast metastases, uncommon sources of, 445–448, 448*f*
  clinical features, 443
  histopathologic evaluation, 443–444
  imaging features, 443
  involving the breast, common sources of, 444–445
    carcinoma of the lung and mesothelioma, 444–445, 444*f*
    gastrointestinal neoplasms, 445, 447*f*
    malignant melanoma, 445, 446*f*
    neoplasms of gynecologic organs, 445, 447*f*, 448*f*
  management, 452–453
  metastatic NMMN in the breast, late presentation of, 449, 449*f*
  metastatic prostatic carcinoma, 448–449, 449*f*
  molecular testing, 453
  occult primary neoplasms, 448
  primary breast carcinoma, use of immunostains to support, 450–452
Nonneoplastic tissue, 513–514
Nottingham system, 513
Nuclear and histologic grade, 513
Nuclear β-catenin, 123

O

Occult primary neoplasms, 448
Ochrocytes, 5
Oncocytic neoplasms, 296
Oncomine, 523
Oncotype ductal carcinoma in situ score, 178, 523
Oncotype Dx test, 523
Osteocartilaginous metaplasia, 257–258, 258*f*
Osteoclast-like giant cells, carcinomas with, 321*f*, 322*f*
Osteoclast-like giant cells, mammary carcinoma with, 321–323
  clinical features, 321

differential diagnosis, 322
histopathologic evaluation, 321–322, 321*f*, 322*f*
immunohistochemistry, 322
prognosis and treatment, 322–323
Osteolipomas, 396, 397*f*

P

p53, phyllodes tumor, 123–124
p63, phyllodes tumor, 123
PALB2 mutation, 523
Pandemic (COVID-19)–related lesions, 30
Pan-endothelial, 491
Papillary carcinoma, 473*f*
  with calcification, 227, 228*f*
  clinical features, 224
  differential diagnosis of, 225*t*
  ductal carcinoma in situ, 226*f*
  with extracellular mucin, 227, 228*f*
  histopathologic evaluation, 224
    apocrine metaplasia, 226
    cells, types of, 224–225, 225*f*
    epithelial proliferations, 227
    glandular pattern, 226
    nuclei, 225–226
    stroma, 226
  immunohistochemistry, 228–230, 229*f*
  with intracytoplasmic mucin, 227, 228*f*
  molecular studies, 238
  patterns of, 230–236
    ductal carcinoma in situ, 230
    encapsulated, 230, 230*f*
    epithelial displacement, 237
    hybrid, 233, 235*f*
    infarction in, 237, 238*f*
    invasive, 233–236, 235*f*
    metastatic, 238
    solid, 230–233, 231–235*f*, 235*t*
  prognosis and treatment, 238–239
  tall cell carcinoma with reversed polarity, 236, 236*f*
Papillary endothelial hyperplasia, 405, 405*f*
Papillary hyperplasia, 41
Papilloma, 41, 42*f*, 476, 477*f*. *See also specific types*
  with adenosis, 43, 43–44*f*
  with apocrine metaplasia, 45, 45*f*
  with atypical ductal hyperplasia, 48, 49–50*f*
  with carcinoma in situ, 48, 50*f*
  with ductal hyperplasia, 43, 43*f*
  fibroepithelial lesion simulating, 46, 48*f*
  with florid adenosis, 43, 44*f*
  with hyperplastic myoepithelial cells, 45, 46*f*
  infarcted, 17, 18*f*
  with infarction, 46, 47–48*f*
  with prominent myoepithelial cells, 45, 46*f*
  with sclerosis, 46, 47*f*
  solid, 43, 44–45*f*
  with squamous metaplasia, 48, 49*f*
Papillomatosis, 41
Parasitic infestation, 37–39, 37–39*f*
PAS. *See* Periodic acid–Schiff
PASH. *See* Pseudoangiomatous stromal hyperplasia
Pathology report, NCB specimen, 513–514
  invasive carcinoma, 513
  nonneoplastic tissue, 513–514
  in situ carcinoma, 513
Patient care, role of the needle core biopsy pathology report in, 514
PAX8, 445
PCM. *See* Plasma cell mastitis
PD-L1. *See* Programmed cell death ligand 1 (PD-L1)
Peau d'orange, 327
Periductal stroma, 5
Periductal stromal tumor, definition of, 106*t*
Perilobular hemangioma, 399, 400*f*
Perineural invasion, 365–366
Perineural/lymphovascular invasion, 302, 303*f*
Periodic acid–Schiff (PAS), 316
PET. *See* Positron emission tomography
PharmDX kit, 524
Phyllodes tumor, 79, 479, 479*f*
  benign. *See* Benign phyllodes tumor
  borderline (low-grade malignant)
    definition of, 106*t*
    differential diagnosis, 116*t*
  clinical presentation, 115
  features of, 118*f*

534 INDEX

Phyllodes tumor (*continued*)
histopathology, 117–119, 117t
imaging, 117
malignant
definition of, 106t
differential diagnosis, 116t
with pseudoangiomatous stromal hyperplasia (PASH), 118, 118f
size, 117
with stromal giant cells, 118–119, 119f
PIK3CA mutations, 325, 523
Plasma cell mastitis (PCM), 22, 22f
Plasma cell neoplasms, 433, 434f
Plasmacytoma, 423t
Pleomorphic adenoma, 75, 77f, 258, 281
Pleomorphic variant of LCIS (P-LCIS), 335–338, 347, 354, 355, 356
Pneumothorax, 494
Polyostotic fibrosing histiocytosis. *See* Erdheim–Chester disease
Positron emission tomography (PET), 505, 506
Postbiopsy excisions
disruption of intraductal carcinoma in, 490f
needle tracks in, 489f
Postbiopsy spindle cell nodule, 485f
Posterior shadowing, 505
Postirradiation angiosarcoma, 411–412, 411f
Postmenopausal hormone replacement therapy, 7
PR. *See* Progesterone receptor
Pregnancy-like change, 7, 9f
with calcification, 10f
Pregnancy-like hyperplasia, 10, 10f
Premature thelarche, 1
breast glandular tissue in, 1
Prepubertal gynecomastia, 468
Primary angiosarcoma, 406–410, 407–410f
Primary breast angiosarcoma, 406–407
Primary breast carcinoma, use of immunostains to support, 450–452
Primary histiocytoid breast carcinoma, diagnosis of, 21
Primary mammary fibromatosis, 256, 257f
Primary mammary sarcoma, 480
Procedural trauma-induced changes, 483
Progesterone, 5
Progesterone receptor (PR), 278, 293, 305, 312, 518–520, 519f, 520t
Programmed cell death 1 (*PD1*), 523
Programmed Death Ligand 1 (PD-L1), 523–525, 524f
Proliferation rate, determination of, 521–523
Proliferative fibrocystic changes, 471
Proliferative phase (days 3-7), 4–5
Prominent myoepithelial cells, papilloma, 45, 46f
Prominent myxoid stroma, squamous cell carcinoma with, 281
Prosigna/PAM50 (56), 523
Pseudoangiomatous stromal hyperplasia (PASH), 105t, 260, 375–379, 376–378f, 479
phyllodes tumor with, 118, 118f
Pseudolactational metaplasia, 7, 9f
Puberty
breast development, 1
estrogen and progesterone, production of, 1
immature breast, 1, 1f
Punctate necrosis, 165t
Pure invasive micropapillary carcinoma, 310
Pure primary small cell carcinoma, 325

R

Radial sclerosing lesions (RSLs), 218, 221f
carcinoma in, 55, 57f
clinical features, 52
differential diagnosis, 55
ductal proliferations in, 55, 57f
excision specimen findings, 55–57
histologic evaluation, 53–55, 53–54f
imaging studies, 52
immunohistochemistry, 55
prognosis, 57–58
treatment, 57
Radiation atrophy of lobules, 455f
and vascular changes, 456f
Radiation atypia
in apocrine duct hyperplasia, 458f
in small duct, 456f
of stromal fibroblasts, 457f

in terminal ducts with atypical lobular hyperplasia, 459f
Radiation/breast-conserving therapy, 455–460, 455–460f, 457t
Radiation changes, 295–296, 295f
Radiotherapy
recurrent carcinoma, 459f
recurrent ductal carcinoma in situ, 458f
Recurrent infiltrating carcinoma, 460f
Requisition form, 501, 501t, 502f
Retraction artifact, 493
Robbins Basic Pathology, 412
Roman arch, 318
Rosai-Dorfman disease, 30, 437, 437–438f
Rosen Triad, 148t, 215t, 341–342, 343f
RSL. *See* I radioactive seed localization
RSLs. *See* Radial sclerosing lesions

S

Salivary glands, 79
Sarcoidosis, 25–26, 25f
SCC. *See* Squamous cell carcinoma
Schwannoma, 391, 391f
Sclerosing adenosis, 82–84, 83–84f
with apocrine ductal carcinoma in situ, 92, 92f
with calcifications, 84, 86f
with dispersed and compact patterns, 83, 85f
with ductal carcinoma in situ, 92, 92f
in fibroadenoma, 93, 93f
with lobular carcinoma in situ, 90–92, 90–91f
mistaken for carcinoma, 96f
with myoid metaplasia, 83, 85f
tubular carcinoma, 217–218, 221f
with variable appearances, 84, 85–86f
Sclerosing lesion mimics invasive carcinoma, apocrine ductal carcinoma in situ in, 294–295, 295f
Sclerosing lesions, 266
Sclerosing lobular hyperplasia, 105–106, 106f
definition of, 105t
Sclerosing lymphocytic mastitis, 24
Sclerosing non-Langerhans cell histiocytosis. *See* Erdheim–Chester disease
Sclerosing papillary proliferation. *See* Radial sclerosing lesions
Sclerosing papilloma, 477f
Sclerosis, papilloma, 46, 47f
Sebaceous pattern, 327
Secretory carcinoma, 281, 314–318, 315f, 480f
clinical features, 315
differential diagnosis, 316
histopathologic evaluation, 315–316, 315–317f
immunohistochemistry/molecular studies, 316–318
prognosis and treatment, 318
Secretory phase (days 21-27), 5
SEER database. *See* Surveillance, Epidemiology, and End Results database
Selective estrogen receptor modulators (SERMs), 518
SERMs. *See* Selective estrogen receptor modulators
SFT. *See* Solitary fibrous tumor
Signet ring cell MC, 273
16q, 214
Small cell carcinoma, 306, 323–326, 444
clinical features, 323
differential diagnosis, 325, 325t
histopathologic evaluation, 323, 324f
immunohistochemistry, 323–325
prognosis and treatment, 325–326
Small cell DCIS, 157, 159f
Small cell neuroendocrine carcinoma, 324f
Small tubular proliferations, 307
Smooth muscle, 394–396
leiomyoma, 394, 395f
leiomyosarcoma, 395–396
Snail (SNAI1)/EMT-related proteins, 262
Solid basaloid morphology, 301, 302f
Solid DCIS, 161, 163f
Solid papillary carcinoma (SPC), 230–233, 231–232f, 273
differential diagnosis of, 235t
with invasion, 234f
with mucinous differentiation and invasion, 234–235f
with neuroendocrine differentiation, 232–233f
Solid papilloma, 43, 44–45f
Solitary fibrous tumor (SFT), 388–389, 389f

Solitary papilloma, 41
Somatic *BRCA1/2* mutation, 523
Sonographic examination, 475
SOX-10 (Sry-related HMg-Box gene 10), 262, 305, 452
SPC. *See* Solid papillary carcinoma
Specimen processing, 503–505, 503–504f
Specimen radiograph, 505
Spindle cell DCIS, 156, 159f
Spindle cell lipomas, 396
Sporadic angiosarcoma, 406
Squamous cell carcinoma (SCC), 251, 251f
in hyperplastic duct, 252f
invasive, 252f
in situ, 252f
Squamous metaplasia, 12f, 13, 17
papilloma, 48, 49f
SSDH. *See* Subareolar sclerosing duct hyperplasia
Standardized reporting, NCB specimen, 514
Staphylococcus aureus, 34, 34f
Stereotactic guidance, 498
Stereotactic NCB, 505
Steroids, for granulomatous lobular mastitis, 24
Storiform growth pattern, 414
Stromal elastosis, 195, 196f
Stromal sarcoma, 375
Subareolar sclerosing duct hyperplasia (SSDH), 58, 58f
Surveillance, Epidemiology, and End Results (SEER) database, 51, 313, 338, 375, 460
Syncytial growth pattern, 244–245
Syringoma, 266
Syringomatous adenoma of nipple
clinical features, 64
differential diagnosis, 65
imaging studies, 65
immunohistochemistry, 65
microscopic pathology, 64–65, 64f
with myxochondroid stroma, 79
prognosis, 65
treatment, 65
Systemic B-cell lymphomas, 427–428, 427f, 428f

T

Taenia solium, 37
Tall cell carcinoma with reversed polarity, 236, 236f, 296
Tattoo pigment, 509
TC. *See* Tubular carcinoma
T-cell lymphomas, 428, 429f
T-cell receptor γ chain gene (*TRG*), 431
TDLU. *See* Terminal duct lobular units
Terminal duct lobular units (TDLU), 2
Therapy, pathologic effects of, 455–466
ablation methods, 465–466
chemotherapy, 460–465, 461–466f, 462t, 463t, 465t
irradiation, 455–460
radiation/breast-conserving therapy, 455–460, 455–460f, 457t
Third National Cancer survey, 61
Thyroid transcription factor (TTF1), 444
TIC. *See* Touch imprint cytology
TILs. *See* Tumor-infiltrating lymphocytes
Tissue, artifactual defects in, 512f
Tissue fixation, 499–501, 503
Tissue processing/ancillary studies, 439–440
TNBC. *See* Triple-negative breast carcinoma
Topoisomerase II, phyllodes tumor, 124
Touch imprint cytology (TIC), 512
Touton-type giant cells, 16
Traumatic neuroma, 392f
Trichinella infection, 38
Triple-negative breast carcinoma (TNBC), 248, 248f
TruSight Oncology 500, 523
Tuberculous mastitis, 35–36, 35f
Tubular adenoma, 107, 109
definition of, 105t
Tubular adenosis, 84, 86, 87–88f
with lobular carcinoma in situ, 90–92, 90–91f
with perineural invasion, 86, 88f
Tubular carcinoma (TC)
age, ethnicity, and gender, 208
biomarkers, 215
clinical presentation, 208
and columnar cell change, 209, 213f
with atypia, 209, 214f
contralateral carcinoma, 209

differential diagnosis of, 215–218
    epithelial features in, 219*t*
    glandular features in, 219*t*
    immunohistochemistry in, 220*t*
    microglandular adenosis, 217, 220–221*f*
    radial scar/radial sclerosing lesion, 218, 221*f*
    sclerosing adenosis, 217–218, 221*f*
    tubulolobular carcinoma, 216–217, 220*f*
    well-differentiated invasive ductal carcinoma, 215–216, 218–219*f*
and estrogen receptor, 218*f*
family history, 208
histopathology, 209, 209*t*, 210–213*f*
imaging, 208
immunohistochemistry, 215, 216–218*f*
with intracytoplasmic mucin, 209, 211*f*
with intraductal carcinoma, 209, 213*f*
lesions associated with, 209–214, 213–214*f*
and lobular carcinoma in situ, classic type, 214, 214*f*
mimics of, 221*f*
molecular pathology, 222
multifocality, 208–209
size, 208
and stromal desmoplasia, 209, 212*f*
    and stromal elastosis, 209, 212*f*
    treatment and prognosis, 218, 221–222
Tubular morphology, 299
Tubulolobular carcinoma, 216–217, 220*f*, 365
Tumoral circumscription, 243
Tumor-infiltrating lymphocytes (TILs), 200–201, 200*f*, 250, 524, 524*f*
Tumors. *See specific types*

U

UDH. *See* Usual Ductal Hyperplasia
Ultrasound (US) imaging, 505
Undifferentiated pleomorphic sarcoma, 414–415, 415*f*
University of Southern California/Van Nuys Prognostic Index (USC/VNPI), 177
US imaging. *See* Ultrasound imaging
USP6 gene, 257
Usual Ductal Hyperplasia (UDH), 130–137
    and breast carcinoma risk, 151–152
    pathologic features, 130, 130*t*
    WHO definition of, 129*t*

V

Vacuum-assisted needle core biopsy (VA-NCB), 498, 498*t*

Vascular, 399–412
    angiomatosis, 403–405, 404*f*
    atypical vascular lesion, 405–406, 406*f*
    hemangioma, 399–403, 400–404*f*
    papillary endothelial hyperplasia, 405, 405*f*
    postirradiation angiosarcoma, 411–412, 411*f*
    primary angiosarcoma, 406–410, 407–410*f*
Vascular AVLs, 405
Vasculitis, 28–30, 29*f*
    giant cell arteritis, 28–30
    lupus mastitis, 30
Venous hemangioma, 401, 402–403*f*

W

Warfarin (Coumadin), for fat necrosis, 14
WHO. *See* World Health Organization
Wire/seed localization, 487, 489*f*
World Health Organization (WHO)
    classification of breast tumours, 241*t*, 285, 310, 325
    intraductal lesions, definitions of, 129*t*
WT1 (Wilms tumor suppressor gene 1), 278, 445
Wuchereria bancrofti infection, 37, 37*f*